Contemporary Theatre, Film, and Television

ISSN 0749-064X

Contemporary Theatre, Film, and Television

A Biographical Guide Featuring Performers, Directors, Writers, Producers, Designers, Managers, Choreographers, Technicians, Composers, Executives, Dancers, and Critics in the United States and Great Britain

A Continuation of

Who's Who in the Theatre

Linda S. Hubbard
Owen O'Donnell
Editors

Sara J. Steen
Associate Editor

Volume 7

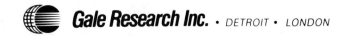 **Gale Research Inc.** · DETROIT · LONDON

STAFF

Linda S. Hubbard and Owen O'Donnell, *Editors*

Sara J. Steen, *Associate Editor*

Sharon Gamboa, *Assistant Editor*

Michael Atkinson, Lillie Balinova, Mel Cobb, Erin McGrath, James R. Kirkland, *Sketchwriters*

June Barnett, Vincent Henry, *Editorial Assistants*

Anne Janette Johnson, Thomas Kozikowski, Sharon Malinowski, Rahadyan T. Sastrowardoyo,
Contributing Editors

Mary Beth Trimper, *Production Manager*
Anthony J. Scolaro, *Production Assistant*

Arthur Chartow, *Art Director*
C. J. Jonik, *Keyliner*

Laura Bryant, *Production Supervisor*
Louise Gagné, *Internal Production Associate*
Shelly Andrews, *Internal Production Assistant*

The paper used in this publication meets the minimum requirements
of American National Standard for Information Sciences—Permanence
Paper for Printed Library Materials, ANSI Z39.48-1984.

Library of Congress Catalog Card Number 84-649371
ISBN 0-8103-2070-3
ISSN 0749-064X

Printed in the United States of America.

Published simultaneously in the United Kingdom
by Gale Research International Limited
(An affiliated company of Gale Research Inc.)

Contents

Preface

The worlds of theatre, film, and television hold an undeniable appeal, and the individuals whose careers are devoted to these fields are subjects of great interest. The people both behind the scenes and in front of the lights and cameras—writers, directors, producers, performers, and others—all have a significant impact on our lives, for they enlighten us as they entertain.

Contemporary Theatre, Film, and Television Provides Broad Coverage in the Entertainment Field

Contemporary Theatre, Film, and Television (CTFT) is a comprehensive biographical series designed to meet the need for information on theatre, film, and television personalities. Prior to the publication of *CTFT*, biographical sources covering entertainment figures were generally limited in scope; for more than seventy years *Who's Who in the Theatre (WWT),* for example, provided reliable information on theatre people. But today few performers, directors, writers, producers, or technicians limit themselves to the stage. And there are also growing numbers of people who, though not active in the theatre, make significant contributions to other entertainment media. With its broad scope, encompassing not only stage notables but also film and/or television figures, *CTFT* is a more comprehensive and, the editors believe, more useful reference tool. Its clear entry format, allowing for the quick location of specific facts, combines with hundreds of photographs to further distinguish *CTFT* from other biographical sources on entertainment personalities.

Moreover, since *CTFT* is a series, new volumes can cover the steady influx of fresh talent into the entertainment media. The majority of the entries in each *CTFT* volume present information on people new to the series, but *CTFT* also includes updated versions of previously published *CTFT* sketches on especially active figures as well as complete revisions of *WWT* entries. The *CTFT* cumulative index makes all listings easily accessible.

Scope

CTFT is a biographical series covering not only performers, directors, writers, and producers but also designers, managers, choreographers, technicians, composers, executives, dancers, and critics from the United States and Great Britain. With nearly 700 entries in *CTFT,* Volume 7, the series now provides biographies for more than 4,200 people involved in all aspects of the theatre, film, and television industries.

Primary emphasis is given to people who are currently active. *CTFT* includes major, established figures whose positions in entertainment history are assured, such as French film director Jean-Luc Godard, actress Audrey Hepburn, playwright Tina Howe, television journalist Bill Moyers, and character actor M. Emmet Walsh. Individuals who are beginning to garner acclaim for their work are represented in *CTFT* as well—people such as Academy Award nominated actress Joan Cusack; playwright and actor Eric Bogosian, who has received critical attention for his Off-Broadway work and for his performance in the film version of his play *Talk Radio;* dancer and clown Bill Irwin, who appeared with Steve Martin and Robin Williams in the heralded 1988 Off-Broadway revival of *Waiting for Godot* and received four Antoinette Perry Award nominations as well as a special New York Drama Critics' Circle Award for his 1989 Broadway play *Largely/New York;* and Willem Dafoe, who has become a leading film actor with his roles in *Platoon, The Last Temptation of Christ,* and *Mississippi Burning.*

Selected sketches also record the achievements of theatre, film, and television personalities who have recently passed away but whose work commands lasting interest. Among such notables with listings in this volume are screenwriter I. A. L. Diamond, who collaborated with Billy Wilder on some of Hollywood's finest films of the late 1950s and early 1960s including *Some Like It Hot, The Apartment,* and *Irma La Douce;* theatre producer Richard Barr, who first presented the plays of Edward Albee on the New York stage; and British actor Maurice Evans, best remembered for his stage and television portrayals of Shakespearean characters.

With its broad coverage and detailed entries, *CTFT* is designed to assist a variety of users—a student preparing for a class, a teacher drawing up an assignment, a researcher seeking a specific fact, a librarian searching for the answer to a question, or a general reader looking for information about a favorite personality.

Compilation Methods

Every effort is made to secure information directly from biographees. The editors consult industry directories, biographical dictionaries, published interviews, feature stories, and film, television, and theatre reviews to identify people not previously covered in *CTFT*. Questionnaires are mailed to prospective listees or, when addresses are unavailable, to their agents, and sketches are compiled from the information they supply. The editors also select major figures included in *WWT* whose entries require updating and send them copies of their previously published entries for revision. *CTFT* sketches are then prepared from the new information submitted by these well-known personalities or their agents. Among the notable figures whose *WWT,* seventeenth edition, entries have been completely revised for this volume of *CTFT* are Rachel Kempson, Walter Matthau, Patrick Stewart, and Melvin Van Peebles. If people of special interest to *CTFT* users are deceased or fail to reply to requests for information, materials are gathered from reliable secondary sources. Sketches prepared solely through research are clearly marked with an asterisk (*) at the end of the entries.

Revised Entries

Each volume of *CTFT* is devoted primarily to people currently active in theatre, film, and television who are not already covered in the series or in *WWT*. However, to ensure *CTFT*'s timeliness and comprehensiveness, in addition to the updates of *WWT* sketches mentioned above, the editors also select *CTFT* listees from earlier volumes who have been active enough to require revision of their previous biographies. Such individuals will merit revised entries as often as there is substantial new information to provide. For example, the update of Academy Award winning actress Olympia Dukakis's entry from *CTFT,* Volume 1, included in this volume adds her most recent stage and film work; moreover, research has brought to light information about television appearances and earlier work in theatre and movies that was not included in her previous sketch. Similarly, Volume 7 provides revised entries containing significant new information on David Dukes, Jane Fonda, Angela Lansbury, Stanley Kubrick, Leonard Nimoy, Jason Robards, and Gene Wilder, among others.

Format

CTFT entries, modeled after those in Gale Research's highly regarded *Contemporary Authors* series, are written in a clear, readable style with few abbreviations and no limits set on length. So that a reader needing specific information can quickly focus on the pertinent portion of an entry, typical *CTFT* listings are clearly divided into the following sections:

Entry heading—Cites the form of the name by which the listee is best known followed by birth and death dates, when available.

Personal—Provides the biographee's full or original name if different from the entry heading, date and place of birth, family data, and information about the listee's education (including professional training), politics, religion, and military service.

Vocation—Highlights the individual's primary fields of activity in the entertainment industry.

Career—Presents a comprehensive listing of principal credits or engagements. The career section lists theatrical debuts (including Broadway and London debuts), principal stage appearances, and major tours; film debuts and principal films; television debuts and television appearances; and plays, films, and television shows directed and produced. Related career items, such as professorships and lecturing, are also included as well as non-entertainment career activities.

Writings—Lists published and unpublished plays, screenplays, and scripts along with production information. Published books and articles, often with bibliographical data, are also listed.

Recordings—Cites album and single song releases with recording labels, when available.

Awards—Notes theatre, film, and television awards and nominations as well as writing awards, military and civic awards, and fellowships and honorary degrees received.

Member—Highlights professional, union, civic, and other association memberships, including official posts held.

Sidelights—Cites favorite roles, recreational activities, and hobbies. Frequently this section includes portions of agent-prepared biographies or personal statements from the listee. In-depth sidelights providing an overview of an individual's career achievements are compiled on selected personalities of special interest.

Other Sources—Indicates periodicals, serials, or books where interviews, criticism, and additional types of information can be found. Not intended as full bibliographies, these citations are provided on brief entries, sketches with sidelights, and a small number of other entries.

Addresses—Notes home, office, and agent addresses, when available. (In those instances where an individual prefers to withhold his or her home address from publication, the editors make every attempt to include at least one other address in the entry.)

Enlivening the text in many instances are large, clear photographs. Often the work of theatrical photographers, these pictures are supplied by the biographees to complement their sketches. This volume, for example, contains nearly 200 such portraits received from various individuals profiled in the following pages.

Brief Entries

CTFT users have indicated that having some information, however brief, on individuals not yet in the series would be preferable to waiting until full-length sketches can be prepared as outlined above under "Compilation Methods." Therefore, *CTFT* includes abbreviated listings on notables who presently do not have sketches in *CTFT*. These short profiles, identified by the heading "Brief Entry," highlight the person's career in capsule form.

Brief entries are not intended to replace sketches. Instead, they are designed to increase *CTFT*'s comprehensiveness and thus better serve *CTFT* users by providing pertinent and timely information about well-known people in the entertainment industry, many of whom will be the subjects of full sketches in forthcoming volumes.

This volume, for example, includes brief entries on such up-and-coming people as Emily Lloyd, David Leisure, and B. D. Wong.

Cumulative Index

To facilitate locating sketches on the thousands of notables profiled in *CTFT,* each volume contains a cumulative index to the entire series. As an added feature, this index also includes references to all seventeen editions of *WWT* and to the four-volume compilation *Who Was Who in the Theatre* (Gale, 1978). Thus by consulting only one source—the *CTFT* cumulative index—users have easy access to the tens of thousands of biographical sketches in *CTFT, WWT,* and *Who Was Who in the Theatre.*

Suggestions Are Welcome

If readers would like to suggest people to be covered in future *CTFT* volumes, they are encouraged to send these names (along with addresses, if possible) to the editors. Other suggestions and comments are also most welcome and should be addressed to: The Editors, *Contemporary Theatre, Film, and Television,* Gale Research Inc., 835 Penobscot Bldg., Detroit, MI 48226-4094.

Contemporary Theatre, Film, and Television

Contemporary Theatre, Film, and Television

* Indicates that a listing has been compiled from secondary sources believed to be reliable.

AAMES, Willie   1960-

PERSONAL: Born William Upton, July 15, 1960, in Newport Beach, CA.

VOCATION: Actor.

CAREER: PRINCIPAL FILM APPEARANCES—Kenny Stevens, *Scavenger Hunt*, Twentieth Century-Fox, 1979; David, *Paradise*, Embassy, 1982; Peyton Nichols, *Zapped!*, Embassy, 1982; Tommy, *Cut and Run* (also known as *Inferno in Diretta*), New World, 1986; Tony, *Killing Machine*, Embassy Home Entertainment, 1986. Also appeared in *Hog Wild* and *Bull from the Sky*.

PRINCIPAL TELEVISION APPEARANCES—Series: Kenny Platt, *We'll Get By*, CBS, 1975; Fred Robinson, *Swiss Family Robinson*, ABC, 1975-76; Tommy Bradford, *Eight Is Enough*, ABC, 1977-81; voice of Hank, *Dungeons and Dragons* (animated), CBS, 1983-87; Buddy Lembeck, *Charles in Charge*, CBS, 1984-85, then syndicated, 1987-88; also Robbie, *The Edge of Night*, NBC. Mini-Series: Wesley Jordache, *Rich Man, Poor Man*, ABC, 1976. Pilots: Adam Morgan, *Doctor Dan*, CBS, 1974; Tom Swift, *The Tom Swift and Linda Craig Mystery Hour*, ABC, 1983. Episodic: Leonard Unger, *The Odd Couple*, ABC, 1973; T.J. Latimer, *Family*, ABC, 1976; Chip, *The New Love, American Style*, ABC, 1985; also voice characterization, *Wait 'til Your Father Gets Home* (animated), syndicated; *The Courtship of Eddie's Father*, ABC. Movies: William Frankenstein, *Frankenstein*, ABC, 1973; Gum, *Unwed Father*, ABC, 1974; Donny, *The Family Nobody Wanted*, ABC, 1975; Tommy Bradford, *Eight Is Enough: A Family Reunion*, NBC, 1987. Specials: *Battle of the Network Stars*, ABC, 1979 and 1980; *Bob Hope's All-Star Look at Television's Prime Time Wars*, NBC, 1980; *We're Movin'*, syndicated, 1982; *Circus of the Stars*, CBS, 1985.

SIDELIGHTS: RECREATIONS—Surfing, skin-diving, and speed-boat racing.

ADDRESSES: AGENT—The Light Company, 113 N. Robertson Boulevard, Los Angeles, CA 90048. PUBLICIST—Jeff Ballard Public Relations, 4814 Lemonia Avenue, Sherman Oaks, CA 91403.*

ACKERMAN, Leslie

PERSONAL: Married Jeff Altman (a comedian and actor).

VOCATION: Actress.

CAREER: PRINCIPAL STAGE APPEARANCES—Abigail, *Mourning Pictures*, Lyceum Theatre, New York City, 1974.

PRINCIPAL FILM APPEARANCES—Karen, *Law and Disorder*, Columbia, 1974; Susie, *The First Nudie Musical*, Paramount, 1976; Felice, *Hardcore* (also known as *The Hardcore Life*), Columbia, 1979; Shelly, *Blame It on the Night*, Tri-Star, 1984. Also appeared in *Cracking Up*, American International, 1977; *Joy Ride to Nowhere*, 1978; and *Baby Dolls*, 1984.

PRINCIPAL TELEVISION APPEARANCES—Series: Barbara Skagska, *Skag*, NBC, 1980. Mini-Series: Helen Borax, *Studs Lonigan*, NBC, 1979. Pilots: Sylvia Hagopian, *Roxy Page*, NBC, 1976; girl at hospital, *The City*, NBC, 1977; Barbara Skagska, *Skag*, NBC, 1980; Faith Newkit, *Washingtoon*, Showtime, 1985; Becky Buxton, *Royal Match*, CBS, 1985. Episodic: *Moonlighting*, ABC, 1986. Movies: Prudy Cass, *The Last Hurrah*, NBC, 1977; Sharon, *Young Love, First Love*, CBS, 1979; Molly Dahl, *Women at West Point*, CBS, 1979; Judith Rosenus, *Missing Pieces*, CBS, 1983; Bonnie, *Shattered Vows*, NBC, 1984; Harriet Parsons, *Malice in Wonderland*, CBS, 1985.

ADDRESSES: AGENT—Abrams Artists and Associates, 9200 Sunset Boulevard, Suite 625, Los Angeles, CA 90025.*

*   *   *

ADAMS, Polly

PERSONAL: Born August 30, in Nashville, TN; married John Klausz (an architect), September 29, 1979; children: Zachary, Jesse. EDUCATION: Stanford University, B.A., 1968; Columbia University, M.F.A., acting, 1971; New York University, M.S.W., 1981.

VOCATION: Actress.

CAREER: BROADWAY DEBUT—Nina, *Zalmen, or the Madness of*

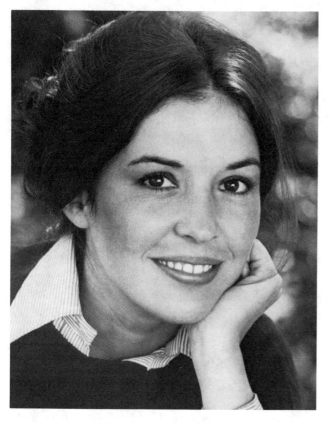

POLLY ADAMS

God, Lyceum Theatre, 1976. PRINCIPAL STAGE APPEARANCES—Hilda and Nancy, *Any Woman Can't,* Playwrights Horizons, New York City, 1973; Lieutenant Mayshank, *Trees in the Wind,* Ham and Clov Stage Company, AMDA Theatre, New York City, 1974; Jane Sloat Shannigan, *The Shortchanged Review,* Ensemble Studio Theatre, New York City, 1975; Amy Herbert, *Porch,* Encompass Theatre, New York City, 1976. Also appeared in *Mother Ryan,* New Dramatists, New York City, 1977; as Amanda, *Private Lives,* Mona, *Want,* Elizabeth, *Deja Vu,* Mary, *Pieces,* Belle Wonder, *The Man-Killer,* Miss Subways, *Miss Subways Meets the Sex Machine,* Marion, *The Ginger Man,* and in *Ord-way Ames-gay,* all Off-Broadway productions, New York City; as Honor, *The Wager,* Henriette, *Learned Ladies,* Alkmene, *Mourning Hercules,* Faye Precious, *Who's Happy Now,* Katerina Prolomnaya, *Journey of the Fifth Horse,* Stella Kowalski, *A Streetcar Named Desire,* Corie Bratter, *Barefoot in the Park,* Brenda, *Lovers and Other Strangers,* Elizabeth, *Catch Me If You Can,* Ruth, *My Sister Eileen,* and Anne Sullivan, *The Miracle Worker,* all in repertory at Stanford University, Stanford, CA, and Dartmouth College, Hanover, NH.

PRINCIPAL FILM APPEARANCES—Receptionist, *Never Put It in Writing,* Allied Artists, 1964; also appeared as Pia Schmeel, *Malachi McNultey Plays for You.*

PRINCIPAL TELEVISION APPEARANCES—Mini-Series: Host, *The Tourists Are Coming.* Episodic: Louisa Dorsey, *All My Children,* ABC; Carole Barclay, *The Edge of Night,* ABC.

RELATED CAREER—Founding member, Ensemble Studio Theatre, New York City; founding member, New York Writers Bloc;

newscaster and host of annual fund raising campaign, WNET-TV (Channel 13), New York City, 1975-82.

MEMBER: Actors' Equity Association, Screen Actors Guild, American Federation of Television and Radio Artists.

ADDRESSES: AGENT—Don Buchwald and Associates, 10 E. 44th Street, New York, NY 10017.

*   *   *

AKINS, Claude   1926-

PERSONAL: Born May 25, 1926, in Nelson, GA; son of Ernest Marion (a police officer) and Anna Maude (Howell) Akins; married Therese Marie Fairfield (a registered nurse), August 30, 1952; children: Claude Marion, Wendy Marie, Michelle Marion. EDUCATION: Received B.S. in speech from Northwestern University. MILITARY: U.S. Army, Signal Corps, master sergeant, 1944-46.

VOCATION: Actor.

CAREER: BROADWAY DEBUT—Salesman, *The Rose Tattoo,* Martin Beck Theatre, New York City, 1951, for one hundred ninety-two performances. PRINCIPAL STAGE APPEARANCES—Everett, *Traveler in the Dark,* Center Theatre Group, Mark Taper Forum, Los Angeles, CA, 1985. Also appeared in *The Comedy of Errors, The Hasty Heart, The Heiress,* and *The Show Off,* all Barter

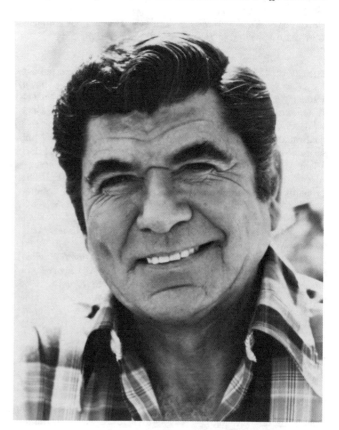

CLAUDE AKINS

Theatre, Abingdon, VA, 1950-51; with Drury Lane South Theatre, Chicago, IL; Windmill Dinner Theatre, Houston, TX; and the Alhambra Dinner Theatre, Jacksonville, FL.

MAJOR TOURS—Salesman, *The Rose Tattoo,* U.S. cities, 1951-52.

FILM DEBUT—Sergeant Baldy Thom, *From Here to Eternity,* Columbia, 1953. PRINCIPAL FILM APPEARANCES—Vance Morgan, *Butter Creek,* Allied Artists, 1954; Horrible, *The Caine Mutiny,* Columbia, 1954; Lieutenant Ramsey, *The Raid,* Twentieth Century-Fox, 1954; Matty Pavelich, *Down Three Dark Streets,* United Artists, 1954; Mandy, *The Human Jungle,* Allied Artists, 1954; Fat Michaels, *Shield for Murder,* United Artists, 1954; Winkler, *The Sea Chase,* Warner Brothers, 1955; Ben Hindeman, *The Burning Hills,* Warner Brothers, 1956; Marty Brennan, *Battle Stations,* Columbia, 1956; Lem, *Johnny Concho,* United Artists, 1956; big soldier, *The Proud and the Profane,* Paramount, 1956; Chief "Gordy" Gordon, *The Sharkfighters,* United Artists, 1956; truck driver, *Hot Summer Night,* Metro-Goldwyn-Mayer (MGM), 1957; Aaron Grant, *Joe Dakota,* Universal, 1957; Pete Logan, *The Kettles on Old MacDonald's Farm,* Universal, 1957; Blackburn, *The Lonely Man,* Paramount, 1957; Mac, *The Defiant Ones,* United Artists, 1958; Poznicki, *Onionhead,* Warner Brothers, 1958; Lieutenant Commander Farber, *Don't Give Up the Ship,* Paramount, 1959; Hog Peyson, *Hound-Dog Man,* Twentieth Century-Fox, 1959; detective, *Porgy and Bess,* Columbia, 1959; Joe Burdette, *Rio Bravo,* Warner Brothers, 1959; sergeant, *Yellowstone Kelly,* Warner Brothers, 1959.

Ben Lane, *Comanche Station,* Columbia, 1960; Reverend Brown, *Inherit the Wind,* United Artists, 1960; S.T. Crawford, *Claudelle Inglish* (also known as *Young and Eager*), Warner Brothers, 1961; Sergeant Kolowicz, *Merrill's Marauders,* Warner Brothers, 1962; Chick Carrington, *Black Gold,* Warner Brothers, 1963; Earl Sylvester, *The Killers* (also known as *Ernest Hemingway's "The Killers"*), Universal, 1964; Krausman, *Incident at Phantom Hill,* Universal, 1966; Frank, *Return of the Seven,* United Artists, 1966; Elwood Coates, *Ride beyond Vengeance* (also known as *Night of the Tiger*), Columbia, 1966; Captain Mason, *First to Fight,* Warner Brothers, 1967; Sergeant Henry Foggers, *Waterhole No. 3,* Paramount, 1967; Rocky Rockman, *The Devil's Brigade,* United Artists, 1968; Slade, *The Great Bank Robbery,* Warner Brothers, 1969; Lobo, *Flap* (also known as *The Last Warrior, Nobody Loves a Drunken Indian,* and *Nobody Loves a Flapping Eagle*), Warner Brothers, 1970; Hooker, *A Man Called Sledge,* Columbia, 1971; Sergeant Ben Puzo, *Sky-jacked* (also known as *Sky Terror*), MGM, 1972; Aldo, *Battle for the Planet of the Apes,* Twentieth Century-Fox, 1973; Captain Robards, *Tentacoli* (also known as *Tentacles*), American International/Twentieth Century-Fox, 1977; Nathan Hayes, *The Curse* (also known as *The Farm*), Trans World, 1987; Sheriff Ketchum, *Monster in the Closet,* Troma, 1987. Also appeared in *Timber Tramps,* Howco, 1973.

TELEVISION DEBUT—Sailor, *Suspense,* CBS, 1951. PRINCIPAL TELEVISION APPEARANCES—Series: Regular, *You Are There,* CBS, 1953-57; Sonny Pruitt, *Movin' On,* NBC, 1974-76; Detective Lieutenant Stonewall Huff, *Nashville 99,* CBS, 1977; Sheriff Elroy P. Lobo, *B.J. and the Bear,* NBC, 1979; Sheriff Elroy P. Lobo, *The Misadventures of Sheriff Lobo,* NBC, 1979-80, renamed *Lobo,* NBC, 1980-81; Tom Bannon, *Legmen,* NBC, 1984. Mini-Series: Walter Kendall, *The Rhinemann Exchange,* NBC, 1977; Uncle Ben Luther, *Celebrity,* NBC, 1984; Tom Fitzpatrick, *Dream West,* CBS, 1986. Pilots: Gus Gardner, *Belle Starr,* CBS, 1958; title role, *Sam Hill,* NBC, 1961; Sergeant Ben Thompson,

Outpost, NBC, 1962; Sergeant Michael Lujack, *The Hat of Sergeant Martin,* ABC, 1963; Punch Logan, *Lock, Stock, and Barrel,* NBC, 1971; Sheriff Warren Butcher, *The Night Stalker,* ABC, 1972; Sheriff Tom Hartley, *The Norliss Tapes,* NBC, 1973; Sonny Pruett, *In Tandem,* NBC, 1974; Dr. Matthews, *Medical Story,* NBC, 1975; Harry Gant, *Kiss Me . . . Kill Me,* ABC, 1976; Sheriff Lobo, *B.J. and the Bear,* NBC, 1978; Joe Blair, *Ebony, Ivory, and Jade,* CBS, 1979.

Episodic: Steve Brand, "The Monsters Are Due on Maple Street," *The Twilight Zone,* CBS, 1960; William Fletcher, "The Little People," *The Twilight Zone,* CBS, 1962; Ethan Cragg, *Murder, She Wrote,* CBS, 1984; Homer Clements, *Crazy Like a Fox,* CBS, 1986; Grandpa, "Pecos Bill, King of the Cowboys," *Shelley Duvall's Tall Tales and Legends,* Showtime, 1986; Charlie, *The New Mike Hammer,* CBS, 1987; also "Desert Island," *I Love Lucy,* CBS, 1956; *Hotel,* ABC, 1985; as Ranger Cotton Buckmeister, *Laredo,* NBC; *Jane Wyman Presents the Fireside Theatre,* NBC; *Zane Grey Theatre* (also known as *Dick Powell's Zane Grey Theatre*), CBS; *The Loretta Young Show,* NBC; *Police Story,* NBC; *Mannix,* CBS; *McCloud,* NBC; *Marcus Welby, M.D.,* ABC; *Cannon,* CBS; *The Streets of San Francisco,* ABC; *Fantasy Island,* ABC. Movies: Ernie Dorata, *River of Mystery,* NBC, 1971; Connie Brennan, *The Death Squad,* ABC, 1974; Stanley Swenson, *Eric,* NBC, 1975; Bert Springer, *Tarantulas: The Deadly Cargo,* CBS, 1977; Cliff Henley, *Yesterday's Child,* NBC, 1977; Oscar Billingham, *Killer on Board,* NBC, 1977; Gus Berste, *Little Mo,* NBC, 1978; Woody Stone, *The Concrete Cowboys,* CBS, 1979; Billy West, *Murder in Music City* (also known as *The Country-Western Murders*), NBC, 1979; Carl, *Desperate Intruder,* syndicated, 1983; Darlin' Harley Medford, *The Baron and the Kid,* CBS, 1984; Bill Pogue, *Manhunt for Claude Dallas,* CBS, 1986; Mo Wyshocki, *If It's Tuesday, It Still Must Be Belgium,* NBC, 1987. Specials: *Bob Hope's All-Star Look at Television's Prime Time Wars,* NBC, 1980; *The All-Star Salute to Mother's Day,* NBC, 1981; *The Way They Were,* syndicated, 1981; Sheriff Will Masters, *Bus Stop,* HBO, 1982; *Academy of Country Music's Twentieth Anniversary Reunion,* NBC, 1986; announcer and host, *Willie Nelson's Picnic,* syndicated, 1987.

RELATED CAREER—Actor in television commercials; host of golf events including the Claude Akins/Julius Boros Kansas City Shrine Classic, Kansas City, MO (1978), the $100,000 Ladies Professional Golf Association Sunstar Classic, Los Angeles, CA (1979), and the $150,000 Olympia Gold Ladies Professional Golf Association Classic, Industry Hills, CA.

NON-RELATED CAREER—Salesman.

MEMBER: Actors' Equity Association, American Federation of Television Arts and Sciences, Screen Actors Guild, Hollywood Hackers, Braemar Country Club, Industry Hill Country Club.

ADDRESSES: OFFICE—13418 Ventura Boulevard, Suite B, Sherman Oaks, CA 91423. AGENT—Sol Leon, William Morris Agency, 151 El Camino Drive, Beverly Hills, CA 90212. PUBLICIST—Hanson & Schwam Public Relations, 9200 Sunset Boulevard, Suite 307, Los Angeles, CA 90069.

ALBERT, Edward 1951-

PERSONAL: Full name, Edward Laurence Albert; born February 20, 1951, in Los Angeles, CA; son of Eddie (an actor) and Margo (an actress, singer, and dancer; full name, Maria Margarita Guadalupe Bolado Castilla y O'Donnell) Albert; married Kate Woodville; children: Thais Carmen Woodville. EDUCATION: Attended the University of California, Los Angeles, and Oxford University; studied acting in Stratford-on-Avon, England.

VOCATION: Actor.

CAREER: LONDON DEBUT—Don, *Terribly Strange Bed.* PRINCIPAL STAGE APPEARANCES—Fortinbras, *Hamlet,* Mark Taper Forum, Los Angeles, CA; Jim O'Connor, *The Glass Menagerie,* Manhattan Theater Club, New York City.

PRINCIPAL FILM APPEARANCES—George Mellish, *The Fool Killer* (also known as *Violent Journey*), Allied Artists, 1965; Don Baker, *Butterflies Are Free,* Columbia, 1972; Peter Latham, *Forty Carats,* Columbia, 1973; Lieutenant Tom Garth, *Midway* (also known as *The Battle of Midway*), Universal, 1976; Jerry, *Un Taxi mauve* (also known as *The Purple Taxi*), Parafrance, 1977; Ross Pine, *The Domino Principle* (also known as *The Domino Killings*), AVCO-Embassy, 1977; Nico Tomasis, *The Greek Tycoon,* Universal, 1978; Michael Rogan, *A Time to Die,* Almi, 1979; Jeff, *The Squeeze,* Maverick, 1980; Brian, *When Time Ran Out,* Warner Brothers, 1980; Cabren, *Galaxy of Terror* (also known as *Mindwarp, An Infinity of Terror,* and *Planet of Horrors*), New World, 1981; Wash Gillespie, *Butterfly,* Analysis, 1982; Ted, *The House Where Evil Dwells,* Metro-Goldwyn-Mayer/United Artists (MGM/UA), 1982; Tom, *Ellie,* Film Ventures, 1984; "Tag" Taggar, *Getting Even* (also known as *Hostage: Dallas*), American Distribution Group, 1986; Danny Warren, *The Underachievers,* Lightning, 1988; Commander Merrill, *The Rescue,* Buena Vista, 1988; Dana Lund, *Mind Games,* MGM/UA, 1989. Also appeared in *Distortions,* Cori/Academy Entertainment, 1988.

PRINCIPAL FILM WORK—Production assistant, *Patton,* Twentieth Century-Fox, 1970.

PRINCIPAL TELEVISION APPEARANCES—Series: Quisto Champion, *The Yellow Rose,* NBC, 1983-84; Jeff Wainwright, *Falcon Crest,* CBS, 1986. Mini Series: Ron "Dal" Dalrymple, *The Last Convertible,* NBC, 1979. Pilots: Paul Matthews, *The Millionaire,* CBS, 1978. Episodic: Oliver Alden, *The New Mike Hammer,* CBS, 1987; Lester Farnum, *Houston Knights,* CBS, 1987; Elliot Burch, *Beauty and the Beast* (three episodes), CBS, 1987-88; also *Gibbsville,* NBC, 1976; *Walking Tall,* NBC, 1981; "Man at the Window," *The Hitchhiker,* HBO, 1985; *The Rookies,* ABC; *Kung Fu,* ABC; *Ellery Queen,* NBC; *Medical Story,* NBC; *Police Story,* NBC; *Orson Welles' Great Mysteries.* Movies: Edward Van Bohlen, *Killer Bees,* ABC, 1974; James Radney, *Death Cruise,* ABC, 1974; Lewis Barry, *Black Beauty,* NBC, 1978; Tom Buchanan, *Silent Victory: The Kitty O'Neil Story,* CBS, 1979; Phil Wharton, *Blood Feud,* syndicated, 1983. Specials: *Battle of the Network Stars,* ABC, 1983.

RELATED CAREER—Pop musician and composer.

NON-RELATED CAREER—Photographer and freelance writer; has had exhibits of his photography in Los Angeles.

AWARDS: Golden Globe Award, Most Promising Male Newcomer, 1972; Nosostros Golden Eagle Award for Highest Career Achievement.

SIDELIGHTS: RECREATIONS—Ranching and raising horses, raising organic fruits and vegetables.

ADDRESSES: AGENTS—Jay Bernstein, P.O. Box 1148, Beverly Hills, CA 90213; Triad Artists, 10100 Santa Monica Boulevard, 16th Floor, Los Angeles, CA 90067. PUBLICIST—Michael Levine Public Relations, 8730 Sunset Boulevard, 6th Floor, Los Angeles, CA 90069.*

*   *   *

ALBERY, Donald 1914-1988

PERSONAL: Full name, Donald Arthur Rolleston Albery; born June 19, 1914, in London, England; died September 14, 1988, in Monte Carlo, Monaco; son of Bronson James (a stage producer and theatre owner) and Una Gwynn (Rolleston) Albery; married Heather Boys, 1946 (marriage ended); children: four. EDUCATION: Attended Alpine College (Switzerland).

VOCATION: Stage producer and theatre owner.

CAREER: FIRST STAGE WORK—Producer, *Birthday Honours,* Q Theatre, London, 1953. FIRST BROADWAY WORK—Producer (with Gilbert Miller), *The Living Room,* Henry Miller's Theatre, 1954. PRINCIPAL STAGE WORK—Producer: *The Living Room,* Wyndham's Theatre, London, 1953; *I Am a Camera,* New Theatre, London, 1954; *Lucky Strike,* Q Theatre, London, 1955; *The Remarkable Mr. Pennypacker,* New Theatre, 1955; *Waiting for Godot,* Arts Theatre, London, 1955; *The Waltz of the Toreadors,* Arts Theatre, 1956; *Gigi,* New Theatre, 1956; *Grab Me a Gondola,* Lyric Hammersmith Theatre, London, 1956; *Zuleika,* Saville Theatre, London, 1957; *Tea and Sympathy,* Comedy Theatre, London, 1957; *Paddle Your Own Canoe,* Criterion Theatre, London, 1957; *Dinner with the Family,* New Theatre, 1957; *The Potting Shed,* Globe Theatre, London, 1958; *Epitaph for George Dillon,* Royal Court Theatre, London, 1958, then retitled *George Dillon,* Comedy Theatre, 1958; *Irma La Douce,* Lyric Theatre, London, 1958; *The Rose Tattoo* and *Make Me an Offer,* both New Theatre, 1959; *A Taste of Honey* and *The Hostage,* both Wyndham's Theatre, 1959; *The Complaisant Lover,* Globe Theatre, 1959; *One to Another,* Lyric Hammersmith Theatre, 1959; *The Ring of Truth,* Savoy Theatre, London, 1959; *The World of Suzie Wong,* Prince of Wales' Theatre, London, 1959.

Fings Ain't Wot They Used t' Be, Garrick Theatre, London, 1960; *A Passage to India* and *The Tinker,* both Comedy Theatre, 1960; *Call It Love,* Wyndham's Theatre, 1960; *Oliver!,* New Theatre, 1960, then (with David Merrick) Imperial Theatre, New York City, 1963, later (with Merrick) Martin Beck Theatre, New York City, 1964; *The Art of Living,* Criterion Theatre, 1960; *The Miracle Worker,* Royalty Theatre, London, 1961; *Beyond the Fringe,* Fortune Theatre, London, 1961; *Blitz!,* Adelphi Theatre, London, 1961; *A Severed Head,* Criterion Theatre, 1963, then (with Merrick) Royale Theatre, New York City, 1964; (with Richard Barr and Clinton Wilder) *Who's Afraid of Virginia Woolf?* and (with Brian Rix) *Instant Marriage,* both Piccadilly Theatre, London, 1964; *Poker Session,* Globe Theatre, 1964; *Beyond the Fringe,* May Fair Theatre, London, 1964; (with Rix) *Diplomatic Baggage,* Wyndham's Theatre, 1964; *Entertaining Mr. Sloane,* New Arts Theatre, London, 1964, then (with Slade Brown, Tanya Chasman, E.A. Gilbert, and Michael Codron) Lyceum Theatre, New York City, 1965; *Jorrocks,* New Theatre, 1965; (with H. Clay Blaney) *Portrait of a Queen,* Vaudeville Theatre, London, 1965; *The Prime of Miss Jean Brodie,* Wyndham's Theatre, 1966; *The Restoration of Arnold Middleton* and (with Perry Raffles) *Mrs. Wilson's Diary,* both Criterion Theatre, 1967; *Spring and Port Wine,* New Theatre, 1967; *The Italian Girl,* Wyndham's Theatre, 1968; *Man of La Mancha,* Piccadilly Theatre, 1968; *Conduct Unbecoming,* Queen's Theatre, London, 1969, then (with Roger Stevens) Ethel Barrymore Theatre, New York City, 1970.

(With Michael Codron) *It's a Two Foot Six Inches above the Ground World,* Wyndham's Theatre, 1970; *Poor Horace,* Lyric Theatre, 1970; *Mandrake,* Criterion Theatre, 1970; *Popkiss,* Globe Theatre, 1972. Also produced *Sparrers Can't Sing, Celebration, Bonne Soupe,* and *Heartbreak House,* all in London 1961; *Not to Worry, Semi-Detached,* and *Fiorello!,* all in London, 1962; *Le Mariage de Figaro* and *License to Murder,* both in London, 1963; *The Time of the Barracudas,* 1963; *The Fourth of June* and *Carving a Statue,* both in London, 1964; *Very Good Eddie* and *The Family Dance,* both in London, 1976; *Candida,* London, 1977.

MAJOR TOURS—Producer: *The Perils of Scobie Prilt,* U.K. cities, 1963; *A Little Winter Love,* U.K. cities, 1964; *Oliver!,* U.S. cities, 1965.

RELATED CAREER—General manager, Sadler's Wells Ballet, 1941-45; managing director, Wyndham Theatres, Ltd., 1950-78; director and administrator, Festival Ballet, London, 1964-68; managing director, Donmar Productions, Ltd.; managing director, Piccadilly Theatre, Ltd.; managing director, Calabash Productions, Ltd.; director, Independent Plays, Ltd.; director, Anglia Television, Ltd.; executive council member, Society of West End Managers.

AWARDS: Knighted in 1977.

SIDELIGHTS: In honor of Douglas Albery, the New Theatre in London was renamed the Albery Theatre in 1972.

OBITUARIES AND OTHER SOURCES: *Variety,* September 21, 1988.*

*   *   *

ALDRICH, Janet   1956-

PERSONAL: Born Janet Wallerich, October 16, 1956, in Chicago, IL; daughter of George Mueller (a business executive) and Frances Marion (Harper) Wallerich; married Carlos R. Valdes Dapenza (a photography stock company manager), April 9, 1989. EDUCATION: University of Miami, B.F.A., theatre, 1978; trained for the stage at the Actors Institute and with Dan Fauci and Warren Robertson.

VOCATION: Actress.

CAREER: BROADWAY DEBUT—Star to Be, *Annie,* Uris Theatre, 1982. PRINCIPAL STAGE APPEARANCES—Exerciser, nurse, and Joan, *American Princess,* INTAR Theatre, New York City, 1982; courtesan, *The Comedy of Errors,* Equity Library Theatre, New York City, 1985; ensemble, *Godspell,* Ford's Theatre, Washington, DC, 1985; Prudie, *Pump Boys and Dinettes,* GeVa Theatre,

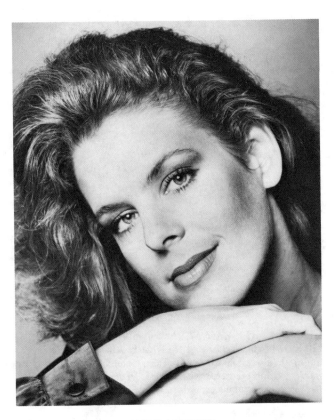

JANET ALDRICH

Rochester, NY, 1986; ensemble, *Forbidden Broadway* (revue), Shoreham Hotel, Washington, DC, 1986; Sonia, *They're Playing Our Song,* Downtown Cabaret Theatre, Bridgeport, CT, 1987; Ruby, *Broadway,* Royale Theatre, New York City, 1987. Also appeared in *The Men's Group,* Equity Library Theatre, Bruno Walter Auditorium, New York City, 1983; *The Three Musketeers,* Broadway Theatre, New York City, 1984; *Starmites,* Criterion Theatre, New York City, 1989; and in productions of *A Funny Thing Happened on the Way to the Forum* and *Wanted Dead or Alive,* both in New York City.

MAJOR TOURS—Cecile and Bonnie Boylan, then Star to Be, *Annie,* U.S. cities, 1981; Sally Bowles, *Cabaret,* European cities, 1987-89.

FILM DEBUT—Blossom, *Ringers,* Orion, 1986. PRINCIPAL FILM APPEARANCES—Judy, *Une Femme ou deux* (also known as *One Woman or Two*), Orion Classics, 1985.

TELEVISION DEBUT—Courtney, *As The World Turns,* CBS, 1984. PRINCIPAL TELEVISION APPEARANCES—Episodic: Suzi, *The Guiding Light,* CBS, 1985; Karen, *The Guiding Light,* CBS, 1987.

AWARDS: Helen Hayes Award, Outstanding Actress in a Musical, 1986, for *Forbidden Broadway;* Victoire de la Musique, 1987, for *Cabaret.*

MEMBER: Actors' Equity Association, American Federation of Television and Radio Artists, Screen Actors Guild, American Guild of Variety Artists, SACEM, Conges Spectacles.

SIDELIGHTS: Janet Aldrich told *CTFT* that she has appeared in productions of *Cabaret* in seven countries and three languages, adding, ''It was the film *Cabaret* that originally inspired me to become an actress and Bob Fosse, coincidentally, was the first person I met when I moved to New York.''

ADDRESSES: AGENT—Agents for the Arts, Inc., 1650 Broadway, New York, NY 10019.

*   *   *

ALLEN, Jay Presson   1922-

PERSONAL: Born Jacqueline Presson, March 3, 1922, in Ft. Worth, TX; daughter of Albert Jeffrey (a merchant) and May (a buyer; maiden name, Miller) Presson; married second husband, Lewis Maitland Allen (a producer), March 12, 1955; children: Anna Brooke. EDUCATION: Attended Miss Hackaday's School, Dallas, TX.

VOCATION: Writer and producer.

CAREER: Also see *WRITINGS* below. PRINCIPAL FILM WORK— Executive producer: *Just Tell Me What You Want,* Warner Brothers, 1980; (also producer) *It's My Turn,* Columbia, 1980; *Prince of the City,* Orion/Warner Brothers, 1981; *Deathtrap,* Warner Brothers, 1982. Also producer, *Stone,* 1984.

PRINCIPAL TELEVISION WORK—Series: Creator and story consultant, *Family,* ABC, 1976-80; creator and executive producer, *Hothouse,* ABC, 1988.

WRITINGS: STAGE—*The Prime of Miss Jean Brodie,* Princess Theatre, Torquay, U.K., then Wyndham's Theatre, London, both 1966, later Helen Hayes Theatre, New York City, 1968, published by Samuel French, Inc., 1969; *Forty Carats,* Morosco Theatre, New York City, 1968, published by Random House, 1969; *I and Albert,* Piccadilly Theatre, London, 1972; *A Little Family Business,* Center Theatre Group, Ahmanson Theatre, Los Angeles, CA, then Martin Beck Theatre, New York City, both 1982. Also *The First Wife.*

FILM—*Marnie,* Universal, 1964; *The Prime of Miss Jean Brodie,* Twentieth Century-Fox, 1969; *Cabaret,* Allied Artists, 1972; (with Hugh Wheeler) *Travels with My Aunt,* Metro-Goldwyn-Mayer, 1972; (with Arnold Schulman) *Funny Lady,* Columbia, 1975; *Just Tell Me What You Want,* Warner Brothers, 1980; (with Sidney Lumet) *Prince of the City,* Orion/Warner Brothers, 1981; *Deathtrap,* Warner Brothers, 1982. Also *Stone,* 1984.

TELEVISION—Episodic: *Playhouse 90,* CBS; *Philco Playhouse,* NBC. Specials: ''The Borrowers,'' *Hallmark Hall of Fame,* NBC, 1973.

OTHER—*Spring Riot* (novel), Rinehart, 1948; *Just Tell Me What You Want* (novel), Dutton, 1975.

AWARDS: Humanities Award, 1976; David DiDonatello Award, Best Script, 1980, for *Just Tell Me What You Want;* also received three Screen Writers Guild awards.

MEMBER: Writers Guild of America, Dramatists Guild, Academy of Motion Picture Arts and Sciences.

ADDRESSES: OFFICE—Lewis Allen Productions, 1500 Broadway, New York, NY 10036. AGENTS—International Creative Management, 40 W. 57th Street, New York, NY 10019; International Creative Management, 8899 Beverly Boulevard, Los Angeles, CA 90069.*

*   *   *

ALLEN, Joan   1956-

PERSONAL: Born August 20, 1956, in Rochelle, IL; father, a gas station operator. EDUCATION: Attended Eastern Illinois University and Western Illinois University.

VOCATION: Actress.

CAREER: OFF-BROADWAY DEBUT—Helen Stott, *And a Nightingale Sang,* Steppenwolf Theatre Company, Mitzi E. Newhouse Theatre, 1983. PRINCIPAL STAGE APPEARANCES—Helen Stott, *And a Nightingale Sang,* Steppenwolf Theatre Company, Hartford Stage Company, Hartford, CT, 1983; Bette, *The Marriage of Bette and Boo,* New York Shakespeare Festival, Public Theatre, New York City, 1985; Anna Mann, *Burn This!,* Centre Theatre Group, Mark Taper Forum, Los Angeles, CA, then Plymouth Theatre, New York City, both 1987; Dr. Heidi Holland, *The Heidi Chronicles,* Playwrights Horizons, New York City, 1988, then Plymouth Theatre, 1989. Also appeared in productions of *A Lesson from Aloes, The Three Sisters, The Miss Firecracker Contest, Cloud 9, Balm in Gilead,* and *The Fifth of July,* all with the Steppenwolf Theatre Company, Chicago, IL.

PRINCIPAL FILM APPEARANCES—Mary Alice Mahoney, *Compromising Positions,* Paramount, 1985; Lala, *Fat Guy Goes Nutzoid!!,* Troma, 1986; Reba, *Manhunter,* De Laurentiis Entertainment Group, 1986; Maddy Nagle, *Peggy Sue Got Married,* Tri-Star, 1986; Vera Tucker, *Tucker: The Man and His Dream,* Paramount, 1988.

PRINCIPAL TELEVISION APPEARANCES—Mini-Series: Iris Friedman, *Evergreen,* NBC, 1985. Episodic: Ann Deever, ''All My Sons,'' *American Playhouse,* PBS, 1987; also ''Robert Frost,'' *Voices and Visions,* PBS, 1988. Movies: Ellie, *The Room Upstairs,* CBS, 1987.

RELATED CAREER—Founding member, Steppenwolf Theatre Company, Chicago, IL.

NON-RELATED CAREER—Secretary at an educational film company.

AWARDS: Theatre World Award, Clarence Derwent Award, Drama Desk Award, and Outer Critics Circle Award, all 1984, for *And a Nightingale Sang;* Antoinette Perry Award, Best Actress in a Play, 1988, for *Burn This!.*

ADDRESSES: AGENT—Brian Mann, International Creative Management, 8899 Beverly Boulevard, Los Angeles, CA 90048.*

ALLEN, Jonelle 1944-

PERSONAL: Born July 18, 1944, in New York, NY. EDUCATION: Attended the Professional Children's School.

VOCATION: Actress.

CAREER: BROADWAY DEBUT—*The Wisteria Trees*, Martin Beck Theatre, 1950. PRINCIPAL STAGE APPEARANCES—Dionne, *Hair*, New York Shakespeare Festival (NYSF), Public Theatre, New York City, 1967; living statue and secretary in the Cohan and Harris office, *George M!*, Palace Theatre, New York City, 1968; Tamara Bissy, *Someone's Comin' Hungry*, Pocket Theatre, New York City, 1969; Sara Jane, *The House of Leather*, Ellen Stewart Theatre, New York City, 1970; Silvia, *Two Gentlemen of Verona*, NYSF, Delacorte Theatre, then St. James Theatre, both New York City, 1971; Sandi, *Mail*, Pasadena Playhouse, Pasadena, CA, 1987; Sheri, *Etta Jenks*, Los Angeles Theatre Center, Los Angeles, CA, 1988. Also appeared in *Five on the Backhand Side*, Theatre at St. Clement's Church, New York City, 1969; *The All Night Strut!*, Ford's Theatre Society, Washington, DC, 1976; *Tintypes*, South Coast Repertory Theatre, Costa Mesa, CA, 1981; and in *Bury the Dead* and *Moon on a Rainbow Shawl*, both in New York City.

MAJOR TOURS—*Two Gentlemen of Verona*, U.S. and Canadian cities, 1973.

PRINCIPAL FILM APPEARANCES—Bishop Deb, *The Cross and the Switchblade*, Dick Ross Associates, 1970; Carol, *Come Back Charleston Blue*, Warner Brothers, 1972; Ann Vanderguild, *The River Niger*, Cine Artists, 1976; Sabrina Jones, *The Hotel New Hampshire*, Orion, 1984.

PRINCIPAL TELEVISION APPEARANCES—Series: Bessie Freeman, *Palmerstown, U.S.A.*, CBS, 1980-81; Stacey Russell, *Berrengers*, NBC, 1985. Pilots: Dory, *Sparrow*, CBS, 1978; Lulu, *After Midnight*, ABC, 1988. Episodic: *Barney Miller*, ABC, 1975; *All in the Family*, CBS, 1978; also Claudia Petrie, *Cagney and Lacey*, CBS; Maxine, *Police Woman*, NBC. Movies: Tommy, *Cage without a Key*, CBS, 1975; Jacqueline Foster, *Foster and Laurie*, CBS, 1975; Brandy, *Vampire*, ABC, 1979; Fanny Crowne, *Brave New World*, NBC, 1980; Maydene Jarriott, *Victims*, NBC, 1982; Lucinda Cavender, *The Midnight Hour*, ABC, 1985; Susan Jansen, *Penalty Phase*, CBS, 1986. Specials: *Cotton Club '75*, NBC, 1974; *Opryland USA*, ABC, 1975; *Battle of the Network Stars*, ABC, 1980; also "Green Pastures," *Hallmark Hall of Fame*.

RELATED CAREER—Child actress in theatre and television during the 1950s.

AWARDS: Theatre World Award, 1971-72.*

*   *   *

ALONSO, Maria Conchita 1957-

PERSONAL: Born in 1957 in Cuba.

VOCATION: Actress and singer.

CAREER: PRINCIPAL FILM APPEARANCES—Lucia Lombardo, *Moscow on the Hudson*, Columbia, 1984; Claudia Pazzo, *A Fine Mess*, Columbia, 1986; Denise DeLeon, *Touch and Go*, Tri-Star, 1986; Sarita Cisneros, *Extreme Prejudice*, Tri-Star, 1987; Amber Mendez, *The Running Man*, Tri-Star, 1987; Louisa Gomez, *Colors*, Orion, 1988. Also appeared in *Vampire's Kiss* (also known as *Vampire Kiss*), Hemdale, 1989.

PRINCIPAL TELEVISION APPEARANCES—Series: Maria, *One of the Boys*, NBC, 1989—. Movies: Caterina Ammirati, *Blood Ties*, Showtime, 1986.

RELATED CAREER—Miss Teenager of the World, 1971; Miss Venezuela, 1975; appeared in four Venezuelan films and ten Spanish-language soap operas.

RECORDINGS: ALBUMS—*Maria Conchita*, A&M International, 1984; *O ella o yo*, A&M International, 1985.

AWARDS: Grammy Award nomination, Best Latin Artist, 1985, for *Maria Conchita*.

ADDRESSES: AGENT—Hildy Gottlieb, International Creative Management, 8899 Beverly Boulevard, Los Angeles, CA 90048. PUBLICIST—Susan Geller, Guttman and Pam, Ltd., 8500 Wilshire Boulevard, Suite 801, Beverly Hills, CA 90211.*

*   *   *

ALTMAN, Robert 1925-

PERSONAL: Born February 20, 1925, in Kansas City, MO; third wife's name, Kathryn Reed; children: Christine (first marriage); Michael, Stephen (second marriage); Robert, Matthew (third marriage). EDUCATION: Attended the University of Missouri. MILITARY: U.S. Army, bomber pilot, 1943-47.

VOCATION: Director, producer, and screenwriter.

CAREER: Also see *WRITINGS* below. FIRST STAGE WORK—Director, "Precious Blood" and "Rattlesnake in a Cooler" in *Two by South*, Actors Theatre, Los Angeles, CA, 1981. PRINCIPAL STAGE WORK—Director, "Precious Blood" and "Rattlesnake in a Cooler" in *Two by South*, Theatre at St. Clement's Church, New York City, 1981; director, *Come Back to the 5 & Dime, Jimmy Dean, Jimmy Dean*, Martin Beck Theatre, New York City, 1982; producer, *Secret Honor: The Last Testament of Richard M. Nixon*, Provincetown Playhouse, New York City, 1983.

PRINCIPAL FILM APPEARANCES—Bob, *Events*, Grove Press, 1970; also appeared in *Endless Love*, Universal, 1981.

PRINCIPAL FILM WORK—All as director, unless indicated: (Also producer) *The Delinquents*, United Artists, 1957; (with George W. George; also producer and editor with George) *The James Dean Story* (documentary), Warner Brothers, 1957; *Nightmare in Chicago*, Universal, 1967; *Countdown* (documentary), Warner Brothers-Seven Arts, 1968; *That Cold Day in the Park*, Commonwealth United, 1969; *M*A*S*H*, Twentieth Century-Fox, 1970; *Brewster McCloud*, Metro-Goldwyn-Mayer, 1970; *McCabe and Mrs. Miller*, Warner Brothers, 1971; *Images*, Columbia, 1972; *The Long Goodbye*, United Artists, 1973; *Thieves Like Us*, United Artists, 1974; (also producer with Joseph Walsh) *California Split*, Columbia, 1974; (also producer) *Nashville*, Paramount, 1975; (also producer) *Buffalo Bill and the Indians, or Sitting Bull's History Lesson*, United Artists, 1976; producer, *Welcome to L.A.*, United

Artists, 1976; producer, *The Late Show,* Warner Brothers, 1977; (also producer) *Three Women,* Twentieth Century-Fox, 1977; (also producer) *A Wedding,* Twentieth Century-Fox, 1978; producer, *Remember My Name,* Columbia, 1978; (also producer) *Quintet,* Twentieth Century-Fox, 1979; (also producer) *A Perfect Couple,* Twentieth Century-Fox, 1979; producer, *Rich Kids,* United Artists, 1979; *Health* (also known as *H.E.A.L.T.H.*), Twentieth Century-Fox, 1980; *Popeye,* Paramount, 1980; *Come Back to the 5 & Dime, Jimmy Dean, Jimmy Dean,* Viacom, 1982; (also producer with Nick J. Mileti) *Streamers,* United Artists Classics, 1983; (also producer) *Secret Honor* (also known as *Secret Honor: The Last Testament of Richard M. Nixon* and *Secret Honor: A Political Myth*), Cinecom, 1984; *Fool for Love,* Cannon, 1985; "Les Boreades" in *Aria,* Virgin Vision, 1987; *Beyond Therapy,* New World, 1987; (also producer with Peter Newman) *O.C. and Stiggs,* Metro-Goldwyn-Mayer/United Artists, 1987. Also *The Builders* (industrial film), 1954; *The Party* (short film), 1964; *Pot au feu* (short film), 1965; *The Kathryn Reed Story* (short film), 1965; *The Easter Egg Hunt,* 1981; and *The Diviners,* 1983.

PRINCIPAL TELEVISION WORK—All as director. Mini-Series: (Also producer) *Tanner '88: The Dark Horse,* HBO, 1988. Pilots: *Sam Hill,* NBC, 1961; *County General,* ABC, 1962; (also producer with Raymond Wagner) *A Walk in the Night,* CBS, 1968. Episodic: *Alfred Hitchcock Presents,* CBS, 1957; *The Roaring Twenties,* ABC, 1960; also *Kraft Mystery Theatre,* NBC; *The Desilu Playhouse,* CBS; *Bonanza,* NBC; *M Squad,* NBC; *The Millionaire,* CBS; *Maverick,* ABC; *Route 66,* CBS; *Sugarfoot,* ABC; *Surfside 6,* ABC; *The Long Hot Summer,* ABC; *The Gallant Men,* ABC; *Bronco,* ABC; *Lawman,* ABC; *Bus Stop,* ABC; *Combat,* ABC; *Peter Gunn.* Movies: *The Caine Mutiny Court-Martial,* CBS, 1988. Specials: (Also producer) *The Laundromat,* HBO, 1985; (also producer) *The Dumb Waiter,* ABC, 1987; (also producer) *The Room,* ABC, 1987.

RELATED CAREER—Writer, photographer, editor, and director of industrial films, Calvin Company, Kansas City, MO; founder, Lion's Gate Productions (a film production company) and Westwood Editorial Services (a film post-production facility); founder, Sandcastle 5 Productions (a film production company).

WRITINGS: See production details above. FILM—*The Delinquents,* 1957; (with George W. George) *The James Dean Story* (documentary), 1957; (with Brian McKay) *McCabe and Mrs. Miller,* 1971; *Images,* 1972; (with Calder Willingham and Joan Tewkesbury) *Thieves Like Us,* 1974; *Three Women,* 1977; (with John Considine, Patricia Resnick, and Allan Nicholls) *A Wedding,* 1978; (with Frank Barhydt and Resnick) *Quintet,* 1979; (with Nicholls) *A Perfect Couple,* 1979; (with Barhydt and Paul Dooley) *Health,* 1980; (with Christopher Durang) *Beyond Therapy,* 1987. Also co-songwriter, "The Day I Looked Jesus in the Eye" in *Nashville,* Paramount, 1975.

TELEVISION—Episodic: *Kraft Television Theatre,* NBC; *The Long Hot Summer,* ABC; *Combat,* ABC.

AWARDS: Golden Palm from the Cannes International Film Festival, 1970, and Academy Award nomination, Best Director, 1971, both for *M*A*S*H;* New York Film Critics Circle Awards, Best Picture and Best Director, 1975, and Academy Award nominations, Best Picture and Best Director, 1976, all for *Nashville;* Golden Bear from the Berlin International Film Festival, 1976, for *Buffalo Bill and the Indians, or Sitting Bull's History Lesson.*

MEMBER: Directors Guild of America.

ADDRESSES: OFFICE—1861 S. Bundy Drive, Los Angeles, CA 90025. AGENT—International Creative Management, 40 W. 57th Street, New York, NY 10019.*

*   *   *

ALVARADO, Trini   1967-

PERSONAL: Full name, Trinidad Alvarado; born in 1967 in New York, NY.

VOCATION: Actress.

CAREER: BROADWAY DEBUT—Melinda, *Runaways,* New York Shakespeare Festival, Plymouth Theatre, 1978. PRINCIPAL STAGE APPEARANCES—Melinda, *Runaways,* New York Shakespeare Festival, Public Theatre, New York City, 1978; Anne Frank, *Yours, Anne,* Playhouse 91, New York City, 1985; Maggie, *Maggie Magalita,* Lamb's Theatre, New York City, 1986.

PRINCIPAL FILM APPEARANCES—Franny Phillips, *Rich Kids,* United Artists, 1979; Pamela Pearl, *Times Square,* Associated Film Distribution, 1980; Irene Soffel, *Mrs. Soffel,* Metro-Goldwyn-Mayer/United Artists, 1984; Molly, *Sweet Lorraine,* Angelika, 1987; May "Mooch" Stark, *Satisfaction,* Twentieth Cetury-Fox, 1988; Lisa Titus, *The Chair,* Angelika, 1988.

PRINCIPAL TELEVISION APPEARANCES—Episodic: Mindy, *Kate and Allie,* CBS, 1986; Sarah, *Kay O'Brien,* CBS, 1986; Laurie Kincaid, *Spenser: For Hire,* ABC, 1987. Movies: Teresa, *Dreams Don't Die,* ABC, 1982; Lisa Castello, *Jacobo Timerman: Prisoner without a Name, Cell without a Number,* NBC, 1983; Anna Rogna, *Frank Nitti: The Enforcer,* ABC, 1988. Specials: Dena McKain, "A Movie Star's Daughter," *ABC Afterschool Special,* ABC, 1979; Alicia Marin, "Starstruck," *ABC Afterschool Special,* ABC, 1981; also *Private Contentment,* PBS, 1982.*

*   *   *

AMECHE, Don   1908-

PERSONAL: Born Dominic Felix Amici, May 31, 1908, in Kenosha, WI; son of Felix (a bartender) and Barbara Etta (Hertle) Amici; married Honore Prendergast, 1932 (separated); children: Dominic Felix, Ronald John, Thomas Anthony, Lawrence Michael, Barbara, Cornelia. EDUCATION: Attended Columbia College (now known as Loras College), 1926-28; studied law at Marquette University, Georgetown University, and the University of Wisconsin. POLITICS: Republican. RELIGION: Roman Catholic.

VOCATION: Actor.

CAREER: STAGE DEBUT—With the Al Jackson Stock Company, Madison, WI, 1928. BROADWAY DEBUT—Perkins, *Jerry-for-Short,* Waldorf Theatre, 1929. PRINCIPAL STAGE APPEARANCES—Steve Canfield, *Silk Stockings,* Imperial Theatre, New York City, 1955; Robert Dean, *Holiday for Lovers,* Longacre Theatre, New York City, 1957; Max Grady, *Goldilocks,* Lunt-Fontanne Theatre, New York City, 1958; Chun, *13 Daughters,* 54th Street Theatre, New York City, 1961; Henry Orient, *Henry, Sweet Henry,* Palace Theatre, New York City, 1967; Jimmy Smith, *No, No, Nanette,*

State Fair Music Hall, Dallas, TX, 1972, then Westbury Music Fair, Westbury, NY, 1974; Stage Manager, *Our Town,* Lyceum Theatre, New York City, 1989. Also appeared in *Excess Baggage,* Greenwich, CT, 1930; *Illegal Practice,* Chicago, IL, 1930; and *Never Get Smart with an Angel,* Country Dinner Playhouse, Austin, TX, 1976.

MAJOR TOURS—Steve Canfield, *Silk Stockings,* U.S. cities, 1956; Oscar Madison, *The Odd Couple,* U.S. cities, 1968; Jimmy Smith, *No, No, Nanette,* U.S. cities, 1973; also with Texas Guinan's vaudeville show, U.S. cities, 1930; and in *I Married an Angel,* U.S. cities, 1964.

PRINCIPAL FILM APPEARANCES—Black Hole of Calcutta prisoner, *Clive of India,* United Artists, 1935; Dr. Rudy Imre, *Ladies in Love,* Twentieth Century-Fox, 1936; Ned Sparks, *One in a Million,* Twentieth Century-Fox, 1936; Allesandro, *Ramona,* Twentieth Century-Fox, 1936; Karl Freyman and Mario Singarelli, *Sins of Man,* Twentieth Century-Fox, 1936; Peter Nostrand, *Fifty Roads to Town,* Twentieth Century-Fox, 1937; Martin Canavan, *Love Is News,* Twentieth Century-Fox, 1937; Tracy Egan, *Love under Fire,* Twentieth Century-Fox, 1937; George Macrea, *You Can't Have Everything,* Twentieth Century-Fox, 1937; Charlie Dwyer, *Alexander's Ragtime Band,* Twentieth Century-Fox, 1938; Dick, *Gateway,* Twentieth Century-Fox, 1938; Jimmy Hall, *Happy Landing,* Twentieth Century-Fox, 1938; Jack O'Leary, *In Old Chicago,* Twentieth Century-Fox, 1938; David Brossard, Jr., *Josette,* Twentieth Century-Fox, 1938; Michael Linnett Connors, *Hollywood Cavalcade,* Twentieth Century-Fox, 1939; Tibor Czerny, *Midnight,* Paramount, 1939; title role, *The Story of Alexander Graham Bell* (also known as *The Modern Miracle*), Twentieth Century-Fox, 1939; Stephen Foster, *Swanee River,* Twentieth Century-Fox, 1939; D'Artagnan, *The Three Musketeers* (also known as *The Singing Musketeer*), Twentieth Century-Fox, 1939.

Ricardo Quintana, *Down Argentine Way,* Twentieth Century-Fox, 1940; Chris, *Four Sons,* Twentieth Century-Fox, 1940; Edward Solomon, *Lillian Russell,* Twentieth Century-Fox, 1940; Mitch, *Confirm or Deny,* Twentieth Century-Fox, 1941; John Hathaway, *The Feminine Touch,* Metro-Goldwyn-Mayer, 1941; Lloyd Lloyd, *Kiss the Boys Goodbye,* Paramount, 1941; Phil O'Neil, *Moon over Miami,* Twentieth Century-Fox, 1941; Larry Martin and Baron Duarte, *That Night in Rio,* Twentieth Century-Fox, 1941; Don Pedro Sullivan, *Girl Trouble,* Twentieth Century-Fox, 1942; Dawson, *The Magnificent Dope,* Twentieth Century-Fox, 1942; Lew Marsh, *Happy Land,* Twentieth Century-Fox, 1943; Henry Van Cleve, *Heaven Can Wait,* Twentieth Century-Fox, 1943; Ken Douglas, *Something to Shout About,* Columbia, 1943; Kenneth Harvey, *Greenwich Village,* Twentieth Century-Fox, 1944; Flight Commander Bingo Harper, *Wing and a Prayer,* Twentieth Century-Fox, 1944; Joe, *Guest Wife,* United Artists, 1945; as himself, *It's in the Bag* (also known as *The Fifth Chair*), United Artists, 1945; Hiram Stephen Maxim, *So Goes My Love* (also known as *A Genius in the Family*), Universal, 1946; Joe Grange, *That's My Man,* Republic, 1947; Richard Courtland, *Sleep, My Love,* United Artists, 1948; John Gayle, *Slightly French,* Columbia, 1949.

Senator A.S. Simon, *A Fever in the Blood,* Warner Brothers, 1961; Edward Shelley, *Picture Mommy Dead,* Embassy, 1966; Commander Taylor, *The Boatniks,* Buena Vista, 1970; Colonel Flanders, *Suppose They Gave a War and Nobody Came?* (also known as *War Games*), Cinerama, 1970; Mortimer Duke, *Trading Places,* Paramount, 1983; Art Selwyn, *Cocoon,* Twentieth Century-Fox, 1985; Dr. Wallace Wrightwood, *Harry and the Hendersons,* Universal, 1987; Art Selwyn, *Cocoon: The Return,* Twentieth Century-

Fox, 1988; Mortimer Duke, *Coming to America,* Paramount, 1988; Gino, *Things Change,* Columbia, 1988. Also appeared as himself, *Rings around the World,* 1966.

PRINCIPAL TELEVISION APPEARANCES—Series: Host, *Take a Chance,* NBC, 1950; host, *Startime,* Dumont, 1950-51; manager, *Holiday Hotel,* ABC, 1950-51, renamed *Don Ameche's Musical Playhouse,* ABC, 1951; host, *The Frances Langford-Don Ameche Show,* ABC, 1951-52; host, *Coke Time with Eddie Fisher,* NBC, 1953; regular, *The Jack Carson Show,* NBC, 1954-55; host, *The Don Ameche Theater,* syndicated, 1958; host, *International Showtime,* NBC, 1961-65. Pilots: Harry Graves, *Junior Miss,* CBS, 1957; Dr. Hewitt, *Shepherd's Flock,* CBS, 1971; Otis Ramsey, *Gidget Gets Married,* ABC, 1972; Armand Beller, *Boston and Kilbride,* CBS, 1979; Ben Rosen, *Not in Front of the Kids,* ABC, 1984. Episodic: Tom Blake, *Too Young to Go Steady,* NBC, 1959; also *Climax,* CBS, 1958; *The Love Boat,* ABC; *Fantasy Island,* ABC. Movies: Justin Petit, *Shadow over Elveron,* NBC, 1968; Frank Aherne, *A Masterpiece of Murder,* NBC, 1986; Art Riddle, *Pals,* CBS, 1987. Specials: Henry Longstreet, *High Button Shoes,* NBC, 1956; *The Frances Langford Show,* NBC, 1960; *Kennedy Center Honors: A Celebration of the Performing Arts,* CBS, 1985; *The American Film Institute Salute to Billy Wilder,* NBC, 1986; *Kennedy Center Honors: A Celebration of the Performing Arts,* CBS, 1987.

PRINCIPAL RADIO APPEARANCES—Series: *The Empire Builder,* 1930; *The Chase and Sanborn Hour,* 1937-39; *The Old Gold Don Ameche Show,* 1940; *The Morgan-Ameche-Langford Show,* 1947-48; *Don Ameche's Real Life Stories,* 1958; also host, *Grand Hotel;* host, *The First Nighter;* John Bickerson, *The Bickersons.* Episodic: *The Charlie McCarthy Show,* 1940; also in *The Little Theatre Off Times Square* and *Rin Tin Tin.*

AWARDS: Academy Award, Best Supporting Actor, 1986, for *Cocoon.* Honorary degrees: Loras College, 1960.

SIDELIGHTS: RECREATIONS—Breeding and racing thoroughbred horses.

ADDRESSES: AGENT—Harris/Goldberg, 2121 Avenue of the Stars, Suite 950, Los Angeles, CA 90067.*

*   *   *

ANDERSSON, Bibi   1935-

PERSONAL: Full name, Birgitta Andersson; born November 11, 1935, in Stockholm, Sweden; daughter of Josef and Karin Andersson; married Kjell Grede (a director), 1960 (divorced, 1973); married Per Ahlmark (a politician, journalist, and poet), 1978 (divorced); children: Jennifer Matilda (first marriage). EDUCATION: Attended the Royal Dramatic Theatre School, Stockholm, Sweden, 1954-56; also studied at the Malmo Theatre School and at the Terserus Drama School.

VOCATION: Actress.

CAREER: BROADWAY DEBUT—Anna, *Full Circle,* American National Theatre Academy Theatre, 1973. PRINCIPAL STAGE APPEARANCES—Siri von-Essen-Strindberg, *The Night of the Tribades,* Helen Hayes Theatre, New York City, 1977. Also appeared in productions of *Erik XIV,* 1956; *Tre systrar, King John,* and *Le Balcon* (also known as *The Balcony*), all 1961; *La Grotte* and *Uncle Vanya*, both 1962; *Who's Afraid of Virginia Woolf?*, 1963; *As You Like It* and *After the Fall*, both 1964; *The Archbishop's Ceiling*, both 1973; *Twelfth Night*, 1975 and 1980; *Antigone*, *A Streetcar Named Desire*, and *L'Oiseau bleu*, all 1981; *Prisoners of Altona*, 1982; with the Malmo Theatre, Malmo, Sweden, 1956-59; with the Royal Dramatic Theatre, Stockholm, Sweden, 1959-1962; and with the Uppsala Theatre, Uppsala, Sweden, 1962.

PRINCIPAL FILM APPEARANCES—Actress, *Sommarnattens leende* (also known as *Smiles of a Summer Night*), 1955, released in the United States by Rank, 1957; Mia, *Det sjunde inseglet* (also known as *The Seventh Seal*), Svenska Filminstitutet, 1957, released in the United States in 1958; Sara, *Smultronstallet* (also known as *Wild Strawberries*), 1957, released in the United States by Janus, 1959; Sara, *Ansiktet* (also known as *The Magician* and *The Face*), 1958, released in the United States by Janus, 1959; Hjordis, *Nara livet* (also known as *Brink of Life* and *So Close to Life*), Nordisk ToneFilm, 1958, released in the United States in 1960; Britt-Marie, *Djavulens oga* (also known as *The Devil's Eye*), ABSF, 1960; Maria, *Nasilje na Trgu* (also known as *Square of Violence*), 1961, released in the United States by Metro-Goldwyn-Mayer, 1963; girl, *Alskarinnan* (also known as *The Mistress* and *The Swedish Mistress*), 1962, released in the United States by Janus, 1964; Edvarda Mack, *Kort ar Sommaren* (also known as *Short Is the Summer* and *Pan*), 1962, released in the United States by Shaw, 1968; Humian, *For att inte tala om alla dessa kvinnor* (also known as *Not to Mention All These Women*, *Now about These Women*, and *All These Women*), Janus, 1964; Ellen Grange, *Duel at Diablo*, United Artists, 1965; Charlotte, *Syskonbadd 1782* (also known as *My Sister, My Love*), 1965, released in the United States by Sigma III, 1967; Nurse Alma, *Persona* (also known as *Masks*), 1966, released in the United States by Lopert, 1967; Marianne Pescourt, *Le Viol* (also known as *Overgreppet*, *Le Viol ou un amour fou*, *A Question of Rape*, and *The Rape*), 1967, released in the United States by GG Productions, 1968; Karin Ullman, *Story of a Woman* (also known as *Storia di una donna*), 1969, released in the United States by Universal, 1970; Eva Vegerus, *The Passion of Anna* (also known as *A Passion* and *En passion*), 1969, released in the United States by United Artists, 1970.

Erika Boeck, *The Kremlin Letter*, Twentieth Century-Fox, 1970; Karin Vergerus, *Beroringen* (also known as *The Touch*) Cinerama-Twentieth Century-Fox, 1971; as herself, *Ingmar Bergman* (documentary), Svenska Filminstitutet, 1971; Britt Stagenlius, *Mannen fran andra sidan* (also known as *Chelovek s drugoi storoni* and *The Man from the Other Side*), Columbia, 1972; Katerina, *Scener ur ett aktenskap* (also known as *Scenes from a Marriage*), 1973, released in the United States by Cinema V, 1974; Blanche, *La Rivale* (also known as *The Rival*), Lugo, 1974; Mitta, *Blondy* (also known as *Vortex*), Lugo, 1975; Monique, *Il pleut sur Santiago* (also known as *It Is Raining on Santiago*), Films Marquise/Bulgarofilm, 1975; Dr. Fried, *I Never Promised You a Rose Garden*, New World, 1977; as herself, *A Look at Liv* (also known as *Norway's Liv Ullmann* and *Liv Ullmann's Norway*), W.K. Kap Productions, 1977; Catherine Dumais, *L'Amour en question* (also known as *Love in Question*), Exportacion Francaise Cinematographiqe/Silenes, 1978; Catherine Stockmann, *An Enemy of the People*, Warner Brothers, 1978; Ambrosia, *Quintet*, Twentieth Century-Fox, 1979; Francine, *The Concorde—Airport '79* (also known as *Airport '80—The Concorde*), Universal, 1979; mother, *Barnforbjudet* (also known as *The Elephant Walk*, *Not for Children*, and *The Elephant*), Svenska Filminstitutet, 1979; Laura, *Twee vrouwen* (also known as *Two Women*, *Twice a Woman*, and *Second Touch*), Actueel, 1979.

Anna-Berit, *Marmeladupproret* (also known as *The Revolution Marmalade* and *The Marmalade Revolution*), Svenska Filminstitutet, 1980; Siv Andersson, *Jag rodnar* (also known as *I Blush* and *I'm Blushing*), Svenska Filminstitutet, 1981; Ann-Charlotte Leffler, *Berget pa manens baksida* (also known as *A Hill on the Dark Side of the Moon*), 1982, released in the United States by Crystal, 1983; Margaret Carlson, *Exposed*, Metro-Goldwyn-Mayer/United Artists, 1983; Simone Cambral, *Svarte fugler* (also known as *Black Crows*), Europa, 1983; Viktor's wife, *Sista leken* (also known as *The Last Summer*), Jorn Donner, 1984; singer, *Huomenna* (also known as *Tomorrow*), Kinosto, 1986; Gertrud, *Pobre mariposa* (also known as *Poor Butterfly*), Instituto Nacional de Cinematografia, 1986; flower seller, *Matador*, Cinevista/World Artists, 1986; ambassador, *Svart gryning* (also known as *Los duenos del silencio*, *The Owners of Silence*, *Why*, *Black Dawn*, and *Y*), Hem Films, 1987; Swedish court lady-in-waiting, *Babette's gastebud* (also known as *Babette's Feast*), Walter Manley, 1987.

Also *Dom-Bom* (also known as *Stupid Bomb*), 1953; *En natt pa Glimmingehus* (also known as *A Night at Glimminge Castle*), 1954; *Herr Arnes penningar* (also known as *Sir Arne's Treasure*), 1954; *Flickan i regnet* (also known as *Girl in the Rain*), 1955; narrator, *Staden vid vattnen* (also known as *Town by the Sea*), 1955; *Sista paret ut* (also known as *Last Pair Out* and *The Last Couple Out*), 1956; *Egen ingang* (also known as *Private Entrance*), 1956; *Sommarnoje sokes* (also known as *Summer House* and *A Summer Place Is Wanted*), 1957; *Du ar mitt aventyr* (also known as *You Are My Adventure*), 1958; *Den kara leken* (also known as *The Love Game*), 1959; *Brollopsdagen* (also known as *Wedding Day*), 1960; *Karneval* (also known as *Carnival*), 1961; *Lustgarden* (also known as *The Pleasure Garden*), 1961; *On* (also known as *The Island*), 1964; *Juninatt* (also known as *June Night*), 1965; *Scusi, lei e favorevole o contrario* (also known as *Scusi lei e contrario o favorevole*), 1966; *Svarta palmkronor* (also known as *Black Palm Trees*), 1968; *The Girls* (also known as *Flickorna*), 1968, released in the United States by Lindgren-Sandrews, 1972; *Una estate in quattro* (also known as *L'Isola*), 1969; *Taenk pa ett tal* (also known as *Think of a Number*), 1969; *Afskedens timme* (also known as *The Hour of Parting*), A/S Constantin, 1973; *Justices*, 1978; and *Prosperous Times*, 1981.

PRINCIPAL TELEVISION APPEARANCES—Movies: Major von Dardel, *Wallenberg: A Hero's Story*, NBC, 1985; also Katerina, *Scener ur ett aktenskap* (also known as *Scenes from a Marriage*), Swedish television, 1973; *En dares forsvartal* (also known as *A Madman's Defense*), Swedish television. Plays: Holga, *After the Fall*, NBC, 1974; also *Miss Julie*, Swedish television.

RELATED CAREER—Movie extra, 1949-51; appeared in a soap commercial directed by Ingmar Bergman, 1951.

AWARDS: Cannes International Film Festival Award, Best Actress, 1958, for *Nara livet* (also known as *Brink of Life* and *So Close to Life*); Silver Bear Award from the Berlin International Film Festival, Best Actress, 1963, for *Alskarinnan* (also known as *The Mistress* and *The Swedish Mistress*); Etoile de Cristal from the French Film Academy, Best Actress, 1967, for *Syskonbadd 1782* (also known as *My Sister, My Love*); British Academy Award, Best Foreign Actress, 1971, for *Beroringen* (also known as *The Touch*).

ADDRESSES: OFFICES—Tykovagen 28, Lidingo 18161, Sweden; 11 W. 81st Street, New York, NY 10024.*

ANDREWS, Anthony 1948-

PERSONAL: Born January 12, 1948, in London, England; married Georgina Simpson; children: one son and one daughter.

VOCATION: Actor.

CAREER: PRINCIPAL STAGE APPEARANCES—Chief Stoat and Mr. Turkey, *Toad of Toad Hall,* Duke of York's Theatre, London, 1970; Mustardseed, *A Midsummer Night's Dream,* and Balthasar, *Romeo and Juliet,* both Regent's Park Open Air Theatre, London, 1971; Douglas Blake, *The Dragon Variation,* Duke of York's Theatre, 1977; Neville, *Coming In to Land,* National Theatre Company, Lyttelton Theatre, London, 1987. Also appeared in *Forty Years On,* New Shakespeare Company, Chichester Festival Theatre, Chichester, U.K., then Apollo Theatre, London, 1968; and in *One of Us,* 1986.

PRINCIPAL FILM APPEARANCES—Joseph Gabcik, *Operation Daybreak* (also known as *Price of Freedom*), Warner Brothers, 1976; Hugh Firmin, *Under the Volcano,* Universal, 1984; Johann Tennyson von Tiebolt, *The Holcroft Covenant,* EMI/Universal, 1985; Major Hanlon, *The Second Victory,* J&M, 1986; Major Meinertzhagen, *The Lighthorsemen,* Cannon, 1987; McCormack, *Hanna's War,* Cannon, 1988. Also appeared in *Take Me High,* EMI, 1973; *Les Adolescentes,* 1976; *Observations under the Volcano* (documentary), Teleculture, 1983; and *Notes from under the Volcano* (documentary), 1983.

PRINCIPAL TELEVISION APPEARANCES—Series: Paul Richard, *Dixon of Dock Green,* BBC, 1972. Mini-Series: Lord Silverbridge, *The Pallisers,* BBC, 1974, then PBS, 1977; Nero, *A.D.,* NBC, 1985; Sebastian Flyte, *Brideshead Revisited,* Granada, 1980, then PBS, 1982; Lord Stockbridge, *Upstairs Downstairs,* London Weekend Television (LWT), then PBS, 1975; also *Fortunes of Nigel,* BBC, 1973; "Danger UXB," *Masterpiece Theatre,* PBS, 1978. Episodic: Johnnie Aysgarth, "Suspicion," *American Playhouse,* PBS, 1988. Movies: Reg Hogg, *A War of Children,* CBS, 1972; Stephen Kelno, *QB VII,* ABC, 1974; Buckley, *Mistress of Paradise,* ABC, 1981; Sir Percy Blakeney/title role, *The Scarlet Pimpernel,* CBS, 1982; title role, *Ivanhoe,* CBS, 1982; Tony Browne, *Agatha Christie's "Sparkling Cyanide,"* CBS, 1983; Edward VII, *The Woman He Loved,* CBS, 1988; Michael Fitzgerald, *Bluegrass,* CBS, 1988. Plays: Mercutio, *Romeo and Juliet,* PBS, 1979; also *Much Ado about Nothing,* 1977; *The Country Wife,* 1977; *French without Tears,* 1977; as the school prefect, "Alma Mater," *Play for Today,* BBC; in "The Beast with Two Backs," *Wednesday Play,* BBC; and in *Play of the Month* and *London Assurance.* Also appeared as Carlos, *A Day Out,* 1973; Steerforth, *David Copperfield,* 1974; Basil and actor, "As the Actress Said to the Bishop," *Mating Machine,* LWT; in *Doomwatch,* 1972; *Woodstock,* 1972; *Follyfoot,* 1973; *Z for Zachariah,* 1983; *The Judge's Wife;* and *A Superstition.*

RELATED CAREER—Founder (with Derek Granger and Jeffrey Taylor), Stagescreen Productions, 1984—.

ADDRESSES: AGENTS—International Creative Management, 388-396 Oxford Street, London W1, England; Tom Chasin, The Chasin Agency, 190 N. Canon Drive, Beverly Hills, CA 90212. PUBLICIST—Marcia Newberger, Rogers and Cowan Public Relations, 10000 Santa Monica Boulevard, Suite 400, Los Angeles, CA 90067.*

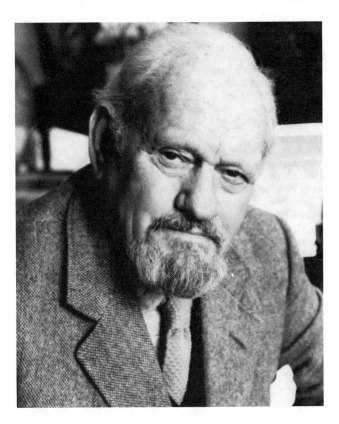

HARRY ANDREWS

ANDREWS, Harry 1911-1989

PERSONAL: Full name, Harry Fleetwood Andrews; born November 10, 1911, in Tonbridge, England; died as the result of a viral infection, March 7, 1989, in Salehurst, England; son of Henry Arthur and Amy Diana Frances (Horner) Andrews. EDUCATION: Attended Tonbridge College and Wrekin College. MILITARY: British Army, Royal Artillery, 1939-45.

VOCATION: Actor.

CAREER: STAGE DEBUT—John, *The Long Christmas Dinner,* Liverpool Repertory Company, Liverpool Playhouse, Liverpool, U.K., 1933. LONDON DEBUT—John, *Worse Things Happen at Sea,* St. James' Theatre, 1935. BROADWAY DEBUT—Horatio, *Hamlet,* Empire Theatre, 1936. PRINCIPAL STAGE APPEARANCES—Christopher, *Snow in Summer,* Whitehall Theatre, London, 1935; Lion, *Noah,* then Abraham and captain, *Romeo and Juliet,* both New Theatre, London, 1935; Francis, *He Was Born Gay,* Queen's Theatre, London, 1937; Queen's gentleman, *Victoria Regina,* Lyric Theatre, London, 1937; Diomedes, *Troilus and Cressida,* Westminster Theatre, London, 1938; Demetrius, *A Midsummer Night's Dream,* Old Vic Theatre, London, 1938; Charlie Glover, *Hundreds and Thousands,* Garrick Theatre, London, 1939; John, *We at the Crossroads,* Globe Theatre, London, 1939; Laertes, *Hamlet,* Lyceum Theatre, London, then Kronborg Castle, Elsinore, Denmark, both 1939; Sir Walter Blunt, *Henry IV, Part I,* Scroop, *Henry IV, Part II,* Creon, *Oedipus,* and Sneer, *The Critic,* all Old Vic Company, Old Vic Theatre, 1945, then Century Theatre, New York City, 1946; Cornwall, *King Lear,* Gerald Croft, *An Inspector Calls,* De Castel-Jaloux, *Cyrano de Bergerac,* Bolingbroke, *Richard II,* Hortensio, *The Taming of the Shrew,* Earl of Warwick, *Saint*

Joan, Osip, *The Government Inspector*, Tullus Aufidius, *Coriolanus*, Orsino, *Twelfth Night*, Lucifer, *Dr. Faustus*, Mirabel, *The Way of the World*, and Epihodov, *The Cherry Orchard*, all New Theatre, 1946-49; Macduff, *Macbeth*, Don Pedro, *Much Ado about Nothing*, Theseus, *A Midsummer Night's Dream*, Pisanio, *Cymbeline*, and Cardinal Wolsey, *King Henry VIII*, all Shakespeare Memorial Theatre Company, Shakespeare Memorial Theatre, Stratford-on-Avon, U.K., 1949.

Vincentio, *Measure for Measure*, Brutus, *Julius Caesar*, Edgar, *King Lear*, and Benedick, *Much Ado about Nothing*, all Shakespeare Memorial Theatre Company, Shakespeare Memorial Theatre, 1950; Bolingbroke, *Henry IV*, Shakespeare Memorial Theatre Company, Shakespeare Memorial Theatre, 1951; Lucius Septimus, *Caesar and Cleopatra*, and Enobarbus, *Antony and Cleopatra*, both Ziegfeld Theatre, New York City, 1951; Antonio, *The Merchant of Venice*, Buckingham, *Richard III*, Enobarbus, *Antony and Cleopatra*, and Kent, *King Lear*, all Shakespeare Memorial Theatre Company, Shakespeare Memorial Theatre, 1953; Claudius, *Hamlet*, title role, *Othello*, and Don Adriano de Armado, *Love's Labour's Lost*, all Shakespeare Memorial Theatre Company, Shakespeare Memorial Theatre, 1956; Casanova, *Camino Real*, Phoenix Theatre, London, 1957; title role, *King Henry VIII*, Old Vic Theatre, 1958; Menenius, *Coriolanus*, Shakespeare Memorial Theatre Company, Shakespeare Memorial Theatre, 1959; General Allenby, *Ross*, Haymarket Theatre, London, 1960; Robert Rockhart, *The Lizard on the Rock*, Phoenix Theatre, 1962; Ekart, *Baal*, Haymarket Theatre, 1963; Crampton, *You Never Can Tell*, Haymarket Theatre, 1966; title role, *King Lear*, Royal Court Theatre, London, 1971; Ivan Kilner, *A Family*, Haymarket Theatre, 1978; Von Hotzendorf, *A Patriot for Me*, Chichester Festival Theatre, Chichester, U.K., then Haymarket Theatre, both 1983, later Los Angeles, CA, 1984. Also appeared in *Richard II*, *The School for Scandal*, *The Three Sisters*, and *The Merchant of Venice*, all Queen's Theatre, 1937-38; and *Uncle Vanya*, Haymarket Theatre, 1982.

MAJOR TOURS—Macduff, *Macbeth*, Don Pedro, *Much Ado about Nothing*, Theseus, *A Midsummer Night's Dream*, Pisanio, *Cymbeline*, and Cardinal Wolsey, *King Henry VIII*, all with the Shakespeare Memorial Theatre Company, Australian cities, 1949; title role, *King Henry VIII*, European cities, 1958.

FILM DEBUT—R.S.M., *Paratrooper* (also known as *The Red Beret*), Columbia, 1954. PRINCIPAL FILM APPEARANCES—Earl of Yeonil, *The Black Knight*, Columbia, 1954; Williams, *The Man Who Loved Redheads*, United Artists, 1955; Darius, *Alexander the Great*, United Artists, 1956; Hector, *Helen of Troy*, Warner Brothers, 1956; Sergeant Payne, *Hell in Korea* (also known as *A Hill in Korea*), British Lion, 1956; Stubb, *Moby Dick*, Warner Brothers, 1956; John de Stognumber, *Saint Joan*, United Artists, 1957; M.S.M. Pugh, *Desert Attack* (also known as *Ice Cold in Alex*), Twentieth Century-Fox, 1958; Major Henry, *I Accuse!* (also known as *Dreyfus*), Metro-Goldwyn-Mayer (MGM), 1958; Baltor, *Solomon and Sheba*, United Artists, 1959; Major Swindon, *The Devil's Disciple*, United Artists, 1959.

Chief Officer Williams, *In the Nick*, Columbia, 1960; Captain Graham, *A Touch of Larceny*, Paramount, 1960; Captain Rawson, *Circle of Deception*, Twentieth Century-Fox, 1961; Peter, *Barabbas*, Columbia, 1962; Captain Rootes, *The Best of Enemies*, Columbia, 1962; Ayoob, *Lisa* (also known as *The Inspector*), Twentieth Century-Fox, 1962; General Singh, *Nine Hours to Rama* (also known as *Nine Hours to Live*), Twentieth Century-Fox, 1963; Captain Curlew, *Reach for Glory*, Columbia, 1963; Father de Bearn, *55 Days at Peking*, Allied Artists, 1963; Mr. Horton,

Nothing but the Best, Royal, 1964; Air Marshal Davis, *Squadron 633*, United Artists, 1964; Bramante, *The Agony and the Ecstasy*, Twentieth Century-Fox, 1965; R.S.M. Bert Wilson, *The Hill*, MGM, 1965; Grimmelman, *Sands of the Kalahari*, Paramount, 1965; Sellers, *The Truth about Spring*, Universal, 1965; Superintendent Bestwick, *Underworld Informers* (also known as *The Informers* and *The Snout*), Rank-Continental Distributing, 1965; Larsey, *The Girl Getters* (also known as *The System*), American International, 1966; Sir Gerald Tarrant, *Modesty Blaise*, Twentieth Century-Fox, 1966; Inspector Mendel, *The Deadly Affair*, Columbia, 1967; Gerald Sater, *I'll Never Forget What's 'is Name*, Regional Films, 1967; Inspector Marryatt, *The Jokers*, Universal, 1967; Superintendent Stafford, *The Long Duel*, Paramount, 1967; Governor Stupnagel, *The Night of the Generals* (also known as *La Nuit de generaux*), Columbia, 1967; Lord Lucan, *The Charge of the Light Brigade*, United Artists, 1968; Intelligence Chief Fraser, *A Dandy in Aspic*, Columbia, 1968; Canning, *Dangerous Route*, United Artists, 1968; Jacob Schpitendavel, *The Night They Raided Minsky's* (also known as *The Night They Invented Striptease*), United Artists, 1968; Sorin, *The Sea Gull*, Warner Brothers, 1968; senior civil servant, *The Battle of Britain*, United Artists, 1969; Savage, *A Nice Girl Like Me*, AVCO-Embassy, 1969; Brigadier Blore, *Play Dirty* (also known as *Written in the Sand*), United Artists, 1969; Kramer, *The Southern Star* (also known as *L'Etoile du sud*), Columbia, 1969.

Brigadier Crieff, *Brotherly Love* (also known as *Country Dance*), MGM, 1970; Ed, *Entertaining Mr. Sloan*, Warner Pathe, 1970; Lieutenant Colonel Thompson, *Too Late the Hero* (also known as *Suicide Run*), Cinerama, 1970; Mr. Earnshaw, *Wuthering Heights*, American International, 1970; Grand Duke Nicholas, *Nicholas and Alexandra*, Columbia, 1971; master of the house, *The Nightcomers*, AVCO-Embassy, 1971; Father, *I Want What I Want*, Cinerama, 1972; governor and innkeeper, *Man of La Mancha*, United Artists, 1972; 13th Earl of Gurney, *The Ruling Class*, AVCO-Embassy, 1972; title role, *The Mackintosh Man*, Warner Brothers, 1973; Lord Ackerman, *Man at the Top*, Anglo-EMI, 1973; Trevor Dickman, *Theatre of Blood*, United Artists, 1973; Albert Parsons, *The Internecine Project*, Allied Artists, 1974; John, *The Last Days of Man on Earth* (also known as *The Final Programme*), New World, 1975; Oak, *The Blue Bird*, Twentieth Century-Fox, 1976; Yohanan the Baptist, *The Passover Plot*, Atlas, 1976; Carl Auerbach, *Sky Riders*, Twentieth Century-Fox, 1976; Harry Dalton, *Equus*, United Artists, 1977; Butler Norris, *The Big Sleep*, United Artists, 1978; Hertford, *Crossed Swords* (also known as *The Prince and the Pauper*), Warner Brothers, 1978; Barnstaple, *Death on the Nile*, Paramount, 1978; Assistant Commissioner, *The Medusa Touch*, Warner Brothers, 1978; second elder, *Superman*, Warner Brothers, 1978; voice of General Woundwort, *Watership Down* (animated), AVCO-Embassy, 1978; high abbot, *Hawk the Slayer*, ITC, 1980; Old Thompson, *Mesmerized*, Thorn-EMI, 1985. Also appeared in *Play It Cooler*, 1961; *Night Hair Child* (also known as *Child of the Night*), Towers, 1971; *Burke and Hare*, Armitage, 1972.

PRINCIPAL TELEVISION APPEARANCES—Series: Tom Carrington, *Dynasty*, ABC, 1985; also *Clayhanger*. Mini-Series: Lord Bellinger, *The Return of Sherlock Holmes*, Granada, then *Mystery*, PBS, 1987; Lord Glenross, *Inside Story*, ABC, 1988; Francis Rattenbury, "Cause Celebre," *Mystery*, PBS, 1988; Wynn Baxter, *Jack the Ripper*, CBS, 1988; Mr. Fitzgeorge, "All Passion Spent," *Masterpiece Theatre*, PBS, 1989; also *A Woman of Substance*, syndicated, 1984. Episodic: "Clowns," *The Play on One*, BBC, 1989. Movies: General Kirk, *Destiny of a Spy*, NBC, 1969; Isaac, *The Story of Jacob and Joseph*, ABC, 1974; General David Feversham, *The Four Feathers*, NBC, 1978; Captain Edward J. Smith, *S.O.S.*

Titanic, ABC, 1979; Lord George Carnarvon, *The Curse of King Tut's Tomb*, NBC, 1980. Specials: General William Howe, "Valley Forge," *The Hallmark Hall of Fame*, NBC, 1975; Superintendent Battle, *The Seven Dials Mystery*, syndicated, 1981. Also appeared in *Edward VII*, 1974; as Tolstoy, *A Question of Faith;* title role, *Othello;* and in *An Affair of Honor, Two Gentle People,* and *Closing Ranks.*

RELATED CAREER—Company member, Liverpool Repertory Theatre, Liverpool, U.K., 1933-35.

AWARDS: National Board of Review of Motion Pictures Award, Best Supporting Actor, 1965, for *The Hill;* Commander of the British Empire.

OBITUARIES AND OTHER SOURCES: New York Times, March 8, 1989; *Variety,* March 15-21, 1989.*

*   *   *

ANDREWS, Julie   1935-
(Julie Edwards)

PERSONAL: Born Julia Elizabeth Wells, October 1, 1935, in Walton-on-Thames, England; daughter of Edward C. (a teacher) and Barbara (a pianist; maiden name, Ward) Wells; took her stepfather's surname when her mother married Ted Andrews (a music hall singer); married Tony Walton (a theatrical designer), May 10, 1959 (divorced, 1968); married Blake Edwards (a film producer, director, and screenwriter), November 12, 1969; children: Emma Kate (first marriage); Amy Leigh, Joanna Lynne (adopted). EDUCATION: Studied singing with Ted Andrews and Madame Stiles-Allen.

VOCATION: Actress, singer, and writer.

CAREER: STAGE DEBUT—Singer, *Starlight Roof* (revue), Hippodrome Theatre, London, 1947. BROADWAY DEBUT—Polly, *The Boyfriend*, Royale Theatre, 1954. PRINCIPAL STAGE APPEARANCES—Title role, *Humpty Dumpty* (pantomime), Casino Theatre, London, 1948; title role, *Red Riding Hood* (pantomime), Nottingham Theatre Royal, Nottingham, U.K., 1950; Princess Balroulbadour, *Aladdin,* Casino Theatre, 1951; title role, *Cinderella* (pantomime), Palladium Theatre, London, 1953; ensemble, *Caps and Belles* (revue), Empire Theatre, Nottingham, 1953; Becky Dunbar, *Mountain of Fire,* Royal Court Theatre, Liverpool, U.K., 1954; Eliza Doolittle, *My Fair Lady,* Shubert Theatre, New Haven, CT, then Mark Hellinger Theatre, New York City, 1956, later Drury Lane Theatre, London, 1958; Guinevere, *Camelot,* Majestic Theatre, New York City, 1960. Also appeared in a Royal Command Performance, Palladium Theatre, 1948; and in *Jack and the Beanstalk* (pantomime), Coventry Hippodrome, Coventry, U.K., 1952.

FILM DEBUT—Title role, *Mary Poppins,* Buena Vista, 1964. PRINCIPAL FILM APPEARANCES—Emily Barham, *The Americanization of Emily,* Metro-Goldwyn-Mayer (MGM), 1964; Maria, *The Sound of Music,* Twentieth Century-Fox, 1965; Jerusha, *Hawaii,* United Artists, 1966; Sarah Sherman, *Torn Curtain,* Universal, 1966; voice of Princess Zeila, *The Singing Princess* (also known as *La rosa di Bagdad;* animated), Trans-National, 1967; Millie Dillmount, *Thoroughly Modern Millie,* MGM, 1967; Gertrude Lawrence, *Star!* (also known as *Those Were the Happy*

Times), Twentieth Century-Fox, 1968; Lili Smith, *Darling Lili,* Paramount, 1970; Judith Farrow, *The Tamarind Seed,* AVCO-Embassy, 1974; Sam, *10,* Warner Brothers, 1979; Amanda, *Little Miss Marker,* Universal, 1980; Sally Miles, *S.O.B.,* Paramount, 1981; title roles, *Victor/Victoria,* Metro-Goldwyn-Mayer/United Artists, 1982; Marianna, *The Man Who Loved Women,* Columbia, 1983; Stephanie Anderson, *Duet for One,* Cannon, 1986; Gillian Fairchild, *That's Life,* Columbia, 1986.

TELEVISION DEBUT—Lise, *High Tor,* CBS, 1956. PRINCIPAL TELEVISION APPEARANCES—Series: Host, *The Julie Andrews Hour,* ABC, 1972-73. Specials: *The Jack Benny Hour,* CBS, 1959; *The Fabulous 50's,* CBS, 1960; *Julie and Carol at Carnegie Hall,* CBS, 1962; *The Julie Andrews Show,* NBC, 1965; *The Julie Andrews Special,* ABC, 1968; *The Julie Andrews Special,* ABC, 1969; host, *An Evening with Julie Andrews and Harry Belafonte,* NBC, 1969; *A World of Love,* CBS, 1970; *Disney World—A Gala Opening: Disneyland East,* NBC, 1971; *Julie and Carol at Lincoln Center,* CBS, 1971; host, *Julie!* (documentary), ABC, 1972; *Julie on Sesame Street,* ABC, 1973; *Julie and Dick in Covent Garden,* ABC, 1974; *Julie—My Favorite Things,* ABC, 1975; *America Salutes the Queen,* NBC, 1977; *Julie Andrews: One Step into Spring,* CBS, 1978; *Merry Christmas . . . With Love, Julie,* syndicated, 1979; *Bob Hope's Pink Panther Thanksgiving Gala,* NBC, 1982; *Julie Andrews: The Sound of Music,* ABC, 1987; host, *The 16th Annual American Film Institute Life Achievement Award: A Salute to Jack Lemmon,* CBS, 1988; also *Julie and Jackie: How Sweet It Is,* 1974; *Julie and Perry and the Muppets,* 1974; *The Puzzle Children,* 1976; sang "Once Upon a Bedtime" in "Peter Pan," *Hallmark Hall of Fame,* NBC, 1976; *ABC's Silver Anniversary Special,* 1978; and appeared in *Julie Andrews' Invitation to the Dance with Rudolf Nureyev.*

WRITINGS: (As Julie Edwards) *Mandy* (children's book), Harper & Row, 1971; (as Julie Edwards) *The Last of the Really Great Whangdoodles* (children's book), Harper & Row, 1974.

RECORDINGS: ALBUMS—*My Fair Lady* (original Broadway cast recording), Columbia Special Projects, 1956; *My Fair Lady* (original London cast recording), Columbia, 1959; *Camelot* (original cast recording), Columbia, 1960; also *Christmas with Julie Andrews,* Columbia; *Tell It Again, Broadway's Fair Julie, Lion's Cage,* and *Julie Andrews and Carol Burnett at Carnegie Hall.*

AWARDS: Theatre World Award, 1955, for *The Boyfriend;* New York Drama Critics Award, Best Actress in a Musical, 1956, and Antoinette Perry Award nomination, Best Actress in a Musical, 1957, both for *My Fair Lady;* Antoinette Perry Award nomination, Best Actress in a Musical, 1961, for *Camelot;* Academy Award, Best Actress, Golden Globe Award, Best Motion Picture Actress in a Musical or Comedy, and British Academy of Film and Television Arts Award, Most Promising Newcomer to Leading Film Roles, all 1964, for *Mary Poppins;* Woman of the Year Award from the *Los Angeles Times,* 1965; Golden Globe Award, Best Motion Picture Actress in a Musical or Comedy, and Academy Award nomination, Best Actress, both 1965, for *The Sound of Music;* Golden Globe Award, World's Film Favorite, 1967; Star of the Year Award from the Theatre Owners of America, 1967; Emmy Award, Outstanding Variety and Musical Series, and Silver Rose Montreux award, both 1973, for *The Julie Andrews Hour;* Academy Award nomination and Golden Globe Award nomination, both Best Actress, 1982, and Golden David Award, Rome, Italy, 1983, all for *Victor/Victoria;* Woman of the Year from the B'nai B'rith Anti-Defamation League, 1983; Hasty Pudding Woman of the Year Award from the

Harvard Hasty Pudding Theatricals, 1983. Honorary degrees: University of Maryland, D.F.A., 1970.

MEMBER: Actors' Equity Association, Screen Actors Guild, American Federation of Television and Radio Artists.

SIDELIGHTS: RECREATIONS—Boating, skiing, and horseback riding.

ADDRESSES: HOME—Gstaad, Switzerland. OFFICE—P.O. Box 666, Beverly Hills, CA 90213. AGENT—Triad Artists, 10100 Santa Monica Boulevard, 16th Floor, Los Angeles, CA 90067. PUBLICIST—Hanson and Schwam Public Relations, 9200 Sunset Boulevard, Suite 307, Los Angeles, CA 90069.*

*   *   *

ARKIN, Adam   1956-

PERSONAL: Born August 19, 1956, in Brooklyn, NY; son of Alan Arkin (an actor, director, and writer).

VOCATION: Actor and screenwriter.

CAREER: PRINCIPAL STAGE APPEARANCES—Nikolai Kaminisi, *Nanawatai,* Los Angeles Theatre Center, Los Angeles, CA, 1985. Also appeared in *The Sorrows of Stephen,* Burt Reynolds Dinner Theatre, Jupiter, FL, 1984; and with the Asolo State Theater, Sarasota, FL, 1985-86.

FILM DEBUT—*The Monitors,* Commonwealth United Entertainment, 1969. PRINCIPAL FILM APPEARANCES—Teenage Gig, *Made for Each Other,* Twentieth Century-Fox, 1971; Charlie, *Chu Chu and the Philly Flash,* Twentieth Century-Fox, 1981; Henry Hudson, *Under the Rainbow,* Orion/Warner Brothers, 1981; Tony Walker, *Full Moon High,* Filmways, 1982; Jeremy, *Personal Foul,* Personal Foul, Ltd., 1987. Also appeared in *Baby Blue Marine,* Columbia, 1976.

PRINCIPAL TELEVISION APPEARANCES—Series: Lenny Markowitz, *Busting Loose,* CBS, 1977; Michael Dreyfus, *Teachers Only,* NBC, 1982; Danny Polchek, *Tough Cookies,* CBS, 1986; Jim Eisenberg, *A Year in the Life,* NBC, 1987-88. Mini-Series: Private Zylowski, *Pearl,* ABC, 1978. Pilots: Ralph, *Mo and Jo,* CBS, 1974; Max, *Between the Lines,* ABC, 1980; Jim Eisenberg, *A Year in the Life,* NBC, 1986. Episodic: Doug Zajk, *St. Elsewhere,* NBC. Movies: Jerry, *All Together Now,* ABC, 1975; Ken Walters, *It Couldn't Happen to a Nicer Guy,* ABC, 1974.

WRITINGS: FILM—(With Morrie Ruvinsky and Ian Sutherland) *Improper Channels,* Crown International, 1979.

ADDRESSES: AGENT—Donna Perricone, Smith-Freedman and Associates, 121 N. San Vicente Boulevard, Beverly Hills, CA 90211. PUBLICIST—Nan Sumski, Sumski, Green, and Company, 8380 Melrose Avenue, Suite 200, Los Angeles, CA 90069.*

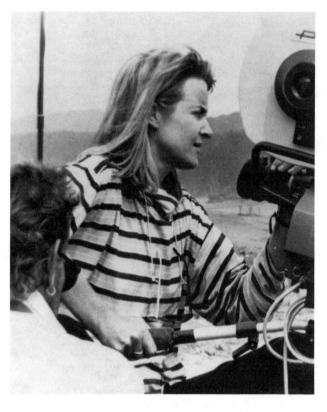

GILLIAN ARMSTRONG

ARMSTRONG, Gillian   1950-

PERSONAL: Full name, Gillian May Armstrong; born in 1950 in Melbourne, Australia. EDUCATION: Attended Swinbourne College and the Australian Film and Television School.

VOCATION: Director, producer, art director, and screenwriter.

CAREER: PRINCIPAL FILM APPEARANCES—Nurse, *Promised Woman,* BC Productions, 1974. PRINCIPAL FILM WORK—Art director, *Promised Woman,* BC Productions, 1974; art director, *The Trespassers,* Filmways, 1975; producer and director, *The Singer and the Dancer,* Columbia, 1977; director, *My Brilliant Career,* Analysis, 1980; director, *Starstruck,* Cinecom, 1982; director, *Mrs. Soffel,* Metro-Goldwyn-Mayer/United Artists, 1984; director, *High Tide,* Hemdale, 1987; producer and director, *Bingo, Bridesmaids, and Braces,* Big Picture, 1988. Also director of the short films *Old Man and Dog,* 1970; *Roof Needs Mowing,* 1971; *Gretel,* 1973; *Satdee Night,* 1973; *One Hundred a Day,* 1973; and *Storytime;* and of the documentaries *Smokes and Lollies,* 1975; (also producer) *Fourteen's Good, Eighteen's Better,* 1980; *Touch Wood,* 1980; *Having a Go,* 1983; *A Time and a Place;* and *Tassie Wood.*

PRINCIPAL TELEVISION WORK—Specials: Producer and director, *Bob Dylan in Concert,* HBO, 1986.

RELATED CAREER—Director of television commercials.

WRITINGS: FILM—(With John Pleffer) *The Singer and the Dancer,* Columbia, 1977.

AWARDS: FACTS Award, Best Travel Commercial, 1982, for an American Express television commercial.

ADDRESSES: AGENT—Judy Scott-Fox, William Morris Agency, 151 El Camino Drive, Beverly Hills, CA 90212.

*   *   *

ATKINSON, Don   1940-

PERSONAL: Born June 4, 1940, in Louisville, OH; son of Donald Joseph and Harriet Eunice (Sluss) Atkinson; married wife, Margaret (an actress and director), October 11, 1970. EDUCATION: Trained for the stage with David Le Grant, Nikos Psacharopoulos, and at the Herbert Berghof Studios.

VOCATION: Actor and director.

CAREER: BROADWAY DEBUT—Dancer, *Greenwillow,* Alvin Theatre, 1960, for eighty-five performances. PRINCIPAL STAGE APPEARANCES—Mercury, *The Happiest Girl in the World,* Martin Beck Theatre, New York City, 1961; Glen, *Sail Away,* Broadhurst Theatre, New York City, 1961; Larry, *Mr. President,* St. James Theatre, New York City, 1962; Larry, *All American,* Winter Garden Theatre, New York City, 1962; Jimmy, *110 in the Shade,* Broadhurst Theatre, 1963; Fyedka, *Fiddler on the Roof,* Imperial Theatre, New York City, 1964; Otto, *Love Me, Love My Children,* Mercer-O'Casey Theatre, New York City, 1971; Overnight Guest, *The Faggot,* Judson Poets' Theatre, New York City, 1973; Earl of Rochester, *Charles the Second,* Classic Theatre, New York City, 1977; Clarence Fountain, *The Impossible* and Clarence Fountain, *The Night before Christmas: A Morality,* both Classic Theatre, 1982. Also appeared as S.S. Captain Meuller, *The Grand Tour,* Jewish Repertory Theatre, New York City; Nathan Detroit, *Guys and Dolls,* State University of New York at Binghamton, Binghamton, NY; press secretary, *The Future,* Judson Poets' Theatre; St. Just, *Danton's Death,* and Dauphine, *The Epicoene,* both Classic Theatre; Fritz, *Anatol,* ensemble, *Ben Franklin in Paris,* Lenny, *Naomi Court,* Rio-Rita, *The Hostage,* and Robbie Ross, *Masque of Wilde,* all in New York City; Count Falcone, *Tortesa the Usrer;* McFarland, *Poor Richard;* Felix, *The Owl and The Pussycat;* Paul Bratter, *Barefoot in the Park;* Starbuck, *The Rainmaker;* Henry II, *Becket;* Harold, *Strictly Dishonorable;* Hod O'Flynn, *Lame Duck Party;* John Howard Payne, *Ever So Humble;* John Charles Fremont, *A Brave Man's Part;* and in *The Decline and Fall of the World as Seen through the Eyes of Cole Porter.*

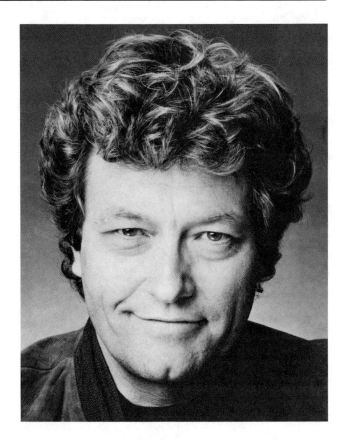

DON ATKINSON

PRINCIPAL STAGE WORK—Director, *Berlin to Broadway,* Light Opera of Riverdell, Riverdell, NJ; also directed productions of *Jesus Christ Superstar, Leaves of Grass, Mame,* and *The Mikado.*

PRINCIPAL TELEVISION APPEARANCES—Series: Greg, *Love of Life,* CBS, 1970-73.

RELATED CAREER—Perfomer in industrial and trade shows.

MEMBER: Actors' Equity Association, Screen Actors Guild, American Federation of Television and Radio Artists.

ADDRESSES: HOME—New York, NY.

B

BACALL, Lauren   1924-

PERSONAL: Born Betty Joan Perske, September 16, 1924, in New York, NY; daughter of William and Natalie (Bacall) Perske; married Humphrey Bogart (an actor), May 21, 1945 (died, January 14, 1957); married Jason Robards, Jr. (an actor), July 4, 1961 (divorced, September 10, 1969); children: Stephen, Leslie (first marriage); Sam (second marriage). EDUCATION: Studied acting at the American Academy of Dramatic Arts, 1941.

VOCATION: Actress.

CAREER: BROADWAY DEBUT—*Johnny Two-by-Four,* Longacre Theatre, 1942. LONDON DEBUT—Margo Channing, *Applause,* Her Majesty's Theatre, 1972. PRINCIPAL STAGE APPEARANCES—Title role, *Goodbye, Charlie,* Lyceum Theatre, New York City, 1959; Stephanie, *Cactus Flower,* Royale Theatre, New York City,

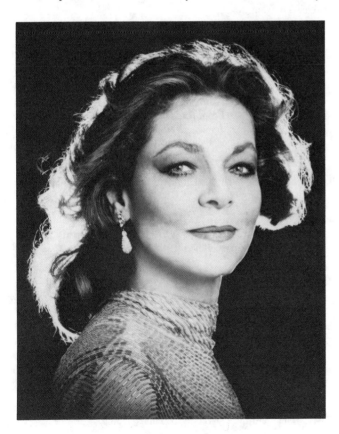

LAUREN BACALL

1965; Margo Channing, *Applause,* Palace Theatre, New York City, 1970, then Civic Auditorium, Toronto, ON, Canada, 1971; Tess Harding, *Woman of the Year,* Palace Theatre, 1981; Princess Kosmonopolis, *Sweet Bird of Youth,* Royal Haymarket Theatre, London, 1985, then Center Theatre Group, Ahmanson Theatre, Los Angeles, CA, 1987. Also appeared in *Wonderful Town,* 1977; and in "Applause" and "Woman of the Year" segments, *Parade of Stars Playing the Palace,* Palace Theatre, 1983.

MAJOR TOURS—Margo Channing, *Applause,* U.S., Canadian, and U.K. cities, 1972; Tess Harding, *Woman of the Year,* U.S. cities, 1983-84; Princess Kosmonopolis, *Sweet Bird of Youth,* U.S. and Australian cities, 1986; also in *Franklin Street,* U.S. cities, 1942.

FILM DEBUT—Marie Browning, *To Have and Have Not,* Warner Brothers, 1944. PRINCIPAL FILM APPEARANCES—Rose Cullen, *Confidential Agent,* Warner Brothers, 1945; Vivian Sternwood Rutledge, *The Big Sleep,* Warner Brothers, 1946; as herself, *Two Guys from Milwaukee* (also known as *Royal Flush*), Warner Brothers, 1946; Irene Jansen, *Dark Passage,* Warner Brothers, 1947; Nora Temple, *Key Largo,* Warner Brothers, 1948; Sonia Kovac, *Bright Leaf,* Warner Brothers, 1950; Amy North, *Young Man with a Horn,* Warner Brothers, 1950; Elizabeth, *Woman's World,* Twentieth Century-Fox, 1953; Schatze Page, *How to Marry a Millionaire,* Twentieth Century-Fox, 1954; Cathy, *Blood Alley,* Warner Brothers, 1954; Meg Paversen Rinehart, *The Cobweb,* Metro-Goldwyn-Mayer (MGM), 1955; Lucy Moore Hadley, *Written on the Wind,* Universal, 1956; Marilla Hagen, *Designing Woman,* MGM, 1957; Julie Beck, *The Gift of Love,* Twentieth Century-Fox, 1958; Catherine Wyatt, *Flame over India* (also known as *North West Frontier*), Twentieth Century-Fox, 1960; Sylvia Broderick, *Sex and the Single Girl,* Warner Brothers, 1964; Dr. Edwina Beighley, *Shock Treatment,* Twentieth Century-Fox, 1964; Mrs. Sampson, *Harper* (also known as *The Moving Target*), Warner Brothers, 1966; Mrs. Hubbard, *Murder on the Orient Express,* Paramount, 1974; Bond Rogers, *The Shootist,* Paramount, 1976; Sally Ross, *The Fan,* Paramount, 1981; Lady Westholme, *Appointment with Death,* Cannon, 1988; as herself, *John Huston* (documentary), Point Blank, 1988; Mrs. Amelia Cranston, *Mr. North,* Samuel Goldwyn, 1988. Also appeared in *Health* (also known as *H.E.A.L.T.H.*), Twentieth Century-Fox, 1980; and *The Great Muppet Caper,* Universal, 1981.

PRINCIPAL TELEVISION APPEARANCES—Episodic: Gabrielle Maple, "The Petrified Forest," *Producers' Showcase,* NBC, 1955; also *The Dupont Show of the Week,* NBC, 1963; *Dr. Kildare,* NBC, 1963; *Stage 67,* ABC, 1967; *The Rockford Files,* NBC. Movies: Lizzie Martin, *Perfect Gentlemen,* CBS, 1978. Specials: *Light's Diamond Jubilee,* ABC, CBS, DuMont, and NBC, 1954; Elvira Condomine, "Blithe Spirit," *Hallmark Hall of Fame,* CBS, 1956;

host, *The Light Fantastic, or How to Tell Your Past, Present, and Maybe Your Future through Social Dancing,* ABC, 1967; Margo Channing, *Applause,* CBS, 1973; Catherine, "A Commercial Break," *Happy Endings,* ABC, 1975; *The American Film Institute Tenth Anniversary Special,* CBS, 1977; *CBS: On the Air,* CBS, 1978; *The Night of the Empty Chairs,* PBS, 1978; *Circus of the Stars,* CBS, 1979; *The Wayne Newton Special,* ABC, 1982; *Parade of Stars,* ABC, 1983; host and narrator, "Bacall on Bogart," *Great Performances,* PBS, 1987; *The American Film Institute Salute to John Huston,* CBS, 1983; *Secrets Women Never Share,* NBC, 1987; "Gregory Peck—His Own Man," *Crazy about the Movies,* Showtime, 1988; also *A Dozen Deadly Roses,* 1963; and *The Paris Collections,* 1968.

PRINCIPAL RADIO APPEARANCES—Series: *Bold Venture,* syndicated, 1951-52. Episodic: Marie Browning, "To Have and Have Not," *Lux Radio Theatre.*

RELATED CAREER—Fashion model, *Harper's Bazaar,* 1943; also appeared in television commercials.

WRITINGS: *Lauren Bacall, By Myself* (autobiography), Knopf, 1979.

AWARDS: American Academy of Dramatic Arts Award for Achievement, 1963; Medallion of Recognition for Contribution to International Fashion from *Harper's Bazaar,* 1966; New York Drama Critics Award, Best Female Lead in a Musical, Antoinette Perry Award, Best Actress in a Musical, and Drama Desk Award, Best Actress in a Musical, all 1970, for *Applause;* Antoinette Perry Award, Best Actress in a Musical, 1981, for *Woman of the Year.*

MEMBER: Actors' Equity Association, Screen Actors Guild, American Federation of Television and Radio Artists, Players Club.

SIDELIGHTS: RECREATIONS—Fashion, tennis, swimming, and needlepoint.

ADDRESSES: AGENT—Johnnie Planco, William Morris Agency, 1350 Avenue of the Americas, New York, NY 10019.*

*   *   *

BAKULA, Scott

PERSONAL: Born in St. Louis, MO.

VOCATION: Actor.

CAREER: BROADWAY DEBUT—Joe DiMaggio, *Marilyn: An American Fable,* Minskoff Theatre, 1983. PRINCIPAL STAGE APPEARANCES—Ted Klausterman, *3 Guys Naked from the Waist Down,* Minetta Lane Theatre, New York City, 1985, and at the Pasadena Playhouse, Los Angeles, CA; Alfred Von Wilmers, "The Little Comedy," and Sam, "Summer Share," in *Romance/Romance,* Helen Hayes Theatre, New York City, 1988. Also appeared in *Keystone,* GeVa Theatre, Rochester, NY, 1981; *It's Better with a Band,* Don't Tell Mama, then Sardi's Club Room, both New York City, 1983; *Broadway Babylon—The Musical That Never Was!,* Paper Moon Cabaret, New York City, 1984; *Accentuate the Positive,* Bottom Line, New York City; *Godspell,* Equity Library Theatre, New York City; *The Baker's Wife,* Cincinnati Playhouse, Cincinnati, OH; as Buck Holden, *Nite Club Confidential,* Tiffany

Theatre, Los Angeles, CA; and in productions of *Shenandoah, The Pirates of Penzance, Magic to Do,* and *I Love My Wife.*

PRINCIPAL TELEVISION APPEARANCES—Series: Hunt Stevenson, *Gung Ho,* ABC, 1986; Bud Lutz, Jr., *Eisenhower and Lutz,* CBS, 1988; Sam Beckett, *Quantum Leap,* NBC, 1989—. Pilots: Jeffrey Wilder, *I-Man,* ABC, 1986. Episodic: Ted Shively, *Designing Women,* CBS, 1986; Peter Strickland, *My Sister Sam,* CBS, 1986; Paul Sanderson, "Infiltrator," *CBS Summer Playhouse,* CBS, 1987; also *Matlock,* NBC; *On Our Own,* CBS. Movies: Drew, *The Last Fling,* ABC, 1987.

AWARDS: Drama Desk Award nomination, Best Ensemble Performance (with Jerry Colker and John Kassir), 1985, for *3 Guys Naked from the Waist Down;* Antoinette Perry Award nomination, Best Actor in a Musical, 1988, for *Romance/Romance;* also *Drama-Logue* Award for *Nite Club Confidential.*

ADDRESSES: AGENT—Jerry Hogan, Henderson/Hogan Agency, 405 W. 44th Street, New York, NY 10036. PUBLICIST—Jay Schwartz, Baker/Winokur/Ryder Public Relations, 9348 Civic Center Drive, Suite 407, Beverly Hills, CA 90210.*

*   *   *

BALDWIN, Adam   1962-

PERSONAL: Born in 1962 in Chicago, IL.

VOCATION: Actor.

CAREER: PRINCIPAL FILM APPEARANCES—Linderman, *My Bodyguard,* Twentieth Century-Fox, 1980; Stillman, *Ordinary People,* Paramount, 1980; Albert, *D.C. Cab,* Universal, 1983; Bobo McKenzie, *Hadley's Rebellion,* ADI, 1984; Randy Daniels, *Reckless,* Metro-Goldwyn-Mayer/United Artists, 1984; Jeff Hannah, *3:15, the Moment of Truth* (also known as *3:15*), Dakota Entertainment, 1986; Skip Jackson, *Bad Guys,* InterPictures, 1986; Animal Mother, *Full Metal Jacket,* Warner Brothers, 1987; Carter, *The Chocolate War,* Management Company Entertainment Group, 1988.

PRINCIPAL TELEVISION APPEARANCES—Movies: Mickey South, *Off Sides,* NBC, 1984; Ike Dimick, *Poison Ivy,* NBC, 1985; Cleary Biggs, *Welcome Home, Bobby,* CBS, 1986. Specials: Otto Frommer, "Out of Time," *NBC Special Treat,* NBC, 1987.

ADDRESSES: AGENT—Cary Woods, William Morris Agency, 151 El Camino Drive, Beverly Hills, CA 90212.*

*   *   *

BALLARD, Lucien   1908-1988

PERSONAL: Born May 6, 1908 (some sources say 1904), in Miami, OK; died as the result of a bicycling accident, October 1, 1988, in Rancho Mirage, CA; married second wife, Merle Oberon (an actress), 1945 (divorced, 1949); third wife's name, Inez (died, 1982); children: two sons. EDUCATION: Attended the University of Oklahoma and the University of Pennsylvania.

VOCATION: Cinematographer.

CAREER: FIRST FILM WORK—Second cameraman (with Lee Garmes), *Morocco*, Paramount, 1930. PRINCIPAL FILM WORK—All as cinematographer, unless indicated: Second cameraman (with Josef von Sternberg), *The Devil Is a Woman*, Paramount, 1935; *Crime and Punishment*, Columbia, 1935; *Craig's Wife*, Columbia, 1936; *The Final Hour*, Columbia, 1936; *The King Steps Out*, Columbia, 1936; *Devil's Playground*, Columbia, 1937; *Girls Can Play* (also known as *Fielder's Field*), Columbia, 1937; *I Promise to Pay*, Columbia, 1937; *Life Begins with Love*, Columbia, 1937; *Racketeers in Exile*, Columbia, 1937; *The Shadow*, Columbia, 1937; *Venus Makes Trouble*, Columbia, 1937; *From Bad to Worse* (short film), Columbia, 1937; *Violent Is the Word for Curly* (short film), Columbia, 1938; *Home on the Rage* (short film), Columbia, 1938; *Three Little Sew and Sews* (short film), Columbia, 1938; *Flight to Fame*, Columbia, 1938; *Highway Patrol*, Columbia, 1938; *The Lone Wolf in Paris*, Columbia, 1938; *Penitentiary*, Columbia, 1938; *Squadron of Honor*, Columbia, 1938; *Blind Alley*, Columbia, 1939; *Coast Guard*, Columbia, 1939; *Let Us Live*, Columbia, 1939; *Outside These Walls*, Columbia, 1939; *Rio Grande*, Columbia, 1939; *Texas Stampede*, Columbia, 1939; *The Thundering West*, Columbia, 1939; *A Star Is Shorn* (short film), Columbia, 1939; *The Villain Still Pursued Her* (also known as *She Done Him Wrong*), RKO, 1940; *Wild Geese Calling*, Twentieth Century-Fox, 1941; (with Charles Clarke) *Moontide*, Twentieth Century-Fox, 1942; *Orchestra Wives*, Twentieth Century-Fox, 1942; *The Undying Monster* (also known as *The Hammond Mystery*), Twentieth Century-Fox, 1942; *Whispering Ghosts*, Twentieth Century-Fox, 1942; *Bomber's Moon*, Twentieth Century-Fox, 1943; *Holy Matrimony*, Twentieth Century-Fox, 1943; *Tonight We Raid Calais*, Twentieth Century-Fox, 1943; *The Lodger*, Twentieth Century-Fox, 1944; co-cinematographer (uncredited), *Laura*, Twentieth Century-Fox, 1944; *Sweet and Lowdown*, Twentieth Century-Fox, 1944; *This Love of Ours*, Universal, 1945; *Temptation*, Universal, 1946; *Night Song*, RKO, 1947; *Berlin Express*, RKO, 1948.

Fixed Bayonets, Twentieth Century-Fox, 1951; *Let's Make It Legal*, Twentieth Century-Fox, 1951; *The House on Telegraph Hill*, Twentieth Century-Fox, 1951; *Diplomatic Courier*, Twentieth Century-Fox, 1952; *Don't Bother to Knock*, Twentieth Century-Fox, 1952; *Night without Sleep*, Twentieth Century-Fox, 1952; "The Clarion Call" in *O. Henry's Full House* (also known as *Full House*), Twentieth Century-Fox, 1952; *Return of the Texan*, Twentieth Century-Fox, 1952; *The Desert Rats*, Twentieth Century-Fox, 1953; *The Glory Brigade*, Twentieth Century-Fox, 1953; *Inferno*, Twentieth Century-Fox, 1953; *New Faces*, Twentieth Century-Fox, 1954; *Prince Valiant*, Twentieth Century-Fox, 1954; *The Raid*, Twentieth Century-Fox, 1954; *The Magnificent Matador* (also known as *The Brave and the Beautiful*), Twentieth Century-Fox, 1955; *Seven Cities of Gold*, Twentieth Century-Fox, 1955; *White Feather*, Twentieth Century-Fox, 1955; *The Killer Is Loose*, United Artists, 1956; *The Killing*, United Artists, 1956; *The King and Four Queens*, United Artists, 1956; *A Kiss before Dying*, United Artists, 1956; *The Proud Ones*, Twentieth Century-Fox, 1956; *Band of Angels*, Warner Brothers, 1957; *The Unholy Wife*, Universal, 1957; *Anna Lucasta*, United Artists, 1958; *Buchanan Rides Alone*, Columbia, 1958; *I Married a Woman*, Universal, 1958; *Murder by Contract*, Columbia, 1958; *City of Fear*, Columbia, 1959; *Al Capone*, Allied Artists, 1959.

The Bramble Bush, Warner Brothers, 1960; *Desire in the Dust*, Twentieth Century-Fox, 1960; *Pay or Die*, Allied Artists, 1960; *The Rise and Fall of Legs Diamond*, Warner Brothers, 1960; *Marines, Let's Go*, Twentieth Century-Fox, 1961; *The Parent Trap*, Buena Vista, 1961; *Susan Slade*, Warner Brothers, 1961; *Ride the High Country* (also known as *Guns in the Afternoon*),

Metro-Goldwyn-Mayer (MGM), 1962; *The Caretakers* (also known as *Borderlines*), United Artists, 1963; *Take Her, She's Mine*, Twentieth Century-Fox, 1963; *Wall of Noise*, Warner Brothers, 1963; *Wives and Lovers*, Paramount, 1963; *The New Interns*, Columbia, 1964; *Roustabout*, Paramount, 1964; *Boeing Boeing*, Paramount, 1965; *Dear Brigette*, Twentieth Century-Fox, 1965; *The Sons of Katie Elder*, Paramount, 1965; *An Eye for an Eye*, Embassy, 1966; *Nevada Smith*, Paramount, 1966; *Hour of the Gun*, United Artists, 1967; *How Sweet It Is*, National General, 1968; *The Party*, United Artists, 1968; *Will Penny*, Paramount, 1968; *True Grit*, Paramount, 1969; *The Wild Bunch*, Warner Brothers, 1969.

The Ballad of Cable Hogue, Warner Brothers, 1970; (with Philip Lathrop) *The Hawaiians* (also known as *Master of the Islands*), United Artists, 1970; *Elvis—That's the Way It Is*, MGM, 1970; *A Time for Dying*, Etoile Distribution, 1971; *What's the Matter with Helen?*, United Artists, 1971; *The Getaway*, National General, 1972; *Junior Bonner*, Cinerama, 1972; *Lady Ice*, National General, 1973; *Thomasine and Bushrod*, Columbia, 1974; *Three the Hard Way*, Allied Artists, 1974; *Breakout*, Columbia, 1975; *Breakheart Pass*, United Artists, 1976; *Drum*, United Artists, 1976; *Mikey and Nicky* (end sequence only), Paramount, 1976; *From Noon to Three*, United Artists, 1976; *St. Ives*, Warner Brothers, 1976; *Rabbit Test*, AVCO-Embassy, 1978. Also *Arruza*, 1968.

PRINCIPAL TELEVISION WORK—Cinematographer, *Six-Gun Law*, 1962.

RELATED CAREER—Assistant cinematographer and film cutter.

NON-RELATED CAREER—In the lumber business.

AWARDS: Academy Award nomination, Best Cinematography (black and white), 1964, for *The Caretakers*.

OBITUARIES AND OTHER SOURCES: Variety, October 5, 1988.*

*   *   *

BALSAM, Martin   1919-

PERSONAL: Full name, Martin Henry Balsam; born November 4, 1919, in New York, NY; son of Albert (a manufacturer) and Lillian (Weinstein) Balsam; married Pearl L. Somner (an actress), October, 1952 (divorced, 1954); married Joyce Van Patten (an actress), August, 1959 (divorced, 1962); married Irene Miller (a television production assistant), November, 1963; children: Talia (second marriage). EDUCATION: Attended the New School of Social Research, 1946-48. MILITARY: U.S. Army, 1941-45.

VOCATION: Actor.

CAREER: STAGE DEBUT—The villain, *Pot Boiler*, Playground Theatre, New York City, 1935. BROADWAY DEBUT—Mr. Blow, *Ghost for Sale*, Daly's Theatre, 1941. PRINCIPAL STAGE APPEARANCES—Johann, *The Play's the Thing*, Red Barn Theatre, Locust Valley, NY, 1941; Sizzi, *Lamp at Midnight*, New Stages Theatre, New York City, 1947; Eddie, *The Wanhope Building*, Princess Theatre, New York City, 1947; murderer, *Macbeth*, National Theatre, New York City, 1948; Merle, *Sundown Beach*, Belasco Theatre, New York City, 1948; ambulance driver, *The Closing Door*, Empire Theatre, New York City, 1949; servingman, *The*

Liar, Broadhurst Theatre, New York City, 1950; man, *The Rose Tattoo*, Martin Beck Theatre, New York City, 1951; pilot of the "Fugitivo" and various roles, *Camino Real*, National Theatre, 1953; Bernie Dodd, *The Country Girl*, Westchester Playhouse, Mt. Kisco, NY, 1953; gangster, *Detective Story*, Westchester Playhouse, then Playhouse-in-the-Park, Philadelphia, PA, both 1953; Bernie Dodd, *The Country Girl*, John Drew Theatre, Easthampton, NY, 1954; Golux, *Thirteen Clocks*, Westport Country Playhouse, Westport, CT, 1954; son-in-law, *Middle of the Night*, American National Theatre and Academy Theatre, New York City, 1956; Eddie Carbone, *A View from the Bridge*, La Jolla Playhouse, La Jolla, CA, 1958.

Hickey, *The Iceman Cometh*, Theatre Group, University of California, Los Angeles, CA, 1961; Moe Smith, *Nowhere to Go but Up*, Winter Garden Theatre, New York City, 1962; Richard Pawling, George, and Chuck, *You Know I Can't Hear You When the Water's Running*, Ambassador Theatre, New York City, 1967; Willie Loman, *Death of a Salesman*, Walnut Street Theatre, Philadelphia, 1974; Joseph Parmigian, *Cold Storage*, American Place Theatre, then Lyceum Theatre, both New York City, 1977. Also appeared in *High Tor*, 1945; *A Sound of Hunting*, Equity Library Theatre, New York City, 1946; *Three Men on a Horse*, Monticello Playhouse, Kiamesha Lake, NY, 1949; *A Letter from Harry*, Putnam County Playhouse, New York, 1949; *Home of the Brave*, Straw Hat Players, West Newbury, MA, 1949; *With Respect to Joey*, Westport Country Playhouse, 1957.

MAJOR TOURS—Norman, *Wedding Breakfast*, U.S. cities, 1955; Jules Walker, *The Porcelain Year*, U.S. cities, 1965.

FILM DEBUT—Gillette, *On the Waterfront*, Columbia, 1954. PRINCIPAL FILM APPEARANCES—Foreman, *Twelve Angry Men*, United Artists, 1957; Sergeant Baker, *Time Limit*, United Artists, 1957; Dr. David Harris, *Marjorie Morningstar*, Warner Brothers, 1958; Kelly, *Al Capone*, Allied Artists, 1959; Jack, *Middle of the Night*, Columbia, 1959; Milton Arbogast, *Psycho*, Paramount, 1960; Steve Jackson, *Ada*, Metro-Goldwyn-Mayer, 1961; O.J. Berman, *Breakfast at Tiffany's*, Paramount, 1961; Mark Dutton, *Cape Fear*, Universal, 1962; Corporal Fornaciari, *Everybody Go Home!* (also known as *Tutti a casa*, *La grande pagaille*, and *All at Home*), Davis-Royal Films, 1962; Feinberg, *The Captive City* (also known as *La citta' prigioniera*), Paramount, 1963; Stanford Kaufman, *Who's Been Sleeping in My Bed?*, Paramount, 1963; Bernard B. Norman, *The Carpetbaggers*, Paramount, 1964; Paul Girard, *Seven Days in May*, Paramount, 1964; Lieutenant Commander Chester Potter, *The Bedford Incident*, Columbia, 1965; Everett Redman, *Harlow*, Paramount, 1965; Arnold Burns, *A Thousand Clowns*, United Artists, 1965; Harry, *After the Fox*, United Artists, 1966; Mendez, *Hombre*, Twentieth Century-Fox, 1967; Mayor Wilker, *The Good Guys and the Bad Guys*, Warner Brothers, 1969; Uncle Harold, *Me, Natalie*, National General, 1969; Ivor Belli, "Among the Paths to Eden" in *Truman Capote's Trilogy*, Allied Artists, 1969.

Colonel Cathcart, *Catch 22*, Filmways, 1970; Allardyce T. Merriweather, *Little Big Man*, National General, 1970; Admiral Husband E. Kimmel, *Tora! Tora! Tora!*, Twentieth Century-Fox, 1970; Haskins, *The Anderson Tapes*, Columbia, 1971; Commander Bonavia, *Confessions of a Police Captain*, Euro International, 1971; Jim Talley, *The Man*, Paramount, 1972; Vescari, *The Stone Killer*, Columbia, 1973; Harry Walden, *Summer Wishes, Winter Dreams*, Columbia, 1973; Green, *The Taking of Pelham One, Two, Three*, United Artists, 1974; Bianchi, *Murder on the Orient Express*, Paramount, 1974; James Arthur Cummins, *Mitchell*, Allied

Artists, 1975; Howard Simons, *All the President's Men*, Warner Brothers, 1976; professor, *The Sentinel*, Universal, 1977; Joe Fiore, *Silver Bears*, Columbia, 1978; General Bello, *Cuba*, United Artists, 1979; Mr. Babcock, *There Goes the Bride*, Vanguard, 1980; Stefanelli, *The Salamander*, ITC, 1983; Max Silverman, *The Goodbye People*, Embassy, 1984; Bennett, *Death Wish III*, Cannon, 1985; Mr. Beamish, *St. Elmo's Fire*, Columbia, 1985; Ben Kaplan, *The Delta Force*, Cannon, 1986; Hap Perchicksky, *Whatever It Takes*, Aquarius, 1986; Cliff Dowling, *P.I. Private Investigations*, Metro-Goldwyn-Mayer/United Artists, 1987. Also appeared in *Youngblood Hawke*, Warner Brothers, 1964; *Eyes behind the Stars*, 1972; *Two Minute Warning*, Universal, 1976; *Death Race*, S.J. International, 1978; and *Innocent Play*, 1983.

TELEVISION DEBUT—*Philco Television Playhouse*, NBC, 1948. PRINCIPAL TELEVISION APPEARANCES—Series: Murray Klein, *Archie Bunker's Place*, CBS, 1979-81. Mini-Series: Senator Michael Glancey, *James A. Michener's "Space"* (also known as *Space*), CBS, 1985; also *Queenie*, ABC, 1987. Pilots: Francis Toohey, "The Defender," *Studio One*, CBS, 1957; Dr. Gillespie, "The Time Element," *Westinghouse Desilu Playhouse*, CBS, 1958; Dr. Rudy Wells, *The Six Million Dollar Man*, ABC, 1973; Buckner, *Death among Friends* (also known as *Mrs. R—Death among Friends*), NBC, 1975; Arthur Haines, *The Millionaire*, CBS, 1978; David Franklin, *The Love Tapes*, ABC, 1980.

Episodic: Harold Matthews, *The Greatest Gift*, NBC, 1954; Danny Weiss, "The Sixteen-Millimeter Shrine," *The Twilight Zone*, CBS, 1959; Martin Lombard Senescu, "The New Exhibit," *The Twilight Zone*, CBS, 1963; also *Goodyear TV Playhouse*, NBC; *Hollywood Screen Test*, ABC; *Dupont Show of the Month*, CBS; *The Alcoa Hour*, NBC; *T-Men in Action*, NBC; *Actors Studio Theatre*, CBS; *The Goldbergs*, CBS; *Captain Video*, ABC; *Crime Photographer*, CBS; *Danger*, CBS; *U.S. Steel Hour*, ABC, CBS, and NBC; *Mr. Peepers*, NBC; *Search for Tomorrow*, CBS; *Valiant Lady*, CBS; *Colonel Flack*, NBC; *Inner Sanctum*, NBC; *Magic Cottage*, CBS; *Robert Montgomery Presents*, NBC; *The Eternal Light*, NBC; *The Stranger*, NBC; *American Inventory*, NBC; *Frontiers of Faith*, NBC; *The Ed Sullian Show*, CBS; *Alfred Hitchcock Presents*, CBS; *Father Knows Best*, CBS; *Desilu Playhouse*, NBC; *The Untouchables*, ABC; *Playhouse 90*, CBS; *Have Gun, Will Travel*, CBS; *Rawhide*, CBS; *The Naked City*, ABC; *Ellery Queen*, NBC; *Westinghouse Theatre*, CBS; *Rendezvous*, CBS; *Five Fingers*, NBC; *Cain's Hundred*, ABC; *Dr. Kildare*, NBC; *Target Corruptors*, syndicated; *Zane Grey Theatre*, CBS; *The New Breed*, ABC; *Route 66*, CBS; *Eleventh Hour*, NBC; *Breaking Point*, ABC; *Arrest and Trial*, NBC; *Espionage*, NBC; *Chrysler Show*, NBC; *Armstrong Circle Theatre*, NBC. *The Defenders*, CBS; *Mr. Broadway*, CBS; *Decoy*, CBS; *The Man from U.N.C.L.E.*, NBC; *The Fugitive*, ABC; *Name of the Game*, NBC.

Movies: Ivor Belli, *Among the Paths to Eden*, ABC, 1967; Stanley Pulska, *The Old Man Who Cried Wolf!*, ABC, 1970; Wade Hamilton, *Hunters Are for Killing*, CBS, 1970; Captain Caleb Sark, *Night of Terror*, ABC, 1972; Jim Douglas, *A Brand New Life*, ABC, 1973; T.C. Hollister, *Trapped beneath the Sea*, ABC, 1974; Ben Montgomery, *Miles to Go before I Sleep*, CBS, 1975; Edward J. Reilly, *The Lindbergh Kidnapping Case*, NBC, 1976; Ira Davidson, *The Storyteller*, NBC, 1977; Captain Ernie Weinberg, *Contract on Cherry Street*, NBC, 1977; Daniel Cooper, *Raid on Entebbe*, NBC, 1977; Louis B. Mayer, *Rainbow*, NBC, 1978; Henry Fancher, *Siege*, CBS, 1978; Dr. Samuel Melman, *The Seeding of Sarah Burns*, CBS, 1979; Isser Harel, *The House on Garibaldi Street*, ABC, 1979; Harry Strasberg, *Aunt Mary*, CBS, 1979; Joel Aurnou, *The People vs. Jean Harris*, NBC, 1981;

Nathan Burkan, *Little Gloria . . . Happy at Last,* NBC, 1982; Jack Brady, *I Want to Live,* ABC, 1983; Alexander Rostov, *Murder in Space,* Showtime, 1985; Dr. Stone, *Second Serve,* CBS, 1986; also *Kids Like These,* CBS, 1987; *The Child Saver,* NBC, 1988. Specials: Garth, *Winterset,* NBC, 1959; also *Hallmark Hall of Fame,* NBC; *The Time Element.* Plays: Doc Delaney, *Come Back, Little Sheba,* ITV (England), 1965.

RELATED CAREER—Member, Town Hall Players, Newbury, MA, 1947; appeared in nightclub act, *The Skeptics,* Cafe Society Uptown, Cafe Society Downtown, Spivy's Roof, and the Blue Angel, all New York City, 1947; member, board of directors, Actors Studio, New York City.

NON-RELATED CAREER—Salesman, radio operator, mechanic, commentator, waiter, usher, and announcer.

AWARDS: Academy Award, Best Supporting Actor, 1965, for *A Thousand Clowns;* Antoinette Perry Award, Outer Critics Circle Award, and Variety poll citation, all Best Actor in a Play, 1967, for *You Know I Can't Hear You When the Water's Running;* Emmy Award nomination, 1977, for *Raid on Entebbe;* Obie Award from the *Village Voice* and Outer Critics Circle Award, Outstanding Performance, both 1978, for *Cold Storage.*

MEMBER: Actors' Equity Association, American Federation of Television and Radio Artists, Screen Actors Guild.

SIDELIGHTS: RECREATIONS—Golf and photography.

ADDRESSES: AGENT—Don Buchwald and Associates, 10 E. 44th Street, New York, NY 10017.*

* * *

BALSAM, Talia

PERSONAL: Daughter of Martin Balsam (an actor) and Joyce Van Patten (an actress).

VOCATION: Actress.

CAREER: PRINCIPAL STAGE APPEARANCES—*The Taking Away of Little Willie,* Center Theatre Group, Mark Taper Forum, Los Angeles, 1979; *Sally's Gone, She Left Her Name,* Center Stage Theatre, Baltimore, MD, 1980.

PRINCIPAL FILM APPEARANCES—Ann Rosario, *Sunnyside,* American International, 1979; Liz Dolson, *Mass Appeal,* Universal, 1984; Lori Bancroft, *Crawlspace,* Empire, 1986; Judy Cusimano, *In the Mood,* Lorimar, 1987; Sharon Raymond, *The Kindred,* F-M Entertainment, 1987; Jenny Fox, *P.I. Private Investigations,* Metro-Goldwyn-Mayer/United Artists, 1987; Private Angela Lejune, *The Supernaturals,* Republic Entertainment International, 1987.

PRINCIPAL TELEVISION APPEARANCES—Series: Randi Mitchell, *Punky Brewster,* NBC, 1983. Pilots: Doreen, *The Millionaire,* CBS, 1978; Grace Geary, *Sticking Together,* ABC, 1978; Eve, *Crazy Times,* ABC, 1981; Princess Nicole, *Fit for a King,* NBC, 1982; Linda Taylor, *The Ladies,* NBC, 1987. Episodic: Cathy Consuelos, "Like Father, Like Daughter" and "Father of the Bride," *Taxi,* ABC, 1978; Sharon Jenkins, *When the Whistle Blows,* ABC, 1980. Movies: Allison, *The Initiation of Sarah,*

ABC, 1978; Rona Sims, *Survival of Dana,* CBS, 1979; Noranne Wing, *Ohms,* CBS, 1980; Sandy Scheuer, *Kent State,* NBC, 1981; Marta Karolyi, *Nadia,* syndicated, 1984; Jean, *Calamity Jane,* CBS, 1984; Margie, *Consenting Adults,* ABC, 1985; also *Alexander: The Other Side of Dawn,* NBC, 1977.

ADDRESSES: AGENT—Leslie Larkin, The Gersh Agency, 222 N. Canon Drive, Suite 202, Beverly Hills, CA 90210.*

* * *

BANCROFT, Anne 1931-
(Anne Italiano)

PERSONAL: Born Anna Maria Luisa Italiano, September 17, 1931, in Bronx, NY; daughter of Michael (a dress pattern maker) and Mildred (a telephone operator; maiden name, DiNapoli) Italiano; married Martin A. May (a building contractor), July 1, 1953 (divorced, February 13, 1957); married Mel Brooks (a director, screenwriter, actor, and producer), 1964; children: Maximilian (second marriage). EDUCATION: Trained for the stage at the American Academy of Dramatic Arts, 1948-50, with Herbert Berghof, 1957, and at the Actors Studio, 1958; studied film directing at the Woman's Directing Workshop of the American Film Institute.

VOCATION: Actress, director, producer, and screenwriter.

CAREER: BROADWAY DEBUT—Gittel Mosca, *Two for the Seesaw,* Booth Theatre, 1958. PRINCIPAL STAGE APPEARANCES—

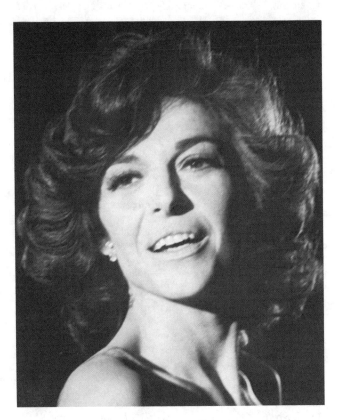

ANNE BANCROFT

Annie Sullivan, *The Miracle Worker*, Playhouse Theatre, New York City, 1959; Mother Courage, *Mother Courage and Her Children*, Martin Beck Theatre, New York City, 1963; Prioress, *The Devils*, Broadway Theatre, New York City, 1965; Regina Giddens, *The Little Foxes*, Vivian Beaumont Theatre, New York City, 1967; Anne, *A Cry of Players*, Vivian Beaumont Theatre, 1968; Golda Meir, *Golda*, Morosco Theatre, New York City, 1977; Stephanie Abrahams, *Duet for One*, Royale Theatre, New York City, 1981.

FILM DEBUT—Lyn Leslie, *Don't Bother to Knock*, Twentieth Century-Fox, 1952. PRINCIPAL FILM APPEARANCES—Marian, *The Kid from Left Field*, Twentieth Century-Fox, 1953; Emma Hurok, *Tonight We Sing*, Twentieth Century-Fox, 1953; Marie, *Treasure of the Golden Condor*, Twentieth Century-Fox, 1953; Paula, *Demetrius and the Gladiators*, Twentieth Century-Fox, 1954; Laverne Miller, *Gorilla at Large*, Twentieth Century-Fox, 1954; Katy Bishop, *The Raid*, Twentieth Century-Fox, 1954; Corinna Marston, *The Last Frontier* (also known as *Savage Wilderness*), Columbia, 1955; Maria Ibinia, *A Life in the Balance*, Twentieth Century-Fox, 1955; Rosalie Regalzyk, *The Naked Street*, United Artists, 1955; Kathy Lupo, *New York Confidential*, Warner Brothers, 1955; Marie Gardner, *Nightfall*, Columbia, 1956; Tianay, *Walk the Proud Land*, Universal, 1956; Beth Dixon, *Girl in Black Stockings*, United Artists, 1957; Angelita, *The Restless Breed*, Twentieth Century-Fox, 1957.

Annie Sullivan, *The Miracle Worker*, United Artists, 1962; Jo Armitage, *The Pumpkin Eater*, Columbia, 1964; Inga Dyson, *The Slender Thread*, Paramount, 1965; Dr. D.R. Cartwright, *Seven Women*, Metro-Goldwyn-Mayer, 1966; Mrs. Robinson, *The Graduate*, Embassy, 1967; Lady Jennie Churchill, *Young Winston*, Columbia, 1972; the Countess, *The Hindenburg*, Universal, 1975; Edna Edison, *The Prisoner of Second Avenue*, Warner Brothers, 1975; as herself, *Silent Movie*, Twentieth Century-Fox, 1976; Carla Bondi, *Lipstick*, Paramount, 1976; Emma Jacklin, *The Turning Point*, Twentieth Century-Fox, 1977; Madge Kendal, *The Elephant Man*, Paramount, 1980; Antoinette, *Fatso*, Twentieth Century-Fox, 1980; Anna Bronski, *To Be or Not to Be*, Twentieth Century-Fox, 1983; Estelle Rolfe, *Garbo Talks*, Metro-Goldwyn-Mayer/United Artists, 1984; Mother Miriam Ruth, *Agnes of God*, Columbia, 1985; Thelma Cates, *'night Mother*, Universal, 1986; Helene Hanff, *84 Charing Cross Road*, Columbia, 1987; Ma, *Torch Song Trilogy*, New Line Cinema, 1988; Mrs. Perlestein, *Bert Rigby, You're a Fool*, Warner Brothers, 1989. Also appeared in *The Brass Ring*, 1955; and in *Arthur Penn* (documentary), 1970.

FIRST FILM WORK—Director, *The August* (unreleased). PRINCIPAL FILM WORK—Choreographer, "Anna Karenina" dance sequence, *The Turning Point*, Twentieth Century-Fox, 1977; producer and director, *Fatso*, Twentieth Century-Fox, 1980.

TELEVISION DEBUT—(As Anne Italiano) "The Torrents of Spring," *Studio One*, CBS, 1950. PRINCIPAL TELEVISION APPEARANCES—Series: *The Goldbergs*, CBS, 1950-51. Mini-Series: Mary Magdalene, *Jesus of Nazareth*, NBC, 1977; Signora Polo, *Marco Polo*, NBC, 1982. Episodic: Virginia, "I'm Getting Married," *ABC Stage '67*, ABC, 1967; also "So Soon to Die" and "Invitation to a Gunfighter," both *Playhouse 90*, CBS, 1957; "Hostages to Fortune," *The Alcoa Hour*, NBC, 1957; "A Time to Cry," *The Frank Sinatra Show*, ABC, 1958; *The Perry Como Show*, NBC, 1960; *Climax!*, CBS; *The Lux Video Theater*, CBS; *Danger*, CBS; *Suspense*, CBS; *Omnibus*, CBS; *Philco-Goodyear Playhouse*, NBC; *Kraft Music Hall*, NBC; and *The Tom Jones Show*, ABC. Specials: *The Bob Hope Show*, NBC, 1964; *The Perry Como*

Special, NBC, 1964; *The Bob Hope Show*, NBC, 1968; host, *Annie, the Women in the Life of a Man*, CBS, 1970; host, *Annie and the Hoods*, ABC, 1974; *The Stars Salute Israel at Thirty*, ABC, 1978; *Variety '77—The Year in Entertainment*, CBS, 1978; *Bob Hope's Women I Love—Beautiful but Funny*, NBC, 1982; host, *That Was the Week That Was*, ABC, 1985.

PRINCIPAL TELEVISION WORK—Director, *Annie, the Women in the Life of a Man*, CBS, 1970.

RELATED CAREER—Member, Actors' Studio.

NON-RELATED CAREER—Drug store clerk, English tutor, and receptionist.

WRITINGS: FILM—*Fatso*, Twentieth Century-Fox, 1980. TELEVISION—Specials: *Annie, the Women in the Life of a Man*, CBS, 1970.

AWARDS: Antoinette Perry Award, Best Supporting or Featured Actress (Dramatic), *Variety* New York Drama Critics Poll Award, and Theatre World Award, all 1958, for *Two for the Seesaw;* New York Drama Critics Award, Best Performance by a Straight Actress, 1959, Antoinette Perry Award, Best Actress (Dramatic), 1960, American National Theatre and Academy Award, 1960, and New York Philanthropic League Award, 1960, all for *The Miracle Worker;* Academy Award, Best Actress, and British Academy Award, Best Foreign Actress, both 1962, for *The Miracle Worker;* Best Actress Award from the Cannes Film Festival, Academy Award nomination, Best Actress, and British Academy Award, Best Foreign Actress, all 1964, for *The Pumpkin Eater;* Academy Award nomination, Best Actress, 1967, and Golden Globe Award, Best Motion Picture Actress in a Musical or Comedy, 1968, both for *The Graduate;* Academy Award nomination, Best Actress, 1977, for *The Turning Point;* Academy Award nomination, Best Actress, 1985, for *Agnes of God;* Golden Globe Award nomination, Best Actress in a Drama, 1987, for *'night Mother;* British Academy of Film and Television Arts Award, Best Actress, 1988, for *84 Charing Cross Road*.

MEMBER: Actors' Equity Association, Screen Actors Guild, American Federation of Television and Radio Artists.

ADDRESSES: AGENT—Toni Howard, William Morris Agency, 151 El Camino Drive, Beverly Hills, CA 90212.*

*   *   *

BANKS, Jonathan

VOCATION: Actor.

CAREER: PRINCIPAL STAGE APPEARANCES—Bob and M.P., *Black Angel*, Center Theatre Group, Mark Taper Forum, Los Angeles, CA, 1977; also appeared in *Safe House*, Center Theatre Group, Mark Taper Forum, 1977; *The Idol Makers*, Center Theatre Group, Mark Taper Forum, 1979.

MAJOR TOURS—Frid, *A Little Night Music*, U.S. cities, 1974-75.

PRINCIPAL FILM APPEARANCES—Party marine, *Coming Home*, United Artists, 1978; marine, *Who'll Stop the Rain?*, United Artists, 1978; television promoter, *The Rose*, Twentieth Century-

Fox, 1979; Jack Graham, *Stir Crazy,* Columbia, 1980; Gunderson, *Airplane!,* Paramount, 1980; hitchhiker, *Frances,* Universal, 1982; Algren, *48 Hours,* Paramount, 1982; Lizardo hospital guard, *The Adventures of Buckaroo Banzai: Across the Eighth Dimension,* Twentieth Century-Fox, 1984; Zack, *Beverly Hills Cop,* Paramount, 1984; Deputy Brent, *Gremlins,* Warner Brothers, 1984; Clyde Klepper, *Armed and Dangerous,* Columbia, 1986; Iceman, *Cold Steel,* Cinetel, 1987. Also appeared in *The Cheap Detective,* Columbia, 1978.

PRINCIPAL TELEVISION APPEARANCES—Series: Dutch Schultz, *The Gangster Chronicles,* NBC, 1981; Vinnie, *Report to Murphy,* CBS, 1982; Kommander Nuveen Kroll, *Otherworld,* CBS, 1985; Frank McPike, *Wiseguy,* CBS, 1987—. Mini-Series: First sergeant, *Ike,* ABC, 1979. Pilots: Courtland Gates, *The Girl in the Empty Grave,* NBC, 1977; patient number one, *The Fighting Nightingales,* CBS, 1978; Sergeant John Vitella, *G.I.'s,* CBS, 1980; Janos Saracen, *Mickey Spillane's Mike Hammer: Murder Me, Murder You,* CBS, 1983; Slick Slim, *The Boys in Blue,* CBS, 1984; Captain Jackson, *The Rowdies,* ABC, 1986. Episodic: Kolinski, *Falcon Crest,* CBS, 1987; also *Designing Women,* CBS, 1987; Krewson, *Police Woman,* NBC. Movies: Woodward, *The Macahans,* ABC, 1976; Buck, *The Night They Took Miss Beautiful,* NBC, 1977; Pato, *The Ordeal of Patty Hearst,* ABC, 1979; Rudy, *She's Dressed to Kill,* NBC, 1979; first heckler, *Wild Times,* syndicated, 1980; Louis, *Desperate Voyage,* CBS, 1980; second resident, *Rage,* NBC, 1980; Darren, *The Invisible Woman,* NBC, 1983; Gheorghe Comaneci, *Nadia,* syndicated, 1984; Earl Dickman, *Assassin,* CBS, 1986; Ray Olson, *The Fifth Missile,* NBC, 1986; Jack Beaudine, *Who Is Julia?,* CBS, 1986; Detective McKenzie, *Downpayment on Murder,* NBC, 1987; Luck Dickson, *Perry Mason: The Case of the Lost Love,* NBC, 1987; also *Alexander: The Other Side of Dawn,* NBC, 1977.

ADDRESSES: AGENT—Dick Dunne, Brooke-Dunne-Oliver, 9165 Sunset Boulevard, Suite 202, Los Angeles, CA 90069.*

*   *   *

BARAKA, Amiri   1934-
(Imamu Amiri Baraka, LeRoi Jones)

PERSONAL: Born Everett LeRoi Jones, October 7, 1934, in Newark, NJ; son of Coyette LeRoi (a postal supervisor) and Anna Lois (a social worker; maiden name, Russ) Jones; changed name to Imamu Amiri Baraka, 1968; dropped honorific title, Imamu (spiritual leader), 1974; married Hettie Roberta Cohen, October 13, 1958 (divorced, August 1965); married Sylvia Robinson (later called Bibi Amina Baraka and Amina Baraka), August, 1966; children: Kellie Elisabeth, Lisa Victoria (first marriage); Obalaji Malik Ali, Ras Jua Al Aziz, Shani Isis Makeda, Amiri Seku Musa, Ahi Mwenge (second marriage). EDUCATION: Howard University, B.A., English, 1954; received M.A. from Columbia University; also attended Rutgers University, 1951-52, and the New School for Social Research. MILITARY: U.S. Air Force, sergeant, 1954-57.

VOCATION: Writer and director.

CAREER: Also see *WRITINGS* below. PRINCIPAL STAGE WORK—Director: *Madheart,* Black Arts Alliance, San Francisco State College, San Francisco, CA, 1967; *Sidnee Poet Heroical,* New

Federal Theatre, New York City, 1975; *S-1,* Afro-American Studio, New York City, 1976; *The Motion of History,* New York Theatre Ensemble, New York City, 1977.

RELATED CAREER—(With Hettie Roberta Cohen) Founder, publisher, and editor, *Yugen* (magazine), New York City, 1958-62; (with Cohen) founder and editor, Totem Press, New York City, 1958; poetry editor, Corinth Books, New York City, early 1960s; founder, American Theatre for Poets, 1961; contributing editor, *Kulchur* (magazine), 1961; (with Diane DiPrima) founder and editor, *The Floating Bear* (magazine), 1961-63; poetry instructor, New School for Social Research, New York City, 1961-64; visiting professor of literature, State University of New York, Buffalo, NY, 1964; founder and director, Black Arts Repertory Theatre/School, New York City, 1964-66; visiting professor of drama, Columbia University, New York City, 1964, then 1966-67; founder, Spirit House (also known as Heckalu Community Center; a black community theatre), Newark, NJ, 1966; visiting professor, San Francisco State College, San Francisco, CA, 1967-68; visiting professor of Afro-American studies, Yale University, New Haven, CT, 1977-78; member, New Jersey Council for the Arts, 1982; associate professor of African studies, 1983-85, then professor, 1985, State University of New York, Stony Brook, NY; (with Amina Baraka) poetry reading, *Poets in the Bars* series, Village Gate, New York City, 1989; member, Second International World Festival of Black Arts; publications director, Jihad Press and Peoples War Publications; editor, *Black New Ark* (monthly newspaper), renamed *Unity and Struggle;* editor, *The Black Nation.*

NON-RELATED CAREER—Organizer, On Guard for Freedom Committee, New York City, 1961; president, Fair Play for Cuba Committee, 1961; organizer, United Brothers, Newark, NJ, 1967; organizer, Committee for a United Newark, 1968; founder, Black Community Development and Defense Organization, Newark, 1968; coordinator of creativity workshops, Black Power Conference, 1968; organizer, Pan-African Congress, Atlanta, GA, 1970; organizer, later chairman, Congress of African Peoples, 1970; organizer, Black American Congress, Gary, IN, 1972; secretary-general, National Black Political Assembly, 1972; chairman, Congress of Afrikan People, renamed the Revolutionary Communist League, Newark, 1974; co-governor, National Black Political Convention; head of advisory group, Treat Elementary School, Newark; member: All African Games, African Liberation Day Committee, African Liberation Day Support Committee, Pan African Federation Groups, Political Prisoners Relief Fund, IFCO International Force.

WRITINGS: STAGE—As LeRoi Jones: *A Good Girl Is Hard to Find,* Sterington House, Montclair, NJ, 1958; *Dante,* Off Bowery Theatre, New York City, 1964, revised as *The Eighth Ditch,* New Bowery Theatre, New York City, 1964, published in *The System of Dante's Hell,* Grove, 1965, then MacGibbon & Kee, 1966; *Dutchman,* Village South Theatre, then Cherry Lane Theatre, both New York City, 1964, then London, 1967, published by Grove, 1967, then Faber and Faber, 1967, and in *Dutchman [and] The Slave,* Morrow, 1964, then Faber and Faber, 1965; *The Baptism,* Writer's Stage Theatre, New York City, 1964, then London, 1971, published in *The Baptism [and] The Toilet,* Grove, 1967; *The Slave,* St. Mark's Playhouse, New York City, 1964, then London, 1972, published in *Dutchman [and] The Slave,* 1964, then Faber and Faber, 1965; *The Toilet,* St. Mark's Playhouse, 1964, published in *The Baptism [and] The Toilet,* 1967; *J-E-L-L-O,* Black Arts Repertory Theatre, New York City, 1965, published (as Imamu Amiri Baraka) by Third World Press, 1970; *Experimental Death Unit #1,* Black Arts Repertory Theatre, St. Mark's Playhouse,

1965, published in *Four Black Revolutionary Plays: All Praises to the Black Man*, Bobbs-Merrill, 1969, then as *Four Black Revolutionary Plays*, Calder and Boyars, 1971; *A Black Mass*, Black Arts Repertory Theatre, Proctor's Theatre, Newark, NJ, 1966, published in *Four Black Revolutionary Plays*, 1969 and 1971; *Slave Ship: A Historical Pageant*, Spirit House Movers, Newark, 1967, then Chelsea Theatre Center, Brooklyn Academy of Music, Brooklyn, NY, 1969, later Washington Square Methodist Church, New York City, 1970, published by Jihad, 1969, and in *The Motion of History and Other Plays*, Morrow, 1978; *Madheart*, Black Arts Alliance, San Francisco State College, San Francisco, CA, 1967, published in *Four Black Revolutionary Plays*, 1969 and 1971; *Arm Yourself, or Harm Yourself!*, Spirit House Theatre, Newark, 1967, published by Jihad, 1967; *Great Goodness of Life (A Coon Show)*, Spirit House Theatre, 1967, then on a bill as *A Black Quartet*, Gate Theatre, New York City, 1969, published in *Four Black Revolutionary Plays*, 1969 and 1971.

As Amiri Baraka: *Home on the Range*, Spirit House Theatre, then Town Hall, New York City, both 1968, published in *Drama Review*, summer, 1968; *Police*, published in *Drama Review*, summer, 1968; *Resurrection in Life*, first produced in Harlem, NY, 1969; *The Death of Malcolm X*, published in *New Plays from the Black Theatre*, Bantam, 1969; *Junkies Are full of (SHH. . .)* and *Bloodrites*, both Spirit House Theatre, then Henry Street Playhouse, New York City, 1970, published in *Black Drama Anthology*, New American Library, 1971; *BA-RA-KA*, published in *Spontaneous Combustion: Eight New American Plays*, Morrow, 1972; *A Recent Killing*, New Federal Theatre, New York City, 1973; *The New Ark's a Moverin*, Spirit House Theatre, 1974; *Sidnee Poet Heroical or If in Danger of Suit, the Kid Poet Heroical*, New Federal Theatre, 1975, published as *The Sidney Poet Heroical*, Reed and Cannon, 1979; *S-1*, Afro-American Studios, New York City, 1976, published in *The Motion of History and Other Plays*, Morrow, 1978; *The Motion of History*, New York Theatre Ensemble, New York City, 1977, published in *The Motion of History and Other Plays*, 1978; *What Was the Lone Ranger to the Means of Production?*, Ladies Fort Theatre, New York City, 1979; *Boy and Tarzan Appear in a Clearing*, New Federal Theatre, 1981. Plays also appear in *Selected Plays and Prose of Amiri Baraka/LeRoi Jones* (contains *Dutchman*, *The Slave*, *Great Goodness of Life*, and *What Was the Relationship of the Lone Ranger to the Means of Production?*), Morrow, 1979.

FILM—(As LeRoi Jones) *Dutchman*, Continental, 1966; *Black Spring*, Black Arts Alliance, 1968; *A Fable* (also known as *The Slave*), MFR, 1971; *Supercoon* (animated short film), Gene Persson, 1971.

OTHER—Poetry: (As LeRoi Jones) *Preface to a Twenty Volume Suicide Note*, Totem/Corinth, 1961; (as LeRoi Jones) *The Dead Lecturer*, Grove, 1964; (as LeRoi Jones) *Black Art*, Jihad, 1966; (as LeRoi Jones) *A Poem for Black Hearts*, Broadside Press, 1967; (as LeRoi Jones) *Black Magic: Sabotage; Target Study; Black Art; Collected Poetry, 1961-1967*, Bobbs-Merrill, 1969, then MacGibbon & Kee, 1969; *It's Nation Time*, Third World Press, 1970; (as *Spirit Reach*, Jihad, 1972; *Afrikan Revolution: A Poem*, Jihad, 1973; *Hard Facts*, People's War Publishing, 1975; *Selected Poetry of Amiri Baraka/LeRoi Jones*, Morrow, 1979. Fiction: (As LeRoi Jones) *The System of Dante's Hell*, Grove, 1965, then MacGibbon & Kee, 1966; (as LeRoi Jones) *Tales* (short stories), Grove, 1967, then MacGibbon & Kee, 1969; *Three Books by Imamu Amiri Baraka* (contains *The System of Dante's Hell*, *Tales*, and *The Dead Lecturer*), Grove, 1975.

Essays and non-fiction: (As LeRoi Jones) *Cuba Libre*, Fair Play for Cuba Committee, 1961; (as LeRoi Jones) *Blues People . . . Negro Music in White America*, Morrow, 1963, then as *Negro Music in White America*, MacGibbon & Kee, 1965; (as LeRoi Jones) *Home: Social Essays*, Morrow, 1966, then MacGibbon and Kee, 1968; (as LeRoi Jones) *Black Music*, Morrow, 1967, then MacGibbon & Kee, 1969; (with Fundi; also known as Billy Abernathy) *In Our Terribleness (Some Elements and Meaning in Black Style)*, Bobbs-Merrill, 1970; *Strategy and Tactics of a Pan-African Nationalist Party*, Jihad, 1971; *A Black Value System*, Jihad, 1970; *Raise Race Rays Raze: Essays Since 1965*, Random House, 1971; *The Life and Times of John Coltrane*, 1971; *The Creation of the New Ark*, Spirit Reach, 1972; *Kawaida Studies: The New Nationalism*, Third World Press, 1972; *Crisis in Boston*, Vita Wa Watu—Peoples War Publishing, 1974; *Reggae or Not!*, Contact Two, 1982; *The Autobiography of Leroi Jones-Amiri Baraka*, Freundlich, 1984; *Daggers and Javelins, Essays, 1974-79*, Morrow, 1984; *The Music: Reflections on Jazz and Blues*, Morrow, 1987.

All as editor, unless indicated: (As LeRoi Jones) Compiler, *January 1st 1959: Fidel Castro*, Totem, 1959; (as LeRoi Jones) *Four Young Lady Poets*, Corinth, 1962; (as LeRoi Jones) contributor, *Soon, One Morning*, Knopf, 1963; (as LeRoi Jones; also writer of introduction) *The Moderns: An Anthology of New Writing in America*, Corinth, 1963, then MacGibbon & Kee, 1965, also published as *The Moderns: New Fiction in America*, 1964; (as LeRoi Jones; also co-author) *Information*, Totem, 1965; (as LeRoi Jones) *Black and White*, Corinth, 1965; (as LeRoi Jones) *Hands Up!*, Corinth, 1965; (as LeRoi Jones; also contributor) *Afro-American Festival of the Arts Magazine*, Jihad, 1966, then as *Anthology of Our Black Selves*, 1969; (as LeRoi Jones) writer of introduction, *Felix of the Silent Forest*, Poets Press, 1967; (as LeRoi Jones, with Larry Neal; also contributor) *Black Fire: An Anthology of Afro-American Writing*, Morrow, 1968; (with Neal and A.B. Spellman) *The Cricket: Black Music in Evolution*, Jihad, 1968, then as *Trippin': A Need for Change*, New Ark, 1969; writer of preface, *Black Boogaloo (Notes on Black Liberation)*, Journal of Black Poetry Press, 1969; (also writer of introduction) *African Congress: A Documentary of the First Modern Pan-African Congress*, Morrow, 1972; (with Amina Baraka) *Confirmation: An Anthology of African American Women*, Morrow, 1983. Also contributer of articles to journals, magazines, and periodicals.

RECORDINGS: ALBUMS—*New Music/New Poetry*, India Navigation.

AWARDS: Longview Foundation Award, 1961, for *Cuba Libre;* John Whitney Foundation Fellowship for Poetry and Action, 1962; Guggenheim Fellowship, 1965; Obie Award from the *Village Voice*, Best American Play, 1964, for *Dutchman;* Yoruba Academy Fellowship, 1965; Second Prize from the First World Festival of Negro Arts in Dakar (Senegal), 1966, for *The Slave;* National Endowment for the Arts grant, 1966; Rockefeller Foundation Fellowship, 1981; National Endowment for the Arts Poetry Award, 1981; Drama Award, 1985. Honorary degrees: Malcolm X College, Doctor of Humane Letters, 1977.

MEMBER: Black Academy of Arts and Letters.

ADDRESSES: OFFICES—Congress of African People, 13 Belmont Avenue, Newark, NJ 07103; William Morrow and Company, 105 Madison Avenue, New York, NY 10016. AGENT—Ronald Hobbs Literary Agency, 516 Fifth Avenue, New York, NY 10036.*

BARAKA, Imamu Amiri
See BARAKA, Amiri

* * *

BARKER, Ronnie 1929-

PERSONAL: Born September 25, 1929, in Bedford, England; son of Leonard William and Edith Eleanor (Carter) Barker; married Joy Tubb.

VOCATION: Actor and comedian.

CAREER: STAGE DEBUT—Lieutenant Spicer, *Quality Street,* Aylesbury Repertory Theatre, Aylesbury, U.K., 1948. LONDON DEBUT—Chantyman and Joe Silva, *Mourning Becomes Electra,* Apollo Theatre, 1955. PRINCIPAL STAGE APPEARANCES—Farmer, *Summertime,* Apollo Theatre, London, 1955; gypsy man, *Listen to the Wind,* Arts Theatre, London, 1955; Mr. Thwaites, *Double Image,* Savoy Theatre, London, 1956; various roles, *Camino Real,* Phoenix Theatre, London, 1957; Perigord, *Nekrassov,* Royal Court Theatre, London, 1957; Robertoles-Diams, *Irma La Douce,* Lyric Theatre, London, 1958; Nikolai Triletski, *Platonov,* Royal Court Theatre, 1960; ensemble, *On the Brighter Side* (revue), Phoenix Theatre, then Comedy Theatre, both London, 1961; Quince, *A Midsummer Night's Dream,* Royal Court Theatre, 1962; Bob Acres, *All in Love,* May Fair Theatre, London, 1964; Lord Slingsby-Craddock, *Mr. Whatnot,* Arts Theatre, 1964; Alf Always, *Sweet Fanny Adams,* Stratford Theatre Royal, Stratford-on-Avon, U.K., 1966; Birdboot, *The Real Inspector Hound,* Criterion Theatre, London, 1968; Sir John, *Good-Time Johnny,* Birmingham Repertory Theatre, Birmingham, U.K., 1971; as himself, *The Two Ronnies* (two-man show with Ronnie Corbett), Bristol, U.K., then London Palladium, London, both 1978. Also appeared in *Lysistrata,* Royal Court Theatre, 1957.

MAJOR TOURS—As himself, *The Two Ronnies* (two-man show with Ronnie Corbett), U.K. and Australian cities, both 1979.

PRINCIPAL FILM APPEARANCES—Burton, *Kill or Cure,* Metro-Goldwyn-Mayer, 1962; Ronnie, *The Bargee,* Warner Brothers-Pathe, 1964; Mr. Galore, *Runaway Railway,* Children's Film Fund, 1965; George Venaxas, *The Man Outside,* Allied Artists, 1968; Friar Tuck, *Robin and Marian,* Columbia, 1976; Norman Fletcher, *Porridge* (also known as *Doing Time*), ITC Film Distributors, 1979. Also appeared in *Wonderful Things!,* Associated British-Pathe, 1958; *Futtock's End;* and *Picnic.*

PRINCIPAL TELEVISION APPEARANCES—Series: As himself, *The Two Ronnies,* PBS, 1978; Arkwright, *Open All Hours,* Entertainment Channel, 1982. Also appeared in *Sorry.*

NON-RELATED CAREER—Bank clerk.

WRITINGS: FILM—*Picnic.* TELEVISION—*The Two Ronnies,* PBS, 1978.

AWARDS: Order of the British Empire.*

BARR, Richard 1917-1989

PERSONAL: Born Richard Baer, September 6, 1917, in Washington, DC; died of liver failure resulting from the HIV virus associated with AIDS, January 9, 1989, in New York, NY; son of David Alphonse (a builder) and Ruth Nanette (Israel) Baer. EDUCATION: Princeton University, A.B., 1938. MILITARY: U.S. Army Air Forces, captain and head of motion picture unit, 1941-46.

VOCATION: Producer, director, and actor.

CAREER: STAGE DEBUT—Convention attendant, *Danton's Death,* Mercury Theatre Company, Mercury Theatre, New York City, 1938. PRINCIPAL STAGE WORK—Director, *Volpone, Angel Street,* and *The Bear,* all City Center Theatre, New York City, 1948; director and lighting designer, *Richard III,* Booth Theatre, New York City, 1949; director, *Deirdre of the Sorrows,* Master Institute Theatre, New York City, 1949; director, *Arms and the Man,* Arena Theatre, New York City, 1950; producer (with Charles Bowden) and director, *At Home with Ethel Waters,* 48th Street Theatre, New York City, 1953; producer (with Bowden), *Ruth Draper and Her Company of Characters,* Vanderbilt Theatre, New York City, 1954; director, *The Boy with a Cart,* Broadway Tabernacle Church, New York City, 1954; producer (with Bowden), *Ruth and Paul Draper,* Bijou Theatre, New York City, 1954; producer (with Bowden), "Trouble in Tahiti," "Paul Draper," and "27 Wagons Full of Cotton," in *All in One,* Playhouse Theatre, New York City, 1955; producer (with Bowden), *Ruth Draper,* Playhouse Theatre, 1956; producer (with Bowden and H. Ridgely Bullock), *Fallen Angels,* Playhouse Theatre, 1956; producer (with Bowden, Bullock, Richard Myers, and Julius Fleischmann), *Hotel Paradiso,* Henry Miller's Theatre, New York City, 1957; producer (with Bowden and Bullock), *Season of Choice,* Barbizon-Plaza Theatre, New York City, 1959.

Producer (with H.B. Lutz and Harry J. Brown, Jr.), as "Theatre 1960": *Krapp's Last Tape* and *The Zoo Story* (double-bill), Provincetown Playhouse, New York City, 1960; (also director) *The Killer,* Seven Arts Theatre, New York City, 1960; (also director) *Nekros, Embers,* and *Fam and Yam* (triple-bill), American National Theatre and Academy (ANTA) Matinee Series, Theatre De Lys, New York City, 1960.

Producer, as "Theatre 1961": *The Sudden End of Anne Cinquefoil,* East End Theatre, New York City, 1961; (with Clinton Wilder) *The American Dream* and *Bartleby* (double-bill), York Theatre, New York City, 1961 (*Bartleby* was replaced by the Valerie Bettis Dance Theatre and later by *The Death of Bessie Smith*); (with Wilder) *Gallows Humor,* Gramercy Arts Theatre, New York City, 1961.

Producer (with Wilder), as "Theatre 1962": *Happy Days,* Cherry Lane Theatre, New York City, 1961; *The Theatre of the Absurd* (a repertory program consisting of of *Endgame, Bertha, Gallows Humor, The Sandbox, Deathwatch, Picnic on the Battlefield, The American Dream,* [also director] *The Zoo Story,* and [also director] *The Killer*), Cherry Lane Theatre, 1962.

Producer (with Wilder), as "Theatre 1963": *Mrs. Dally Has a Lover* and *Whisper into My Good Ear* (double-bill), Cherry Lane Theatre, 1962; *Who's Afraid of Virginia Woolf?,* Billy Rose Theatre, New York City, 1962; *Like Other People,* Village South Theatre, New York City, 1963; *The American Dream* and *The Zoo Story* (double-bill), Cherry Lane Theatre, 1963.

Producer (with Wilder and Edward Albee), as "Theatre 1964": *Corruption in the Palace of Justice*, Cherry Lane Theatre, 1963; *Play* and *The Lover* (double-bill), then *Play, The Two Executioners*, and *The Dutchman* (triple-bill), then *The Zoo Story* and *The Dutchman* (double-bill), all Cherry Lane Theatre, 1964; *Funnyhouse of a Negro*, East End Theatre, 1964; *Who's Afraid of Virginia Woolf?*, Picadilly Theatre, London, 1964. Also producer (with Wilder), *The Giants' Dance*, Cherry Lane Theatre, 1964.

Producer (with Albee and Wilder), as "Theatre 1965": *Tiny Alice*, Billy Rose Theatre, 1964; New Playwrights Series I, II, and III, including *Up to Thursday, Balls,* and *Home Free!* (Series I), *Pigeons* and *Conerico Was Here to Stay* (Series II), and *Hunting the Jingo Bird* and *Lovey* (Series III), then (with Frith Banbury) *Do Not Pass Go*, later *The Zoo Story* and *Krapp's Last Tape* (double-bill), all Cherry Lane Theatre, 1965. Also producer (with Wilder), *That Thing at the Cherry Lane* (revue), Cherry Lane Theatre, 1965.

Producer (with Albee and Wilder), as "Theatre 1966": *Happy Days*, Cherry Lane Theatre, 1965; *Malcolm*, Shubert Theatre, New York City, 1966.

Producer (with Albee and Wilder, unless noted), as "Theatre 1967": *A Delicate Balance*, Martin Beck Theatre, New York City, 1966; *Thornton Wilder's Triple Bill* (a program consisting of *The Long Christmas Dinner, Queens of France,* and *The Happy Journey to Trenton and Camden*), then *The Butter and Egg Man*, later *Night of the Dunce*, all Cherry Lane Theatre, 1966; *The Rimers of Eldritch*, then *The Party on Greenwich Avenue*, both Cherry Lane Theatre, 1967; (with Wilder and Michael Kasdan) *Match-Play* and *A Party for Divorce* (double-bill), Provincetown Playhouse, New York City, 1966; Paul Taylor Dance Company, ANTA Theatre, 1966.

Producer (with Wilder and Charles Woodward, Jr., unless noted), as "Theatre 1968": *Johnny No-Trump*, Cort Theatre, New York City, 1967; (with Wilder) *Everything in the Garden*, Plymouth Theatre, New York City, 1967. Also producer (with Woodward), *The Boys in the Band*, Theatre Four, New York City, 1968; director, *Private Lives*, Theatre De Lys, 1968.

Producer (with Albee), as "Theatre 1969 Playwrights Repertory": *Box* and *Quotations from Chairman Mao Tse-Tung* (double-bill), *The Death of Bessie Smith* and *The American Dream* (double-bill), (also director) *Krapp's Last Tape* and *The Zoo Story* (double-bill), and *Happy Days*, all Studio Arena Theatre, Buffalo, NY, then Billy Rose Theatre, 1968. Also producer (with Albee and Woodward), as "Theatre 1969," *The Front Page*, Ethel Barrymore Theatre, New York City, 1969.

Producer (with Albee and Woodward), as "Playwrights Unit of Theatre 1970" (also with ANTA), *Watercolor* and *Criss-Crossing* (double-bill), ANTA Theatre, 1970; producer (with Woodward and Albee), as "Theatre 1971," *All Over*, Martin Beck Theatre, 1971; producer (with Woodward), as "Theatre 1972," *Drat!*, McAlpin Rooftop Theatre, New York City, 1971, and (also with Michael Harvey) *The Grass Harp*, Martin Beck Theatre, 1971; producer, as "Theatre 1973" (also with Woodward and ANTA), *The Last of Mrs. Lincoln*, ANTA Theatre, 1972, and (with Woodward) *Detective Story*, Paramus Playhouse, Paramus, NJ, then Shubert Theatre, Philadelphia, PA, both 1973. Also producer (with Woodward), *Noel Coward in Two Keys*, Ethel Barrymore Theatre, 1974.

Producer (with Woodward and Terry Spiegel), *P.S.: Your Cat Is Dead!*, Studio Arena Theatre, then John Golden Theatre, New York City, both 1975; producer (with Woodward and Wilder), *Seascape*, Shubert Theatre, 1975, then in Los Angeles; producer, *I Was Sitting on My Patio This Guy Appeared I Thought I Was Hallucinating*, Cherry Lane Theatre, 1977; producer (with Woodward, Robert Fryer, Mary Lea Johnson, and Martin Richards), *Sweeney Todd*, Uris Theatre, New York City, 1979; producer (with Lester Osterman, Roger Berlind, Marc Howard, Spencer H. Berlin, and Hale Matthews), *The Lady from Dubuque*, Morosco Theatre, New York City, 1980; producer (with Woodward and David Bixler), *Home Front*, Royale Theatre, New York City, 1985.

MAJOR TOURS—Producer: *Auntie Mame* (two companies), U.S. cities, 1957-59; (with Clinton Wilder and Sometimes, Inc.) *Who's Afraid of Virginia Woolf?*, U.S. and Canadian cities, 1964-65; *A Delicate Balance*, U.S. cities, 1967; (with Charles Woodward, Jr.) *The Boys in the Band* (two companies), U.S. cities, 1969; (with Woodward) *Noel Coward in Two Keys*, U.S. cities, 1974.

PRINCIPAL FILM WORK—Executive assistant, *Citizen Kane*, RKO, 1941; also served as dialogue director for several films, including *The Voice of the Turtle*, Warner Brothers, 1947.

PRINCIPAL RADIO APPEARANCES—Series: Regular, *Mercury Theatre on the Air*, CBS, 1938.

RELATED CAREER—Member, Mercury Theatre Company, New York City, 1938-41; director, summer theatre productions, 1946-49; producer and director of various theatrical productions, 1950-52; co-founder, Playwrights Unit (a workshop for American playwrights), during the 1960s; producer and director (with Edward Albee), John Drew Theatre, Easthampton, NY, 1972; director, American National Theatre and Academy, New York City, 1969-71; president, League of American Theatres and Producers, New York City, 1967-89.

WRITINGS: STAGE—Adaptor (with Richard Whorf and Jose Ferrer), *Volpone*, City Center Theatre, New York City, 1948.

AWARDS: (With Clinton Wilder) Vernon Rice Award, 1962, for "Theatre 1961" productions; (with Wilder) Antoinette Perry Award and New York Drama Critics Circle Award, both Best Play, 1963, for *Who's Afraid of Virginia Woolf?*; (with Wilder and Edward Albee, as "Theatre 1965") Margo Jones Award, 1965, for encouragement given to new plays and playwrights; (with Wilder) Antoinette Perry Award nomination, Best Play, 1967, for *A Delicate Balance;* (with Charles Woodward, Jr., Robert Fryer, Mary Lea Johnson, and Martin Richards) Antoinette Perry Award, Best Musical, 1979, for *Sweeney Todd*.

SIDELIGHTS: Rather than stage out-of-town tryouts for their 1962 production of *Who's Afraid of Virginia Woolf?*, Richard Barr and his partner, Clinton Wilder, elected to preview the drama on Broadway. The success of these advance showings helped establish the practice of New York previews and, according to Barr's *New York Times* obituary, he and Wilder "were credited with changing the way Broadway plays were produced."

OBITUARIES AND OTHER SOURCES: New York Times, January 10, 1989; *Variety*, January 18-24, 1989.*

BARRY, Michael 1910-1988

PERSONAL: Born James Barry Jackson, May 15, 1910, in London, England; died June 27, 1988, in Brighton, England; son of Archie and Helen (Callaghan) Jackson; married Judith Gick (divorced); married Rosemary Corbett (deceased); married Pamela Corbett; children: one daughter. EDUCATION: Attended the Hertfordshire Agricultural Institute; trained for the stage at the Royal Academy of Dramatic Arts, 1929-30. MILITARY: Royal Marines.

VOCATION: Actor, designer, director, producer, stage manager, and writer.

CAREER: Also see *WRITINGS* below. PRINCIPAL STAGE APPEARANCES—In repertory at Northampton, U.K., and Birmingham, U.K., 1932-34; also appeared on stage in London. PRINCIPAL STAGE WORK—Designer and stage manager, Northampton and Birmingham repertory theatres, 1932-34; director, Hull Repertory Theatre, Hull, U.K., 1934-35; director, Croydon Repertory Theatre, Croyden, U.K., 1935-38.

PRINCIPAL FILM WORK—Director, *Stop Press Girl,* General Films Distributors, 1949.

PRINCIPAL TELEVISION WORK—Mini-Series: Executive producer, *The Wars of the Roses,* 1966. Also producer, *Promise of Tomorrow;* producer, *The Passionate Pilgrim;* producer, *Shout Aloud Salvation;* executive producer, *1984;* executive producer, *An Age of Kings.*

RELATED CAREER—Producer, BBC, 1938; head of Television Drama department, BBC, 1951-61; member, Arts Council Drama Pancl, 1955-68; program controller, Telefis Eirann, 1961-63; professor of drama and head of drama department, Stanford University, 1968-72; council member, Royal Academy of Dramatic Arts, 1966-69; director, Royal Exchange Theatre, Manchester, U.K., 1972-1978; principal, London Academy of Music and Dramatic Arts, 1973-78; member, National Council for Drama Training, 1976-78.

WRITINGS: TELEVISION—*Promise of Tomorrow, The Passionate Pilgrim,* and *Shout Aloud Salvation.*

AWARDS: Order of the British Empire, 1956, for services to television drama.

OBITUARIES AND OTHER SOURCES: Variety, July 6, 1988.*

*   *   *

BASS, Kingsley B., Jr.
See BULLINS, Ed

*   *   *

BATES, Alan 1934-

PERSONAL: Full name, Alan Arthur Bates; born February 17, 1934, in Allestree, England; son of Harold Arthur (an insurance salesman) and Florence Mary (Wheatcroft) Bates; married Victoria

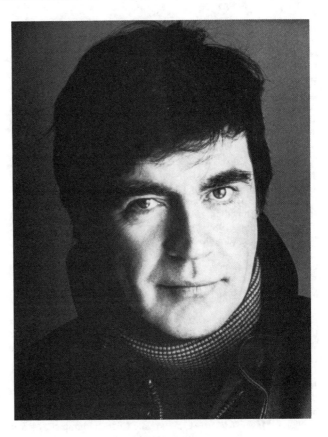

ALAN BATES

Valerie Ward (an actress), 1970; children: Benedick, Tristan (twins). EDUCATION: Trained for the stage at the Royal Academy of Dramatic Art and with Claude W. Gibson; studied voice with Gladys Lea. RELIGION: Church of England. MILITARY: Royal Air Force.

VOCATION: Actor.

CAREER: STAGE DEBUT—*You and Your Wife,* Midland Theatre Company, Coventry, U.K., 1955. LONDON DEBUT—Simon Fellowes, *The Mulberry Bush,* Royal Court Theatre, 1956. BROADWAY DEBUT—Cliff Lewis, *Look Back in Anger,* Lyceum Theatre, 1958. PRINCIPAL STAGE APPEARANCES—Hopkins, *The Crucible,* Cliff Lewis, *Look Back in Anger,* Mr. Harcourt, *The Country Wife,* and Stapleton, *Cards of Identity,* all English Stage Company, Royal Court Theatre, London, 1956; Monsieur le Cracheton, *The Apollo de Bellac,* and Dr. Brock, *Yes—and After,* both English Stage Company, Royal Court Theatre, 1957; Cliff Lewis, *Look Back in Anger,* English Stage Company, World Youth Festival, Moscow, U.S.S.R., 1957, then Edinburgh Festival, Edinburgh, Scotland, 1958; Edmund Tyrone, *Long Day's Journey into Night,* Edinburgh Festival, Lyceum Theatre, Edinburgh, then Globe Theatre, London, both 1958.

Mick, *The Caretaker,* Arts Theatre, then Duchess Theatre, both London, 1960, later Lyceum Theatre, New York City, 1961; Richard Ford, *Poor Richard,* Helen Hayes Theatre, New York City, 1964; Adam, *The Four Seasons,* Saville Theatre, London, 1965; Ford, *The Merry Wives of Windsor,* and title role, *Richard III,* both Stratford Shakespearean Festival, Stratford, ON, Canada, 1967; Andrew Shaw, *In Celebration,* Royal Court Theatre, 1969;

Jaffer, *Venice Preserved*, Bristol Old Vic Company, Royale Theatre, Bristol, U.K., 1969; title role, *Hamlet*, Nottingham Playhouse, Nottingham, U.K., 1971; title role, *Butley*, Criterion Theatre, London, 1971, then Morosco Theatre, New York City, 1972; Petruchio, *The Taming of the Shrew*, Royal Shakespeare Company, Royal Shakespeare Theatre, Stratford-on-Avon, U.K., 1973; Allott, *Life Class*, Royal Court Theatre, then Duke of York's Theatre, London, both 1974; Simon, *Otherwise Engaged*, Queen's Theatre, London, 1975; Boris Trigorin, *The Seagull*, Duke of York's Theatre, 1976; Robert, *Stage Struck*, Vaudeville Theatre, London, 1979; Alfred Redl, *A Patriot for Me*, Chichester Festival Theatre, Chichester, U.K., then London, both 1983, later Center Theatre Group, Ahmanson Theatre, Los Angeles, CA, 1984; title role, *Melon*, Royal Haymarket Theatre, London, 1987; title role, *Ivanov*, and Benedick, *Much Ado about Nothing*, both Strand Theatre, London, 1989. Also appeared in *One for the Road* and *Victoria Station* (double-bill), 1984; *Dance of Death*, London, 1985; *Yonadab*, National Theatre, London, 1985; and (with Patrick Garland) *Down Cemetery Road* (poetry recital), 1986.

MAJOR TOURS—Title role, *Butley*, U.S. cities, 1975.

FILM DEBUT—Frank Rice, *The Entertainer*, Bryanston/British Lion, 1960. PRINCIPAL FILM APPEARANCES—Arthur Blakey, *Whistle Down the Wind*, Pathe, 1961; Vic Brown, *A Kind of Loving*, Governor, 1962; Mick, *The Guest* (also known as *The Caretaker*), Janus, 1963; Stephen Maddox, *The Running Man*, Columbia, 1963; Jimmy Brewster, *Nothing But the Best*, Royal, 1964; Basil, *Zorba the Greek*, International Classics, 1964; Jos, *Georgy Girl*, Columbia, 1966; Gabriel Oak, *Far from the Madding Crowd*, Metro-Goldwyn-Mayer (MGM), 1967; Private Charles Plumpick, *Le Roi de coeur* (also known as *King of Hearts* and *Tutti pazzio meno lo*), Lopert/United Artists, 1967; Yakov Bok, *The Fixer*, MGM, 1968; Rupert Birkin, *Women in Love*, United Artists, 1969.

Ted Burgess, *The Go-Between*, Columbia, 1971; Bri, *A Day in the Death of Joe Egg*, Columbia, 1972; Harry, *L'Impossible objet* (also known as *Impossible Object* and *Story of a Love Story*), Valoria, 1973; title role, *Butley*, American Film Theatre, 1974; Colonel Vershinin, *Three Sisters*, American Film Theatre, 1974; Andrew Shaw, *In Celebration*, American Film Theatre, 1975; Rudi von Starnberg, *Royal Flash*, Twentieth Century-Fox, 1975; Charles Crossley, *The Shout*, Films, Inc., 1978; Saul Kaplan, *An Unmarried Woman*, Twentieth Century-Fox, 1978; Rudge, *The Rose*, Twentieth Century-Fox, 1979; Sergei Diaghilev, *Nijinsky*, Paramount, 1980; H.J. Heidler, *Quartet*, New World, 1981; Mr. Macready, *Brittania Hospital*, Universal, 1982; Captain Chris Baldry, *Return of the Soldier*, Twentieth Century-Fox, 1983; Captain Jerry Jackson, *The Wicked Lady*, Metro-Goldwyn-Mayer-United Artists, 1983; David Cornwallis, *Duet for One*, Cannon, 1986; Dandy Jack Meehan, *A Prayer for the Dying*, Goldwyn, 1987; Frank Meadows, *We Think the World of You*, Cinecom, 1988. Also appeared as narrator, *Insh'Allah*, 1965; in *Second Best* (short film), 1972; and in *Mikis Theodorakis: A Profile of Greatness*, 1974.

PRINCIPAL FILM WORK—Co-producer, *Second Best* (short film), 1972.

PRINCIPAL TELEVISION APPEARANCES—Mini-Series: Michael Henchard/title role, *The Mayor of Casterbridge*, BBC, then *Masterpiece Theatre*, PBS, 1978. Movies: Narrator, *The Story of Jacob and Joseph*, ABC, 1974. Specials: John Malcolm and Major Pollack, *Separate Tables*, HBO, 1983; Guy Burgess, *An Englishman Abroad*, BBC, then PBS, 1983; Jones, "Dr. Fischer of

Geneva," *Great Performances*, PBS, 1985; Stewart, "Pack of Lies," *Hallmark Hall of Fame*, CBS, 1987; also *A Voyage 'round My Father*, PBS, 1982. Also appeared in *Duel for Love*, ABC, 1959; *Three on a Gas Ring*, ABC, 1959; *The Wind and the Rain*, Granada, 1959; *The Square Ring*, AR-TV, 1959; *The Juke Box*, AR-TV, 1959; *A Memory of Two Mondays*, Granada, 1959; *The Thug*, ABC, 1959; as Cliff Lewis, *Look Back in Anger*; Mick, *The Caretaker*; in *Very Like a Whale*, 1981; *The Tresspasser*, 1981; *One for the Road*, 1986; *The Collection*, 1987; *The Dog It Was That Died*, 1988; *Two Sundays*; *Plaintiff and Defendent*; and *A Hero for Our Time*.

AWARDS: Forbes Robinson Award from the Royal Academy of Dramatic Art and Clarence Derwent Award, both 1959, for *Long Day's Journey into Night*; Academy Award nomination, Best Actor, 1968, for *The Fixer*; Evening Standard Award, Best Actor, 1972, for London performance of *Butley*; Antoinette Perry Award, Best Actor (Dramatic), and Drama Desk Award, both 1973, for New York performance of *Butley*; Best Actor Award from the Variety Club of Great Britain, 1975, for *Otherwise Engaged*; Best Actor Award from the Variety Club of Great Britain and Society of West End Theatre Managers Award, Best Actor in a Revival, both 1983-84, for *A Patriot for Me*; British Academy of Film and Television Arts Award, Best Actor, 1983, for *An Englishman Abroad*.

SIDELIGHTS: RECREATIONS—Tennis, squash, swimming, traveling, driving, and reading.

MEMBER: Actors' Equity Association, British Actors' Equity Association.

ADDRESSES: AGENT—Chatto and Linnit, Prince of Wales Theatre, Coventry Street, London SW7, England.

*   *   *

BEASLEY, Allyce   1954-

PERSONAL: Born Allyce Tannenberg, July 6, 1954, in Brooklyn, NY; daughter of Marvin (a cartoonist) and Harriet (a bookkeeper) Tannenberg; married Christopher Sansocie (a photographer; divorced); married Vincent Schiavelli (an actor), 1985. EDUCATION: Attended State University of New York, Brockport; trained for the stage with Lee Strasberg and Wynn Handman.

VOCATION: Actress.

CAREER: PRINCIPAL STAGE APPEARANCES—Nurse, *Romeo and Juliet*, Ensemble Studio Theatre, New York City, 1988; also appeared with the Santa Fe Open Theatre, Santa Fe, NM.

PRINCIPAL TELEVISION APPEARANCES—Series: Agnes DiPesto, *Moonlighting*, ABC, 1985—. Episodic: Lisa Pantusso, "The Coach's Daughter," *Cheers*, NBC, 1982; also "Scenskees from a Marriage," *Taxi*, NBC, 1982; *Remington Steele*, NBC; *King's Crossing*, ABC. Movies: Mrs. Cutler, *One Cooks, the Other Doesn't*, CBS, 1983; Paisan receptionist, *The Ratings Game*, Movie Channel, 1984. Specials: *Walt Disney Celebrity Circus*, NBC, 1987; *The Ice Capades with Kirk Cameron* (also known as *Kirk Cameron at*

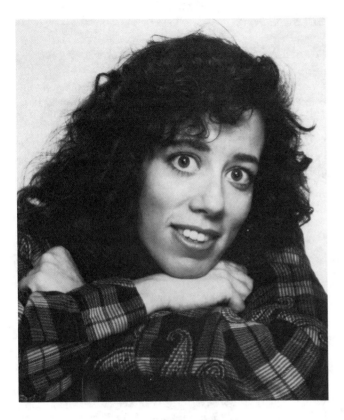

ALLYCE BEASLEY

the Ice Capades), ABC, 1988; *Battle of the Network Stars,* ΛBC, 1988.

RELATED CAREER—Actress in television commercials.

NON-RELATED CAREER—Waitress.

AWARDS: Golden Globe nomination, Best Performance by an Actress in a Supporting Role in a Series, Mini-Series, or Motion Picture Made for Television, 1988, for *Moonlighting.*

ADDRESSES: AGENT—Belle Zwerdling, Progressive Artists Agency, 400 S. Beverly Drive, Suite 216, Beverly Hills, CA 90212. PUBLICIST—George Freeman, P/M/K Public Relations, 8436 W. Third Street, Suite 650, Los Angeles, CA 90048.

*   *   *

BELMONDO, Jean-Paul   1933-

PERSONAL: Born April 9, 1933, in Neuilly-sur-Seine, France; son of Paul Belmondo (a sculptor); married wife, Elodie, 1952 (divorced, 1967); children: Patricia, Florence, Paul. EDUCATION: Attended College Pascal, Paris; trained for the stage at the National Conservatory of Dramatic Art, Paris, and with Raymond Girard.

VOCATION: Actor and producer.

CAREER: PRINCIPAL STAGE APPEARANCES—*Moliere,* 1955;

Caesar and Cleopatra, 1958; *Tresor-Party* (also known as *Treasure Party*), 1958; *Oscar,* 1958; also *L'Hotel du libre-echange, Medee,* and *La Megere apprivoisee.*

PRINCIPAL FILM APPEARANCES—Michel Poiccard, *Breathless* (also known as *A bout de souffle*), Imperia, 1959; Michel Barrot, *Ein Engel auf Erden* (also known as *Mademoiselle Ange* and *Angel on Earth*), 1959, released in United States by Comet, 1966; Stark, *Classe tous risques* (also known as *The Big Risk*), 1960, released in the United States by United Artists, 1963; Lou, *Les Tricheurs* (also known as *The Cheaters, Youthful Sinners,* and *Peccator in Blue Jeans*), Continental, 1961; Gil, ''L'adultere'' in *La Francaise et l'amour* (also known as *Love and the Frenchwoman*), Auerbach-Kingsley, 1961; Michele, *La Ciociara* (also known as *Two Women*), Embassy, 1961; Alfred Lubitsch, *Une Femme est une femme* (also known as *A Woman Is a Woman*), Pathe-Contemporary, 1961; Laszlo Kovacs, *A Double Tour* (also known as *Web of Passion, A doppia mandator,* and *Leda*), Times, 1961; title role, *Cartouche* (also known as *Swords of Blood*), Vides, 1962; Amerigo Casamunti, *La viaccia* (also known as *The Love Makers*), Embassy, 1962; Gabriel Fouquet, *Un singe en hiver* (also known as *A Monkey in Winter* and *It's Hot in Hell*), Metro-Goldwyn-Mayer (MGM), 1962; Silien, *Le Doulos* (also known as *Doulos—The Finger Man*), Pathe-Contemporary, 1962; Giuliano Verdi, *Lettere di una novizia* (also known as *Rita, La Novice,* and *Letter from a Novice*), Colorama Features, 1963; Chauvin, *Moderato cantabile* (also known as *Seven Days . . . Seven Nights*), Royal Films International, 1964; Raymond, *Dragees au poivre* (also known as *Sweet and Sour* and *Confetti al pepe*), Pathe-Contemporary, 1964; Adrien Dufourquet, *L'homme de Rio* (also known as *That Man from Rio* and *L'uomo di Rio*), Lopert, 1964.

David Ladislas, *Enchappement libre* (also known as *Backfire*), Royal Films International 1965; Michel, *Peau de banane* (also known as *Banana Peel*), Pathe-Contemporary, 1965; Rocco, *Cent mille dollars au soleil* (also known as *Greed in the Sun* and *Centamila dollari al sole*), Gaumont/MGM, 1965; Fernand, *La Chasse a l'homme* (also known as *The Gentle Art of Seduction, Male Hunt,* and *Caccia al maschio*), Pathe-Contemporary, 1965; Morandat, *Is Paris Burning?* (also known as *Paris brule-t-il?*), Paramount, 1966; Arthur Lempereur, *Les Tribulations d'un chinois en Chine* (also known as *Up to His Ears* and *L'uomo di Hong Kong*), Lopert, 1966; Sergeant Maillat, *Week-end a Zuydcoote* (also known as *Weekend at Dunkirk*), Twentieth Century-Fox, 1966; French legionnaire, *Casino Royale,* Columbia, 1967; Tony Marechal, *Tendre voyou* (also known as *Tender Scoundrel* and *Un avventuriero a Tahiti*), Embassy, 1967; George Rondal, *Le Voleur* (also known as *The Thief of Paris*), Lopert, 1967; title role, *Ho!,* Cocinor, 1968; Ferdinand Griffon/title role, *Pierrot le Fou,* Pathe-Contemporary/Corinth, 1968; Arthur, *Le Cerveau* (also known as *The Brain*), Paramount, 1969.

Capella, *Borsalino,* Paramount, 1970; Henri, *Histoire d'aimer* (also known as *Love Is a Funny Thing, Again a Love Story, Un tipo chi mi piace, Un homme qui me plait,* and *A Man I Like*), United Artists, 1970; Louis Mahe, *La sirene du Mississippi* (also known as *Mississippi Mermaid* and *La mia droga si chiama Julie*), Lopert-United Artists, 1970; husband, *Les Maries de l'an deux* (also known as *The Married Couple of Year Two* and *The Scoundrel*), Gaumont International, 1971; Azad, *La Casse* (also known as *The Burglars*), Columbia, 1972; Dr. Paul Simay, *Docteur Popaul* (also known as *Scoundrel in White*), CIC, 1972; Cordell, *L'Heritier* (also known as *The Inheritor* and *The Heir*), Valoria, 1972; title role, *La Scoumoune* (also known as *Killer Man*), Fox-Lira, 1972; Francois,

Le Magnifique (also known as *The Magnificent One* and *How to Destroy the Reputation of the Greatest Secret Agent*), Cine III, 1974; title role, *Stavisky*, Cinemation, 1974; title role, *L'Alpagueur* (also known as *The Predator*), AMLF, 1975; Tellier, *Peur sur la ville* (also known as *Fear over the City* and *The Night Caller*), AMLF, 1975; Francois, *Le Corps de mon ennemi* (also known as *The Body of the Enemy*), AMLF, 1976; Fechner, *L'Animal*, AMLF-Roissy, 1977; Stan Borowitz, *Flic ou voyou* (also known as *Cop or Hood*), Gaumont International, 1979.

Victor, *L'Incorrigible*, EDP, 1980; Jo Cavlier, *L'As des as* (also known as *Ace of Aces*), Gaumont International/Cerito-Rene Chateau, 1982; Grimm, *Hold-Up*, AMLF, 1985; Commissioner Stan Jalard, *Le Solitaire*, AMLF/Cerito, 1987; Sam Lion, *Itineraire d'un enfant gate* (also known as *Itinerary of a Spoiled Child*), AFDM/Films 13, 1988. Also appeared in *Dimanche nous volerons*, 1956; *A pied, a cheval, et en voiture*, 1957; *Drole du dimanche*, 1958; *Les copains du dimanche*, 1958; *Charlotte et son Jules* (short film), 1958; *Sois belle et tais-toi* (also known as *Blonde for Danger* and *Look Pretty and Shut Up*), 1958; *Les Distractions* (also known as *Trapped by Fear*), 1960; *Leon Morin, pretre* (also known as *Leon Morin, Priest*), 1961; "Lauzon" in *Amours celebres*, 1961; *Un nomme la rocca*, 1961; *I Don Giovanni della costa azzurra*, 1962; *L'Aine des Ferchaux*, 1962; *Mare matto*, 1963; *Il giorno piu corto* (also known as *The Shortest Day*), 1963; *Par un beau matin d'ete* (also known as *Crime on a Summer Morning*), 1965; *La Bande a Bebel*, 1967; *Dieu a choisi Paris*, 1969; *Le Guignolo*, 1980; *I piccioni di Piazza San Marco*, 1980; *Le Professionnel*, 1981; *Le Marginal* (also known as *The Outsider*), Roissy/Gaumont, 1983; *Les Morfalous* (also known as *The Vultures*), AAA/Roissy/Cerito-Rene Chateau, 1983; *Joyeuses paques*, Sara/Cerito, 1984.

PRINCIPAL FILM WORK—Producer: *L'As des as* (also known as *Ace of Aces*), Gaumont International/Cerito-Rene Chateau, 1982; *Joyeuses paques*, Sara/Cerito, 1984; *Itineraire d'un enfant gate* (also known as *Itinerary of a Spoiled Child*), AFDM/Films 13, 1988.

PRINCIPAL TELEVISION APPEARANCES—*The Three Musketeers*, French television.

RELATED CAREER—Founder (with Annie Girardot and Guy Bedos) of a traveling theatre group, 1956-57; founder, Cerito Films, during the 1960s; also appeared with Comedie Francaise and as a performer in Parisian cafes.

NON-RELATED CAREER—Welterweight boxer, 1949; part-owner, Les Polymuscles (soccer team).

WRITINGS: Trente ans et vingt-cinq films (autobiography), 1963.

AWARDS: Prix Citron, 1972; Chevalier de la Legion d'honneur; Chevalier l'Ordre national du Merite et des Arts et des Lettres.

MEMBER: Syndicat Francais des Acteurs (president, 1963-66).

SIDELIGHTS: RECREATIONS—Sports.

ADDRESSES: AGENT—Artmedia, 10 Avenue Georges V, 75008 Paris, France.*

BELSON, Jerry

VOCATION: Producer, director, screenwriter, and actor.

CAREER: Also see *WRITINGS* below. PRINCIPAL FILM APPEARANCES—Television producer, *Semi-Tough*, United Artists, 1977; Jerry, *Modern Romance*, Columbia, 1981; voice of Yuri, *The Couch Trip*, Orion, 1988.

PRINCIPAL FILM WORK—Producer (with Gary Marshall), *How Sweet It Is*, National General, 1968; producer (with Marshall), *The Grasshopper*, National General, 1970; executive producer, *Student Bodies*, Paramount, 1981; director, *Jekyll and Hyde—Together Again*, Paramount, 1982; director, *Surrender*, Warner Brothers, 1987; producer (with Walter Coblenz), *For Keeps* (also known as *Maybe Baby*), Tri-Star, 1988.

PRINCIPAL TELEVISION WORK—Series: Producer (with Gary Marshall), *Hey, Landlord*, NBC, 1966-67; executive producer (with Marshall, Harvey Miller, and Sheldon Keller), *The Odd Couple*, ABC, 1970-75; creator and executive producer (with James L. Brooks, Heide Perlman, and Ken Estin), *The Tracey Ullman Show*, Fox, 1987—. Pilots: Producer (with Marshall), *Sheriff Who?*, NBC, 1967; executive producer (with Marshall), *The Murdocks and the McClays*, ABC, 1970; creator and director, *Cops*, CBS, 1973; producer (with Marshall), *Evil Roy Slade*, NBC, 1972; director, *Pete 'n' Tillie*, CBS, 1974; executive producer (with Mark Carliner), *Mixed Nuts*, ABC, 1977; producer (with Michael Leeson), *Young Guy Christian*, ABC, 1979. Episodic: Director, *The Odd Couple*, ABC, 1970-75; director, "What Is Mary Richards Really Like?" and "You've Got a Friend," both *The Mary Tyler Moore Show*, CBS, 1972; director, "Rhoda's Sister Gets Married," *The Mary Tyler Moore Show*, CBS, 1973; director, *Rhoda*, CBS, 1974-78.

WRITINGS: FILM—(With Gary Marshall) *How Sweet It Is*, National General, 1968; (with Marshall) *The Grasshopper*, National General, 1970; *Smile*, United Artists, 1975; (with David Giler and Mordecai Richler) *Fun with Dick and Jane*, Columbia, 1977; *The End*, United Artists, 1978; (with Brock Yates) *Smokey and the Bandit II* (also known as *Smokey and the Bandit Ride Again*), Universal, 1980; (with Michael Leeson, Monica Johnson, and Harvey Miller) *Jekyll and Hyde—Together Again*, Paramount, 1982; *Surrender*, Warner Brothers, 1987.

TELEVISION—Series: (With Gary Marshall, Harvey Miller, and Bill Idelson) *Barefoot in the Park*, ABC, 1970-71; (with Dale McRaven and James Parker) *The Texas Wheelers*, ABC, 1974-75. Pilots: (With Marshall) *Sheriff Who?*, NBC, 1967; (with Marshall) *The Murdocks and the McClays*, ABC, 1970; (with Marshall) *Evil Roy Slade*, NBC, 1972; *Cops*, CBS, 1973; (with Michael Leeson) *Mixed Nuts*, ABC, 1977; (with Leeson) *Young Guy Christian*, ABC, 1979. Episodic: (With Marshall) *The Dick Van Dyke Show* (eleven episodes), CBS, 1964-66; *I Spy*, NBC, 1965-68; *The New Odd Couple*, ABC, 1982-83; *The Tracey Ullman Show*, Fox, 1987—. Specials: (With Marshall) *Think Pretty*, NBC, 1964; (with Marshall) *The Danny Thomas Special*, NBC, 1966; (with Marshall) *Danny Thomas: The Road to Lebanon*, NBC, 1967; (with Marshall) *The Dick Van Dyke Special*, CBS, 1968.

ADDRESSES: AGENT—Creative Artists Agency, 1888 Century Park E., Los Angeles, CA 90067.*

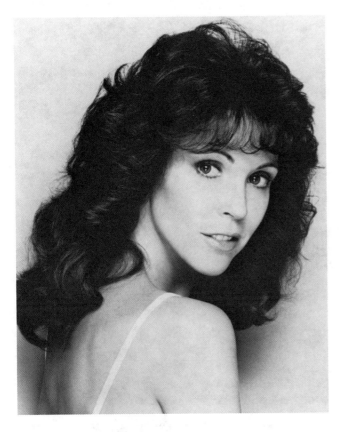

MEG BENNETT

BENNETT, Meg 1948-

PERSONAL: Born October 4, 1948, in Los Angeles, CA; daughter of Harold McQuairie (a sales executive) and Margaret Cooper (a family counselor) Bennett. EDUCATION: Received B.S. in theatre from Northwestern University.

VOCATION: Actress and screenwriter.

CAREER: Also see *WRITINGS* below. STAGE DEBUT—Ensemble, *Godspell*, Promenade Theatre, New York City, 1971. BROADWAY DEBUT—Marty, *Grease*, Broadhurst Theatre, then Royale Theatre, both 1972. Also appeared in *The Wizard of Oz*, Pasadena Playhouse, Pasadena, CA; *Romeo and Juliet*, *Hamlet*, and *Twelfth Night*, all University of California at Los Angeles Shakespeare Festival, Los Angeles, CA; *Barefoot in the Park*, Louisville, KY; and in *Cabaret*, *Mame*, *Picnic*, *George M!*, *The Apple Tree*, and *The Pajama Game*, all summer theatre productions.

FILM DEBUT—*Loving Couples*, Rank/Twentieth Century-Fox, 1980.

TELEVISION DEBUT—Liza, *Search for Tomorrow*, CBS, 1975. PRINCIPAL TELEVISION APPEARANCES—Series: Julia Newman, *The Young and the Restless*, CBS, 1980-88; Megan, *Santa Barbara*, NBC, 1989. Episodic: *The Paper Chase: The Second Year*, Showtime, 1983; *The New Love, American Style*, ABC, 1986. Specials: *After Hours: Getting to Know Us*, CBS, 1977.

RELATED CAREER—Member of Daytime Emmy Awards committee of the Academy of Television Arts and Sciences.

WRITINGS: TELEVISION—Pilots: *You Are the Jury*, NBC, 1986. Episodic: *The Young and the Restless*, CBS, 1981-87; *The Bold and the Beautiful*, CBS, 1987-88; *Family Medical Center*, syndicated, 1988; *Generations*, NBC, 1989. Specials: *You Are the Jury*, NBC, 1987.

AWARDS: Emmy Award nomination, Best Writing for a Daytime Serial, 1986, for *The Young and the Restless*.

MEMBER: Writers Guild of America, American Federation of Television and Radio Artists, Screen Actors Guild, Academy of Television Arts and Sciences, American Film Institute.

ADDRESSES: HOME—1670 Malcolm Avenue, Los Angeles, CA 90024. AGENT—Jim Sarnoff, Sarnoff Company, 8489 W. Third Street, Los Angeles, CA 90048.

*   *   *

BENNETT, Ruth

VOCATION: Television producer and screenwriter.

CAREER: Also see *WRITINGS* below. PRINCIPAL TELEVISION WORK—Series: Producer, *Family Ties*, NBC, 1982-86; creator and supervising producer, *Sara*, NBC, 1985; production supervisor, *The All New Newlywed Game*, syndicated, 1985; creator and executive producer, *Duet*, Fox, 1987—. Pilots: Executive producer, *Taking It Home*, NBC, 1986.

WRITINGS: TELEVISION—Pilots: *Taking It Home*, NBC, 1986. Episodic: "Louie Sees the Light," *Taxi*, ABC, 1979; *Family Ties*, NBC, 1982-89; *Sara*, NBC, 1985; *Duet*, Fox, 1987—; also *Laverne and Shirley*, ABC.

ADDRESSES: OFFICE—c/o Paramount Television, 5555 Melrose Avenue, Los Angeles, CA 90038.*

*   *   *

BERENSON, Marisa 1948-

PERSONAL: Born February 15, 1948, in New York, NY; married Jim Randall (in business; divorced); married Richard Golub (an attorney; divorced); children: Starlite (first marriage).

VOCATION: Actress.

CAREER: PRINCIPAL STAGE APPEARANCES—Julia Seton, *Holiday*, Center Theatre Group, Ahmanson Theatre, Los Angeles, CA, 1980.

PRINCIPAL FILM APPEARANCES—Frau von Aschenbach, *Death in Venice* (also known as *Morte a Venezia*), Warner Brothers, 1971; Natalie Landauer, *Cabaret*, Allied Artists, 1972; Lady Lyndon, *Barry Lyndon*, Warner Brothers, 1975; Ann, *Killer Fish* (also known as *Treasure of the Piranha* and *Deadly Treasure of the Piranha*), Associated Film Distribution, 1979; Caliph of Shiraz, *Some Like It Cool* (also known as *Casanova and Company* and *The*

Rise and Rise of Casanova), PRO International, 1979; Mavis, *S.O.B.*, Paramount, 1981; Emma Herrmann, *The Secret Diary of Sigmund Freud*, Twentieth Century-Fox/TLC, 1984; Vera, *La Tete dans le sac* (also known as *The Head in a Bag*), Parafrance, 1984; Jeanne Barnac, *Flagrant Desire* (also known as *A Certain Desire*), Hemdale, 1986; Fabrizio's mother, *Via Montenapoleone*, Columbia, 1987. Also appeared in *L'Arbalete* (also known as *The Cross-Bow*), ACM/CCFC, 1984.

PRINCIPAL TELEVISION APPEARANCES—Mini-Series: Luba Tcherina, *Sins*, CBS, 1986; Pauline Pfeiffer, *Hemingway*, syndicated, 1988. Pilots: Marian, *Tourist*, syndicated, 1980. Episodic: Andrea Brown, *The Equalizer*, CBS, 1986; also *Who's the Boss?*, ABC, 1986. Movies: Elzvieta, *Playing for Time*, CBS, 1980. Specials: Liz Childs, "Getting Even: A Wimp's Revenge," *ABC Afterschool Special*, ABC, 1986.

RELATED CAREER—Model.

ADDRESSES: AGENT—Dick Heckenkamp, Film Artists Associates, 470 San Vicente Boulevard, Suite 104, Los Angeles, CA 90048.*

*   *   *

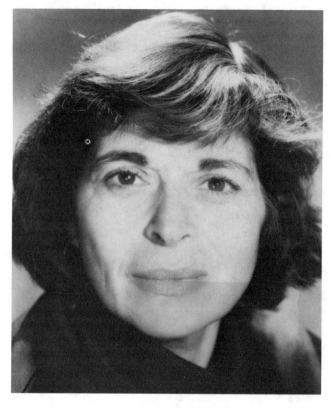

ANNA BERGER

BERGER, Anna

PERSONAL: Born July 28, in New York, NY; daughter of William and Bella (Heller) Berger; married Robert Malatzky (a board of education administrator), December 22, 1957; children: Joanne, Susan. EDUCATION: Attended George Washington University and the New School for Social Reseach; trained for the stage at the Actors Studio.

VOCATION: Actress.

CAREER: STAGE DEBUT—*Diamond Lil*, Blackstone Theatre, Chicago, IL. BROADWAY DEBUT—Mrs. Kramer, *Twilight Walk*, Fulton Theatre, 1951. PRINCIPAL STAGE APPEARANCES—(As Anna Vita Berger) Golde, *Tevya and His Daughters*, Carnegie Hall Playhouse, New York City, 1957; Goldie, "Epstein" in *Unlikely Heroes*, Plymouth Theatre, New York City, 1971; Filomena, *The Mute Who Sang*, New Dramatists, New York City, 1977. Also appeared in *The Flowering Peach*, Belasco Theatre, New York City, 1954; *A Very Special Baby*, Playhouse Theatre, New York City, 1956; *Gideon*, Plymouth Theatre, New York City, 1961; *Him*, Circle Repertory Theatre, New York City, 1974; in *Paradise Lost*, Center Stage, Baltimore, MD; and in productions of *Come Blow Your Horn, Community Property, Juno and the Paycock, The Silver Tassie, The Last Analysis, Golden Boy, Bye Bye Birdie, A Majority of One, Enter Laughing, Midnight Ride of Alvin Blum, The World of Sholom Aleichem, The Rose Tattoo, Scuba-Duba, And Miss Reardon Drinks a Little, Lovers and Other Strangers, Prisoner of Second Avenue, God's Favorite, Torch Song Trilogy, Within the Gates*, and *The Dog beneath the Skin*.

MAJOR TOURS—*Diamond Lil*, U.S. cities, 1950-51; Mother, *Torch Song Trilogy*, U.S. cities, 1984-85.

FILM DEBUT—Caroline, *Middle of the Night*, Columbia, 1959. PRINCIPAL FILM APPEARANCES—Mother, *The Taking of Pelham One, Two, Three*, United Artists, 1974; nurse, *Endless Love*, Universal, 1981; analyst, *Lovesick*, Warner Brothers, 1983; funeral woman, *The House on Carroll Street*, Orion, 1988; also appeared in *Hester Street*, Midwest, 1975; *Brothers*; and *God's Payroll*.

PRINCIPAL TELEVISION APPEARANCES—Mini-Series: Celia Blackman, *Seventh Avenue*, NBC, 1977. Pilots: Louise, *Street Killing*, ABC, 1976; Mrs. Goldman, *Cagney and Lacey*, CBS, 1981. Episodic: *Philco Playhouse*, NBC, 1953; *Barney Miller*, ABC, 1977 and 1981; also *Naked City*, ABC; *East Side, West Side*, CBS; *One Life to Live*, ABC; *Ryan's Hope*, ABC; *The Doctors*, NBC; *As the World Turns*, NBC; *Rhoda*, CBS; *Kojak*, CBS; *Baretta*, ABC; *CHiPS*, NBC; *Harry-O*, ABC; *The Blue Knight*, CBS; *Popi*, CBS; *Doc*, CBS; *The Goldbergs*, NBC; *Leg Work*, CBS; *Snip*; and *Clinic*. Movies: Mrs. Moore, *Contract on Cherry Street*, NBC, 1977; Mrs. Berg, *Raid on Entebbe*, NBC, 1977; real estate agent, *Terrible Joe Moran*, CBS, 1984.

RELATED CAREER—Drama teacher, New York City public schools; private drama teacher, New York City.

ADDRESSES: HOME—875 West End Avenue, New York, NY 10025. AGENT—Fifi Oscard, 19 W. 44th Street, New York, NY

10036. MANAGER—Michael Greene, 225 Central Park W., New York, NY 10025.

* * *

BERGMAN, Sandahl

VOCATION: Actress and dancer.

CAREER: PRINCIPAL STAGE APPEARANCES—Liane d'Exelmans, *Gigi,* Uris Theatre, New York City, 1973; ensemble, *Dancin',* Broadhurst Theatre, New York City, 1978; also appeared as Judy, *A Chorus Line,* Shubert Theatre, New York City.

MAJOR TOURS—Ensemble, *Dancin',* U.S. cities, 1979.

PRINCIPAL FILM APPEARANCES—Dancer, *All That Jazz,* Twentieth Century-Fox, 1979; Muse, *Xanadu,* Universal, 1980; officer, *Airplane II: The Sequel,* Paramount, 1982; Valeria, *Conan the Barbarian,* Universal, 1982; title role, *She,* American National Enterprises, 1985; Queen Gedren, *Red Sonja,* Metro-Goldwyn-Mayer/United Artists, 1985; Wanda Polanski, *Stewardess School,* Columbia, 1987; Samira, *Programmed to Kill* (also known as *Retaliator*), Trans World Entertainment, 1987; Spangle, *Hell Comes to Frogtown,* New World, 1988; Harlow, *Kandyland,* New World, 1988.

PRINCIPAL TELEVISION APPEARANCES—Episodic: Daniel, *Hard Time on Planet Earth,* CBS, 1989. Movies: Blonde jogger, *How to Pick Up Girls,* ABC, 1978; Nadine Cawley, *Getting Physical,* CBS, 1984. Specials: *Getting the Last Laugh,* ABC, 1985; *Happy Birthday Hollywood,* ABC, 1987; *Don Johnson's Music Video Feature: "Heartbeat,"* HBO, 1987.

ADDRESSES: AGENT—Light/Gordon/Rosson Agency, 901 Bringham Avenue, Los Angeles, CA 90049.*

* * *

BERNSEN, Corbin 1954-

PERSONAL: Born September 7, 1954, in North Hollywood, CA; son of Harry Bernsen (a producer) and Jeanne Cooper (an actress); married Amanda Pays (an actress), November 19, 1988; children: Oliver Miller. EDUCATION: University of California, Los Angeles, B.A., theatre, 1973, then M.F.A., playwriting.

VOCATION: Actor.

CAREER: PRINCIPAL FILM APPEARANCES—Boy, *Three the Hard Way,* Allied Artists, 1974; Roy Puir, *Eat My Dust,* New World, 1976; Dr. Jason Chadman, *Hello Again,* Buena Vista, 1987; Webster, *Mace,* Double Helix, 1987; Jim Shirley, *Bert Rigby, You're a Fool,* Warner Brothers, 1989; Roger Dorn, *Major League,* Paramount, 1989; Frank Salazar, *Disorganized Crime,* Touchstone, 1989. Also appeared in *King Kong,* Paramount, 1976; and *S.O.B.,* Paramount, 1981.

PRINCIPAL TELEVISION APPEARANCES—Series: Arnold Becker, *L.A. Law,* NBC, 1986—; also Ken Graham, *Ryan's Hope,* ABC. Pilots: Steve Malloy, *Allison Sidney Harrison,* NBC, 1983. Epi-

sodic: *Police Story,* NBC; *The Waltons,* CBS; *Police Woman,* NBC. Movies: Tennis pro, *Doubletake,* CBS, 1985. Specials: Lifeguard, "Blind Sunday," *ABC Holiday Weekend Special,* ABC, 1976; *Jay Leno Family Comedy Special,* NBC, 1987.

RELATED CAREER—Founder, Team Cherokee Productions; also appeared in television commercials.

NON-RELATED CAREER—Carpenter.

SIDELIGHTS: RECREATIONS—Marathon running, writing, and traveling.

ADDRESSES: AGENT—John Carraro, Agency for the Performing Arts, 9000 Sunset Boulevard, Suite 1200, Los Angeles, CA 90069. MANAGER—Miles Levy/Randall James, 17712 Margate Street, Suite 5365, Encino, CA 91316.

* * *

BILLINGSLEY, Peter 1972-

PERSONAL: Born in 1972 in New York, NY.

VOCATION: Actor.

CAREER: PRINCIPAL FILM APPEARANCES—Child, *If Ever I See You Again,* Columbia, 1978; Tad, *Paternity,* Paramount, 1981; Billy Kramer, *Honky Tonk Freeway,* Universal/Associated Film Distribution, 1981; Billy, *Death Valley,* Universal, 1982; Ralphie, *A Christmas Story,* Metro-Goldwyn-Mayer/United Artists, 1983; Jack Simmons, *The Dirt Bike Kid,* Concorde/Cinema Group, 1985; Adam, *Russkies,* New Century/Vista, 1987.

PRINCIPAL TELEVISION APPEARANCES—Series: *Real People,* NBC, 1982-84. Pilots: Host, *Real Kids,* NBC, 1981; Christopher ("the Brain"), *Massarati and the Brain,* ABC, 1982; Roland Krantz, Jr., *Carly's Web,* NBC, 1987. Episodic: Kevin, "Pecos Bill, King of the Cowboys," *Shelley Duvall's Tall Tales and Legends,* Showtime, 1986l Richmond Matzie, *Punky Brewster,* NBC, 1986. Movies: Shawn Tilford, *Memories Never Die,* CBS, 1982; Marty Adamson, *The Last Frontier,* CBS, 1986.

RELATED CAREER—Actor in television commercials.*

* * *

BISHOP, Joey 1918-

PERSONAL: Born Joseph Abraham Gottlieb, February 3, 1918 (some sources say 1919), in Bronx, NY; children: Larry.

VOCATION: Comedian and actor.

CAREER: BROADWAY DEBUT—*Sugar Babies,* Mark Hellinger Theatre, New York City, 1981.

PRINCIPAL FILM APPEARANCES—Ski Krakowski, *The Deep Six,* Warner Brothers, 1958; Roth, *The Naked and the Dead,* Warner Brothers, 1958; Gutsell, *Onionhead,* Warner Brothers, 1958; "Mushy" O'Conners, *Ocean's Eleven,* Warner Brothers, 1960; as

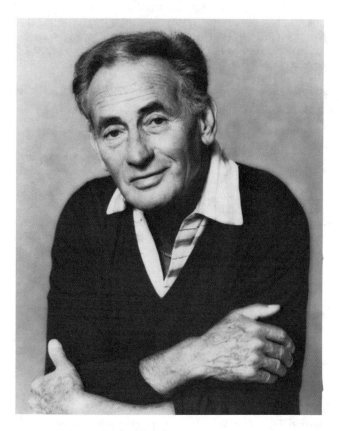

JOEY BISHOP

himself, *Pepe,* Columbia, 1960; Sergeant Major Roger Boswell, *Sergeants Three,* United Artists, 1962; used car salesman, *Johnny Cool,* United Artists, 1963; Kronk, *Texas across the River,* Universal, 1966; technical advisor, *A Guide for the Married Man,* Twentieth Century-Fox, 1967; emcee at telethon, *Valley of the Dolls,* Twentieth Century-Fox, 1967; Ralph Randazzo, *Who's Minding the Mint?,* Columbia, 1967; Harry Goldman, *The Delta Force,* Cannon, 1986.

PRINCIPAL TELEVISION APPEARANCES—Series: Regular, *Keep Talking,* CBS, 1959, then ABC, 1959-60; Joey Barnes, *The Joey Bishop Show,* NBC, 1961-65; host, *The Joey Bishop Show,* ABC, 1967-69; regular, *Celebrity Sweepstakes,* NBC, 1974-76; panelist, *The Liar's Club,* syndicated, 1976-78. Mini-Series: Sid Rosen, *Glory Years,* HBO, 1987. Pilots: Joey Barnes, *Everything Happens to Me* (broadcast as an episode of *The Danny Thomas Show*), CBS, 1961; coach, *Sorority '62,* syndicated, 1978. Episodic: *The Jack Paar Show,* NBC, 1958-62; also *The Tonight Show,* NBC. Specials: *The Frank Sinatra Timex Show,* ABC, 1960; *Esther Williams at Cypress Gardens,* NBC, 1960; *Romp,* ABC, 1968; *The Andy Williams Special,* NBC, 1971; *City vs. Country,* ABC, 1976; *Dean Martin Celebrity Roast: Jack Klugman,* NBC, 1978; *A Tribute to "Mr. Television," Milton Berle,* NBC, 1978.

RELATED CAREER—As a stand-up comedian, has appeared in nightclubs throughout the United States.

SIDELIGHTS: Joey Bishop told *CTFT* that he is currently writing a book entitled *I Was a Mouse in the Rat-Pack.*

ADDRESSES: MANAGER—Abby Greshler, 9200 Sunset Boulevard, Los Angeles, CA 90069.

*   *   *

BISHOP, John
  See WILLIS, Ted

*   *   *

BLAKLEY, Ronee   1946-

PERSONAL: Born in 1946 in Stanley, ID.

VOCATION: Actress, singer, and composer.

CAREER: Also see *WRITINGS* below. PRINCIPAL STAGE APPEARANCES—Rhetta Cupp, *Pump Boys and Dinettes,* Princess Theatre, New York City, 1982; Marta Gibson, *Sunset,* Village Gate Theatre, New York City, 1983.

FILM DEBUT—Barbara Jean, *Nashville,* Paramount, 1975. PRINCIPAL FILM APPEARANCES—Connection, *The Driver,* Twentieth Century-Fox, 1978; Carrie DeWitt, *The Private Files of J. Edgar Hoover,* American International, 1978; Mrs. Dylan, *Renaldo and Clara,* Circuit, 1978; Betsy, *Good Luck, Miss Wyckoff* (also known as *The Sin*), Bel-Air/Gradison, 1979; Carolina Red, *The Baltimore Bullet,* AVCO-Embassy, 1980; Marge Thompson, *A Nightmare on Elm Street,* New Line Cinema, 1984; Sally, *A Return to Salem's Lot,* Warner Brothers, 1987; Jenny Selden, *Student Confidential,* Troma, 1987. Also appeared in *Lightning over Water* (also known as *Nick's Movie*), Pari, 1980; *I Played It for You,* Fox International, 1985; *Someone to Love,* International Rainbow, 1987; and *She Came to the Valley,* 1979.

PRINCIPAL FILM WORK—Producer and director, *I Played It for You,* Fox International, 1985.

PRINCIPAL TELEVISION APPEARANCES—Episodic: Ginny, *Vega$,* ABC. Movies: Selena Watson, *Desperate Women,* NBC, 1978; Valene Burns, *The Oklahoma City Dolls,* ABC, 1981. Specials: Gina Sherman, "Divorced Kids' Blues," *ABC Afterschool Special,* ABC, 1987.

WRITINGS: All as composer. FILM—*Welcome Home, Soldier Boys,* Twentieth Century-Fox, 1971; *Lightning over Water* (also known as *Nick's Movie*), Pari, 1980; (also screenplay) *I Played It for You,* Fox International 1985.

AWARDS: Academy Award nomination, Best Supporting Actress, 1975, for *Nashville.**

*   *   *

BLOOM, Verna

PERSONAL: Born August 7, in Lynn, MA. EDUCATION: Graduated from Boston University; trained for the stage at the Uta Hagen-Herbert Berghof School.

VOCATION: Actress.

CAREER: BROADWAY DEBUT—Charlotte Corday, *The Persecution and Assassination of Marat as Performed by the Inmates of the Asylum of Charenton under the Direction of the Marquis de Sade* (also known as *Marat/Sade*), Majestic Theatre, 1967. PRINCIPAL STAGE APPEARANCES—Mona, "The Street Koans," *Kool Aid*, Forum Theatre, New York City, 1971; Blanche, *Brighton Beach Memoirs*, Alvin Theatre, New York City, 1983; Rebecca, *Messiah*, Manhattan Theatre Club, City Center Theatre, New York City, 1984. Also appeared in *Bits and Pieces*, Plaza 9 Room, New York City, 1964; *Barbary Shore*, New York Shakespeare Festival, Public Theatre, New York City, 1974; *The Cherry Orchard*, Off-Broadway production; and in repertory in Denver, CO.

FILM DEBUT—Eileen Horton, *Medium Cool*, Paramount, 1969. PRINCIPAL FILM APPEARANCES—The girl, *Children's Games*, Welebit, 1969; Hannah Collings, *The Hired Hand*, Universal, 1971; Maureen, *Badge 373*, Paramount, 1973; Sarah Belding, *High Plains Drifter*, Universal, 1973; waitress, *Heroes*, Universal, 1977; Marion Wormer, *National Lampoon's Animal House*, Universal, 1978; Emmy, *Honkytonk Man*, Warner Brothers, 1982; June, *After Hours*, Warner Brothers, 1985; farm woman, *The Journey of Natty Gann*, Buena Vista, 1985; Mary, the mother of Jesus, *The Last Temptation of Christ*, Universal, 1988.

PRINCIPAL TELEVISION APPEARANCES—Pilots: Mary Beth Hickey, *Doc Elliot*, ABC, 1973; Moody Larkin, *The Blue Knight*, CBS, 1975; Bertha, *Rivkin: Bounty Hunter*, CBS, 1981. Episodic: Joan Torvec, *Cagney and Lacey*, CBS, 1987; Marian Grey, *The Equalizer*, CBS, 1988. Movies: Jenny, *Where Have All the People Gone?*, NBC, 1974; Jean Hodges, *Sarah T.: Portrait of a Teenage Alcoholic*, NBC, 1975; Emily Hovannes, *Contract on Cherry Street*, NBC, 1977; Paulette, *Playing for Time*, CBS, 1980.

ADDRESSES: OFFICE—9130 Sunset Boulevard, Los Angeles, CA 90069.*

*   *   *

BLOUNT, Lisa

VOCATION: Actress.

CAREER: PRINCIPAL FILM APPEARANCES—Billie Jean, *9/30-55*, Universal, 1977; girl on the beach, *Dead and Buried*, AVCO-Embassy, 1981; Lynette Pomeroy, *An Officer and a Gentleman*, Paramount, 1982; Paula Murphy, *Cease Fire*, CineWorld, 1985; Fran Hudson, *Cut and Run* (also known as *Inferno in Diretta*), New World, 1986; Miles, *Radioactive Dreams*, De Laurentiis Entertainment Group, 1986; Leslie Peterson, *What Waits Below* (also known as *Secrets of the Phantom Caverns*), Blossom, 1986; Audrey Zale, *Nightflyers*, Vista/New Century, 1987; Catherine, *Prince of Darkness*, Universal, 1987; Anette, *South of Reno* (also known as *Darkness, Darkness*), Castle Hill, 1987; Phyllis, *Out Cold*, Hemdale, 1989. Also appeared in *Sam's Song* (also known as *The Swap*), Cannon, 1979; *Great Balls of Fire*, Orion, 1989; and *Blind Fury*, 1989.

PRINCIPAL TELEVISION APPEARANCES—Pilots: Michelle Jameson, *Mickey Spillane's Mike Hammer: Murder Me, Murder You*, CBS, 1983; Cindy, *The Annihilator*, NBC, 1986; Sissy Rigetti, *Stormin' Home*, CBS, 1985; Pat Yaraslovsky, "Off Duty," *CBS Summer*

Playhouse, CBS, 1988. Episodic: Toby, *Moonlighting*, ABC, 1986.

ADDRESSES: AGENT—J.J. Harris, William Morris Agency, 151 El Camino Drive, Beverly Hills, CA 90212.

*   *   *

BOCHNER, Lloyd   1924-

PERSONAL: Born July 29, 1924, in Toronto, ON, Canada; children: Hart.

VOCATION: Actor.

CAREER: PRINCIPAL STAGE APPEARANCES—George, *Richard III*, and Longaville, *All's Well That Ends Well*, both Stratford Shakespearean Festival, Stratford, ON, Canada, 1953; Vincentio, the Duke, *Measure for Measure*, and Vincentio, *The Taming of the Shrew*, both Stratford Shakespearean Festival, 1954; Cassius, *Julius Caesar*, and Salanio, *The Merchant of Venice*, both Stratford Shakespearean Festival, 1955; Callapine, *Tamburlaine the Great*, Stratford Shakespearean Festival, then Winter Garden Theatre, New York City, both 1956; Rugby, *The Merry Wives of Windsor*, and Duke of Burgundy, *Henry V*, both Stratford Shakespearean Festival, 1956; Horatio, *Hamlet*, and Orsino, *Twelfth Night*, both Stratford Shakespearean Festival, 1957; Protheus, *Two Gentlemen of Verona*, Stratford Shakespearean Theatre, then Phoenix Theatre, New York City, both 1958.

PRINCIPAL FILM APPEARANCES—David Moore, *Drums of Africa*, Metro-Goldwyn-Mayer (MGM), 1963; man in the dream, *The Night Walker*, Universal, 1964; Marc Peters, *Harlow*, Magna, 1965; Bruce Stamford III, *Sylvia*, Paramount, 1965; Frederick Carter, *Point Blank*, MGM, 1967; Vic Rood, *Tony Rome*, Twentieth Century-Fox, 1967; Dr. Roberts, *The Detective*, Twentieth Century-Fox, 1968; Archer Madison, *The Horse in the Gray Flannel Suit*, Buena Vista, 1968; Raymond Marquis Allen, *The Young Runaways*, MGM, 1968; Dr. Cory, *The Dunwich Horror*, American International, 1970; Del Ware, *Tiger by the Tail*, Commonwealth, 1970; Captain Gates, *Ulzana's Raid*, Universal, 1972; Burton, *It Seemed Like a Good Idea at the Time*, Ambassador, 1975; Churchill, *The Man in the Glass Booth*, American Film Theatre, 1975; Severo, *Hot Touch*, Astral, 1982; Walter, *The Lonely Lady*, Universal, 1983; Frank Newley, *Crystal Heart*, New World, 1987.

PRINCIPAL TELEVISION APPEARANCES—Series: Captain Nicholas Lacey, *One Man's Family*, NBC, 1952; regular, *Star Tonight*, ABC, 1955-56; Police Commissioner Neil Campbell, *Hong Kong*, ABC, 1960-61; regular, *General Electric True*, CBS, 1962-63; regular, *The Richard Boone Show*, NBC, 1963-64; Cecil Colby, *Dynasty*, ABC, 1981-82; C.C. Capwell, *Santa Barbara*, NBC, 1984. Pilots: Joseph Campbell, *Arena* (broadcast as an episode of *The Richard Boone Show*), NBC, 1964; John Pendennis, *Scalplock*, ABC, 1966; Lawrence, *Braddock*, CBS, 1968; A.B. Carr, *They Call It Murder*, NBC, 1971; David, *Rex Harrison Presents Short Stories of Love*, NBC, 1974; Davenport, *Richie Brockelman: Missing 24 Hours*, NBC, 1976; Hank's aide, *The Eyes of Texas*, NBC, 1980; Ritter, *Crazy Dan*, NBC, 1986. Episodic: Chambers, "To Serve Man," *The Twilight Zone*, CBS, 1962; Logan Rinewood, *Dynasty*, ABC, 1981; Vincent Mulligan, *Crazy Like a Fox*, CBS, 1986; Cameron Wheeler, *Hotel*, ABC, 1986; Charles Linney, *Fall*

Guy, ABC, 1986; also "The Prisoner in the Mirror," *Thriller,* NBC, 1961; "The Fear Makers," *Voyage to the Bottom of the Sea,* ABC, 1964; "The Deadliest Game," *Voyage to the Bottom of the Sea,* ABC, 1965; *The Man from U.N.C.L.E.,* NBC; *Mission: Impossible,* CBS; *Mannix,* CBS; *Charlie's Angels,* ABC; *Daniel Boone,* NBC.

Movies: Mr. Gorman, *Stranger on the Run,* NBC, 1967; Kevin Pierce, *Crowhaven Farm,* ABC, 1970; Professor Delacroix, *Satan's School for Girls,* ABC, 1973; Dr. Roger Cabe, *Terraces,* NBC, 1977; Paul Gilliam, *A Fire in the Sky,* NBC, 1978; Chris Noel, *The Immigrants,* syndicated, 1978; Bob Stockwood, *The Best Place to Be,* NBC, 1979; Dr. Hamill, *The Golden Gate Murders,* CBS, 1979; Matthew, *Mary and Joseph: A Story of Faith,* NBC, 1979; Hall, *Rona Jaffe's "Mazes and Monsters,"* CBS, 1982; Adrien Damvilliers, *Louisiana,* Cinemax, 1984; Special Agent Vaughn, "Double Agent," *Disney Sunday Movie,* ABC, 1987. Specials: Orsino, *Twelfth Night,* NBC, 1957; Jack Favall, *Rebecca,* NBC, 1962; Sam Hall, *A Mouse, A Mystery, and Me,* NBC, 1987.

RELATED CAREER—Actor in radio and stage productions in Canada.

ADDRESSES: AGENT—David Shapira and Associates, 15301 Ventura Boulevard, Sherman Oaks, CA 91403.*

*　　　*　　　*

BOERS, Jr., Frank
See BONNER, Frank

*　　　*　　　*

BOGOSIAN, Eric　1953-

PERSONAL: Born April 24, 1953, in Boston, MA; son of Henry (an accountant) and Edwina (a hairdresser) Bogosian; married Jo Anne Bonney (a graphic designer), October, 1980; children: Harris Wolf. EDUCATION: Attended the University of Chicago for two years; Oberlin College, B.A., theatre, 1976.

VOCATION: Actor, performance artist, and writer.

CAREER: Also see *WRITINGS* below. OFF-BROADWAY DEBUT—*Men Inside* and *Voices of America* (a double-bill of one-man plays), New York Shakespeare Festival, Public Theatre, 1982. PRINCIPAL STAGE APPEARANCES—*Careful Moment* (one-man play), St. Mark's Church, New York City, 1977; *FunHouse* (one-man play), New York Shakespeare Festival (NYSF), Public Theatre, then Actors Playhouse, both New York City, 1983; *Drinking in America* (one-man play), American Place Theatre, New York City, 1986; Barry Champlain, *Talk Radio,* New York Shakespeare Festival, Public Theatre, 1987; *Sex, Drugs, and Rock 'n' Roll* (one-man play), Performance Space 122, New York City, 1988. Also appeared in *Men in Dark Times, Sheer Heaven, The New World,* and in the title role, *The Ricky Paul Show.*

PRINCIPAL STAGE WORK—Director and design supervisor, *FunHouse* (one-man play), Actors Playhouse, New York City, 1983.

MAJOR TOURS—Has appeared in his one-man plays throughout the United States and Great Britain.

PRINCIPAL FILM APPEARANCES—CBS technician, *Born in Flames,* COW Films, 1982; Chris Neville, *Special Effects,* New Line Cinema, 1984; Barry Champlain, *Talk Radio,* Universal, 1988. Also appeared as the Entertainer, *Arena Brains* (short film), 1987.

PRINCIPAL TELEVISION APPEARANCES—Episodic: Jackie Thompson, "The Healer," *The Twilight Zone,* CBS, 1985; DeWitt Morton, *Crime Story,* NBC, 1986; also *Miami Vice,* NBC. Movies: Lieutenant Barney Greenwald, *The Caine Mutiny Court Martial,* CBS, 1988. Specials: *Eric Bogosian—Drinking in America,* Cinemax, 1986; *Ann Magnuson's Vandemonium,* Cinemax, 1987.

RELATED CAREER—Founder of a contemporary dance program and director at the Kitchen (a performance space), New York City.

WRITINGS: STAGE—*Careful Moment* (one-man play), St. Mark's Church, New York City, 1977; *Men Inside* and *Voices of America* (a double-bill of one-man plays), New York Shakespeare Festival (NYSF), Public Theatre, New York City, 1982; *FunHouse* (one-man play), NYSF, Public Theatre, then Actors Playhouse, New York City, 1983; *Drinking in America* (one-man play), American Place Theatre, New York City, 1986, published by Vintage, 1987; *Talk Radio,* NYSF, Public Theatre, 1987. Also *Men in Dark Times, Sheer Heaven, The New World,* and *The Ricky Paul Show.* FILM—(With Oliver Stone) *Talk Radio,* Universal, 1988; also *Arena Brains* (short film), 1987; *Blue Smoke,* upcoming. TELEVISION—Specials: *Eric Bogosian—Drinking in America,* Cinemax, 1986.

AWARDS: Obie Award from the *Village Voice,* Playwriting category, and Drama Desk Award, Outstanding Solo Performance, both 1986, for *Drinking in America.*

SIDELIGHTS: Described as "part standup comic and part dramatist of obsessions" by Samuel G. Freedman in the *New York Times* (September 30, 1983), Eric Bogosian insists that, "I'm not a fun guy. . . . I'm not the type of person who will do anything to have people laugh, to have someone run up to you and ask for your autograph. I try to do nice characters sometimes, but they change on me. So the challenge is to do the dark guys, the very dark guys."

It is with these "dark guys" that Bogosian has gained a reputation as a writer and actor of keen insight into the culture and mores of American society. In his one-man plays such as *FunHouse* and *Drinking in America,* Bogosian offers a series of a dozen or more character monologues, according to *Women's Wear Daily's* David Lida. "His people tend to be from the sleazier side of life: a coke-snorting Hollywood agent; a Southern preacher who talks his congregation into torching abortion clinics; a traveling salesman sweet-talking a hooker; a bum hustling spare change." Bogosian described these works to Lida as being similar to "concept albums—there's 12 or 15 cuts, they're each between three and seven minutes, and they're all related in a theme, sort of."

In *Talk Radio,* his first full-length play, Bogosian plays Barry Champlain, an acerbic, audience-baiting late-night radio talk show host. As he explained to Lida, Barry has "built his reputation being extremely difficult and nasty to his callers. His show is about to go national and the producer's putting pressure on him to keep it lively. The callers give him more than he can handle and he unravels progressively, until he's confused reality with the part he plays on the air." After repeating the role in the 1988 film version directed by and co-written with Oliver Stone, Bogosian told *Rolling Stone's*

Anthony DeCurtis (January 12, 1989), "Barry is me. I'm not writing about anybody over there. I'm writing about myself. . . . I do believe that if you keep looking at the nasty stuff you don't want to look at, you can live with it better. It's better than just ignoring it."

OTHER SOURCES: New York Times, September 30, 1983, February 14, 1986, August 26, 1988; *Rolling Stone,* January 12, 1989; *Women's Wear Daily,* May 6, 1987.

ADDRESSES: AGENT—George Lane, William Morris Agency, 1350 Avenue of the Americas, New York, NY 10019.*

*   *   *

BONHAM CARTER, Helena   1966-

PERSONAL: Born May 26, 1966, in London, England; daughter of Raymond (a merchant banker) and Elena (a psychotherapist; maiden name, Propper de Allejon) Bonham Carter.

VOCATION: Actress.

CAREER: STAGE DEBUT—Laura Fairlie, *The Woman in White,* Greenwich Theatre, London, 1988.

FILM DEBUT—Lady Jane Grey, *Lady Jane,* Paramount, 1986. PRINCIPAL FILM APPEARANCES—Lucy Honeychurch, *A Room*

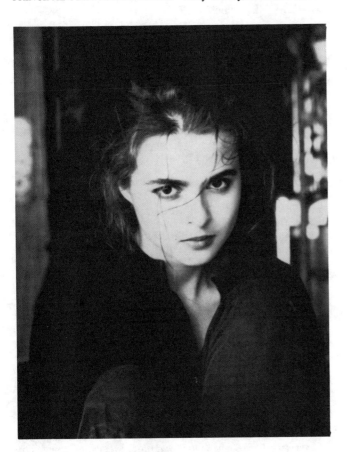

HELENA BONHAM CARTER

with a View, Cinecom, 1986; young lady at cricket match, *Maurice,* Cinecom, 1987; Iris, *La Maschera* (also known as *The Mask*), Italnoleggio Cinematografica, 1987; Chiara, *Francesco* (also known as *St. Francis*), Niccon/Filmtrust, 1988. Also appeared in *Getting It Right,* Manson International, 1989.

TELEVISION DEBUT—Netty, *A Pattern of Roses,* Channel Four, 1982. PRINCIPAL TELEVISON APPEARANCES—Episodic: Dr. Theresa Lyons, *Maimi Vice,* NBC, 1987. Movies: Jo Marriner, *The Vision,* BBC, 1987; Serena Staverly, *A Hazard of Hearts,* CBS, 1987. Plays: *Arms and the Man,* BBC, 1988.

SIDELIGHTS: RECREATIONS—Travel.

Helena Bonham Carter told *CTFT* that she speaks French, Italian, and Spanish.

ADDRESSES: AGENT—Robert Lantz, The Lantz Office, 888 Seventh Avenue, New York, NY 10106.

*   *   *

BONNER, Frank   1942-

PERSONAL: Born Frank Boers, Jr., February 28, 1942, in Little Rock, AR; son of Frank Woodrow and Grace Marie (Dobbins) Boers; married Lilliana Carmen Van Groag, September 24, 1977; children: Desiree.

VOCATION: Actor.

CAREER: STAGE DEBUT—*The Only Bathtub in Oasis,* Gallery Theatre, West Hollywood, CA. PRINCIPAL STAGE APPEARANCES— In productions of *The Sign in Sidney Brustein's Window, The Lion in Winter, Twelve Angry Men, Measure for Measure, Auntie Mame, A Majority of One, The Crucible,* and *The Balcony.* Also appeared with the Arkansas Repertory Theatre, Little Rock, AR, 1985-86.

PRINCIPAL FILM APPEARANCES—(As Frank Boers, Jr.) Jim, *Equinox,* VIP, 1970; Cleta Dempsey, *The Hoax,* All-Scope International, 1972; realtor, *The Longshot,* Orion, 1986; Chuck Hayes, *You Can't Hurry Love,* Lightening, 1988. Also appeared in *Hearts of the West* (also known as *Hollywood Cowboy*), Metro-Goldwyn-Mayer/United Artists, 1975; *Swiss Bank Account,* American Films, 1975; and *Las Vegas Lady,* Crown International, 1976.

PRINCIPAL TELEVISION APPEARANCES—Series: Herb Tarlek, *WKRP in Cincinnati,* CBS, 1978-82; Detective P.J. Mooney, *Sidekicks,* ABC, 1986; Father Robert Hargis, *Just the Ten of Us,* ABC, 1988. Pilots: Howard, *Sutters Bay,* CBS, 1983. Episodic: Buck, *Scarecrow and Mrs. King,* CBS, 1986; also *Sweepstakes,* NBC, 1979; *George Burns Comedy Week,* NBC, 1985; also *Mannix,* CBS; *Emergency,* NBC; *Police Woman,* NBC; *The Man from Atlantis,* NBC; *Cannon,* CBS. Movies: Compton, *Fer de Lance,* CBS, 1974; Peter, *Sex and the Single Parent,* CBS, 1979; Garth Kiley, *The Facts of Life Goes to Paris,* NBC, 1982; Deputy Thad Prouty, *No Man's Land,* NBC, 1984; also *The Lives of Jenny Dolan,* NBC, 1975; *The Amazing Howard Hughes,* CBS, 1977; *Rainbow,* NBC, 1978.

PRINCIPAL TELEVISION WORK—All as director. Episodic: *WKRP*

in Cincinnati, CBS, 1978; *Family Ties*, NBC, 1982; *Head of the Class*, ABC, 1986.

NON-RELATED CAREER—Karate teacher.

AWARDS: Los Angeles Drama Critics Award for *The Sign in Sidney Brustein's Window*.

MEMBER: Screen Actors Guild, American Federation of Television and Radio Artists, Actors' Equity Association, Directors Guild of America.

ADDRESSES: AGENT—Jack Fields, Gores/Fields Agency, 10100 Santa Monica Boulevard, Suite 700, Los Angeles, CA 90067.*

*   *   *

BONO, Sonny   1935-

PERSONAL: Full name, Salvatore Phillip Bono; born February 16, 1935, in Detroit, MI; married Donna Rankin (divorced); married Cher (an actress and singer), October 27, 1964 (divorced, 1974); married Susie Coehlo (divorced); married Mary Whitaker, March 1986; children: Santo, Jean (first marriage); Chastity (second marriage); one son (third marriage).

VOCATION: Singer, actor, producer, and composer.

CAREER: Also see *WRITINGS* below. PRINCIPAL FILM APPEARANCES—As himself, *Good Times*, Columbia, 1967; Rotelli, *Escape to Athena*, Associated Film Distributors, 1969; Salucci, *Airplane II: The Sequel*, Paramount, 1982; spaced-out guest, *The Vals*, Sundowner, 1985; Peter Dickenson, *Troll*, Empire, 1986; Terry Carlo, *Balboa*, Vestron Video, 1986; Maurice, *Dirty Laundry*, Skouras, 1987; Franklin Von Tussle, *Hairspray*, New Line Cinema, 1988. Also appeared in *Special Delivery*, American International, 1976; and *Under the Boardwalk*, New World, 1988.

PRINCIPAL FILM WORK—Producer, *Chastity*, American International, 1969.

PRINCIPAL TELEVISION APPEARANCES—Series: *The Sonny and Cher Comedy Hour*, CBS, 1971-74; *The Sonny Comedy Revue*, ABC, 1974; *The Sonny and Cher Show*, CBS, 1976-77. Episodic: *Our Time*, NBC, 1985; *Late Night with David Letterman*, NBC, 1987; *Later with Bob Costas*, NBC, 1988; also *Hullabaloo*, NBC; *Shindig*, ABC; *Love, American Style*, ABC; *Fantasy Island*, ABC; *The Love Boat*, ABC; *Switch*, CBS. Movies: Jack Marshall, *Murder on Flight 502*, ABC, 1975; Sonny Hunt, *Murder in Music City* (also known as *The Country-Western Murders*), NBC, 1979; Bobby Antoine, *The Top of the Hill*, syndicated, 1980. Specials: Third husband, *The First Nine Months Are the Hardest*, NBC, 1971; *How to Handle a Woman*, NBC, 1972; *Battle of the Network Stars*, ABC, 1977; co-host, *The Sensational, Shocking, Wonderful, Wacky 70s*, NBC, 1980.

RELATED CAREER—Songwriter for Specialty Records, 1950s; arranger and background vocalist for record producer Phil Spector, early 1960s; appeared with Cher as a singing duo (originally named Caesar and Cleo, then as Sonny and Cher), 1964-74.

NON-RELATED CAREER—Mayor of Palm Springs, CA, 1988—; restaurant owner, Palm Springs, CA.

WRITINGS: FILM—Soundtrack composer, *Good Times*, Columbia, 1967; soundtrack composer, *Chastity*, American International, 1969. OTHER—Songs: (With Jack Nitzsche) "Needles and Pins," 1963; "Baby, Don't Go," 1965; "But You're Mine," 1965; "I Got You Babe," 1965; "Just You," 1965; "Laugh at Me," 1965; "Where Do You Go?," 1965; "Bang, Bang (My Baby Shot Me Down)," 1966; "Have I Stayed Too Long?," 1966; "The Beat Goes On," 1967; "It's the Little Things," 1967; "You'd Better Sit Down Kids," 1967; "A Cowboy's Work Is Never Done," 1972.

RECORDINGS: All with Cher, unless indicated. ALBUMS—*Look at Us*, Atco, 1965; *Wonderful World*, Atco, 1966. SINGLES—"Baby, Don't Go," Reprise, 1965; "But You're Mine," Atco, 1965; "I Got You Babe," Atco, 1965; "Just You," Atco, 1965; (solo) "Laugh at Me," Atco, 1965; "Have I Stayed Too Long?," Atco, 1966; "The Beat Goes On," Atco, 1967; "It's the Little Things," Atco, 1967; "A Cowboy's Work Is Never Done," Kapp, 1972.

MEMBER: Screen Actors Guild, American Federation of Television and Radio Artists, American Society of Composers, Authors, and Publishers.

ADDRESSES: MANAGER—Denis Pregnolato, Anonymous Management Company, 804 Broom Way, Los Angeles, CA 90049.*

*   *   *

BORGNINE, Ernest   1917-

PERSONAL: Born Ermes Effron Borgnino, January 24, 1917 (some sources say 1915 or 1918), in Hamden, CT; son of Charles B. and Anna (Bosselli) Borgnino; married Rhoda Kemins (divorced, 1959); married Katy Jurado (an actress), 1959 (divorced); married Ethel Merman (an actress and singer), July, 1964 (divorced, 1964); married Donna Rancourt, 1964 (divorced); married Tove Newman (a cosmetics entrepreneur), 1972; children: Nancy (first marriage); Sharon, Christopher (fourth marriage). EDUCATION: Studied acting at the Randall School of Dramatic Art, Hartford, CT. MILITARY: U.S. Navy, gunner's mate, 1935-45.

VOCATION: Actor.

CAREER: BROADWAY DEBUT—*Mrs. McThing*, American National Theatre and Academy Theatre, 1952. PRINCIPAL STAGE APPEARANCES—*Harvey*, American National Theatre and Academy Theatre, New York City. Also appeared in repertory at the Barter Theatre, Abingdon, VA, 1946-50.

FILM DEBUT—Hu Chang, *China Corsair*, Columbia, 1951. PRINCIPAL FILM APPEARANCES—Joe Castro, *The Mob*, Columbia, 1951; Bill Street, *Whistle at Eaton Falls*, Columbia, 1951; Sergeant "Fatso" Judson, *From Here to Eternity*, Columbia, 1953; Bull Slager, *The Stranger Wore a Gun*, Columbia, 1953; Rachin, *The Bounty Hunter*, Warner Brothers, 1954; Strabo, *Demetrius and the Gladiators*, Twentieth Century-Fox, 1954; Bart Lonergan, *Johnny Guitar*, Republic, 1954; Donnegan, *Vera Cruz*, United Artists, 1954; Coley Trimble, *Bad Day at Black Rock*, Metro-Goldwyn-Mayer (MGM), 1955; Mike Radin, *The Last Command*, Republic, 1955; title role, *Marty*, United Artists, 1955; Morgan, *Run for Cover*, Paramount, 1955; Bernie Browne, *The Square Jungle*, Universal, 1955; Stadt, *Violent Saturday*, Twentieth Century-Fox, 1955; Lew Brown, *The Best Things in Life Are Free*, Twentieth

Century-Fox, 1956; Tom Hurley, *The Catered Affair* (also known as *Wedding Breakfast*), MGM, 1956; Shep Horgan, *Jubal*, Columbia, 1956; Bernie Goldsmith, *Three Brave Men*, Twentieth Century-Fox, 1957; John McBain, *The Badlanders*, MGM, 1958; Lieutenant Archer Sloan, *Torpedo Run*, MGM, 1958; King Ragnar, *The Vikings*, United Artists, 1958; Eddie Colt, *The Rabbit Trap*, United Artists, 1959.

Boris Mitrov, *Man on a String* (also known as *Confessions of a Counterspy*), Columbia, 1960; Lieutenant Joseph Petrosino, *Pay or Die*, Allied Artists, 1960; Pete Stratton, *Go Naked in the World*, MGM, 1961; Roo, *Season of Passion* (also known as *Summer of the Seventeenth Doll*), United Artists, 1961; Lucius, *Barabbas*, Columbia, 1962; Lieutenant Commander Quinton McHale, *McHale's Navy*, Universal, 1964; Trucker Cobb, *The Flight of the Phoenix*, Twentieth Century-Fox, 1965; Barney Yale, *The Oscar*, Embassy, 1966; Sergeant Otto Hansbach, *Chuka*, Paramount, 1967; General Worden, *The Dirty Dozen*, MGM, 1967; Boris Vaslov, *Ice Station Zebra*, Filmways/MGM, 1968; Barney Sheehan, *The Legend of Lylah Clare*, MGM, 1968; Bert Clinger, *The Split*, MGM, 1968; Dutch Engstrom, *The Wild Bunch*, Warner Brothers, 1969.

Fat Cat, *The Adventurers*, Paramount, 1970; Don Pedro Sandoval, *A Bullet for Sandoval* (also known as *Los desperados*), Universal, 1970; Sheriff Harve, *Suppose They Gave a War and Nobody Came?* (also known as *War Games*), Cinerama, 1970; Bill Green, *Bunny O'Hare*, American International, 1971; Emmett Clemens, *Hannie Caulder*, Paramount, 1971; Dictator, *Rain for a Dusty Summer*, Do-Bar, 1971; Al Martin, *Willard*, Cinerama, 1971; Mike Rogo, *The Poseidon Adventure*, Twentieth Century-Fox, 1972; Hoop, *The Revengers*, National General, 1972; Shack, *Emperor of the North Pole* (also known as *Emperor of the North*), Twentieth Century Fox, 1973; Don "Mack" Mackay, *The Neptune Factor* (also known as *Underwater Odyssey* and *The Neptune Disaster*), Twentieth Century-Fox, 1973; Cy, *Law and Disorder*, Columbia, 1974; Corbis, *The Devil's Rain*, Bryanston, 1975; Santoro, *Hustle*, Paramount, 1975; Adam Smith, *Sunday in the Country*, American International, 1975; Lou, *Shoot*, AVCO-Embassy, 1976; Angelo Dundee, *The Greatest*, Columbia, 1977; Lyle Wallace, *Convoy*, United Artists, 1978; John Canty, *Crossed Swords* (also known as *The Prince and the Pauper*), Warner Brothers, 1978; Harry Booth, *The Black Hole*, Buena Vista, 1979; Rann, *The Ravagers*, Columbia, 1979; Firat, *The Double McGuffin*, Mulberry Square, 1979.

Tom Conti, *When Time Ran Out* (also known as *Earth's Final Fury*), Warner Brothers, 1980; Isaiah, *Deadly Blessing*, United Artists, 1981; cabby, *Escape from New York*, AVCO-Embassy, 1981; Clint, *High Risk*, American Cinema, 1981; Willy Dunlop, *Super Fuzz* (also known as *Supersnooper*), AVCO-Embassy, 1981; Lieutenant Bob Carrigan, *Young Warriors*, Cannon, 1983; Ben Robeson, *The Manhunt*, Samuel Goldwyn, 1986. Also appeared in *The Last Judgement* (also known as *Il giudizio universale*), 1961; *Vengeance Is Mine* (also known as *Quei dispe rati che puzzano di sudore et di morte*), Atlantida, 1969; *Ripped Off* (also known as *Un uomo dalla pelle dura* and *The Boxer*), Cinema Shares, 1971; and *Codename: Wild Geese* (also known as *Geheimecode Wildganse*), Entertainment, 1985.

PRINCIPAL TELEVISION APPEARANCES—Series: Lieutenant Commander Quinton McHale, *McHale's Navy*, ABC, 1962-66; Officer Joe Cleaver, *Future Cop*, ABC, 1977; Dominic Santini, *Air Wolf*, CBS, 1984-85. Mini-Series: Centurion, *Jesus of Nazareth*, NBC, 1977; Marcus, *The Last Days of Pompeii*, ABC, 1984; Billy Bones, *Treasure Island*, RAI-2 (Italian television), 1987. Pilots: Lieutenant Commander Quinton McHale, "Seven against the Sea," *Alcoa*

Premiere, ABC, 1962; Deputy Sam Hill, *Sam Hill: Who Killed the Mysterious Mr. Foster?*, NBC, 1971; Sam Paxton, *The Trackers*, ABC, 1971; Vince Boselli, *Twice in a Lifetime*, NBC, 1974; Joe Cleaver, *Future Cop*, ABC, 1976; Joe Cleaver, *The Cops and Robin*, NBC, 1978; *Take One Starring Jonathan Winters*, NBC, 1981. Episodic: Nargola, *Captain Video and His Video Rangers*, Dumont; also *The Bob Hope Chrysler Theatre*, NBC; *Fireside Theatre*, NBC; *The General Electric Theatre*, CBS; *Zane Grey Theatre*, CBS; *Philco TV Playhouse*, NBC; *Laramie*, NBC; *Little House on the Prairie*, NBC; *Navy Log;* and *Wagon Train*.

Movies: Sam Brisbane, *Fire!*, NBC, 1977; Dom Cimoli, *The Ghost of Flight 401*, NBC, 1978; Stanislaus Katczinskyk, *All Quiet on the Western Front*, CBS, 1979; J. Edgar Hoover, *Blood Feud*, syndicated, 1983; Mickey Doyle, *Carpool*, CBS, 1983; Senator Brighton, *Love Leads the Way*, Disney Channel, 1984; Lion, *Alice in Wonderland*, CBS, 1985; General Worden, *The Dirty Dozen: The Next Mission*, NBC, 1985; General Worden, *The Dirty Dozen: The Deadly Mission*, NBC, 1987; General Worden, *The Dirty Dozen: The Fatal Mission*, NBC, 1988. Specials: *The General Motors 50th Anniversary Show*, NBC, 1957; *The Andy Williams Show*, NBC, 1963; *The Bob Hope Show*, NBC, 1967; *What's Up, America?*, NBC, 1971; *The Rowan and Martin Special*, NBC, 1973; *Sandy in Disneyland*, CBS, 1974; *The Funniest Joke I Ever Heard*, ABC, 1984.

NON-RELATED CAREER—Truck driver.

AWARDS: New York Film Critics Award, Best Actor, 1955, Academy Award, Best Actor, 1955, British Academy Award, Best Foreign Actor, 1955, and Golden Globe Award, Best Motion Picture Actor—Drama, 1956, all for *Marty;* Emmy Award nomination, Outstanding Supporting Actor, 1980, for *All Quiet on the Western Front*.

ADDRESSES: PUBLICIST—Harry Flynn, The Flynn Company, 1110 Hortense Street, North Hollywood, CA 91602.*

*   *   *

BOSSON, Barbara   1939-

PERSONAL: Born November 1, 1939, in Belle Vernon, PA; father, a tennis coach; married Steven Bochco (a television producer and writer), 1969; children: Melissa, Jesse. EDUCATION: Attended the Carnegie Institute of Technology.

VOCATION: Actress.

CAREER: PRINCIPAL FILM APPEARANCES—Alva Leacock, *Capricorn One*, Warner Brothers, 1977; Jane Rogan, *The Last Starfighter*, Universal, 1984; Mom, *Little Sweetheart* (also known as *Poison Candy*), Nelson Entertainment, 1988.

PRINCIPAL TELEVISION APPEARANCES—Series: Sharon Peterson, *Richie Brockelman, Private Eye*, NBC, 1978; Fay Furillo, *Hill Street Blues*, NBC, 1981-85; Captain C.Z. Stern, *Hooperman*, ABC, 1987—. Episodic: Ms. Cox, *Sunshine*, NBC, 1975; Marie Rizon, *Crazy Like a Fox*, CBS, 1986; Stacey Gill, *L.A. Law*, NBC, 1986. Pilots: Sharon Peterson, *Richie Brockelman: Missing 24 Hours*, NBC, 1976. Movies: Esther Crowley, *The Impatient Heart*, NBC, 1971; Nancy, *The Calendar Girl Murders*, ABC, 1984; Roberta Spooner, *Hostage Flight*, NBC, 1985. Specials: Donna

Crandall, ''Supermom's Daughter,'' *ABC Afterschool Special*, ABC, 1987; also ''Words to Live By,'' *Schoolbreak Special*, CBS, 1989.

RELATED CAREER—Member, the Committee (an improvisational comedy group), San Francisco, CA; also appeared in summer theatre productions.

NON-RELATED CAREER—Playboy Club bunny.

WRITINGS: TELEVISION—Episodic: *Family*, ABC, 1976.

AWARDS: Emmy Award nomination, Outstanding Supporting Actress in a Drama Series, 1981, for *Hill Street Blues*.

SIDELIGHTS: RECREATIONS—Skiing.

ADDRESSES: AGENT—Writers and Artists Agency, 11726 San Vicente Boulevard, Suite 300, Los Angeles, CA 90049.*

*   *   *

BOVASSO, Julie   1930-

PERSONAL: Full name, Julia Anne Bovasso; born August 1, 1930, in Brooklyn, NY; daughter of Bernard Michael (a truck driver) and Angela Ursula (Padovani) Bovasso; married George Ortman (an artist), February 4, 1951 (divorced, 1958); married Leonard Wayland (an actor), August 12, 1959 (divorced, 1964). EDUCATION: Graduated from the High School of Music and Art, 1948; attended City College of New York, 1948-51; trained for the stage with Herbert Berghof, 1950-51, Uta Hagen, 1951-53, Mira Rostova, 1953-55, and Harold Clurman, 1961.

VOCATION: Actress, director, producer, and playwright.

CAREER: Also see *WRITINGS* below. STAGE DEBUT—Maid, *The Bells*, Davenport Free Theatre, New York City, 1943. PRINCIPAL STAGE APPEARANCES—Gwendolyn, *The Importance of Being Earnest*, title role, *Salome*, and title role, *Hedda Gabler*, all Rolling Players, New York City, 1947-49; Belissa, *Don Perlimplin*, Studio Theatre of Komissarjevski, New York City, 1949; Lona Hessel, *Pillars of Society*, Globe Repertory Theatre, New York City, 1949; Emma, *Naked*, and Countess Geschwitz, *Earth Spirit*, both Provincetown Playhouse, New York City, 1950; Zinida, *He Who Gets Slapped*, Theatre Workshop, New York City, 1950; title role, *Faustina*, Living Theatre, Cherry Lane Theatre, New York City, 1952; Anna Petrovna, *Ivanov*, San Francisco Repertory Theatre, San Francisco, CA, 1952; Margot, *The Typewriter*, Tempo Playhouse, New York City, 1953; Madeleine, *Amedee*, and Claire, *The Maids*, both Tempo Playhouse, 1955; Solange, *The Maids*, and the Student, *The Lesson*, both Tempo Playhouse, 1956; Henriette, *Monique*, John Golden Theatre, New York City, 1957; Luella, *Dinny and the Witches*, Cherry Lane Theatre, 1959.

Wife, *Victims of Duty*, Theatre de Lys, New York City, 1960; Lucy and Martha, *Gallows Humor*, Gramercy Arts Theatre, New York City, 1961; Mistress Quickly, *Henry IV, Part I*, American Shakespeare Festival, Stratford, CT, 1962; Madame Rosepettle, *Oh Dad, Poor Dad, Mamma's Hung You in the Closet and I'm Feelin' So Sad*, Playhouse in the Park, Cincinnati, OH, 1964; Mrs. Prosser, *Minor Miracle*, Henry Miller's Theatre, New York City, 1965; Esmeralda, *The Skin of Our Teeth*, Playhouse in the Park, 1966; Madame Irma, *The Balcony*, Center Stage, Baltimore, MD, 1967;

Agata, *Island of Goats*, and Constance, *The Madwoman of Chaillot*, both Playhouse in the Park, 1968; Gloria B. Gilbert, *Gloria and Esperanza*, La Mama Experimental Theatre Club, New York City, 1969, then American National Theatre Academy Theatre, New York City, 1970; Mother, *The Screens*, Brooklyn Academy of Music, Brooklyn, NY, 1971. Also appeared and in *What I Did Last Summer*, New York City.

PRINCIPAL STAGE WORK—Director: (Also producer) *The Typewriter*, Tempo Playhouse, New York City, 1953; (also producer) *The Maids*, *Amedee* and *Three Sisters Who Are Not Sisters*, all Tempo Playhouse, 1955; (also producer) *The Lesson*, Tempo Playhouse, 1956; *The Moon Dreamers*, La Mama Experimental Theatre Club (E.T.C.), New York City, 1968, then (revised version) Ellen Stewart Theatre, New York City, 1969; *Gloria and Esperanza*, La Mama E.T.C., 1969, then American National Theatre Academy Theatre, New York City, 1970; *Monday on the Way to Mercury Island*, La Mama E.T.C., 1971; *Schubert's Last Serenade*, La Mama E.T.C., 1971, then Manhattan Theatre Club, New York City, 1973; *The Boom Boom Room*, New York Shakespeare Festival, Vivian Beaumont Theatre, New York City, 1973; *The Nothing Kid* and *Standard Safety*, both La Mama E.T.C., 1974; *Super Lover*, *Schubert's Last Serenade*, and *The Final Analysis*, all La Mama E.T.C., 1975.

PRINCIPAL FILM APPEARANCES—Ramona, *Tell Me That You Love Me, Junie Moon*, Paramount, 1970; Flo, *Saturday Night Fever*, Paramount, 1977; Mrs. D'Amico, *Willie and Phil*, Twentieth Century-Fox, 1980; Maureen Rooney, *The Verdict*, Twentieth Century-Fox, 1982; Frieda Stein, *Daniel*, Paramount, 1983; Mrs. Manero, *Staying Alive*, Paramount, 1983; Mrs. Wareham, *Off Beat*, Silver Screen Partners II, 1986; Lil Dickstein, *Wise Guys*, Metro-Goldwyn-Mayer/United Artists (MGM/UA), 1986; Rita Cappomaggi, *Moonstruck*, MGM/UA, 1988.

PRINCIPAL FILM WORK—Dialect coach and technical advisor, *Prizzi's Honor*, Twentieth Century-Fox, 1985; dialogue coach, *Moonstruck*, Metro-Goldwyn-Mayer/United Artists, 1988.

PRINCIPAL TELEVISION APPEARANCES—Series: Rose Fraser, *From These Roots*, NBC, 1958-60. Pilots: Aunt Rosa, *Daughters*, NBC, 1977. Episodic: Pearl, ''The Iceman Cometh,'' *Play of the Week*, WNTA, 1960; bag lady, *Miami Vice*, NBC, 1986; Violetta DeScarfo, *Cagney and Lacey*, CBS, 1987; also ''Man on a Mountain'' and ''Two Black Kings,'' both *U.S. Steel Hour*, CBS, 1961; ''The Colossus,'' *The Defenders*, CBS, 1963. Movies: Marie, *The Last Tenant*, ABC, 1978; waitress, *Just Me and You*, NBC, 1978; Mrs. Campana, *King Crab*, ABC, 1980; Doris, *The Gentleman Bandit*, CBS, 1981; Lou DiMona, *Doubletake*, CBS, 1985; Jackie, *A Time to Triumph*, CBS, 1986; Mrs. Zeffirelli, *Hot Paint*, CBS, 1988.

RELATED CAREER—Founder, manager, producer, and director, Tempo Playhouse, New York City, 1953-56; drama instructor, New School for Social Research, 1965-71, Brooklyn College of the City University of New York, 1968-69, and Sarah Lawrence College, 1969-74; former president, New York Theatre Strategy, Inc.

WRITINGS: See production details above, unless indicated. STAGE—*The Moon Dreamers*, 1968, revised, 1969, published as *The Moon Dreamers: A Play in Two Acts with Music*, Samuel French, Inc., 1969; *Gloria and Esperanza*, 1969, revised, 1970, published as *Gloria and Esperanza: A Play in Two Acts*, Samuel French, Inc., 1969; *Monday on the Way to Mercury Island*, 1971; *Schubert's Last*

Serenade, 1971, published in *Spontaneous Combustion: Eight New American Plays*, Winter House, 1972; *Down by the River Where the Water Lilies Are Disfigured Every Day*, Trinity Square Repertory Company, Bridgham Street Theatre, Providence, RI, 1971, then Circle Repertory Company, New York City, 1975; *The Nothing Kid* 1974; *Standard Safety*, 1974, published by Samuel French, Inc., 1976; *Super Lover*, 1975; *The Final Analysis*, 1975; *Angelo's Wedding*, Circle Repertory Company, New York City, 1985.

AWARDS: Obie Awards from the *Village Voice*, Best Actress, for *The Maids*, and Best Experimental Theatre, for Tempo Playhouse, both 1956; Triple Obie Award, Best Playwright-Director-Actress, 1969, for *Gloria and Esperanza*; Drama Desk Award and Outer Critics Circle Award, both 1972, for *The Screens*; Public Broadcasting Award, 1972, for *Shubert's Last Serenade;* also Rockefeller Foundation Grant for Playwriting, 1969; Guggenheim Fellowship in Drama, 1971; and New York State Council on the Arts Public Service grants, 1971 and 1973.

MEMBER: Actors' Equity Association, American Federation of Television and Radio Artists, Screen Actors Guild, Dramatists Guild, Author's League of America.*

*   *   *

BOWEN, Roger   1932-

PERSONAL: Born May 25, 1932, in Attleboro, MA.

VOCATION: Actor.

CAREER: PRINCIPAL FILM APPEARANCES—Warren, *Petulia*, Warner Brothers, 1968; Colonel Henry Blake, *M*A*S*H*, Twentieth Century-Fox, 1970; rabbi, *Move*, Twentieth Century-Fox, 1970; Lester, *Funnyman*, New Yorker, 1971; manager, *Wicked, Wicked*, Metro-Goldwyn-Mayer, 1973; Kissinger, *Tunnelvision*, World Wide, 1976; newspaperman, *Heaven Can Wait*, Paramount, 1978; owner of Sinthia Cosmetics, *The Main Event*, Warner Brothers, 1979; counsellor, *Foxes*, United Artists, 1980; Mr. Springboro, *Zapped!*, Embassy, 1982; Dr. Cabot, *Morgan Stewart's Coming Home* (also known as *Home Front*), New Century/Vista, 1987.

PRINCIPAL TELEVISION APPEARANCES—Series: Hamilton Majors, Jr., *Arnie*, CBS, 1970-72; Dr. Austin Chaffee, *The Brian Keith Show*, NBC, 1973-74; Dr. Floyd Beiderbeck, *House Calls*, CBS, 1980-82; Colonel Clapp, *At Ease*, ABC, 1983; Donny Bauer, *Suzanne Pleshette Is Maggie Briggs*, CBS, 1984. Pilots: Ski, *Deadlock*, NBC, 1969; Alfred Blunt, *Hunter*, CBS, 1973; Sam, *The Rangers*, NBC, 1974; fire chief, *Where's the Fire?*, ABC, 1975; Thomas N. Tibbles, *Duffy*, CBS, 1977; Dr. Frosman, *Good Penny*, NBC, 1977; Coach Spaulding, *The Murder That Wouldn't Die*, NBC, 1980; U.S. ambassador, *Bulba*, ABC, 1981. Episodic: Lindquist, "The Arsonist," *Barney Miller*, ABC, 1975; also "Archie and the Ku Klux Klan," *All in the Family*, CBS, 1977; *Kate and Allie*, CBS, 1987. Movies: Stu Dotney, *It Couldn't Happen to a Nicer Guy*, ABC, 1974; Fergus Gatwick, *Arthur Hailey's "The Moneychangers*," NBC, 1976; landlord, *The Bastard* (also known as *The Kent Family Chronicles*), syndicated, 1978; Mr. Stit, *Last of the Good Guys*, CBS, 1978; man in kiddieland, *Playmates*, ABC, 1979; Prime Minister Gibson, *Damien: The Leper Priest*, NBC, 1980; Scott Durkin, *Goldie and the Boxer Go to Hollywood*, NBC, 1981; Mr. Gore, *Sharing Richard*, CBS, 1988.

ADDRESSES: AGENT—J. Carter Gibson Agency, 9000 Sunset Boulevard, Suite 801, Los Angeles, CA 90069.*

*   *   *

BRAGA, Sonia   1951-

PERSONAL: Born in 1951 in Maringa, Parana, Brazil; daughter of Zeze Braga (a seamstress); father, a realtor.

VOCATION: Actress.

CAREER: STAGE DEBUT—*Jorge Dandin*, in Brazil. PRINCIPAL STAGE APPEARANCES—*Hair*, in Sao Paulo, Brazil.

PRINCIPAL FILM APPEARANCES—Title role, *Dona Flor e sues dois maridos* (also known as *Dona Flor and Her Two Husbands*), Gaumont/Coline, 1977; title role, *Gabriela*, Metro-Goldwyn-Mayer/United Artists Classics, 1984; Leni Lamaison/Marta/the Spider Woman, *Kiss of the Spider Woman*, Island Alive, 1985; Ruby Archuleta, *The Milagro Beanfield War*, Universal, 1988; Madonna, *Moon over Parador*, Universal, 1988. Also appeared in *A moreninha*, 1969; *Captain Bandeira versus Doctor Moura Brasil*, 1970; *Mestica, The Indomitable Slave*, 1972; *The Couple*, 1974; as Maria, *Eu te amo* (also known as *I Love You*), 1982; and in *The Main Road* and *A Lady on the Bus*.

TELEVISION DEBUT—Princess, *Gardin encatado* (also known as *The Enchanted Garden*), Brazilian television. PRINCIPAL TELEVISION APPEARANCES—Series: *Gabriela*, TV Globo, 1974; *Dancin' Days*, TV Globo, 1978; also *The Girl of the Blue Sailboat*, 1968. Episodic: Anna Maria Westlake, *The Cosby Show* (two episodes), NBC, 1986. Movies: Emily, *The Man Who Broke 1,000 Chains*, HBO, 1987. Specials: *Women of the World*, 1986; also *Sesame Street* (Brazilian production).

RELATED CAREER—Jury member, Cannes International Film Festival, Cannes, France.

AWARDS: Golden Globe Award nomination, Best Supporting Actress, 1985, for *Kiss of the Spider Woman*.

ADDRESSES: AGENT—Michael Black, International Creative Management, 8899 Beverly Boulevard, Los Angeles, CA 90048.*

*   *   *

BRANDON, Michael

PERSONAL: Born in Brooklyn, NY; married Lindsay Wagner (an actress), December, 1976 (divorced).

VOCATION: Actor.

CAREER: PRINCIPAL STAGE APPEARANCES—*The Lady and the Clarinet*, Long Wharf Theatre, New Haven, CT, 1983.

PRINCIPAL FILM APPEARANCES—Mike Vecchio, *Lovers and Other Strangers*, Cinerama, 1970; Marcus, *Jennifer on My Mind*, United Artists, 1971; Robert, *Four Flies on Grey Velvet* (also known as *Quarto mosche di velluto gris*), Paramount, 1972; voice characterization, *Heavy Traffic* (animated), American International, 1973; Jeff Dugan, *FM* (also known as *Citizen's Band*), Universal, 1978; Dr. Jim Sandman, *Promises in the Dark,* Warner Brothers, 1979; Pete Lachapelle, *A Change of Seasons,* Twentieth Century-Fox, 1980; Max, *Rich and Famous,* Metro-Goldwyn-Mayer/United Artists, 1981.

PRINCIPAL TELEVISION APPEARANCES—Series: David Marquette, *Emerald Point, N.A.S.,* CBS, 1983-84; Lieutenant James Dempsey, *Dempsey and Makepeace,* syndicated, 1984. Pilots: Kirk, *Man in the Middle,* CBS, 1972; Tony Scott, *Scott Free,* NBC, 1976; Dr. Pete Marcus, *Venice Medical,* ABC, 1983; Bryan Dobbs, *Divided We Stand,* ABC, 1988. Movies: Frank Pescadero, *The Impatient Heart,* NBC, 1971; Billy, *The Strangers in 7-A,* CBS, 1972; David, *The Third Girl from the Left,* ABC, 1973; Jim Conklin, *The Red Badge of Courage,* NBC, 1974; Keith Miles, *Hitchhike!,* ABC, 1974; Ben Holian, *Cage without a Key,* CBS, 1975; Davis Asher, *Queen of the Stardust Ballroom,* CBS, 1975; Bill Bast, *James Dean,* NBC, 1976; Carl Wyche, *Red Alert,* CBS, 1977; Paul Lester, *The Comedy Company,* CBS, 1978; Alan, *A Vacation in Hell,* NBC, 1979; Steve Triandos, *A Perfect Match,* CBS, 1980; Bob Frazer, *Between Two Brothers,* CBS, 1982; Keith Sindell, *The Seduction of Gina,* CBS, 1984; Michael Krasnick, *Deadly Messages,* ABC, 1985; Jeff Robins, *Rock 'n' Roll Mom,* ABC, 1988. Specials: *Lindsay Wagner—Another Side of Me,* ABC, 1977.

MEMBER: Actors' Equity Association, Screen Actors Guild, American Federation of Television and Radio Artists.

ADDRESSES: MANAGER—Herb Nanas, Moress/Nanas Entertainment, 2128 Pico Boulevard, Santa Monica, CA 90069.*

*　　*　　*

BREST, Martin 1951-

PERSONAL: Born in 1951 in Bronx, NY. EDUCATION: Attended New York University.

VOCATION: Director, producer, screenwriter, editor, and actor.

CAREER: Also see *WRITINGS* below. PRINCIPAL FILM APPEARANCES—Dr. Miller, *Fast Times at Ridgemont High,* Universal, 1982; drive-in security guard, *Spies Like Us,* Warner Brothers, 1985. PRINCIPAL FILM WORK—All as director: (Also producer and editor) *Hot Tomorrows,* American Film Institute, 1978; *Going in Style,* Warner Brothers, 1979; *Beverly Hills Cop,* Paramount, 1984; producer, *Midnight Run,* Universal, 1988.

WRITINGS: See production details above. FILM—*Hot Tomorrows,* 1978; *Going in Style,* 1979.

SIDELIGHTS: Early in his career, Martin Brest made an award-winning short subject film entitled *Hot Dogs for Gauguin.*

ADDRESSES: AGENT—Jack Rapke, Creative Artists Agency, 1888 Century Park E., Suite 1400, Los Angeles, CA 90067.*

BRITTANY, Morgan 1951-
(Suzanne Cupito)

PERSONAL: Born Suzanne Cupito, December 5, 1951, in Hollywood, CA; married Jack Gill.

VOCATION: Actress.

CAREER: PRINCIPAL FILM APPEARANCES—(As Suzanne Cupito) "Baby" June, *Gypsy,* Warner Brothers, 1962; (as Suzanne Cupito) Sandy Swope, *Stage to Thunder Rock,* Paramount, 1964; (as Suzanne Cupito) Louise Beardsley, *Yours, Mine, and Ours,* United Artists, 1968; Vivien Leigh, *Gable and Lombard,* Universal, 1976; Mary, *In Search of Historic Jesus,* Sunn Classic, 1980; Sheila Holt-Browning, *The Prodigal,* World-Wide, 1984. Also appeared in *The Birds,* Universal, 1963; and *Marnie,* Universal, 1964.

PRINCIPAL TELEVISION APPEARANCES—Series: Katherine Wentworth, *Dallas,* CBS, 1981-84; Kate Simpson, *Glitter,* ABC, 1984-85; host, *Star Games,* syndicated, 1986. Pilots: Doris Ann, *Delta County, U.S.A.,* ABC, 1977; Cathy Berman, *Samurai,* ABC, 1979; Elena Sweet, *Stunt Seven,* CBS, 1979. Episodic: (As Suzanne Cupito) Little girl, "Nightmare as a Child," *The Twilight Zone,* CBS, 1960; (as Suzanne Cupito) girl, "Valley of the Shadow," *The Twilight Zone,* CBS, 1963; (as Suzanne Cupito) Susan, "Caesar and Me," *The Twilight Zone,* CBS, 1964; also *The New Love, American Style,* ABC, 1985; *Fame, Fortune, and Romance,* syndicated, 1986; *True Confessions,* syndicated, 1986. Movies: Ella Hughes, *The Amazing Howard Hughes,* CBS, 1977; Patti, *The Initiation of Sarah,* ABC, 1978; Becky Lyons, *Death Car on the Freeway,* CBS, 1979; Vivien Leigh, *Moviola: The Scarlett O'Hara War,* NBC, 1980; Astrid James, *The Dream Merchants,* syndicated, 1980; Lannie, *The Wild Women of Chastity Gulch,* ABC, 1982; voice of Princess Niamh, *Faeries* (animated), CBS, 1982; Alice Glass, *LBJ: The Early Years,* NBC, 1987; Marianne Clayman, *Perry Mason: The Case of the Scandalous Scoundrel,* NBC, 1987; also *Going Home Again.* Specials: *Hollywood Stars' Screen Tests,* NBC, 1984; *The Funniest Joke I Ever Heard,* ABC, 1984; *Bob Hope's Comedy Salute to the Soaps,* NBC, 1985; host, *On Top All Over the World,* syndicated, 1985; host, *Miss Teen U.S.A.,* CBS, 1986; *Bob Hope's Tropical Comedy Special from Tahiti,* NBC, 1987; *Happy Birthday Hollywood,* ABC, 1987; *Lifetime Salutes Mom,* Lifetime, 1987; *The World's Greatest Stunts: A Tribute to Hollywood's Stuntmen,* ABC, 1988.

ADDRESSES: AGENT—Steven Sauer Entertainment, 2029 Century Park E., Suite 3250, Los Angeles, CA 90067.*

*　　*　　*

BROLIN, James 1941-

PERSONAL: Born July 18, 1941 (some sources say 1940), in Los Angeles, CA; father, a builder; married Jane Agee, 1967 (divorced, 1985); married Jan Smithers (an actress), 1986; children: two sons (first marriage); Molly Elizabeth (second marriage). EDUCATION: Attended the University of California, Los Angeles.

VOCATION: Actor.

CAREER: PRINCIPAL FILM APPEARANCES—Student, *Dear Brigette,* Twentieth Century-Fox, 1965; Private Aames, *Von Ryan's Express,* Twentieth Century-Fox, 1965; technician, *Fan-*

tastic Voyage (also known as *Microscopia* and *Strange Journey*), Twentieth Century-Fox, 1966; technician, *Our Man Flint*, Twentieth Century-Fox, 1966; Ted Robertson, *Way . . . Way Out*, Twentieth Century-Fox, 1966; Sergeant Lisi, *The Boston Strangler*, Twentieth Century-Fox, 1968; Jerome K. Weber, *Skyjacked* (also known as *Sky Terror*), Metro-Goldwyn-Mayer (MGM), 1972; John Blane, *Westworld*, MGM, 1973; Clark Gable, *Gable and Lombard*, Universal, 1976; Wade Parent, *The Car*, Universal, 1977; Charles Brubaker, *Capricorn One*, Warner Brothers, 1978; George Lutz, *The Amityville Horror*, American International, 1979; Sean Boyd, *Night of the Juggler*, Columbia, 1980; Stone, *High Risk*, American Cinema, 1981; P.W., *Pee-Wee's Big Adventure*, Warner Brothers, 1985. Also appeared in *Take Her She's Mine*, Twentieth Century-Fox, 1963; *Goodbye, Charlie*, Twentieth Century-Fox, 1964; *Morituri*, Twentieth Century-Fox, 1965; *Capetown Affair*, Twentieth Century-Fox, 1967; and *The Gringos*, Warner Brothers, 1980.

PRINCIPAL TELEVISION APPEARANCES—Series: Dalton Wales, *The Monroes*, ABC, 1966-67; Dr. Steven Kiley, *Marcus Welby, M.D.*, ABC, 1969-76; Peter McDermott, *Hotel*, ABC, 1983-88. Pilots: Dr. Steven Kiley, *Marcus Welby, M.D.*, ABC, 1969. Episodic: *Bus Stop*, CBS, 1961; "Ring around the Riddler," *Batman*, ABC, 1967. Movies: Tom Phelan, *Short Walk to Daylight*, ABC, 1972; Joe Hart, *Class of '63*, ABC, 1973; Chuck Brenner, *Trapped*, ABC, 1973; Clayton Pfanner, *Steel Cowboy*, NBC, 1978; Paul Marshall, *The Ambush Murders*, CBS, 1982; Jim Timony, *Mae West*, ABC, 1982; Mike McKay, *White Water Rebels*, CBS, 1983; Ward McNally, *Cowboy*, CBS, 1983; Harry Wild, *Beverly Hills Cowgirls Blues*, CBS, 1985; Nick Atkins, *Intimate Encounters*, NBC, 1986; Ross Nelson, *Hold That Dream*, syndicated, 1986; Michael Wakefield, *Deep Dark Secrets*, NBC, 1987; Martin Shrevelowe, *Finishing Line*, TNT, 1988. Specials: *City vs. Country*, ABC, 1976.

AWARDS: Most Promising Actor poll winner, *Fame* and *Photoplay* magazines, both 1970; Emmy Award, Outstanding Performance by an Actor in a Supporting Role in Drama, 1970, for *Marcus Welby, M.D.*

MEMBER: Screen Actors Guild, American Federation of Television and Radio Artists.

ADDRESSES: AGENT—Audrey Caan, Triad Artists, 10100 Santa Monica Boulevard, 16th Floor, Los Angeles, CA 90067.*

*   *   *

BROOKES, Jacqueline   1930-

PERSONAL: Full name, Jacqueline Victoire Brookes; born July 24, 1930, in Montclair, NJ; daughter of Frederick Jack (an investment banker) and Maria Victoire (Zur Haar) Brookes. EDUCATION: University of Iowa, B.F.A., 1951; trained for the stage at the Royal Academy of Dramatic Art, 1953; studied acting with Michael Howard and singing with Raymond J.D. Buckingham, both in New York City.

VOCATION: Actress.

CAREER: STAGE DEBUT—*La Boheme* (opera), Metropolitan Opera House, New York City, 1943. OFF-BROADWAY DEBUT—Emilia, *Othello*, Shakespeare Guild, Jan Hus Playhouse, 1953.

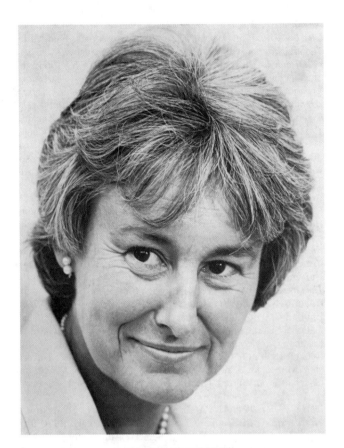

JACQUELINE BROOKES

PRINCIPAL STAGE APPEARANCES—Phaedra, *The Cretan Woman*, Provincetown Playhouse, New York City, 1954; Gelda, *The Dark Is Light Enough*, American National Theatre and Academy (ANTA) Theatre, New York City, 1955; Vittoria Corombona, *The White Devil*, Phoenix Theatre, New York City, 1955; second woman, *Medea*, Theatre Sarah Bernhardt, Paris, France, 1955; Lady Macbeth, *Macbeth*, the Queen, *Cymbeline*, and the Jailer's Daughter, *Two Noble Kinsmen*, all Antioch Shakespeare Festival, Yellow Springs, OH, 1955; woman, *Tiger at the Gates*, Plymouth Theatre, New York City, 1955; Blanche of Spain, then Constance, *King John*, and Juliet, *Measure for Measure*, both American Shakespeare Festival, Stratford, CT, 1956; Celimene, *The Misanthrope*, Theatre East, New York City, 1956; title role, *The Duchess of Malfi*, Phoenix Theatre, 1957; Desdemona, *Othello*, and Ursula, *Much Ado about Nothing*, both American Shakespeare Festival, 1957; Sheila, *Dial M for Murder*, Cape Playhouse, Dennis, MA, 1958; Anna Petrovna, *Ivanov*, Renata Theatre, New York City, 1958; Lady Macbeth, *Macbeth*, University of Michigan Drama Festival, Lydia Mendelssohn Theatre, Ann Arbor, MI, 1959; Mother, *Kinderspiel*, Boston University, Boston, MA, 1959.

Portia, *Julius Caesar*, Rosalind, *As You Like It*, and Gertrude, *Hamlet*, all National Shakespeare Festival, Old Globe Theatre, San Diego, CA, 1960; Ilona, *Anatol*, Zerbinette, *Scapin*, Goneril, *King Lear*, Helena, *A Midsummer Night's Dream*, and Ophelia, *Hamlet*, all Association of Producing Artists, McCarter Theatre, Princeton, NJ, 1960; Viola, *Twelfth Night*, Portia, *The Merchant of Venice*, and Elizabeth, *Richard III*, all National Shakespeare Festival, Old Globe Theatre, 1961; Mrs. Molloy, *The Matchmaker*, the Stepdaughter, *Six Characters in Search of an Author*, Katherine, *The Taming of* the Shrew, Elizabeth Proctor, *The Crucible,* and Dona Lucia, *Charley's Aunt,* all Association of Producing Artists, Fred Miller Theatre, Milwaukee, WI, 1961-62; Madame Ranevsky, *The Cherry Orchard,* University of Kansas, Lawrence, KS, 1963; the Stepdaughter, *Six Characters in Search of an Author,* Martinique Theatre, New York City, 1963; Helena, *A Midsummer Night's Dream,* Hermione, *The Winter's Tale,* and Cleopatra, *Antony and Cleopatra,* all National Shakespeare Festival, Old Globe Theatre, 1963; title role, *Saint Joan at the Stake* (opera), City Center Theatre, New York City, 1963; Elizabeth, *Richard III,* and Beatrice, *Much Ado about Nothing,* both American Shakespeare Festival, 1964; Katherine, *The Taming of the Shrew,* Queen Elizabeth Theatre, Vancouver, BC, Canada, 1964.

Mistress Page, *The Merry Wives of Windsor,* Katherine of Aragon, *Henry VIII,* and Volumnia, *Coriolanus,* all National Shakespeare Festival, Old Globe Theatre, 1965; Elinor Frost, *An Evening's Frost,* Lydia Mendelssohn Theatre, then Theatre De Lys, New York City, both 1965; title role, *White Widow,* Florida State University, Tallahassee, FL, 1966; Athene and Leader of Chorus, *The Oresteia,* Ypsilanti Greek Festival, Ypsilanti, MI, 1966; Lavinia, *Come Slowly, Eden,* Theatre De Lys, 1966; Maria, *Twelfth Night,* Emilia, *Othello,* and Helena, *All's Well That Ends Well,* all National Shakespeare Festival, Old Globe Theatre, 1967; Gertrude Eastman Quevas, *In the Summer House,* Dublin Festival, Dublin, Ireland, 1969; title role, *Mother Courage,* Morehead State University, Morehead, KY, 1969; Renata, *The Increased Difficulty of Concentration,* Forum Theatre, New York City, 1969.

Diane, *Watercolor,* ANTA Theatre, New York City, 1970; Atossa, *The Persians,* St. George's Church, New York City, 1970; title role, *Herodiade,* Little Orchestra Society, Alice Tully Hall, New York City, 1970; Estella, *Sunday Dinner,* American Place Theatre, Theatre at St. Clement's Church, New York City, 1970; Abbess of Argenteuil, *Abelard and Heloise,* Brooks Atkinson Theatre, New York City, 1971; Countess Tolstoy, *Body and Soul,* and Elizabeth Bruce, *Bruce,* both Eugene O'Neill Theatre Center, Waterford, CT, 1971; Bunny, *The House of Blue Leaves,* Truck and Warehouse Theatre, New York City, 1971; Carrie, *The Silent Partner,* Actors Studio, New York City, 1972; Julie English, *And the Old Man Had Two Sons,* and Lena and the Old Woman, *Tales of the Revolution and Other American Fables,* both Eugene O'Neill Theatre Center, 1972; Mother, *A Meeting by the River,* Edison Theatre, New York City, 1972; Marion, *Owners,* Mercer-Shaw Theatre, New York City, 1973; Marion Akers, *Hallelujah!,* Central Arts Theatre, New York City, 1973; Kath, *Entertaining Mr. Sloan,* URGENT, New York City, 1974.

Grace Dunning, *Knuckle,* Playhouse II, New York City, 1975; Jocasta, *Oedipus,* Cathedral of St. John the Divine, New York City, 1977; Agave, *The Bacchae,* Cathedral of St. John the Divine, 1978; Halie, *Buried Child,* Theatre De Lys, 1978; Dorothea Merz, *On Mount Chimborazo,* Brooklyn Academy of Music, Brooklyn, NY, 1979; Betsy Hunt, *The Winter Dancers,* Phoenix Theatre, 1979; Gertrude, *Hamlet,* and Norma, *The Diviners,* both Circle Repertory Theatre, New York City, 1980; Duchess of York, *Richard II,* Entermedia Theatre, New York City, 1982; Mrs. Wire, *Vieux Carre,* WPA Theatre, New York City, 1983; Anna Trumbull, *What I Did Last Summer,* Circle Repertory Theatre, 1983; Rosie, *Full Hookup,* Circle Repertory Theatre, 1984; Amanda Wingfield, *The Glass Menagerie,* Actors Studio, 1985. Also appeared in *Dear Liar,* ANTA Regional Conference, St. Paul, MN, 1967; *Immoral Husband,* Dublin Festival, 1969; *American Roulette,* 1969; *The Plebians Rehearse the Uprising,* Actors Studio, 1969; *Dream of a Blacklisted Actor,* Ensemble Studio, New York City, 1975; *Old Flames,* 1981; *Seascape,* Coconut Grove Playhouse, Miami, FL, 1985; *Seagull,* Thirteenth Street Theatre, New York City, 1986; and in *Home Sweet Home* and *Crack,* both Ohio Theatre, 1988.

MAJOR TOURS—Gelda, *The Dark Is Light Enough,* U.S. cities, 1955; Ursula, *Much Ado about Nothing,* U.S. cities, 1957-58; also *Dear Liar,* U.S. cities, 1967.

PRINCIPAL FILM APPEARANCES—Dr. Immelman, *The Hospital,* United Artists, 1971; publisher, *Werewolf of Washington,* Diplomat, 1973; Naomi, *The Gambler,* Paramount, 1973; Becky, *Looking Up,* Levitt-Pickman, 1977; Dr. Coopersmith, *Last Embrace,* United Artists, 1979; Mrs. Novak, *The Line,* Enterprise, 1980; Milly, *Ghost Story,* Universal, 1981; Aunt Ethel, *Paternity,* Paramount, 1981; Mrs. Paultz, *Love and Money,* Paramount, 1982; Dr. Cooley, *The Entity,* Twentieth Century-Fox, 1982; Margaret Mayo, *Without a Trace,* Twentieth Century-Fox, 1983; Mrs. Connaloe, *Stacking* (also known as *Season of Dreams*), Spectrafilm, 1987.

TELEVISION DEBUT—*Adventure,* NBC, 1955. PRINCIPAL TELEVISION APPEARANCES—Series: Liz Conroy, *Love of Life,* CBS, 1962; Flora Perkins, *A Time for Us,* ABC, 1964; Miss Thompson, *As the World Turns,* CBS, 1970; Ursula Winthrop, *Secret Storm,* CBS, 1972; Nora Adler, *Jack and Mike,* ABC, 1986-87; also *Direction,* CBS, 1968-70; Beatrice Gordon, *Another World,* NBC; *Ryan's Hope,* ABC. Pilots: Frances Hollander, *One of Our Own,* NBC, 1975. Episodic: Title role, "Antigone," *Look Up and Live,* CBS, 1956; Mary Magdalene, *Frontiers of Faith,* CBS, 1958; Athena, "The Oresteia," *Omnibus,* CBS, 1959; second woman, "Medea," *Play of the Week,* NTA, 1959; citizen, "Fall of a City," *Accent,* CBS, 1962; also "Elizabethan Miscellany," *Camera Three,* CBS, 1956; *Lamp Unto My Feet,* CBS, 1958; *You Are There,* CBS, 1971; *Look Up and Live,* CBS, 1971. Movies: Mildred Carston, *A Death in Canaan,* CBS, 1978; Stella Botsford, *Hardhat and Legs,* CBS, 1980; Charlene, *Rodeo Girl,* CBS, 1980; Eugenia Cybulkowski, *Act of Love,* NBC, 1980; Spinner, *Word of Honor,* CBS, 1981; Charlotte Beach, *An Invasion of Privacy,* CBS, 1983; Judge Miriam Roth, *License to Kill,* CBS, 1984; Ma Dunne, *Silent Witness,* NBC, 1985; Professor Hobbs, *Starcrossed,* ABC, 1985; Doris Perlman, *Unholy Matrimony,* CBS, 1988.

RELATED CAREER—Member, Actors Studio, New York City, 1969—; acting teacher, Circle in the Square, New York City, 1973-74.

AWARDS: Fulbright fellow, 1953; Temperly Prize from the Royal Academy of Dramatic Art, 1953; Theatre World Award, 1955, for *The Cretan Woman;* Obie Award from the *Village Voice,* 1963, for *Six Characters in Search of an Author;* Actress of the Year Award from the [Dublin, Ireland] *Times,* 1969, for *In the Summer House;* Downtowner Award, 1981, for *Old Flames.*

MEMBER: Actors' Equity Association, Screen Actors Guild, American Federation of Television and Radio Artists.

SIDELIGHTS: RECREATIONS—Tennis and bridge.

Jacqueline Brookes told *CTFT* that she is a three-time winner of the Broadway Show League Tennis Championship.

ADDRESSES: AGENT—Triad Artists, 10100 Santa Monica Boulevard, 16th Floor, Los Angeles, CA 90067.

BROUGHTON, Bruce 1945-

PERSONAL: Born March 8, 1945, in Los Angeles, CA. EDUCATION: University of Southern California, B.M., 1967.

VOCATION: Composer and music director.

CAREER: Also see *WRITINGS* below. PRINCIPAL FILM WORK—Music director, *The Presidio,* Paramount, 1988.

WRITINGS: All as composer. FILM—*The Ice Pirates,* Metro-Goldwyn-Mayer/United Artists, 1984; *The Prodigal,* World Wide, 1984; *Silverado,* Columbia, 1985; *Young Sherlock Holmes,* Paramount, 1985; *Sweet Liberty,* Universal, 1986; (also lyricist with Stephen Bishop) *The Boy Who Could Fly,* Twentieth Century-Fox, 1986; *Square Dance* (also known as *Home Is Where the Heart Is*), Island, 1987; *Harry and the Hendersons,* Universal, 1987; *The Monster Squad,* Tri-Star, 1987; *Big Shots,* Twentieth Century-Fox, 1987; *Cross My Heart,* Universal, 1987; *The Rescue,* Buena Vista, 1988; *The Presidio,* Paramount, 1988; *Jacknife,* Cineplex Odeon, 1989.

TELEVISION—Series: *Hawaii Five-O,* CBS, 1968-80; *Barnaby Jones,* CBS, 1973-80; *Police Woman,* NBC, 1974-78; *Khan!,* CBS, 1975; *Spencer's Pilots,* CBS, 1976; *Quincy, M.E.,* NBC, 1976-83; *Logan's Run,* CBS, 1977-78; *The Oregon Trail,* NBC, 1977; *How the West Was Won,* ABC, 1977-79; *Dallas,* CBS, 1978—; *The Runaways,* NBC, 1979; *Buck Rogers in the Twenty-Fifth Century,* NBC, 1979-81; *Two Marriages,* ABC, 1983; also *Gunsmoke,* CBS. Mini-Series: *The Blue and the Gray,* CBS, 1983. Pilots: *The Paradise Connection,* CBS, 1979. Movies: *Desperate Voyage,* CBS, 1980; *The Return of Frank Cannon,* CBS, 1980; *Killjoy,* CBS, 1981; *Desperate Lives,* CBS, 1982; *One Shoe Makes It Murder,* CBS, 1982; *M.A.D.D.: Mothers against Drunk Drivers,* NBC, 1983; *Cowboy,* CBS, 1983; *This Girl for Hire,* CBS, 1983; *The Master of Ballantrae,* CBS, 1984; *The Cowboy and the Ballerina,* CBS, 1984; *The First Olympics—Athens 1896,* NBC, 1984; *The Thanksgiving Promise,* ABC, 1986; *George Washington II: The Forging of a Nation,* CBS, 1986.

RELATED CAREER—Music supervisor, CBS television, 1967-77.

AWARDS: Emmy Award, 1981, for *Buck Rogers in the Twenty-Fifth Century;* Emmy Awards, 1983 and 1984, both for *Dallas;* Emmy Award, 1984, for *The First Olympics—Athens 1896;* Emmy Award nominations, Best Music Score, 1982, for *Killjoy* and 1983, for *The Blue and the Gray;* Academy Award nomination, Best Original Score, 1986, for *Silverado.*

MEMBER: Academy of Television Arts and Sciences, Society of Composers and Lyricists, Academy of Motion Picture Arts and Sciences.

ADDRESSES: MANAGER—Milt Kahn, 9229 Sunset Boulevard, Suite 305, Los Angeles, CA 90069.*

*   *   *

BROWN, Bryan 1950-

PERSONAL: Born in 1950 (some sources say 1947) in Sydney, Australia; married Rachel Ward (an actress).

VOCATION: Actor.

CAREER: PRINCIPAL STAGE APPEARANCES—Samson and watch, *Romeo and Juliet,* Old Vic Theatre, London, 1979; also appeared in repertory at the National Theatre Company, London, and with Theatre Australia.

FILM DEBUT—Len, *Love Letters from Teralba Road,* Scala, 1977. PRINCIPAL FILM APPEARANCES—Eric Haywood, *The Irishman,* Greater Union, 1978; Bennett, *Weekend of Shadows,* Roadshow, 1978; Mark, *Third Person Plural,* Abraxas, 1978; Brian Jackson, *Money Movers,* Roadshow, 1978; Nicko, *Cathy's Child,* Roadshow, 1979; Geoff, *Newsfront,* Roadshow, 1979; Rogers, *The Odd Angry Shot,* Roadshow, 1979; Paul Kite, *Palm Beach,* Albie Thoms, 1979; Lieutenant Peter Handcock, *Breaker Morant,* New World, 1980; Kelly, *The Chant of Jimmie Blacksmith,* New Yorker, 1980; China, *Stir,* Hoyts, 1980; Brian Shields, *Blood Money,* Greg Lynch Film Distributors/J.C. Williamson Film Distributors, 1980; Rob, *Winter of Our Dreams,* Enterprises/Satori, 1982; Morgan Keefe, *Far East,* Roadshow/Virgin Vision, 1982; Steve, *Give My Regards to Broad Street,* Twentieth Century-Fox, 1984; Cliff Hardy, *The Empty Beach,* Jethro, 1985; Tiger Kelly, *Rebel,* Vestron, 1985; David Parker, *Parker,* Virgin, 1985; Rollie Tyler, *F/X,* Orion, 1986; Dirk Struan/title role, *Tai-Pan,* De Laurentiis Entertainment Group, 1986; Sonny Hills, *The Good Wife* (also known as *The Umbrella Woman*), Atlantic, 1987; Doug Coughlin, *Cocktail,* Buena Vista, 1988; Bob Campbell, *Gorillas in the Mist,* Universal, 1988.

PRINCIPAL TELEVISION APPEAREANCES—Mini-Series: Michael Connor, *Against the Wind,* syndicated, 1979; John Harmon, ''A Town Like Alice,'' *Masterpiece Theatre,* PBS, 1981; Luke O'Neill, *The Thorn Birds,* ABC, 1983. Movies: Mahbub Ali, *Kim,* CBS, 1984.

ADDRESSES: AGENT—Fred Specktor, Creative Artists Agency, 1888 Century Park E., Suite 1400, Los Angeles, CA 90067.*

*   *   *

BROWN, Georg Stanford 1943-

PERSONAL: Born June 24, 1943, in Havana, Cuba; married Tyne Daly (an actress), June 1966; children: Alisabeth, Kathryne, Alyxandra.

VOCATION: Actor, director, and producer.

CAREER: PRINCIPAL FILM APPEARANCES—Henri Philipot, *The Comedians,* Metro-Goldwyn-Mayer, 1967; Dr. Willard, *Bullitt,* Warner Brothers, 1968; Theon Gibson, *Dayton's Devils,* Cue, 1968; Fisher, *Colossus: The Forbin Project* (also known as *The Forbin Project* and *Colossus*), Universal, 1969; Robert Wheeler, *The Man,* Paramount, 1972; Lynch, *Black Jack* (also known as *Wild in the Sun*), American International, 1973; Rory Schultebrand, *Stir Crazy,* Columbia, 1980.

PRINCIPAL TELEVISION APPEARANCES—Series: Officer Terry Webster, *The Rookies,* ABC, 1972-76. Mini-Series: Tom Harvey, *Roots,* ABC, 1977; Tom Harvey, *Roots: The Next Generation,* ABC, 1979; Grady, *North and South,* ABC, 1985. Pilots: Officer Terry Webster, *The Rookies,* ABC, 1972; Police Chief Otis Pittman, *The City,* ABC, 1986; also *The Young Lawyers,* ABC, 1969.

Episodic: *Police Squad!*, ABC, 1982. Movies: Larry Richmond, *Ritual of Evil*, NBC, 1970; Donald Umber, *Dawn: Portrait of a Teenage Runaway*, NBC, 1976; Charles Neville, *The Night the City Screamed*, ABC, 1980; Rudy Desautel, *The Kid with the Broken Halo*, NBC, 1982; Ben Humphries, *In Defense of Kings*, CBS, 1983; Lew Gilbert, *The Jesse Owens Story*, syndicated, 1984; Sergeant Clevon Jackson, *Alone in the Neon Jungle* (also known as *Neon Jungle* and *Command in Hell*), CBS, 1988. Specials: *Variety '77—The Year in Entertainment*, CBS, 1978.

PRINCIPAL TELEVISION WORK—All as director, unless indicated. Mini-Series: *Roots: The Next Generation*, ABC, 1979; executive producer, *Vietnam War Story*, HBO, 1987. Episodic: *The Rookies*, ABC, 1972-76; *Starsky and Hutch*, ABC, 1975-79; *Family*, ABC, 1976-80; *Charlie's Angels*, ABC, 1976-81; *The Fitzpatricks*, CBS, 1977-78; *Lucan*, ABC, 1977-78; *Lou Grant*, CBS, 1977-82; *The Lazarus Syndrome*, ABC, 1979; *Paris*, CBS, 1979-80; *Tenspeed and Brown Shoe*, ABC, 1980; *Palmerstown, U.S.A.*, CBS, 1980-81; *The Fall Guy*, ABC, 1981; *The Greatest American Hero*, ABC, 1981-83; *Hill Street Blues*, NBC, 1981-87; *Dynasty*, ABC, 1981-89; *Police Squad!*, ABC, 1982; *Fame*, NBC, 1982-83, then syndicated, 1983-87; *Trauma Center*, ABC, 1983; *Finder of Lost Loves*, ABC, 1984; *Call to Glory*, ABC, 1984-85; *Miami Vice*, NBC, 1984—; *Cagney and Lacey*, CBS, 1986. Movies: *Grambling's White Tiger*, NBC, 1981; *Miracle of the Heart: A Boystown Story*, syndicated, 1986; (also executive producer) *Kids Like These*, CBS, 1987; *Alone in the Neon Jungle* (also known as *Neon Jungle* and *Command in Hell*), CBS, 1988.

AWARDS: Emmy Award, Best Directing for a Drama Series, 1986, for *Cagney and Lacey;* Emmy Award nomination, Best Directing for a Drama Series, for *Hill Street Blues.*

MEMBER: Actors' Equity Association, Screen Actors Guild, Directors Guild of America, American Federation of Television and Radio Artists.

ADDRESSES: MANAGER—Jules Sharr, Sharr Enterprises, P.O. Box 69453, Los Angeles, CA 90069-0153.*

*   *   *

BRYCELAND, Yvonne

PERSONAL: Born Yvonne Heilbuth, November 18, in Cape Town, South Africa; daughter of Adolphus Walter and Clara Ethel (Sanderson) Heilbuth; married Daniel Bryceland (divorced); married Brian Astbury.

VOCATION: Actress.

CAREER: STAGE DEBUT—Movie actress, *Stage Door*, Rondebosch Theatre, Cape Town, South Africa, 1947. LONDON DEBUT—Lena, *Boesman and Lena*, Theatre Upstairs, 1971. PRINCIPAL STAGE APPEARANCES—Madame Desmortes, *Ring round the Moon*, Cape Town Performing Arts Board, Cape Town, South Africa, 1964; Georgie, *Winter Journey*, Cape Town Performing Arts Board, 1966; Miss Madrigal, *The Chalk Garden*, Cape Town Performing Arts Board, 1968; Madame Ranevskaya, *The Cherry Orchard*, Cape Town Performing Arts Board, 1970; Frieda, *Statements after an Arrest under the Immorality Act*, Space Theatre, Cape Town, 1972; Mary Tyrone, *Long Day's Journey into Night*, Space Theatre, 1973; Amanda Wingfield, *The Glass Menagerie*,

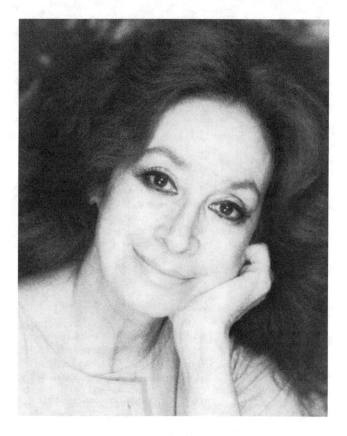

YVONNE BRYCELAND

Space Theatre, 1974; Frieda, *Statements after an Arrest under the Immorality Act*, Royal Court Theatre, London, 1974 and 1975; Sophia, *Dimetos*, Edinburgh Festival, Edinburgh, Scotland, 1975, then Comedy Theatre, London, 1976; Bananas, *The House of Blue Leaves*, Anne, *Ashes*, and title role, *The Bitter Tears of Petra von Kant*, all Space Theatre, 1976; title role, *Mother Courage and Her Children*, and title role, *Medea*, both Space Theatre, 1977; Hester, *Hello and Goodbye*, Riverside Studios, London, 1978; Witch, *Macbeth*, and Hecuba, *The Woman*, both National Theatre Company, Olivier Theatre, London, 1978; Queen Margaret, *Richard III*, and Gina Ekdal, *The Wild Duck*, both National Theatre Company, Olivier Theatre, 1979; Miss Helen, *The Road to Mecca*, Promenade Theatre, New York City, 1988. Also appeared as Millie, *People Are Living There*, Lena, *Boesman and Lena*, and Clytemnestra and Iris, *Orestes*, all in South Africa, 1971; and as Emilia, *Othello*, National Theatre Company, 1980.

MAJOR TOURS—Frieda, *Statements after an Arrest under the Immorality Act*, European cities, 1974.

PRINCIPAL FILM APPEARANCES—Bertha, *A World Apart*, Atlantic Releasing, 1988. Also appeared as Lena, *Boesman and Lena*, 1972; and in *Stealing Heaven*, FilmDallas, 1988.

PRINCIPAL TELEVISION APPEARANCES—Episodic: Darlene, *The Equalizer*, CBS, 1988. Plays: Millie, *People Are Living There;* Hester, *Hello and Goodbye.*

RELATED CAREER—Founder (with Brian Astbury), Space Theatre, Cape Town, South Africa, 1972.

NON-RELATED CAREER—Newspaper librarian.

AWARDS: Obie Award from the *Village Voice,* 1988, for *The Road to Mecca.*

SIDELIGHTS: FAVORITE ROLES—Millie in *People Are Living There,* Lena in *Boesman and Lena,* Hester in *Hello and Goodbye,* and Clytemnestra and Iris in *Orestes.*

ADDRESSES: AGENT—Ronnie Waters, International Creative Management, 388 Oxford Street, London W1, England.*

*   *   *

BULLINS, Ed 1935-
(Kingsley B. Bass, Jr.)

PERSONAL: Born July 2, 1935, in Philadelphia, PA; son of Edward and Bertha Marie (Queen) Bullins; wife's name, Trixie. EDUCATION: Attended Los Angeles City College, 1961-63, and San Francisco State College (now known as San Francisco State University). MILITARY: U.S. Navy, 1952-55.

VOCATION: Playwright and producer.

CAREER: See *WRITINGS* below. RELATED CAREER—Writer in residence, New Lafayette Theatre, New York City, 1968-73, and associate director, 1971-73; producing director, Surviving Theatre, New York City, 1974; writers unit coordinator, New York Shakespeare Festival, New York City, 1975-82; public relations director, Berkeley Black Repertory, Berkeley, CA, 1982; promotion director, Magic Theatre, San Francisco, CA, 1982-83; group sales coordinator, Julian Theatre, San Francisco, 1983; also co-founder, Black Arts West; co-founder, Black Arts Alliance; playwright in residence, American Place Theatre, New York City; editor, *Black Theatre* (magazine); writing and English instructor: Fordham University, Columbia University, University of Massachusetts, Bronx Community College, Manhattan Community College, People's School of Dramatic Arts (San Francisco), City College of San Francisco, Antioch University, Sonoma State University, and Bay Area Playwrights Festival; lecturer: Dartmouth College, Talladega College, Clark College, Amherst College, and University of California, Berkeley.

NON-RELATED CAREER—Co-founder, Black House (Black Panther Party headquarters), San Francisco, CA; cultural director, then Minister of Culture of the Party, Black Panther Party.

WRITINGS: STAGE—*How Do You Do?,* Firehouse Repertory Theatre, San Francisco, CA, 1965, then La Mama Experimental Theatre Club (E.T.C.), New York City, 1972, published by Illuminations Press, 1967; *Clara's Ole Man,* Firehouse Repertory Theatre, 1965, then on a bill as *The Electronic Nigger and Others,* American Place Theatre, New York City, 1968, published in *Five Plays by Ed Bullins,* Bobbs-Merrill, 1969; *The Rally, or Dialect Determinism,* Firehouse Repertory Theatre, 1965, then La Mama E.T.C., 1972, published in *The Theme Is Blackness and Other Plays,* Morrow, 1972; *It Has No Choice* and *A Minor Scene,* both Black Arts/West Repertory Theatre/School, San Francisco, CA, 1966, then La Mama E.T.C., 1972, both published in *The Theme Is*

Blackness and Other Plays; (with Shirley Tarbell) *The Game of Adam and Eve,* Playwrights Theatre, Los Angeles, CA, 1966; *The Theme Is Blackness,* San Francisco State College, San Francisco, CA, 1966, published in *The Theme Is Blackness and Other Plays.*

The Electronic Nigger, on a bill as *The Electronic Nigger and Others,* American Place Theatre, then Ambiance Lunch Hour Theatre, London, both 1968, published in *Five Plays by Ed Bullins; A Son Come Home,* on a bill as *The Electronic Nigger and Others,* American Place Theatre, 1968, published in *Negro Digest,* April, 1968, then in *Five Plays by Ed Bullins; Goin' a Buffalo,* American Place Theatre, 1968, published in *Five Plays by Ed Bullins; In the Wine Time,* New Lafayette Theatre, New York City, 1968, published in *Five Plays by Ed Bullins; The Corner,* Theatre Company of Boston, Boston, MA, 1969, then Public Theatre, New York City, 1972, published in *The Theme Is Blackness and Other Plays; The Man Who Dug Fish,* Theatre Company of Boston, 1969, published in *The Theme Is Blackness and Other Plays;* (as Kingsley B. Bass, Jr.) *We Righteous Bombers* (adapted from *The Just Assassins* by Albert Camus), New Lafayette Theatre, 1969; *The Gentleman Caller* on a bill as *A Black Quartet,* Chelsea Theatre Center, Brooklyn Academy of Music, Brooklyn, NY, 1969, published in *A Black Quartet,* New American Library, 1970.

The Duplex, New Lafayette Theatre, 1970, then Forum Theatre, Lincoln Center, New York City, 1972, published by Morrow, 1971; *A Ritual to Raise the Dead and Foretell the Future* and *The Devil Catchers,* both New Lafayette Theatre, 1970; *The Pig Pen* and *Night of the Beast,* both American Place Theatre, 1970, both published in *Four Dynamite Plays,* Morrow, 1973; *The Helper,* New Dramatists Workshop, New York City, 1970, published in *The Theme Is Blackness and Other Plays; It Bees Dat Way,* Ambiance Lunch Hour Theatre, then ICA Theatre, New York City, both 1970, published in *Four Dynamite Plays; Death List,* Theatre Black, New York City, 1970, published in *Four Dynamite Plays; Street Sounds,* La Mama E.T.C., 1970, published in *The Theme Is Blackness and Other Plays; In New England Winter,* New Federal Theatre, Henry Street Playhouse, New York City, 1971, published in *New Plays from the Black Theatre,* Bantam, 1969; *The Fabulous Miss Marie,* New Lafayette Theatre, 1971, then Mitzie E. Newhouse Theatre, New York City, 1979; *Next Time,* on a bill as *City Stops,* Bronx Community College, Bronx, NY, 1972; *Ya Gonna Let Me Take You Out Tonight, Baby?,* New York Shakespeare Festival, Public Theatre, 1972, published in *Black Arts,* Black Arts Publishing, 1969.

The Psychic Pretenders (A Black Magic Show), New Lafayette Theatre, 1972; (book and lyrics for musical) *House Party, a Soul Happening,* American Place Theatre, 1973; *The Taking of Miss Janie,* New Federal Theatre, Henry Street Playhouse, 1975, published in *Famous American Plays of the 1970s,* Dell, 1981; *The Mystery of Phyllis Wheatley,* New Federal Theatre, Henry Street Playhouse, 1976; *I Am Lucy Terry,* American Place Theatre, 1976; (book and lyrics for musical) *Home Boy,* Perry Street Theatre, New York City, 1976; *Jo Anne!,* Theatre Riverside Church, New York City, 1976; (book for musical) *Storyville,* Mandeville Theatre, University of California, La Jolla, CA, 1977; *DADDY!,* New Federal Theatre, Henry Street Playhouse, 1977; (book for musical) *Sepia Star,* Stage 73, New York City, 1977; *Michael,* New Heritage Repertory Theatre, New York City, 1978; *C'mon Back to Heavenly House,* Amherst College Theatre, Amherst, MA, 1978; *Leavings,* Syncopation, New York City, 1980; *Steve and Velma,* New African Company, Boston, 1980. Also *Black Commercial #2, The American Flag Ritual, State Office Bldg. Curse, One Minute Commercial, A Street Play, A Short Play for a Small*

Theatre, and *The Play of the Play,* all published in *The Theme Is Blackness; Malcolm '71, or Publishing Blackness,* published in *Black Scholar,* June, 1975.

OTHER—(Editor and contributor) *New Plays from the Black Theatre* (anthology), Bantam, 1969; *The Hungered One* (short stories), Morrow, 1971; *The Reluctant Rapist* (novel), Harper & Row, 1973; (editor) *The New Lafayette Theatre Presents the Complete Plays and Aesthetic Comments by Six Black Playwrights* (anthology), Doubleday-Anchor, 1973.

AWARDS: Vernon Rice Award, 1968, for *The Electronic Nigger and Others;* Obie Award from the *Village Voice,* Distinguished Playwrighting, and Black Arts Alliance Award, both 1971, for *In New England Winter* and *The Fabulous Miss Marie;* New York Drama Critics Circle Award and Obie Award, Distinguished Playwriting, both 1975, for *The Taking of Miss Janie;* also American Place Theatre grant, 1967; Rockefeller Foundation grants for playwriting, 1968, 1970, and 1973; Black Arts Alliance Award, 1971; Guggenheim Fellowship grants, 1971 and 1976; Creative Artists Program Service grant, 1973; and National Endowment for the Arts grant. Honorary degrees: Columbia College (Chicago), L.L.D., 1976.

MEMBER: Dramatists Guild, P.E.N.

ADDRESSES: HOME—2128-A Fifth Street, Berkeley, CA 94710. AGENT—Helen Merrill, 435 W. 23rd Street, Apartment 1-A, New York, NY 10011.*

*   *   *

BURKE, Delta   1956-

PERSONAL: Full name, Delta Ramona Leah Burke; born July 30, 1956, in Orlando, FL; daughter of Jean and Frederick Burke. EDUCATION: Attended the London Academy of Music and Dramatic Arts.

VOCATION: Actress.

CAREER: PRINCIPAL TELEVISION APPEARANCES—Series: Bonnie Sue Chisholm, *The Chisholms,* CBS, 1980; Kathleen Beck, *Filthy Rich,* CBS, 1982-83; Diane Barrow, *1st and Ten,* HBO, 1985-87; Suzanne Sugarbaker, *Designing Women,* CBS, 1986—. Pilots: Angela Spinelli, *The Home Front,* CBS, 1980; Laura De Vega, *Rooster,* ABC, 1982; Paula Corey, *Mickey Spillane's Mike Hammer: Murder Me, Murder You,* CBS, 1983; Joanne Kruger, *Johnny Blue,* CBS, 1983; Diane Barrow, *1st and Ten,* HBO, 1984. Episodic: Diane Barrow, *Training Camp: The Bulls Are Back,* HBO, 1986; Linda Stone, *Mickey Spillane's Mike Hammer,* CBS, 1986; Sherry Keegan, *Hotel,* ABC, 1986; Kristy Keaton, *Simon and Simon,* CBS, 1987; also *Hollywood Squares,* syndicated, 1987. Movies: Terri, *Zuma Beach,* NBC, 1978; Elizabeth Fletcher, *The Seekers,* syndicated, 1979; Stella Farrell, *Charleston,* NBC, 1979; Carol, *A Last Cry for Help,* ABC, 1979; Margie, *A Bunny's Tale,* ABC, 1985; Germany, *Where the Hell's That Gold?!!?* CBS, 1988. Specials: *Battle of the Network Stars,* ABC, 1982; *Circus of the Stars,* CBS, 1987.

ADDRESSES: AGENT—Karg/Weissenbach, 329 N. Wetherly, Suite 101, Beverly Hills, CA 90211. PUBLICIST—Phil Paladino,

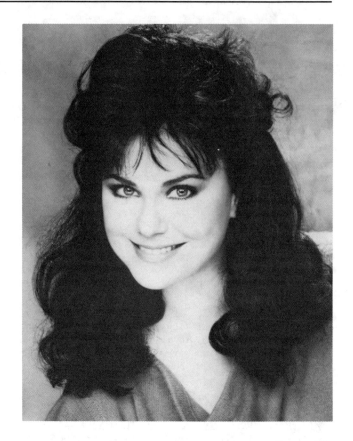

DELTA BURKE

Paladino and Associates, 9200 Sunset Boulevard, Los Angeles, CA 90069.

*   *   *

BURTON, Levar   1957-

PERSONAL: Full name, Levardis Robert Martyn Burton, Jr.; born February 16, 1957, in Landstuhl, Germany; son of Levardis Robert (a photographer in the U.S. Army Signal Corps) and Erma (an educator, social worker, and administrator; maiden name, Christian) Burton. EDUCATION: Attended the University of Southern California.

VOCATION: Actor.

CAREER: PRINCIPAL FILM APPEARANCES—Cap Jackson, *Looking for Mr. Goodbar,* Paramount, 1977; Tommy Price, *The Hunter,* Paramount, 1980; Private Michael Osgood, *The Supernaturals,* Republic Entertainment International, 1987.

TELEVISION DEBUT—Kunte Kinte, *Roots,* ABC, 1977. PRINCIPAL TELEVISION APPEARANCES—Series: Host, *Reading Rainbow,* PBS, 1983—; Lieutenant Geordi La Forge, *Star Trek: The Next Generation,* syndicated, 1987-88. Episodic: Dave Robinson, *Murder, She Wrote,* CBS, 1987; Evans, *Houston Knights,* CBS, 1987. Movies: Billy Peoples, *Billy: Portrait of a Street Kid,* CBS, 1977; Andrew Sinclair, *Battered,* NBC, 1978; title role, *One in a Million: The Ron LeFlore Story,* CBS, 1978; Donald Lang, *Dum-*

my, CBS, 1979; Richard Jefferson, *Guyana Tragedy: The Story of Jim Jones*, CBS, 1980; Charles "Tank" Smith, *Grambling's White Tiger*, NBC, 1981; Rodney, *The Acorn People*, NBC, 1981; Ray Walden, *Emergency Room*, syndicated, 1983; Professor Slade Preston, *The Jesse Owens Story*, syndicated, 1984; Vinnie Davis, *The Midnight Hour*, ABC, 1985; Ben Sumner, *A Special Friendship*, CBS, 1987; Kunte Kinte, *A Roots Christmas: Kunte Kinte's Gift*, ABC, 1988. Specials: *Battle of the Network Stars*, ABC, 1976 and 1977; *The Paul Lynde Comedy Hour*, ABC, 1977; *Celebrity Challenge of the Sexes*, CBS, 1977 and 1979; *Celebrity Football Classic*, NBC, 1979; *I Love Liberty*, ABC, 1982.

AWARDS: Emmy Award nomination, Best Actor, 1977, for *Roots*.

ADDRESSES: MANAGER—Delores Robinson Management, 7319 Beverly Boulevard, Los Angeles, CA 90036.*

*   *   *

BUTKUS, Dick   1942-

PERSONAL: Born December 9, 1942, in Chicago, IL; wife's name, Helen; children: Nicole, Richard, Matthew. EDUCATION: Attended the University of Illinois.

VOCATION: Actor.

CAREER: PRINCIPAL FILM APPEARANCES—Rob Cargil, *Gus*, Buena Vista, 1976; Rodeo, *Mother, Jugs, and Speed*, Twentieth Century-Fox, 1976; Joe, *Who Fell Asleep?*, Twentieth Century-Fox, 1979; Arthur, *Johnny Dangerously*, Twentieth Century-Fox, 1984; Drootin, *Hamburger . . . The Motion Picture*, Entertainment Inc., 1986. Also appeared in *Smorgasbord* (also known as *Cracking Up*), Warner Brothers, 1983.

PRINCIPAL TELEVISION APPEARANCES—Series: Sports analyst, *NFL Today*, CBS, 1988—. Mini-Series: Al Fanducci, *Rich Man, Poor Man*, ABC, 1976. Pilots: Heavy, *A Matter of Wife . . . and Death*, NBC, 1976; Officer Alvin Dimsky, *Cass Mallot*, CBS, 1982; Dick Kowalski, *Time Out for Dad*, NBC, 1987. Episodic: Richard "Ski," Butowski, *Blue Thunder*, ABC, 1984; Kurt, *Half Nelson*, ABC, 1985; Ruston, *Blacke's Magic*, NBC, 1986; Stanley, *Night Court*, NBC, 1986; also in "The Apartment," *Taxi*, ABC, 1979; *Growing Pains*, ABC, 1987. Movies: As himself, *Brian's Song*, ABC, 1971; Hennerson, *Superdome*, ABC, 1978; Brom Bones, *The Legend of Sleepy Hollow*, NBC, 1980; Tom Wilcox, *The Stepford Children*, NBC, 1987; Smilin' Ed Konner, *Crash Course*, NBC, 1988. Specials: *Dynamic Duos*, NBC, 1978; Tank McNamara, *Sunday Funnies*, NBC, 1983; *The Dean Martin Celebrity Roast*, NBC, 1984; *Rodney Dangerfield: Exposed*, ABC, 1985; commissioner, *Star Games*, syndicated, 1985.

PRINCIPAL RADIO APPEARANCES—Sports commentator, WGN-Radio, Chicago, IL, 1986—.

RELATED CAREER—Actor in television commercials.

NON-RELATED CAREER—Professional football player with the Chicago Bears, 1965-73.

AWARDS: Elected to the Professional Football Hall of Fame, Canton, OH, 1979.

ADDRESSES: AGENT—Mark Teitelbaum, William Morris Agency, 151 El Camino Drive, Beverly Hills, CA 90212.*

*   *   *

BYNER, John

VOCATION: Actor and comedian.

CAREER: PRINCIPAL FILM APPEARANCES—Head, *What's Up Doc?*, Warner Brothers, 1972; disc jockey, *The Great Smokey Roadblock* (also known as *The Last of the Cowboys*), Dimension, 1978; Doc Seegle, *Stroker Ace*, Universal/Warner Brothers, 1983; voices of Gurgli and Dolil, *The Black Cauldron*, Buena Vista, 1985; Radu, *Transylvania 6-5000*, New World, 1985. Also appeared in *A Pleasure Doing Business*, 1979.

PRINCIPAL TELEVISION APPEARANCES—Series: Regular, *The Garry Moore Show*, CBS, 1966-67; regular, *The Steve Allen Comedy Hour*, CBS, 1967; regular, *The Kraft Music Hall*, NBC, 1968; co-host, *Something Else*, syndicated, 1970; host, *The John Byner Comedy Hour*, CBS, 1972; Dr. Roland Caine, *The Practice*, NBC, 1976-77; Detective George Donahue, *Soap*, ABC, 1978-80; host, *The Best of Sullivan*, syndicated, 1980-82; host, *Bizarre*, Showtime, 1980; host, *Relatively Speaking*, syndicated, 1988—; also voice characterization, "The Ant and the Aardvark," *The Pink Panther Show* (animated), NBC. Pilots: Freddy, *Singles*, CBS, 1972; Dr. David Froelich, *The Nancy Dussault Show*, CBS, 1973; Johnny McNamara, *McNamara's Band* (two episodes), ABC, 1977; Jack Sheehy, *Sheehy and the Supreme Machine*, ABC, 1977; also voice characterization, *Aesop's Fables*, 1971. Episodic: *The Peter Marshall Variety Show*, syndicated, 1976; *ABC Monday Night Comedy Special*, ABC, 1977; Arthur Burkley, *The Love Boat*, ABC, 1986; *Evening at the Improv*, Arts and Entertainment, 1988; also Bert, *The Odd Couple*, ABC; *The Bobby Vinton Show*, syndicated. Movies: Elevator man, *A Guide for the Married Woman*, ABC, 1978; Donald Lumis, *Three on a Date*, ABC, 1978; Stan Summerville, *The Man in the Santa Claus Suit*, NBC, 1979; Hatch, *Murder Can Hurt You!*, ABC, 1980; voice of Richard Nixon, *Will: G. Gordon Liddy*, NBC, 1982. Specials: *A Last Laugh at the Sixties*, ABC, 1970; *Bing Crosby's Sun Valley Christmas Show*, NBC, 1973; *The Captain and Tennille in New Orleans*, ABC, 1978; *Pat Boone and Family Easter Special*, ABC, 1979; *Life's Most Embarrassing Moments*, ABC, 1984 and 1985; *World's Funniest Commercial Goofs*, ABC, 1985; voice of man with the dog, "The Mouse and the Motorcycle" (animated), *ABC Weekend Special*, ABC, 1986; host, *A Whole Lotta Fun*, NBC, 1988; *Circus of the Stars*, CBS, 1988.

RELATED CAREER—As a stand-up comedian, has appeared in nightclubs and colleges throughout the United States.

WRITINGS: TELEVISION—Series: *The John Byner Comedy Hour*, CBS, 1972; *Bizarre*, Showtime, 1980.

ADDRESSES: OFFICE—5863 Ramirez Canyon Road, Malibu, CA 90265.*

C

CAAN, James 1940-

PERSONAL: Born March 26, 1940 (some sources say 1939), in Bronx, NY; son of Arthur (a meat dealer) and Sophie Caan; married DeeJay Mathis, 1961 (divorced, 1966); married Sheila Ryan, 1976; children: Tara (first marriage), Scott Andrew (second marriage). EDUCATION: Attended Michigan State University and Hofstra University; trained for the stage at the Neighborhood Playhouse and with Wynn Handman.

VOCATION: Actor.

CAREER: OFF-BROADWAY DEBUT—(As Jimmy Caan) The Soldier, *La Ronde,* Theatre Marquee, 1960. BROADWAY DEBUT—*Blood, Sweat, and Stanley Poole,* Morosco Theatre, 1961. PRINCIPAL STAGE APPEARANCES—*Mandingo,* Lyceum Theatre, New York City, 1961.

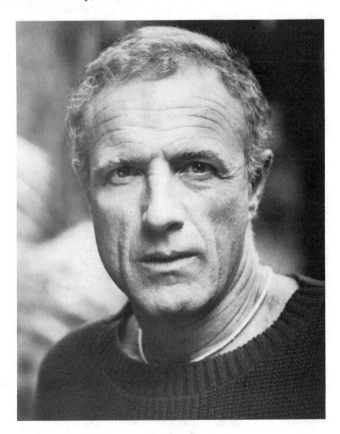

JAMES CAAN

FILM DEBUT—*Irma La Douce,* United Artists, 1963. PRINCIPAL FILM APPEARANCES—Randall, *Lady in a Cage,* Paramount, 1964; Mike Marsh, *Red Line 7000,* Paramount, 1965; Dugan, *The Glory Guys,* United Artists, 1965; Paul, *Games,* Universal, 1967; Alan "Mississippi" Bourdillon, *El Dorado,* Paramount, 1967; Buck Burnett, *Journey to Shiloh,* Universal, 1968; Lee, *Countdown,* Warner Brothers, 1968; Jimmie "Killer" Kilgannon, *The Rain People,* Warner Brothers, 1969; Lieutenant Commander Bolton, *Submarine X-1,* United Artists, 1969.

Rabbit Angstrom, *Rabbit, Run,* Warner Brothers, 1970; Larry Moore, *T.R. Baskin* (also known as *A Date with a Lonely Girl*), Paramount, 1971; Sonny Corleone, *The Godfather,* Paramount, 1972; Dick Kanipsia, *Slither,* Metro-Goldwyn-Mayer, 1973; Sonny Corleone, *The Godfather, Part II,* Paramount, 1974; Alex Freed, *The Gambler,* Paramount, 1974; Freebie, *Freebie and the Bean,* Warner Brothers, 1974; John Baggs, Jr., *Cinderella Liberty,* Twentieth Century-Fox, 1975; Jonathan E., *Rollerball,* United Artists, 1975; Mike Locken, *The Killer Elite,* United Artists, 1975; Billy Rose, *Funny Lady,* Columbia, 1975; as himself, *Silent Movie,* Twentieth Century-Fox, 1976; Harry Dighby, *Harry and Walter Go to New York,* Columbia, 1976; David Williams, *Un Autre homme, une autre chance* (also known as *Another Man, Another Chance*), United Artists, 1977; Sergeant Dohun, *A Bridge Too Far,* United Artists, 1977; Jud McGraw, *Little Moon and Jud McGraw,* Prism Entertainment, 1978; Frank Athearn, *Comes a Horseman,* United Artists, 1978; George Schneider, *Chapter Two,* Columbia, 1979.

Thomas Hacklin, Jr. *Hide in Plain Sight,* Metro-Goldwyn-Mayer-United Artists (MGM/UA), 1980; Frank, *Thief* (also known as *Violent Streets*) United Artists, 1981; Glen, Sr. and Glen, Jr., *Les Uns et les autres* (also known as *Bolero*), Double 13, 1982; Jolly Villano, *Kiss Me Goodbye,* Twentieth Century-Fox, 1982; Clell Hazard, *Gardens of Stone,* Tri-Star, 1988; Matthew Sykes, *Alien Nation,* Twentieth Century-Fox, 1988. Also appeared in *Gone with the West* (also known as *Man without Mercy*), 1976.

PRINCIPAL FILM WORK—Director, *Hide in Plain Sight,* Metro-Goldwyn-Mayer/United Artists, 1980.

PRINCIPAL TELEVISION APPEARANCES—Movies: Brian Piccolo, *Brian's Song,* ABC, 1972. Episodic: *Naked City,* ABC; *Route 66,* CBS; *Ben Casey,* ABC; *Combat,* ABC; *The Untouchables,* ABC; also *Alfred Hitchcock Presents* and *Wagon Train.* Specials: *Rickles,* CBS, 1975; *Superstunt,* NBC, 1977; *Celebration: The American Spirit,* ABC, 1976; *Playboy's Twenty-Fifth Anniversary Celebration,* ABC, 1979.

AWARDS: Emmy Award nomination, 1972, for *Brian's Song;*

Academy Award nomination, Best Supporting Actor, 1972, for *The Godfather*.

ADDRESSES: AGENT—Triad Artists, 10100 Santa Monica Boulevard, 16th Floor, Los Angeles, CA 90067. PUBLICIST—Rogers and Cowan, Inc., 10000 Santa Monica Boulevard, Los Angeles, CA 90067-7007.

* * *

CAMP, Joe 1939-

PERSONAL: Full name, Joseph Shelton Camp, Jr.; born April 20, 1939, in St. Louis, MO; son of Joseph Shelton and Ruth Wilhelmena (McLaulin) Camp; married Andrea Carolyn Hopkins, August 7, 1960; children: Joseph Shelton III, Brandon Andrew. EDUCATION: University of Mississippi, B.B.A., 1961.

VOCATION: Director, producer, and screenwriter.

CAREER: Also see *WRITINGS* below. PRINCIPAL FILM APPEARANCES—Voice of television director, *Benji the Hunted*, Buena Vista, 1987. PRINCIPAL FILM WORK—Director: (Also producer) *Benji*, Mulberry Square Productions, 1973; (also producer) *Hawmps!*, Mulberry Square Productions, 1976; (also producer) *For the Love of Benji*, Mulberry Square Productions, 1977; (also producer) *The Double McGuffin*, Mulberry Square Productions, 1979; (also producer) *Oh, Heavenly Dog*, Twentieth Century-Fox, 1980; *Benji the Hunted*, Buena Vista, 1987.

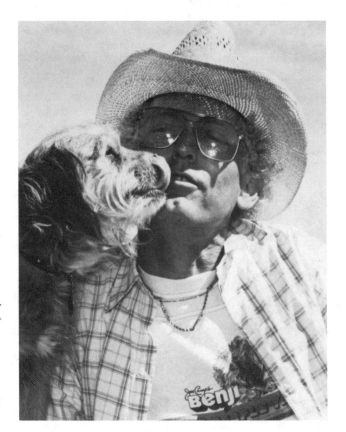

JOE CAMP

PRINCIPAL TELEVISION WORK—Series: Director, *Benji, Zax, and the Alien Prince*, CBS, 1983-84. Specials: Executive producer, *The Phenomenon of Benji*, NBC, 1978; also producer and director, *Benji's Very Own Christmas Story*, 1978; executive producer, *Benji at Work*, 1980; director, *Benji (Takes a Dive) at Marineland*, 1981.

RELATED CAREER—Director of television commercials, Jamieson Film Company, Dallas, TX, 1969-71; founder and president, Mulberry Square Productions, Inc., Dallas, TX, 1971—.

NON-RELATED CAREER—Junior account executive, McCann-Erickson, Houston, TX, 1961-62; account executive, Norsworthy-Mercer, Dallas, TX, 1964-69; owner, Joe Camp Real Estate, Houston, TX, 1962-64.

WRITINGS: See production details above. FILM—*Benji*, 1973; co-writer, *Hawmps!*, 1976; *For the Love of Benji*, 1977; *The Double McGuffin*, 1979; *Oh, Heavenly Dog*, 1980; *Benji the Hunted*, 1987. TELEVISION—*The Phenomenon of Benji*, 1978; *Benji's Very Own Christmas Story*, 1978; *Benji at Cannes*, 1980; *Benji at Work*, 1980; *Benji (Takes a Dive) at Marineland*, 1981.

AWARDS: Recipient of two Emmy Award nominations.

MEMBER: Directors Guild of America, Writers Guild of America, Academy of Television Arts and Sciences, American Society of Composers, Authors, and Publishers.

ADDRESSES: OFFICE—Mulberry Square Productions, Inc., 8140 Walnut Hill Lane, Suite 301, Dallas, TX 75231.

* * *

CANNELL, Stephen J. 1941-

PERSONAL: Full name, Stephen Joseph Cannell; born February 5, 1941, in Los Angeles, CA; son of Joseph Knapp and Carolyn (Baker) Cannell; married Marcia C. Finch, August 8, 1964; children: Derek (deceased), Tawnia, Chelsea, Cody. EDUCATION: University of Oregon, B.A., 1964. RELIGION: Episcopalian.

VOCATION: Television producer, director, and writer.

CAREER: PRINCIPAL TELEVISION APPEARANCES—Pilots: Host, *On Top All Over the World*, syndicated, 1983; Rosco Tanner, *Charley Hannah*, ABC, 1986. Specials: *Today at Night, Volume II*, NBC, 1986.

PRINCIPAL TELEVISION WORK—Series: Creator and associate producer, *Chase*, NBC, 1973; producer (with Jo Swerling, Jr.), *Toma*, ABC, 1973-74; creator (with Roy Huggins), executive producer (with Meta Rosenberg), and supervising producer, *The Rockford Files*, NBC, 1974-80; creator and executive producer, *Baa-Baa Blacksheep*, NBC, 1976-77, renamed *The Black Sheep Squadron*, NBC, 1977-78; creator (with Steven Bochco) and executive producer (with Bochco), *Richie Brockelman, Private Eye*, NBC, 1978; executive producer, *The Duke*, NBC, 1979; executive producer, *Tenspeed and Brownshoe*, ABC, 1980; executive producer (with Donald P. Bellisario), *Stone*, ABC, 1980; executive producer (with Juanita Bartlett), *The Greatest American Hero*, ABC, 1981-83; executive producer, *The Quest*, ABC, 1982; executive producer, *The Rousters*, NBC, 1983-84; executive producer (with Patrick Harsburgh), *Hardcastle and McCormick*, ABC, 1983-86; executive producer (with Frank Lupo), *The A-Team*, NBC, 1983-87; executive producer (with Swerling and Lupo), *Riptide*, NBC, 1984-86; executive producer, *Hunter*, NBC, 1984—; executive producer (with Lupo), *The Last Precinct*, NBC, 1986; creator and executive producer (with Lawrence Hertzog), *Stingray*, NBC, 1986-87; creator and executive producer (with Hertzog and Babs Greyhosky), *J.J. Starbuck*, NBC, 1987-88; creator and executive producer (with Hasburgh and Steven Beers), *21 Jump Street*, Fox, 1987—; creator and executive producer (with Lupo), *Wiseguy*, CBS, 1987—; creator and executive producer, *Sonny Spoon*, NBC, 1988.

Pilots: Producer, *The Rockford Files*, NBC, 1974; executive producer (with Bochco), *Richie Brockelman: Missing 24 Hours*, NBC, 1976; executive producer (with Rosenberg), *Scott Free*, NBC, 1976; executive producer, *Dr. Scorpion*, ABC, 1978; executive producer, *The Gypsy Warriors*, CBS, 1978; executive producer, *Stone*, ABC, 1979; executive producer (with Alex Beaton), *The Night Rider*, ABC, 1979; executive producer, *Boston and Kilbride*, CBS, 1979; executive producer (with Glen A. Larson), *Nightside*, ABC, 1980; executive producer, *Brothers-in-Law*, ABC, 1985; executive producer, *Stingray*, NBC, 1985; executive producer (with Lupo), *The Last Precinct*, NBC, 1986; executive producer (with Harsburgh), *Destination: America*, ABC, 1987; executive producer, "Sirens," *CBS Summer Playhouse*, CBS, 1987. Episodic: Director, *Jigsaw*, ABC, 1972; director, *Chase*, NBC, 1973; director, *The Rockford Files*, NBC, 1974; director, *Tenspeed and Brownshoe*, ABC, 1980; director, *Stone*, ABC, 1980. Movies: Executive producer (with Bartlett), *Midnight Offerings*, ABC, 1981.

RELATED CAREER—Chief executive officer, Stephen J. Cannell Productions, 1979—.

WRITINGS: See production details above, unless indicated. FILM—*The November Plan*, Universal/CIC, 1976. TELEVISION—Pilots: *The Rockford Files*, 1974; (with Steven Bochco) *Richie Brockelman: Missing 24 Hours*, 1976; *Scott Free*, 1976; *Dr. Scorpion*, 1978; (with Philip DeGuere) *The Gypsy Warriors*, 1978; *The Jordan Chance*, CBS, 1978; *Stone*, 1979; *The Night Rider*, 1979; *Boston and Kilbride*, 1979; (with Glen A. Larson) *Nightside*, 1980; *Brothers-in-Law*, 1985; (with Herbert Wright) *Stingray*, 1985. Episodic: *Columbo*, NBC, 1971; *Chase*, 1973; *Toma*, 1973; *The Rockford Files*, 1974; *Baa-Baa Blacksheep*, 1976; *Baretta*, ABC, 1978; *Richie Brockelman, Private Eye*, 1978; *The Greatest American Hero*, 1981; *The Quest*, 1982; *The Rousters*, 1983; *Harcastle and McCormick*, 1983; *The A-Team*, 1983; *Riptide*, 1983; *Hunter*, 1984; *Brothers-in-Law*, 1985; (with Frank Lupo) *The Last Precinct*, 1986; *Stingray*, 1987; *J.J. Starbuck*, 1987; *21 Jump Street*, 1987; *Wiseguy*, 1987—; *Sonny Spoon*, 1988.

AWARDS: Mystery Writers Award, 1975; Emmy Award, Outstanding Drama Series, 1978, for *The Rockford Files;* also received Emmy awards in 1979, 1980, and 1981, and four Writers Guild awards.

MEMBER: Writers Guild of America, Producers Guild, Directors Guild.

ADDRESSES: OFFICE—Stephen J. Cannell Productions, 7083 Hollywood Boulevard, Los Angeles, CA 90028.*

CANTOR, Arthur   1920-

PERSONAL: Born March 12, 1920, in Boston, MA; son of Samuel S. (a salesman) and Lillian (Landsman) Cantor; married Deborah Rosmarin, November 18, 1951 (died, September 22, 1970); children: David Jonathan, Jacqueline Hope, Michael Stephen. EDUCATION: Harvard University, B.A., 1940. MILITARY: U.S. Army Air Forces, first lieutenant, 1942-46.

VOCATION: Producer and press representative.

CAREER: PRINCIPAL STAGE WORK—All as producer, unless indicated: (With Saint Subber) *The Tenth Man*, Booth Theatre, New York City, 1959; (with Fred Coe) *All the Way Home*, Belasco Theatre, New York City, 1960; *Gideon*, Plymouth Theatre, New York City, 1961; *A Thousand Clowns*, Eugene O'Neill Theatre, New York City, 1962; *The Golden Age*, Lyceum Theatre, New York City, 1963; *Put It in Writing*, Theatre De Lys, New York City, 1963; *The Passion of Josef D.*, Ethel Barrymore Theatre, New York City, 1964; (with Committee Productions) *The Committee*, Henry Miller's Theatre, New York City, 1964; (also director) *The Trigon*, Stage 73, New York City, 1965; associate producer, *La Grosse Valise*, 54th Street Theatre, New York City, 1965; *The World of Gunter Grass*, Pocket Theatre, New York City, 1966; company manager, *The Threepenny Opera*, Stockholm Marionette Theatre of Fantasy, Billy Rose Theatre, New York City, 1966; (with Nicholas Vanoff) *Of Love Remembered*, American National Theatre Academy Theatre, New York City, 1967; *People Is the Thing That the World Is Fullest Of*, Bil Baird Theatre, New York City, 1967; *By George*, Lyceum Theatre, 1967; director, *The Tenth Man*, City Center Theatre, New York City, 1967; (with the Theatre of Genoa) *The Venetian Twins*, Henry Miller's Theatre, 1968; (with Mortimer Levitt) *The Concept*, Daytop Theatre Company, Sheridan Square Playhouse, New York City, 1968; (with Bil and Cora Baird) *Tango*, Pocket Theatre, 1969; *The Wizard of Oz* and *Winnie the Pooh*, both Bil Baird Marionettes, Bil Baird Theatre, 1969; *The Concept*, Gramercy Arts Theatre, New York City, 1969; then Pocket Theatre, 1970.

Golden Bat, Sheridan Square Playhouse, 1970; (with David Merrick) *Vivat! Vivat Regina!*, London, 1970, then Broadhurst Theatre, New York City, 1972; co-producer, *Old Times*, Montparnasse Theatre, Paris, France, 1971; *Promenade, All!*, Alvin Theatre, New York City, 1972; (with H.M. Tennant, Ltd.) *Captain Brassbound's Conversion*, Cambridge Theatre, London, 1971, then (with Roger L. Stevens) Ethel Barrymore Theatre, 1972; *The Little Black Book*, Helen Hayes Theatre, New York City, 1972; *Davy Jones' Locker*, Bil Baird Marionettes, Bil Baird Theatre, 1972; *Band Wagon, The Whistling Wizard*, and *The Sultan of Tuffet*, all Bil Baird Marionettes, Bil Baird Theatre, 1973; *Forty-Two Seconds from Broadway*, Playhouse Theatre, New York City, 1973; (with H.M. Tennant, Ltd.) *In Praise of Love*, Morosco Theatre, New York City, 1974; *Pinocchio*, Bil Baird Marionettes, Bil Baird Theatre, 1974; *Private Lives*, 46th Street Theatre, New York City, 1975; *The Constant Wife*, Shubert Theatre, New York City, 1975; (with Rose Teed) *The Innocents*, Morosco Theatre, 1976; *Dylan Thomas Growing Up*, Theatre Four, New York City, 1976; (with Leonard Friedman) *A Party with Betty Comden and Adolph Green*, Morosco Theatre, 1977; (with Michael White) *Housewife! Superstar!*, Theatre Four, 1977; (with Greer Garson) *The Playboy of the Weekend World*, Playhouse Theatre, 1978; (with Garson) *St. Mark's Gospel*, Marymount Manhattan Theatre, then Playhouse Theatre, both 1978; *My Astonishing Self*, Astor Place Theatre, New York City, 1978; *The Biko Inquest*, Theatre Four, 1978; (with Garson) *On Golden Pond*, New Apollo Theatre, New York City, 1979, then

Center Theatre Group, Mark Taper Forum, Los Angeles, CA, 1980.

(With Garson) *St. Mark's Gospel,* Playhouse Theatre, 1981; (also company manager) *Emlyn Williams as Charles Dickens,* Century Theatre, New York City, 1981; (with Jonathan Reinis; also general manager) *Shay Duffin as Brendan Behan,* Astor Place Theatre, 1981; (with Garson) *Jitters,* Walnut Street Theatre, Philadelphia, PA, 1981; (with Dorothy Cullman) *The Hothouse,* Playhouse Theatre, 1982; (with Brad Hall, Bruce Ostler, Paul Barrosse, and Bonnie Nelson Schwartz) *Babalooney,* Provincetown Playhouse, New York City, 1984; (with Schwartz and Rebecca Kuehn) *Ian McKellen Acting Shakespeare,* Ritz Theatre, New York City, 1984; (with Schwartz) *Pack of Lies,* Royale Theatre, New York City, 1985; (with Schwartz) *Jerome Kern Goes to Hollywood,* Ritz Theatre, 1986; (with Edwin W. Schloss) *Elisabeth Welch: Time to Start Living,* Lucille Lortel Theatre, New York City, 1986; (with Caroline Hirsch, Peter Wilson, and Tony Aljoe) *Rowan Atkinson at the Atkinson,* Brooks Atkinson Theatre, New York City, 1986; production adviser, *Starlight Express,* Gershwin Theatre, New York City, 1987. Also *A Matter of Position,* Philadelphia, PA, 1962; *Man in the Moon,* New York City, 1963; *Blithe Spirit, Bequest to the Nation, The Winslow Boy, Butterflies Are Free,* and *The Patrick Pearse Motel,* all in London, 1970-71; and *Souvenir,* Los Angeles, 1975.

MAJOR TOURS—All as producer, unless indicated: (With Fred Coe) *A Thousand Clowns,* U.S. cities, 1963-64; co-producer, *Three Cheers for the Tired Businessman,* U.S. cities, 1963-64; co-producer, *Camelot,* U.S. cities, 1963-64; (with Henry Guettel) *Camelot,* U.S. cities, 1964; *Oliver!,* U.S. cities, 1965; *The Day after the Fair,* U.S. cities, 1972; *The Bed Before Yesterday,* U.S. cities, 1976. Also supervised the stage arrangements for a U.S. State Department tour of European and Middle Eastern cities with Florence Eldridge and Frederic March, 1965.

PRINCIPAL TELEVISION WORK—Specials: Producer, *The Thirteen Stars,* PBS.

RELATED CAREER—Assistant press representative, Playwright's Company, New York City, 1945, then publicist, 1947-51; president, Advance Public Relations, New York City, 1953—; president, Arthur Cantor, Inc., 1953—; managing director, H.M. Tennant, Ltd., 1973—; executive producer, American Puppet Arts Council.

Press representative: *Hook 'n' Ladder,* Royale Theatre, New York City, 1952; *Inherit the Wind,* National Theatre, New York City, 1955; *The Most Happy Fella,* Imperial Theatre, New York City, 1956; *Long Day's Journey into Night,* Helen Hayes Theatre, New York City, 1956; *Auntie Mame,* Broadhurst Theatre, New York City, 1956; *Two for the Seesaw,* Booth Theatre, New York City, 1958; *The Miracle Worker,* Playhouse Theatre, New York City, 1959; *Three Cheers for the Tired Businessman,* tour of U.S. cities, 1963-64; *Follies Bergere,* Broadway Theatre, New York City, 1964; (with Artie Solomon) *The Great Western Union,* Bouwerie Lane Theatre, New York City, 1965; *Matty and the Moron and Madonna,* Orpheum Theatre, New York City, 1965; *Bugs and Veronica,* Pocket Theatre, New York City, 1965; (with Soloman) *Man of La Mancha,* American National Theatre Academy, Washington Square Theatre, New York City, 1965; *La Grosse Valise,* 54th Street Theatre, New York City, 1965; *The World of Gunter Grass,* Pocket Theatre, 1966; *Fitz* and *Biscuit,* both Circle in the Square, New York City, 1966; *Kicking the Castle Down,* Gramercy Arts Theatre, New York City, 1967; *People Is the Thing That the World Is Fullest Of,* Bil Baird Theatre, New York City, 1967; *Diary*

of a Madman, Orpheum Theatre, 1967; *Darling of the Day,* George Abbott Theatre, New York City, 1968; *Le Tartuffe* and *Waiting for Godot,* both Barbizon-Plaza Theatre, New York City, 1968; "The Picnic on the Battlefield" and "Guernica," on a double-bill as *Two Plays by Fernando Arrabal,* Barbizon-Plaza Theatre, 1969; *The House of Atreus* and *Arturo Ui,* both Tyrone Guthrie Theatre Company, New York City, 1968; *L'Amante Anglaise,* Barbizon-Plaza Theatre, 1971; *St. Mark's Gospel,* Playhouse Theatre, 1981; *A Little Family Business,* Martin Beck Theatre, New York City, 1982; *A Little Madness,* Provincetown Playhouse, New York City, 1983; *Ian McKellen Acting Shakespeare,* Ritz Theatre, New York City, 1984; *Jerome Kern Goes to Hollywood,* Ritz Theatre, 1986; *Rowan Atkinson at the Atkinson,* Brooks Atkinson Theatre, New York City, 1986. Also press representative for tours by the Gate Theatre of Dublin, Ireland, and the Habimah Theatre of Tel-Aviv, Israel, both 1948.

WRITINGS: (With Stuart W. Little) *The Playmakers* (nonfiction), Norton, 1970.

AWARDS: American Jewish Congress Award, 1969; New York Drama Critics Circle Award for *All the Way Home.*

MEMBER: League of New York Theatres (board of governors, 1967), Harvard Club, Coffee House Club, Players Club, Association of Theatrical Producers, Agents and Managers.

ADDRESSES: HOME—1 W. 72nd Street, New York, NY 10023. OFFICE—Arthur Cantor, Inc., 234 W. 44th Street, New York, NY 10036.*

*   *   *

CARLIN, George   1937-

PERSONAL: Full name, George Denis Patrick Carlin; born May 12, 1937, in New York, NY; son of Patrick and Mary Carlin; married Brenda Hosbrook, 1961; children: Kelly. MILITARY: U.S. Air Force.

VOCATION: Comedian, actor, and writer.

CAREER: Also see WRITINGS below. PRINCIPAL FILM APPEARANCES—Herbie Fleck, *With Six You Get Egg Roll* (also known as *A Man in Mommy's Bed*), National General, 1968; taxi driver, *Car Wash,* Universal, 1976; Frank, *Outrageous Fortune,* Buena Vista, 1987; Rufus, *Bill and Ted's Excellent Adventure,* Orion, 1989.

PRINCIPAL TELEVISION APPEARANCES—Series: Regular, *The Kraft Summer Music Hall,* NBC, 1966; George Lester, *That Girl,* ABC, 1966-67; co-host, *Away We Go,* CBS, 1967; regular, *Tony Orlando and Dawn,* CBS, 1976. Episodic: *The Tonight Show,* NBC, 1967—; *Talent Scouts,* CBS, 1968; *The Burns and Schreiber Comedy Hour,* ABC, 1973; *Saturday Night Live,* NBC, 1975; *The Late Show,* Fox, 1986; also *On Broadway Tonight,* CBS; *The Merv Griffin Show,* syndicated; *The Flip Wilson Show,* NBC. Movies: Title role, *Justin Case,* ABC, 1988. Specials: *The Perry Como Springtime Show,* NBC, 1967; *The Flip Wilson Comedy Show,* NBC, 1975; *Perry Como's Hawaiian Holiday,* NBC, 1976; *The Mad Mad Mad Mad World of the Super Bowl,* NBC, 1977; "University of Southern California," *On Location,* HBO, 1977; "Phoenix," *On Location,* HBO, 1978; *Mac Davis . . . Sounds Like Home,* NBC, 1977; *A Tribute to "Mr. Television"* Milton

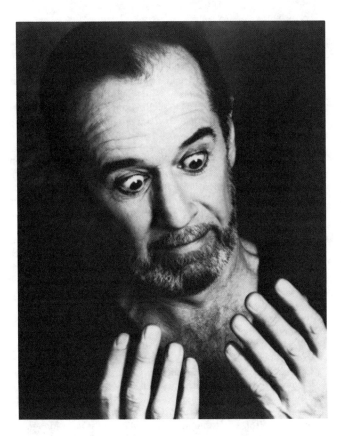

GEORGE CARLIN

Berle, NBC, 1978; *Make 'em Laugh*, CBS, 1979; *Carlin at Carnegie*, HBO, 1983; *Carlin on Campus*, HBO, 1984; *Apartment 2-C, Starring George Carlin*, HBO, 1985; *George Carlin—Playin' with Your Head*, HBO, 1986; *George Carlin: What Am I Doing in New Jersey?*, HBO, 1988; *What's Alan Watching?*, CBS, 1989.

PRINCIPAL RADIO APPEARANCES—Disc jockey: KJOE, Shreveport, LA; WEZE, Boston, MA; KXOL, Fort Worth, TX; and KDAY, Los Angeles, CA.

RELATED CAREER—As a comedian, appeared in nightclubs, theatres, concert halls, and colleges throughout the United States.

WRITINGS: See above for production details. TELEVISION—Specials: "University of Southern California," *On Location*, 1977; "Phoenix," *On Location*, 1978; *Carlin at Carnegie*, 1983; *Carlin on Campus*, 1984; *Apartment 2-C, Starring George Carlin*, 1985; *George Carlin—Playin' with Your Head*, 1986; *George Carlin: What Am I Doing in New Jersey?*, 1988. OTHER—*Sometimes a Little Brain Damage Can Help*.

RECORDINGS: ALBUMS—*Burns and Carlin at the Playboy Club Tonight*, ERA Records, 1960; *FM and AM*, Little David, 1972; *Class Clown*, Little David, 1972; *Occupation: Foole*, Little David, 1973; *Toledo Window Box*, Little David, 1974; *An Evening with Wally Londo Featuring Bill Slazo*, Little David, 1975; *On the Road*, Little David, 1977; *Indecent Exposure*, Little David, 1978; *A Place for My Stuff*, Atlantic, 1982; *The George Carlin Collection*, Little David, 1984; *Carlin on Campus*, Eardrum, 1984; *Playin' with Your Head*, Eardrum, 1986; *What Am I Doing in New Jersey?*, Eardrum, 1988.

AWARDS: Grammy Award, Best Comedy Album, 1972, for *FM and AM*.

MEMBER: Screen Actors Guild, American Federation of Television and Radio Artists, American Guild of Variety Artists, Writers Guild of America.

ADDRESSES: OFFICE—Carlin Productions, 901 Bringham Avenue, Los Angeles, CA 90049.

*   *   *

CARRADINE, John   1906-1988
(John Peter Richmond, Peter Richmond)

PERSONAL: Born Richmond Reed Carradine, February 5, 1906, in New York, NY; changed his name in 1935; died November 27, 1988, in Milan, Italy; son of William Reed (an Associated Press correspondent) and Genevieve Winifred (a surgeon; maiden name, Richmond) Carradine; married Ardanelle McCool, 1935 (divorced, 1944); married Sonia Sorel (an actress), 1945 (divorced, 1955); married Doris Irving Rich, 1957 (died, 1971); married Emily Cisneros, 1975; children: (first marriage) Bruce John, John Arthur (known as David); (second marriage) Christopher John, Keith Ian, Robert Reed.

VOCATION: Actor.

CAREER: STAGE DEBUT—*Camille*, St. Charles Theatre, New Orleans, LA, 1925. PRINCIPAL STAGE APPEARANCES—Allan Manville, *My Dear Children*, Brighton Theatre, New York City, 1945; Jonathan Brewster, *Arsenic and Old Lace*, Town Hall, New York City, 1946; the Cardinal, *The Duchess of Malfi*, Ethel Barrymore Theatre, New York City, 1946; Rupert Cadell, *Rope*, Toledo Theatre, New York City, 1946; the Inquisitor, *Galileo*, Maxine Elliot's Theatre, New York City, 1947; Voltore, *Volpone*, City Center Theatre, New York City, 1948; Nyunin, *The Wedding*, City Center Theatre, 1948; Walter Fowler, *The Cup of Trembling*, Music Box Theatre, New York City, 1948; Benjy, *The Leading Lady*, National Theatre, New York City, 1948; the Ragpicker, *The Madwoman of Chaillot*, Belasco Theatre, New York City, 1948; Kit Carson, *The Time of Your Life*, City Center Theatre, 1955; Lycus, *A Funny Thing Happened on the Way to the Forum*, Alvin Theatre, New York City, 1962; Jeeter Lester, *Tobacco Road*, Alhambra Dinner Theatre, Jacksonville, FL, 1970; Sir Thomas More, *A Man for All Seasons*, Episcopal Academy, Philadelphia, PA, 1974; DeLacey, *Frankenstein*, Palace Theatre, New York City, 1981. Also appeared in *Window Panes*, Egan Theatre, Los Angeles, CA, 1927; as Louis XI, *The Vagabond King*, Los Angeles and San Francisco, CA, 1941; as Matthew, *Murder without Crime*, Bridgeport, CT, 1945; in *The Royal Family*, Long Beach, CA, 1946; as Dr. Austin Sloper, *The Heiress*, 1949; as Brutus, *Julius Caesar*, 1950; as Sir Robert, *The Winslow Boy*, 1950; in *Shadow and Substance*, 1950; in *Silver Whistle*, 1951; as Mephistopheles, *Dr. Faustus*, 1951; as Jeeter Lester, *Tobacco Road*, 1951; in *The Fantasticks* and *You Never Can Tell*, both Arlington Park, IL, 1973; in *Boo*, 1984; and in *Rain*.

PRINCIPAL STAGE WORK—Director, *A Man for All Season*, Episcopal Academy, Philadelphia, PA, 1974.

MAJOR TOURS—Shylock, *The Merchant of Venice*, title role and Iago, *Othello*, and title role, *Hamlet* (in repertory), U.S. cities,

1943-44; the Ragpicker, *The Madwoman of Chaillot*, U.S. cities, 1949-50; Nickles, *JB*, U.S. cities, 1960-61; Fagin, *Oliver!*, U.S. cities, 1966; Jonathan Brewster, *Arsenic and Old Lace*, U.S. cities, 1974.

FILM DEBUT—(As Peter Richmond) Buzzard, *Tol'able David*, Columbia, 1930. PRINCIPAL FILM APPEARANCES—As John Peter Richmond or Peter Richmond until 1935: Captain Chicken Sam, *Heaven on Earth*, Universal, 1931; leader of the gladiators and a Christian, *The Sign of the Cross*, Paramount, 1932; the informer, *The Invisible Man*, Universal, 1933; courtroom spectator, *The Story of Temple Drake*, Paramount, 1933; Pete Garon, *To the Last Man*, Paramount, 1933; cult member, *The Black Cat*, Universal, 1934; Roman citizen, *Cleopatra*, Paramount, 1934.

Drunken-faced clerk, *Clive of India*, United Artists, 1935; Enjolras, *Les Miserables*, United Artists, 1935; customer, *She Gets Her Man*, Universal, 1935; Simon Girty, *Daniel Boone*, RKO, 1936; Richards, *Dimples*, Twentieth Century-Fox, 1936; sand diviner, *The Garden of Allah*, United Artists, 1936; David Rizzio, *Mary of Scotland*, RKO, 1936; voice of President McKinley, *A Message to Garcia*, Twentieth Century-Fox, 1936; Sergeant Rankin, *The Prisoner of Shark Island*, Twentieth Century-Fox, 1936; Jim Farrar, *Ramona*, Twentieth Century-Fox, 1936; Cafard, *Under Two Flags*, Twentieth Century-Fox, 1936; Beauty Smith, *White Fang*, Twentieth Century-Fox, 1936; Romagna, *Winterset*, RKO, 1936; Ishak, *Ali Baba Goes to Town*, Twentieth Century-Fox, 1937; Long Jack, *Captains Courageous*, Metro-Goldwyn-Mayer (MGM), 1937; Herbert Pemberton, *Danger—Love at Work*, Twentieth Century-Fox, 1937; the jailer, *The Hurricane*, United Artists, 1937; Casper, *The Last Gangster*, MGM, 1937; Alec Brady, *Laughing at Trouble* (also known as *Laughing at Death*), Twentieth Century-Fox, 1937; Captain Delmar, *Love Under Fire*, Twentieth Century-Fox, 1937; Harry Wilkins, *Nancy Steele Is Missing*, Twentieth Century-Fox, 1937; Pereira, *Thank You, Mr. Moto*, Twentieth Century-Fox, 1937; Ed, *This Is My Affair* (also known as *His Affair*), Twentieth Century-Fox, 1937; taxi driver, *Alexander's Ragtime Band*, Twentieth Century-Fox, 1938; General Adolfo Arturo Sebastian, *Four Men and a Prayer*, Twentieth Century-Fox, 1938; leader of the refugees, *Gateway*, Twentieth Century-Fox, 1938; Kopelpeck, *I'll Give a Million*, Twentieth Century-Fox, 1938; Murdock, *International Settlement*, Twentieth Century-Fox, 1938; Reef Hatfield, *Kentucky Moonshine* (also known as *Three Men and a Girl*), Twentieth Century-Fox, 1938; President Abraham Lincoln, *Of Human Hearts*, MGM, 1938; McAllison, *Submarine Patrol*, Twentieth Century-Fox, 1938; Gordon, *Kidnapped*, Twentieth Century-Fox, 1938; Coughy, *Captain Fury*, United Artists, 1939; Caldwell, *Drums Along the Mohawk*, Twentieth Century-Fox, 1939; Crimp, *Five Came Back*, RKO, 1939; Ben Carter, *Frontier Marshal*, Twentieth Century-Fox, 1939; Barryman, *The Hound of the Baskervilles*, Twentieth Century-Fox, 1939; Bob Ford, *Jesse James*, Twentieth Century-Fox, 1939; Danforth and Richard Burke, *Mr. Moto's Last Warning*, Twentieth Century-Fox, 1939; Hatfield, *Stagecoach*, United Artists, 1939; Naveau, *The Three Musketeers* (also known as *The Singing Musketeers*), Twentieth Century-Fox, 1939.

Porter Rockwell, *Brigham Young—Frontiersman* (also known as *Brigham Young*), Twentieth Century-Fox, 1940; Bisbee, *Chad Hanna*, Twentieth Century-Fox, 1940; Jim Casey, *The Grapes of Wrath*, Twentieth Century-Fox, 1940; Bob Ford, *The Return of Frank James*, Twentieth Century-Fox, 1940; El Nacional, *Blood and Sand*, Twentieth Century-Fox, 1941; Mr. Jones, *Manhunt*, Twentieth Century-Fox, 1941; Jesse Wick, *Swamp Water* (also known as *The Man Who Came Back*), Twentieth Century-Fox,

1941; Doc Murdoch, *Western Union*, Twentieth Century-Fox, 1941; Martin Caswell, *Northwest Rangers*, MGM, 1942; Ulrich Windler, *Reunion in France* (also known as *Mademoiselle France* and *Reunion*), MGM, 1942; Caleb Green, *Son of Fury*, Twentieth Century-Fox, 1942; Nobert and Long Jack, *Whispering Ghosts*, Twentieth Century-Fox, 1942; Doctor Sigmund Walters, *Captive Wild Woman*, Universal, 1943; Wellington, *Gangway for Tomorrow*, RKO, 1943; Heydrich, *Hitler's Madman* (also known as *Hitler's Hangman*), MGM, 1943; Martin, *I Escaped from the Gestapo* (also known as *No Escape*), Monogram, 1943; Clancy, *Isle of Forgotten Sins*, Producers Releasing Corporation, 1943; Von Altermann, *Revenge of the Zombies* (also known as *The Corpse Vanished*), Monogram, 1943; Lucky Miller, *Silver Spurs*, Republic, 1943; Bret Harte, *The Adventures of Mark Twain*, Warner Brothers, 1944; Duke Cleat, *Barbary Coast Gent*, MGM, 1944; General von Bodenbach, *The Black Parachute*, Columbia, 1944; Gaston, *Bluebeard*, Producers Releasing Corporation, 1944; Count Dracula, *House of Frankenstein*, Universal, 1944; Doctor Peter Drury, *The Invisible Man's Revenge*, Universal, 1944; Doctor Walters, *Jungle Woman*, Universal, 1944; Yousef Bey and Egyptian Priest, *The Mummy's Ghost*, Universal, 1944; Professor Gilmore, *Return of the Ape Man*, Monogram, 1944; Job, *Voodoo Man*, Monogram, 1944; Victor Marlowe, *Waterfront*, Producers Releasing Coporation, 1944.

Orange Povey, *Captain Kidd*, United Artists, 1945; Professor Madley, *Fallen Angel*, Twentieth Century-Fox, 1945; Count Dracula, *House of Dracula*, Universal, 1945; Pike, *It's in the Bag* (also known as *The Fifth Chair*), United Artists, 1945; Thorndyke P. Dunning, *Down Missouri Way*, Producers Releasing Corporation, 1946; Professor Randolph, *The Face of Marble*, Monogram, 1946; Charles Forestier, *The Private Affairs of Bel Ami*, United Artists, 1947; Doc Spencer, *C-Man*, Film Classics, 1949; Minister Foressi, *Casanova's Big Night*, Paramount, 1954; grave robber, *The Egyptian*, Twentieth Century-Fox, 1954; Old Tom, *Johnny Guitar*, Republic, 1954; Bergstron, *Thunder Pass*, Lippert, 1954; Arab Jala, *Desert Sands*, United Artists, 1955; Claude Almstead, *The Female Jungle*, American International, 1955; Doctor John Raybourn, *Half Human* (also known as *Jujin Yukiotoko*), DCA, 1955; Fletcher, *The Kentuckian*, United Artists, 1955; Colonel Streeter, *Stranger on Horseback*, United Artists, 1955; Colonel Proctor Stamp, *Around the World in 80 Days*, United Artists, 1956; Borg, *The Black Sleep* (also known as *Dr. Cadman's Secret*), United Artists, 1956; Giacomo, *The Court Jester*, Paramount, 1956; Snipe Harding, *Hidden Guns*, Republic, 1956; Aaron, *The Ten Commandments*, Paramount, 1956; Malone, *Hell Ship Mutiny*, Republic, 1957; Pharaoh Khufu, *The Story of Mankind*, Warner Brothers, 1957; Reverend Jethro Bailey, *The True Story of Jesse James*, Twentieth Century-Fox, 1957; Professor Charles Conway, *The Unearthly*, Republic, 1957; Amos Force, *The Last Hurrah*, Columbia, 1958; traveling salesman, *The Proud Rebel*, Buena Vista, 1958; Doc Weber, *Showdown at Boot Hill*, Twentieth Century-Fox, 1958; title role, *The Cosmic Man*, Allied Artists, 1959; Doctor Wyman, *The Incredible Petrified World*, Governor Films, 1959; Doctor Karol Noymann, *Invisible Invaders*, United Artists, 1959; Zachariah Garrison, *The Oregon Trail*, Twentieth Century-Fox, 1959.

Slave catcher, *The Adventures of Huckleberry Finn*, MGM, 1960; Professor Watts, *Sex Kittens Go to College* (also known as *Beauty and the Robot* and *Beauty and the Brain*), Allied Artists, 1960; Abel Banton, *Tarzan the Magnificent*, Paramount, 1960; Doctor Frederick Wilson and narrator, *Invasion of the Animal People* (also known as *Rymdinvasion I Lappland*, *Terror in the Midnight Sun*, *Space Invasion from Lappland*, and *Horror in the Midnight Sun*), Agnes

DeLahaie, 1962; Major Cassius Starbuckle, *The Man Who Shot Liberty Valance*, Paramount, 1962; Major Jeff Blair, *Cheyenne Autumn*, Warner Brothers, 1964; Bruce Alden, *The Patsy*, Paramount, 1964; title role, *The Wizard of Mars*, American General, 1964.

Hypnotist, *Curse of the Stone Hand*, Associated Distributors, 1965; Andre Desade, *House of the Black Death* (also known as *Blood of the Man Devil* and *Night of the Beast*), Medallion-Taurus, 1965; Doctor Vanard, *Psycho a Go-Go!* (also known as *Blood of Ghastly Horror*, *The Fiend with the Electric Brain*, *The Man with the Synthetic Brain*, and *The Love Maniac*), Hemisphere-American General, 1965; Dracula, *Billy the Kid vs. Dracula*, Embassy, 1966; Otis Lovelace, *The Hostage*, Crown International, 1966; Cruikshank, *Munster, Go Home!*, Universal, 1966; train engineer, *Night Train to Mundo Fine*, Hollywood Star Pictures, 1966; George, *Blood of Dracula's Castle* (also known as *Dracula's Castle*), Paragon, 1967; Tristam Halbin and narrator, "The Witch's Clock," *Dr. Terror's Gallery of Horrors* (also known as *Blood Suckers*, *Return from the Past*, and *Gallery of Horrors*), American General, 1967; Doctor Himmil, *Hillbillys in a Haunted House*, Woolner, 1967; Doctor Diabolo, *La senora muerte* (also known as *Madame Death*, *Mrs. Death*, and *The Death Woman*), Filmica Vergara, 1967; Laslow, *They Ran for Their Lives*, Color Vision, 1968; Doctor DeMarco, *The Astro-Zombies*, Geneni, 1968; narrator, *Genesis*, Genesis I-R.B. Childs, 1968; Preacher Sims, *Cain's Way* (also known as *Cain's Cutthroats*, *The Blood Seekers*, and *Justice Cain*), Fanfare, 1969; Ticker, *The Good Guys and the Bad Guys*, Warner Brothers, 1969; Mr. Drewcolt, *The Trouble with Girls*, MGM, 1969; Boone Hawkins, *The Gun Riders* (also known as *Five Bloody Graves*, *The Lonely Man*, and *Five Bloody Days to Tombstone*), Independent International, 1969.

Shop owner, *Hell's Bloody Devils* (also known as *The Fakers*, *Smashing the Crime Syndicate*, *Swastika Savages*, and *Operation M*), Independent-International, 1970; Doctor Rynning, *Horror of the Blood Monsters* (also known as *Creatures of the Prehistoric Planet*, *Horror Creatures of the Red Planet*, *Flesh Creatures of the Red Planet*, *The Flesh Creatures*, *Space Mission of the Lost Planet*, and *Vampire Men of the Lost Planet*), Independent-International, 1970; preacher, *The McMasters* (also known as *The Blood Crowd* and *The McMasters . . . Tougher Than the West Itself*), Chevron, 1970; surgeon, *Myra Breckinridge*, Twentieth Century-Fox, 1970; Sean O'Flanagan, *The Seven Minutes*, Twentieth Century-Fox, 1971; voice of Tyrone T. Tattersall, *Shinbone Alley* (animated), Allied Artists, 1971; H. Buckram Sartoris, *Boxcar Bertha*, American International, 1972; Doctor Bernardo, *Everything You Always Wanted to Known About Sex** (**but were afraid to ask), United Artists, 1972; Reverend Harper, *The Gatling Gun*, Ellman International, 1972; the walker, *Moonchild* (also known as *Full Moon*), Filmmakers, 1972; plastic surgeon, *Richard*, Aurora City Group, 1972; voice of the judge, *Portnoy's Complaint*, Warner Brothers, 1972; reporter, *Bad Charleston Charlie*, International Cinema, 1973; Jasper B. Hawks, *Bigfoot*, Ellman International, 1973; old gunfighter, *Hex*, Twentieth Century-Fox, 1973; Christopher Dean, *Legacy of Blood* (also known as *Blood Legacy*), Universal, 1973; narrator, *The Legend of Sleepy Hollow* (animated short), Pyramid, 1973; Igor Smith, *Superchick*, Crown International, 1973; Claude Dupree, *Terror in the Wax Museum*, Cinerama, 1973; towman, *Silent Night, Bloody Night* (also known as *Night of the Dark Full Moon*, *Death House*, and *Zora*), Cannon, 1974.

Mary's father, *Mary, Mary, Bloody Mary*, Translor-Proa, 1975; Doctor Smith, *The Killer Inside Me*, Warner Brothers, 1976; studio guide, *The Last Tycoon*, Paramount, 1976; Hezekiah Beckum, *The Shootist*, Paramount, 1976; drunk, *Won Ton Ton, the Dog Who Saved Hollywood*, Paramount, 1976; Doctor Edwards, *Crash!*, Group I, 1977; Fairweather, *Golden Rendezvous*, Golden Rendezvous, 1977; bum, *Satan's Cheerleaders*, World Amusements, 1977; Halliran, *The Sentinel*, Universal, 1977; Captain Ben, *Shock Waves* (also known as *Death Corps* and *Almost Human*), Cinema Shares, 1977; Amos Briggs, *The White Buffalo*, United Artists, 1977; Doctor Sigmund Hummel, *The Bees*, New World, 1978; Adonijah, "The Judgement of Solomon," *Greatest Heroes of the Bible* (video), Lucerne Media, 1979; Judge Winslow, *Sunset Cove* (also known as *Save Our Beach*), Cal-AM, 1978; Count Dracula, *Nocturna* (also known as *Nocturna, Grandaughter of Dracula*), Compass International, 1979.

Doctor, *The Boogeyman*, Jerry Roos, 1980; Erle Kenton, *The Howling*, AVCO-Embassy, 1981; Ronald Chetwynd-Haynes, *The Monster Club*, ITC, 1981; Colonel LeBrun, *The Nesting* (also known as *Phobia*), Feature Films, 1981; Father Stratten, *Satan's Mistress* (also known as *Fury of the Succubus*, *Demon Rage*, and *Dark Eyes*), Motion Picture Marketing, 1982; Salter, *The Scarecrow*, Oasis, 1982; voice of the Great Owl, *The Secret of NIMH* (animated), Metro-Goldwyn-Mayer/United Artists (MGM/UA), 1982; doctor, *Boogeyman II*, New West, 1983; Lord Grisbane, *The House of Long Shadows*, Cannon, 1983; the supreme commander, *The Ice Pirates*, MGM/UA, 1984; Doctor Kozmar, *Evils of the Night*, Shapiro, 1985; Soothsayer, *The Tragedy of Antony and Cleopatra* (video), Kultur, 1985; Mr. Stanton, *The Vals*, Sundowner, 1985; narrator, *Hollywood Ghost Stories* (documentary), Caidin Film, 1986; Leo, *Peggy Sue Got Married*, Tri-Star, 1986; Senator Bradford, *Revenge* (video), United Entertainment, 1986; Mr. Androheb, *The Tomb*, Trans World, 1986; Doctor Zeitman, *Evil Spawn* (also known as *Deadly Sting* and *Alive by Night*), American Independent, 1987; old Joe, *Monster in the Closet*, Troma, 1987; the justice, *Prison Ship*, Worldwide, 1987.

Also appeared (as John Peter Richmond or Peter Richmond until 1935) in: *Bright Lights*, First National, 1931; *Forgotten Commandments*, Paramount, 1932; *This Day and Age*, Paramount, 1933; *The Meanest Gal in Town*, RKO, 1934; *Alias Mary Dow*, Universal, 1935; *Bad Boy*, Twentieth Century-Fox, 1935; *The Bride of Frankenstein*, Universal, 1935; *Cardinal Richelieu*, United Artists, 1935; *The Crusades*, Paramount, 1935; *The Man Who Broke the Bank at Monte Carlo*, Twentieth Century-Fox, 1935; *Transient Lady* (also known as *False Witness*), Universal, 1935; *Anything Goes* (also known as *Tops Is the Limit*), Paramount, 1936; *Half Angel*, Twentieth Century-Fox, 1936; *The Devil and Daniel Webster* (also known as *All That Money Can Buy*, *Here Is a Man*, and *A Certain Mr. Scratch*), RKO, 1941; *Information Please (Number 5)* (short), RKO, 1942; *Alaska*, Monogram, 1944; *Gangway for Tomorrow*, 1944; *Dark Venture*, First National, 1956; *Something for Mrs. Gibbs* (short), 1965; *Broken Sabre* (unreleased), 1966; *The Emperor's New Clothes* (unreleased), 1966; *The Helicopter Spies*, MGM, 1968; Satan, *Autopsia de un fantasma* (also known as *Autopsy on a Ghost*), 1968; *Pacto diabolico* (also known as *Pact with the Devil*), 1968; *Dracula vs. Frankenstein* (also known as *Blood of Frankenstein* and *The Blood Seekers*), 1969; *Las vampiras* (also known as *The Vampires* and *The Vampire Girls*), Columbia, 1969; *Is This Trip Really Necessary?* (also known as *Trip to Terror* and *Blood of the Iron Maiden*), Hollywood Star, 1970; *Red Zone Cuba*, 1972; *Shadow House* (short), 1972; *Dracula's Daughter* (also known as *House of Dracula's Daughter*), 1973; *1,000,000 A.D.* (unreleased), 1973; *The House of Seven Corpses*, International Amusements, 1974; narrator, *Journey into the Beyond*, 1977; *The Lady and the Lynchings*, 1977; *Frankenstein Island*, 1977; *Monster* (also known as *Monster: The Legend That*

Became a Terror), 1979; *The Vampire Hookers* (also known as *Sensuous Vampires* and *Cemetery Girls*), Capricorn Three, 1979; *Teheran Incident* (also known as *Missle X, The Neutron Bomb Incident*, and *Cruise Missile*), 1979; *The Mandate of Heaven*, 1979; *Carradines in Concert* (documentary), 1980; *Monstroid*, 1980; *Blood of Dracula's Castle*, Independent-International; and *Dr. Dracula, Imps, Star Slammer, Demented Death Farm Massacre,* and *The Coven.*

PRINCIPAL TELEVISION APPEARANCES—Series: Host, *Trapped*, syndicated, 1951; Mr. Corday, *My Friend Irma*, CBS, 1953-54. Mini-Series: Father Hale, *Captains and the Kings*, NBC, 1976. Pilots: Title role, *The Adventures of Dr. Fu Manchu*, NBC, 1950; Llwellyn Crossbinder, *The Night Strangler*, ABC, 1973; also *Decisions! Decisions!*, NBC, 1971. Movies: Mr. Bosch, *Daughter of the Mind*, ABC, 1969; Nate Cheever, *Crowhaven Farm*, ABC, 1970; hotel clerk, *The Cat Creature*, ABC, 1973; Jacob Avril, *Stowaway to the Moon*, CBS, 1975; Conan Carroll, *Death at Love House* (also known as *The Shrine of Lorna Love*), ABC, 1976; Grampa, *Christmas Miracle in Caulfield, U.S.A.* (also known as *The Christmas Coal Mine Miracle*), NBC, 1977; Wisconsin farmer, *Tail Gunner Joe*, NBC, 1977; Avery Mills, *The Seekers*, HBO, 1979; Ronald Bentley, *Goliath Awaits*, syndicated, 1981.

Episodic: *NBC Repertory Theatre*, NBC, 1949; *Crimson Circle*, syndicated, 1950; *The Secrets of Wu Sin*, syndicated, 1950; *Sure As Fate*, CBS, 1950; "The Half-Pint Flask," *Lights Out*, NBC, 1950; "Stone Cold Dead," *The Web*, CBS, 1950; *Faith Baldwin's Theater of Romance* (also known as *The Faith Baldwin Playhouse*), ABC, 1951; "Meddlers," *Lights Out*, NBC, 1951; "Come into My Parlor," *Suspense*, CBS, 1953; *So This Is Hollywood*, NBC, 1955; "The First and the Last," *Climax*, CBS, 1955; "The Adventures of Huckleberry Finn," *Climax*, CBS, 1955; *Gunsmoke*, CBS, 1955; "Appointment of Eleanor," *Alfred Hitchcock Presents*, CBS, 1956; "The Hanging Judge," *Climax*, CBS, 1956; "Deadlock," *Front Row Center*, CBS, 1956; "The Rarest Stamp," *Studio 57*, syndicated, 1956; "Miracle Jones," *Damon Runyon Theatre*, CBS, 1956; "The House of the Seven Gables," *Matinee Theatre*, NBC, 1956; "Shoes," *Playhouse 90*, CBS, 1957; "The Star," *Navy Log*, ABC, 1957; "Switch Station," *Schlitz Playhouse of Stars*, CBS, 1957; "The Prince and the Pauper," *Dupont Show of the Month*, CBS, 1957; "Please Report Any Odd Characters," *Studio One*, CBS, 1957; "Novel Appeal," *Telephone Time*, ABC, 1957; "Daniel Webster and the Sea Serpent," *Matinee Theatre*, NBC, 1957; "The Deacon Whitehall Case," *Lineup*, CBS, 1958; "The Dora Gray Story," *Wagon Train*, NBC, 1958; "A Touch of Evil," *Suspicion*, NBC, 1958; "More Than Kin," *Restless Gun*, NBC, 1958; "All Our Yesterdays," *77 Sunset Strip*, ABC, 1958; "Tumbleweed Trail," *Bat Masterson*, NBC, 1959; "Tumbleweed Wagon," *Bat Masterson*, NBC, 1959; "The Fugitive," *The Life and Legend of Wyatt Earp*, ABC, 1959; "Millionaire Karl Miller," *The Million-aire*, CBS, 1959; *The Rebel*, ABC, 1959; "The Photographer," *The Rifleman*, ABC, 1959; "The Mindreader," *The Rifleman*, ABC, 1959; "The End of Nowhere," *Rough Riders*, ABC, 1959; *Gunsmoke*, CBS, 1959; "The Rain Man," *Johnny Ringo*, CBS, 1959; "A Matter of Dignity," *Harrigan and Son*, ABC, 1960; "The Reckoning," *Overland Trail*, NBC, 1960; "Bequest," *The Rebel*, ABC, 1960; "The Howling Man," *The Twilight Zone*, CBS, 1960; "The Colter Craven Story," *Wagon Train*, NBC, 1960; "Tolliver Bender," *Wanted Dead or Alive*, CBS, 1960; "Springtime," *Bonanza*, NBC, 1961; "Red Dog," *Maverick*, ABC, 1961; "Masquerade," *Thriller*, NBC, 1961; "The Remark-able Mrs. Hawks," *Thriller*, NBC, 1962; "Lucy Goes to Art Class," *The Lucy Show*, CBS, 1964; "Death Scene," *Alfred Hitchcock Theatre*, NBC, 1965; Jason's Grandfather, *Branded*,

NBC, 1965; Mr. Gateman, "Herman's Raise," *The Munsters*, CBS, 1965; "The Great Jethro Spring," *The Beverly Hillbillies*, CBS, 1966; "The Montori Device Affair," *The Girl from U.N.C.L.E.*, NBC, 1966; "As Far as the Sea," *Jesse James*, ABC, 1966; "Sound of Terror," *Laredo*, NBC, 1966; Mr. Gateman, *The Munsters*, CBS, 1966; *The Green Hornet*, ABC, 1967; "The Galaxy Gift," *Lost in Space*, CBS, 1967; "The Prince of Darkness Affair," *The Man from U.N.C.L.E.*, NBC, 1967; *Hondo*, ABC, 1967; *Daniel Boone*, NBC, 1968; "Town of No Exit," *Big Valley*, ABC, 1969; *Bonanza*, NBC, 1969; "Comeback," *Land of the Giants*, ABC, 1969; "Gentle Oaks," *Ironside*, NBC, 1971; farm-er, "The Big Surprise," *Night Gallery*, NBC, 1971; *Kung Fu*, ABC, 1972; *Love, American Style*, ABC, 1973; *The Cowboys*, ABC, 1974; *Emergency!*, ABC, 1974; "The Lady's Not for Burn-ing," *Hollywood Television Theatre*, syndicated, 1974; *Kung Fu*, ABC, 1974; *Mobile One*, ABC, 1975; *Westwind*, NBC, 1975; *Kung Fu*, ABC, 1975; *The Rookies*, ABC, 1975; *McCoy*, NBC, 1976; "The Whistle," *Fantasy Island*, ABC, 1982; "October the 31st," *The Fall Guy*, ABC, 1984; "Leroy and the Kid," *Fame*, syndicated, 1985; also *The Chevrolet Tele-Theater*, NBC; *Chey-enne*, ABC; *Vega$*, ABC; *Beany and Cecil; The Misunderstood Monsters; Pantomine Quiz.* Specials: *The Horror of It All*, PBS, 1983; *Umbrella Jack*, syndicated, 1984.

RELATED CAREER—Sketch artist and scenery painter; founder and actor, Shakespearean Repertory Company; appeared in summer stock and West Coast theatrical productions; performed readings throughout the United States.

AWARDS: Emmy Award, Best Performer in a Children's Program, 1985, for *Umbrella Jack.*

MEMBER: Actors' Equity Association, American Federation of Television and Radio Artists, Screen Actors Guild, Players Club, Channel Island Yacht Club.

OBITUARIES AND OTHER SOURCES: Films and Filming, De-cember, 1981; *Films in Review*, October, 1979, and January, 1980; *New York Times*, November 29, 1988; *Variety*, November 30, 1988.*

*   *   *

CASEY, Bernie   1939-

PERSONAL: Born June 8, 1939, in Wyco, WV.

VOCATION: Actor.

CAREER: PRINCIPAL FILM APPEARANCES—Cassie, *Guns of the Magnificent Seven*, United Artists, 1969; George Harley, *. . . Tick . . . Tick . . . Tick . . .*, Metro-Goldwyn-Mayer (MGM), 1970; Seth, *Black Gunn*, Columbia, 1972; Maurice Stokes, *Maurie* (also known as *Big Mo*), National General, 1973; Von Morton, *Boxcar Bertha*, American International, 1972; Tyrone Tackett, *Hit Man*, MGM, 1972; Reuben, *Cleopatra Jones*, Warner Brothers, 1973; Atkins, *Cornbread, Earl, and Me*, American International, 1975; Peters, *The Man Who Fell to Earth*, Cinema V, 1976; Dr. Pride-Hyde, *Dr. Black and Mr. Hyde* (also known as *The Watts Monster*), Dimension, 1976; David Thomas, *Brothers*, Warner Brothers, 1977; Arch, *Sharky's Machine*, Warner Brothers, 1982; Felix Leiter, *Never Say Never Again*, Warner Brothers, 1983; U.N. Jefferson, *Revenge of the Nerds*, Twentieth Century-Fox, 1984;

Colonel Rhombus, *Spies Like Us,* Warner Brothers, 1985; Reese, *Steele Justice,* Atlantic, 1987; Clinton James, *Backfire,* ITC, 1987; Lemar, *Rent-a-Cop,* Kings Road Entertainment, 1988; John Slade, *I'm Gonna Git You Sucka,* United Artists, 1989. Also appeared in *Black Chariot,* Goodwin, 1971.

PRINCIPAL TELEVISION APPEARANCES—Series: Mike Harris, *Harris and Company,* NBC, 1979; Ozzie Peoples, *Bay City Blues,* NBC, 1983. Mini-Series: Bubba Haywood, *Roots: The Next Generations,* ABC, 1979; Major Jeff Spender, *The Martian Chronicles,* NBC, 1980. Pilots: Mike Harris, *Love Is Not Enough,* NBC, 1978; Monday, *Hear No Evil,* CBS, 1982; Captain Bernie Rollins, *Pros and Cons,* ABC, 1986. Episodic: Bernie Taylor, *Alfred Hitchcock Presents,* NBC, 1985; also Johnson, *Police Woman,* NBC. Movies: J.C. Caroline, *Brian's Song,* ABC, 1971; head gargoyle, *Gargoyles,* CBS, 1972; Wendell Weaver, *Panic on the 5:22,* ABC, 1974; Vince, *It Happened at Lakewood Manor,* ABC, 1977; Dave Williams, *Mary Jane Harper Cried Last Night,* CBS, 1977; Joe Louis, *Ring of Passion,* NBC, 1978; Shurley Walker, *The Sophisticated Gents,* NBC, 1981; J.T. Collins, *The Fantastic World of D.C. Collins,* NBC, 1984. Specials: Guard, "First Offender," *HBO Family Playhouse,* HBO, 1987.

NON-RELATED CAREER—Professional football player with the San Francisco Forty-Niners and the Los Angeles Rams.

ADDRESSES: AGENT—Nicole David, Triad Artists, 10100 Santa Monica Boulevard, 16th Floor, Los Angeles, CA 90067.*

*   *   *

CASSAVETES, John   1929-1989

PERSONAL: Born December 9, 1929, in New York, NY; died of cirrhosis of the liver, February 3, 1989, in Los Angeles, CA; married Gena Rowlands (an actress), March 19, 1958; children: Nicholas, Alexandra, Zoe. EDUCATION: Graduated from Colgate University; also attended Mohawk College; studied acting at the American Academy of Dramatic Arts.

VOCATION: Actor, director, playwright, and screenwriter.

CAREER: Also see *WRITINGS* below. PRINCIPAL STAGE APPEARANCES—Appeared with a theatrical repertory company in Providence, RI, 1950-52. PRINCIPAL STAGE WORK—Assistant stage manager, *The Fifth Season,* Cort Theatre, New York City, 1953; producer, "Love Streams," "Knives," and "The Third Day Comes," in *Three Plays of Love and Hate,* Center Theatre, Hollywood, CA, 1981.

FILM DEBUT—*Fourteen Hours,* Twentieth Century-Fox, 1951. PRINCIPAL FILM APPEARANCES—Robert Batsford, *The Night Holds Terror,* Columbia, 1955; Frankie Dane, *Crime in the Streets,* Allied Artists, 1956; Nick, *Affair in Havana,* Allied Artists, 1957; Axel North, *Edge of the City* (also known as *A Man Is Ten Feet Tall*), Metro-Goldwyn-Mayer (MGM), 1957; Tony Sinclair, *Saddle the Wind,* MGM, 1958; Evan, *Virgin Island* (also known as *Our Virgin Island*), Films-around-the-World, 1960; Vance Miller, *The Webster Boy* (also known as *Middle of Nowhere*), Regal, 1962; Johnny North, *The Killers* (also known as *Ernest Hemingway's The Killers*), Universal, 1964; Cody, *The Devil's Angels,* American International, 1967; Victor Franko, *The Dirty Dozen,* MGM, 1967; Guy Woodhouse, *Rosemary's Baby,* Para-

mount, 1968; card player, *If It's Tuesday, This Must Be Belgium,* United Artists, 1969; Gus, *Husbands,* Columbia, 1970; Hank McCain, *Machine Gun McCain* (also known as *Gli intoccabili*), Columbia, 1970; Jim, *Minnie and Moskowitz,* Universal, 1971; Frankie Yale, *Capone,* Twentieth Century-Fox, 1975; Nicky, *Mikey and Nicky,* Paramount, 1976; Sergeant Chris Button, *Two-Minute Warning,* Universal, 1976; Maurice Aarons, *Opening Night,* Faces Distribution, 1977; Major Joe DeLuca, *Brass Target,* United Artists, 1978; Childress, *The Fury,* Twentieth Century-Fox, 1978; Dr. Michael Emerson, *Whose Life Is It Anyway?,* Metro-Goldwyn-Mayer/United Artists (MGM/UA), 1981; Dr. Sam Cordell, *The Incubus,* Artists Releasing, 1982; Phillip Dimitrious, *Tempest,* Columbia, 1982; Marvin Stewart, *Marvin and Tige,* Major, 1983; Robert Harmon, *Love Streams,* MGM/UA, 1984. Also appeared in *Taxi,* Twentieth Century-Fox, 1953; *Bandits in Rome* (also known as *Roma coma Chicago*), 1969; *Heroes,* Universal, 1977; *I'm Almost Not Crazy . . . John Cassavetes: The Man and His Work* (documentary), Cannon Releasing, 1983; and *Movies Are My Life: Martin Scorsese* (documentary).

FIRST FILM WORK—Director, *Shadows,* Lion, 1960. PRINCIPAL FILM WORK—Director: (Also producer) *Too Late Blues,* Paramount, 1962; *A Child Is Waiting,* Paramount, 1963; (also editor with Maurice McEndree and Al Ruban) *Faces,* Continental Distributing, 1968; *Husbands,* Columbia, 1970; *Minnie and Moskowitz,* Universal, 1971; *A Woman under the Influence,* Faces International, 1974; *The Killing of a Chinese Bookie,* Faces Distribution, 1976; *Opening Night,* Faces Distribution, 1977; (also producer) *Gloria,* Columbia, 1980; *Love Streams,* MGM/UA, 1984; *Big Trouble,* Columbia, 1986.

TELEVISION DEBUT—*Omnibus,* CBS, 1953. PRINCIPAL TELEVISION APPEARANCES—Series: Title role, *Johnny Staccato,* NBC, 1959-60. Pilots: Sergeant Lee Harmon, "The Fliers," *Bob Hope Presents the Chrysler Theatre,* NBC, 1965; Paul Chandler, "Won't It Ever Be Morning?," *Kraft Suspense Theatre,* NBC, 1965; General Karonos, *Alexander the Great,* ABC, 1968; Carmine Kelly, *Nightside,* ABC, 1973. Episodic: "Crime in the Streets," *The Elgin Television Hour,* ABC, 1955; *Columbo,* NBC, 1972; "The Haircut," *Shortstories,* Arts and Entertainment, 1988; also "Combat Medics," *The Elgin Television Hour,* ABC; *Alcoa Theatre,* NBC; *Danger,* CBS; *Philco Television Playhouse,* NBC; *Goodyear Television Playhouse,* NBC; "Winter Dreams," *Playhouse 90,* CBS; *Studio One,* CBS; *General Electric Theatre,* CBS; *Lux Playhouse,* CBS; *Rawhide,* CBS; *Dr. Kildare,* NBC; *The Lloyd Bridges Show,* CBS; *Channing,* ABC; *The Breaking Point,* ABC; *Burke's Law,* ABC; *Profiles in Courage,* NBC; *Combat,* ABC; *The Legend of Jesse James,* ABC; *Voyage to the Bottom of the Sea,* ABC; *The Virginian,* NBC; *The Long, Hot Summer,* ABC; *Climax,* CBS; "The Death of Socrates," *You Are There,* CBS; *Appointment with Adventure,* CBS; *Kraft Mystery Theatre,* NBC; *Pursuit,* CBS; *Kraft Television Theatre; Alfred Hitchcock Presents; Armstrong Circle Theatre; U.S. Steel Hour.* Movies: Gus Caputo, *Flesh and Blood,* CBS, 1979. Specials: *Hedda Hopper's Hollywood,* NBC, 1960. Also appeared in *The Expendable House,* 1963; *There Are the Hip and There Are the Square,* 1963; and *Murder Case,* 1964.

RELATED CAREER—Method acting instructor, Burt Lane's Drama Workshop, New York City, 1959-60; founder, Center Theatre, Hollywood, CA, 1981.

NON-RELATED CAREER—Sports announcer.

WRITINGS: STAGE—*The East/West Game,* produced in Los Angeles, CA, 1980; "Knives" in *Three Plays of Love and Hate,*

Center Theatre, Hollywood, CA, 1981; *A Woman of Mystery,* Court Theatre, Los Angeles, 1987. FILM—(Improvisation written with cast members) *Shadows,* Lion, 1960; (with Richard Carr) *Too Late Blues* Paramount, 1962; *Faces,* Continental Distributing, 1968, published by New American Library, 1970; *Husbands,* Columbia, 1970, published by Scripts Limited; *Minnie and Moskowitz,* Universal, 1971, published by Black Sparrow Press, 1973; *A Woman under the Influence,* Faces International, 1974; *The Killing of a Chinese Bookie,* Faces Distribution, 1976; *Opening Night,* Faces Distribution, 1977; *Gloria,* Columbia, 1980; (with Ted Allan; also songwriter) *Love Streams,* Metro-Goldwyn-Mayer-United Artists, 1984.

AWARDS: Critics Award from the Venice Film Festival, 1960, for *Shadows;* Academy Award nomination, Best Supporting Actor, 1967, for *The Dirty Dozen;* Academy Award nomination, Best Screenplay, National Society of Film Critics Award, Best Screenplay, and five awards from the Venice Film Festival, all 1968, for *Faces;* Academy Award nomination, Best Director, and National Board of Review Award, Best Picture, both 1974, for *A Woman under the Influence;* Emmy Award nomination, Best Supporting Actor, 1979, for *Flesh and Blood;* Golden Lion Award from the Venice Film Festival, 1980, for *Gloria;* Golden Bear Award from the Berlin Film Festival, Best Picture, 1984, for *Love Streams;* Los Angeles Film Critics Career Achievement Award, 1986.

OBITUARIES AND OTHER SOURCES: New York Times, February 4, 1989; *Variety,* February 8-14, 1989.*

*   *   *

CASTELLANO, Richard   1933-1988

PERSONAL: Born September 4, 1933, in New York, NY; died of a heart attack, December 10, 1988, in North Bergen, NJ; married Ardell Sheridan (an actress and writer); children: one daughter. EDUCATION: Attended Columbia University.

VOCATION: Actor.

CAREER: PRINCIPAL STAGE APPEARANCES—Louis and Eddie, *A View from the Bridge,* Sheridan Square Playhouse, New York City, 1965; one of the accused, *The Investigation,* Ambassador Theatre, New York City, 1966; Victor, *That Summer—That Fall,* Helen Hayes Theatre, New York City, 1967; first guard, *Antigone,* and first murderer, *Macbeth,* both American Shakespeare Festival, Stratford, CT, 1967; Sam, *Mike Downstairs,* Hudson Theatre, New York City, 1968; Frank Vecchio, *Lovers and Other Strangers,* Brooks Atkinson Theatre, New York City, 1968; Prince Gow, *Sheep on the Runway,* Helen Hayes Theatre, 1970. Also appeared with the New Yiddish Theatre, New York City, 1963.

PRINCIPAL FILM APPEARANCES—Frank Vecchio, *Lovers and Other Strangers,* Cinerama, 1970; Clemenza, *The Godfather,* Paramount, 1972; Lieutenant Tonelli, *Night of the Juggler,* Columbia, 1980. Also appeared in *A Fine Madness,* Warner Brothers, 1966.

PRINCIPAL TELEVISION APPEARANCES—Series: Joe Girelli, *The Super,* ABC, 1972; Joe Vitale, *Joe and Sons,* CBS, 1975-76; Giuseppe "Joe the Boss" Masseria, *The Gangster Chronicles,* NBC, 1981. Pilots: Frank Romeo, *Incident on a Dark Street,* NBC, 1973. Episodic: *NYPD,* ABC. Movies: Frank Labruzzo, *Honor Thy Father,* CBS, 1973.

NON-RELATED CAREER—Construction company owner and construction consultant.

AWARDS: Antoinette Perry Award, 1968, for *Lovers and Other Strangers;* Academy Award nomination, Best Supporting Actor, 1970, for *Lovers and Other Strangers.*

OBITUARIES AND OTHER SOURCES: Variety, December 21-27, 1988.*

*   *   *

CHAIKIN, Joseph   1935-

PERSONAL: Born September 16, 1935, in Brooklyn, NY. EDUCATION: Attended Drake University, 1950-53; trained for the stage at the Herbert Berghof Studio and with Nola Chilton and Mira Rostova.

VOCATION: Actor, director, and writer.

CAREER: Also see *WRITINGS* below. OFF-BROADWAY DEBUT—Mr. Atkins, *Dark of the Moon,* Carnegie Hall Playhouse, New York City, 1958. PRINCIPAL STAGE APPEARANCES—Serafina's boy friend and real estate agent, *Many Loves,* Ephron, *The Cave at Machpelah,* Leach, *The Connection,* and Mangini, *Tonight We Improvise,* all Living Theatre, New York City, 1959; title role, *Santa Claus,* Lazarus, *Calvary,* and Folial, *Escurial,* all Gate Theatre, New York City, 1960; Serafina's boy friend and real estate agent, *Many Loves,* Living Theatre, 1961; Galy Gay, *Man Is Man,* Living Theatre, 1962; Leach, *The Connection,* and C. Maynes, *In the Jungle of Cities,* both Living Theatre, 1963; furniture mover, "The New Tenant," and detective, "Victims of Duty," in *Two by Ionesco,* Writers' Stage Theatre, New York City, 1964; the Clown, *Sing to Me through Open Windows,* Players Theatre, New York City, 1965; Coolie, *The Exception and the Rule,* Greenwich Mews Theatre, New York City, 1965; Hamm, *Endgame,* Open Theatre, Washington Square Methodist Church, New York City, 1970; title role, *Woyzeck,* New York Shakespeare Festival (NYSF), Public Theatre, New York City, 1976; *Tongues* (one-man show), Magic Theatre, San Francisco, CA, 1978; man, "Tongues" and "Savage-Love" in *Tongues* (one-man show), Eureka Theatre, San Francisco, CA, then NYSF, Public Theatre, both 1979, later Center Theatre Group, Mark Taper Forum, Los Angeles, CA, 1981; *Texts* (one-man show), NYSF, Public Theatre, 1981; title role, *Uncle Vanya,* La Mama Experimental Theatre Club Annex, New York City, 1983. Also appeared in *Captain Fantastic Meets the Ectomorph,* New Theatre Workshop, New York City, 1966; *Is This Real?,* Kennedy Center for the Performing Arts, Washington, DC, 1985.

FIRST LONDON STAGE WORK—Director, "Interview" in *America Hurrah,* Open Theatre of New York, Royal Court Theatre, 1967. PRINCIPAL STAGE WORK—All as director, unless indicated. "Interview" in *America Hurrah,* Pocket Theatre, New York City, 1966; *The Serpent: A Ceremony,* Open Theatre of New York, Public Theatre, New York City, 1969, then Washington Square Methodist Church, New York City, 1970; *Terminal,* Open Theatre of New York, Washington Square Methodist Church, then Theatre at St. Clement's Church, New York City, both 1970, later Theatre at St. Clement's Church, 1973; *The Mutation Show,* Open Theatre of New York, Space for Innovative Development, New York City, then Theatre at St. Clement's Church, both 1973; *Nightwalk,* Open Theatre of New York, Theatre at St. Clement's Church, 1973; (also producer) *Electra,* Theatre at St. Clement's Church, 1974; *The Seagull,* Manhattan Theatre Club, New York City, 1975; producer (with the Theatre of Latin America), *Chile, Chile,* Washington Square Methodist Church, 1975; *A Fable,* Exchange Theatre, Westbeth, New York City, 1975; *Electra,* Mark Taper Forum, Los Angeles, CA, 1976; *The Dybbuk,* New York Shakespeare Festival, Public Theatre, 1977, then Habimah Theatre, Tel Aviv, Israel, 1979; (with Sam Shepard) *Antigone,* NYSF, Public Theatre, 1982; *Solo Voyages,* Interart Theatre, New York City, 1985. Also served as assistant to Peter Brook on productions of *US* and *The Tempest,* both 1966.

MAJOR TOURS—Leach, *The Connection,* Living Theatre, European cities, 1961-1962; also appeared with the Open Theatre of New York, U.S., Canadian, European, and Middle Eastern cities.

PRINCIPAL FILM APPEARANCES—Julius Orlovsky, *Me and My Brother,* New Yorker, 1969.

RELATED CAREER—Member, Living Theatre, New York City, 1959-63; founder, president, and director, Open Theatre of New York, New York City, 1963-73; director, Winter Project (a workshop with writers and performers), 1976—.

WRITINGS: See production details above. STAGE—All as collaborator, unless indicated: *The Serpent: A Ceremony,* 1969; *Terminal,* 1970; *The Mutation Show,* 1973; *Nightwalk,* 1973; *Electra,* 1974; *Chile, Chile,* 1975; *A Fable,* 1975; (with Mira Rafalowicz) *The Dybbuk* (new version), 1977; (with Sam Shepard) *Tongues,* 1978; (with Shepard) *Savage/Love,* 1979; (adaptor) *Texts* (from the works of Samuel Beckett), 1981. OTHER—*The Presence of the Actor,* Atheneum, 1972.

AWARDS: Obie Award from the *Village Voice,* Distinguished Performance, 1963, for *The Connection* and *Man Is Man;* Obie Award, Outstanding Achievement, 1969, for *The Serpent: A Ceremony;* Obie Award, Best Theatre Piece of the Season, 1972, and Drama Desk Award, Best Director, 1973, both for *The Mutation Show;* Guggenheim Fellowship in Stage Design and Production, 1969; received grants from the National Endowment for the Arts, the Ford Foundation, and the New York Council on the Arts. Honorary degrees: Drake University, Ph.D., 1972.

Awards presented to the Open Theatre of New York include: Obie Award, Special Citation, 1967; Vernon Rice Award, Outstanding Contribution to the Broadway Theatre, 1969; Brandeis University Creative Arts Citation, 1970; and New England Theatre Conference Award, 1971.

MEMBER: Actors' Equity Association.

ADDRESSES: OFFICE—c/o Artservices, 463 W. Street, New York, NY, 10014.*

*   *   *

CHANCELLOR, John   1927-

PERSONAL: Full name, John William Chancellor; born July 14, 1927, in Chicago, IL; son of Estil Marion (in real estate and hotels) and Mollie (Barrett) Chancellor; married Constance Herbert, 1950 (divorced, 1956); married Barbara Upshaw (a graphic designer), January 25, 1958; children: Mary (first marriage); Laura Campbell,

Barnaby John (second marriage). EDUCATION: Studied history and philosophy at the University of Illinois, 1947-48. MILITARY: U.S. Army, public relations specialist, 1945-47.

VOCATION: Journalist, television news anchor, commentator, and writer.

CAREER: PRINCIPAL TELEVISION APPEARANCES—Reporter, WMAQ-TV, Chicago, IL, 1950; Midwest news correspondent based in Chicago, NBC, 1950-58; foreign correspondent based in Vienna, 1958, London, 1959-60, and Moscow, 1960-61, NBC, 1958-61; host, *Today Show,* NBC, 1961-62; news correspondent based in New York City, NBC, 1961-63; foreign correspondent based in Brussels, NBC, 1963-64; White House correspondent based in Washington, DC, NBC, 1964-65; national news correspondent based in Washington, DC, NBC, 1967-70; anchor, *NBC Nightly News,* NBC, 1970-82; news commentator, *NBC Nightly News,* NBC, 1982—.

PRINCIPAL RADIO APPEARANCES—Series: Host, *The Chancellor Report,* NBC, 1970-82.

RELATED CAREER—Copy boy, reporter, and feature writer, *Chicago Times* (now known as the *Chicago Sun-Times*), 1947-50; director, Voice of America, Washington, DC, 1965-67.

NON-RELATED CAREER—Tugboat deckhand, bookstore clerk.

WRITINGS: RADIO—Series: *The Chancellor Report,* NBC, 1970-82. OTHER—(Contributor) *Memo to JFK from NBC News,* Putnam, 1961; (with Walter R. Mears) *The News Business,* Harper, 1983.

AWARDS: Distinguished Service Award from Sigma Delta Chi, Radio Spot-News Recording, 1955; Emmy Award, 1970; News Broadcaster of the Year Award from the International Radio and Television Society, 1982; Paul White Award from the Radio-Television News Directors Association, 1983; Sol Taishoff Award from the National Press Foundation, 1985, for Excellence in Broadcasting.

MEMBER: American Federation of Television and Radio Artists, Council on Foreign Relations, Century Association, Federal City Club (Washington, DC).

SIDELIGHTS: RECREATIONS—Classical music, tennis, photography, walking, and bicycling.

OTHER SOURCES: *Contemporary Authors,* Volume 109, Gale, 1983.

ADDRESSES: OFFICE—NBC News, 30 Rockefeller Plaza, New York, NY 10020. AGENT—Esther Newberg, International Creative Management, 40 W. 57th Street, New York, NY 10019.*

*   *   *

CHANNING, Stockard   1944-

PERSONAL: Born Susan Stockard, February 13, 1944, in New York, NY; daughter of Lester Napier (a shipping executive) and Mary Alice (English) Stockard; married Walter Channing, Jr. (in business; divorced); married Paul Schmidt (a college professor;

divorced); married David Debin (a screenwriter), 1976 (divorced). EDUCATION: Radcliffe College, B.A., 1965.

VOCATION: Actress.

CAREER: STAGE DEBUT—Candy Coke, *The Investigation,* Theatre Company of Boston, Boston, MA, 1966. OFF-BROADWAY DEBUT—*Adaptation/Next,* Theatre Company of Boston, Greenwich Mews Theatre, 1969. BROADWAY DEBUT—Chorus, *Two Gentlemen of Verona,* St. James Theatre, 1971. PRINCIPAL STAGE APPEARANCES—Alice, *Play Strindberg,* Theatre Company of Boston, Boston, MA, 1972; Joanna Wilkins, *No Hard Feelings,* Martin Beck Theatre, New York City, 1973; Julia, *Two Gentlemen of Verona,* Ahmanson Theatre, Los Angeles, CA, 1973; Mary, *Vanities,* Center Theatre Group, Mark Taper Forum, Los Angeles, 1976; Jane, *Absurd Person Singular,* Center Theatre Group, Ahmanson Theatre, 1978; Sonia Walsk, *They're Playing Our Song,* Imperial Theatre, New York City, 1980; Sheila, *A Day in the Death of Joe Egg,* Long Wharf Theatre, New Haven, CT, 1982; Luba, *The Lady and the Clarinet,* Long Wharf Theatre, then Lucille Lortel Theatre, New York City, both 1983; Angel, *The Rink,* Martin Beck Theatre, 1984; Virginia, *The Golden Age,* Jack Lawrence Theatre, New York City, 1984; Sheila, *A Day in the Death of Joe Egg,* Roundabout Theatre, New York City, 1985, then retitled *Joe Egg,* Longacre Theatre, New York City, 1985; Bunny Flingus, *The House of Blue Leaves,* Mitzi E. Newhouse Theatre, then Vivian Beaumont Theatre, both New York City, 1986; Susan, *Woman in Mind,* Manhattan Theatre Club, City Center Theatre, New York City, 1988; Melissa Gardner, *Love Letters,* Promenade Theatre, New York City, 1989. Also appeared as Rosalind, *As You Like It,* Long Beach, CA, 1979.

PRINCIPAL FILM APPEARANCES—Judy Stanley, *Up the Sandbox,* National General, 1972; Freddie, *The Fortune,* Columbia, 1975; Kitty Baxter, *The Big Bus,* Paramount, 1976; title role, *Dandy, the All American Girl* (also known as *Sweet Revenge*), Metro-Goldwyn-Mayer (MGM), 1976; Bess, *The Cheap Detective,* Columbia, 1978; Rizzo, *Grease,* Paramount, 1978; Mona Mondieu, *The Fish That Saved Pittsburgh,* United Artists, 1979; J.J. Dalton, *Safari 3000,* MGM, 1982; Jocelyn Norris, *Without a Trace,* Twentieth Century Fox, 1983; Julie, *Heartburn,* Paramount, 1986; Nancy, *The Men's Club,* Atlantic, 1986; Margaret, *A Time of Destiny,* Columbia, 1988. Also appeared in *Comforts of Home,* 1970; *The Hospital,* United Artists, 1971; and *The Boys* (also known as *Staying the Same, Boy's Life,* and *A Boy's Life*), Hemdale Releasing, 1989.

PRINCIPAL TELEVISION APPEARANCES—Series: Susan Hughes, *Stockard Channing in Just Friends,* CBS, 1979; Susan Goodenow, *The Stockard Channing Show,* CBS, 1980. Pilots: Mickey, *Lucan,* ABC, 1977. Movies: Miriam Knight, *The Girl Most Likely To . . . ,* ABC, 1973; title role, *Silent Victory: The Kitty O'Neil Story,* CBS, 1979; Helen Bower, *Not My Kid,* CBS, 1985; Susan Reinert, *Echoes in the Darkness,* CBS, 1987; Leah Lazenby, *The Room Upstairs,* CBS, 1987. Specials: *The Eddie Rabbitt Special,* NBC, 1980; Marion, "Tidy Endings," *HBO Showcase,* HBO, 1988.

AWARDS: Antoinette Perry Award, Best Actress in a Play, 1985, for *Joe Egg;* Antoinette Perry Award nomination and Drama Desk Award nomination, both Best Featured Actress in a Play, 1986, for *The House of Blue Leaves;* Drama Desk Award, Best Actress in a Play, 1988, for *Woman in Mind.*

ADDRESSES: AGENT—Andrea Eastman, International Creative Management, 8899 Beverly Boulevard, Los Angeles, CA 90048.*

CHAPMAN, David 1938-

PERSONAL: Born November 11, 1938, in Atlanta, GA; son of R.S. and Ellen (Graham) Chapman; married Dianne Finn (a costume designer; divorced); married Carol Oditz (a costume designer). EDUCATION: Georgia Institute of Technology, B.S., 1960, B. Architecture, 1963. MILITARY: U.S. Navy.

VOCATION: Designer.

CAREER: PRINCIPAL STAGE WORK—All as set designer: *Red, White, and Maddox,* Cort Theatre, New York City, 1969; *Lulu,* Sheridan Square Playhouse, New York City, 1970; *Leaves of Grass,* Theatre Four, New York City, 1971; *Where Has Tommy Flowers Gone?,* Eastside Playhouse, New York City, 1971; *Soon,* Ritz Theatre, New York City, 1971; *Promenade All,* Alvin Theatre, New York City, 1972; *God Says There Is No Peter Ott,* McAlpin Rooftop Theatre, New York City, 1972; *Alpha Beta,* Eastside Playhouse, 1973; *Nash at Nine,* Helen Hayes Theatre, New York City, 1973; *Creeps,* Playhouse Theatre, New York City, 1973; *The Magic Show,* Cort Theatre, 1974; *Music! Music!,* City Center Theatre, New York City, 1974; *Once I Saw a Boy Laughing,* Westside Theatre, New York City, 1974; *Finn Mackool, the Grand Distraction,* Theatre De Lys, New York City, 1975; *Fixed,* Theatre of the Riverside Church, New York City, 1977; *White Pelicans,* Theatre De Lys, 1978; *The First,* Martin Beck Theatre, New York City, 1981; *Booth,* South Street Theatre, New York City, 1982; *Othello,* Winter Garden Theatre, New York City, 1982; *Play Me a Country Song,* Virginia Theatre, New York City, 1982; *Zorba,* Broadway Theatre, New York City, 1983; (also costume designer) *Henry IV, Part I* and *Hamlet,* both American Shakespeare Theatre, Stratford, CT, 1982; *Oliver!,* Mark Hellinger Theatre, New York City, 1984; *Harlem Nocturne,* Latin Quarter Theatre, New York City, 1984; *Cabaret,* Palace Theatre, New York City, 1987. Also set designer, *Le Bellybutton,* New York City, 1975; and at the Asolo State Theatre, Sarasota, FL, Theatre Atlanta, Atlanta, GA, Folger Theatre, Washington, DC, Pittsburgh Public Theatre, Pittsburgh, PA, PAF Playhouse, Long Island, NY, and Syracuse Stage, Syracuse, NY.

MAJOR TOURS—Set designer: *Zorba,* U.S. cities, 1983-86; *Stop the World . . . I Want to Get Off,* U.S. cities, 1986-87; *Cabaret,* U.S. cities, 1986-87.

PRINCIPAL FILM WORK—Art director, *Somebody Killed Her Husband,* Columbia, 1978; art director, *The Seduction of Joe Tynan,* Universal, 1979; production designer, *Four Friends* (also known as *Georgia's Friends*), Filmways, 1981; art director, *Wolfen,* Warner Brothers, 1981; art director, *The Cotton Club,* Orion, 1984; art director (New York locale), *Legal Eagles,* Universal, 1986; production designer, *Dirty Dancing,* Vestron, 1987; production designer, *Mystic Pizza,* Samuel Goldwyn, 1988.

PRINCIPAL TELEVISION WORK—Series: Production designer, *The Dick Cavett Show.* Pilots: Production designer, *Stunt Seven,* CBS, 1979. Movies: Art director, *You Can't Go Home Again,* CBS, 1979; production designer, *Into the Homeland* (also known as *When the Swallows Come Back* and *Swallows Come Back*), HBO, 1987. Specials: Production designer, *The Annie Christmas Show.*

RELATED CAREER—Theatre consultant: Westbeth Theatre, Westbeth, NY; Folger Theatre, Washington, DC; and Theatre Atlanta, Atlanta, GA.

NON-RELATED CAREER—Professional architect.

MEMBER: United Scenic Artists.

ADDRESSES: OFFICE—c/o Alfred Geller, 122 E. 42nd Street, New York, NY 10017.*

*   *   *

CHAYKIN, Maury

VOCATION: Actor.

CAREER: PRINCIPAL STAGE APPEARANCES—Ton, ''Gotcha'' in *Gimme Shelter,* Brooklyn Academy of Music, Brooklyn, NY, 1978; Thompson, *Leave It to Beaver Is Dead,* New York Shakespeare Festival, Public Theatre, New York City, 1979. Also appeared in *After the Rain,* Public Theatre, 1974.

PRINCIPAL FILM APPEARANCES—Harvey Cannon, *The Kidnapping of the President,* Crown International, 1980; Clarence, *Death Hunt,* Twentieth Century-Fox, 1981; Monty, *Curtains,* Jensen Farley, 1983; Dan Errol, *Of Unknown Origin,* Warner Brothers, 1983; Jim Sting, *Wargames,* Metro-Goldwyn-Mayer/United Artists (MGM/UA), 1983; Lawrence, *Harry and Son,* Orion, 1984; Falco, *Highpoint,* New World, 1984; Guard Reynolds, *Mrs. Soffel,* MGM/UA, 1984; Burt, *The Vindicator* (also known as *Frankenstein '88*), Twentieth Century-Fox, 1984; Vinny, *Def-Con 4,* New World, 1985; man in wheelchair, *Turk 182!,* Twentieth Century-Fox, 1985; title role, *Canada's Sweetheart: The Saga of Hal C. Banks,* National Film Board of Canada/Canadian Broadcasting Company, 1986; pool player, *The Bedroom Window,* De Laurentiis Entertainment Group, 1987; Charlie Kelso, *Hearts of Fire,* Lorimar, 1987; Guido, *Higher Education,* Norstar, 1987; Detective Trask, *Wild Thing,* Atlantic, 1987; Marchais, *Nowhere to Hide,* New Century, 1987; Freeborn, *Stars and Bars,* Columbia, 1988; Captain Burdoch, *Caribe,* Miramax, 1988; Downs, *Iron Eagle II* (also known as *Iron Eagle II—The Battle Beyond the Flag*), Tri-Star, 1988. Also appeared in *Soup for One,* Warner Brothers, 1982.

PRINCIPAL TELEVISION APPEARANCES—Movies: Williams, *In Like Flynn,* CBS, 1980; Bruno, *Jimmy B. and Andre,* CBS, 1980; Rudy Simbro, *The Guardian,* HBO, 1984; Claude Vealy, *Act of Vengeance,* HBO, 1986; Wilensky, *Hot Paint,* CBS, 1988. Specials: *Overdrawn at the Memory Bank,* PBS, 1985.

AWARDS: Association of Canadian Television and Radio Artists Award, Best Actor in a Leading Role, 1986, for *Canada's Sweetheart: The Saga of Hal C. Banks.*

ADDRESSES: AGENT—Smith-Freedman and Associates, 121 N. San Vicente Boulevard, Beverly Hills, CA 90211.

*   *   *

CHILES, Lois

PERSONAL: Born in Alice, TX.

VOCATION: Actress.

CAREER: PRINCIPAL STAGE APPEARANCES—Maggie, *Cat on a Hot Tin Roof,* Coconut Grove Playhouse, Coconut Grove, FL,

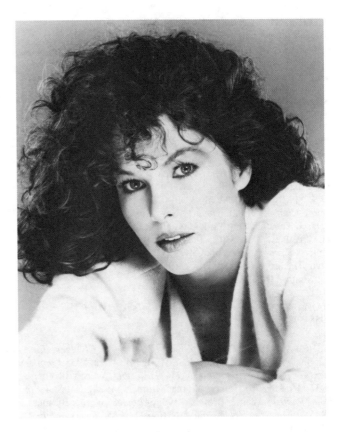

LOIS CHILES

1984; Mom, reporter, and Darlene, *The Incredibly Famous Willy Rivers,* WPA Theatre, New York City, 1984; Mabel Cantwell, *The Best Man,* Ahmanson Theatre, Los Angeles, CA, 1987.

PRINCIPAL FILM APPEARANCES—Shelley, *Together for Days* (also known as *Black Cream*), Olas, 1972; Carol Ann, *The Way We Were,* Columbia, 1973; Jordan Baker, *The Great Gatsby,* Paramount, 1974; Nancy Greenly, *Coma,* United Artists, 1978; Linnet Ridgeway, *Death on the Nile,* Paramount, 1978; Holly Goodhead, *Moonraker,* United Artists, 1979; Ruth, *Raw Courage* (also known as *Courage*), New World, 1984; Leslie, *Sweet Liberty,* Universal, 1986; Annie Lansing, *Creepshow 2,* New World, 1987; Jennifer Mack, *Broadcast News,* Twentieth Century-Fox, 1987; Miss Virginia, *Twister,* Vestron, 1988.

PRINCIPAL TELEVISION APPEARANCES—Series: Holly Harwood, *Dallas,* CBS, 1982-84. Pilots: Jessica Drake, *Dark Mansions,* ABC, 1986. Episodic: Scottie, *Hart to Hart,* ABC. Specials: Lita Nathan, ''Tales from the Hollywood Hills: A Table at Ciro's,'' *Great Performances,* PBS, 1987.

MEMBER: Actors' Equity Association, Screen Actors Guild, American Federation of Television and Radio Artists, Academy of Motion Picture Arts and Sciences.

ADDRESSES: AGENT—Audrey Caan, Triad Artists, 10100 Santa Monica Boulevard, 16th Floor, Los Angeles, CA 90067. OFFICE—Kindel and Kosberg, 16055 Ventura Boulevard, Suite 535, Encino, CA 91436-2601.

CHODOROV, Edward   1904-1988

PERSONAL: Born April 17, 1904 (some sources say 1914), in New York, NY; died October 9, 1988, in New York, NY; son of Harry (an actor and businessman) and Lena (Simmons) Chodorov; married Marjorie Roth (divorced); married Rosemary Pettit, June 16, 1954; children: one son, two daughters. EDUCATION: Attended Brown University.

VOCATION: Playwright, screenwriter, producer, and director.

CAREER: Also see *WRITINGS* below. FIRST STAGE WORK—Stage manager, *Abie's Irish Rose,* Fulton Theatre, New York City, 1922. PRINCIPAL STAGE WORK—Director: *Those Endearing Young Charms,* Booth Theatre, New York City, 1944; *Decision,* Belasco Theatre, New York City, 1944; *Common Ground,* Fulton Theatre, New York City, 1945; *Oh, Men! Oh, Women!,* Henry Miller's Theatre, New York City, 1953; *Monsieur Lautrec,* Belgrade Civic Theatre, Coventry, U.K., 1959. Also stage manager, *Is Zat So,* South Africa, 1928.

MAJOR TOURS—Director, *Listen to the Mocking Bird,* U.S. cities, 1958-59.

PRINCIPAL FILM WORK—Producer: *The World Changes,* First National, 1933; *The Mayor of Hell,* Warner Brothers, 1933; *Gentlemen Are Born,* First National, 1934; *Desirable,* Warner Brothers, 1934; *Madame Du Barry,* Warner Brothers, 1934; *The Story of Louis Pasteur,* Warner Brothers, 1935; *Alibi Ike,* Warner Brothers, 1935; *Living on Velvet,* First National, 1935; *Sweet Adeline,* Warner Brothers, 1935; *Craig's Wife,* Columbia, 1936; *Yellow Jack,* Metro-Goldwyn-Mayer (MGM), 1938; *Rich Man, Poor Girl,* MGM, 1938; *Woman against Woman,* MGM, 1938; *Spring Madness,* MGM, 1938; *Tell No Tales,* MGM, 1939; *The Man from Dakota,* MGM, 1940; *Road House,* Twentieth Century-Fox, 1948.

RELATED CAREER—Writer, director, and producer, Horizon Pictures, 1961-63, A.C.E. Productions, London, 1964, Columbia Pictures, 1965, and Twentieth Century-Fox, 1966-67; writer and producer, Warner Brothers-Seven Arts, 1968-69; writer and director, Dowling, Whitehead & Stevens, 1971-72, Cheryl Crawford Productions, 1973, Universal Pictures, 1974-75, and Theatre Guild, 1976; instructor in film and television writing, California State University, 1976-78; lecturer, New York University, 1979; instructor in stage directing, Actors and Directors Lab, Los Angeles, CA, 1980; film publicist, Columbia Pictures.

WRITINGS: STAGE—(With Arthur Barton) *Wonder Boy,* Alvin Theatre, New York City, 1931; *Kind Lady,* Booth Theatre, New York City, 1935, published by Samuel French, Inc., 1936, and in *Three Plays about Crime and Criminals,* Pocket Books, 1979; (with H.S. Kraft) *Cue for Passion,* Royale Theatre, New York City, 1940, published by Samuel French, Inc., 1941; *Those Endearing Young Charms,* Booth Theatre, 1943, published by Samuel French, Inc., 1943; *Decision,* Belasco Theatre, New York City, 1944, published by Samuel French, Inc., 1946; *Common Ground,* Fulton Theatre, New York City, 1945, published by Samuel French, Inc., 1946; *Signor Chicago,* first produced in 1947; *Oh, Men! Oh, Women!,* Henry Miller's Theatre, New York City, 1953, published by Samuel French, Inc., 1955; *The Spa,* first produced in 1955, published by Dramatists Play Service, 1957; *Listen to the Mocking Bird,* Colonial Theatre, Boston, MA, 1958; *Monsieur Lautrec,* Belgrade Civic Theatre, Coventry, U.K., 1959. Also wrote *Erskine, The Clubwoman,* and *Irrational Knot,* all unproduced.

FILM—See production details above, unless indicated. *The Mayor of Hell,* 1933; *Captured,* Warner Brothers, 1933; *The World Changes,* 1933; *Madame Du Barry,* 1934; (with Mary C. McCall) *Craig's Wife,* 1936; (with F. Hugh Herbert and Brown Holmes) *Snowed Under,* First National, 1936; *Yellow Jack,* 1938; *Woman against Woman,* 1938; *Spring Madness,* 1939; (with Marguerite Roberts and George Oppenheimer) *Undercurrent,* Metro-Goldwyn-Mayer (MGM), 1946; (with Luther Davis and George Wells) *The Hucksters,* MGM, 1947; (with Margaret Gruen, Oscar Saul, and David Hertz) *Road House,* 1948; (with Jerry Davis and Charles Bennett) *Kind Lady,* MGM, 1951; (uncredited with Nunnally Johnson) *Oh, Men! Oh, Women!,* Twentieth Century-Fox, 1957.

TELEVISION—Series: *The Billy Rose Show,* ABC, 1952.

OBITUARIES AND OTHER SOURCES: Variety, October 19, 1988.*

*   *   *

CHONG, Rae Dawn

PERSONAL: Born in Vancouver, BC, Canada; daughter of Tommy Chong (a comedian, actor, writer, and director); married Owen Baylis (a stockbroker; divorced); children: Morgan.

VOCATION: Actress.

CAREER: PRINCIPAL FILM APPEARANCES—Janetta, *Stony Island* (also known as *My Main Man from Stony Island*), World-Northal, 1978; Ika, *Quest for Fire,* Twentieth Century-Fox, 1982; Tracy, *Beat Street,* Orion, 1984; gypsy, *Cheech and Chong's "The Corsican Brothers,"* Orion, 1984; Pearl Antoine, *Choose Me,* Island Alive, 1984; Liela, *Fear City,* Chevy Chase Distribution, 1984; Sarah, *American Flyers,* Warner Brothers, 1985; Yogi, *City Limits,* Atlantic Releasing, 1985; Squeak, *The Color Purple,* Warner Brothers, 1985; Cindy, *Commando,* Twentieth Century-Fox, 1985; slave girl, *Running out of Luck,* CBS Records Group, 1986; Sarah Walker, *Soul Man,* New World, 1986; Rachel Dobs, *The Squeeze,* Tri-Star, 1987; Hilary Orozco, *The Principal,* Tri-Star, 1987. Also appeared in *Walking after Midnight,* Kay, 1988; *The Borrower,* Vision; *Far Out, Man!,* Cinetel; and *Loon.*

PRINCIPAL TELEVISION APPEARANCES—Pilots: Diane Miller, *Friends,* CBS, 1978. Episodic: Circe La Femme, "Casey at the Bat," *Shelley Duvall's Tall Tales and Legends,* Showtime, 1986. Movies: Rita, *The Top of the Hill,* syndicated, 1980; Christine Horn, *Badge of the Assassin,* CBS, 1985.

RELATED CAREER—Narrator of *Sex, Drugs, and AIDS,* an educational documentary for high school students.

MEMBER: Screen Actors Guild, American Federation of Television and Radio Artists.

ADDRESSES: AGENT—Kevin Huvane, Creative Artists Agency, 1888 Century Park E., Suite 1400, Los Angeles, CA 90067. PUBLICIST—Nancy Seltzer Public Relations, 8845 Ashcroft Avenue, Los Angeles, CA 90048.

CLARK, Bob 1941-

PERSONAL: Born August 5, 1941, in New Orleans, LA. EDUCA-TION: Attended Hillsdale College.

VOCATION: Director, producer, and screenwriter.

CAREER: Also see *WRITINGS* below. PRINCIPAL FILM APPEAR-ANCES—*Meat Cleaver Massacre*, Group 1, 1977. PRINCIPAL FILM WORK—Director: *The She Man*, Southeastern, 1967; (also producer) *Dead of Night*, Alpha, 1972; (also producer and make-up) *Deathdream*, Europix, 1972; (also producer) *Black Christmas*, Ambassador, 1974; (also producer) *Breaking Point*, Twentieth Century-Fox, 1976; (also producer) *Murder by Decree*, AVCO-Embassy, 1979; *Tribute*, Twentieth Century-Fox, 1980; (also producer) *Porky's*, Twentieth Century-Fox, 1982; (also producer) *A Christmas Story*, Metro-Goldwyn-Mayer/United Artists, 1983; (also producer) *Porky's II: The Next Day*, Twentieth Century-Fox, 1983; *Rhinestone*, Twentieth Century-Fox, 1984; *Turk 182!*, Twentieth Century-Fox, 1985; (also producer) *From the Hip*, De Laurentiis Entertainment Group, 1987.

WRITINGS: See production details above. FILM—*The She Man*, 1967; *Murder by Decree*, 1979; *Porky's*, 1982; *Porky's II: The Next Day*, 1983; *A Christmas Story*, 1983; (composer and lyricist) *Rhinestone*, 1984; *From the Hip*, 1987.

ADDRESSES: AGENT—Harold Cohen Associated Management, 9200 Sunset Boulevard, Los Angeles, CA 90069.*

*   *   *

CLARK, Roy 1933-

PERSONAL: Full name, Roy Linwood Clark; born April 15, 1933, in Meherrin, VA; father, a tobacco farmer; wife's name, Barbara Joyce.

VOCATION: Singer, writer, actor, and recording artist.

CAREER: PRINCIPAL FILM APPEARANCES—Wild Bill Wildman, *Matilda*, American International, 1978; Ben Hooker, *Uphill All the Way*, New World, 1986. PRINCIPAL FILM WORK—Executive producer, *Uphill All the Way*, New World, 1986.

PRINCIPAL TELEVISION APPEARANCES—Series: Regular, *The George Hamilton IV Show*, ABC, 1959; host, *Swinging Country*, NBC, 1966; host, *Hee Haw*, CBS, 1969-71, then syndicated, 1971-86. Pilots: Harvey, *Pioneer Spirit*, NBC, 1969; also *Star Search*, syndicated, 1983. Episodic: Mr. Bailey, *In the Heat of the Night*, NBC, 1988; also *Arthur Godfrey's Talent Scouts*, CBS, 1956; Roy, *The Beverly Hillbillies*, CBS; *The Nashville Palace*, NBC; *Hollywood Squares*, NBC; *The Jimmy Dean Show*. Specials: *Bing and Carol Burnett—Together Again for the First Time*, NBC, 1969; *Movin'*, CBS, 1970; *Sing Out, Sweet Land*, NBC, 1971; *Country Music Hit Parade*, CBS, 1975; *The Mac Davis Christmas Special*, NBC, 1975; *The Bob Hope Comedy Special*, NBC, 1976; *Jubilee*, NBC, 1976; *The Johnny Cash Christmas Special*, CBS, 1976; *Mitzi . . . Zings into Spring*, CBS, 1977; *The Johnny Cash Christmas Special*, CBS, 1977; *Kraft 75th Anniversary Special*, NBC, 1978; *Country Stars of the 70s*, NBC, 1979; *A Country Christmas*, CBS, 1979; *The Sensational, Shocking, Wonderful, Wacky 70s*, NBC, 1980; *Country Comes Home*, CBS, 1981; *Fifty*

Years of Country Music, NBC, 1981; *Country Galaxy of Stars*, syndicated, 1981; *A Country Christmas*, CBS, 1981; *USA Country Music*, HBO, 1982; *Disneyland's 30th Anniversary Celebration*, ABC, 1985; *Life's Most Embarrasing Moments*, NBC, 1986; *The Hee Haw 20th Anniversary Show*, syndicated, 1988.

RELATED CAREER—As a singer and musician, has appeared in concert halls throughout the world; also partner, Jim Halsey Proper-ties/Halark Music Publishing Company; board of directors and vice-president, American Entertainment Corporation.

NON-RELATED CAREER—Part owner, Tulsa Drillers (baseball team).

RECORDINGS: ALBUMS—*Back to the Country*, MCA; *Classic Clark*, Dot; *Do You Believe This?*, Dot; *The Entertainer*, Dot; *Entertainer of the Year*, Capitol; *Everlovin' Soul*, Dot; *Family and Friends*, Dot; *Greatest Hits—Volume 1*, MCA; *Guitar Spectacu-lar*, Capitol; *Heart to Heart*, MCA; *Hockin' It*, MCA; *I Never Picked Cotton*, Dot; *In Concert*, MCA; *Incredible*, Dot; *Lightening Fingers of Roy Clark*, Capitol; *Live!*, Dot; *Live with Me*, Dot; *Magnificent Sanctuary Band*, Dot; *The Other Side of Roy Clark*, Dot; *Pair of Fives*, Dot; *Roy Clark Country*, Dot; *Roy Clark Sings Gospel*, Word; *Silver Threads and Golden Needles*, Hilltop; *Sin-cerely Yours*, Paramount; *So Much to Remember*, Capitol; *Superpicker*, MCA; *Take Me As I Am*, Hilltop; *Urban, Suburban*, Dot; *Yesterday When I Was Young*, Dot.

SINGLES—"The Tip of My Fingers," Capitol, 1963; "Yesterday When I Was Young," Dot, 1969; "I Never Picked Cotton," Dot, 1970; "Thank God and Go Greyhound," Dot, 1970; "A Simple Thing Called Love," Dot, 1971; "Magnificent Sanctuary Band," Dot, 1971; "The Lawrence Welk Counter Revolutionary Polka," Dot, 1972; "Come Live with Me," Dot, 1973; "Honeymoon Feeling," Dot, 1974; "Somewhere Between Love and Tomor-row," Dot, 1974; "If I Had to Do It All Over Again," Dot, 1976.

AWARDS: Entertainer of the Year Award from the Country Music Association, 1973; Entertainer of the Year Award from the Acade-my of Country Music, 1974; Guitarist of the Year Award from *Player* magazine, 1978; Instrumentalist of the Year awards from the Country Music Association, 1978 and 1980. Honorary degrees: Doctor of Humane Letters, Baker University, 1978.

MEMBER: American Federation of Television and Radio Artists, American Society of Composers, Authors, and Publishers, Ameri-can Country Music Association.

ADDRESSES: OFFICE—Jim Halsey Company, Inc., 3225 S. Norwood Avenue, Tulsa, OK, 74135.*

*   *   *

COBB, Randall "Tex"

VOCATION: Actor.

CAREER: PRINCIPAL FILM APPEARANCES—Bowers, *The Champ*, Metro-Goldwyn-Mayer/United Artists, 1979; sailor, *Uncommon Valor*, Paramount, 1983; Til, *The Golden Child*, Paramount, 1986; Leonard Smalls, *Raising Arizona*, Twentieth Century-Fox, 1987; Box, *Critical Condition*, Paramount, 1987; Zach, *Police Academy 4: Citizens on Patrol*, Warner Brothers, 1987; Wolf, *Buy and Cell*,

Empire, 1988; Ben Dover, *Fletch Lives,* Universal, 1989. Also appeared in *Blind Fury.*

PRINCIPAL TELEVISION APPEARANCES—Pilots: R.E. Packard, *Braker,* ABC, 1985; Willard Singleton, *Code of Vengeance,* NBC, 1985. Episodic: Dennis ''Corky'' Conklyn, *Hardcastle and Mc-Cormick,* ABC, 1985; Willard Singleton, *Dalton's Code of Vengeance* (two episodes), NBC, 1986; ''Moon'' McAllister, *Miami Vice,* NBC, 1987; Cyrus Litt, *Frank's Place,* CBS, 1987; ''Earthquake'' Toberman, *MacGyver,* ABC, 1988. Movies: Eric ''Swede'' Wallan, *The Dirty Dozen: The Deadly Mission,* NBC, 1987.

NON-RELATED CAREER—Professional boxer; competed in WBC Heavyweight Championship, 1982, and PKA Heavyweight Championship, 1984.

ADDRESSES: AGENT—Merritt Blake, Camden Artists, 2121 Avenue of the Stars, Suite 410, Los Angeles, CA 90067.*

*   *   *

COEN, Ethan   1958-
(Roderick James, a joint pseudonym)

PERSONAL: Born in 1958 in St. Louis Park, MN. EDUCATION: Attended Princeton University.

VOCATION: Producer and screenwriter.

CAREER: Also see *WRITINGS* below. PRINCIPAL FILM WORK—Producer and editor (with Joel Cohen, under the joint pseudonym Roderick James), *Blood Simple,* Circle, 1984; producer, *Raising Arizona,* Twentieth Century-Fox, 1987.

WRITINGS: FILM—(With Joel Coen) *Blood Simple,* Circle, 1984; (with Joel Coen and Sam Raimi) *Crimewave* (also known as *The XYZ Murders* and *Broken Hearts and Noses*), Embassy, 1985; (with Joel Coen) *Raising Arizona,* Twentieth Century-Fox, 1987.

ADDRESSES: AGENT—Jim Berkus, Leading Artists Agency, 445 N. Bedford Drive, Penthouse, Beverly Hills, CA 90210.*

*   *   *

COEN, Joel   1955-
(Roderick James, a joint pseudonym)

PERSONAL: Born in 1955 in St. Louis Park, MN. EDUCATION: Attended Simon's Rock College; studied film at New York University.

VOCATION: Director, film editor, and screenwriter.

CAREER: Also see *WRITINGS* below. PRINCIPAL FILM APPEARANCES—Security guard, *Spies Like Us,* Warner Brothers, 1985. PRINCIPAL FILM WORK—Assistant editor, *The Evil Dead,* New Line Cinema, 1980; assistant editor, *Fear No Evil,* AVCO-Embassy, 1981; director and editor (with Ethan Coen, under the joint pseudonym Roderick James), *Blood Simple,* Circle, 1984; director, *Raising Arizona,* Twentieth Century-Fox, 1987.

WRITINGS: FILM—(With Ethan Coen) *Blood Simple,* Circle,

1984; (with Ethan Coen and Sam Raimi) *Crimewave* (also known as *The XYZ Murders* and *Broken Hearts and Noses*), Embassy, 1985; (with Ethan Coen) *Raising Arizona,* Twentieth Century-Fox, 1987.

ADDRESSES: AGENT—Jim Berkus, Leading Artists Agency, 445 N. Bedford Drive, Penthouse, Beverly Hills, CA 90210.*

*   *   *

COHEN, Larry   1947-

PERSONAL: Born April 20, 1947, in Chicago, IL. EDUCATION: Attended the University of Wisconsin.

VOCATION: Director, producer, and writer.

CAREER: Also see *WRITINGS* below. PRINCIPAL STAGE WORK—Director, *Trick,* Playhouse Theatre, New York City, 1979.

PRINCIPAL FILM APPEARANCES—Ace Tomato agent, *Spies Like Us,* Warner Brothers, 1985. PRINCIPAL FILM WORK—All as director, unless indicated: *Bone,* Jack H. Harris Enterprises, 1972; (also producer) *Black Caesar,* American International, 1973; (also producer) *Hell up in Harlem,* American International, 1973; (also producer) *It's Alive,* Warner Brothers, 1974; (also producer) *God Told Me To* (also known as *Demon*), New World, 1976; (also producer) *It Lives Again* (also known as *It's Alive II*), Warner Brothers, 1978; (also producer) *The Private Files of J. Edgar Hoover,* American International, 1978; (also producer) *Full Moon High,* Filmways, 1982; (also producer) *Q* (also known as *The Winged Serpent*), United Film Distribution, 1982; *Special Effects,* New Line Cinema, 1984; (also producer) *Perfect Strangers* (also known as *Blind Alley*), New Line Cinema, 1984; (also executive producer) *The Stuff,* New World Cinema, 1985; (with William Tanne) *Deadly Illusion,* Cinetel, 1987; (also producer) *It's Alive III: Island of the Alive,* Warner Brothers, 1987; (also executive producer) *A Return to Salem's Lot,* Warner Brothers, 1987; producer, *Maniac Cop,* Shapiro/Glickenhaus Entertainment, 1988; (also executive producer) *Wicked Stepmother,* Metro-Goldwyn-Mayer-United Artists, 1989.

WRITINGS: See production details above, unless indicated. STAGE—*Trick,* 1979; *Washington Heights,* Jewish Repertory Theatre, New York City, 1988.

FILM—*I Deal in Danger,* Twentieth Century-Fox, 1966; *Return of the Seven,* United Artists, 1966; *Daddy's Gone A-Hunting,* National General, 1969; (with Steven Carabatsos) *El Condor,* National General, 1970; *Black Caesar,* 1973; *Hell Up in Harlem,* 1973; *It's Alive,* 1974; *God Told Me To,* 1976; *It Lives Again,* 1978; *The Private Files of J. Edgar Hoover,* 1978; (with William Richert) *The American Success Company,* Columbia, 1980; *Full Moon High,* 1982; *I, the Jury,* Twentieth Century-Fox, 1982; *Q,* 1982; *Special Effects,* 1984; *Perfect Strangers,* 1984; (story, with John Byrum) *Scandalous,* Orion, 1984; *The Stuff,* 1985; *Best Seller,* Orion, 1987; (with William Tanne) *Deadly Illusion,* 1987; *It's Alive III: Island of the Alive,* 1987; (co-writer) *A Return to Salem's Lot,* 1987; *Maniac Cop,* 1988; *Wicked Stepmother,* 1989.

TELEVISION—Pilots: *Man on the Outside,* ABC, 1975. Movies: *In Broad Daylight,* ABC, 1971; *Cool Million,* NBC, 1972; (with Dick Nelson) *Shootout in a One-Dog Town,* ABC, 1974; (story, with Mark Rodgers) *Women of San Quentin,* NBC, 1983; *Desperado:*

Avalanche at Devil's Ridge (also known as *Desperado: Avalanche*), NBC, 1988.

ADDRESSES: ATTORNEY—Skip Brittenham, 2049 Century Park E., Los Angeles, CA 90067.*

*   *   *

COLIN, Margaret   1957-

PERSONAL: Born in 1957 in New York, NY; married Justin Deas (an actor). EDUCATION: Attended Hofstra University.

VOCATION: Actress.

CAREER: PRINCIPAL STAGE APPEARANCES—Debbie, "House" in *Marathon '84*, Ensemble Studio Theatre, New York City, 1984; Tina, *Planet Fires*, GeVa Theatre, Rochester, NY, 1985; Alice, *Aristocrats*, Manhattan Theatre Club, Theatre Four, New York City, 1989.

PRINCIPAL FILM APPEARANCES—English teacher, *Pretty in Pink*, Paramount, 1986; Irene, *Something Wild*, Orion, 1986; Ginnie Armbruster, *Like Father, Like Son*, Tri-Star, 1987; Rebecca, *Three Men and a Baby*, Buena Vista, 1987; Kitty Greer, *True Believer*, Columbia, 1989.

PRINCIPAL TELEVISION APPEARANCES—Series: Assistant District Attorney Alex Harrigan, *Foley Square*, CBS, 1985-86; Claire McCarron, *Leg Work*, CBS, 1987; also Paige Madison, *The Edge of Night*, ABC; Margo, *As the World Turns*, CBS. Pilots: Claire McCarron, *Leg Work*, CBS, 1987. Episodic: *Magnum, P.I.*, CBS, 1988. Movies: Jane Watson, *The Return of Sherlock Holmes*, CBS, 1987; Amy, *Warm Hearts, Cold Feet*, CBS, 1987.

MEMBER: Actors' Equity Association, Screen Actors Guild, American Federation of Television and Radio Artists.

ADDRESSES: AGENT—Dick Berman, The Agency, 10351 Santa Monica Boulevard, Suite 211, Los Angeles, CA 90025.*

*   *   *

CONNELLY, Christopher   1941-1988

PERSONAL: Born September 8, 1941, in Wichita, KS; died of cancer, December 7, 1988, in Burbank, CA; children: two sons. EDUCATION: Attended Regis College; studied acting at the Pasadena Playhouse.

VOCATION: Actor.

CAREER: PRINCIPAL FILM APPEARANCES—Executive seaman, *Move Over, Darling*, Twentieth Century-Fox, 1963; John the cop, *They Only Kill Their Masters*, Metro-Goldwyn-Mayer (MGM), 1972; Billy, *Corky* (also known as *Lookin' Good*), MGM, 1972; Henry, *Benji*, Mulberry Square, 1974; Uriah Tibbs, *Hawmps!*, Mulberry Square, 1976; Rolf, *The Norseman*, American International, 1978; Zef, *Earthbound*, Taft International, 1981; Hot Dog, *1990 i guerrieri del Bronx* (also known as *1990: The Bronx Warriors*), United Film Distribution Company, 1982; Mrs. King's

man, *Strikebound*, Mainline, 1983; Captain Yankee, *Jungle Raiders* (also known as *La legenda del Rudio Malese* and *Captain Yankee*), Cannon, 1986; Professor George Hacker, *L'occhio del male* (also known as *Possessed* and *Manhattan Baby*), Fulvia, 1986; John Thomas, *Foxtrap*, Snizzlefritz, 1986; Colonel Radek, *Strike Commando*, Flora, 1987; FBI Agent Parker, *The Messenger*, Snizzlefritz, 1987. Also appeared in *Liar's Moon*, Crown International, 1982; *Raiders of Atlantis*, 1983; *Cobra Mission* (also known as *The Rainbow Professional*), VIP-Delta, 1986; and *Le miniere del Kilimangiaro* (also known as *The Mines of Kilimanjaro*), Filmexport Group, 1986.

PRINCIPAL TELEVISION APPEARANCES—Series: Norman Harrington, *Peyton Place*, ABC, 1964-69; Moses Pray, *Paper Moon*, ABC, 1974-75. Mini-Series: Ben Driscoll, *The Martian Chronicles*, NBC, 1980. Pilots: Jeff Marshall, *Incident in San Francisco*, ABC, 1971; Waco, *Charlie Cobb: Nice Night for a Hanging*, NBC, 1977; Hill Singleton, *Stunt Seven*, CBS, 1979; Steve Ward, *Skyward Christmas*, NBC, 1981. Episodic: Saint John Hawke, *Airwolf*, CBS, 1984; also Taylor, *Eight Is Enough*, ABC; *The Lieutenant*, NBC; *Voyage to the Bottom of the Sea*, ABC; *The Eleventh Hour*, NBC; *Sam Benedict*, NBC; *Mr. Novak*, NBC; *Gunsmoke*, CBS; *Police Story*, NBC; *My Three Sons*; *Alfred Hitchcock Presents*. Movies: Tony Caruso, *In Name Only*, ABC, 1969; Dick Broadwell, *The Last Day*, NBC, 1975; Mark Twain, *The Incredible Rocky Mountain Race*, NBC, 1977; Norman Harrington, *Murder in Peyton Place*, NBC, 1977; Mike Tagliarino, *Crash*, ABC, 1978; Jay Arnold Wayne, *Return of the Rebels*, CBS, 1981; Norman Harrington, *Peyton Place: The Next Generation*, NBC, 1985.

OBITUARIES AND OTHER SOURCES: Variety, December 14-20, 1988.*

*   *   *

CONVERSE-ROBERTS, William

VOCATION: Actor.

CAREER: PRINCIPAL STAGE APPEARANCES—Lycaste, "The Forced Marriage," Lelie, "Sganarelle," and ensemble, "A Dumb Show," all in *Sganarelle: An Evening of Moliere Farces*, New York Shakespeare Festival (NYSF), Public Theatre, New York City, 1978; Victor Frankenstein, *Frankenstein*, Palace Theatre, New York City, 1981; Bryan, *The Chisholm Trail Went Through Here*, Manhattan Theatre Club In-the-Works, Upstage Theatre, New York City, 1981; John, *Monday after the Miracle*, Eugene O'Neill Theatre, New York City, 1982; Eugene, *Lumiere*, Ark Theatre Company, Ark Theatre, New York City, 1983; Don Kane, *Buried Inside Extra*, NYSF, Public Theatre, 1983; Henry David Thoreau and George Armstrong Custer, *Romance Language*, Playwrights Horizons, New York City, 1984; Frank Gardner, *Mrs. Warren's Profession*, Roundabout Theatre, New York City, 1985; Willie, *Walk the Dog, Willie*, Production Company, New York City, 1985; Berowne, *Love's Labor's Lost*, NYSF, Public Theatre, 1989. Also appeared in *Romeo and Juliet* and *As You Like It*, both Dallas Shakespeare Festival, Dallas, TX, 1981; and in *The Common Pursuit*, Long Wharf Theatre, New Haven, CT, 1984.

PRINCIPAL FILM APPEARANCES—Horace Robedaux, *1918*, Cinecom International, 1985; Horace Robedaux, *On Valentine's Day*, Cinecom International, 1986.

PRINCIPAL TELEVISION APPEARANCES—Series: Fred C. Dodd, *The Days and Nights of Molly Dodd*, NBC, 1986-88, then Lifetime, 1989—. Pilots: Artist, *Private Sessions*, NBC, 1985. Episodic: Horace Robedaux, "Story of a Marriage Courtship," *American Playhouse*, PBS, 1987; Harry, "The Fig Tree," *Wonderworks*, PBS, 1987; Will Rattigan, *The Equalizer*, CBS, 1987; Steve Altman, *Crime Story* (two episodes), NBC, 1987; Clay Roper, *Spenser: For Hire*, ABC, 1987; John Kelly, *The Equalizer*, CBS, 1989. Movies: Stephen Hopkins, *Mayflower: The Pilgrim's Adventure*, CBS, 1979; Max, *Stone Pillow*, CBS, 1985.

ADDRESSES: AGENT—Jonathan Howard, 10100 Santa Monica Boulevard, 16th Floor, Los Angeles, CA 90067.*

*   *   *

COOPER, Chris 1951-

PERSONAL: Full name, Christopher W. Cooper; born July 9, 1951, in Kansas City, MO; father, an Air Force doctor and rancher; married Marianne Leone (a writer, actress, and comedienne), 1985. EDUCATION: Graduated from the University of Missouri. MILITARY: National Guard Reserves.

VOCATION: Actor.

CAREER: BROADWAY DEBUT—Ben Mercer, *Of the Fields, Lately*, Century Theatre, 1980. PRINCIPAL STAGE APPEARANCES—Tyler Biars, *A Different Moon*, WPA Theatre, New York City, 1983; Paul Anthony MacAleer, *The Ballad of Soapy Smith*, Seattle Repertory Theatre, Seattle, WA, 1983, then New York Shakespeare Festival, Public Theatre, New York City, 1984; Ty, *Cobb*, Yale Repertory Theatre, New Haven, CT, 1989. Also appeared as Stuff, *Sweet Bird of Youth*, London, 1985; and with the Actors Theatre of Louisville, Louisville, KY, 1980-81.

PRINCIPAL FILM APPEARANCES—Joe Kenehan, *Matewan*, Cinecom, 1987; also appeared in *Bad Timing* (also known as *A Sexual Obsession* and *Bad Timing: A Sexual Obsession*), Rank, 1980; and *Undertow*.

PRINCIPAL TELEVISION APPEARANCES—Series: Sam Cranshaw, *The Edge of Night*, ABC. Mini-Series: July Johnson, *Lonesome Dove*, CBS, 1989. Episodic: Michael, *The Equalizer*, CBS, 1987; Yagovitch, *Miami Vice*, NBC, 1988; Louis Halliday, "Journey into Genius," *American Playhouse*, PBS, 1988.

RELATED CAREER—Set builder and designer for community theatre.

NON-RELATED CAREER—Janitor, carpenter, and construction worker.

ADDRESSES: AGENT—Katy Rothacker, William Morris Agency, 1350 Avenue of the Americas, New York, NY 10019.*

COPELAND, Joan 1922-

PERSONAL: Born Joan Maxine Miller, June 1, 1922, in New York, NY; daughter of Isidore (a women's clothing manufacturer) and Augusta (Barnett) Miller; married George J. Kupchik (an engineer); children: Eric. EDUCATION: Attended Brooklyn College; trained for the stage at the American Academy of Dramatic Arts and the Actors Studio; studied voice with Jack Harrold and John Wallowitch.

VOCATION: Actress and singer.

CAREER: STAGE DEBUT—Juliet, *Romeo and Juliet*, Brooklyn Academy of Music, Brooklyn, NY, 1945. BROADWAY DEBUT—Nadine, *Sundown Beach*, Belasco Theatre, 1948. PRINCIPAL STAGE APPEARANCES—Desdemona, *Othello*, Equity Library Theatre, New York City, 1946; title role, *Claudia*, Hempstead Summer Theatre, Hempstead, NY, 1946; Susan Carmichael, *The Detective Story*, Hudson Theatre, New York City, 1949; Evangeline Orth, *Not for Children*, Coronet Theatre, New York City, 1951; Ann Deever, *All My Sons*, Robin Hood Theatre, Arden, DE, 1953; Betty Shapiro, *The Grass Is Always Greener*, and Elise, *The Miser*, both Downtown National Theatre, New York City, 1955; Melanie, *Conversation Piece*, Barbizon-Plaza Theatre, New York City, 1957; Maria, *Handful of Fire*, Martin Beck Theatre, New York City, 1958; Raina, *Arms and the Man*, Westport Country Playhouse, Westport, CT, 1959; Mrs. Erlynne, *Delightful Season*, Gramercy Arts Theatre, New York City, 1960; Tatiana, *Tovarich*, Winter Garden Theatre, New York City, 1963; Marchesa Valentina Crespi, *Something More!*, Eugene O'Neill Theatre, New York City, 1964; Esther Franz, *The Price*, Morosco Theatre, New York City, 1968.

Esther, *Two by Two*, Imperial Theatre, New York City, 1970; Leonie Frothingham, *End of Summer*, Manhattan Theatre Club, New York City, 1974; Vera, *Pal Joey*, Circle in the Square, New York City, 1976; Florence Grayson, *Checking Out*, Longacre Theatre, New York City, 1976; Lillian Hellman, *Are You Now or Have You Ever Been?*, Promenade Theatre, New York City, 1978; title role, *Candida*, Roundabout Theatre, New York City, 1979; Rose Baum, *The American Clock*, Biltmore Theatre, New York City, 1980; Esther Franz, *The Price*, American Jewish Theatre, 92nd Street YM-YWHA, New York City, 1981; Tasha Blumberg, *Isn't It Romantic?*, Playwrights Horizons, New York City, 1983, then Lucille Lortel Theatre, New York City, 1984; Mrs. Thompson, *Hunting Cockroaches*, Manhattan Theatre Club, 1987. Also appeared in *The Servant of Two Masters*, Equity Library Theatre, 1946; *How I Wonder*, Hudson Theatre, 1947; *There's Always Juliet*, Equity Library Theatre, 1947; *The Tender Trap*, Longacre Theatre, 1954; *The Diary of Anne Frank*, Cort Theatre, New York City, 1955; *Coco*, Mark Hellinger Theatre, New York City, 1969; and *Mame*, 1979.

MAJOR TOURS—Eliza Doolittle, *My Fair Lady*, U.S. cities, 1964; Kate, *Brighton Beach Memoirs*, U.S. cities, 1983.

FILM DEBUT—Aunt, *The Goddess*, Columbia, 1958. PRINCIPAL FILM APPEARANCES—Lillian Kingsley, *Middle of the Night*, Columbia, 1959; Pauline, *Roseland*, Cinema Shares International, 1977; Rita, *It's My Turn*, Columbia, 1980; Mrs. Harrison, *A Little Sex*, Universal, 1982; Sunny, *Happy New Year*, Columbia, 1987; Ruth Weiss, *The Laser Man*, ADN Associates, 1987.

PRINCIPAL TELEVISION APPEARANCES—Series: Maggie Porter, *Love of Life*, CBS; Andrea Whiting, *Search for Tomorrow*, CBS.

Pilots: Mrs. Friedlander, *Cagney and Lacey,* CBS, 1981; Marion, "Baby on Board," *CBS Summer Playhouse,* CBS, 1988. Episodic: Cora, "The Iceman Cometh," *Play of the Week,* WNTA-TV; also "New Year's Wedding," *All in the Family,* CBS, 1976; *Nurse,* NBC; *As the World Turns,* CBS; and *One Life to Live,* ABC. Movies: Monica Courtland, *How to Survive a Marriage,* NBC, 1974. Specials: *Kennedy Center Honors: A Celebration of the Performing Arts,* CBS, 1984.

RELATED CAREER—Charter member, Actors Studio, 1947—; appeared as a singer in cabaret at Upstairs at the Duplex and The Showcase, both New York City, 1963, and in concert at Town Hall, New York City, 1964; concert pianist.

NON-RELATED CAREER—Secretary.

AWARDS: Drama Desk Award nomination, Outstanding Actress in a Musical, 1976, for *Pal Joey;* Drama Desk Award, Best Leading Actress in a Play, 1981, for *The American Clock;* Hollywood Drama Critics Award and Los Angeles Drama Critics Award, both 1984, for *Brighton Beach Memoirs.*

MEMBER: Actors' Equity Association, Screen Actors Guild, American Federation of Television and Radio Artists.

SIDELIGHTS: FAVORITE ROLES—Eliza Doolittle in *My Fair Lady,* Melanie in *Conversation Piece,* and Vera in *Pal Joey.* RECREATIONS—Tennis, sewing, piano, swimming, and snorkeling.

ADDRESSES: HOME—88 Central Park W., New York, NY 10023.*

* * *

COPPERFIELD, David   1957-

PERSONAL: Born David Kotkin, 1957 (some sources say 1956) in Metuchen, NJ. EDUCATION: Attended Fordham University.

VOCATION: Magician, producer, and director.

CAREER: PRINCIPAL STAGE APPEARANCES—Illusionist, *The Magic Man,* First Chicago Center, Chicago, IL, 1974.

PRINCIPAL FILM APPEARANCES—The Magician, *Terror Train* (also known as *Train of Terror*), Twentieth Century-Fox, 1980.

PRINCIPAL TELEVISION APPEARANCES—Specials: Host, *The Magic of David Copperfield,* CBS, 1981; *The All Star Salute to Mother's Day,* NBC, 1981; *Magic with the Stars,* NBC, 1982; host, *The Magic of David Copperfield,* CBS, 1983; Dave, *Mr. T and Emmanuel Lewis in a Christmas Dream,* NBC, 1984; host, *The Magic of David Copperfield,* CBS, 1984; *The Magic of David Copperfield,* CBS, 1985; *Kraft Salutes the Magic of David Copperfield . . . In China,* CBS, 1986; *All-Star Gala at Ford's Theatre,* ABC, 1987; *Kraft Salutes the Magic of David Copperfield IX: The Escape from Alcatraz,* CBS, 1987; host, *The Magic of David Copperfield X: The Bermuda Triangle,* CBS, 1988; judge, *Super Model Search: Look of the Year,* ABC, 1988; host, *The Magic of David Copperfield XI: The Explosive Encounter,* CBS, 1989.

PRINCIPAL TELEVISION WORK—Specials: Producer and director, *The Magic of David Copperfield,* CBS, 1981; producer, *Magic with the Stars,* NBC, 1982; director, *The Magic of David Copperfield,* CBS, 1983; director (with Jeff Margolis), *The Magic of David Copperfield,* CBS, 1984; director, *The Magic of David Copperfield,* CBS, 1985; director, *Kraft Salutes the Magic of David Copperfield . . . In China,* CBS, 1986; executive producer, co-producer, and co-director, *Kraft Salutes the Magic of David Copperfield IX: The Escape from Alcatraz,* CBS, 1987; executive producer and director, *The Magic of David Copperfield X: The Bermuda Triangle,* CBS, 1988; executive producer, *The Magic of David Copperfield XI: The Explosive Encounter,* CBS, 1989.

RELATED CAREER—Instructor of magic, New York University, 1972; founder, Project Magic, 1982.

ADDRESSES: PUBLICIST—Michael Sterling Company, 455 Leftmount Drive, Angeles, CA 90048.*

*   *   *

COPPOLA, Carmine   1910-

PERSONAL: Born June 11, 1910, in New York, NY; son of August and Maria (Zasa) Coppola; married Italia Pennino, April 30, 1934; children: August, Francis Ford, Talia. EDUCATION: Studied flute and composition at the Juilliard School of Music, 1933; Manhattan School of Music, Mus.M., 1950.

VOCATION: Composer, conductor, and musician.

CAREER: Also see *WRITINGS* below. PRINCIPAL STAGE WORK—Musician in pit orchestra, *The Great Waltz,* Center Theatre, New York City, 1934; *Kismet,* Ziegfeld Theatre, New York City, 1953; *La Plume de Ma Tante,* Royale Theatre, New York City, 1958; *Once Upon a Mattress,* Phoenix Theatre, New York City, 1959; *Stop the World—I Want to Get Off,* Shubert Theatre, New York City, 1962; *110 in the Shake,* Broadhurst Theatre, New York City, 1963.

PRINCIPAL FILM APPEARANCES—Conductor, *Harry and Walter Go to New York,* Columbia, 1976; (with Italia Coppola) couple in elevator, *One from the Heart,* Columbia, 1982; street musician, "Life Without Zoe," *New York Stories,* Touchstone, 1989. PRINCIPAL FILM WORK—Music director, *The Godfather, Part II,* Paramount, 1974; conductor of live orchestral performance, *Napoleon,* Metro-Goldwyn-Mayer, 1980.

RELATED CAREER—Orchestra musician, Radio City Music Hall, during the 1930s; member of musical staff at WTIC, Hartford, CT; first flutist, Detroit Symphony, Detroit, MI; musician, NBC Symphony Orchestra; music director, Los Angeles Civic Opera; music director, Merrick Productions.

WRITINGS: All as composer of musical score. STAGE—*Escorial* (opera), 1979. FILM—(With Nino Rota) *The Godfather, Part II,* Paramount, 1974; (also songwriter) *Mustang . . . The House That Joe Built,* United Artists, 1975; *Apocalypse Now,* United Artists, 1979; *The Black Stallion,* United Artists, 1979; (score for restored version) *Napoleon,* Metro-Goldwyn-Mayer (originally released in 1927), 1980; *The Outsiders,* Warner Brothers, 1983; *Gardens of Stone,* Tri-Star, 1987; "Life without Zoe," *New York Stories,* Touchstone, 1989; also *Tonight for Sure,* 1980. TELEVISION—

Movies: *The People,* ABC, 1972; *The Last Day,* NBC, 1975; also *Rip Van Wrinkle,* 1987.

AWARDS: Academy Award, Best Musical Score, 1975, for *The Godfather, Part II;* Arts and Letters Medal of France, 1985; California Arts Council grant.

MEMBER: American Society of Composers, Authors, and Publishers, Academy of Motion Picture Arts and Sciences, Beta Gamma.

*   *   *

CORMAN, Roger   1926-

PERSONAL: Full name, Roger William Corman; born April 5, 1926, in Detroit, MI; son of William (an engineer) Corman; married Julie Halloran (a film producer), 1969; children: Catherine Ann, Roger Martin, Brian, Mary. EDUCATION: Stanford University, B.S., industrial engineering, 1947; graduate work, Oxford University, 1950. MILITARY: U.S. Navy, 1944.

VOCATION: Director, producer, and film executive.

CAREER: PRINCIPAL FILM APPEARANCES—Technician, *War of the Satellites,* Allied Artists, 1958; senator, *The Godfather, Part II,* Paramount, 1974; lawyer, *The State of Things,* Artificial Eye, 1983; Mr. MacBride, *Swing Shift,* Warner Brothers, 1984. Also appeared in *The Wasp Woman,* Allied Artists, 1959; *The Last Woman on Earth,* Filmgroup, 1960; *Ski Troop Attack,* Filmgroup,

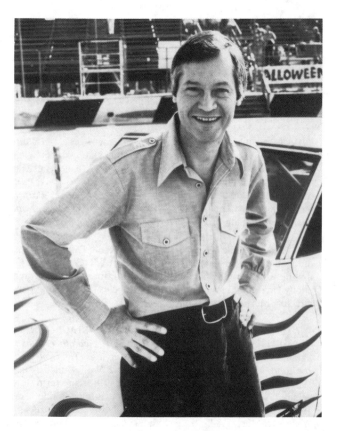

ROGER CORMAN

1960; *Creature from the Haunted Sea,* Filmgroup, 1961; *The Little Shop of Horrors,* Filmgroup, 1961; *The Young Racers,* American International, 1963; *Cannonball* (also known as *Carquake*), New World, 1976; *Roger Corman: Hollywood's Wild Angel* (documentary), 1978; and *The Howling,* AVCO-Embassy, 1981.

FIRST FILM WORK—Associate producer, *Highway Dragnet,* Allied Artists, 1954. PRINCIPAL FILM WORK—Producer, *The Fast and the Furious,* American Releasing, 1954; producer, *The Monster from the Ocean Floor* (also known as *It Stalked the Ocean Floor* and *Monster Maker*), Lippert, 1954; executive producer, *The Beast with a Million Eyes,* American Releasing, 1955; producer and director, *Apache Woman,* Associated Releasing, 1955; producer and director, *Five Guns West,* American Releasing, 1955; producer and director, *The Day the World Ended,* American International, 1956; producer and director, *Gunslinger,* Associated Releasing, 1956; producer and director, *It Conquered the World,* American International, 1956; producer and director, *The Oklahoma Woman,* American Releasing, 1956; producer and director, *Swamp Woman* (also known as *Swamp Diamonds* and *Cruel Swamp*), Favorite Films of California, 1956; producer and director, *Attack of the Crab Monsters,* Allied Artists, 1957; producer and director, *Carnival Rock,* Howco, 1957; producer and director, *Naked Paradise* (also known as *Thunder Over Hawaii*), American International, 1957; producer and director, *Not of This Earth,* Allied Artists, 1957; producer and director, *Rock All Night,* American International, 1957; producer and director, *The Saga of the Viking Women and Their Voyage to the Waters of the Great Sea Serpent* (also known as *The Viking Women and the Sea Serpent*), American International, 1957; producer and director, *Sorority Girl* (also known as *The Bad One* and *Confessions of a Sorority Girl*), American International, 1957; producer and director, *Teenage Doll* (also known as *The Young Rebels*), Allied Artists, 1957; producer and director, *The Undead,* American International, 1957.

Producer and director, *Machine Gun Kelly,* American International, 1958; producer and director, *She-Gods of Shark Reef* (also known as *Shark Reef*), American International, 1958; producer and director, *Teenage Caveman* (also known as *Out of the Darkness* and *Prehistoric World*), American International, 1958; producer (with Jack Rabin and Irving Block) and director, *War of the Satellites,* Allied Artists, 1958; executive producer, *Stake Out on Dope Street,* Warner Brothers, 1958; executive producer, *The Cry Baby Killer,* Allied Artists, 1958; executive producer, *Hot Car Girl,* Allied Artists, 1958; executive producer, *Night of the Blood Beast,* American International, 1958; executive producer, *The Brain Eaters,* American International, 1958; executive producer, *Paratroop Command,* American International, 1958; executive producer, *The Wild Ride,* Filmgroup, 1958; producer and director, *A Bucket of Blood,* American International, 1959; producer (with Edward L. Alperson and Gene Corman) and director, *I, Mobster* (also known as *The Mobster*), Twentieth Century-Fox, 1959; producer, *T-Bird Gang* (also known as *The Pay-Off*), Filmgroup, 1959; producer and director, *The Wasp Woman,* Allied Artists, 1959; executive producer, *Tank Commandos* (also known as *Tank Commando*), American International, 1959; executive producer, *Crime and Punishment U.S.A.,* Allied Artists, 1959; executive producer, *High School Big Shot* (also known as *The Young Sinners*), Filmgroup, 1959; executive producer, *Attack of the Giant Leeches* (also known as *The Giant Leeches* and *Demons of the Swamp*), American International, 1959.

Producer and director, *Atlas,* Filmgroup, 1960; producer and director, *The House of Usher* (also known as *The Fall of the House of Usher*), American International, 1960; producer and director, *The Last Woman on Earth,* Filmgroup, 1960; producer and director, *Ski*

Troop Attack, Filmgroup, 1960; executive producer, *Beast from the Haunted Cave*, Filmgroup, 1960; executive producer, *Battle of Blood Island*, Filmgroup, 1960; producer and director, *Creature from the Haunted Sea*, Filmgroup, 1961; producer and director, *The Little Shop of Horrors*, Filmgroup, 1961; producer and director, *The Pit and the Pendulum*, American International, 1961; executive producer, *Night Tide*, American International, 1961; executive producer, *The Mermaids of Tiburon* (also known as *The Aqua Sex*), Filmgroup, 1961; producer and director, *The Intruder* (also known as *I Hate Your Guts, Shame,* and *The Stranger*), Pathe-America, 1962; producer and director, *The Premature Burial*, American International, 1962; producer and director, *Tower of London*, United Artists, 1962; executive producer, *The Magic Voyage of Sinbad*, Filmgroup, 1962; producer and director, *Tales of Terror* (also known as *Poe's Tales of Terror*), American International, 1962; producer and director, *"X"—The Man with the X-Ray Eyes* (also known as *The Man with the X-Ray Eyes* and *X*), American International, 1963; producer (with Charles Hannawalt and R. Wright Campbell), *Dementia 13* (also known as *The Haunted and the Hunted*), American International, 1963; producer and director, *The Haunted Palace*, American International, 1963; producer and director, *The Raven*, American International, 1963; producer and director, *The Terror* (also known as *Lady of the Shadows*), American International, 1963; producer and director, *The Young Racers*, American International, 1963; executive producer, *Battle Beyond the Sun*, American International, 1963; producer and director, *The Masque of the Red Death*, American International, 1964; producer and director, *The Secret Invasion*, United Artists, 1964.

Producer and director, *The Tomb of Ligeia* (also known as *Tomb of the Cat*), American International, 1965; executive producer, *The Girls on the Beach*, Paramount, 1965; executive producer, *Ski Party*, American International, 1965; executive producer, *Beach Ball*, Paramount, 1965; executive producer (uncredited), *The Shooting*, filmed in 1965, released by Proteus/Favorite Films, 1971; producer (with Norman D. Wells), *Voyage to the Planet of Prehistoric Women* (also known as *Gill Woman* and *Gill Women of Venus*), Filmgroup, 1966; producer and director, *The Wild Angels*, American International, 1966; executive producer, *Blood Bath* (also known as *Track of the Vampire*), American International, 1966; executive producer, *Queen of Blood* (also known as *Planet of Blood*), American International, 1966; executive producer (uncredited), *Ride in the Whirlwind*, Favorite Films/Jack H. Harris, 1966; producer and director, *The St. Valentine's Day Massacre*, Twentieth Century-Fox, 1967; producer and director, *The Trip*, American International, 1967; executive producer, *Targets*, Paramount, 1967; executive producer, *Devil's Angels*, American International, 1967; director (uncredited, with Phil Karlson), *A Time for Killing* (also known as *The Long Ride Home*), Columbia, 1967; executive producer, *Wild Racers*, American International, 1967; executive producer, *The Dunwich Horror*, American International, 1969; executive producer, *Naked Angels*, Crown International, 1969; executive producer, *Pit Stop*, Crown International, 1969; director (uncredited, with Cy Endfield) *De Sade*, American International-Transcontinental, 1969.

Producer and director, *Bloody Mama*, American International, 1970; producer and director, *Gas-s-s-s!* (also known as *Gas-s-s-s, or It Became Necessary to Destroy the World in Order to Save It*), American International, 1970; executive producer and director, *Von Richthofen and Brown* (also known as *The Red Baron*), United Artists, 1970; executive producer, *Paddy* (also known as *Goodbye to the Hill*), Allied Artists, 1970; executive producer, *Student Nurses*, New World, 1970; executive producer, *Angels Die Hard!*, New World, 1970; executive producer, *Angels Hard as They Come*,

New World, 1971; executive producer, *Private Duty Nurses*, New World, 1971; executive producer, *The Big Doll House*, New World, 1971; executive producer, *The Velvet Vampire* (also known as *Through the Looking Glass* and *Cemetery Girls*), New World, 1971; executive producer, *Women in Cages*, New World, 1971; producer, *Boxcar Bertha*, American International, 1972; executive producer, *The Big Bird Cage*, New World, 1972; executive producer, *The Unholy Rollers* (also known as *Leader of the Pack*), American International, 1972; executive producer, *Night Call Nurses*, New World, 1972; executive producer, *Fly Me*, New World, 1972; executive producer, *The Hot Box*, New World, 1972; executive producer, *Night of the Cobra Woman*, New World, 1972; executive producer, *The Final Comedown*, New World, 1972; producer (with Gene Corman), *I Escaped from Devil's Island*, United Artists, 1973; executive producer, *The Young Nurses*, New World, 1973; executive producer, *The Arena*, New World, 1973; executive producer, *The Student Teachers*, New World, 1973; executive producer, *Tender Loving Care* (also known as *Naughty Nurses*), New World, 1973; producer, *Big Bad Mama*, New World, 1974; executive producer, *TNT Jackson*, New World, 1974; executive producer, *The Woman Hunt* (also known as *The Highest Bidder*), New World, 1974; executive producer, *Candy Stripe Nurses*, New World, 1974; executive producer, *Caged Heat* (also known as *Renegade Girls*), New World, 1974; executive producer, *Street Girls*, New World, 1974.

Producer (with Sam Gellman), *Born to Kill* (also known as *Cockfighter*), New World, 1975; producer, *Capone*, Twentieth Century-Fox, 1975; producer, *Death Race 2000*, New World, 1975; executive producer, *Summer School Teachers*, New World, 1975; executive producer, *Darktown Strutters* (also known as *Get Down and Boogie*), New World, 1975; executive producer, *Crazy Mama*, New World, 1975; executive producer, *Cover Girl Models*, New World, 1975; executive producer, *Cannonball* (also known as *Carquake*), New World, 1976; producer, *Eat My Dust*, New World, 1976; producer (with Evelyn Purcell), *Fighting Mad*, Twentieth Century-Fox, 1976; executive producer, *Hollywood Boulevard*, New World, 1976; executive producer, *Jackson County Jail*, New World, 1976; executive producer, *Nashville Girl* (also known as *New Girl in Town* and *Country Music Daughter*), New World, 1976; executive producer, *Moving Violation*, Twentieth Century-Fox, 1976; executive producer, *God Told Me To* (also known as *Demon*), New World, 1976; executive producer, *Dynamite Women* (also known as *The Great Texas Dynamite Chase*), New World, 1976; producer, *Thunder and Lightning*, Twentieth Century-Fox, 1977; producer, *I Never Promised You a Rose Garden*, New World, 1977; executive producer, *Black Oak Conspiracy*, New World, 1977; executive producer, *Grand Theft Auto*, New World, 1977; executive producer, *Moonshine County Express*, New World, 1977; executive producer, *Maniac* (also known as *Ransom, The Town That Cried Terror,* and *Assault on Paradise*), New World, 1977; executive producer, *A Hero Ain't Nothin' But a Sandwich*, New World, 1977; producer, *Avalanche*, New World, 1978; producer, *Deathsport*, New World, 1978; executive producer, *Piranha*, New World, 1978; executive producer, *The Bees*, New World, 1978; producer (with Saul Krugman), *Fast Charlie . . . The Moonbeam Rider* (also known as *Fast Charlie and the Moonbeam*), Universal, 1979; producer, *Saint Jack*, New World, 1979.

Executive producer, *Battle Beyond the Stars*, New World, 1980; producer (with Marc Siegler), *Galaxy of Terror* (also known as *Mindwarp, An Infinity of Terror,* and *Planet of Horrors*), New World, 1981; producer (with Gale Hurd), *Smokey Bites the Dust*, New World, 1981; producer (with Mary Ann Fisher), *Forbidden World* (also known as *Mutant*), New World, 1982; producer, *Love*

Letters (also known as *My Love Letters*), New World, 1983; producer, *Space Raiders* (also known as *Star Child*), New World, 1983; executive producer, *Barbarian Queen,* Concorde, 1985; executive producer, *Streetwalkin',* Concorde, 1985; producer (with Alex Sessa), *Cocaine Wars,* Concorde, 1986; producer, *Big Bad Mama II,* Concorde, 1986; producer (with Ginny Nugent), *Munchies,* Metro-Goldwyn-Mayer/United Artists, 1987; executive producer, *Stripped to Kill,* Concorde, 1987; producer, *The Drifter,* Concorde, 1988; producer, *Daddy's Boys,* Concorde, 1988. Also producer and director, *The Little Guy* (uncompleted), 1957; producer and director, *Reception* (uncompleted), 1957.

PRINCIPAL TELEVISION APPEARANCES—Specials: *The Horror of It All,* PBS, 1983.

PRINCIPAL TELEVISION WORK—Pilots: Executive producer, *The Georgia Peaches,* CBS, 1980. Movies: Executive producer, *Outside Chance,* CBS, 1978.

RELATED CAREER—Messenger, Twentieth Century-Fox, Hollywood, CA, 1948, then script reader, 1948-49; television stagehand; founder and president, Roger Corman Productions and Filmgroup; founder and president, New World Pictures, 1970-83; founder and president, Concorde-New Horizons Corporation (a film production and distribution company), 1983—.

NON-RELATED CAREER—Literary agent, 1951-52.

MEMBER: Producers Guild of America, Directors Guild of America.

SIDELIGHTS: As a producer and director for American International Pictures and founder of such production companies as New World and New Horizons, Roger Corman has been responsible for a long string of films which, although derided or virtually ignored by critics, have consistently found an audience for more than thirty years. Working outside the mainstream of the Hollywood film community, Corman's exploitation films have, according to Ed Lowry in *The International Dictionary of Films and Filmmakers,* cultivated the ''drive-in/inner city audience by developing specialized sub-genres (women's prison pictures; soft-core nurse/teacher films; hard-core action and horror movies) and a strict formula, requiring given amounts of violence, nudity, humor, and social commentary. The social element not only reflected Corman's own attitudes . . . but also an understanding of the politically disfranchised groups which comprised [his] audience.''

Although his films are notorious for their meagre budgets, Corman has been responsible for some of the earliest career work of directors Francis Ford Coppola, Martin Scorsese, Jonathan Demme, Peter Bogdanovich, and Ron Howard, screenwriters Robert Towne and John Sayles, and actors Jack Nicholson, Robert DeNiro, Bruce Dern, and Ellen Burstyn, as well as for the U.S. release of such acclaimed foreign films as Ingmar Bergman's *Cries and Whispers* and *Autumn Sonata,* Federico Fellini's *Amarcord,* Francois Truffaut's *Small Change* and *The Story of Adele H.,* and Volker Schlondorff's *The Tin Drum.*

OTHER SOURCES: *The International Dictionary of Films and Filmmakers,* Vol. 4—''Writers and Production Artists,'' St. James Press, 1987.

ADDRESSES: OFFICE—New Horizons Production Company, 11600 San Vicente Boulevard, Los Angeles, CA 90049.*

CORREIA, Don   1951-

PERSONAL: Born August 28, 1951, in San Jose, CA; married Sandy Duncan (an actress); children: Jeffrey, Michael. EDUCATION: Attended San Jose State University.

VOCATION: Actor and dancer.

CAREER: BROADWAY DEBUT—Mike, *A Chorus Line,* Shubert Theatre, 1980. PRINCIPAL STAGE APPEARANCES—Frankie Polo, *Little Me,* Eugene O'Neill Theatre, New York City, 1982; Vernon Castle, *Parade of Stars Playing the Palace,* Palace Theatre, New York City, 1983; Captain Billy Buck Chandler, *My One and Only,* St. James Theatre, New York City, 1984; Don Lockwood, *Singin' in the Rain,* Gershwin Theatre, New York City, 1985. Also appeared in *Perfectly Frank,* Helen Hayes Theatre, New York City, 1980; *Sophisticated Ladies,* Lunt-Fontanne Theatre, New York City, 1981; *5-6-7-8 . . . Dance!,* Radio City Music Hall, New York City, 1983; *Waitin' in the Wings: The Night the Understudies Take Centerstage,* Triplex Theatre, New York City, 1986.*

*   *   *

CORSARO, Frank   1924-

PERSONAL: Full name, Francesco Andrea Corsaro; born December 22, 1924, in New York, NY; son of Joseph (a tailor) and Marie (Quarino) Corsaro; married Mary Cross Lueders (an actress), May 30, 1971; children: Andrew. EDUCATION: Graduated from Yale University, 1947; also attended City College (now City University of New York); trained for the stage at the Actors Studio, 1954-67.

VOCATION: Director, actor, and writer.

CAREER: Also see *WRITINGS* below. PRINCIPAL STAGE APPEARANCES—Professor of philosophy, *The Would-Be Gentleman,* Cherry Lane Theatre, New York City, 1949; Tapster and Petruchio's servant, *The Taming of the Shrew,* City Center Theatre, New York City, 1951; Dirty Joe, *Mrs. McThing,* American National Theatre and Academy Theatre, New York City, 1952; Launcelot Gobbo, *The Merchant of Venice,* City Center Theatre, 1953.

FIRST STAGE WORK—Director, *No Exit,* Cherry Lane Theatre, New York City, 1947. PRINCIPAL STAGE WORK—Director: *Family Reunion,* Cherry Lane Theatre, 1947; *Creditors,* Cherry Lane Theatre, 1949; *Heartbreak House,* Bleecker Street Playhouse, New York City, 1950; *Naked,* Provincetown Playhouse, New York City, 1950; *The Curtain Rises,* Olney Theatre, Olney, MD, 1951; *Rain,* Pocono Playhouse, Mountainhome, PA, 1951; *The Voice of the Turtle, For Love or Money, Legend of Sarah,* and *Holiday,* all Rooftop Theatre, Atlanta, GA, 1951; *The Scarecrow,* Theatre De Lys, New York City, 1953; *The Honeys,* Longacre Theatre, New York City, 1955; *A Hatful of Rain,* Lyceum Theatre, New York City, 1955; *The Making of Moo,* Rita Allen Theatre, New York City, 1958; *The Night Circus,* John Golden Theatre, New York City, 1958; *The Night of the Iguana* and *The Tiny Closet,* both Spoleto Festival of Two Worlds, Teatro Caio Melisso, Spoleto, Italy, 1959; *A Piece of Blue Sky,* Fort Lee Playhouse, Fort Lee, NJ, 1958, then Westport Country Playhouse, Westport, CT, 1959; *The Night of the Iguana,* Coconut Grove Playhouse, Coconut Grove, FL, 1960, then Royale Theatre, New York City, 1961; *Oh Dad, Poor Dad, Mama's Hung You in the Closet and I'm Feelin' So Sad,* Lyric Hammersmith Theatre, London, 1961; *Baby Want a Kiss,*

Little Theatre, New York City, 1964; *The Sweet Enemy,* Actors Playhouse, New York City, 1965; *Cold Storage,* Lyceum Theatre, 1977; *Knockout,* Helen Hayes Theatre, New York City, 1979; *Whoopee!,* American National Theatre and Academy Theatre, New York City, 1979; *It's So Nice to Be Civilized,* Martin Beck Theatre, New York City, 1980; *Master Class,* Roundabout Theatre, New York City, 1986. Also directed *Fitz and Biscuit,* 1966.

Director of the following operas: *Susannah,* City Center Theatre, New York City, 1956, then Brussels World's Fair, Brussels, Belgium, 1958; *Angel of Fire,* Spoleto Festival of Two Worlds, Teatro Caio Melisso, 1959; *La Traviata,* New York City Opera Company, State Theatre, New York City, 1966; *Madama Butterfly,* New York City Opera Company, State Theatre, 1967; *Cavalleria rusticana, I Pagliacci, The Crucible, Carry Nation,* and *Faust,* all New York City Opera Company, State Theatre, 1968; *Rigoletto* and *Prince Igor,* both New York City Opera Company, State Theatre, 1969; *Pelleas et Melisande* and *The Makropoulos Case,* both New York City Opera Company, State Theatre, 1970; *Of Mice and Men,* Seattle Opera Company, Seattle, WA, 1970; *Hugh the Drover,* Houston Grand Opera, Houston, TX, 1970; *Koanga,* Opera Society of Washington, Lisner Auditorium, Washington, DC, 1970; *Summer and Smoke,* St. Paul Opera Company, St. Paul, MN, 1971; *A Village Romeo and Juliet,* Opera Society of Washington, Opera House, Kennedy Center for the Performing Arts, Washington, DC, 1972; *Summer and Smoke* and *Don Giovanni,* both New York City Opera Company, State Theatre, 1972; *L'Histoire du soldat* and *Lulu,* both Houston Grand Opera, 1973; *Cervantes,* American Opera Company, Washington, DC, 1973; *L'Incoronazione di Poppea* (also known as *The Coronation of Poppea*), Opera Society of Washington, Opera House, 1973; *La Boheme,* Municipal Opera, Atlanta, GA, 1973; *Impresario* and *Prima la musica,* both Caramoor Music Festival, Katonah, NY, 1974; *The Sea Gull,* Houston Grand Opera, 1974; *Medea* and *Manon Lescaut,* both New York City Opera Company, State Theatre, 1974.

Die Tote Stadt, New York City Opera Company, State Theatre, 1975; *Rinaldo,* Houston Grand Opera, 1975; *L'Ormindo,* Caramoor Music Festival, 1975; *Treemonisha,* Uris Theatre, New York City, 1975; *La Fanciulla del West,* Deutches Oper, Berlin, Germany, 1983; *Rinaldo,* Metropolitan Opera Company, Metropolitan Opera House, New York City, 1983; *Fennimore and Gerda,* Edinburgh Festival, Edinburgh, Scotland, 1983; *Love for Three Oranges,* Glyndebourne Festival, Glyndebourne, U.K., 1985; also *Katerina Ismailova,* 1965; *The Flaming Angel,* 1965; *The Flower* and *Hawk,* both Jacksonville, FL, 1972; at Glyndebourne Festival, U.K., 1982-85; Chicago Lyric Opera, Chicago, IL, 1984; Covent Garden, London, 1984; Metropolitan Opera House, 1984; Spitalfields Festival, London, 1985; Den Norske Opera, Oslo, Norway, 1985; and the Australian Opera, 1986.

MAJOR TOURS—Director: *Peter Pan,* U.S. cities, 1951; *A Short Happy Life,* U.S. cities, 1961.

FILM DEBUT—Marquess, *Emperor Waltz,* Paramount, 1948. PRINCIPAL FILM APPEARANCES—Hector Jonas, *Rachel, Rachel,* Warner Brothers, 1968.

FIRST TELEVISION WORK—Stage director, "A Piece of Blue Sky," *Play of the Week,* WNEW, 1960. PRINCIPAL TELEVISION WORK—All as stage director. Episodic: "On the Outskirts of Town," *Bob Hope Chrysler Theatre,* NBC, 1964. Specials: *Treemonisha,* PBS, 1986; also stage director for a broadcast of the opera *Prince Igor* from the Cincinnati Academy of Music, Cincinnati, OH, 1966.

RELATED CAREER—Resident stage director, New York City Opera Company, New York City, 1966—; artistic director, Actors Studio, New York City, 1988—; artistic adviser and principal stage director, Houston Grand Opera, Houston, TX; acting teacher, University of Houston, Houston, TX; head of music and drama division, New Jersey Institute of Opera and Music Theatre; trustee, National Opera Institute; teacher of acting for singers.

WRITINGS: STAGE—(Adaptor) *Naked,* Provincetown Playhouse, New York City, 1950; *A Piece of Blue Sky,* Fort Lee Playhouse, Fort Lee, NJ, 1958; (adaptor) *L'Histoire du soldat* (opera), Houston Grand Opera, Houston, TX, 1973, published by Belwin-Mills, 1975; (adaptor) *Love for Three Oranges* (opera), Glyndebourne Festival, Glyndebourne, U.K., 1985; (adaptor) *Where the Wild Things Are, Higgeldy Piggelby Pop* (opera), Los Angeles Opera, Los Angeles, CA, then Netherlanders Opera, Amsterdam, Netherlands, later Montreal Opera, Montreal, PQ, Canada, all 1986; also libretto, *Before Breakfast,* published by Belwin-Mills. OTHER— *Maverick: A Director's Personal Experience in Opera and Theatre,* Vanguard, 1978.

MEMBER: Actors' Equity Association, Society of Stage Directors and Choreographers, Dramatists Guild, American Guild of Musicians and Artists, Screen Directors Guild, National Endowment for the Arts.

SIDELIGHTS: RECREATIONS—Piano, tennis, ice-skating, music, and painting.

ADDRESSES: HOME—33 Riverside Drive, New York, NY 10023. OFFICES—Actors Studio, 432 W. 44th Street, New York, NY 10036; New York City Opera, Lincoln Center Plaza, New York, NY 10023.*

*   *   *

COX, Courteney   1964-

PERSONAL: Born June 15, 1964, in Birmingham, AL; daughter of Richard Lewis (a contractor) and Courteney (Bass-Copland) Cox. EDUCATION: Attended Mt. Vernon College for one year.

VOCATION: Actress.

CAREER: FILM DEBUT—*Down Twisted,* Cannon, 1986. PRINCIPAL FILM APPEARANCES—Julie Winston, *Masters of the Universe,* Cannon, 1987; Sara, *Cocoon: The Return,* Twentieth Century-Fox, 1988.

PRINCIPAL TELEVISION APPEARANCES—Series: Gloria Dinallo, *Misfits of Science,* NBC, 1985-86; Lauren Miller, *Family Ties,* NBC, 1987-88. Pilots: Lucy, *Sylvan in Paradise,* NBC, 1986. Episodic: Carol, *Murder, She Wrote* (two episodes), CBS, 1986; also "Daredevil," *The Love Boat,* ABC, 1986; *The Tonight Show,* NBC, 1988. Movies: Hana Wyshocki, *If It's Tuesday, It Still Must Be Belgium,* NBC, 1987; Nora Bundy, *I'll Be Home for Christmas,* NBC, 1988. Special: *Inside Family Ties: Behind the Scenes of a Hit,* PBS, 1988.

RELATED CAREER—Actress in the music video for the Bruce Springsteen song "Dancing in the Dark."

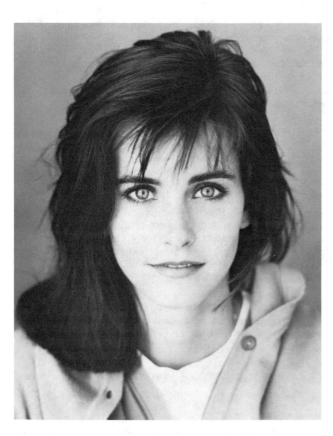

COURTENEY COX

ADDRESSES: PUBLICIST—Susan Culley, P/M/K Public Relations, 8436 W. Third Street, Suite 650, Los Angeles, CA 90048.

*   *   *

CRONYN, Hume   1911-

PERSONAL: Born July 18, 1911, in London, ON, Canada; immigrated to the United States, 1931; son of Hume Blake (a financier and member of Canadian Parliament) and Frances Amelia (Labatt) Cronyn; married Jessica Tandy (an actress), September 27, 1942; children: Susan, Christopher Hume, Tandy. EDUCATION: Graduated from Ridley College, 1930; graduate work at McGill University, 1930-31; graduated from the American Academy of Dramatic Arts, 1934; also trained for the stage with Harold Kreutzberg at the Mozarteum, Salzburg, Austria, 1932-33, and at the New York School of the Theatre.

VOCATION: Actor, director, producer, and writer.

CAREER: Also see *WRITINGS* below. STAGE DEBUT—Paper boy, *Up Pops the Devil*, Cochran's Stock Company, National Theatre, Washington, DC, 1931. BROADWAY DEBUT—Janitor, *Hipper's Holiday*, Maxine Elliot's Theatre, 1934. LONDON DEBUT—Jimmy Luton, *Big Fish, Little Fish*, Duke of York's Theatre, 1962. PRINCIPAL STAGE APPEARANCES—Austin Lowe, *The Second Man*, Dr. Haggett, *The Late Christopher Bean*, Jim Hipper, *He Knew Dillinger* (also known as *Hipper's Holiday*), and Doke Odum, *Mountain Ivy*, all Barter Theatre, Abingdon, VA, 1934;

Green, *Boy Meets Girl,* and Erwin Trowbridge, *Three Men on a Horse,* both Cort Theatre, New York City, 1936; Elkus, *High Tor,* Martin Beck Theatre, New York City, 1937; Leo Davis, *Room Service,* Cort Theatre, 1937; Abe Sherman, *There's Always a Breeze,* Windsor Theatre, New York City, 1938; Steve, *Escape This Night,* 44th Street Theatre, New York City, 1938; Harry Quill, *Off to Buffalo,* Ethel Barrymore Theatre, New York City, 1939; Andrei Prozoroff, *The Three Sisters,* Longacre Theatre, New York City, 1939; Hutchens Stubbs, *Susan and God,* Toby Cartwright, *Ways and Means,* George Davies, "We Were Dancing" in *Tonight at 8:30,* Francis O'Connor, *Shadow and Substance,* Christy Dudgeon, *The Devil's Disciple,* Lloyd Lloyd, *Kiss the Boys Goodbye,* Judas, *Family Portrait,* Stage Manager, *Our Town,* Denis Dillon, *The White Steed,* Karl Baumer, *Margin for Error,* and Joe Bonaparte, *Golden Boy,* all Lakewood Theatre, Skowhegan, ME, 1939-40; Peter Mason, *The Weak Link,* John Golden Theatre, New York City, 1940; Lee Tatnall, *Retreat to Pleasure,* Group Theatre Company, Belasco Theatre, New York City, 1940; Joe Bonaparte, *Golden Boy,* Bucks County Playhouse, New Hope, PA, 1941; Harley L. Miller, *Mr. Big,* Lyceum Theatre, New York City, 1941; Jodine Decker, *The Survivors,* Plymouth Theatre, New York City, 1948.

Gandersheim, *The Little Blue Light,* Brattle Theatre, Cambridge, MA, 1950; Michael, *The Fourposter,* Ethel Barrymore Theatre, 1951; Dr. Brightlee, *Madam, Will You Walk?,* Phoenix Theatre, New York City, 1953; Michael, *The Fourposter,* City Center Theatre, New York City, 1955; Curtis and Bennett Honey, *The Honeys,* Longacre Theatre, 1955; Julian Anson, *A Day by the Sea,* American National Theatre and Academy (ANTA) Theatre, New York City, 1955; Oliver Walling, *The Man in the Dog Suit,* Coronet

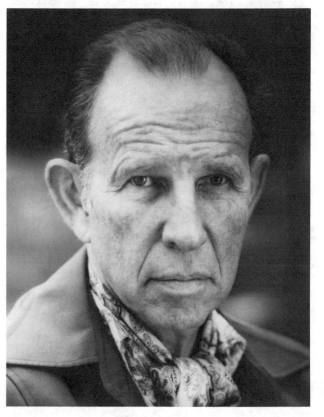

HUME CRONYN

Theatre, New York City, 1958; Professor Ivan Ivanovitch Nyukhin, "Some Comments on the Harmful Effects of Tobacco" (monologue), Doctor, "Portrait of a Madonna," Jerry, "A Pound on Demand," and John Jo Mulligan, "Bedtime Story," all in *Triple Play*, Playhouse Theatre, New York City, 1959; Jimmy Luton, *Big Fish, Little Fish*, ANTA Theatre, 1961; Harpagon, *The Miser*, Tchebutkin, *The Three Sisters*, and Willie Loman, *Death of a Salesman*, all Tyrone Guthrie Theatre, Minneapolis, MN, 1963; Polonius, *Hamlet*, Lunt-Fontanne Theatre, New York City, 1964; Newton, *The Physicists*, Martin Beck Theatre, 1964; title role, *Richard III*, Yephikodov, *The Cherry Orchard*, and Harpagon, *The Miser*, all Tyrone Guthrie Theatre, 1965; Tobias, *A Delicate Balance*, Martin Beck Theatre, 1966; Harpagon, *The Miser*, Mark Taper Forum, Los Angeles, CA, 1968; Frederick William Rolfe, *Hadrian VII*, Stratford Shakespearean Festival, Stratford, ON, Canada, 1969.

Captain Queeg, *The Caine Mutiny Court Martial*, Ahmanson Theatre, Los Angeles, 1971; Grandfather and Willie, *Promenade, All!*, Alvin Theatre, New York City, 1972; title role, "Krapp's Last Tape," Willie, "Happy Days," and Player, "Act without Words I," all in *Samuel Beckett Festival*, Forum Theatre, New York City, 1972; Verner Conklin and Sir Hugo Latymer, *In Two Keys*, Ethel Barrymore Theatre, 1973; Shylock, *The Merchant of Venice*, and Bottom, *A Midsummer Night's Dream*, both Stratford Shakespearean Festival, 1976; Weller Martin, *The Gin Game*, Long Wharf Theatre, New Haven, CT, then John Golden Theatre, both 1977; Hector Nations, *Foxfire*, Stratford Shakespearean Festival, 1980, then Tyrone Guthrie Theatre, 1981, later Ethel Barrymore Theatre, 1982, then Center Theatre Group, Ahmanson Theatre, 1986; General Sir Edmund Milne, *The Petition*, John Golden Theatre, 1986. Also appeared in *The Adding Machine*, *Dr. Faustus*, *From Morn to Midnight*, *The Road to Rome*, *Alice in Wonderland*, and *Red and White Revue*, all with the Montreal Repertory Theatre and McGill University Players Club, Montreal, PQ, Canada, 1930-31; *Hear America Speaking* (revue with Jessica Tandy), special performance at the White House, Washington, DC, 1965; and in *Traveler in the Dark*, American Repertory Theatre, Cambridge, MA, 1984.

PRINCIPAL STAGE WORK—Director, *Portrait of a Madonna*, Actors Laboratory Theatre, Las Palmas Theatre, Los Angeles, CA, 1946; director, *Now I Lay Me Down to Sleep*, Stanford University, Stanford, CA, 1949, then Broadhurst Theatre, New York City, 1950; director, *Hilda Crane*, Coronet Theatre, New York City, 1950; director (with Norman Lloyd), *Madam, Will You Walk?*, Phoenix Theatre, New York City, 1953; director, *The Egghead*, Ethel Barrymore Theatre, New York City, 1957; director, *Triple Play*, Playhouse Theatre, New York City, 1959; producer, *Slow Dance on the Killing Ground*, Plymouth Theatre, New York City, 1964; producer (with Mike Nichols), *The Gin Game*, John Golden Theatre, New York City, 1977; producer, *Salonika*, New York Shakespeare Festival, Public Theatre, New York City, 1985.

MAJOR TOURS—Stingo and Sir Charles Marlowe, *She Stoops to Conquer*, and Gideon Bloodgood, *The Streets of New York*, both Jitney Players, U.S. cities, 1935; Erwin Trowbridge, *Three Men on a Horse*, U.S. cities, 1935-36; Green, *Boy Meets Girl*, U.S. cities, 1936; Leo Davis, *Room Service*, U.S. cities, 1937; Tommy Turner, *The Male Animal*, Actors Laboratory Theatre, U.S. military bases in California, 1944; title role, *Hamlet*, American National Theatre and Academy, U.S. cities, 1949; Oliver Walling, *The Man in the Dog Suit*, U.S. cities, 1957; director and appeared as Doctor, "Portrait of a Madonna," Jerry, "A Pound on Demand," John Jo Mulligan, "Bedtime Story," and Professor Ivan Ivanovitch Nyukhin, "Some Comments on the Harmful Effects of Tobacco" (a mono-

logue), all in *Triple Play*, U.S. cities, 1958; Tobias, *A Delicate Balance*, U.S. cities, 1967; William Rolfe, *Hadrian VII*, U.S. cities, 1970; director and appeared as Grandfather and Willie, *Promenade, All!*, U.S. cities, 1972 and 1973; title role, *Krapp's Last Tape*, U.S. and Canadian cities, 1973; Verner Conklin and Sir Hugo Latymer, *In Two Keys*, U.S. cities, 1974; *The Many Faces of Love* (dramatic reading), U.S. cities, 1974-75; producer (with Mike Nichols), and appeared as Weller Martin, *The Gin Game*, U.S., Canadian, U.K., and Soviet cities, 1978-1979. Also producer, director, and appeared in a revue with the Canadian Active Service Canteen, 1941; co-producer and appeared in *It's All Yours* (revue), USO tour, 1942; producer, *Junior Miss* (revue), USO tour, 1942; appeared in vaudeville sketch for Victory Loan, Canadian cities, 1944; *Face to Face* (concert reading), U.S. cities, 1954.

FILM DEBUT—Herbie Hawkins, *Shadow of a Doubt*, Universal, 1943. PRINCIPAL FILM APPEARANCES—Duval, *The Cross of Lorraine*, Metro-Goldwyn-Mayer (MGM), 1943; Gerard, *The Phantom of the Opera*, Universal, 1943; Stanley Garrett, *Lifeboat*, Twentieth Century-Fox, 1944; Keller, *Main Street after Dark*, MGM, 1944; Paul Roeder, *The Seventh Cross*, MGM, 1944; John Phineas McPherson, *A Letter for Evie*, MGM, 1945; Monty, "The Sweepstakes Ticket" in *Ziegfeld Follies*, MGM, 1945; Papa Leckie, *The Green Years*, MGM, 1946; Arthur Keats, *The Postman Always Rings Twice*, MGM, 1946; Freddie, *The Sailor Takes a Wife*, MGM, 1946; man's voice, *The Secret Heart*, MGM, 1946; Dr. J. Robert Oppenheimer, *The Beginning or the End*, MGM, 1947; Captain Munsey, *Brute Force*, Universal, 1947; John McGrath, *The Bride Goes Wild*, MGM, 1948; Hughie Devine, *Top o' the Morning*, Paramount, 1949; Professor Elwell, *People Will Talk*, Twentieth Century-Fox, 1951; George Heath, *Crowded Paradise*, Tudor, 1956.

Louis Howe, *Sunrise at Campobello*, Warner Brothers, 1960; Sosigenes, *Cleopatra*, Twentieth Century-Fox, 1963; Polonius, *Hamlet*, Warner Brothers, 1964; Arthur, *The Arrangement*, Warner Brothers, 1969; "Honest" Tim Grogan, *Gaily, Gaily* (also known as *Chicago, Chicago*), United Artists, 1969; Dudley Whinner, *There Was a Crooked Man*, Warner Brothers, 1970; Skeffington, *Conrack*, Twentieth Century-Fox, 1974; Editor Edgar Rintels, *The Parallax View*, Paramount, 1974; Sherm Schaefler, *Honky Tonk Freeway*, Universal/Associated Film Distributors, 1981; Maxwell Emery, *Rollover*, Warner Brothers, 1981; Mr. Fields, *The World According to Garp*, Warner Brothers, 1982; Dr. Carr, *Impulse*, Twentieth Century-Fox, 1984; Rupert Horn, *Brewster's Millions*, Universal, 1985; Joe Finley, *Cocoon*, Twentieth Century-Fox, 1985; Frank Riley, **batteries not included*, Universal, 1987; Joe Finley, *Cocoon: The Return*, Twentieth Century-Fox, 1988. Also appeared in *Hitchcock, Il brivido del genio* (documentary; also known as *The Thrill of Genius*), RAI-TV Channel 1, 1985.

TELEVISION DEBUT—Ned Farrar, *Her Master's Voice*, NBC, 1939. PRINCIPAL TELEVISION APPEARANCES—Series: Ben Marriott, *The Marriage*, NBC, 1954. Pilots: Dr. Paul Jaffe, *The Oath: Thirty-Three Hours in the Life of God*, ABC, 1976. Episodic: Polonius, *Hamlet*, Electronovision, 1964; Weller Martin, "The Gin Game," *American Playhouse*, PBS, 1984; also *Ben Hecht's Tales of the City* (also known as *Tales of the City*), CBS, 1953; *The Motorola Television Hour*, CBS, 1954; *The Great Adventure*, CBS, 1956; *The Confidence Man*, NBC, 1956; *The Big Wave*, NBC, 1956; *The Five Dollar Bill*, CBS, 1957; *Member of the Family*, CBS, 1957; "The Bridge of San Luis Rey," *DuPont Show of the Month*, CBS, 1958; "Juno and the Paycock," *Play of the Week*, WNTA, 1960; *The Kaiser Aluminum Hour*, NBC; *Studio One*, CBS; *The Alcoa Hour*, NBC; *The Ed Sullivan Show*, CBS; *Omni-*

bus, CBS; "One Sunday Afternoon," *Ford Theatre.* Movies: Hector Nations, *Foxfire,* CBS, 1987; James F. Byrnes, *Day One,* CBS, 1989. Specials: Michael, *The Fourposter,* NBC, 1955; Nils Krogstad, "A Doll's House," *Hallmark Hall of Fame,* NBC, 1959; Dirk Stroeve, *The Moon and Sixpence,* NBC, 1959; *John F. Kennedy Memorial Broadcast,* NBC, 1963; *The Many Faces of Love,* CBC, 1977; *Kennedy Center Honors: A Celebration of the Performing Arts,* CBS, 1986 and 1987; "Everybody's Doing It" (documentary), *Summer Showcase,* NBC, 1988; *Onstage: Twenty-Five Years at the Guthrie,* syndicated, 1988.

PRINCIPAL TELEVISION WORK—Series: Producer (with Donald Davis) and director (with Fred Carr and Ralph Warren), *Actors Studio,* ABC, 1948-49, then CBS, 1949-50; producer, *The Marriage,* NBC, 1954. Episodic: Producer and director, "Portrait of a Madonna," *Actors Studio,* ABC, 1948; producer, *The Fourposter,* NBC, 1955.

PRINCIPAL RADIO APPEARANCES—Series: Ben Marriott, *The Marriage,* NBC, 1953.

RELATED CAREER—Production director, Barter Theatre Company, Abingdon, VA, 1934; lecturer in drama, American Academy of Dramatic Arts, 1938-39, then trustee; lecturer in drama, Actors Lab, Los Angeles, CA, 1945-46; board of governors, Stratford Shakespearean Festival, Stratford, ON, Canada; board of directors, Tyrone Guthrie Theatre, Minneapolis, MN.

WRITINGS: STAGE—(With Susan Cooper) *Foxfire,* Stratford Shakespearean Festival, Stratford, ON, Canada, then Ethel Barrymore Theatre, New York City, both 1980, published by Samuel French, Inc., 1983. FILM—(With Arthur Laurents) *Rope,* Warner Brothers, 1948; (with James Bridie) *Under Capricorn,* Warner Brothers, 1949; also *Dinner at the Homesick Restaurant* (unproduced). TELEVISION—(With Cooper) *The Dollmaker,* ABC, 1985. OTHER—Contributor of articles and short stories to journals and periodicals.

AWARDS: Academy Award nomination, Best Supporting Actor 1944, for *The Seventh Cross;* Comoedia Matinee Club Award, 1952, for *The Fourposter;* Barter Theatre Award for Outstanding Contribution to the Theatre, 1961; Antoinette Perry Award nomination, Best Actor (Dramatic), and New York Drama League Delia Austria Medal, both 1961, for *Big Fish, Little Fish;* Antoinette Perry Award, Best Supporting or Featured Actor (Dramatic), and *Variety* New York Drama Critics Poll Award, both 1964, for *Hamlet;* American Academy of Dramatic Arts Award for Achievement by Alumni, 1964; Antoinette Perry Award nomination, Best Actor (Dramatic), and Herald Theatre Award, both 1967, for *A Delicate Balance;* Los Angeles Drama Critics Circle Award, Best Actor, 1972, for *The Caine Mutiny Court Martial;* Straw Hat Award, Best Director, 1972, for *Promenade, All!;* Obie Award from the *Village Voice,* Distinguished Performance, 1973, for *Krapp's Last Tape;* inducted into the Theatre Hall of Fame, 1974; Brandeis University Creative Arts Award for Distinguished Achievement, 1978; Antoinette Perry Award nomination, Best Actor in a Play, and Los Angeles Critics Circle Award, both 1979, for *The Gin Game;* National Press Club Award, 1979; Commonwealth Award for Distinguished Service in Dramatic Arts, 1983; Humanitas Prize from the Human Family Institute, Emmy Award, Best Television Script One Hour or Longer, Christopher Award, and Writers Guild Award, all 1985, for *The Dollmaker;* Kennedy Center Honors, 1986; Alley Theatre Award in Recognition of Significant Contributions to the Theatre Arts, 1987; Antoinette Perry Award nomination, Best Actor in a Play, 1986, for *The Petition.* Honorary

degrees: University of Western Ontario, LLD, 1974; Fordham University, LHD, 1985.

MEMBER: Actors' Equity Association, Screen Actors Guild, American Federation of Television and Radio Artists, Writers Guild of America, Dramatists Guild, Society of Stage Directors and Choreographers, Screen Writers Guild, Theatre Development Fund.

SIDELIGHTS: RECREATIONS—Skin diving and fishing.

ADDRESSES: HOME—Route 137, Box 85-A, Pound Ridge, NY 10576. OFFICE—62-23 Carlton Street, Rego Park, New York, NY 11374. AGENTS—Sam Cohn, International Creative Management, 40 W. 57th Street, New York, NY 10019; Martha Luttrell, International Creative Management, 8899 Beverly Boulevard, Los Angeles, CA 90048.*

*   *   *

CROSBY, Gary   1933-

PERSONAL: Born June 25, 1933, in California; son of Bing (an actor and singer) and Dixie Lee Crosby.

VOCATION: Actor.

CAREER: PRINCIPAL FILM APPEARANCES—As himself, *Star Spangled Rhythm,* Paramount, 1942; as himself, *Duffy's Tavern,* Paramount, 1945; child in the audience, *Out of This World,* Paramount, 1945; Tony Runkle, *Mardi Gras,* Twentieth Century-Fox, 1958; Paul Gattling, *Holiday for Lovers,* Twentieth Century-Fox, 1959; Mike, *A Private's Affair,* Twentieth Century-Fox, 1959; Rip Hulett, *The Right Approach,* Twentieth Century-Fox, 1961; Marty Sackler, *Battle at Bloody Beach* (also known as *Battle on the Beach*), Twentieth Century-Fox, 1961; Gary, *Two Tickets to Paris,* Columbia, 1962; Seaman Floyd Givens, *Operation Bikini,* American International, 1963; Andy, *Girl Happy,* Metro-Goldwyn-Mayer, 1965; Ensign Sloan, *Morituri* (also known as *The Saboteur: Code Name Morituri* and *The Saboteur*), Twentieth Century-Fox, 1965; SS guard, *Which Way to the Front?,* Warner Brothers, 1970; Vic Gallegher, *The Night Stalker,* Almi, 1987.

TELEVISION DEBUT—*The Jack Benny Show,* CBS, 1955. PRINCIPAL TELEVISION APPEARANCES—Series: Eddie, *The Bill Dana Show,* NBC, 1963-64; Officer Ed Wells, *Adam-12,* NBC, 1968-75; Officer Ed Rice, *Chase,* NBC, 1973-74; Bruce Daniels, *Mobile One,* ABC, 1975; Officer Gene Cody, *Sam,* CBS, 1978; Officer Dabney Smith, *Hunter,* NBC, 1984-85. Pilots: Harry Fish, *O'Hara, United States Treasury: Operation Cobra,* CBS, 1971; Officer Gene Cody, *Sam,* CBS, 1977. Episodic: Floyd Burney, "Come Wander with Me," *The Twilight Zone,* CBS, 1964; Ted Stully, *Murder, She Wrote,* CBS, 1986; Virgil Fedderson, *Blacke's Magic,* NBC, 1986; Master Sergeant Dixon, *Matlock* (two episodes), NBC, 1987; also *The Hollywood Palace,* ABC, 1964. Movies: Scott, *Wings of Fire,* NBC, 1967; Frank Watson, *Sandcastles,* CBS, 1972; Trooper, *Partners in Crime,* NBC, 1973; Leonard, *Three on a Date,* ABC, 1978. Specials: Eddie Davis, *Time Out for Ginger,* CBS, 1955; *The Bob Hope Show,* NBC, 1957.

RELATED CAREER—Participated in a musical act with his brothers, Dennis, Phillip, and Lindsay.

WRITINGS: (With Ross Firestone) *Going My Own Way* (autobiography), Doubleday, 1983.

RECORDINGS: SINGLES—(With Bing Crosby) ''Play a Simple Melody'' and ''Sam's Song,'' both 1950.

ADDRESSES: AGENT—Thomas Jennings and Associates, 427 N. Canon Drive, Suite 205, Beverly Hills, CA 90210.*

*   *   *

CRUICKSHANK, Andrew   1907-1988

PERSONAL: Full name, Andrew John Cruickshank; born December 25, 1907, in Aberdeen, Scotland; died April 28, 1988, in London, England; son of Andrew and Mary Evelyn Grace Burnett (Cadger) Cruickshank; married Curigwen Lewis; children: one son, two daughters. MILITARY: Royal Welsh Fusiliers, major, 1940-45.

VOCATION: Actor.

CAREER: LONDON DEBUT—*Othello,* Savoy Theatre, 1930. BROADWAY DEBUT—Maudelyn, *Richard of Bordeaux,* Empire Theatre, 1934. PRINCIPAL STAGE APPEARANCES—Prince Ernest, General Grey, and John Brown, *Victoria Regina,* Gate Theatre, London, 1935; Lord Clinton, *Mary Tudor,* Playhouse Theatre, London, 1935; Spartan herald, *Lysistrata,* Sir Edward Clarke, *Oscar Wilde,* and Parnell, *Mr. Gladstone,* all Gate Theatre, 1936; Banquo, *Macbeth,* Theseus, *A Midsummer Night's Dream,* and Ludovico and Cassio, *Othello,* all Old Vic Company, Old Vic Theatre, London, 1937; Dr. Forbes, *The Painted Smile,* New Theatre, London, 1938; O'Dwyer, *Trelawny of the Wells,* Roebuck Ramsden, *Man and Superman,* Claudius, *Hamlet,* and Sir Lucius O'Trigger, *The Rivals,* all Old Vic Company, Old Vic Theatre, 1938; Rosencrantz, *Hamlet,* Lyceum Theatre, London, then Elsinor, Denmark, both 1939; Duke of Marlborough, *Viceroy Sarah,* and chorus, *Escalus,* both Old Vic Company, Buxton Festival, Buxton, U.K., 1939; Apothecary, *Romeo and Juliet,* Titus, *The Devil's Disciple,* Sir William Honeywood, *The Good Natured Man,* and Warwick, *Saint Joan,* all Old Vic Company, Buxton Festival, then Streatham Hill, U.K., 1939; Cornwall, *King Lear,* and Sebastian, *The Tempest,* both Old Vic Company, Old Vic Theatre, 1940; Richard Burbage, *Spring 1600,* Lyric Hammersmith Theatre, London, 1945; Mark, *The Nineteenth Hole of Europe,* title role, *Fortunato,* and Archie, *Cellar,* all Granville Theatre, London, 1946; Duke of Florence, *The White Devil,* Duchess Theatre, London, 1947; Hugh Wigmore, *The Indifferent Shepherd,* Criterion Theatre, London, 1948.

Title role, *Julius Caesar,* Wolsey, *Henry VIII,* Leonato, *Much Ado about Nothing,* Earl of Kent, *King Lear,* and Angelo, *Measure for Measure,* all Memorial Theatre, Stratford-on-Avon, U.K., 1950; Reverend James Mavor Morrell, *Candida,* and Claudius, *Hamlet,* both New Boltons Theatre, London, 1951; Lord Angus, *The Thistle and the Rose,* Vaudeville Theatre, London, 1951; Earl of Warwick, *Saint Joan,* Cort Theatre, New York City, 1951; Chief Inspector Hubbard, *Dial M for Murder,* Westminster Theatre, London, 1952; Agamemnon, *Sacrifice to the Winds,* Arts Theatre, London, 1955; Richard Farrow, *Dead on Nine,* Westminster Theatre, 1955; Maurice, *The House by the Lake,* Duke of York's Theatre, London, 1956; Henry Drummond, *Inherit the Wind,* Pembroke Theatre, Croydon, U.K., then St. Martin's Theatre, London, both 1960;

W.O. Gant, *Look Homeward, Angel,* Pembroke Theatre, 1960; Dr. Wangle, *The Lady from the Sea,* Queen's Theatre, London, 1961; Tom Howard, *Unfinished Journey,* Pembroke Theatre, 1961; W.O. Gant, *Look Homeward, Angel,* Phoenix Theatre, London, 1962; Halvard Solness, *The Master Builder,* Ashcroft Theatre, Croydon, U.K., 1962; Cornelius Melody, *A Touch of the Poet,* Ashcroft Theatre, 1963; Mr. Justice Carstairs, *Alibi for a Judge,* Grand Theatre, Leeds, U.K., 1964, then Savoy Theatre, London, 1965; Henry Oldershaw, *The Crunch,* St. Martin's Theatre, 1969.

Judge, *The Douglas Cause,* Duke of York's Theatre, 1971; title role, *Noah,* Yvonne Arnaud Theatre, Guildford, U.K., 1973; Sir William Boothroyd, *Lloyd George Knew My Father,* Savoy Theatre, 1973; Rubek, *When We Dead Awaken,* Haymarket Theatre, Leicester, U.K., 1976; Nestor, *The Women,* John Anthony, *Strife,* and leading peasant, *The Fruits of Enlightenment,* all National Theatre, London, 1978; Duke Senior, *As You Like It,* Derby, *Richard III,* and Count Orsini-Rosenberg, *Amadeus,* all National Theatre, 1979; Old Ekdal, *The Wild Duck,* National Theatre, 1980; Justice Treadwell, *Beyond Reasonable Doubt,* Queen's Theatre, 1987. Also appeared with numerous repertory companies early in his career.

MAJOR TOURS—Lot Johnson, *Mountain Fire,* U.K. cities, 1954; Solness, *The Master Builder,* U.K. cities, 1972; also with the Arts League Travelling Theatre, U.K. cities, early 1930s; and with the Old Vic Company, European and Egyptian cities, 1939.

FILM DEBUT—Robert Burns, *Auld Lang Syne,* Metro-Goldwyn-Mayer, 1937. PRINCIPAL FILM APPEARANCES—Prince Nicholas, *Idol of Paris,* Warner Brothers, 1948; Sir Jonathan Dockwra, *The Mark of Cain,* General Films Distributors, 1948; Baxter, *Forbidden,* British Lion, 1949; Inspector Clement Pill, *Paper Orchid,* Columbia, 1949; Sir Adrian Horth, *Eye Witness* (also known as *Your Witness*), Warner Brothers, 1950; Lord Bedlington, *The Reluctant Widow,* Fine Arts, 1951; trustee, *John Wesley,* Radio and Film Commission of the Methodist Church, 1954; Brankenbury, *Richard III,* Lopert, 1956; Inspector Thornton, *The Secret Tent,* British Lion, 1956; Uncle Ben, *John and Julie,* British Lion, 1957; Captain Stubs, *Pursuit of the Graf Spee* (also known as *The Battle of the River Plate*), Rank, 1957; Dr. Stein, *The Story of Esther Costello* (also known as *Golden Virgin*), Columbia, 1957; doctor, *Innocent Sinners,* Rank, 1958; Doctor Cameron, *A Question of Adultery* (also known as *The Case of Mrs. Loring*), Eros, 1959; Colin Roy Campbell, *Kidnapped,* Buena Vista, 1960; Colonel Henderson, *The Stranglers of Bombay,* Columbia, 1960; Count Gomez, *El Cid,* Allied Artists, 1961; lord provost, *Greyfriars Bobby,* Buena Vista, 1961; vicar, *Live Now—Pay Later,* Regal Films, 1962; McKillup, *There Was a Crooked Man,* Lopert/United Artists, 1962; Admiral Filmer, *We Joined the Navy* (also known as *We Are in the Navy Now*), Warner Brothers/Pathe, 1962; Cardwell, *Come Fly with Me,* Metro-Goldwyn-Mayer (MGM), 1963; Justice Crosby, *Murder Most Foul,* MGM, 1964; Minister Bar, *Wagner,* Alan Landsburg, 1983. Also appeared in *Ivory Hunter* (also known as *The Ivory Hunters* and *Where No Vultures Fly*), Universal, 1952; and *The Cruel Sea,* General Films Distributors, 1953.

PRINCIPAL TELEVISION APPEARANCES—Series: Dr. Cameron, *Dr. Finlay's Casebook.* Mini-Series: John Jarndyce, *Bleak House.* Episodic: *The Lilli Palmer Theatre,* syndicated, 1956.

WRITINGS: STAGE—*Unfinished Journey,* Pembroke Theatre, Croydon, U.K., 1961; *Games,* Edinburgh Festival, Edinburgh, Scotland, 1975.

AWARDS: Honorary degrees: D.Litt., St. Andrew's University (Scotland), 1977.

OBITUARIES AND OTHER SOURCES: Variety, May 11, 1988.*

*   *   *

CUPITO, Suzanne
See BRITTANY, Morgan

*   *   *

CURRY, Tim

VOCATION: Actor.

CAREER: PRINCIPAL STAGE APPEARANCES—Peter, *Lie Down, I Think I Love You,* Strand Theatre, London, 1970; Sexton, *Man Is Man,* English Stage Company, Royal Court Theatre, London, 1971; Jesse, *The Baby Elephant,* Theatre Upstairs, London, 1971; Bassianus, *Titus Andronicus,* Round House Theatre, London, 1971; Dr. Frank N. Furter, *The Rocky Horror Show,* Theatre Upstairs, then Kings Row Theatre, both London, 1973, later Belasco Theatre, New York City, 1975; Tristan Tzara, *Travesties,* Royal Shakespeare Company, Ethel Barrymore Theatre, New York City, 1975; title role, *Amadeus,* Broadhurst Theatre, New York City, 1980; Bill Snibson, *Me and My Girl,* Pantages Theatre, Los Angeles, CA, 1988. Also appeared in *England's Ireland,* Round House Theatre, 1972; *Once Upon a Time,* Duke of York's Theatre, London, 1972; as Puck in *A Midsummer Night's Dream,* as the pirate king in *The Pirates of Penzance,* and in *Hair,* all London productions.

PRINCIPAL FILM APPEARANCES—Dr. Frank N. Furter, *The Rocky Horror Picture Show,* Twentieth Century-Fox, 1975; Robert Graves, *The Shout,* Films Inc., 1978; Johnny La Guardia, *Times Square,* Associated, 1980; Rooster, *Annie,* Columbia, 1982; Jeremy Hancock, *The Ploughman's Lunch,* Samuel Goldwyn, 1984; Larry Gormley, *Blue Money,* London Weekend Television/Blue Money Productions, 1984; Wadsworth, *Clue,* Paramount, 1985; Lord of Darkness, *Legend,* Universal, 1985; Ray Porter, *Pass the Ammo,* New Century, 1988.

PRINCIPAL TELEVISION APPEARANCES—Episodic: Winston Newquay, *Wiseguy,* CBS, 1989. Movies: Bill Sikes, *Oliver Twist,* CBS, 1982. Also appeared as the grand wizard, *The Worst Witch,* 1986.

RECORDINGS: ALBUMS—*Fearless,* A & M. SINGLES—"I Do the Rock," A & M.

AWARDS: Antoinette Perry Award nomination, Best Actor in a Play, 1981, for *Amadeus;* Royal Variety Club Award for *The Pirates of Penzance.*

ADDRESSES: AGENTS—William Morris Agency, 31/32 Soho Square, London W1, England; David Schiff, Creative Artists Agency, 1888 Century Park E., Suite 1400, Los Angeles, CA 90067.*

CURTIN, Valerie

PERSONAL: Born March 31, in Jackson Heights, NY; daughter of Joseph Curtin (a radio actor).

VOCATION: Actress and screenwriter.

CAREER: Also see *WRITINGS* below. PRINCIPAL STAGE APPEARANCES—Edna Klein, *Children of a Lesser God,* Center Theatre Group, Ahmanson Theatre, Los Angeles, CA, 1979; also appeared in productions with New Theatre for Now, Center Theatre Group, Mark Taper Forum, Los Angeles, 1983.

PRINCIPAL FILM APPEARANCES—Vera, *Alice Doesn't Live Here Anymore,* Warner Brothers, 1975; Naomi Fishbine, *Mother, Jugs, and Speed,* Twentieth Century-Fox, 1976; intensive care nurse, *Silent Movie,* Twentieth Century-Fox, 1976; Plain Jane, *Silver Streak,* Twentieth Century-Fox, 1976; Miss Milland, *All the President's Men,* Warner Brothers, 1976; Phyllis, *A Different Story,* AVCO-Embassy, 1978; Mrs. Bok, *Why Would I Lie?,* Metro-Goldwyn-Mayer/United Artists, 1980; Miss Sheffer, Maxie, Orion, 1985; Arlene Hoffman, *Big Trouble,* Columbia, 1986; Pearl Waxman, *Down and Out in Beverly Hills,* Buena Vista, 1986. Also appeared in *The Great Smokey Roadblock* (also known as *The Last of the Cowboys*), Dimension, 1978.

PRINCIPAL TELEVISION APPEARANCES—Series: Regular, *The Jim Stafford Show,* ABC, 1975; Judy Bernly, *9 to 5,* ABC, 1982-83, then syndicated, 1986-87. Pilots: Sandy Lambert, *The Primary English Class,* ABC, 1977. Episodic: *Barney Miller,* ABC, 1976. Movies: Miss Goldfarb, *The Greatest Thing That Almost Happened,* CBS, 1977; Kitty, *A Love Affair: The Eleanor and Lou Gehrig Story,* NBC, 1978; Chief Warden Stelina Shell, *Brave New World,* NBC, 1980; Muriel, *A Christmas without Snow,* CBS, 1980. PRINCIPAL TELEVISION WORK—Series: Co-creator, *Square Pegs,* CBS, 1982-83.

WRITINGS: FILM—(With Barry Levinson) *. . . And Justice for All,* Columbia, 1979; (with Levinson) *Inside Moves,* Associated, 1980; (with Levinson) *Best Friends,* Warner Brothers, 1982; (with Levinson and Robert Klane) *Unfaithfully Yours,* Twentieth Century-Fox, 1984. TELEVISION—Episodic: "Mary's Delinquent," *The Mary Tyler Moore Show,* CBS, 1975; *Phyllis,* CBS, 1975-77.

ADDRESSES: AGENT—Creative Artists Agency, 1888 Century Park E., Suite 1400, Los Angeles, CA 90067.*

*   *   *

CUSACK, Cyril   1910-

PERSONAL: Full name, Cyril James Cusack; born November 26, 1910, in Durban, Natal, South Africa; son of James Walter (a member of the Natal mounted police) and Alice Violet (an actress; maiden name, Cole) Cusack; married Maureen Kiely (an actress), April 5, 1945 (deceased); children: two sons, four daughters. EDUCATION: Attended Dominican College, Droichead Nua, Ireland, 1922-26, and the National University of Ireland, 1928-32.

VOCATION: Actor, manager, producer, and playwright.

CAREER: Also see *WRITINGS* below. STAGE DEBUT—Little Willie Carlyle, *East Lynne,* Clonmel, Ireland, 1916. LONDON

DEBUT—Richard, *Ah, Wilderness!*, Westminster Theatre, 1936. BROADWAY DEBUT—Phil Hogan, *A Moon for the Misbegotten*, Bijou Theatre, 1957. PRINCIPAL STAGE APPEARANCES—Indian student, *Tilly of Bloomsbury*, and Carruthers, *Mr. Wu*, both Norwich Repertory Company, Norwich, U.K., 1928; Richard, *Ah, Wilderness!*, Ambassadors Theatre, London, 1936; Christy Mahon, *The Playboy of the Western World*, Mercury Theatre, London, 1939; the Covey, *The Plough and the Stars*, Q Theatre, London, 1939; Michel, *Les Parents terribles*, Gate Theatre, Dublin, Ireland, 1940; Streeter, *Thunder Rock*, St. Martin's Theatre, London, 1941; Louis Dubedat, *The Doctor's Dilemma*, Haymarket Theatre, London, 1942; Christy Mahon, *The Playboy of the Western World*, Theatre Sarah Bernhardt, Paris, France, 1954; Nosey, *Pommy*, People's Palace Theatre, London, 1950; Roger Casement, *Casement*, Theatre Royal, Waterford, Ireland, 1958; Seumas O'Beirne, *Goodwill Ambassador*, Olympia Theatre, Dublin, Ireland, 1959, then Shubert Theatre, New Haven, CT, later Wilbur Theatre, Boston, MA, both 1960.

Krapp, *Krapp's Last Tape*, Empire Theatre, Belfast, Ireland, 1960; Bluntschli, *Arms and the Man*, Empire Theatre, then Queen's Theatre, Dublin, Ireland, both 1960; title role, *The Temptation of Mr. O*, Dublin Theatre Festival, Olympia Theatre, 1961; Johann Wilhelm Stettler, *The Physicists*, Royal Shakespeare Company, Aldwych Theatre, London, 1963; Cassius, *Julius Caesar*, Royal Shakespeare Company, Shakespeare Memorial Theatre, Stratford-on-Avon, U.K., 1963; Can, *Andorra*, National Theatre Company, Old Vic Theatre, London, 1964; Conn, *The Shaughraun*, Abbey Theatre Company, Aldwych Theatre, 1968; Gaev, *The Cherry Orchard*, Dublin Theatre Festival, 1968; Menenius, *Coriolanus*, John F. Kennedy Theatre, Honolulu, HI, then Old Vic Theatre, both 1970; Antonio, *The Tempest*, and the Masked Man, *Spring Awakening*, both National Theatre Company, Old Vic Theatre, 1974; Fluther Good, *The Plough and the Stars*, National Theatre, London, 1977; Drumm, *A Life*, Old Vic Theatre, 1980. Also appeared in *Milestones*, *The Promised Land*, and *Ambrose Applejohn's Adventure*, all Norwich Repertory Company, 1928; *Tareis an Aifrinn (After Mass)*, Gate Theatre, 1942; and *You Never Can Tell*, Malvern Theatre Festival, Malvern, U.K., 1978; and with the Liverpool Shakespeare Theatre, Liverpool, U.K., 1958.

With the Abbey Theatre, Dublin, Ireland: The Boy, *The Vigil*, and Hughie Boyle, *Wrack*, both 1932; Michael, *Drama at Inish*, 1933; Irish countryman, *Parnell of Avondale*, Malcolm, *Macbeth*, the Son, *Six Characters in Search of an Author*, and Colin Langford, *At Mrs. Beams'*, all 1934; Marchbanks, *Candida*, Japhet, *Noah*, and Curran, *Summer's Day*, all 1935; Titus Larius, *Coriolanus*, Andy, *Boyd's Shop*, Jo Mahony, *Katie Roche*, Hind, *The Passing Day*, John Joseph Barrett, *The Silver Jubilee*, and Mr. Bunton, *The Jailbird*, all 1936; O'Flingsley, *Shadow and Substance*, Quin, *Quin's Secret*, Loftus de Lury, *Killycreggs in Twilight*, Dan Cusack, *The Patriot*, Mangan, *The Man in the Cloak*, Kelly, *The Invincibles*, Cartney, *Cartney and Kevney*, and Neddy, *She Had to Do Something*, all 1937; Adam, *Neal Maquade*, Ned Hegarty, *Moses Rock*, Hyacinth, *Bird's Nest*, the Fool, *On Baile's Strand*, the Covey, *The Plough and the Stars*, Christy Mahon, *The Playboy of the Western World*, and O'Flingsley, *Shadow and Substance*, all 1938; Pat Hooey, *Give Him a House*, and John Joe Martin, *They Went by Bus*, both 1939; Kevin McMorna, *The Spanish Soldier*, 1940; Dewis, *The Whiteheaded Boy*, 1942; title role, *The O'Cuddy*, and Michael, *The Old Road*, both 1943; Francis, *The Wise Have Not Spoken*, and Seuman, *The End House*, both 1944; Dawson, *Tenants at Will*, 1945; Conn, *The Shaughraun*, 1967; title role, *Hadrian VII*, 1969; title role, *The Vicar of Wakefield*, 1974; Fluther Good, *The Plough and the Stars*, 1976. Also appeared in *Margaret Gillan*, 1933;

Gallant Cassian, 1934; *The King of Spain's Daughter*, *The Silver Tassie*, *A Deuce of Jacks*, and *A Saint in a Hurry*, all 1935; *The Grand House in the City* and *Blind Man's Buff*, both 1936; *A Spot in the Sun*, *The Great Adventure*, and *Pilgrims*, all 1938; *William John Mawhinney*, 1940; *An Apple a Day*, 1942; *Faustus Kelly* and *Poor Man's Miracle*, both 1943; *The New Regime*, 1944; *Rossa*, 1945; *You Never Can Tell*, 1978.

With the Gaiety Theatre, Dublin, Ireland: John, *The Barrell Organ*, 1942; Romeo, *Romeo and Juliet*, 1944; Tom, *The Last of Summer*, and Sid Hunt, *Hell Bent for Heaven*, both 1945; Dick Dudgeon, *The Devil's Disciple*, Louis Dubedat, *The Doctor's Dilemma*, and Bluntschli, *Arms and the Man*, all 1947; Christy Mahon, *The Playboy of the Western World*, and Bluntschli, *Arms and the Man*, both 1953; Codger, *The Bishop's Bonfire*, 1955; Do-the-Right, *The Golden Cuckoo*, Androcles, *Androcles and the Lion*, and the Man, *The Rising of the Moon*, all 1956; title role, *Hamlet*, 1957; Roger Casement, *Casement*, 1958; Doolin, *The Voices of Doolin*, 1960; title role, *The Temptation of Mr. O*, 1961; Fox Melarkey, *Crystal and Fox*, 1968.

PRINCIPAL STAGE WORK—All as producer with Cyril Cusack Productions, unless indicated. Director, *Tareis an Aifrinn (After Mass)*, Gate Theatre, Dublin, Ireland, 1942; (with Shelah Richards) *Romeo and Juliet*, Gaiety Theatre, Dublin, 1944; *The Last of Summer*, Gaiety Theatre, 1945; *Arms and the Man*, Gaiety Theatre, 1953; *The Playboy of the Western World*, Gaiety Theatre, 1953, then Theatre Sarah Bernhardt, Paris, France, 1954; *The Bishop's Bonfire*, Gaiety Theatre, 1955; *Androcles and the Lion* and *The Rising of the Moon*, both Gaiety Theatre, 1956; *Hamlet*, Gaiety Theatre, 1957; *Casement*, Gaiety Theatre, 1958; *Arms and the Man* and *Krapp's Last Tape*, tours of European cities, both 1960; co-producer, *Goodwill Ambassador*, Olympia Theatre, Dublin, 1960; *The Voices of Doolin*, Gaiety Theatre, 1961; (also director) *The Temptation of Mr. O*, Dublin Theatre Festival, Olympia Theatre, 1961.

MAJOR TOURS—The Cat, *Dick Whittington*, Irish cities, 1920; the Donkey, *Ali Baba*, and Babe, *The Babes in the Wood*, Irish cities, both 1922; the Boy, *Irish and Proud of It*, U.K. cities, 1924; Christy Mahon, *The Playboy of the Western World*, Irish cities, 1954; Doolin, *The Voices of Doolin*, Irish cities, 1960; Seumas O'Beirne, *Goodwill Ambassador*, U.S. cities, 1960; Bluntschli, *Arms and the Man*, and Krapp, *Krapp's Last Tape*, European cities, both 1960; title role, *Hadrian VII*, Abbey Theatre Company, U.K. cities, 1969-70. Also appeared in *Arrah-na-Pogue*, Irish cities, 1918; *The Sign of the Cross* and *Shot at Dawn*, Irish cities, both 1920; *The Terror*, U.K. cities, 1928.

FILM DEBUT—Young O'Brien, *Knocknagow, or The Homes of Tipperary* (silent), Film Company of Ireland, 1916. PRINCIPAL FILM APPEARANCES—Jules, *Late Extra*, Twentieth Century-Fox, 1935; Bill Hopkins, *Once a Crook*, Twentieth Century-Fox, 1941; Pat, *Odd Man Out* (also known as *Gang War*), Universal, 1947; Rogers, *Escape*, Twentieth Century-Fox, 1948; Fred Parsons, *Esther Waters*, General Film Distributors, 1948; Gerald Vane, *All Over the Town*, General Film Distributors, 1949; James Carter, *The Blue Lagoon*, Universal, 1949; Corporal Taylor, *Hour of Glory* (also known as *The Small Back Room*), British Lion, 1949; Chauvelin, *The Fighting Pimpernel* (also known as *The Elusive Pimpernel*), British Lion, 1950; Frank Hutchins, *The Blue Veil*, RKO, 1951; Duggie Lewis, *Maniacs on Wheels* (also known as *Once a Jolly Swagman*), International Releasing, 1951; Limey, *The Secret of Convict Lake*, Twentieth Century-Fox, 1951; Private Dennis Malloy, *Soldiers Three*, Metro-Goldwyn-Mayer (MGM), 1951;

Edward Marston, *The Wild Heart* (also known as *Gone to Earth* and *Gypsy Blood*), RKO/Selznick, 1952; Khadir, *Saadia*, MGM, 1953; Bohannon, *Passage Home*, General Film Distributors, 1955; Mr. Flannagan, *Jacqueline*, Rank, 1956; taxi driver, *The Man Who Never Was*, Twentieth Century-Fox, 1956; Lazy Mangan, *The March Hare* (also known as *Gamblers Sometimes Win*), British Lion, 1956; Dr. Kelly, *The Man in the Road*, Republic, 1957; Sam Bishop, *Miracle in Soho*, Rank, 1957; Garcia, *The Spanish Gardener*, Rank, 1957; Inspector Michael Dillon, "The Majesty of the Law" in *The Rising of the Moon*, Warner Brothers, 1957; Peebles, *Floods of Fear*, Universal, 1958; Sandy, *Night Ambush* (also known as *Ill Met by Moonlight*), Rank, 1958; Herbert "Birdy" Sparrow, *Gideon of Scotland Yard* (also known as *Gideon's Day*), Columbia, 1959; Chris Noonan, *Shake Hands with the Devil*, United Artists, 1959.

Jimmy Hannafin, *The Night Fighters* (also known as *A Terrible Beauty*), United Artists, 1960; Captain Ferris, *I Thank a Fool*, MGM, 1962; Dr. Grogan, *Waltz of the Toreadors* (also known as *The Amorous General*), Continental Distributing, 1962; Father Maguire, *80,000 Suspects*, Rank, 1963; Control, *The Spy Who Came in from the Cold*, Paramount, 1965; prosecuting counsel, *Johnny Nobody*, Medallion, 1965; Peter Rosser, *Where the Spies Are*, MGM, 1965; captain, *Fahrenheit 451*, Universal, 1966; Hogan, *Time Lost and Time Remembered* (also known as *I Was Happy Here* and *Passage of Love*), Continental Distributing, 1966; Grumio, *The Taming of the Shrew*, Columbia, 1967; title role, *Galileo*, Fenice Cinemato-Grafica/Rizzoli/Kinozenter, 1968; messenger, *Oedipus the King*, Universal, 1968; Dr. Maitland, *Brotherly Love* (also known as *Country Dance*), MGM, 1970; Barkis, *David Copperfield*, Twentieth Century-Fox, 1970; sculptor, *Harold and Maude*, Paramount, 1971; Duke of Albany, *King Lear*, Altura, 1971; Frederick Katzmann, *Sacco e Vanzetti* (also known as *Sacco and Vanzetti*), UMC, 1971; Stolfi, *La polizia ringrazia* (also known as *The Law Enforcers* and *From the Police, with Thanks*), Produzioni Atlas Consorziale, 1972; Julian Ainsley, *The Devil's Widow* (also known as *Tam Lin*), International Pictures, 1972; Matto, *Piu forte ragazzi!* (also known as *All the Way, Boys*), AVCO-Embassy/Seven Keys, 1973; gunsmith, *The Day of the Jackal*, Universal, 1973; Sam, *The Homecoming*, American Film Theatre, 1973; Corso, *La Mala ordina* (also known as *The Italian Connection* and *Manhunt*), International Pictures, 1973; Chancellor Oxenstierna, *The Abdication*, Warner Brothers, 1974; David's father, *Children of Rage*, Emmessee Productions, 1975; poteen maker, *Poitin*, Cinegael, 1979.

Cardinal Danaher, *True Confessions*, United Artists, 1981; Sulzer, *Wagner*, Alan Landsburg, 1983; Myles Keenan, *The Outcasts*, Cinegate, 1983; Charrington, *1984*, Atlantic Releasing, 1984; Frederick Dorritt, *Little Dorrit*, Sands/Cannon Screen Entertainment, 1987. Also appeared in *Guests of the Nation*, 1934; *The Man without a Face*, 1935; *Mail Train* (also known as *Inspector Hornleigh Goes to It*), Twentieth Century-Fox, 1941; as Billy, *Servants All*, 1941; in *Christopher Columbus*, 1949; *Destination Milan*, British Lion, 1954; *The Last Moment*, British Lion, 1954; *Lawrence of Arabia*, Columbia, 1962; *Tristan et Iseult* (also known as *Tristan and Isolde*), Films du soir, 1973; *Juggernaut*, United Artists, 1974; as balloon vendor, *Last Moments* (also known as *Venditore di palloncini*), 1974; in *Run, Run Joe!*, 1974; *The Bloody Hands of the Law* (also known as *La mano spietata della legge* and *Execution Squad*), 1976; *The Temptation of Mr. O*, 1981; *The Kingfisher*, 1982; and in *One Spy Too Many* and *Passport to Oblivion*.

PRINCIPAL TELEVISION APPEARANCES—Mini-Series: Yehuda, *Jesus of Nazareth*, NBC, 1977; Old Mr. Lorimer, *Death of an*

Expert Witness, Anglia Television, then *Mystery!*, PBS, 1985; also *The Golden Bowl*, BBC, then *Masterpiece Theatre*, PBS, 1973. Episodic: Thomas a Becket, "Murder in the Cathedral," and the Father, "Six Characters in Search of an Author," *BBC Festival*, BBC, 1964. Movies: Petley, *The Big Toe*, ITV, 1964; Barkis, *David Copperfield*, NBC, 1970; Father Manus, *Catholics*, CBS, 1973; Fauchelevent, *Les Miserables*, CBS, 1978; Tom Maloney, *Cry of the Innocent*, NBC, 1980; Doc Spencer, *Danny, the Champion of the World*, Disney Channel, 1989. Specials: Dr. Coutras, *The Moon and Sixpence*, ABC, 1957; Krapp, *Krapp's Last Tape*, BBC, 1963; Inspector Hubbard, *Dial M for Murder*, ABC, 1967; Mr. Reese, *The Hands of Cormac Joyce*, NBC, 1972; Steiner, *Dr. Fischer of Geneva*, BBC, 1983, then *Great Performances*, PBS, 1985; Theban citizen, *The Theban Plays*, BBC, then PBS, 1988; parish priest, "The Tenth Man," *Hallmark Hall of Fame*, CBS, 1988. Also appeared in *The Shadow of the Glen*, BBC, 1938; *Ship Day*, Elstree, 1948; *Highland Fling*, Elstree, 1948; *The Sensible Man*, Elstree, 1949; *Oedipus Complex*, BBC, 1953; *What Every Woman Knows*, ABC, 1959; *The Enchanted*, ABC, 1959; *The Power and the Glory*, ABC, 1959; *The Dummy*, ABC, 1962; *The Chairs*, Granada, 1962; *Don Juan in Hell*, Granada, 1962; *The Lotus Eater*, Granada, 1962; as Michael McInerney, *The Workhouse Ward*, 1963; in *The Wedding Dress*, Granada, 1963; *Tryptych*, 1963; *In the Train*, 1963; *The Good and Faithful Servant*, 1974; *Crystal and Fox*, 1975; *No Country for Old Men*, 1981; *One of Ourselves*, 1983; and in *Moon in the Yellow River*, *Deirdre*, *The Hitchhiker*, *Trial of Marshall Petain*, *Uncle Vanya*, *A Time of Wolves and Tigers*, *Passage to India*, *In the Bosom of the Country*, *Them*, *Clochemerie*, *I Stand Well with All Parties*, *The Plough and the Stars*, *You Never Can Tell*, *The Tower*, *St. Francis*, *The Physicists*, and *The Reunion*.

PRINCIPAL RADIO APPEARANCES—Plays: *The Dark Tower*, BBC, 1946; *Troilus and Cressida*, Third Network, 1965; also appeared as Pip, *Great Expectations*, BBC; in *Frederic General*, BBC; *The Dead*, BBC; *The Wild Goose*, BBC; and performed characters from Charles Dickens for Radio-Eireann.

RELATED CAREER—Member, Abbey Theatre, Dublin, Ireland, 1932-35; producer, Gaelic Players, 1935-36; manager, Gaiety Theatre, Dublin, 1944; managing director, Cyril Cusack Productions, 1944-61; associate and stockholder, National Theatre, Dublin, 1966.

WRITINGS: STAGE—*Tareis an Aifrinn (After Mass)*, Gate Theatre, Dublin, Ireland, 1942; *The Temptation of Mr. O*, Dublin Theatre Festival, Olympia Theatre, Dublin, Ireland, 1961. OTHER—*Timepieces* (poetry), 1972; *Poems*, 1976. Also contributor to journals and periodicals.

RECORDINGS: Beckett: *Molloy, Malone Dies, [and] The Unnameable*, Caedmon, 1964.

AWARDS: English Tatler Radio Critics Award, 1954, for *The Dark Tower*; Sylvania Television Citation, 1959, for *The Moon and Sixpence*; International Critics Awards, 1961, for *Arms and the Man* and *Krapp's Last Tape*; Irish Television Critics' Award, Best Actor, 1963. Honorary degrees: LL.D., honoris causa, from National University of Ireland, 1977; Hon D. Litt., University of Ulster, Northern Ireland, 1982.

MEMBER: British Actors' Equity Association, Irish Actors' Equity Association, Screen Actors Guild, American Federation of Television and Radio Artists, United Arts Club (Dublin, Ireland), Irish Club (London), National University of Ireland Club (London).

SIDELIGHTS: FAVORITE ROLES—The Covey in *The Plough and the Stars,* Christy Mahon in *The Playboy of the Western World,* Romeo in *Romeo and Juliet,* and Shavian parts. RECREATIONS—Riding, collecting objets d'art of theatrical interest, rare books, and posters of Irish theatrical interest.

ADDRESSES: HOME—Cluain Chaoin, Br. Sorrento, Deilginis, County Dublin, Ireland.*

*   *   *

CUSACK, Joan 1962-

PERSONAL: Born October 11, 1962, in New York, NY; daughter of Richard (owner of a film production company) and Nancy (owner of a film production company) Cusack. EDUCATION: Graduated from the University of Wisconsin, Madison; trained for the stage at the Piven Theatre Workshop, Chicago, IL.

VOCATION: Actress.

CAREER: PRINCIPAL STAGE APPEARANCES—Louise and Clare, *Road,* LaMama Experimental Theatre Club, New York City, 1988; Rosannah DeLuce, *Brilliant Traces,* Circle Repertory Company, Cherry Lane Theatre, New York City, 1989; Imogen, *Cymbeline,* New York Shakespeare Festival, Public Theatre, New York City, 1989; also appeared in *Bits and Pieces, Connections,* and *Aesop's Greatest Hits,* all Piven Theatre, Chicago, IL.

FILM DEBUT—Shelley, *My Bodyguard,* Twentieth Century-Fox, 1980. PRINCIPAL FILM APPEARANCES—Julia, *Class,* Orion, 1983; Mary, *Grandview, U.S.A.,* Warner Brothers, 1984; first geek girl, *Sixteen Candles,* Universal, 1984; Gina, *The Allnighter,* Universal, 1987; Blair Litton, *Broadcast News,* Twentieth Century-Fox, 1987; Irene Stein, *Stars and Bars,* Columbia, 1988; Rose, *Married to the Mob,* Orion, 1988; Cyn, *Working Girl,* Twentieth Century-Fox, 1988. Also appeared in *Say Anything,* Twentieth Century-Fox, 1989; *Men Don't Leave,* 1989.

PRINCIPAL TELEVISION APPEARANCES—Series: Regular, *Saturday Night Live,* NBC, 1985-86. Pilots: Linda Parker, *All Together Now,* NBC, 1984.

AWARDS: Academy Award nomination, Best Supporting Actress, 1989, for *Working Girl.*

SIDELIGHTS: RECREATIONS—Painting.

ADDRESSES: AGENT—Steve Dontanville, International Creative Management, 8899 Beverly Boulevard, Los Angeles, CA 90048.*

D

D'ABO, Maryam 1961-

PERSONAL: Born 1961, in London, England; mother, head of the UNICEF Greeting Card operation in Europe.

VOCATION: Actress.

PERSONAL: PRINCIPAL FILM APPEARANCES—Analise, *Xtro,* New Line Cinema, 1983; Nathalie, *Until September,* Metro-Goldwyn-Mayer/United Artists, 1984; French girlfriend, *White Nights,* Columbia, 1985; Kara Milovy, *The Living Daylights,* Metro-Goldwyn-Mayer/United Artists, 1987.

PRINCIPAL TELEVISION APPEARANCES—Series: Ta'Ra, *Something Is Out There,* NBC, 1988. Mini-Series: Dominique, *Master of the Game,* CBS, 1984; Solange, *If Tomorrow Comes,* CBS, 1986. Pilots: Claudie DeBrille, *Behind Enemy Lines,* NBC, 1985; Ta'Ra, *Something Is Out There,* NBC, 1988. Movies: Lady of the court, *Arthur the King,* CBS, 1985; also *The Man Who Lived at the Ritz,* syndicated, 1988.

RELATED CAREER—Appeared in television commercials.

ADDRESSES: AGENT—Dennis Selinger, International Creative Management, 388 Oxford Street, London W1, England.*

*   *   *

DAFOE, Willem 1955-

PERSONAL: Born July 22, 1955, in Appleton, WI; father, a surgeon; mother, a nurse; children: Jack (with Elizabeth DeCompte, a stage director).

VOCATION: Actor.

CAREER: PRINCIPAL STAGE APPEARANCES—Lieutenant Buchevski and first customer, *Cop,* Performance Group, Envelope Theatre, New York City, 1978; Arthur, *The Balcony,* Performing Garage, New York City, 1979; Colonel Lloyd Lud, *North Atlantic,* Wooster Group, Kennedy Center for the Performing Arts, Washington, DC, 1985. Also appeared in *Miss Universal Happiness,* Wooster Group, Performing Garage, New York City, 1985.

FILM DEBUT—Vance, *The Loveless,* Mainline, 1982. PRINCIPAL FILM APPEARANCES—Youth in phone booth, *The Hunger,* Metro-Goldwyn-Mayer/United Artists (MGM/UA), 1983; punk boyfriend, *New York Nights,* Bedford Entertainment, 1984; Johnny Harte, *Roadhouse 66,* Atlantic, 1984; Raven, *Streets of Fire,*

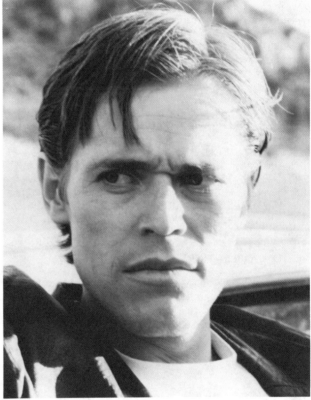

WILLEM DAFOE

Universal/RKO, 1984; Eric Masters, *To Live and Die in L.A.,* MGM/UA, 1985; Sergeant Elias, *Platoon,* Orion, 1986; narrator, *Dear America: Letters Home from Vietnam,* HBO Productions, 1987; Buck McGriff, *Off Limits,* Twentieth Century-Fox, 1988; Jesus Christ, *The Last Temptation of Christ,* Universal, 1988; Ward, *Mississippi Burning,* Orion, 1988. Also appeared in *The Communists Are Comfortable (And Three Other Stories),* 1984.

RELATED CAREER—Actor and set builder, Theatre X, Milwaukee, WI; actor, Wooster Group, New York City.

AWARDS: Academy Award nomination, Best Supporting Actor, 1987, for *Platoon.*

ADDRESSES: AGENT—Michael Menchel, Creative Artists Agency, 1888 Century Park E., Suite 1400, Los Angeles, CA 90067.*

DALTON, Abby   1935-

PERSONAL: Born August 15, 1935 (some sources say 1932), in Las Vegas, NV; children: Matthew.

VOCATION: Actress.

CAREER: FILM DEBUT—Julie, *Rock All Night,* American International, 1957. PRINCIPAL FILM APPEARANCES—Lucy, *Cole Younger, Gunfighter,* Allied Artists, 1958; Agnes Clark, *Girls on the Loose,* Universal, 1958; Kathy, *Stakeout on Dope Street,* Warner Brothers, 1958; Calamity Jane, *The Plainsman,* Universal, 1966; Ann Fields, *A Whale of a Tale,* Luckris, 1977. Also appeared in *The Saga of the Viking Women and Their Voyage to the Waters of the Great Sea Serpent* (also known as *The Viking Women and the Sea Serpent*), American International, 1957.

TELEVISION DEBUT—Belle Starr, "Way of the West," *Schlitz Playhouse of Stars,* CBS, 1958. PRINCIPAL TELEVISION APPEARANCES—Series: Nurse Martha Hale, *Hennessey,* CBS, 1959-62; Ellie Barnes, *The Joey Bishop Show,* NBC, 1962, then CBS, 1962-65; regular, *The Jonathan Winters Show,* CBS, 1967-69; Margaret Kelly, *Adams of Eagle Lake,* ABC, 1975; Julia Cumson, *Falcon Crest,* CBS, 1981-86. Pilots: Augusta Anderson, *Anderson and Company,* NBC, 1969; Elizabeth Miller, *Barney Miller,* ABC, 1975. Episodic: "Dead Man's Walk," *The Chevy Mystery Show,* NBC, 1960; Fran Hendrix, *Hardcastle and McCormick,* ABC, 1986; also Nancy Moore, *The Rifleman,* ABC; showgirl, *Rawhide,* CBS; *Maverick,* ABC; *Have Gun Will Travel,* CBS. Movies: Lucy Kane, *Magic Carpet,* ABC, 1972. Specials: *Battle of the Network Stars,* ABC, 1984; *All Star Blitz,* NBC, 1985; *The Real Trivial Pursuit,* ABC, 1985.

RELATED CAREER—Model.

ADDRESSES: AGENT—David Shapira and Associates, Inc., 15301 Ventura Boulevard, Suite 345, Sherman Oaks, CA 91403. PUBLICIST—Sheri Goldberg, Hanson and Schwam Public Relations, 9200 Sunset Boulevard, Suite 307, Los Angeles, CA 90069.*

*   *   *

DALTON, Timothy   1944-

PERSONAL: Born March 21, 1944, in Colwyn Bay, Wales.

VOCATION: Actor.

CAREER: PRINCIPAL STAGE APPEARANCES—All in London, unless indicated. Bob, *The Samaritan,* Shaw Theatre, 1971; Arthur, *A Game Called Arthur,* Theatre Upstairs, 1971; Edgar, *King Lear,* Prospect Theatre Company, Aldwych Theatre, 1972; Romeo, *Romeo and Juliet,* and Costard, *Love's Labour's Lost,* both Royal Shakespeare Company, Royal Shakespeare Theatre, Stratford-on-Avon, U.K., 1973; Hal, the Prince of Wales, *King Henry IV, Parts I and II,* and title role, *Henry V,* all Prospect Theatre Company, Round House Theatre, 1974; Nicky Lancaster, *The Vortex,* Greenwich Theatre, 1975; Harold Gorringe, "Black Comedy," and Tom, "White Liars," both in *Black Comedy and White Liars,* Dolphin Theatre Company, Shaw Theatre, 1976; Cornelius Melody, *A Touch of the Poet,* Young Vic Theatre, then Royal Haymarket Theatre, both 1988. Also appeared in *Antony and Cleopatra* and *The Taming of the Shrew,* both in 1986.

PRINCIPAL FILM APPEARANCES—King Philip of France, *The Lion in Winter,* AVCO-Embassy, 1968; Prince Rupert, *Cromwell,* Columbia, 1970; Heathcliff, *Wuthering Heights,* American International, 1970; Henry, Lord Darnley, *Mary, Queen of Scots,* Universal, 1971; Charles Lord, *Permission to Kill,* AVCO-Embassy, 1975; John of God, *El Hombre Que Supo Amar* (also known as *The Man Who Knew Love*), General Film Corporation, 1976; Sir Michael Barrington, *Sextette,* Crown International, 1978; Archie Christie, *Agatha,* Warner Brothers, 1979; Prince Barin, *Flash Gordon,* Universal, 1980; Boy Capel, *Chanel Solitaire,* United Film Distribution, 1981; Dr. Thomas Rock, *The Doctor and the Devils,* Twentieth Century-Fox, 1985; James Bond, *The Living Daylights,* Metro-Goldwyn-Mayer/United Artists, 1987; Bancroft, *Hawks,* Skouras, 1988. Also appeared in *Lady Caroline Lamb,* United Artists, 1972; and in *The Voyeur.*

PRINCIPAL TELEVISION APPEARANCES—Mini-Series: Oliver Seccombe, *Centennial,* NBC, 1979; Perry Kilkullen, *Mistral's Daughter,* CBS, 1984; Mr. Rochester, *Jane Eyre,* Arts and Entertainment, 1988. Movies: Marquis de Guaita, *The Flame Is Love,* NBC, 1979; Colonel Francis Blake, *The Master of Ballantrae,* CBS, 1984; Richard Milnes, *Florence Nightingale,* NBC, 1985; Edmund Junot, *Sins,* CBS, 1986.

ADDRESSES: AGENTS—J. Michael Bloom Agency, 9200 Sunset Boulevard, Suite 710, Los Angeles, CA 90069.*

*   *   *

DANNING, Sybil

VOCATION: Actress.

CAREER: PRINCIPAL FILM APPEARANCES—Prostitute, *Bluebeard,* Vulcano, 1972; Eugenie, *The Three Musketeers,* Twentieth Century-Fox, 1974; girl, *Operation Lady Marlene,* AMLF, 1975; visitor, *Les Noces de Porcelaine* (also known as *The Porcelain Anniversary*), Fox/Lira, 1975; secretary, *Folies bourgeoises* (also known as *Twist*), Union Generale Cinematographique/Parafrance, 1976; Mother Canty, *Crossed Swords* (also known as *The Prince and the Pauper*), Warner Brothers, 1978; Sally, *Night of the Askari* (also known as *Whispering Death*), Topar, 1978; Halima, *Operation Thunderbolt* (also known as *Entebbe: Operation Thunderbolt*), Cinema Shares International, 1978; girl skier, *Meteor,* American International, 1979; Amy Sande, *The Concorde—Airport '79* (also known as *Airport '79* and *Airport '80: The Concorde*), Universal, 1979.

St. Exmin, *Battle beyond the Stars,* New World, 1980; Veronica, *Cuba Crossing* (also known as *Kill Castro* and *Assignment: Kill Castro*), Key West, 1980; Charlotte, *How to Beat the High Cost of Living,* American International, 1980; Cynthia, *The Man with Bogart's Face* (also known as *Sam Marlow, Private-Eye*), Twentieth Century-Fox, 1980; Mary, *Separate Ways,* Crown International, 1981; Susan, *Julie Darling,* Tat/ Cinequity, 1982; Julia, *The Seven Magnificent Gladiators,* Cannon, 1982; Ericka, *Chained Heat,* Jensen Farley, 1983; Lili Anders, *The Salamander,* ITC, 1983; Arianna, *Hercules,* Metro-Goldwyn-Mayer/United Artists-Cannon, 1983; Angel, *Jungle Warriors,* Aquarius, 1984; Dianne Stevens, *They're Playing with Fire,* New World, 1984; Stirba, *The Howling II . . . Your Sister Is a Werewolf,* Thorn/EMI, 1985; Brenda, *The Day of the Cobra,* Media Home Entertainment, 1985; Judith, *Young Lady Chatterley II* (also known as *Private Property*),

Cine-Circle Distributors/Park Land, 1985; Katherine, *Private Passions,* Delta/Uranium, 1985; Contessa Luciana, *Malibu Express,* Universal, 1985; Jade, *The Tomb,* Trans World Entertainment, 1986; Ilona, *Panther Squad,* Greenwich International, 1986; Sutter, *Reform School Girls,* New World/Balcor, 1986; Berenice, *Warrior Queen,* Seymour Borde, 1987; Lara, *Amazon Women on the Moon,* Universal, 1987; bathing beauty, *Talking Walls* (also known as *Motel Vacancy*), New World, 1987. Also appeared in *Sam's Song* (also known as *The Swap*), Cannon, 1971; *Gelobt Sei Was Hart Macht* (also known as *Praise Be What Hardens You*), Cinerama Releasing Corporation, 1972; *Naughty Nymphs,* 1974; *Run, Run, Joe!,* 1974; *Hausfrauen-Report* (also known as *God's Gun*), Irwin Yablans, 1977; and *Albino,* 1980.

PRINCIPAL FILM WORK—Producer (with Daniel LeSoeur and Ken Johnston), *Panther Squad,* Greenwich International, 1986.

MEMBER: Screen Actors Guild.*

*   *   *

DANTE, Joe

PERSONAL: Born in Morristown, NJ.

VOCATION: Director and film editor.

CAREER: Also see *WRITINGS* below. PRINCIPAL FILM APPEARANCES—*Cannonball* (also known as *Carquake*) New World, 1976; *Roger Corman: Hollywood's Wild Angel,* Cinegate, 1978.

PRINCIPAL FILM WORK—Director (with Allan Arkush) and editor (with Arkush and Amy Jones), *Hollywood Boulevard,* New World, 1976; editor, *Grand Theft Auto,* New World, 1977; director and editor (with Mark Goldblatt), *Piranha,* New World, 1978; director and editor (with Goldblatt), *The Howling,* AVCO-Embassy, 1981; director, "It's a Good Life," *Twilight Zone—The Movie,* Warner Brothers, 1983; director, *Gremlins,* Warner Brothers, 1984; director, *Explorers,* Paramount, 1985; director, "Hairlooming," "Bullshit or Not," "Critics Corner," "Roast Your Loved One," and "Reckless Youth," *Amazon Women on the Moon,* Universal, 1987; director, *Innerspace,* Warner Brothers, 1987; director, *The Burbs,* Universal, 1989.

PRINCIPAL TELEVISION WORK—Episodic: Director, *Police Squad!,* ABC, 1982; director, *The Twilight Zone,* CBS, 1985; director, *Amazing Stories,* NBC, 1985 and 1986.

RELATED CAREER—Managing editor, *Film Bulletin;* creator of advertising campaigns for films.

ADDRESSES: AGENT—David Gersh, The Gersh Agency, 222 N. Canon Drive, Suite 202, Beverly Hills, CA 90210.

*   *   *

D'ARBANVILLE, Patti

PERSONAL: Born c. 1952; father, a bartender; mother, an artist; married Roger Mirmont (an actor), 1975 (divorced); married Steve Curry (an actor and farmer); children: Jesse Wayne (with Don Johnson). EDUCATION: Trained for the stage with Herbert Berghof.

VOCATION: Actress.

CAREER: PRINCIPAL STAGE APPEARANCES—Janice, *Italian American Reconciliation,* GNU Theatre, Los Angeles, CA, 1987.

FILM DEBUT—*Andy Warhol's "Flesh."* PRINCIPAL FILM APPEARANCES—Patti, *L'Amour,* Altura, 1973; Betty Fargo, *Rancho Deluxe,* United Artists, 1975; title role, *Bilitis,* Societe nouvelle de cinema, 1976; Sally Johnson, *Big Wednesday,* Warner Brothers, 1978; Shirley, *Time after Time,* Warner Brothers/Orion, 1979; Donna Washington, *The Main Event,* Warner Brothers, 1979; Cathy Burke, *The Fifth Floor,* Film Ventures, 1980; Angie Barnes, *Hog Wild,* AVCO-Embassy, 1980; Darcy, *Modern Problems,* Twentieth Century-Fox, 1981; Angie, *The Boys Next Door,* Republic/New World, 1985; Sherry Nugil, *Real Genius,* Tri-Star, 1985; Cori, *Call Me,* Vestron, 1988; Jean, *Fresh Horses,* Columbia, 1988; Cathy Smith, *Wired,* Atlantic Entertainment Group, 1989. Also appeared in *The Crazy American Girl,* 1975; *La Maison;* and *La Soignee.*

PRINCIPAL TELEVISION APPEARANCES—Mini-Series: Michele, *Once an Eagle,* NBC, 1976-77. Episodic: Mrs. Stone, *Miami Vice,* NBC, 1985; Jordan Sims, *Midnight Caller,* NBC, 1988; Amber Twine, *Wiseguy,* CBS, 1989. Movies: Lucy, *Crossing the Mob* (also known as *Philly Boy*), NBC, 1988.

RELATED CAREER—Professional model; disc jockey, Le Figaro Cafe, New York City; appeared in Ivory Soap television commercials at age three.

NON-RELATED CAREER—Boutique worker.*

*   *   *

DAVIDSON, John   1941-

PERSONAL: Born December 13, 1941, in Pittsburgh, PA; father, a minister; wife's name, Rhonda; children: John, Jr., Jennifer, Ashleigh Marie. EDUCATION: Received B.A. in theatre arts from Denison University.

VOCATION: Actor, television host, and singer.

CAREER: BROADWAY DEBUT—Ben, *Foxy,* Ziegfeld Theatre, 1964. PRINCIPAL STAGE APPEARANCES—Curly, *Oklahoma!,* City Center Theatre, New York City, 1965.

MAJOR TOURS—Harold Hill, *The Music Man,* U.S. cities, 1988; also *Camelot, L'il Abner, Paint Your Wagon, The Fantasticks, Oklahoma,* and *I Do, I Do,* all U.S. cities.

PRINCIPAL FILM APPEARANCES—Angie Dule, *The Happiest Millionaire,* Buena Vista, 1967; Joe Carder, *The One and Only Genuine Original Family Band,* Buena Vista, 1968; Robert Palmer, *Concorde—Airport '79* (also known as *Airport '79* and *Airport '80: The Concorde*), Universal, 1979; Honest Tom T. Murray, *The Squeeze,* Tri-Star, 1987.

PRINCIPAL TELEVISION APPEARANCES—Series: Regular, *The Entertainers,* CBS, 1964-65; host, *The Kraft Summer Music Hall,*

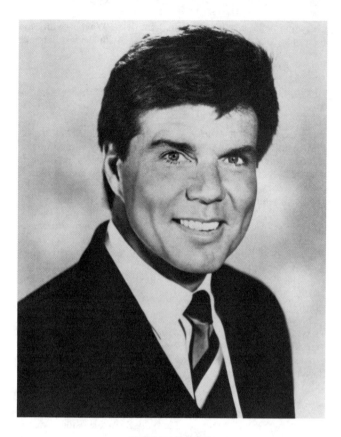

JOHN DAVIDSON

NBC, 1966; host, *The John Davidson Show*, NBC, 1969; John Burton, *The Girl with Something Extra*, NBC, 1973-74; host, *The John Davidson Show*, ABC, 1976; host, *That's Incredible*, ABC, 1980-84; host, *The John Davidson Show*, syndicated, 1980-82; host, *Time Machine*, NBC, 1985; host, *The New Hollywood Squares*, syndicated, 1986-88; host, *Incredible Sunday*, ABC, 1988—. Pilots: Max Castle, *Shell Game*, CBS, 1975; Roger Quentin, *Roger and Harry: The Mitera Target*, ABC, 1977; as himself, *King of the Road*, CBS, 1978; George Erskine, *Goodbye Charlie*, ABC, 1985; also *The NBC Follies*, NBC, 1973. Episodic: *The Ice Palace*, CBS, 1971; *The Golddiggers*, syndicated, 1971; *Spenser: For Hire*, ABC, 1986; guest host, *The Kraft Music Hall*, NBC, 1988; also guest host, *The Tonight Show Starring Johnny Carson* (over eighty-five appearances), NBC; *The Wacky World of Jonathan Winters*, syndicated; *The F.B.I.*, ABC; *The Interns*, CBS; *Owen Marshall, Counselor at Law*, ABC; *The Streets of San Francisco*, ABC.

Movies: Dennis Burnham, *Coffee, Tea or Me?*, CBS, 1973; Terry Killian, *Dallas Cowboys Cheerleaders II*, ABC, 1980. Specials: Matt, *The Fantasticks*, NBC, 1964; *Perry Como's Summer Show*, NBC, 1966; *The Bob Hope Show*, NBC, 1968, then 1969; John Kent, *Roberta*, NBC, 1969; *Sandy in Disneyland*, CBS, 1974; *The Sandy Duncan Show*, CBS, 1974; Star, *Stars and Stripes Show*, NBC, 1975; *The John Davidson Christmas Show*, NBC, 1976; *The John Davidson Christmas Show*, ABC, 1977; *The Carpenters . . . Space Encounters*, ABC, 1978; *The Carpenters—Music, Music, Music*, ABC, 1980; *Battle of the Network Stars*, ABC, 1980, then 1982; co-host, *One Hundred Years of Golden Hits*, NBC, 1981; host, *From Hawaii with Love*, syndicated, 1986; *A Crystal Christmas* (also known as *A Crystal Christmas in Sweden*), syndicated, 1987; *Game Show Biz* (documentary), syndicated, 1987; *That's*

Incredible! Reunion, ABC, 1988; *Friday Night Surprise* (also known as *Surprise*), NBC, 1988; *Life's Most Embarrassing Moments*, syndicated, 1988; host, *The Mother/Daughter U.S.A. Pageant*, syndicated, 1989; also host, *The Golden Globe Awards*, *Miss Hollywood Beauty Pageant*, *Miss World Competition*, *Miss Junior America*, and *Miss Hawaiian Tropics*.

RELATED CAREER—Nightclub performer.

WRITINGS: (With Cort Casady) *The Art of the Singing Entertainer: A Contemporary Study of the Art and Business of Being a Professional* (non-fiction), Alfred, 1982.

RECORDINGS: ALBUMS—*John Davidson*, Columbia Records, 1967; *Kind of Hush*, Columbia Records, 1967; *My Cherie Amour*, Columbia Records, 1969; also *Time of My Life*, 1966; *Everything Is Beautiful*, 1973; *Well Here I Am*, 1973; *Closeup*, Accord; and *Everytime I Sing*.

AWARDS: Theatre World Award, 1966, for *Oklahoma!*.

SIDELIGHTS: RECREATIONS—Yachting, scuba diving, jet skiing, and beachcombing.

ADDRESSES: AGENT—Marcia Resnick, Triad Artists, 10100 Santa Monica Boulevard, 16th Floor, Los Angeles, CA 90067.*

*   *   *

DAVIS, Judy   1956-

PERSONAL: Born in 1956 in Australia. EDUCATION: Attended the National Institute of Dramatic Art.

VOCATION: Actress.

CAREER: PRINCIPAL FILM APPEARANCES—Lynn, *High Rolling* (also known as *High Rolling in a Hot Corvette*), Hexagon Roadshow, 1977; Sybylla Melvyn, *My Brilliant Career*, Analysis, 1980; Sarah, *Hoodwink*, New South Wales, 1981; Kate Dean, *Heatwave*, Roadshow/New Line Cinema, 1981; Lou, *Winter of Our Dreams*, Enterprises/Satori, 1982; Frankie Leith, *The Final Option* (also known as *Who Dares Win*), Metro-Goldwyn-Mayer, 1983; Adela Quested, *A Passage to India*, Columbia, 1984; Harriet Somers, *Kangaroo*, Enterprise/Filmways, 1986; Lilli, *High Tide*, Hemdale, 1987; Nina Bailey/title role, *Georgia*, Contemporary World Cinema, 1988. Also appeared in *Phar Lap*, Twentieth Century-Fox, 1984.

PRINCIPAL FILM WORK—Co-producer, *Global Assembly Line*, 1986.

PRINCIPAL TELEVISION APPEARANCES—Movies: Young Golda, *A Woman Called Golda*, syndicated, 1982. Plays: Cleo Singer, *Rocket to the Moon*, PBS, 1986.

RELATED CAREER—Appeared with theatre companies in Adelaide and Sydney, Australia; also a singer with a rock band.

AWARDS: Emmy Award nomination, 1982, for *A Woman Called Golda*.*

DAVIS, Sammi

PERSONAL: Full name, Samantha Davis; born c. 1964, in Worcestershire, England; daughter of Michael (owner of an advertising company) and Debbie Davis.

VOCATION: Actress.

CAREER: LONDON DEBUT—*A Collier's Friday Night,* 1987. PRINCIPAL STAGE APPEARANCES—*The Home Front, The Apple Club, Nine Days, Databased,* and *Choosey Susie,* all with Big Brum Theatre Company, Birmingham, U.K.; also appeared with the Birmingham Repertory Theatre Company, Birmingham.

FILM DEBUT—May, *Mona Lisa,* Island/Handmade, 1986. PRINCIPAL FILM APPEARANCES—Dawn Rohan, *Hope and Glory,* Columbia, 1987; Anna, *A Prayer for the Dying,* Samuel Goldwyn, 1987; Felicity Stubbs, *Consuming Passions,* Samuel Goldwyn, 1987; Baptista, *Lionheart,* Orion, 1987; Mary Trent, *The Lair of the White Worm,* Vestron, 1988; also appeared as Ursula, *The Rainbow.*

PRINCIPAL TELEVISION APPEARANCES—Movies: Julie Jackson, *Pack of Lies,* CBS, 1987. Episodic: Anna, *The Day after the Fair,* BBC, 1987, then *Masterpiece Theatre,* PBS, 1988. Also appeared in *Auf Wiedersehn Pet.* *

*   *   *

DAVYS, Edmund   1947-

PERSONAL: Born January 21, 1947, in Nashua, NH; son of Robert Charles (a diplomat) and Shirley Eleanor (Chapman) Davis; married third wife, Christal Lockwood Miller (an actress), April 25, 1987; children: Liam, Colm. EDUCATION: Oberlin College, B.A., theatre arts, 1970; trained for the stage with Frederic O'Brady at La Comedie Francaise and with Michael Howard.

VOCATION: Actor.

CAREER: BROADWAY DEBUT—Jonathan Small, *The Crucifer of Blood,* Helen Hayes Theatre, 1978. PRINCIPAL STAGE APPEARANCES—Cassio, *Othello,* Roundabout Theatre, New York City, 1978; Ilya Ilyich Telegin, *Uncle Vanya,* McCarter Theatre, Princeton, NJ, 1986; Paul Verrall, *Born Yesterday,* King's officer, *Tartuffe,* second narrator, *A Christmas Carol,* Bessmertny, *Sarcophagus,* and Son Gordon, *Dividing the Estate,* all McCarter Theatre, 1988-89. Also appeared in *The Miracle Worker,* Merrimack Regional Theatre, Lowell, MA, 1982; *A Christmas Carol,* Merrimack Regional Theatre, 1983 and 1984; *Fanshen,* McCarter Theatre Lab, Princeton, NJ, 1987; as Whorehound, *A Chaste Maid in Cheapside,* Spectrum Theatre, New York City; Man, *Hello Out There,* Pretender's Theatre, New York City; Jamie, *Long Day's Journey into Night,* Branwell, *Glasstown,* Thomas Mendip, *The Lady's Not for Burning,* and Will, *A Cry of Players,* all Manhattan Conservatory, New York City; Treplev, *The Seagull,* Von Berg, *Incident at Vichy,* and John Worthing, *The Importance of Being Earnest,* all Chicago Actors' Repertory Theatre, Chicago, IL; Giles, *The Mousetrap,* and Richard, *The Lion in Winter,* both Merrimack Regional Theatre; Grimaldi, *'Tis Pity She's a Whore,* and Ted Ragg, *Arturo Ui,* both Goodman Theatre, Chicago; Willie, *Will o' Wisp,* Boston Playwrights Theatre, Boston, MA; Laertes, *Hamlet,* and Edmund, *King Lear,* both Court Theatre, Chicago;

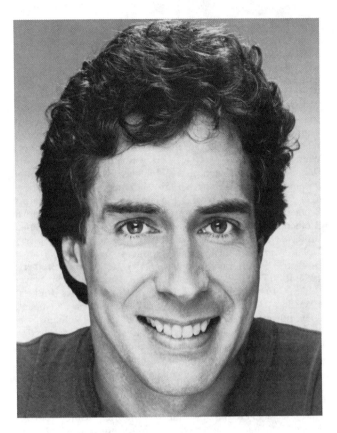

EDMUND DAVYS

Tom Wingfield, *The Glass Menagerie,* Chagrin Valley Little Theatre, Chagrin Falls, OH; Hastings, *She Stoops to Conquer,* and Chorus and Prince, *Romeo and Juliet,* both American Stage Festival, Milford, NH; Acaste, *The Misanthrope,* Theatre Intime; and Feargus O'Connor, *The Hostage,* Academy Playhouse.

RELATED CAREER—Actor in industrial films and commercials.

MEMBER: Actors' Equity Association, Screen Actors Guild, American Federation of Televison and Radio Artists.

SIDELIGHTS: RECREATIONS—Tennis, stage combat, folk guitar, and travel.

ADDRESSES: HOME—476 Central Park W., New York, NY 10021.

*   *   *

DAY, Doris   1924-

PERSONAL: Born Doris von Kappelhoff, April 3, 1924, in Cincinnati, OH; daughter of Frederick Wilhelm and Alma Sophia von Kappellhoff; married Al Jorden (a musician), 1941 (divorced, 1943); married George Weilder (a musician), 1946 (divorced, 1949); married Martin Melcher (an agent), 1951 (died, 1968); married Barry Comden (a restaurateur), 1976 (divorced); children: Terry (first marriage).

VOCATION: Actress and singer.

CAREER: FILM DEBUT—Georgia Garrett, *Romance on the High Seas* (also known as *It's Magic*), Warner Brothers, 1948. PRINCIPAL FILM APPEARANCES—Judy Adams, *It's a Great Feeling,* Warner Brothers, 1949; Martha Gibson, *My Dream Is Yours,* Warner Brothers, 1949; Lucy Rice, *Storm Warning,* Warner Brothers, 1950; Nanette Carter, *Tea for Two,* Warner Brothers, 1950; Jan Wilson, *The West Point Story* (also known as *Fine and Dandy*), Warner Brothers, 1950; Jo Jordan, *Young Man with a Horn,* Warner Brothers, 1950; Grace LeBoy Kahn, *I'll See You in My Dreams,* Warner Brothers, 1951; Melinda Howard, *The Lullaby of Broadway,* Warner Brothers, 1951; Marjorie Winfield, *On Moonlight Bay,* Warner Brothers, 1951; as herself, *Starlift,* Warner Brothers, 1951; Aimee Alexander, *The Winning Team,* Warner Brothers, 1952; Ethel "Dynamite" Jackson, *April in Paris,* Warner Brothers, 1953; Marjorie Winfield, *By the Light of the Silvery Moon,* Warner Brothers, 1953; title role, *Calamity Jane,* Warner Brothers, 1953; Candy Williams, *Lucky Me,* Warner Brothers, 1954; Ruth Etting, *Love Me or Leave Me,* Metro-Goldwyn-Mayer (MGM), 1955; Laurie Tuttle, *Young at Heart,* Warner Brothers, 1955; Jo McKenna, *The Man Who Knew Too Much,* Paramount, 1956; title role, *Julie,* MGM, 1956; Katie "Babe" Williams, *The Pajama Game,* Warner Brothers, 1957; Erica Stone, *Teacher's Pet,* Paramount, 1958; Isolde Poole, *The Tunnel of Love,* MGM, 1958; Jane Osgood, *It Happened to Jane* (also known as *Twinkle and Shine*), Columbia, 1959; Jan Morrow, *Pillow Talk,* Universal, 1959.

Kate Mackay, *Please Don't Eat the Daisies,* MGM, 1960; Kit Preston, *Midnight Lace,* Universal, 1960; Carol Templeton, *Lover Come Back,* Universal, 1961; Kitty Wonder, *Jumbo* (also known as *Billy Rose's "Jumbo"*), MGM, 1962; Cathy Timberlake, *That Touch of Mink,* Universal, 1962; Ellen Wagstaff Arden, *Move Over, Darling,* Twentieth Century-Fox, 1963; Beverly Boyer, *The Thrill of It All,* Universal, 1963; Judy Kimball, *Send Me No Flowers,* Universal, 1964; Janet Harper, *Do Not Disturb,* Twentieth Century-Fox, 1965; Jennifer Nelson, *The Glass Bottom Boat,* MGM, 1966; Patricia Fowler, *Caprice,* Twentieth Century-Fox, 1967; Josie Minick, *The Ballad of Josie,* Universal, 1968; Margaret Garrison, *Where Were You When the Lights Went Out?,* MGM, 1968; Abby McClure, *With Six You Get Eggroll* (also known as *A Man in Mommy's Bed*), National General, 1968. Also appeared in *Yankee Doodle Girl,* 1954.

PRINCIPAL TELEVISION APPEARANCES—Series: Doris Martin, *The Doris Day Show,* CBS, 1968-73; host, *The Pet Set,* syndicated, 1972; host, *Doris Day and Friends,* CBN, 1985. Specials: *The Doris Mary Anne Kappelhoff Special,* CBS, 1971; *The John Denver Special,* ABC, 1974; *Doris Day Today,* CBS, 1975.

PRINCIPAL RADIO APPEARANCES—Series: Singer and leading lady, *The Bob Hope Show,* NBC, 1948-50; host, *The Doris Day Show,* CBS, 1952-53; also singer, *Karlin's Karnival,* WCPO.

RELATED CAREER—Singer with Bob Crosby's band, 1940, then Les Brown's band, 1940-46, also with Barney Rapp and Fred Waring; founder, Arwin Productions, 1955; partner in the dance team Doherty and Kappelhoff; toured in U.S.O. shows with Bob Hope.

NON-RELATED CAREER—Founder, Doris Day Pet Foundation; animal rights activist.

WRITINGS: (With A.E. Hotchner) *The Sentimental Journey: Doris Day's Own Story,* 1976.

RECORDINGS: ALBUMS—*Annie Get Your Gun,* Columbia; *Billy Rose's "Jumbo,"* CBS Special Projects; *By the Light of the Silvery Moon,* CBS Special Projects; *Calamity Jane,* CBS Special Projects; *Doris Day's Greatest Hits,* Columbia; (with the Frank DeVol Orchestra) *Hooray for Hollywood,* CBS Special Projects; *I'll See You in My Dreams,* CBS Special Projects; *Love Me or Leave Me,* CBS Special Projects; *Lullaby of Broadway,* CBS Special Projects; *On Moonlight Bay,* CBS Special Projects; *The Pajama Game,* CBS Special Projects; *Tea for Two,* CBS Special Projects; *Young Man with a Horn,* CSP; *Doris Day with Van Alexander's Orchestra,* Hindsight; (with Andre Previn) *Duet,* DRG. Also recorded numerous albums and singles with Columbia Records, including *Que Sera Sera* and *Secret Love,* 1950—.

AWARDS: Laurel Award, Leading New Female Personality in the Motion Picture Industry, 1950; Academy Award nomination, Best Actress, 1959, for *Pillow Talk;* Laurel Award, Top Audience Attractor, 1962.

ADDRESSES: HOME—Carmel Valley, CA.*

*   *   *

DAY, Linda   1938-

PERSONAL: Born Linda Brickner, August 12, 1938, in Los Angeles, CA; daughter of Roy (a film editor) and Sylvia (Agate) Brickner; children: Heidi, Lorraine. EDUCATION: Attended the University California, Santa Barbara, for three years.

VOCATION: Television director.

CAREER: PRINCIPAL TELEVISION WORK—All as director. Series: *Married with Children,* Fox, 1986-88; *Kate and Allie,* CBS, 1988—. Pilots: *I'd Rather Be Calm,* CBS, 1982; *After George,* CBS, 1983; *Married with Children,* Fox, 1986; *Throb,* syndicated, 1986; "Changing Patterns," *CBS Summer Playhouse,* CBS, 1987; *Mutts* (also known as *Conversations with My Dog*), ABC, 1988; also *Home Improvements,* CBS. Episodic: "Tough Love," *Archie Bunker's Place,* CBS, 1981; *Star of the Family,* ABC, 1982; *Teachers Only,* NBC, 1983; *It's Your Move,* NBC, 1984; *Double Trouble,* NBC, 1984; *The Best Times,* NBC, 1985; *Berrenger's,* NBC, 1985; *Dallas* (four episodes), CBS, 1985 and 1986; *Melba,* CBS, 1986; *The Colbys,* ABC, 1986; *Knots Landing,* CBS, 1986; *What a Country!,* syndicated, 1986; *Sidekicks,* ABC, 1986; *Morningstar/Eveningstar,* CBS, 1986; *Gimme a Break,* NBC, 1986 and 1987; *Harry,* ABC, 1987; *Sweet Surrender,* NBC, 1987; *Down and Out in Beverly Hills,* Fox, 1987; *Women in Prison,* Fox, 1987; also *St. Elsewhere,* NBC; *Who's the Boss?,* ABC; *The Bob Newhart Show,* CBS; *WKRP in Cincinnati,* CBS; *Small Wonder,* syndicated; *Brothers,* Showtime; *Different Strokes,* NBC; *Facts of Life,* NBC; *Benson,* ABC; *Too Close for Comfort,* ABC; *Alice,* CBS; and *Taxi.*

AWARDS: Emmy Award nomination, Best Comedy Director, 1981, for *Archie Bunker's Place;* Scott Newton Award, 1981; Humanitas Certificates for Humanizing Achievement in Television, 1981, 1982, 1984, and 1987.

MEMBER: Caucus.

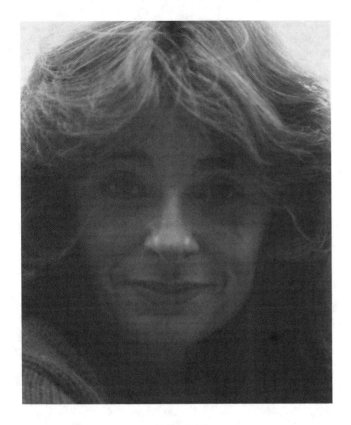

LINDA DAY

ADDRESSES: HOME—3335 Coy Drive, Sherman Oaks, CA 91423. AGENT—Michael Douroux, Lake and Douroux, 445 S. Beverly Drive, Suite 3310, Los Angeles, CA 90212.

* * *

DeCARLO, Yvonne   1924-

PERSONAL: Born Peggy Yvonne Middleton, September 1, 1924 (some sources say 1922), in Vancouver, BC, Canada; married Bob Morgan (a stuntman), 1955 (divorced); children: Bruce, Michael. EDUCATION: Attended the Vancouver School of Drama.

VOCATION: Actress.

CAREER: BROADWAY DEBUT—Carlotta Campion, *Follies,* Winter Garden Theatre, 1971. PRINCIPAL STAGE APPEARANCES—Angela, *Enter Laughing,* Wilbur Theatre, Boston, MA, then Geary Theatre, San Francisco, CA, both 1964; Carlotta Campion, *Follies,* Shubert Theatre, Century City, CA, 1972.

FILM DEBUT—Bathing beauty, *Harvard Here I Come!,* Columbia, 1942. PRINCIPAL FILM APPEARANCES—Girl, *Lucky Jordan,* Paramount, 1942; show girl, *This Gun for Hire,* Paramount, 1942; handmaiden, *The Road to Morocco,* Paramount, 1942; chorus girl, *Rhythm Parade,* Monarch, 1943; secretary, *The Crystal Ball,* United Artists, 1943; student, *Youth on Parade,* Republic, 1943; girl, *True to Life,* Paramount, 1943; Wah-Tah, *The Deerslayer,* Republic, 1943; girl in cafe, *For Whom the Bell Tolls,* Paramount, 1943; girl, *Let's Face It,* Paramount, 1943; singer in quartet, *Salute*

for Three, Paramount, 1943; girl, *Here Come the Waves,* Paramount, 1944; girl, *So Proudly We Hail,* Paramount, 1944; member of Queen's retinue, *Kismet* (also known as *Oriental Dream*), Metro-Goldwyn-Mayer (MGM), 1944; office worker, *Practically Yours,* Paramount, 1944; one of Lona's companions, *Rainbow Island,* Paramount, 1944; secretary, *Standing Room Only,* Paramount, 1944; native girl, *The Story of Dr. Wassell,* Paramount, 1944; Lorena Dumont, *Frontier Gal* (also known as *The Bride Wasn't Willing*), Universal, 1945; hatcheck girl, *Bring on the Girls,* Paramount, 1945; title role, *Salome, Where She Danced,* Universal, 1945; Gina, *Brute Force,* Universal, 1947; Francesca, *Slave Girl,* Universal, 1947; Cara de Talavera, *Song of Scheherazade,* Universal, 1947; Lola Montez, *Black Bart* (also known as *Black Bart, Highwayman*), Universal, 1948; Inez, *Casbah,* Universal, 1948; Sequin, *River Lady,* Universal, 1948; Calamity Jane Canary, *Calamity Jane and Sam Bass,* Universal, 1949; Anna, *Criss Cross,* Universal, 1949; Lillian Marlowe, *The Gal Who Took the West,* Universal, 1949.

Deborah McCoy, *Buccaneer's Girl,* Universal, 1950; Princess Scheherazade, *The Desert Hawk,* Universal, 1950; Yasmin Pallas, *Hotel Sahara,* United Artists, 1951; Candace Surrency, *Silver City* (also known as *High Vermillion*), Paramount, 1951; Julie Madden, *Tomahawk* (also known as *Battle of Powder River*), Universal, 1951; Luana, *Hurricane Smith,* Paramount, 1952; Adelaide McCall, *The San Francisco Story,* Warner Brothers, 1952; Roxy McClanahan, *Scarlet Angel,* Universal, 1952; Nita, *The Captain's Paradise,* British Lion, 1953; Yvette, *Fort Algiers,* United Artists, 1953; Drouette, *Sea Devils,* RKO, 1953; Maria, *Sombrero,* MGM, 1953; Carmelita Caris, *Border River,* Universal, 1954; Rosa and Tonya Melo, *Passion,* RKO, 1954; Serena McGlusky, *Tonight's the Night* (also known as *Happy Every After* and *O'Leary Night*), Pathe, 1954; Rosalind Dee, *Flame of the Islands,* Republic, 1955; Abby, *Shotgun,* Allied Artists, 1955; Bridget Kelly, *Death of a Scoundrel,* RKO, 1956; Minna, *Magic Fire,* Republic, 1956; Hannah Montgomery, *Raw Edge,* Universal, 1956; Sephora, *The Ten Commandments,* Paramount, 1956; Amanda Starr, *Band of Angels,* Warner Brothers, 1957; Natalie Dufort, *Timbuktu,* United Artists, 1959.

Louise Warren, *McLintock!,* United Artists, 1963; Dolores, *A Global Affair,* MGM, 1964; Ellie Irish, *Law of the Lawless,* Paramount, 1964; Lily Munster, *Munster, Go Home,* Paramount, 1966; Laura Mannon, *Hostile Guns,* Paramount, 1967; Jilly Wyler, *Arizona Bushwackers,* Paramount, 1968; Sally Hallson, *The Power,* MGM, 1968; Valerie, *The Delta Factor,* Continental Distributing, 1970; Constance Cumberland, *The Seven Minutes,* Twentieth Century-Fox, 1971; Julia, *It Seemed Like a Good Idea at the Time,* Ambassador, 1975; cleaning woman, *Won Ton Ton, the Dog Who Saved Hollywood,* Paramount, 1976; Emm Bub/high priestess, *Satan's Cheerleaders,* World Amusements, 1977; Jugulia, *Nocturna* (also known as *Nocturna, Granddaughter of Dracula*), Compass International, 1979; Susan Ames, *Guyana, Cult of the Damned,* Universal, 1980; Mrs. Engels, *Silent Scream,* American Cinema Releasing, 1980; Theresa Anastas, *The Man with Bogart's Face* (also known as *Sam Marlow, Private Eye*), Twentieth Century-Fox, 1980; Hester, *Play Dead,* Troma, 1986; Ma, *American Gothic,* Brent Walker, 1987; Mrs. Briggs, *Cellar Dweller,* Empire, 1988. Also appeared in *Cruisin' Down the River,* Columbia, 1953; as Virginia, *La Castiglione* (also known as *The Contessa's Secret*), 1954; Mary Magdalene, *La Spade e la Croce* (also known as *Mary Magdalene*), 1958; in *Tentazioni Proibiti,* 1964; *Blazing Stewardesses,* Independent International, 1975; *Arizona Slim,* 1975; *Liar's Moon,* Crown International, 1982; and *Flesh and Bullets,* Hollywood International Film Corporation, 1985.

PRINCIPAL TELEVISION APPEARANCES—Series: Magda Kolday, *The Greatest Show on Earth*, ABC, 1963-64; Lily Munster, *The Munsters*, CBS, 1964-66. Episodic: Miss Springer, *Murder, She Wrote*, CBS, 1986; also *Lights Out*, NBC; *Star Stage*, NBC. Movies: Lorraine, *The Girl on the Late, Late Show*, NBC, 1974; Isabella Vega, *The Mark of Zorro*, ABC, 1974; Lily Munster, *The Munsters' Revenge*, NBC, 1981; Mrs. Murphy, *A Masterpiece of Murder*, NBC, 1986. Specials: Victoria Johnson, *Backbone of America*, NBC, 1953; Lily Munster, *Marineland Carnival*, CBS, 1965.

RELATED CAREER—Dancer in nightclubs.

ADDRESSES: AGENT—Ruth Webb Enterprises, 7500 De Vista Drive, Los Angeles, CA 90036.*

*   *   *

De CORDOVA, Frederick   1910-

PERSONAL: Full name, Frederick Timmins De Cordova; born October 27, 1910, in New York, NY; son of George (in the theatre business) and Margaret (Timmins) De Cordova; married Janet Thomas (an actress and model), November 27, 1963. EDUCATION: Northwestern University, B.S., 1931; also attended Harvard Law School, 1933.

VOCATION: Director and producer.

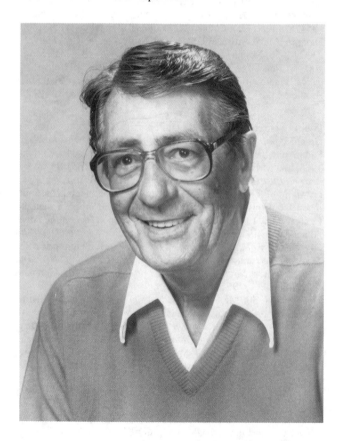

FREDERICK De CORDOVA

CAREER: PRINCIPAL STAGE WORK—All as general stage manager, director, or producer with Shubert Enterprises: *At Home Abroad*, Winter Garden Theatre, New York City, 1935; *The Show Is On* and *Ziegfeld Follies*, both Winter Garden Theatre, 1936; *Between the Devil*, Imperial Theatre, New York City, 1937; *Hellzapoppin*, 46th Street Theatre, New York City, 1938; *Straw Hat Revue*, Ambassador Theatre, New York City, 1939; *Keep Off the Grass*, Broadhurst Theatre, New York City, 1940; *High Kickers*, Broadhurst Theatre, 1941; *Ziegfeld Follies*, Winter Garden Theatre, 1943.

PRINCIPAL FILM APPEARANCES—Bert Thomas, *King of Comedy*, Twentieth Century-Fox, 1983. PRINCIPAL FILM WORK—All as director, unless indicated: Dialogue director, *Janie*, Warner Brothers, 1944; dialogue director, *Between Two Worlds*, Warner Brothers, 1944; dialogue director, *San Antonio*, Warner Brothers, 1945; *Too Young to Know*, Warner Brothers, 1945; *Her Kind of Man*, Warner Brothers, 1946; *Always Together*, Warner Brothers, 1947; *Love and Learn*, Warner Brothers, 1947; *That Way with Women*, Warner Brothers, 1947; *The Countess of Monte Carlo*, Universal, 1948; *For the Love of Mary*, Universal, 1948; *Wallflower*, Warner Brothers, 1948; *The Gal Who Took the West*, Universal, 1949; *Illegal Entry*, Universal, 1949; *Buccaneer's Girl*, Universal, 1950; *The Desert Hawk*, Universal, 1950; *Peggy*, Universal, 1950; *Finders Keepers*, Universal, 1951; *Katie Did It*, Universal, 1951; *Little Egypt* (also known as *Chicago Masquerade*), Universal, 1951; *Bedtime for Bonzo*, Universal, 1951; *Bonzo Goes to College*, Universal, 1952; *Here Come the Nelsons* (also known as *Meet the Nelsons*), Universal, 1952; *Yankee Buccaneer*, Universal, 1952; *Column South*, Universal, 1953; *I'll Take Sweden*, United Artists, 1965; *Frankie and Johnny*, United Artists, 1966.

PRINCIPAL TELEVISION APPEARANCES—Episodic: Fred, *The Jack Benny Program*, CBS, 1960-63. PRINCIPAL TELEVISION WORK—Series: Producer (with Parke Levy), *December Bride*, CBS, 1954-55; producer, *The George Burns and Gracie Allen Show*, CBS, 1955-56; producer (with Howard Duff, William Webb, and Warner Toub, Jr.) and director, *Mr. Adams and Eve*, CBS, 1957-58; producer (with Al Lewis) and director, *The George Gobel Show*, NBC, 1957-59; producer and director, *The Jack Benny Program*, CBS, 1960-63; producer, *The Smothers Brothers Show*, CBS, 1965-66; director, *To Rome with Love*, CBS, 1969-71; executive producer, *The Tonight Show Starring Johnny Carson*, NBC, 1970—. Pilots: Director, *The Barbara Rush Show*, CBS, 1965; director, *Mr. Belevedere*, CBS, 1965. Episodic: All as director. *The Smothers Brothers Show*, CBS, 1965-66; also *The Donna Reed Show*, ABC; *The Doris Day Show*, CBS; *December Bride*, CBS; *The George Burns and Gracie Allen Show*, CBS; *Bewitched*, ABC; *The Farmer's Daughter*, ABC; *The Bob Cummings Show*, CBS; *My Three Sons*, CBS. Specials: Director, *The Bing Crosby Special*, CBS, 1954; director (with Noel Coward), *Blithe Spirit*, CBS, 1956; director, *Have Girls—Will Travel*, NBC, 1964; director, *Her School for Bachelors*, NBC, 1964; producer and director, *The Jack Benny Special*, NBC, 1968; producer and director, *Jack Benny's Birthday Special*, NBC, 1969; executive producer (with Irving Fein), *A Love Letter to Jack Benny*, NBC, 1981; also executive producer of annual specials celebrating the anniversary of *The Tonight Show Starring Johnny Carson*, NBC, 1981—.

RELATED CAREER—Assistant to John Shubert, Shubert Enterprises, New York City, 1932, then general stage manager, director, and producer, Shubert Enterprises, 1932-41; general stage director, Alfred Bloomingdale Productions, New York City, 1942; producer, Louisville Amphitheatre, Louisville, KY, 1943; director of program planning, Screen Gems, 1964.

WRITINGS: Johnny Came Lately (autobiography), Simon & Schuster, 1988.

AWARDS: Emmy Award, Outstanding Program Achievement in the Field of Humor, 1961, for *The Jack Benny Program;* Emmy Awards, 1963 and 1968; Emmy Award, Special Classification of Outstanding Program and Individual Achievement, 1976, for *The Tonight Show Starring Johnny Carson;* Emmy Awards, Special Classificaton of Outstanding Program Achievement, 1977, 1978, and 1979, all for *The Tonight Show Starring Johnny Carson;* also received sixteen Emmy Award nominations.

MEMBER: Bel Air Country Club.

SIDELIGHTS: RECREATIONS—Golf.

ADDRESSES: HOME—1875 Carla Ridge, Beverly Hills, CA 90210. OFFICE—c/o *The Tonight Show,* National Broadcasting Company, 3000 W. Alameda Avenue, Burbank, CA 91505.*

*   *   *

DEHNER, John   1915-

PERSONAL: Full name, John Forkum Dehner; born November 23, 1915, in Staten Island, NY; son of an artist. MILITARY: U.S. Army.

VOCATION: Actor.

CAREER: PRINCIPAL FILM APPEARANCES—Animator, *The Reluctant Dragon,* RKO, 1941; radio announcer, *Lake Placid Serenade,* Republic, 1944; second state trooper, *Christmas in Connecticut* (also known as *Indiscretion*), Warner Brothers, 1945; announcer, *She Went to the Races,* Metro-Goldwyn-Mayer (MGM), 1945; announcer, *State Fair* (also known as *It Happened One Summer*), Twentieth Century-Fox, 1945; Walter Hughes, *The Undercover Woman,* Republic, 1946; German radar captain, *O.S.S.,* Paramount, 1946; Rod Mason, *Out California Way,* Republic, 1946; Jarvis, *The Last Crooked Mile,* Republic, 1946; Georges, *The Catman of Paris,* Republic, 1946; Joe Comstock, *Blonde Savage,* Eagle-Lion, 1947; radio announcer, *Dream Girl,* Columbia, 1947; S.S. man, *Golden Earrings,* Paramount, 1947; Bob Fitzsimmons, *Vigilantes of Boomtown,* Republic, 1947; assistant chief, *He Walked by Night,* Eagle-Lion, 1948; Dempster, *Let's Live a Little,* Eagle-Lion, 1948; Belden, *Mary Ryan, Detective,* Columbia, 1949; Henri Le Clerc, *Kazan,* Columbia, 1949; Murad Reis, *Barbary Pirate,* Columbia, 1949; Couguelat, *The Secret of St. Ives,* Columbia, 1949; oilman, *Tulsa,* Eagle-Lion, 1949.

Sergeant Beluche, *Last of the Buccaneers,* Columbia, 1950; Duke Webster, *Horsemen of the Sierras,* Columbia, 1950; Sir Baldric, *Rogues of Sherwood Forest,* Columbia, 1950; Thurber, *Dynamite Pass,* RKO, 1950; Stanton, *Texas Dynamo* (also known as *Suspected*), Columbia, 1950; Sir Raphael Brokenridge, *Bodyhold,* Columbia, 1950; Hakim, *Captive Girl,* Columbia, 1950; Frank Reynolds, *David Harding, Counterspy,* Columbia, 1950; Robert Reynolds, *Counterspy Meets Scotland Yard,* Columbia, 1950; Frank Niles, *Destination Murder,* RKO, 1950; Tom Marsden, *Al Jennings of Oklahoma,* Columbia, 1951; Charles Bruton, *Bandits of El Dorado* (also known as *Tricked*), Columbia, 1951; Pedro, *China Corsair,* Columbia, 1951; Jefferson Jay, *Corky of Gasoline Alley,* Columbia, 1951; Baron de Wichehalse, *Lorna Doone,* Columbia, 1951; Captain Michael Craydon, *Fort Savage Raiders,* Columbia, 1951;

Turk Thorne, *Hot Lead* (also known as *A Taste of Hot Lead*), RKO, 1951; Jardine, *Ten Tall Men,* Columbia, 1951; John Wesley Hardin, *The Texas Rangers,* Columbia, 1951; John Delmont, *When the Redskins Rode,* Columbia, 1951; Khalil, *Harem Girl,* Columbia, 1952; Emmett Sanderson, *Junction City,* Columbia, 1952; Bokra, *Aladdin and His Lamp,* Monogram, 1952; Fredo Brios, *California Conquest,* Columbia, 1952; Emil Cabeau, *Cripple Creek,* Columbia, 1952; Bronson, *Desert Passage,* RKO, 1952; Gilbert Winslow, *Plymouth Adventure,* MGM, 1952; Doutreval, *Scaramouche,* MGM, 1952; chief, *Man on a Tightrope,* Twentieth Century-Fox, 1953; Harvey Logan, *Powder River,* Twentieth Century-Fox, 1953; Syd Barlow, *The Steel Lady* (also known as *Treasure of Kalifa*), United Artists, 1953; Major Colle, *Fort Algiers,* United Artists, 1953; Matt Ringo, *Gun Belt,* United Artists, 1953; Chief, *Vicki,* Twentieth Century-Fox, 1953; Weddle, *Apache,* United Artists, 1954; Derek, *The Bowery Boys Meet the Monsters,* Allied Artists, 1954; Matt Carrol, *Southwest Passage,* United Artists, 1954.

Ames Luddington, *Tall Man Riding,* Warner Brothers, 1955; Quentin, *Top Gun,* United Artists, 1955; Jules Tulane, *Duel on the Mississippi,* Columbia, 1955; Ranse Jackman, *The Man from Bitter Ridge,* Universal, 1955; Joram, *The Prodigal,* MGM, 1955; Captain Herrick, *The King's Thief,* MGM, 1955; General Nathaniel Greene, *The Scarlet Coat,* MGM, 1955; Mr. Bascombs, *Carousel,* Twentieth Century-Fox, 1956; Preacher Jason, *A Day of Fury,* Universal, 1956; district attorney, *Please Murder Me,* Distributors Corporation of America, 1956; Taylor Swope, *Fastest Gun Alive,* MGM, 1956; Hampton, *Tension at Table Rock,* RKO, 1956; Lew Hanlon, *Terror at Midnight,* Republic, 1956; Major Seth Bradner, *Revolt at Fort Laramie,* United Artists, 1957; Sheriff Holmes, *Girl in Black Stockings,* United Artists, 1957; Pollock, *The Iron Sheriff,* United Artists, 1957; Fred Sutliff, *Trooper Hook,* United Artists, 1957; Pat Garrett, *The Left-Handed Gun,* Warner Brothers, 1958; Grant Kimbrough, *Apache Territory,* Columbia, 1958; Claude, *Man of the West,* United Artists, 1958; Chip Donohue, *Cast a Long Shadow,* United Artists, 1959; Emir, *Timbuktu,* United Artists, 1959.

Viceroy, *The Sign of Zorro,* Buena Vista, 1960; Frank Boone, *The Canadians,* Twentieth Century-Fox, 1961; Geoffrey, *The Chapman Report,* Warner Brothers, 1962; S.P. Champlain, *Critic's Choice,* Warner Brothers, 1963; Scotty Hawke, *Youngblood Hawke,* Warner Brothers, 1964; narrator, *The Hallelujah Trail,* United Artists, 1965; District Attorney Frank Simpson, *Stiletto,* AVCO-Embassy, 1969; Sheriff Chancey Jones, *Tiger by the Tail,* Commonwealth, 1970; Clay Carroll, *The Cheyenne Social Club,* National General, 1970; general, *Dirty Dingus Magee,* MGM, 1970; Colonel Ames, *Support Your Local Gunfighter,* United Artists, 1971; Rumford, *Slaughterhouse-Five,* Universal, 1972; Wallingford, *The Day of the Dolphin,* AVCO-Embassy, 1973; Bob Maples, *The Killer Inside Me,* Warner Brothers, 1976; John Muir, *Guardian of the Wilderness,* Sunn Classic, 1977; Colonel Lafayette C. Baker, *The Lincoln Conspiracy,* Sunn Classic, 1977; Mr. Harper, *Fun with Dick and Jane,* Columbia, 1977; Henry Wheelock, *The Boys from Brazil,* Twentieth Century-Fox, 1978; Commissioner, *Airplane II: The Sequel,* Paramount, 1982; Henry Luce, *The Right Stuff,* Warner Brothers, 1983; Paul, *Creator,* Universal, 1985; Judge Carrigan, *The Jagged Edge,* Columbia, 1985. Also appeared in *Thirty Seconds over Tokyo,* MGM, 1944; *Rendezvous 24,* Twentieth Century-Fox, 1946; *Prejudice,* Motion Picture Sales, 1949.

PRINCIPAL TELEVISION APPEARANCES—Series: Captain, *The Soldiers,* NBC, 1955; regular, *The Betty White Show,* ABC, 1958; Soapie Smith, *The Alaskans,* ABC, 1959-60; John Stearns, *The*

Rebel, ABC, 1959-61; Burgundy Smith, *The Westerner*, NBC, 1960; Jim Duke Williams, *The Roaring Twenties*, ABC, 1960-62; Commodore Cecil Wyntoon, *The Baileys of Balboa*, CBS, 1964-65; regular, *The Don Knotts Show*, NBC, 1970-71; Cy Bennett, *The Doris Day Show*, CBS, 1971-73; Dr. Charles Cleveland Claver, *The New Temperatures Rising*, ABC, 1973-74; Barrett Fears, *Big Hawaii*, NBC, 1977; Marshall Edge Troy, *Young Maverick*, CBS, 1979-80; Lieutenant Jacob Broggi, *Enos*, CBS, 1980-81; Hadden Marshall, *Bare Essence*, CBS, 1983. Mini-Series: Admiral King, *The Winds of War*, ABC, 1983; Admiral Ernest King, *War and Remembrance*, ABC, 1988. Pilots: Frank Jennings, *Forest Ranger* (unaired), 1956; Dr. John Bedford, *Quarantined*, ABC, 1970; Vic Semple, *My Wives Jane*, CBS, 1971; C.J. Bishop, *The Big Ripoff*, NBC, 1975; Barrett Fears, *Danger in Paradise*, NBC, 1977; Hadden Marshall, *Bare Essence*, CBS, 1982.

Episodic: Captain Allenby, "The Lonely," *The Twilight Zone*, CBS, 1959; Alan Richards, "The Jungle," *The Twilight Zone*, CBS, 1961; Jared Garrity, "Mr. Garrity and the Graves," *The Twilight Zone*, CBS, 1964; Colonel Harvey, "Aunt Bee's Medicine Man," *The Andy Griffith Show*, CBS, 1963; Bishop Benjamin, *How the West Was Won*, ABC, 1977; also "The Menfish," *Voyage to the Bottom of the Sea*, ABC, 1967; "The Knightly Murders," *Kolchak: The Night Stalker*, ABC, 1974; *The David Niven Theatre*, NBC, 1979; *Frontier*, NBC, 1955-56; Lieutenant General Armand Bouchard, *Combat!*, ABC; Morgan Starr, *The Virginian*, NBC; Nash, *Hart to Hart*, ABC; *Jane Wyman Presents the Fireside Theatre*, NBC. Movies: High-Spade Johnny Dean, *Winchester '73*, NBC, 1967; Sam Ball, *Something for a Lonely Man*, NBC, 1968; Brazos, *Honky-Tonk*, NBC, 1974; Dean Acheson, *The Missiles of October*, ABC, 1974; Warden Mannering, *The New Daughters of Joshua Cabe*, ABC, 1976; Captain John Sutter, *California Gold Rush*, NBC, 1981; Cyrus, *Help Wanted: Kids*, ABC, 1986. Specials: Commentator, *Tennessee Ernie Ford Meets King Arthur*, NBC, 1960; Mr. Henderson, *The Lucille Ball Comedy Hour*, CBS, 1967; *The Bill Cosby Special, or . . . ?*, NBC, 1971.

PRINCIPAL RADIO APPEARANCES—Series: *Frontier Gentleman* and *Have Gun, Will Travel*.

RELATED CAREER—Stage actor during the 1930s; animator, Walt Disney Studio; radio newscaster.

ADDRESSES: HOME—13951 Shake Ridge Road, Sutter Creek, CA 95685. AGENT—Mishkin Agency, 2355 Benedict Canyon, Beverly Hills, CA 90210.*

*   *   *

DELANEY, Kim   1961-

PERSONAL: Born November 29, 1961, in Philadelphia, PA.

VOCATION: Actress.

CAREER: PRINCIPAL STAGE APPEARANCES—Dory, *Loving Reno*, New York Theatre Studio, AMDA Studio One Theatre, New York City, 1983.

PRINCIPAL FILM APPEARANCES—Cathy Carlson, *That Was Then . . . This Is Now*, Paramount, 1985; Sister Mary, *Delta Force*, Cannon, 1986; Dayna Thomas, *Campus Man*, Paramount, 1987;

Melanie, *Hunter's Blood*, Concorde, 1987; Julia, *The Drifter*, Concorde, 1988.

PRINCIPAL TELEVISION APPEARANCES—Series: Alex Devlin, *Tour of Duty*, CBS, 1988—; also Jenny Gardner, *All My Children*, ABC. Episodic: Kleinberg, *L.A. Law*, NBC, 1987. Movies: Cathy, *First Affair*, CBS, 1983; Jessie, *Christmas Comes to Willow Creek*, CBS, 1987; Jackie, *Cracked Up*, ABC, 1987; Susan Warrenfield, *Perry Mason: The Case of the Sinister Spirit*, NBC, 1987; Mandy Eastabrook, *Something Is Out There*, NBC, 1988; Evan Page, *Take My Daughters, Please* (also known as *All My Darling Daughters*), NBC, 1988.

ADDRESSES: AGENT—John Kimble, Triad Artists, 10100 Santa Monica Boulevard, 16th Floor, Los Angeles, CA 90067.*

*   *   *

De LAURENTIIS, Dino   1919-

PERSONAL: Born August 8, 1919, in Torre Annunziata, Italy; son of Rosario Aurelio (a pasta manufacturer) and Giuseppina (Salvatore) De Laurentiis; came to the United States in 1970; married Silvana Mangano (an actress), July 17, 1949; children: Federico (died, 1981), Veronica, Rafaella, Francesca. EDUCATION: Studied film at the Centro Sperimentale di Cinematografia, Rome, 1937-39. MILITARY: Italian Army.

VOCATION: Producer.

CAREER: FIRST FILM WORK—Producer, *Troppo tardi t' ho conosciuta*, 1939. PRINCIPAL FILM WORK—All as producer, unless indicated: *Riso Amaro* (also known as *Bitter Rice*), 1948, released in the United States by Lux, 1950; (with Carlo Ponti) *Anna*, IFE, 1951; (with Ponti) *Sensualita* (also known as *Barefoot Savage*), Paramount, 1951; executive producer (with Ponti) *Europa '51* (also known as *The Greatest Love*), 1952, released in the United States by Lux, 1954; (with Ponti) *Due notti con Cleopatra* (also known as *Two Nights with Cleopatra*), Ultra, 1953; (with Ponti) *Le infedeli* (also known as *The Unfaithfuls*), 1953, released in the United States by Allied Artists, 1960; executive producer (with Ponti), *La strada* (also known as *The Road*), 1954, released in the United States by Trans-Lux, 1956; *La romana* (also known as *Woman of Rome*), 1954, released in the United States by Distributors Corporation of America, 1956; executive producer (with Ponti), *Un giorno in pretura* (also known as *A Day in Court*), 1954, released in the United States by Ultra, 1965; *Mambo*, Paramount, 1955; (with Ponti and William W. Schorr) *Ulysses* (also known as *Ulisse*), Paramount, 1955; (with Ponti) *L'oro di Napoli* (also known as *Gold of Naples*), 1955, released in the United States by Distributors Corporation of America, 1957; (with Ponti) *La bella mugnaia* (also known as *The Miller's Wife* and *The Miller's Beautiful Wife*), 1955, released in the United States by Distributors Corporation of America, 1957; *War and Peace*, Paramount, 1956; *Le notti di Cabiria* (also known as *Nights of Cabiria* and *Cabiria*), 1956, released in the United States by Lopert, 1957; (with Ponti) *Attila*, Lux, 1958; *La tempesta* (also known as *The Tempest* and *Tempest*), Paramount, 1958; *Barrage contre le Pacifique* (also known as *La diga sul Pacifico*, *This Angry Age*, and *The Sea Wall*), Columbia, 1958; *La grande guerra* (also known as *The Great War* and *La Grande guerre*), 1959, released in the United States by Lopert, 1961.

Under Ten Flags, Paramount, 1960; *Giovanna e le altre* (also known as *Five Branded Women*), Paramount, 1960; *Tutti a cassa* (also known as *Everybody Go Home!*), 1960, released in the United States by Davis-Royal Films International, 1962; *Il gobbo* (also known as *The Hunchback of Rome*), 1960, released in the United States by Royal, 1963; *Crimen* (also known as . . . *and Suddenly It's Murder!*), 1960, released in the United States by Royal, 1964; *I due nemici* (also known as *The Best of Enemies*), 1961, released in the United States by Columbia, 1962; *Io amo, tu ami* (also known as *I Love, You Love*), 1961, released in the United States by Davis-Royal Films International, 1962; executive producer, *Maciste contre il vampiro* (also known as *Goliath and the Vampires*), 1961, released in the United States by American International, 1964; *Barabbas* (also known as *Barabba*), Columbia, 1962; *Mafioso*, 1962, released in the United States by Zenith, 1964; *Il diavalo* (also known as *To Bed or Not to Bed*), Continental Distributing, 1963; *The Flying Saucer* (also known as *Il disco volante*), Dino De Laurentiis, 1964; *Crazy Desire*, Embassy, 1964; *Eighteen in the Sun*, Goldstone, 1964.

The Fascist, Embassy, 1965; *I tre volti* (also known as *Three Faces of a Woman*) Dino De Laurentiis, 1965; *The Hours of Love*, Cinema V, 1965; *The Railroad Man*, Continental Distributing, 1965; *The Bible . . . In the Beginning* (also known as *La Bibbia*), Twentieth Century-Fox, 1966; *Kiss the Girls and Make Them Die* (also known as *Se tutte le donne del mondo* and *Operazione paradiso*), 1966, released in the United States by Columbia, 1967; *The Stranger* (also known as *L'Etranger* and *Lo straniero*), Paramount, 1967; *The Hills Run Red*, United Artists, 1967; *Matchless*, United Artists, 1967; *My Wife's Enemy*, Magna, 1967; *Navajo Joe*, United Artists, 1967; *Barbarella* (also known as *Barbarella, Queen of the Galaxy*), Paramount, 1968; *Diabolik* (also known as *Danger: Diabolik* and *Danger Diabolik*), Paramount, 1968; *The Bride Wore Black*, Lopert, 1968; *Pierrot le fou*, Pathe, 1968; *Banditi a Milano* (also known as *The Violent Four*), Paramount, 1968; *Romeo and Juliet*, Paramount, 1968; *Anzio* (also known as *Lo sbarco di Anzio* and *The Battle for Anzio*), Columbia, 1968; *Fraulein Doktor* (also known as *Gospodjica Doktor—Spijunka Bez Imena*), 1968, released in the United States by Paramount, 1969; *The Brain*, Paramount, 1969; *L'immortelle*, Grove Press, 1969; *Those Daring Young Men in Their Jaunty Jalopies*, Paramount, 1969; *Le streghe* (also known as *The Witches* and *Les sorcieres*), Les Productions Artistes Associes, 1969.

La spina dorsale del diavalo (also known as *The Deserter* and *The Devil's Backbone*), Paramount, 1970; *Waterloo*, Paramount, 1970; *A Man Called Sledge*, Columbia, 1971; *The Valachi Papers* (also known as *Joe Valachi: i segreti di Cosa Nostra*), Columbia, 1972; *The Stone Killer*, Columbia, 1973; *Three Tough Guys*, Paramount, 1974; *Serpico*, Paramount, 1974; *Porgi l'altra guancia* (also known as *Turn the Other Cheek*), Titanus, 1974; *Crazy Joe*, Columbia, 1974; executive producer, *Death Wish*, Paramount, 1974; *Mandingo*, Paramount, 1975; executive producer, *Three Days of the Condor*, Paramount, 1975; *King Kong*, Paramount, 1976; *Casanova* (also known as *Fellini's Casanova*), Universal, 1976; executive producer, *Lipstick*, Paramount, 1976; *The Shootist*, Paramount, 1976; *Drum*, United Artists, 1976; *Face to Face*, Paramount, 1976; *Buffalo Bill and the Indians, or Sitting Bull's History Lesson*, United Artists, 1976; *Mean Frank and Crazy Tony*, Aquarius, 1976; *Das Schlangenei* (also known as *The Serpent's Egg*), Paramount, 1977; executive producer, *The White Buffalo* (also known as *Hunt to Kill*), United Artists, 1977; executive producer, *Orca* (also known as *La orca* and *Orca—The Killer Whale*), Paramount, 1977; executive producer, *King of the Gypsies*, Paramount, 1978;

executive producer, *The Brink's Job*, Universal, 1979; *Hurricane*, Paramount, 1979; *The Great Train Robbery*, United Artists, 1979.

Flash Gordon, Universal, 1980; *Ragtime*, Paramount, 1981; *Halloween II*, Universal, 1981; *Amityville II: The Possession*, Orion, 1982; *Conan the Barbarian*, Universal, 1982; *Amityville 3-D*, Orion, 1983; executive producer, *The Bounty*, Orion, 1983; executive producer, *The Dead Zone*, Paramount, 1983; *Conan the Destroyer*, Universal, 1984; executive producer, *Dune*, Universal, 1984; *Firestarter*, Universal, 1984; *Year of the Dragon*, Metro-Goldwyn-Mayer/United Artists (MGM/UA), 1985; *Stephen King's Silver Bullet* (also known as *Silver Bullet*), Paramount, 1985; *Cat's Eye*, MGM/UA, 1985; *Red Sonja*, MGM/UA, 1985; *Marie*, MGM/UA, 1985; *Maximum Overdrive*, Dino De Laurentiis, 1986; *Crimes of the Heart*, Dino De Laurentiis Entertainment, 1986; *Trick or Treat*, De Laurentiis Entertainment Group (DEG), 1986; *Manhunter*, DEG, 1986; *Raw Deal*, DEG, 1986; *Blue Velvet*, DEG, 1986; *King Kong Lives*, DEG, 1986; *Tai-Pan*, DEG, 1986; *Date with an Angel*, DEG, 1987; *The Bedroom Window*, DEG, 1987; *From the Hip*, DEG, 1987; *Million Dollar Mystery*, DEG, 1987; *Hiding Out* (also known as *Adult Education*), DEG, 1987; *Rampage*, DEG, 1987; *Collision Course*, DEG, 1988; *Weeds*, DEG, 1988; *Traxx* (also known as *Trax*), DEG, 1988; *Pumpkinhead*, MGM/UA, 1988.

Also produced *L'amore canta*, 1941; *Margherita fra i tre*, 1942; *Malombra*, 1942; *La donna della montagna*, 1943; *Il miserie del Signor Travet*, 1946; *Il bandito*, 1946; *La figlia del capitano*, 1947; *Il passatore*, 1947; *Women Trouble* (also known as *Molti sogni per le strade*), 1948; *Il lupo della Sila* (also known as *Lure of the Sila*), 1949; *Il brigante Musolini*, 1950; *Napoli milionaria*, 1950; *Adamo ed Eva*, 1950; *Guardie e ladri* (also known as *Cops and Robbers*), 1951; *Botta e risposta*, 1951; *Romanticismo*, 1951; *Toto a colori* (also known as *Toto in Colour*), 1952; *I tre corsari*, 1952; *La tratta delle bianche* (also known as *Girls Marked Danger*), 1952; *Jolanda, la figlia del Corsaro Nero*, 1952; *Anni facili* (also known as *Easy Years*), 1953; *Dov' e la liberta?*, 1953; *La lupa* (also known as *The She-Wolf*), 1953; *Il coraggio*, 1955; *La donna del fiume*, 1955; *Guendalina*, 1956; *La banda degli honesti*, 1956; *Toto, Peppino, e . . . la malafemmina*, 1956; *Fortunella*, 1958; *Il giudizia universale* (also known as *The Last Judgement*), 1961; *Il boom*, 1963; *Una breve stagione* (also known as *A Brief Season*), 1969; *Striking Back*, 1982; *Dracula's Widow*, 1987.

PRINCIPAL TELEVISION WORK—Mini-Series: Producer, *Noble House*, NBC, 1987.

RELATED CAREER—Founder, Real Cine, Turin, Italy, 1941; executive producer, Lux Film, 1942; founder (with Carlo Ponti), Ponti-De Laurentiis Productions, 1950-57; chairman, board of directors, Embassy Pictures, 1985; founder, chief executive officer, and president, De Laurentiis Entertainment Group (DEG), 1985-88; also actor, propman, unit manager, and assistant director.

NON-RELATED CAREER—Owner, ddl Foodshow (a restaurant), New York City.

AWARDS: Silver Lion Award from the Venice Film Festival, 1952, for *Europa 51;* Italian Film Critics' Silver Ribbon Award, 1954, and Academy Award, Best Foreign Film, 1956, both for *La strada;* Golden David Award and Academy Award, Best Foreign Film, both 1957, for *Le notti di Cabiria;* Golden David Award, 1959, for *The Tempest.*

ADDRESSES: OFFICE—De Laurentiis Entertainment Group, 8670 Wilshire Boulevard, Beverly Hills, CA 90211.*

*   *   *

DELERUE, Georges   1924-

PERSONAL: Born March 12, 1924 (some sources say 1925), in Roubaix, France; married Micheline Gautron, 1959; children: one daughter, one stepdaughter. EDUCATION: Studied music with Henry Busser and Darius Milhaud at the Paris Conservatory.

VOCATION: Composer and conductor.

CAREER: Also see *WRITINGS* below. PRINCIPAL FILM APPEARANCES—Claude's business agent, *Les Deux anglaises et le continent* (also known as *Two English Girls* and *Anne and Muriel*), Janus, 1972. PRINCIPAL FILM WORK—All as music director, unless indicated: *A Man for All Seasons,* Columbia, 1966; *The High Commissioner* (also known as *Nobody Runs Forever*), Cinerama, 1968; *Women in Love,* United Artists, 1969; *A Walk with Love and Death,* Twentieth Century-Fox, 1969; *Day of the Dolphin,* AVCO-Embassy, 1973; *Julia,* Twentieth Century-Fox, 1977; *A Little Romance,* Orion, 1979; music conductor, *All Night Long,* Universal, 1981; *Man, Woman, and Child,* Paramount, 1982; *Silkwood,* Twentieth Century-Fox, 1983; *Exposed,* Metro-Goldwyn-Mayer-United Artists (MGM/UA), 1983; *Salvador,* Hemdale, 1986; music conductor, *Platoon,* Orion, 1986. Also music director for *Marquet* and *Mais ou sont les negres d'antan?,* both 1962; and for short films, including *La Pointe-Courte,* 1954; *Nuit et brouillard,* 1955; *Dimanche a Pekin,* 1956; *Novembre a Paris,* 1956; *Toute la memoire du monde,* 1956; *Les Sorcieres de Salem,* 1956; *Le Mystere de l'atelier 15,* 1957; *La Joconde,* 1957; *Lettre de Siberie,* 1957; *Le Chant du styrene,* 1957; *Notre-Dame, cathedrale de Paris,* 1957; *Andre Masson et les quatre elements,* 1958; *Haim Soutine,* 1959; *Vacances au paradis,* 1959; *L'Ondomane,* 1961; and . . . *a Valparaiso,* 1963.

RELATED CAREER—Conductor, Radio-TV Francais.

WRITINGS: STAGE—Composer of incidental music: *L'Avare* (also known as *The Miser*), City Center Theatre, New York City, 1966; *Diary of a Madman,* Orpheum Theatre, New York City, 1967; *Le Roi se meurt* (also known as *Exit the King*), American Place Theatre, New York City, 1974.

FILM—All as composer. Scores: *Le Farceur* (also known as *The Joker*), Lopert, 1961; *L'Amant de cinq jours* (also known as *The Five Day Lover*), Ariane, 1961; *Cartouche* (also known as *Swords of Blood*), Vides, 1962; *Crime Does Not Pay* (also known as *Le Crime ne paie pas* and *The Gentle Art of Murder*), Embassy, 1962; *Jules and Jim* (also known as *Jules et Jim*), Janus, 1962; *Une aussi longue absence* (also known as *The Long Absence* and *L'inverno ti fara tornare*), Commercial, 1962; (with Cogo Goragher) *Nude in His Pocket* (also known as *Girl in His Pocket*), Madeleine/SNE-Gaumont/Contact Organisation Cosmic, 1962; *La Mort de Belle* (also known as *The Passion of Slow Fire* and *The End of Belle*), Trans-Lux, 1962; *Shoot the Piano Player* (also known as *Tirez sur le pianiste* and *Shoot the Pianist*), Astor, 1962; *L'Amour a vingt ans* (also known as *Love at Twenty*), Embassy, 1963; *Contempt* (also known as *Le Mepris* and *Il Disprezzo*), Embassy, 1963; *Rififi in Tokyo* (also known as *Rififi a Tokyo*), Metro-Goldwyn-Mayer (MGM), 1963; *Le Monte-Charge* (also known as *Paris Pick-Up*

and *La morte sale in ascensore*), Paramount, 1963; *La Morte-Saison des Amours* (also known as *The Season for Love*), Gaston Hakim, 1963; *French Dressing,* Warner Brothers, 1964; *Une Fille pour l'ete* (also known as *A Lover for the Summer* and *A Mistress for the Summer*), American, 1964; *L'Homme de Rio* (also known as *That Man from Rio*), Lopert, 1964; *La Peau douce* (also known as *The Soft Skin, Silken Skin,* and *A Real Double*), Cinema Distributing, 1964; *The Pumpkin Eater,* Columbia, 1964.

Cent mille dollars au soleil (also known as *Greed in the Sun* and *Centomila dollari al sole*) MGM, 1965; *Rapture,* Twentieth Century-Fox, 1965; *Viva Maria,* United Artists, 1965; *Arretez les tambours* (also known as *Women and War* and *Women in War*), Parade Releasing, 1965; *Chair de poule* (also known as *Highway Pickup*), Times, 1965; *Un Monsieur de compagnie* (also known as *Male Companion* and *Poiti Sposero*), International Classics, 1965; *Mata Hari, Agente Segreto H-211* (also known as *Mata Hari* and *Mata Hari Agent H-21*), Magna 1965; *A Man for All Seasons,* Columbia, 1966; *L'Amour a la chaine* (also known as *Tight Skirts, Chainwork Love,* and *Loose Pleasures*), Times, 1966; *Les Tribulations d'un chinois en Chine* (also known as *Up to His Ears* and *L'uomo di Hong Kong*), Lopert, 1966; *Le Corniaud* (also known as *The Sucker* and *The Sucker . . . Or How to Be Glad When You've Been Had*), Royal, 1966; *La Denonciation* (also known as *The Immoral Moment*), Jerand, 1967; *King of Hearts* (also known as *Le Roi de coeur* and *Tutti pazzio meno lo*), United Artists, 1967; *Our Mother's House,* MGM, 1967; *La vingt-cinquieme heure* (also known as *The Twenty-Fifth Hour*), MGM, 1967; *The High Commissioner* (also known as *Nobody Runs Forever*), Cinerama, 1968; *Los pianos mecanicos* (also known as *The Uninhibited*), Peppercorn-Wormser, 1968; *Interlude,* Columbia, 1968; *Le vieil homme et l'enfant* (also known as *The Two of Us, Claude,* and *The Old Man and the Boy*), Cinema V, 1968; *Anne of the Thousand Days,* Universal, 1969; *Le Cerveau* (also known as *The Brain*), Paramount, 1969; *A Walk with Love and Death,* Twentieth Century-Fox, 1969; *Le Diable par la queue* (also known as *The Devil by the Tail* and *Non tirate il diavolo per la coda*), Lopert, 1969; *L'Immortelle,* Grove, 1969.

Les Caprices de Marie (also known as *Give Her the Moon*), United Artists, 1970; *Mira,* City/Cinevog, 1970; *La Promesse de l'aube* (also known as *Promise at Dawn*), AVCO-Embassy, 1970; *The Conformist* (also known as *Il conformista* and *Il Conformist*), Paramount, 1971; *The Horsemen,* Columbia, 1971; *Quelque part, quelque' un* (also known as *Somewhere Someone*), Nouvelles Editions de Film, 1972; *Chere Louise* (also known as *Dear Louise*), Columbia/Warner Distributors, 1972; *Malpertius: Histoire d'une maison maudite* (also known as *Malpertius*), United Artists, 1972; *Les Deux anglaises et le continent* (also known as *Two English Girls* and *Annie and Muriel*), Janus, 1972; *Day for Night* (also known as *La Nuit americaine*), Warner Brothers/Columbia, 1973; *The Day of the Dolphin,* AVCO-Embassy, 1973; *The Day of the Jackal,* Universal, 1973; *Angela,* Unset, 1973; *Une belle fille comme moi* (also known as *Such a Gorgeous Kid Like Me* and *A Gorgeous Bird Like Me*), Columbia, 1973.

L'Incorrigible (also known as *Incorrigible*), EDP, 1975; *L'Important c'est d'aimer* (also known as *The Main Thing Is to Love* and *The Most Important Thing: Love*), CFDC, 1975; *Calmos* (also known as *Cool, Calm, and Collected*), AMLF, 1975; *Police Python .357,* Les Films la Boetie, 1976; *Photo Souvenir,* FR3 Films Production, 1977; *Le Grand Escogriffe,* Gaumont International, 1977; *Julie pot de colle* (also known as *Julie Glue Pot*), Davis/Societe nouvelle prodis, 1977; *Le Point de mire* (also known as *Focal Point*), Warner Brothers/Columbia, 1977; *Julia,* Twentieth Century-Fox, 1977;

Get Out Your Handkerchiefs (also known as *Preparez vos mouchoirs*), Films Ariane/New Line Cinema, 1978; *Va voir Maman, Papa travaille* (also known as *Go See Mother . . . Father Is Working* and *Your Turn, My Turn*), Gaumont International, 1978; *Le Cavaleur* (also known as *The Skirt Chaser* and *Practice Makes Perfect*), Films Ariane, 1978; *La Petite fille en velours bleu* (also known as *Little Girl in Blue Velvet*), Columbia/Warner Distributing, 1978; *Tendre poulet* (also known as *Dear Detective* and *Dear Inspector*), Almi/Cinema V, 1978; *An Almost Perfect Affair*, Paramount, 1979; *Mijn Vriend* (also known as *The Judge's Friend*), Elan, 1979; *Le Mouton noir* (also known as *The Black Sheep*), Parafrance, 1979; *Simone de Beauvoir* (documentary), GMF, 1979; *A Little Romance*, Orion, 1979.

The Case Against Ferro, Specialty, 1980; *Carne: L'Homme a la camera* (documentary; also known as *Carne: The Man Behind the Camera*), Discop, 1980; *Premier Voyage* (also known as *First Voyage*), Planfilm, 1980; *L'Amour en fuite* (also known as *Love on the Run*), Les Films de Carosse, 1980; (with Claude Bolling) *Willie and Phil*, Twentieth Century-Fox, 1980; *The Last Metro* (also known as *Le Dernier Metro*), United Artists, 1981; *Broken English*, Lorimar, 1981; *Richard's Things*, New World, 1981; *Rich and Famous*, MGM/UA, 1981; *True Confessions*, United Artists, 1981; *La Femme d'a cote* (also know as *The Woman Next Door*), United Artists, 1981; *Josepha*, GEF/CCFC, 1981; *The Escape Artist*, Orion/Warner Brothers, 1982; *Partners*, Paramount, 1982; *La Vie continue*, Columbia, 1982; *Man, Woman and Child*, Paramount, 1982; *A Little Sex*, Universal, 1982; *Garde a vue* (also known as *The Inquisitor* and *Under Suspicion*), Gala, 1982; (with Henri Lanoe) *L'Africain* (also known as *The African*), AMLF, 1983; *La Passante* (also known as *La Passante du sans souci*), Cinema V, 1983; *The Black Stallion Returns*, MGM/UA, 1983; *Les Morfalous* (also known as *The Vultures*), AAA/Roissy, 1983; *Liberty Belle*, Films du Scorpion/Gaumont, 1983; *Confidentially Yours* (also known as *Vivement Dimanche!* and *Finally, Sunday*), Artificial Eye, 1983; *Silkwood*, Twentieth Century-Fox, 1983; *Exposed*, MGM/UA, 1983; *Le Bon plaisir*, Marin Karmitz (MK2), 1984; *Mesmerized*, Thorn/EMI, 1984; *L'Ete meurtrier* (also known as *One Deadly Summer*), Universal, 1984.

Agnes of God, Columbia, 1985; *Maxie*, Orion, 1985; *Conseil de Famille* (also known as *Family Council* and *Family Business*), Gaumont International/European Classics, 1986; *Femmes de personne* (also known as *Nobody's Women*), European Classics, 1986; *Crimes of the Heart*, De Laurentiis Entertainment Group, 1986; *Descente aux enfers* (also known as *Descent into Hell*), AAA-World Marketing, 1986; *Salvador*, Hemdale, 1986; (also arranger) *Platoon*, Orion, 1986; *The Pick-Up Artist*, Twentieth Century-Fox, 1987; *Un Homme amoureux* (also known as *A Man in Love*), Cinecom International, 1987; *The Lonely Passion of Judith Hearne*, Island, 1987; *Maid to Order*, New Century-Vista, 1987; *The House on Carroll Street*, Orion, 1988; *A Summer Story*, Atlantic, 1988; *Biloxi Blues*, Universal, 1988; *Memories of Me*, MGM/UA, 1988; *Heartbreak Hotel*, Buena Vista, 1988; *Popielusko* (also known as *To Kill a Priest*, *Le Complot a priest*, and *Le Complot*), Columbia, 1988; *Chouans!*, World Marketing, 1988; *Twins*, Universal, 1988; *Beaches*, Touchstone, 1988; *Her Alibi*, Warner Brothers, 1989.

Also composer: *Le Bel Age*, 1959; *Marche ou creve*, 1959; *Les Jeux de l'amour*, 1960; "La Femme seule" in *La Francaise et l'amour* (also known as *Love and the Frenchwoman*), 1960; *La Recreation*, 1960; *Classe tous risques* (also known as *The Big Risk*), 1960, released in the United States by United Artists, 1963; *L'Ondomane*, 1961; *En plein cirage*, 1961; *Le Petit garcon de l'ascenseur*, 1961; *Marquet*, 1962; *Le Bonheur est pour demain*, 1962; *Jusqu'au bout*

du monde, 1962; *Mais ou sont les negres d'antan?*, 1962; *Vacances portugaises*, 1962; *L'Affaire Nina B.* (also known as *The Nina B. Affair*), 1962; *L'Abominable homme des douanes*, 1963; *Hitler . . . connais pas*, 1963; *Nunca pasa nada*, 1963; *L'Honorable Stanislas, agent secret*, 1963; *L'Aine des Ferchaux*, 1963; *Le Journal d'un fou*, 1963; *Du grabuge chez les veuves*, 1963; *. . . a Valparaiso*, 1963; *Des pissenlits par la racine*, 1964; *Le Gros coup*, 1964; *L'Autre femme*, 1964; *Laissez tirer les tireurs*, 1964; *L'Insoumis*, 1964; *Lucky Jo*, 1964; *L'Age ingrat*, 1964; *Pleins feux sur Stanislas*, 1965; *Le Bestiare d'amour*, 1965; *Mona, l'etoile sans nom*, 1966; *Jeudi on chantera comme dimanche*, 1966; *Derriere la fenetre*, 1966; *Oscar*, 1967; *La Petite vertu*, 1967; *Les Cracks*, 1968; *Les Gommes*, 1968; *Hibernatus*, 1969; *Heureux qui comme Ulysse*, 1970; *Comptes a rebours*, 1970; *Les Aveux les plus doux*, 1971; *L'Ingenu*, 1971; *La Femme de Jean*, 1973; *La Gifle* (also known as *The Slap*), 1974; *Jamais plus toujours*, 1975; *Oublie-moi Mandoline*, 1975; also composed a waltz for *Hiroshima, mon amour*, Zenith, 1959; and a song for *Muriel*, Lopert, 1963.

Composer for the following short films: *Le Mystere du Quai Conti*, 1950; *Les Ingenieurs de la mer*, 1952; "*L'Aventure*" *et ses Terre-Nuevas*, 1953; *Au rythme du siecle*, 1953; *Berre, cite du petrole*, 1953; *Avec les pilotes de porte-avions*, 1953; *La Grande cite*, 1954; *Madagascar*, 1954; *Au pays de Guillaume le Conquerant*, 1954; *Regards sur l'Indochine*, 1954; *La Pointe-Courte*, 1954; *Ame d'argile*, 1955; *La Cite d'argent*, 1955; *Premiere croisiere*, 1955; *Nuit et brouillard*, 1955; *Tu enfanteras sans douleur*, 1956; *La Rue chinoise*, 1956; *Marche francaise*, 1956; *Le Corbusier, l'architecte du bonheur*, 1956; *Dimanche a Pekin*, 1956; *Novembre a Paris*, 1956; *Toute la memoire du monde*, 1956; *Les Sorcieres de Salem*, 1956; *Le Mystere de l'atelier 15*, 1957; *Portrait de la France*, 1957; *Morts en vitrine*, 1957; *Les Surmenes*, 1957; *Courses d'obstacles*, 1957; *Cheres vieilles choses*, 1957; *La Joconde*, 1957; *Lettre de Siberie*, 1957; *Le Chant du styrene*, 1957; *Notre-Dame, cathedrale de Paris*, 1957; (arranger) *Si le roi savait ca*, 1957; *Les Centrales de la mine*, 1958; *L'ile de sein*, 1958; *L'Opera-Mouffe*, 1958; *Mam'zelle Souris series*, 1958; *OCIL*, 1958; *Europe*, 1958; *La Premier nuit*, 1958; *Du cote de la cote*, 1958; *Le Sourire*, 1958; *Images pour Baudelaire*, 1958; *Zinc lamine et architecture*, 1958; *Le Siecle a soif*, 1958; *Le Dragon de Komodo*, 1958; *Des ruines et des hommes*, 1958; *Des ruines et des hommes*, 1958; *Andre Masson et les quatre elements*, 1958; *La Mer et les jours*, 1959; *Le Montreur d'ombres*, 1959; *Images des mondes perdus*, 1959; *L'Age des arteres*, 1959; *Prelude pour orchestre, voix, et camera*, 1959; *L'Etoile de mer*, 1959; *Le Mal des autres*, 1959; *Entre la terre et le ciel*, 1959; *Escale*, 1959; *Une Question d'assurance*, 1959; *Images de Sologne*, 1959; *Le Point de Tancarville*, 1959; *Haim Soutine*, 1959; *Vacances au paradis*, 1959.

Allumorphoses, 1960; *Plaisir de plaire*, 1960; *Dorothea Tanning, ou le regard ebloui*, 1960; *Des hommes . . . une doctrine*, 1960; *La Fleuve invisible*, 1960; *Naissance du plutonium*, 1960; *Diagnostic C.I.V.*, 1960; *Le Vaisseau sur la colline*, 1960; *Picasso, romancero du picador*, 1960; *Architecture et chauffage d'aujourd'hui*, 1960; *Les Etudiants*, 1960; *Sahara an IV*, 1960; *Prenez des gants*, 1960; *Brevet de pilote No. 1: Bleriot*, 1960; *El Gassi*, 1960; *Fruits communs*, 1960; *Des gouts et des couleurs*, 1960; *Neuf etages tout acier*, 1960; *Les Hommes du petrole*, 1961; *Son et lumiere*, 1961; *Les Guepes*, 1961; *L'Amour existe*, 1961; *Enez Eussa* (also known as *L'Ile d'Ouessant*), 1961; *La Parole est au fleuve*, 1961; *Horizons nouveaux*, 1961; *La Balayeur*, 1961; *Les Chevaux de Vaugirard*, 1961; *Defense de fumer*, 1961; *Le Village du milieu des brumes*, 1961; *Une Semaine de bonte, ou les sept elements capitaux*, 1961; *Simon*, 1961; *Les Autogrimpeurs*, 1962; *Les Heros de l'air*, 1962; *Chateaux stop . . . sur la Loire*, 1962; *Le Champ du possible*, 1962;

On a vole la mer, 1962; *La Naturalisee*, 1962; *Le Bureau des mariages*, 1962; *Exemple Entretat*, 1962; *Six petites bougies*, 1962; *Le Chemin de la terre*, 1962; *Le Rendez-vous d'Asnieres*, 1962; *Un Prince belge de l'Europe: Charles-Joseph de Ligne* (also known as *Prince de Ligne*), 1962; *Palissades*, 1962; *La Contrebasse*, 1962; *Le Cousin de Callao*, 1962; *Exposition francaise a Moscou*, 1962; *Route sans sillage*, 1963; *Le Monde des marais*, 1963; *Le Bosphore*, 1963; *Le Soir de notre vie*, 1963; *Corne d'or*, 1963; *Eves futures*, 1962; *Apparances*, 1964; *A*, 1964; *La Rose et le sel*, 1964; *I'Impasse d'un matin*, 1964; *La Montagne vivante*, 1964.

Le Voix d'Orly, 1965; *Vive le Tour!*, 1965; *Le Dernier refuge*, 1965; *Une Alchimie*, 1966; *La Revue blanche*, 1966; *Le Cours d'une vie*, 1966; *Louis Lecoin*, 1966; *Paris au temps des cerises: La Commune*, 1967; *Le Temps redonne*, 1967; *Le Violon du Cremone*, 1968; *Le Jeu de la puce*, 1969; *Au verre de l'amitie*, 1970; *Lautreamont*, 1971.

TELEVISION—All as composer of scores. Mini-Series: *Queenie*, ABC, 1987. Pilots: *Her Secret Life* (also known as *One for the Dancer*), ABC, 1987. Movies: *Silence of the Heart*, CBS, 1984; *Love Thy Neighbor*, ABC, 1984; *Aurora*, NBC, 1984; *Arch of Triumph*, CBS, 1985; *Amos*, CBS, 1985; *A Time to Live*, NBC, 1985; *The Execution*, NBC, 1985; *Stone Pillow*, CBS, 1985; *Sin of Innocence*, CBS, 1986; *Sword of Gideon*, HBO, 1986; *Women of Valor*, CBS, 1986; *Escape from Sobibor*, CBS, 1987. Specials: *Our World*, PBS, 1967; *The Borgias*, BBC, then Arts and Entertainment, 1985.

AWARDS: Emmy Award, Other Outstanding News and Documentary Achievements, 1968; Academy Award nomination, Best Original Score for a Motion Picture (Not a Musical), 1969, for *Anne of the Thousand Days;* Academy Award nomination, Best Original Dramatic Score, 1973, for *The Day of the Dolphin;* Academy Award nomination, Best Original Score, 1977, for *Julia;* Academy Award, Best Original Score, 1979, for *A Little Romance;* Academy Award nomination, Best Original Score, 1986, for *Agnes of God.*

ADDRESSES: OFFICE—8224 Skyline Drive, Los Angeles, CA 90044. AGENT—Al Bart, Bart-Milander Associates, 4146 Lankershim Boulevard, Suite 300, North Hollywood, CA 91602.*

*   *   *

DELL, Gabriel   1919-1988

PERSONAL: Born Gabriel del Vecchio, October 7, 1919 (some sources say 1921 or 1923), in Barbados, British West Indies; died of leukemia, July 3, 1988, in Los Angeles, CA; son of Marcello del Vecchio (a doctor); married Viola Essen (a dancer; divorced, May 14, 1953); married Allyson Daniell (marriage ended); children: one son (first marriage); one son (second marriage). EDUCATION: Studied acting with Lee Strasberg, Etienne Decroux, and Von Heussenstamm. MILITARY: Merchant Marines.

VOCATION: Actor.

CAREER: STAGE DEBUT—Ring Foy, *The Good Earth*, Guild Theatre, New York City, 1932. PRINCIPAL STAGE APPEARANCES—T.B., *Dead End*, Belasco Theatre, New York City, 1935; ensemble, *Tickets, Please* (revue), Coronet Theatre, New York City, 1950; Spud, *Ankles Aweigh*, Mark Hellinger Theatre, New York City, 1955; Boris Adzinidzinadze, *Can-Can*, Theatre in the

Park, New York City, 1959; Emanu, *The Automobile Graveyard*, 41st Street Theatre, New York City, 1961; title role, *Fortuna*, Maidman Theatre, New York City, 1962; Leon V. Kaufenman, *Man Out Loud, Girl Quiet*, and Martino Hacoen Median, *The Spanish Armada*, both Cricket Theatre, New York City, 1962; Boris Adzinidzinadze, *Can-Can*, City Center Theatre, New York City, 1962; Chick Clark, *Wonderful Town*, and Ali Hakim, *Oklahoma!*, both City Center Theatre, 1963; Al Marciano, *Marathon '33*, American National Theatre Academy Theatre, New York City, 1963; Comptroller Schub, *Anyone Can Whistle*, Majestic Theatre, New York City, 1964; Mr. Pinchley, Val Du Val, Fred Poitrine, Otto Schnitzler, Prince Cherney, and Noble, Jr., all in *Little Me*, Melody Top Theatre, Chicago, IL, 1964; Sidney Brustein, *The Sign in Sidney Brustein's Window*, Longacre Theatre, New York City, 1964; Harry Berlin, *Luv*, Booth Theatre, New York City, 1965; Chico, *The Rogues' Trial*, Actors' Studio Theatre, New York City, 1966; Andrew Prale, *Chocolates*, Gramercy Arts Theatre, New York City, 1967; Phil Caponetti, *Something Diff'rent*, Cort Theatre, New York City, 1967; the Contestant, *Adaptation*, Greenwich Mews Theatre, New York City, then Mark Taper Forum, Los Angeles, CA, both 1969; Paul Martino, *Fun City*, Morosco Theatre, New York City, 1972; Mel Edison, *The Prisoner of Second Avenue*, Eugene O'Neill Theatre, New York City, 1973; Remo Weinberger, *Where Do We Go from Here?*, New York Shakespeare Festival, Public Theatre, New York City, 1974; Henry Bech, *Culture Caper*, Playhouse Theatre, Ogunquit, ME, 1975; Fred Santora, *Lamppost Reunion*, Little Theatre, New York City, 1975; Herbert Tucker, *I Ought to Be in Pictures*, Royal Poinciana Playhouse, Palm Beach, FL, 1981. Also appeared in *The Goodbye People*, Berkshire Theatre Festival, Stockbridge, MA, 1971; and in numerous summer theatre productions.

MAJOR TOURS—Sidney Brustein, *The Sign in Sidney Brustein's Window*, U.S. cities, 1965; Tom Gordon, *The Coffee Lover*, U.S. cities, 1966.

FILM DEBUT—T.B., *Dead End* (also known as *Cradle of Crime*), United Artists, 1937. PRINCIPAL FILM APPEARANCES—Patsy, *Angels with Dirty Faces*, Warner Brothers, 1938; Bungs, *Crime School*, Warner Brothers, 1938; String, *Little Tough Guy*, Universal, 1938; Luigi, *Angels Wash Their Faces*, Warner Brothers, 1939; Cadet Georgie Warren, *Dead End Kids on Dress Parade* (also known as *Dead End Kids at Military School*), Warner Brothers, 1939; Bingo, *Hell's Kitchen*, Warner Brothers, 1939; T.B., *They Made Me a Criminal*, Warner Brothers, 1939; String, *Give Us Wings*, Universal, 1940; String, *You're Not So Tough*, Universal, 1940; String, *Hit the Road*, Universal, 1941; String, *Mob Town*, Universal, 1941; Fritz Hienbach, *Let's Get Tough*, Monogram, 1942; Rice Pudding Charlie, *Mr. Wise Guy*, Monogram, 1942; Skid, *'Neath Brooklyn Bridge*, Monogram, 1942; Henry "Hank" Salko, *Smart Alecks*, Monogram, 1942; String, *Tough As They Come*, Monogram, 1942; String, *Keep 'em Slugging*, Universal, 1943; Harry Wyckoff, *Kid Dynamite* (also known as *Queen of Broadway*), Monogram, 1943; Dips Nolan, *Mr. Muggs Steps Out*, Monogram, 1943; String, *Mug Town*, Universal, 1943; Skinny, *Block Busters*, Monogram, 1944; Jim, *Bowery Champs*, Monogram, 1944; W.W. "Fingers" Belmont, *Follow the Leader* (also known as *East of the Bowery*), Monogram, 1944; Lefty, *Million Dollar Kid*, Monogram, 1944.

Pete, *Come Out Fighting*, Monogram, 1945; Gabe Moreno, *Mr. Hex* (also known as *The Pride of the Bowery*), Monogram, 1946; Gabe, *Spook Busters*, Monogram, 1946; Gabe, *Bowery Buckaroos*, Monogram, 1947; Gabe, *Hard Boiled Mahoney*, Monogram, 1947; Gabe, *News Hounds*, Monogram, 1947; Ricky, *Angels Alley*,

Monogram, 1948; Gabe, *Jinx Money*, Monogram, 1948; Gabe, *Smugglers' Cove*, Monogram, 1948; Gabe, *Trouble Makers*, Monogram, 1948; Gabe, *Angels in Disguise*, Monogram, 1949; Gabe, *Fighting Fools*, Monogram, 1949; Gabe, *Hold That Baby!*, Monogram, 1949; Gabe, *Master Minds*, Monogram, 1949; Gabe, *Blonde Dynamite*, Monogram, 1950; Gabe, *Blues Busters*, Monogram, 1950; Gabe, *Lucky Losers*, Monogram, 1950; Gabe, *Triple Trouble*, Monogram, 1950; Colonel Touchenko, *Escape from Terror*, Googan-Rogers, 1960; Henderson, *When the Girls Take Over*, Parade, 1962; Sid, *Who Is Harry Kellerman and Why Is He Saying Those Terrible Things About Me?*, National General, 1971; Wynter, *The 300-Year Weekend*, ABC/Cinerama, 1971; Miles' manager, *Earthquake*, Universal, 1974; Vince, *Framed*, Paramount, 1975; Malcolm, *The Manchu Eagle Murder Caper Mystery*, United Artists, 1975; Uncle Burke, *The Escape Artist*, Orion/Warner Brothers, 1982.

TELEVISION DEBUT—*Broadway Open House*, NBC, 1952. PRINCIPAL TELEVISION APPEARANCES—Series: Regular, *The Steve Allen Show*, NBC, then ABC, 1956-61; Harry Grant, *The Corner Bar*, ABC, 1972; Frederick J. Hanover, *A Year at the Top*, CBS, 1977. Pilots: Leone, *Cutter*, NBC, 1972; Joe Risko, *Risko*, CBS, 1976; Donaldson, *The Jerk, Too*, NBC, 1984. Episodic: *Naked City*, ABC, 1963; *Ben Casey*, ABC, 1965; *Mannix*, CBS, 1967; *Then Came Bronson*, NBC, 1969; *I Dream of Jeannie*, NBC, 1969; *The Governor and J.J.*, CBS, 1969; *The Name of the Game*, NBC, 1971; *McCloud*, NBC, 1971; *Banyon*, NBC, 1972; *Barney Miller*, ABC, 1975.

RELATED CAREER—Teacher, Lee Strasberg Institute; theatre director.

WRITINGS: FILM—(With Dean Hargrove) *The Manchu Eagle Murder Caper Mystery*, United Artists, 1975.

AWARDS: Antoinette Perry Award nomination, Best Featured Actor in a Play, 1976, for *Lamppost Reunion*.

SIDELIGHTS: CTFT learned that Gabriel Dell starred as Fiorello LaGuardia in a special performance of the musical *Fiorello!* staged at the White House for President Lyndon Johnson.

OBITUARIES AND OTHER SOURCES: *Variety*, July 13, 1988.*

*　　　*　　　*

DEMPSEY, Patrick　1966-

PERSONAL: Born in 1966 in Lewiston, ME.

VOCATION: Actor.

CAREER: PRINCIPAL STAGE APPEARANCES—*Torch Song Trilogy*, San Francisco, CA, 1983; also Billy, *On Golden Pond*, Maine Acting Company, ME; and with the Theatre at Monmouth, Monmouth, ME. MAJOR TOURS—Eugene Jerome, *Brighton Beach Memoirs*, U.S. cities.

PRINCIPAL FILM APPEARANCES—Corbet, *Heaven Help Us* (also known as *Catholic Boys*), Tri-Star, 1985; Rudy, *Meatballs III*, Movie Store, 1987; Ellsworth "Sonny" Wisecarver, *In the Mood*, Lorimar, 1987; Ronald Miller, *Can't Buy Me Love*, Buena Vista, 1987; Potter Daventry, *In a Shallow Grave*, Skouras, 1988; Mi-

chael, *Some Girls*, Metro-Goldwyn-Mayer/United Artists, 1988. Also appeared in *Happy Together*, Apollo, 1989; and *Loverboy*, Tri-Star, 1989.

TELEVISION DEBUT—Kellin Taylor, *A Fighting Choice*, ABC, 1986. PRINCIPAL TELEVISION APPEARANCES—Series: Mike Damone, *Fast Times*, CBS, 1986.

RELATED CAREER—Performed as a juggler, magician, and puppeteer for Elks clubs and community organizations.

SIDELIGHTS: RECREATIONS—Skiing.

AWARDS: Emmy Award nomination for *Fast Times*.

ADDRESSES: AGENTS—J.J. Harris, Elaine Goldsmith, William Morris Agency, 151 El Camino Drive, Beverly Hills, CA 90212.*

*　　　*　　　*

De MUNN, Jeffrey　1947-

PERSONAL: Born April 25, 1947, in Buffalo, NY; son of James De Munn; married Ann Sekjaer, October 7, 1974; children: Heather, Kevin. EDUCATION: Graduated from Union College; trained for the stage at the Bristol Old Vic Theatre School, 1969-71.

VOCATION: Actor.

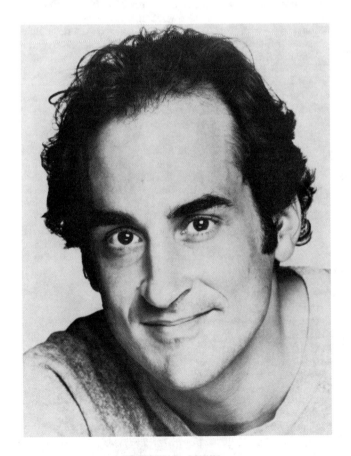

JEFFREY De MUNN

CAREER: OFF-BROADWAY DEBUT—Boyd, *Augusta,* Theatre De Lys, 1975. BROADWAY DEBUT—Phil Murray, *Comedians,* Music Box Theatre, New York City, 1976. LONDON DEBUT—Edmund, *King Lear,* National Theatre Company. PRINCIPAL STAGE APPEARANCES—Escalus and apothecary, *Romeo and Juliet,* and George Hastings, *She Stoops to Conquer,* both National Shakespeare Company, Queens College, Queens, NY, then Jamestown, VA, 1972; Iachimo, *Cymbeline,* Champlain Shakespeare Festival, Burlington, VT, 1975; Aaron Burr, *Founding Father,* Cubiculo Theatre, New York City, 1976; Jack, *A Prayer for My Daughter,* New York Shakespeare Festival (NYSF), Public Theatre, New York City, 1978; title role, *Modigliani,* Astor Place Theatre, New York City, 1979; Horst, *Bent,* New Apollo Theatre, New York City, 1979.

Title role, "The Vagabond," and Savely, "The Witch," on a bill as *The Chekhov Sketchbook,* Harold Clurman Theatre, New York City, 1980; Slimy, *The Carmone Brothers Italian Food Products Corp.'s Annual Pasta Pageant,* Long Wharf Theatre, New Haven, CT, 1981; title role, *Semmelweiss,* Hartman Theatre Company, Stamford, CT, 1981; Lenny Keller, *Total Abandon,* Perry Street Theatre, New York City, 1982; Bottom, *A Midsummer Night's Dream,* NYSF, Delacorte Theatre, New York City, 1982; Taylor, *K2,* Brooks Atkinson Theatre, New York City, 1983; Bernie Dodd, *The Country Girl,* Chelsea Playhouse, New York City, 1984; Howard Bellman, *The Hands of Its Enemy,* Manhattan Theatre Club, City Center Theatre, New York City, 1986; Dancer/Geoffrey, *Sleight of Hand,* Cort Theatre, New York City, 1987; Andrew, *Spoils of War,* Music Box Theatre, New York City, 1988. Also appeared in *La Ronde,* Syracuse Stage, Syracuse, NY, 1974; *The Tavern,* Playwrights Horizons, New York City, 1976; as title role, *Byron's Don Juan* (one-man show), State University of New York, Stonybrook, NY; Tom, *The Glass Menagerie,* American Stage Festival, Milford, NH; Edmund, *King Lear,* National Shakespeare Company, Bristol, U.K.; and with the O'Neill Playwrights Conference, Waterford, CT, 1976-81.

MAJOR TOURS—Edmund, *King Lear,* Demetrius, *A Midsummer Night's Dream,* and chorus, *Antigone,* all National Shakespeare Company, U.S. cities, 1972-73.

PRINCIPAL FILM APPEARANCES—Sergeant Fernandez, *The First Deadly Sin,* Filmways, 1980; Joe McCauley, *Resurrection,* Universal, 1980; Houdini, *Ragtime,* Paramount, 1981; Clifford Odets, *Frances,* Universal, 1982; Dr. Roberts, *I'm Dancing as Fast as I Can,* Paramount, 1982; Bobby, *Windy City,* Warner Brothers, 1984; Ricardo, *Enormous Changes at the Last Minute,* ABC-Ordinary Lives, 1985; Dan Fairchild, *Warning Sign,* Twentieth Century-Fox, 1985; Captain Esteridge, *The Hitcher,* Tri-Star, 1986; Flynn, *Betrayed,* Metro-Goldwyn-Mayer/United Artists, 1988; Sheriff Herb Geller, *The Blob,* Tri-Star, 1988; Georgie, *The Tender,* Trans World Entertainment, 1989.

TELEVISION DEBUT—Vinnie, *The Last Tenant,* ABC, 1978. PRINCIPAL TELEVISION APPEARANCES—Mini-Series: Stanton Rogers, *Sidney Sheldon's "Windmills of the Gods,"* CBS, 1988; Herndon, *Gore Vidal's "Lincoln,"* NBC, 1988; also Adam Brant, *Mourning Becomes Electra,* PBS. Pilots: Whitney Fowler, *Sanctuary of Fear,* NBC, 1979; Carl, *O'Malley,* NBC, 1983; also Nate Goodman, *Elysian Fields,* CBS. Episodic: Raymond Clements, *Moonlighting,* ABC, 1986; George Pierce Baker, "Journey into Genius," *American Playhouse,* PBS, 1988; George Kern, "Pigeon Feathers," *American Playhouse,* PBS, 1988; Brentley Mallard, "The Joy That Kills," *American Playhouse,* PBS, 1985; also "Keeping On," *American Playhouse,* PBS, 1983; Bob Spindler,

The Twilight Zone, CBS. Movies: Sam Campana, *King Crab,* ABC, 1980; Jim Burke, *Word of Honor,* CBS, 1981; Jeff Hammill, *The Face of Rage,* ABC, 1983; Doc Holliday, *I Married Wyatt Earp,* NBC, 1983; Walter Hemmings, *Sessions,* ABC, 1983; Brian Garvey, *When She Says No,* ABC, 1984; Larry Weisman, *A Time to Live,* NBC, 1985; Andrew Lane, *Doubletake,* CBS, 1985; Dr. Matt Matthews, *Who Is Julia?,* CBS, 1986; title role, "Young Harry Houdini," *Disney Sunday Movie,* ABC, 1987; Vincent Marsucci, *Kojak: The Price of Justice* (also known as *Kojak: The Investigation*), CBS, 1987.

AWARDS: Drama Desk Award nomination, 1978, for *A Prayer for My Daughter;* Antoinette Perry Award nomination, Best Actor in a Play, 1983, for *K2.*

ADDRESSES: MANAGER—Harris M. Spylios, Davis Spylios Management, 1650 Broadway, New York, NY 10019. AGENTS—Risa Howard, William Morris Agency, 1350 Avenue of the Americas, New York, NY 10019; Toni Howard and Jeff Witjas, William Morris Agency, 151 El Camino Drive, Beverly Hills, CA 90212.

*   *   *

DENVER, Bob   1935-

PERSONAL: Born January 9, 1935, in New Rochelle, NY; wife's name, Dreama.

VOCATION: Actor.

CAREER: PRINCIPAL STAGE APPEARANCES—*The Foreigner,* Paper Mill Playhouse, Millburn, NJ, 1985.

PRINCIPAL FILM APPEARANCES—(As Robert Denver) MacIntosh, *A Private's Affair,* Twentieth Century-Fox, 1959; (as Robert Denver) Alex, *Take Her, She's Mine,* Twentieth Century-Fox, 1963; Kelp, *For Those Who Think Young,* United Artists, 1964; Willie Owens, *Who's Minding the Mint?,* Columbia, 1967; Bertram, *Did You Hear the One about the Traveling Saleslady?,* Universal, 1968; Choo Choo Burns, *The Sweet Ride,* Twentieth Century-Fox, 1968; Dusty, *The Wackiest Wagon Train in the West,* Topar, 1976. Also appeared in *Back to the Beach,* Paramount, 1987.

PRINCIPAL TELEVISION APPEARANCES—Series: Maynard G. Krebs, *The Many Loves of Dobie Gillis,* CBS, 1959-63; Gilligan, *Gilligan's Island,* CBS, 1964-67; Rufus Butterworth, *The Good Guys,* CBS, 1968-70; Dusty, *Dusty's Trail,* syndicated, 1973; Junior, *The Far Out Space Nuts,* CBS, 1975-77; voice of Gilligan, *The New Adventures of Gilligan* (animated), ABC, 1974-77; voice of Gilligan, *Gilligan's Planet* (animated), CBS, 1982-83. Pilots: Maynard G. Krebs, *Whatever Happened to Dobie Gillis?,* CBS, 1977; Oliver Hopkins, *Scamps,* NBC, 1982; Dr. Dudley Plunkett, *The Invisible Woman,* NBC, 1983; Milton Feld, *High School, U.S.A.,* NBC, 1983; also *Twilight Theatre II,* NBC, 1982.

Episodic: Dudley J. Wash, "The Darlings Are Coming" and "Mountain Wedding," both *The Andy Griffith Show,* CBS, 1963; Dudley J. Wash, "Divorce, Mountain Style," *The Andy Griffith Show,* CBS, 1964; also *The Farmer's Daughter,* ABC; *I Dream of Jeannie,* NBC; *Love, American Style,* ABC. Movies: Gilligan, *Rescue from Gilligan's Island,* NBC, 1978; Gilligan, *The Castaways on Gilligan's Island,* NBC, 1979; Gilligan, *The Harlem Globetrotters on Gilligan's Island,* NBC, 1981; Maynard G. Krebs, *Bring*

Me the Head of Dobie Gillis, CBS, 1988. Specials: *The Bob Goulet Show Starring Robert Goulet,* ABC, 1970; *The All-Star Salute to Mother's Day,* NBC, 1981.*

*   *   *

De SHIELDS, Andre   1946-

PERSONAL: Born January 12, 1946, in Baltimore, MD; son of John Edward (a tailor) and Mary Elizabeth (Gunther) De Shields. EDUCATION: University of Wisconsin, Madison, B.A., English, 1970.

VOCATION: Actor, director, and choreographer.

CAREER: STAGE DEBUT—Hud, *Hair,* Shubert Theatre, Chicago, IL, 1969. BROADWAY DEBUT—Xander the Unconquerable, *Warp,* Ambassador Theatre, 1973, for twelve performances. LONDON DEBUT—The Viper, *Ain't Misbehavin',* Her Majesty's Theatre, 1979, for two hundred twenty-four performances. PRINCIPAL STAGE APPEARANCES—The Old Movie, *2008 1/2,* Truck and Warehouse Theatre, New York City, 1974; title role, *The Wiz,* Majestic Theatre, New York City, 1975; the Viper, *Ain't Misbehavin',* Manhattan Theatre Club, then Longacre Theatre, both New York City, 1978, later Alaska Repertory Theatre, Anchorage, AK, 1983; Billy "Jazzbo" Brown, *Jazzbo Brown,* City Lights Theatre, New York City, 1980; the King and the Snake, *The Little Prince,* Harold Clurman Theatre, New York City, 1982; Nebuchadnezzar, *The Sovereign State of Boogedy Boogedy,* New Federal Theatre, Louis

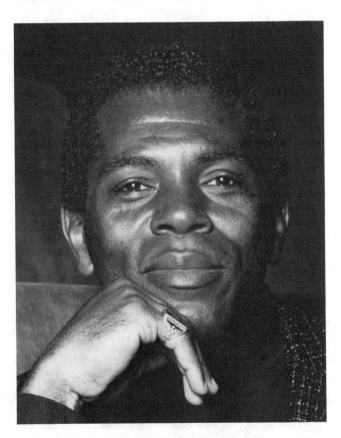

ANDRE De SHIELDS

Abrons Arts for Living Center, New York City, 1986; ensemble, *Stardust* (revue), Theatre Off Park, New York City, 1986, then Biltmore Theatre, New York City, 1987; the Viper, *Ain't Misbehavin',* Ambassador Theatre, New York City, 1988. Also appeared as Xander the Unconquerable, *Warp,* Organic Theatre Company, Chicago, IL; in *L'Historie du Soldat,* Carnegie Hall, New York City; *The Me Nobody Knows,* Chicago; and in *Rachel Lily Rosenbloom* and *Just So,* both in New York City.

PRINCIPAL STAGE WORK—Director and choreographer, *Blackberries,* AMAS Repertory Theatre, New York City, 1984; director and choreographer, *The Colored Museum,* Victory Gardens Theatre, Chicago, IL, then Denver Center Theatre Company, Denver, CO, both 1988; director, *The Trojan Women,* University of Michigan, Ann Arbor, MI, 1988.

MAJOR TOURS—Title role, *The Wiz,* U.S. cities, 1976; the Viper, *Ain't Misbehavin',* U.S. and European cities, 1979-81.

FILM DEBUT—Sandor, *Prison,* Empire, 1988.

TELEVISION DEBUT—The Viper, *Ain't Misbehavin',* NBC, 1982. PRINCIPAL TELEVISION APPEARANCES—Movies: Haji, King of the Genies, *I Dream of Jeannie—15 Years Later,* NBC, 1985. Specials: Tweedledum, *Alice in Wonderland,* PBS; *Ellington: The Music Lives On,* PBS.

RELATED CAREER—Choreographer for the Harlettes (background singers for Bette Midler), 1973-77; president, Black Goat Entertainment and Enlightenment, 1984—; member, Organic Theatre Company, Chicago, IL; director of productions at La Mama Experimental Theatre Club and the Manhattan Theatre Club, both in New York City. Also appeared in nightclub productions, including *Midnight* (one-man show), Reno Sweeney, New York City, 1978; *Haarlem Nocturne,* New Latin Quarter, New York City, 1984.

WRITINGS: STAGE—(With Murray Horwitz) *Haarlem Nocturne,* New Latin Quarter, New York City, 1984.

AWARDS: Emmy Award, Outstanding Individual Achievement, 1982, for *Ain't Misbehavin';* also received two Audelco Recognition awards from the Audience Development Committee, 1984, for *Blackberries.*

MEMBER: Actors' Equity Association, Players Club.

ADDRESSES: AGENT—Dulcina Eisen Associates, 154 E. 61st Street, New York, NY 10021.

*   *   *

DeSOTO, Rosana
(Rosana Soto)

PERSONAL: Born September 2, in San Jose, CA. EDUCATION: Received B.A. from San Jose University.

VOCATION: Actress.

CAREER: PRINCIPAL STAGE APPEARANCES—*Remote Asylum,* Los Angeles, CA; also appeared with the Northern California Light Opera Company.

FILM DEBUT—*The In-Laws,* Warner Brothers, 1979. PRINCIPAL FILM APPEARANCES—Ellen Sedgewick, *Cannery Row,* Metro-Goldwyn-Mayer/United Artists, 1982; Carlotta Munoz, *The Ballad of Gregorio Cortez,* Embassy, 1983; Manuela, *American Justice* (also known as *Jackals*), Movie Store, 1985; Mrs. Lyons, *About Last Night,* Tri-Star, 1986; Connie Valenzuela, *La Bamba,* Columbia, 1987; Fabiola Escalante, *Stand and Deliver,* Warner Brothers, 1987. Also (as Rosana Soto) *Serial,* Paramount, 1980.

TELEVISION DEBUT—*Barney Miller,* ABC. PRINCIPAL TELEVISION APPEARANCES—Series: (As Rosana Soto) Rosa Santiago, *A.E.S. Hudson Street,* ABC, 1978; Diana Olmos, *The Redd Foxx Show,* ABC, 1986. Episodic: *Murder, She Wrote,* CBS; *Punky Brewster,* NBC; *Miami Vice,* NBC. Movies: Lydia, *Three Hundred Miles for Stephanie,* NBC, 1981; Adela Reynosa, *Women of San Quentin,* NBC, 1983.

ADDRESSES: AGENT—Russ Lyster, The Agency, 10351 Santa Monica Boulevard, Suite 211, Los Angeles, CA 90025. PUBLICIST—Ken Amorosano, Sharp and Associates, 9229 Sunset Boulevard, Suite 520, 90069.*

*   *   *

DEWHURST, Keith   1931-

PERSONAL: Born December 24, 1931, in Oldham, England; son of Joseph Frederick and Lily (Carter) Dewhurst; married Eve Pearce, July 14, 1958 (divorced, 1980); married Alexandra Cann, November 4, 1980; children: Alan, Emma, Faith (first marriage). EDUCATION: Cambridge University, B.A., 1953.

VOCATION: Writer.

CAREER: Also see *WRITINGS* below. PRINCIPAL TELEVISION WORK—Presenter, Granada, London, 1968-69; presenter, *Review,* BBC, 1972; presenter, *Extraordinary,* Yorkshire Television, 1978.

RELATED CAREER—Arts columnist, *The Guardian* (newspaper), London, 1969-72.

NON-RELATED CAREER—Yarn tester, Lancashire Cotton Corporation, Romiley, U.K., 1953-55; sportswriter, *Manchester Evening Chronicle* (newspaper), Manchester, U.K., 1955-59.

WRITINGS: STAGE—*Rafferty's Chant,* Mermaid Theatre, London, 1967, published in *Plays of the Year 33,* Elek, 1967; *Pirates,* Royal Court Theatre, London, 1970; *Brecht in '26,* Theatre Upstairs, London, 1971; *Corunna!,* Theatre Upstairs, 1971; (adaptor) *Kidnapped* (from Robert Louis Stevenson's novel), Royal Lyceum Theatre, Edinburgh, Scotland, 1972; (adaptor) *The Miser* (from Moliere's play), Royal Lyceum Theatre, 1973; *The Magic Island,* Birmingham Repertory Theatre, Birmingham, U.K., 1974; *The Bomb in Brewery Street,* Crucible Theatre, Sheffield, U.K., 1975; *One Short,* Crucible Theatre, 1976; *Luggage,* Natural Theatre Platform, London, 1977; (adaptor) *Lark Rise* (from Flora Thompson's novel), Cottesloe Theatre, London, 1978, published by Hutchinson, 1980; (adaptor) *Candleford* (from Thompson's novel), Cottesloe Theatre, 1978, published by Hutchinson, 1980; (adaptor) *The World Turned Upside Down* (from Christopher Miller's novel), Cottesloe Theatre, 1978; (adaptor) *Don Quixote* (from Miguel de

Cervantes's novel), Olivier Theatre, London, 1982. Also wrote *San Salvador,* 1980.

FILM—*The Empty Beach,* Jethro, 1985.

TELEVISON—Episodic: *Z Cars,* 1962-67, published in *Z Cars: Four Scripts from the Televison Series,* Longman, 1968; *Softly, Softly,* 1967; *Just William,* 1976; also *Knight Errant, Skyport, Love Story, Front Page Story, The Villains.* Plays: *Think of the Day,* 1960; *Local Incident,* 1961; *Albert Hope,* 1962; *The Chimney Boy,* 1964; *The Life and Death of Lovely Karen Gilhooley,* 1964; *The Siege of Manchester,* 1965; *The Towers of Manhattan,* 1966; *Last Bus,* 1968; *Men of Iron,* 1969; *Why Danny Misses School,* 1969; *It Calls for a Great Deal of Love,* 1969; (adaptor) *Helen* (from Euripides's play), 1970; *The Sit-In,* 1972; *Lloyd George,* 1973; *End Game,* 1974; *Our Terry,* 1975; *Two Girls and a Millionaire,* 1978.

RADIO—Plays: *Drummer Delaney's Sixpence,* 1971; *That's Charlie George Over There,* 1972; *Dick Turpin,* 1976.

OTHER—(Contributor) *Scene Scripts,* Longman, 1972; *Captain of the Sands* (a novel), Viking, 1982.

AWARDS: Japan Prize for an educational television play, 1968, for *Last Bus.*

ADDRESSES: HOME—2 King Edward's Mansions, Fulham Road, London SW6, England. AGENT—London Management, 235 Regent Street, London W1A 2JT, England.*

*   *   *

DIAMOND, I.A.L.   1920-1988

PERSONAL: Born Itek Domnici, June 27, 1920, in Ungheni, Rumania; immigrated to the United States in 1929; died of cancer, April 21, 1988, in Los Angeles, CA; son of David and Elca (Waldman) Domnici (family changed name to Diamond); married Barbara Bentley (a novelist and screenwriter), July 21, 1945; children: Ann Cynthia, Paul Bentley. EDUCATION: Columbia University, B.A., journalism, 1941.

VOCATION: Screenwriter and producer.

CAREER: Also see *WRITINGS* below. PRINCIPAL FILM WORK—Co-associate producer: *Some Like It Hot,* United Artists, 1959; *The Apartment,* United Artists, 1960; *One, Two, Three,* United Artists, 1961; *Irma La Douce,* United Artists, 1963; *Kiss Me, Stupid,* United Artists, 1964; *The Fortune Cookie* (also known as *Meet Whiplash Willie*), United Artists, 1966; *The Private Life of Sherlock Holmes,* United Artists, 1970; *Fedora,* United Artists, 1978; *Buddy Buddy,* Metro-Goldwyn-Mayer/United Artists, 1981.

RELATED CAREER—Sketchwriter and lyricist (with Lee Wainer), Columbia University varsity shows, New York City, 1941; writer of weekly revues at Catskill and Berkshire Mountain resorts, 1941; junior writer, Paramount Pictures, 1941-43; writer, Twentieth Century-Fox, 1951-55; writer of a skit for the Writers Guild dinner, 1955.

WRITINGS: FILM—(With Stanley Davis) *Murder in the Blue Room,* Universal, 1944; (with James V. Kern) *Never Say Goodbye,*

Warner Brothers, 1946; (with Charles Hoffman) *Two Guys from Milwaukee* (also known as *Royal Flush*), Warner Brothers, 1946; (with Eugene Conrad and Francis Swann) *Love and Learn,* Warner Brothers, 1946; (additional dialogue) *Romance on the High Seas* (also known as *It's Magic*), Warner Brothers, 1948; (with Phoebe Ephron and Henry Ephron) *Always Together,* Warner Brothers, 1948; (with Allen Boretz) *Two Guys from Texas* (also known as *Two Texas Knights*), Warner Brothers, 1948; (story only) *It's a Great Feeling,* Warner Brothers, 1949; *The Girl from Jones Beach,* Warner Brothers, 1949; *Love Nest,* Twentieth Century-Fox, 1951; (with F. Hugh Herbert) *Let's Make It Legal,* Twentieth Century-Fox, 1951; (with Ben Hecht and Charles Lederer) *Monkey Business,* Twentieth Century-Fox, 1952; (with Boris Ingster) *Something for the Birds,* Twentieth Century-Fox, 1952; (with Norman Panama, Melvin Frank, and William Altman) *That Certain Feeling,* Paramount, 1956; (with Billy Wilder) *Love in the Afternoon,* Allied Artists, 1957; (with Isobel Lennart) *Merry Andrew,* MGM, 1958; (with Wilder) *Some Like It Hot,* United Artists, 1959, published by New American Library, 1959.

(With Wilder) *The Apartment,* United Artists, 1960, published in *''The Apartment'' and ''The Fortune Cookie,''* Praeger, 1971; (with Wilder) *One, Two, Three,* United Artists, 1961; (with Wilder) *Irma La Douce,* United Artists, 1963, published by Midwood-Tower, 1963; (with Wilder) *Kiss Me, Stupid,* United Artists, 1964; (with Wilder) *The Fortune Cookie* (also known as *Meet Whiplash Willie*), United Artists, 1966, published in *''The Apartment'' and ''The Fortune Cookie''*; *Cactus Flower,* Columbia, 1969; (with Wilder) *The Private Life of Sherlock Holmes,* United Artists, 1970; (with Wilder) *Avanti!,* United Artists, 1972; (with Wilder) *The Front Page,* Universal, 1974; (with Wilder) *Fedora,* United Artists, 1978; (with Wilder) *Buddy Buddy,* Metro-Goldwyn-Mayer-United Artists, 1981.

OTHER—Writer and editor, *Columbia Daily Spectator,* Columbia University, New York City.

AWARDS: All with Billy Wilder: Writers Guild Award, 1957, for *Love in the Afternoon;* Academy Award nomination, Best Screenplay, and Writers Guild Award, both 1959, for *Some Like It Hot;* Academy Award, Best Screenplay, Writers Guild Award, and New York Film Critics Award, all 1960, for *The Apartment;* Academy Award nomination, Best Screenplay, and Writers Guild Award nomination, both 1966, for *The Fortune Cookie;* Laurel Award, 1980.

SIDELIGHTS: Born Itek Domnici, I.A.L. Diamond adopted the initials of the Interscholastic Algebra League, which he joined as a high school math champion, for his pen name.

OBITUARIES AND OTHER SOURCES: Dictionary of Literary Biography, Vol. 26, *American Screenwriters,* Gale, 1984; *Variety,* April 27, 1988.*

*   *   *

DISPENZA, Joe   1961-

PERSONAL: Born July 18, 1961, in Buffalo, NY; son of Joseph Jerome and Dalia (an X-ray technician; maiden name, Prats) Dispenza. EDUCATION: State University of New York, Fredonia, B.F.A., theatre performance, 1984; trained for the stage in Uta Hagen's master class and with Ron Ross and Joe Totaro; studied

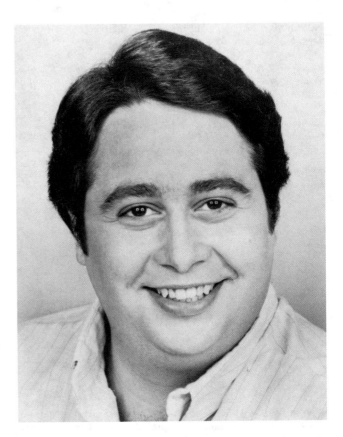

JOE DISPENZA

voice with Bob Wendel, John Wiles, and Frank Pullano; studied dance with Dallett Norris.

VOCATION: Actor.

CAREER: STAGE DEBUT—Melvin P. Thorpe, *The Best Little Whorehouse in Texas,* Palace Theatre, Manchester, NH, 1984, for thirteen performances. OFF-BROADWAY DEBUT—Moose, *Family Obligations,* Circle Repertory Theatre Actors and Directors Lab, then Ensemble Studio Theatre, for twenty performances. PRINCIPAL STAGE APPEARANCES—Big Joe, ''Sleeping Beauty'' in *Festival of Original One-Act Comedies,* Manhattan Punch Line, Judith Anderson Theatre, New York City, 1985; title role, *Fiorello!,* Equity Library Theatre, New York City, 1988. Also appeared as Cyrus Caldwell, *Stampede,* Bruno Walter Auditorium, Lincoln Center, New York City; Lazar Wolf, *Fiddler on the Roof,* and King Charlemagne, *Pippin,* both Palace Theatre, Manchester, NH; as the Justice, *The Miser,* Scrooge, *A Christmas Carol,* and Sir Oliver Surface, *The School for Scandal,* all Marvel Theatre, New York; President, *Dear World,* Mr. McLaren, *Brigadoon,* Sir Joseph Porter, *H.M.S. Pinafore,* and Nathan Detroit, *Guys and Dolls,* all Rockefeller Arts Center, New York; Samuel Chase, *1776,* Cooperstown, NY; and Scrooge, *Merry Christmas, Miami,* Miami, FL.

MAJOR TOURS—Sancho Panza, *Man of La Mancha,* U.S. cities; Mr. Bumble, *Oliver!,* U.S. and Canadian cities.

FILM DEBUT—Sergeant Hoskins, *Deadly Obsessions,* Universal, 1987. PRINCIPAL FILM APPEARANCES—*The Squeeze* (also known as *Skip-Tracer*), Tri-Star, 1987.

PRINCIPAL TELEVISION APPEARANCES—Episodic: *Saturday Night Live*, NBC; *Square One*, PBS.

RELATED CAREER—Appeared as Mr. Gluttone in the exercise video *Skyshapes*, Dylan Enterprises.

NON-RELATED CAREER—Volunteer at a homeless shelter.

MEMBER: Actors' Equity Association, Screen Actors Guild, American Federation of Television and Radio Artists.

ADDRESSES: HOME—235 Seaman Avenue, Apartment A, New York, NY 10034.

*   *   *

DIVINE   1945-1988

PERSONAL: Born Harris Glenn Milstead, October 19, 1945, in Baltimore, MD; died of a heart attack, May 7, 1988, in Los Angeles, CA; son of Harris and Frances Milstead.

VOCATION: Actor and singer.

CAREER: PRINCIPAL STAGE APPEARANCES—Matron, *Women Behind Bars*, Truck and Warehouse Theatre, New York City, 1976, then Whitehall Theatre, London, 1977; Flash Storm, *The Neon Woman*, Hurrah Theatre, New York City, 1978. Also appeared in *Rites of Spring*, La Mama Experimental Theatre Company, New York City, 1975; *The Alternative Miss World* (concert event), Hippodrome, London; *Neon Frame* (concert event); *Restless Underwear* (concert event); and in a revue in San Francisco, CA.

MAJOR TOURS—Flash Storm, *The Neon Woman*, U.S. and Canadian cities.

FILM DEBUT—Divine, *Roman Candles*, 1966. PRINCIPAL FILM APPEARANCES—Hit and run driver, *Mondo Trasho*, Film Makers, 1970; Lady Divine, *Multiple Maniacs*, New Line Cinema, 1971; Babs Johnson and Divine, *Pink Flamingos*, New Line Cinema, 1972; Dawn Davenport and Earl Peterson, *Female Trouble*, New Line Cinema, 1975; guest of honor, *The Alternative Miss World* (documentary), Tigon, 1980; Francine Fishpaw, *Polyester*, New Line Cinema, 1981; Rosie Velez, *Lust in the Dust*, New World, 1984; Hilly Blue, *Trouble in Mind*, Alive, 1985; Edna Turnblad and Arvin Hodgepile, *Hairspray*, New Line Cinema, 1988. Also appeared in *Underground and Emigrants* (documentary), Rosa Von Praunheim/Berliner Festwochen/Sender Freies Berlin, 1976; *Tally Brown, N.Y.* (documentary), Filmwelt Verleigh, 1979; as detective, *Out of the Dark*; and in *Eat Your Makeup*.

PRINCIPAL   TELEVISION   APPEARANCES—Episodic: "Seymourlama," *Tales from the Darkside*, syndicated, 1987.

RELATED CAREER—Appeared with the band Divine Intervention for more than 1,200 performances throughout the world 1979-88.

RECORDINGS: Born to Be Cheap, T-Shirts and Tight Blue Jeans, Jungle Jezebel, You Think You're a Man, Walk Like a Man, and *Little Baby.* VIDEOS—Appeared in six music videos, including *Divine—Live at the Hippodrome.*

SIDELIGHTS: Divine gained a cult following for his transvestite

roles in films made with his high school friend, director John Waters. The actor's trademark elaborate wigs and outlandish make-up were somewhat toned down for his appearance as a housewife in Waters's *Hairspray,* a film that crossed over to attract mainstream audiences.

OBITUARIES AND OTHER SOURCES: [New York] *Daily News,* March 8, 1988, March 9, 1988; *New York Times,* March 8, 1988; *Variety,* March 9, 1988; *Village Voice,* March 15, 1988.*

*   *   *

DIXON, George
See WILLIS, Ted

*   *   *

DONAHUE, Elinor   1937-

PERSONAL: Born April 19, 1937, in Tacoma, WA; daughter of Thomas William and Doris Genevieve (Gelbaugh) Donahue; married Harry Stephen Ackerman, April 21, 1961; children: Brian Patrick, Peter Kyran, James Jay, Christopher Asher. EDUCATION: Received A.A. from the University of California, Los Angeles.

VOCATION: Actress.

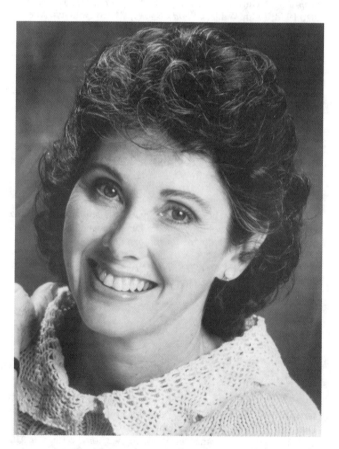

ELINOR DONAHUE

CAREER: FILM DEBUT—(As Mary Eleanor Donahue) Muggsy, *Mr. Big.* Universal, 1943. PRINCIPAL FILM APPEARANCES—Lucille Stewart, *Her First Romance*, Columbia, 1951; Pattie Marie Levoy, *Love Is Better than Ever* (also known as *The Light Fantastic*), Metro-Goldwyn-Mayer (MGM), 1952; Margaret Anderson, *Going Berserk*, Universal, 1983. Also appeared in *Girl's Town* (also known as *The Innocent and the Damned*), MGM, 1959; and in *Unfinished Dance, Three Daring Daughters,* and *Tenth Avenue Angel.*

PRINCIPAL TELEVISION APPEARANCES—Series: Betty "Princess" Anderson, *Father Knows Best*, CBS, 1954-55, then NBC, 1955-58, later CBS, 1958-60; Ellie Walker, *The Andy Griffith Show*, CBS, 1960-61; Joan Randall, *Many Happy Returns*, CBS, 1964-65; Miriam Welby, *The Odd Couple*, ABC, 1972-74; Jane Mulligan, *Mulligan's Stew*, NBC, 1977; Mona Wise, *Doctors' Private Lives*, ABC, 1978; Carol Lambert, *Please Stand By*, syndicated, 1978-79; nurse, *Days of Our Lives*, NBC, 1984-85; Mrs. Baxter, *The New Adventures of Beans Baxter*, Fox, 1987-88. Pilots: Medley Blaine, *Gidget Gets Married*, ABC, 1972; Alice Bennett, *If I Love You, Am I Trapped Forever?*, CBS, 1974; Jane Mulligan, *Mulligan's Stew*, NBC, 1977; Major Oberlin, *Aeromeds*, syndicated, 1978; Mona Wise, *Doctors' Private Lives*, ABC, 1978; Ellie Williams, *The Grady Nutt Show*, NBC, 1981; Mrs. Franklin, *High School, U.S.A.*, NBC, 1983.

Episodic: Nancy Hedford, "Metamorphosis," *Star Trek*, NBC, 1967; Amanda, *The Rookies*, ABC, 1972; Felicia, *One Day at a Time*, CBS, 1981; Elaine Warwick, *Riptide*, NBC, 1986; also "I Want to Be a Star," *Schlitz Playhouse*, CBS, 1952; "No Margin for Error," *Police Story*, NBC, 1978; *$weepstake$*, NBC, 1979; Georgianna Ballinger, *Dennis the Menace*, CBS; Jennifer Ethrington, *The Flying Nun*, ABC; *Alcoa/Goodyear Theatre*, NBC; *Crossroads*, ABC; *The Love Boat*, ABC; *The General Electric Theatre*, CBS; and *Ford Television Theatre*. Movies: Ethel Garrity, *In Name Only*, ABC, 1969; Betty, *The Father Knows Best Reunion*, NBC, 1977; Betty, *Father Knows Best: Home for Christmas*, NBC, 1977; Audrey Ames, *Condominium*, syndicated, 1980. Specials: *Dick Clark's Good Ol' Days: From Bobby Sox to Bikinis*, NBC, 1977; *Battle of the Network Stars*, ABC, 1977; Laura Donovan, "Never Say Goodbye," *CBS Schoolbreak Special*, CBS, 1988.

RELATED CAREER—Singer and dancer, Bert Levy Vaudeville Circuit, 1944-46.

NON-RELATED CAREER—Member of SHARE.

ADDRESSES: AGENT—Fred Amsel and Associates, 6310 San Vicente Boulevard, Los Angeles, CA 90048.

*   *   *

DOUGLAS, Kirk   1916-
(George Spelvin, Jr.)

PERSONAL: Born Issur Danielovitch, December 9, 1916, in Amsterdam, NY; son of Harry (in business) and Bryna (Sanglel) Danielovitch; married Diana Dill (an actress), 1943 (divorced, February, 1950); married Anne Buydens, May 29, 1954; children: Michael, Joel (first marriage); Peter, Eric Anthony (second marriage). EDUCATION: St. Lawrence University, A.B., 1938; trained for the stage at the American Academy of Dramatic Arts, 1939-41. MILITARY: U.S. Navy, lieutenant.

VOCATION: Actor, director, and producer.

CAREER: BROADWAY DEBUT—(As George Spelvin, Jr.) Western Union boy, *Spring Again*, Henry Miller's Theatre, 1941. PRINCIPAL STAGE APPEARANCES—An orderly, *The Three Sisters*, Ethel Barrymore Theatre, New York City, 1942; Lieutenant Lenny Archer, *Kiss and Tell*, Biltmore Theatre, New York City, 1943; Ray Mackenzie, *Trio*, Belasco Theatre, New York City, 1944; Steve, *Alice in Arms*, National Theatre, New York City, 1945; soldier, *The Wind Is Ninety*, Booth Theatre, New York City, 1945; Detective Jim McLeod, *Detective Story*, Sombrero Playhouse, Phoenix, AZ, 1951; Randle F. McMurphy, *One Flew over the Cuckoo's Nest*, Cort Theatre, New York City, 1963. Also appeared in summer theatre productions, 1939-41, and in productions of *Man Bites Dog* and *The Boys of Autumn.*

PRINCIPAL STAGE WORK—Co-producer, *One Flew over the Cuckoo's Nest*, Cort Theatre, New York City, 1963.

FILM DEBUT—Walter O'Neil, *The Strange Love of Martha Ivers*, Paramount, 1946. PRINCIPAL FILM APPEARANCES—Peter Niles, *Mourning Becomes Electra*, RKO, 1947; Whit Sterling, *Out of the Past* (also known as *Build My Gallows High*), RKO, 1947; Noll Turner, *I Walk Alone*, Paramount, 1948; George Phipps, *A Letter to Three Wives*, Twentieth Century-Fox, 1948; Owen Waterbury, *My Dear Secretary*, United Artists, 1948; Tucker Wedge, *Walls of Jericho*, Twentieth Century-Fox, 1948; Midge Kelly, *Champion*, United Artists, 1949.

Jim O'Connor, *The Glass Menagerie*, Warner Brothers, 1950; Rick Martin, *Young Man with a Horn* (also known as *Young Man of Music*), Warner Brothers, 1950; Len Merrick, *Along the Great Divide*, Warner Brothers, 1951; Charles Tatum, *The Big Carnival* (also known as *Ace in the Hole* and *The Human Interest Story*), Paramount, 1951; Detective Jim McLeod, *Detective Story*, Paramount, 1951; Jonathan Shields, *The Bad and the Beautiful*, Metro-Goldwyn-Mayer (MGM), 1952; Deakins, *The Big Sky*, RKO, 1952; John Fallon, *The Big Trees*, Warner Brothers, 1952; Robert Teller, *Act of Love* (also known as *Un Acte d'amour*), United Artists, 1953; Hans Muller, *The Juggler*, Columbia, 1953; Pierre Narval, "Equilibrium" in *The Story of Three Loves*, MGM, 1953; Ned Land, *20,000 Leagues under the Sea*, Buena Vista, 1954; Johnny Hawks, *The Indian Fighter*, United Artists, 1955; Dempsey Rae, *Man without a Star*, Universal, 1955; Gino, *The Racers* (also known as *Such Men Are Dangerous*), Twentieth Century-Fox, 1955; title role, *Ulysses* (also known as *Ulisse*), Paramount, 1955; Vincent Van Gogh, *Lust for Life*, MGM, 1956; John H. "Doc" Holliday, *Gunfight at the O.K. Corral*, Paramount, 1957; Colonel Dax, *Paths of Glory*, United Artists, 1957; Major General Melville Goodwin, *Top Secret Affair* (also known as *Their Secret Affair*), Warner Brothers, 1957; Einar, *The Vikings*, United Artists, 1958; Richard Dudgeon, *The Devil's Disciple*, United Artists, 1959; Matt Morgan, *Last Train from Gun Hill*, Paramount, 1959.

Title role, *Spartacus*, Universal, 1960; Larry Coe, *Strangers When We Meet*, Columbia, 1960; Brendan O'Malley, *The Last Sunset*, Universal, 1961; Major Steve Garrett, *Town without Pity* (also known as *Shocker*), United Artists, 1961; Sergeant P.J. Briscoe, *The Hook*, MGM, 1962; Jack Burns, *Lonely Are the Brave*, Universal, 1962; Jack Andrus, *Two Weeks in Another Town*, MGM, 1962; Deke Gentry, *For Love or Money*, Universal, 1963; George Brougham, *The List of Adrian Messenger*, Universal, 1963; Colonel Martin "Jiggs" Grey, *Seven Days in May*, Paramount, 1964; Dr. Rolf Pedersen, *The Heroes of Telemark*, Columbia, 1965; Commander Paul Eddington, *In Harm's Way*, Paramount,

1965; Colonel David "Mickey" Marcus, *Cast a Giant Shadow,* United Artists, 1966; General George Patton, *Paris brule-t-il?* (also known as *Is Paris Burning?*), Paramount, 1966; Lomax, *The War Wagon,* Universal, 1967; Senator William J. Tadlock, *The Way West,* United Artists, 1967; Frank Ginetta, *The Brotherhood,* Paramount, 1968; Jim Schuyler, *A Lovely Way to Die* (also known as *A Lovely Way to Go*), Universal, 1968; Eddie Anderson and Evangelos, *The Arrangement,* Warner Brothers, 1969.

Paris Pitman, Jr., *There Was a Crooked Man,* Warner Brothers, 1970; Andrej, *Catch Me a Spy,* Rank, 1971; Will Tenneray, *A Gunfight,* Paramount, 1971; Will Denton, *La luz del fin del mondo* (also known as *The Light at the Edge of the World*), National General, 1971; Peg, *Scalawag,* Paramount, 1973; Wallace, *Un uomo da rispettare* (also known as *A Man to Respect, The Master Touch,* and *Hearts and Minds*), Warner Brothers, 1974; Mike Wayne, *Once Is Not Enough* (also known as *Jacqueline Susann's Once Is Not Enough*), Paramount, 1975; Marshal Howard Nightingale, *Posse,* Paramount, 1975; Robert Caine, *The Chosen* (also known as *Holocaust 2000*), American International, 1978; Peter Sandza, *The Fury,* Twentieth Century-Fox, 1978; Dr. Tuttle ("The Maestro"), *Home Movies,* United Artists, 1979; Cactus Jack Slade, *The Villain* (also known as *Cactus Jack*), Columbia, 1979; Captain Matthew Yelland, *The Final Countdown,* United Artists, 1980; Adam, *Saturn 3,* Associated Film Distributors, 1980; Marzack, *Eddie Macon's Run,* Universal, 1983; Harrison and Spur, *The Man from Snowy River,* Twentieth Century-Fox, 1983; Archie Long, *Tough Guys,* Buena Vista, 1986. Also appeared in *Lizzie,* MGM, 1957; and *French Lunch* (short film), 1969.

PRINCIPAL FILM WORK—All as producer, unless indicated: *The Indian Fighter,* United Artists, 1955; *Paths of Glory,* United Artists, 1957; executive producer, *The Vikings,* United Artists, 1958; executive producer, *Spartacus,* Universal, 1960; executive producer, *The Last Sunset,* Universal, 1961; *Lonely Are the Brave,* Universal, 1961; *The List of Adrian Messenger,* Universal, 1963; *Seven Days in May,* Universal, 1963; *The Brotherhood,* Paramount, 1968; *The Light at the Edge of the World,* National General, 1971; *Summertree,* Columbia, 1971; *A Gunfight,* Paramount, 1971; (also director) *Scalawag,* Paramount, 1973; (also director) *Posse,* Paramount, 1975; *Home Movies,* United Artists, 1979; *The Villain* (also known as *Cactus Jack*), Columbia, 1979; (with Peter Vincent Douglas) *The Final Countdown,* United Artists, 1980; executive producer, *Eddie Macon's Run,* Universal, 1983; executive producer, *The Man from Snowy River,* Twentieth Century-Fox, 1983.

PRINCIPAL TELEVISION APPEARANCES—Mini-Series: Alex Vandervoort, *Arthur Hailey's "The Money Changers,"* NBC, 1976; David Konig, *Queenie,* ABC, 1987. Episodic: *This Is Your Life,* NBC, 1958; *The Steve Allen Show,* NBC, 1958 and 1964; *Person to Person,* CBS, 1960; *The Jack Paar Show,* NBC, 1960; *The Best of Paar,* NBC, 1960; *The Tonight Show,* NBC, 1962 and 1963; *Here's Hollywood,* NBC, 1962. Movies: George Anderson, *Mousey* (also known as *Cat and Mouse*), ABC, 1974; Hershel Vilnofsky, *Victory at Entebbe,* ABC, 1976; Joe Rabin, *Remembrance of Love,* NBC, 1982; Harry H. Holland, *Draw!,* HBO, 1984; title role, *Amos,* CBS, 1985; Matthew Harrison Brady, *Inherit the Wind,* NBC, 1988. Specials: *The General Motors Fiftieth Anniversary Show,* NBC, 1957; narrator, *The Legend of Silent Night,* ABC, 1968; *Special London Bridge Special,* NBC, 1972; title role, *Dr. Jekyll and Mr. Hyde,* NBC, 1973; *Show Business Salute to Milton Berle,* NBC, 1973; *The American Film Institute Salute to Henry Fonda,* CBS, 1978; *The Stars Salute Israel at Thirty,* ABC, 1978; *A Tribute to "Mr. Television" Milton Berle,* NBC, 1978; *Johnny Cash: The First Twenty-Five Years,* CBS,

1980; *Celebrity Daredevils,* ABC, 1983; *Salute to Lady Liberty,* CBS, 1984; *Kennedy Center Honors: A Celebration of the Performing Arts,* CBS, 1985; *Bugs Bunny/Looney Tunes All-Star Fiftieth Anniversary,* CBS, 1986; *Circus of the Stars,* CBS, 1987; *America's Tribute to Bob Hope,* NBC, 1988; narrator, *The War in Korea,* TBS, 1988.

RELATED CAREER—Drama coach, Greenwich House Settlement, New York City, 1939-41; founder and president, Bryna Production Company, 1955—; founder and president, Joel Productions, 1962—; actor in radio soap operas.

NON-RELATED CAREER—Director, United Nations Association (Los Angeles chapter).

WRITINGS: *The Ragman's Son* (autobiography), Simon & Schuster, 1988.

AWARDS: Academy Award nomination, Best Actor, 1949, for *Champion;* Laurel Awards, 1951, 1952, 1956, 1960, and 1962; Academy Award nomination, Best Actor, 1952, for *The Bad and the Beautiful;* Academy Award nomination, New York Film Critics Award, and Golden Globe Award, all Best Actor, 1956, for *Lust for Life;* Heart and Torch Award from the American Heart Association, 1956; George Washington Carver Memorial Fund Splendid American Award of Merit, 1957; Golden Scissors Award, 1958; Cecil B. De Mille Award for contributions in the entertainment field, 1968; Presidential Medal of Freedom, 1981; Jefferson Award for public service by a private citizen, 1983; elected to the Cowboy Hall of Fame, 1984; Knight, Legion of Honor, Paris, France, 1985; Emmy Award nomination, Best Actor, 1985, for *Amos;* American Labor Council Distinguished Contribution Award. Honorary degrees: D.F.A., St. Lawrence University, 1958.

MEMBER: Actors' Equity Association, Screen Actors Guild, American Federation of Television and Radio Artists, National Student Federation of America, Heart Committee of the Motion Picture Industry, Friars Club, Honorary Society of Kixioc, Delta Kappa Alpha.

SIDELIGHTS: RECREATIONS—Art collecting, golf, tennis, and swimming.

Kirk Douglas has been cited in the U.S. Congressional Record in 1964 for service as goodwill ambassador to the United Nations. In 1983, he was again appointed goodwill ambassador to the United Nations.

ADDRESSES: OFFICE—The Bryna Company, 141 El Camino Drive, Beverly Hills, CA 90212. AGENT—Fred Specktor, William Morris Agency, 151 El Camino Drive, Beverly Hills, CA 90212.*

*   *   *

DOURIF, Brad   1950-

PERSONAL: Full name, Bradford C. Dourif; born March 18, 1950, in Huntington, WV; son of Jean (an art collector) and Joan (Bradford) Dourif; wife's name, Jonina (an addictions counselor); children: Kristina, Fiona. EDUCATION: Attended Marshall University; trained for the stage with Sanford Meisner.

VOCATION: Actor.

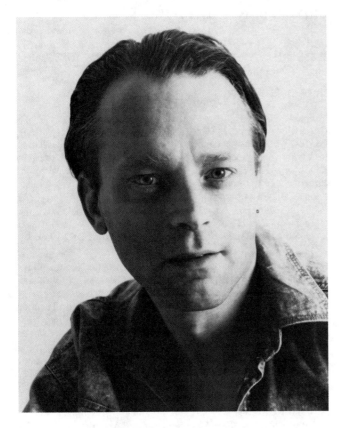

BRAD DOURIF

CAREER: PRINCIPAL STAGE APPEARANCES—Stephen, *When You Comin' Back, Red Ryder?*, Eastside Playhouse, New York City, 1973; also appeared in productions of *The Ghost Sonata, The Doctor in Spite of Himself, Three Sisters, Future Is the Eggs, Time Shadows,* and with the Circle Repertory Company, New York City, for three years.

FILM DEBUT—Billy Bibbit, *One Flew over the Cuckoo's Nest,* United Artists, 1975. PRINCIPAL FILM APPEARANCES—Boris Dourif, *Gruppenbild Mit Dame* (also known as *Group Portrait with Lady*), United Artists, 1977; Tommy Ludlow, *Eyes of Laura Mars,* Columbia, 1978; Hazel Motes, *Wise Blood,* New Line, 1979; Mr. Eggleston, *Heaven's Gate,* United Artists, 1980; younger brother, *Ragtime,* Paramount, 1981; Piter De Vries, *Dune,* Dino De Laurentiis-Universal, 1984; Raymond, *Blue Velvet,* De Laurentiis Entertainment Group, 1986; Kevin Harrington, *Impure Thoughts,* ASA Communications, 1986; Leo Nova, *Fatal Beauty,* Metro-Goldwyn-Mayer/United Artists (MGM/UA), 1987; Charles Lee Ray, *Child's Play,* MGM/UA, 1988; Deputy Pell, *Mississippi Burning,* Orion, 1988. Also appeared in *W.W. and the Dixie Dancekings,* Twentieth Century-Fox, 1975; and *Sonny Boy,* 1988.

PRINCIPAL TELEVISION APPEARANCES—Mini-Series: Danny O'Neill, *Studs Lonigan,* NBC, 1979. Episodic: Max Lyons, *Spencer: For Hire,* ABC, 1986; also *Miami Vice,* NBC; *The Hitchhiker,* HBO; *Moonlighting,* ABC; *Tales of the Unexpected,* syndicated; *The Equalizer,* CBS. Movies: Leonard Matlovich, *Sergeant Matlovich vs. the U.S. Air Force,* NBC, 1978; David Langtree, *Guyana Tragedy: The Story of Jim Jones,* CBS, 1980; Paul, *I Desire,* ABC, 1982; Seymour Bourne, *Rage of Angels: The Story Continues,* NBC, 1986; Lamar Sands, *Vengeance: The Story of*

Tony Cimo, CBS, 1986. Specials: Chad Jasker, "The Mound Builders," *Great Performances,* PBS, 1976; Robert McEvoy, *The Gardener's Son,* PBS, 1977.

RELATED CAREER—Acting and directing teacher, Columbia University, New York City, 1981-86.

AWARDS: Academy Award nomination, British Academy Award, and Golden Globe Award, all Best Supporting Actor, 1975, for *One Flew over the Cuckoo's Nest.*

ADDRESSES: HOME—P.O. Box 491204, Los Angeles, CA 90049. OFFICE—Artist Circle Entertainment, 8957 Norma Place, Los Angeles, CA 90069. AGENT—Nicole Davis, Triad Artists, 10100 Santa Monica Boulevard, 16th Floor, Los Angeles, CA 90067.

*   *   *

DOWNEY, Robert Jr.   1965-

PERSONAL: Born April 4, 1965, in New York, NY; son of Robert Downey (a film director and producer).

VOCATION: Actor.

CAREER: PRINCIPAL STAGE APPEARANCES—Jackson, *American Passion,* Joyce Theatre, New York City, 1983; Rusty, *Fraternity,* Colonnades Theatre, New York City, 1984. Also appeared in *Alms for the Middle Class,* GeVa Theatre, Rochester, NY, 1983.

PRINCIPAL FILM APPEARANCES—Stewart, *Baby It's You,* Paramount, 1983; Thomas Bateman, *To Live and Die in L.A.,* Metro-Goldwyn-Mayer/United Artists, 1985; Jimmy Parker, *Tuff Turf,* New World, 1985; Ian, *Weird Science,* Universal, 1985; Derek, *Back to School,* Orion, 1986; Julian Wells, *Less than Zero,* Twentieth Century-Fox, 1987; Jack Jericho, *The Pick-Up Artist,* Twentieth Century-Fox, 1987; Leo Wiggins, *Johnny Be Good,* Orion, 1988; narrator, *Dear America: Letters Home from Vietnam,* HBO Pictures, 1988; Wolf Dangler, *Rented Lips,* Cineworld, 1988; Ralph, *1969,* Atlantic, 1988; Roger Baron, *True Believer,* Columbia, 1989; Alex Finch, *Chances Are,* Tri-Star, 1989. Also appeared in *Pound,* United Artists, 1970; *America,* ASA, 1986; and *Greaser's Palace.*

PRINCIPAL TELEVISION APPEARANCES—Series: Regular, *Saturday Night Live,* NBC, 1985-86. Mini-Series: Bruno, *Mussolini: The Untold Story,* NBC, 1985.

ADDRESSES: AGENT—Creative Artists Agency, 1888 Century Park E., Los Angeles, CA 90067. MANAGER—Loree Rodkin, Rodkin Management, 8600 Melrose Avenue, Los Angeles, CA 90069. PUBLICIST—Nanci Ryder, Baker/Winokur/Ryder Public Relations, 9348 Civic Center Drive, Suite 407, Beverly Hills, CA 90210.*

*   *   *

DOYLE, David   1925-

PERSONAL: Full name, David Fitzgerald Doyle; born December 1, 1925, in Omaha, NE.

VOCATION: Actor.

CAREER: PRINCIPAL FILM APPEARANCES—Oliver Fisher, *Act One,* Warner Brothers, 1964; housing clerk, *The Tiger Makes Out,* Columbia, 1967; Lieutenant Dawson, *No Way to Treat a Lady,* Paramount, 1968; Oscar, *Paper Lion,* United Artists, 1968; Walters, *The April Fools,* National General, 1969; Will, *Loving,* Columbia, 1970; Mr. Seigbert, *The Sidelong Glances of a Pigeon Kicker* (also known as *Pigeons*), Metro-Goldwyn-Mayer, 1970; Mr. Fanning, *Making It,* Twentieth Century-Fox, 1971; Mel, *A New Leaf,* Paramount, 1971; James Moran, *The Pursuit of Happiness,* Columbia, 1971; Boulting, *Who Killed Mary What's 'er Name?* (also known as *Death of a Hooker*), Cannon, 1971; O'Henry, *Lady Liberty* (also known as *La Mortadella*), United Artists, 1972; Captain Jinks, *Parades* (also known as *Break Loose*), Cinerama, 1972, reedited and rereleased as *The Line,* Enterprise, 1982; Homer Arno, *Vigilante Force,* United Artists, 1976; Walter Loughlin, *Capricorn One,* Warner Brothers, 1978; Webster Jones, *The Comeback* (also known as *The Day the Screaming Stopped*), Lone Star, 1982. Also appeared in *Some Kind of a Nut,* United Artists, 1969.

PRINCIPAL TELEVISION APPEARANCES—Series: Walt Fitzgerald, *Bridget Loves Bernie,* CBS, 1972-73; Ted Atwater, *The New Dick Van Dyke Show,* CBS, 1972-73; John Bosley, *Charlie's Angels,* ABC, 1976-81; Francis Macklin, *Sweet Surrender,* NBC, 1987; also voice characterization, *Foofur* (animated), 1986. Mini-Series: Phineas Wade, *The Blue and the Gray,* CBS, 1982. Pilots: Burton Fairbanks, *Acres and Pains,* CBS, 1965; Kurt Mueller, *Police Story,* NBC, 1973; John Bosley, *Charlie's Angels,* ABC, 1976; Mr. Morgan, *Shaughnessey,* NBC, 1976; Teddy Roosevelt, *Wild and Wooley,* ABC, 1978; John Bosley, *Toni's Boys* (shown as an episode of *Charlie's Angels*), ABC, 1980; Neil Gilmore, *The Invisible Woman,* NBC, 1983. Episodic: Jonathan Harrison, *The Patty Duke Show,* ABC, 1963-66; Professor McCutcheon, *Ozzie's Girls,* syndicated, 1973; also in "The Army-Navy Game," *M*A*S*H,* CBS, 1973; "Et Tu, Archie," *All in the Family,* CBS, 1974; "Ambush," *Taxi,* ABC, 1975; *Fantasy Island,* ABC.

Movies: Mr. Schmidt, *Blood Sport,* ABC, 1973; Luke Burgess, *Incident on a Dark Street,* NBC, 1973; R.H. Macy, *Miracle on 34th Street,* CBS, 1973; Warden Caulfield, *Money to Burn,* ABC, 1973; Bob, *The Stranger Within,* ABC, 1974; Dr. Atkinson, *The First 36 Hours of Dr. Durant,* ABC, 1975; Joseph Carmino, *Black Market Baby,* ABC, 1977; Herman Ohme, *Wait Till Your Mother Gets Home!,* NBC, 1983. Specials: *The Art Carney Show,* NBC, 1959; Fulton, *The Right Man,* CBS, 1960; Harry, *Kiss Me, Kate,* ABC, 1968; Francis X. Gilhooley, *Of Thee I Sing,* CBS, 1972; *The Confessions of Dick Van Dyke,* ABC, 1975; Uncle Ulysses, *Homer and the Wacky Donut Machine,* ABC, 1976; *Jonathan Winters Presents 200 Years of American Humor,* NBC, 1976; *Circus of the Stars,* CBS, 1977; *ABC's Silver Anniversary—25 and Still the One,* ABC, 1978; *Celebrity Football Classics,* NBC, 1979; *John Ritter: Being of Sound Mind and Body,* ABC, 1980.

PRINCIPAL TELEVISION WORK—Episodic: Director, *Charlie's Angels,* ABC, 1976.

RELATED CAREER—Appeared in Broadway stage productions during the 1950s and 60s.

NON-RELATED CAREER—Lawyer.

ADDRESSES: AGENT—David Shapira and Associates, 15301 Ventura Boulevard, Sherman Oaks, CA 91403.*

DRIVER, Donald   c. 1923-1988

PERSONAL: Born c. 1923 in Portland, OR; died of AIDS, June 27, 1988, in New York, NY; children: Dion. EDUCATION: Studied English and art history at Pomona College. MILITARY: U.S. Navy.

VOCATION: Actor, director, and playwright.

CAREER: Also see *WRITINGS* below. PRINCIPAL STAGE APPEARANCES—Chorus dancer, *Guys and Dolls,* 46th Street Theatre, New York City, 1950; chorus dancer, *A Tree Grows in Brooklyn,* Alvin Theatre, New York City, 1951; Private Webster, *Buttrio Square,* Century Theatre, New York City, 1952; Frank, *Show Boat,* City Center Theatre, New York City, 1954; Jerry, *Hit the Trail,* Mark Hellinger Theatre, New York City, 1954; Og the leprechaun, *Finian's Rainbow,* City Center Theatre, 1955; also appeared as Emile, *The Gay Felons,* Wilmington, DE, 1959.

FIRST BROADWAY WORK—Director, *Marat/Sade,* National Players Company, Majestic Theatre, 1967. PRINCIPAL STAGE WORK—Director: *The Taming of the Shrew,* American Shakespeare Festival Theatre, Stratford, CT, 1965; *Your Own Thing,* Orpheum Theatre, New York City, 1968, then Comedy Theatre, London, 1969; *Mike Downstairs,* Hudson Theatre, New York City, 1968; *Jimmy Shine,* Brooks Atkinson Theatre, New York City, 1968; *Our Town,* American National Theatre Academy (ANTA) Theatre, New York City, 1969; *Status Quo Vadis,* Ivanhoe Theatre, Chicago, IL, 1971, then Brooks Atkinson Theatre, 1973; *South Pacific,* Wolf Trap Farm, Vienna, VA, 1977; *Broadway Follies,* Nederlander Theatre, New York City, 1981; (also choreographer) *Oh, Brother!,* ANTA Theatre, 1981; *The Glass Menagerie,* Studio Arena Theatre, Buffalo, NY, 1985.

MAJOR TOURS—Director, *From Paris with Love,* U.S. and Canadian cities, 1962.

PRINCIPAL FILM WORK—Director, *The Naked Ape,* Universal, 1973.

PRINCIPAL TELEVISION APPEARANCES—Specials: Louis D'Arc, *Naughty Marietta,* NBC, 1955.

RELATED CAREER—Dancer with the Ballet Russe de Monte Carlo; also radio announcer in Seattle, WA.

WRITINGS: See production credits above, unless indicated. STAGE—*From Paris with Love,* 1962; (book for musical) *Your Own Thing* (adapted from the play *Twelfth Night* by William Shakespeare), 1968; *Status Quo Vadis,* 1971; *Broadway Follies,* 1981; (book and lyrics for musical) *Oh, Brother!* (adapted from the play *The Comedy of Errors* by Shakespeare), 1981; *In the Sweet Bye and Bye,* Studio Arena Theatre, Buffalo, NY, 1983; *A Walk Out of Water,* Pennsylvania Stage Company, Allentown, PA, 1985. FILM—*The Naked Ape,* 1973. TELEVISION—Specials: *G.I. Jive,* PBS.

AWARDS: Antoinette Perry Award nomination, Best Director of a Play, 1967, for *Marat/Sade.*

MEMBER: Society of Stage Directors and Choreographers.

OBITUARIES AND OTHER SOURCES: Variety, June 29, 1988; *New York Times,* June 28, 1988.*

DRYER, Fred 1946-

PERSONAL: Full name, John Frederick Dryer; born July 6, 1946, in Hawthorne, CA. EDUCATION: Studied acting with Nina Foch.

VOCATION: Actor.

CAREER: PRINCIPAL FILM APPEARANCES—Sergeant Jack Burns, *Death Before Dishonor*, New World, 1987.

PRINCIPAL TELEVISION APPEARANCES—Series: Sergeant Rick Hunter, *Hunter*, NBC, 1984—. Pilots: Lieutenant John LeGarre, *Force Seven* (shown as an episode of *CHiPs*), NBC, 1982; Johnny Paloney, *A Girl's Life*, NBC, 1983; also *The Rousters*, NBC, 1983. Episodic: Sportscaster, "Sam at Eleven" and "Old Flames," both *Cheers*, NBC, 1982 and 1983. Movies: Harvey Denver, *The Star Maker*, NBC, 1981; Mike Bosnick, *Something So Right*, CBS, 1982; Larry Kandal, *The Kid from Nowhere*, NBC, 1982; Barney Daniels, *The Fantastic World of D.C. Collins*, NBC, 1984. Specials: *Super Bloopers and New Practical Jokes*, NBC, 1988.

PRINCIPAL TELEVISION WORK—Episodic: *Hunter* (three episodes), NBC, 1987-88.

RELATED CAREER—Sports commentator, CBS.

NON-RELATED CAREER—Professional football player with the New York Giants, 1969-71, then Los Angeles Rams, 1971-81.

ADDRESSES: PUBLICIST—Howard Brandy, 9507 Santa Monica Boulevard, Suite 211, Beverly Hills, CA 90210.*

*   *   *

DUGGAN, Andrew 1923-1988

PERSONAL: Born December 28, 1923, in Franklin, IN; died of throat cancer, May 15, 1988, in Westwood, CA; son of Edward Dean and Annette (Beach) Duggan; married Elizabeth Logue (a dancer), September 20, 1953; children: Richard, Nancy, Melissa. EDUCATION: Indiana University, B.A., 1943. MILITARY: U.S. Army Air Forces, 1943-46.

VOCATION: Actor.

CAREER: PRINCIPAL STAGE APPEARANCES—Patrolman, *Hey Day*, Shubert Theatre, New Haven, CT, 1947; doctor, *The Rose Tattoo*, Martin Beck Theatre, New York City, 1951; Mike Mooney, *Paint Your Wagon*, Shubert Theatre, New York City, 1952; Philip Mortimer, *Gently Does It*, Playhouse Theatre, New York City, 1953; Chris Steelman and Bud Walters, *Anniversary Waltz*, Broadhurst Theatre, New York City, 1954; Captain Erskine Cooney, *Fragile Fox*, Belasco Theatre, New York City, 1954; Douglas Sayre, *Third Best Sport*, Ambassador Theatre, New York City, 1958. Also appeared in *The Innocents*, Playhouse Theatre, 1949.

MAJOR TOURS—Mike Mooney, *Paint Your Wagon*, U.S. cities, 1952-53; also *Dream Girl*, U.S. cities, 1947.

PRINCIPAL FILM APPEARANCES—Sheriff Swede Hansen, *Decision at Sundown*, Columbia, 1957; Wade Harrington, *Domino Kid*, Columbia, 1957; Browning, *Three Brave Men*, Twentieth Century-Fox, 1957; Padre, *The Bravados*, Twentieth Century-Fox, 1958;

Murray Fallam, *Return to Warbow*, Columbia, 1958; Clay Putnam, *Westbound*, Warner Brothers, 1959; Doctor Chapman, *The Chapman Report*, Warner Brothers, 1962; Warden Cole, *House of Women* (also known as *Ladies of the Mob*), Warner Brothers, 1962; Major "Doc" Nemeny, *Merrill's Marauders*, Warner Brothers, 1962; Chief Dixon, *Palm Springs Weekend*, Warner Brothers, 1963; Alan W. Nichols, *F.B.I. Code 98*, Warner Brothers, 1964; Admiral Harlock, *The Incredible Mr. Limpet*, Warner Brothers, 1964; Colonel "Mutt" Henderson, *Seven Days in May*, Paramount, 1964; General McCabe, *The Glory Guys*, United Artists, 1965; President Trent, *In Like Flint*, Twentieth Century-Fox, 1967; General Armstrong, *The Secret War of Harry Frigg*, Universal, 1968; Calloway, *Skin Game*, Warner Brothers, 1971; Commissioner Gaines, *The Bears and I*, Buena Vista, 1974; professor, *It's Alive*, Warner Brothers, 1974; Doctor Perry, *It Lives Again* (also known as *It's Alive II*), Warner Brothers, 1978; Lyndon B. Johnson, *The Private Files of J. Edgar Hoover*, American International, 1978; Harmon, *Doctor Detroit*, Universal, 1983; the judge, *A Return to Salem's Lot*, Warner Brothers, 1987. Also appeared in *Patterns* (also known as *Patterns of Power*), United Artists, 1954; *Allied Dolphin*, 1964; *Bone*, Jack Harris Enterprises, 1972; and *One Last Ride*, 1980.

PRINCIPAL TELEVISION APPEARANCES—Series: Cal Calhoun, *Bourbon Street Beat*, ABC, 1959-60; George Rose, *Room for One More*, ABC, 1962; Brigadier General Ed Britt, *Twelve O'Clock High*, ABC, 1965-67; Murdoch Lancer, *Lancer*, CBS, 1968-70. Mini-Series: Colonel Deiner, *Rich Man, Poor Man*, ABC, 1976; General McKelvey, *Once an Eagle*, NBC, 1976-77; President Dwight D. Eisenhower, *Backstairs at the White House*, NBC, 1979; Admiral Kimmel, *The Winds of War*, ABC, 1983; also "The Saga of Andy Burnett," *Disneyland*, ABC, 1957-58. Pilots: Alan Nichols, *F.B.I. Code 98* (not broadcast), 1962; Donald Guthrie, "Corridor 400," *The Bob Hope Chrysler Theatre*, NBC, 1963; George Fleming, *You're Only Young Twice*, CBS, 1967; Owen Kerr, *A Walk in the Night*, CBS, 1968; Miller, *Hawaii Five-O*, CBS, 1968; John Walton, *The Homecoming—A Christmas Story*, CBS, 1971; Harrison Delando, *Man on the Move* (also known as *Jigsaw*), ABC, 1972; Captain A.R. Malone, *The Streets of San Francisco*, ABC, 1972; Captain Jim Parr, *Firehouse*, ABC, 1973; Doctor McCabe, *The Last Angry Man*, ABC, 1974; Captain John Shannon, *The Hunted Lady*, NBC, 1977; Captain Ed Wilson, *Pine Canyon Is Burning*, NBC, 1977; Sheriff, *Down Home*, CBS, 1978; Sam Wiggins, *The Long Days of Summer*, ABC, 1980; Andrew McClelland, *M Station: Hawaii*, CBS, 1980; Mace Kaylor, *Jake's Way*, CBS, 1980; Edward Forbes, *Momma the Detective*, NBC, 1981.

Episodic: Red Dawson, "The Restless Guns," *Schlitz Playhouse*, CBS, 1957; Guthrie, "Eye for Eye," *Suspicion*, NBC, 1958; voice of Ernest Hemingway, "Hemingway," *The Dupont Show of the Week*, NBC, 1961; Al "Howitzer" Houlihan, *M*A*S*H*, CBS, 1980; Johnny Cooper, *Remington Steele*, NBC, 1986; also Andersen, *The Fugitive*, ABC; Beaumont, *The Invaders*, ABC; *Great Adventure*, CBS; *The Kaiser Aluminum Hour*, NBC; *Kraft Suspense Theatre*, NBC; *Cannon*, CBS; *Hawaii Five-O*, CBS; *McMillan and Wife*, NBC. Movies: William Forrest, *The Forgotten Man*, ABC, 1971; Burbaker, *Two on a Bench*, ABC, 1971; Congressman, *Pueblo*, ABC, 1973; General Maxwell D. Taylor, *The Missiles of October*, ABC, 1974; Harlan Jack Gardner, *Panic on the 5:22*, ABC, 1974; Inspector Ryder, *Attack on Terror: The F.B.I. versus the Ku Klux Klan*, CBS, 1975; Al Miller, *The Deadliest Season*, CBS, 1977; President Dwight D. Eisenhower, *Tail Gunner Joe*, NBC, 1977; President, *A Fire in the Sky*, NBC, 1978; Dugan, *Overboard*, NBC, 1978; Bean Worthington, *The Time Machine*,

NBC, 1978; Judge Adamson, *The Incredible Journey of Doctor Meg Laurel,* CBS, 1979; Dwight D. Eisenhower, *J. Edgar Hoover,* Showtime, 1987. Specials: Paul Jones, ''The Cat and the Canary,'' *The Dow Hour of Great Mysteries,* NBC, 1960.

RELATED CAREER—Commercial spokesman and voiceover actor on television.

OBITUARIES AND OTHER SOURCES: New York Times, May 18, 1988; [New York] *Newsday,* May 18, 1988; *Variety,* May 18, 1988.*

*   *   *

DUKAKIS, Olympia   1931-

PERSONAL: Born June 20, 1931, in Lowell, MA; daughter of Constantine S. (a manager) and Alexandra (Christos) Dukakis; married Louis Zorich (an actor); children: Christina, Peter, Stefan. EDUCATION: Received B.A. and M.F.A. from Boston University. POLITICS: Democrat.

VOCATION: Actress, producer, and director.

CAREER: STAGE DEBUT—Mrs. Cleveden-Brooks, *Outward Bound,* Rangeley, ME. OFF-BROADWAY DEBUT—Madelena, *The Breaking Wall,* St. Mark's Playhouse, 1960. BROADWAY DEBUT—*The Aspern Papers,* Playhouse Theatre, 1962. PRINCIPAL STAGE APPEARANCES—Widow Leocadia Begbick, *A Man's*

a Man, Masque Theatre, New York City, 1962; Mary Tyrone, *Long Day's Journey into Night,* McCarter Theatre, Princeton, NJ, 1962; Henriette, *Crime and Crime,* Cricket Theatre, New York City, 1963; Anne Dowling, *Abraham Cochrane,* Belasco Theatre, New York City, 1964; Chrysothemis, *Electra,* New York Shakespeare Festival (NYSF), Delacorte Theatre, New York City, 1964; Madama Irma, *The Balcony,* Gertrude, *Hamlet,* and title role, *Mother Courage and Her Children,* all Charles Street Playhouse, 1967; Tamora, *Titus Andronicus,* NYSF, Delacorte Theatre, 1967; Mrs. Bethnal-Green, the Mother, Stepney Green, and Debden, *Father Uxbridge Wants to Marry,* American Place Theatre, Theatre at St. Clement's Church, New York City, 1967; Helena, *The Memorandum,* Public Theatre, New York City, 1968; Ingrid, *Peer Gynt,* Delacorte Theatre, 1969; Goya, *Baba Goya,* American Place Theatre, New York City, 1973, retitled *Nourish the Beast,* Cherry Lane Theatre, New York City, 1973; Ilse, *Who's Who in Hell,* Lunt-Fontanne Theatre, New York City, 1974; title role, *Mother Ryan,* New Dramatists, New York City, 1977; Ella, *Curse of the Starving Class,* Public Theatre, 1978; Nurse Ratched, *One Flew Over the Cuckoo's Nest,* Whole Theatre Company, Upper Montclair, NJ, 1978.

Madame Ranevskaya, *The Cherry Orchard,* Whole Theatre Company, 1981; Filumena, *Snow Orchid,* Circle Repertory Company, New York City, 1982; Soot Hudlocke, *The Marriage of Bette and Boo,* NYSF, Public Theatre, 1985; Sophie Greengrass, *Social Security,* Ethel Barrymore Theatre, New York City, 1986. Also appeared in *The New Tenant,* Royal Playhouse, New York City, 1960; *The Opening of a Window,* Theatre Marquee, New York City, 1961; *Six Characters in Search of an Author,* Charles Street Playhouse, Boston, MA, 1964; *The Rose Tattoo,* Studio Arena Theatre, Buffalo, NY, 1965; *The Rose Tattoo,* Whole Theatre Company, 1976; *Blithe Spirit,* Whole Theatre Company, 1984; *Ghosts,* Whole Theatre Company, 1985; *The Seagull,* Whole Theatre Company, 1986; in summer theatre productions, Williamstown Theatre Festival, Williamstown, MA; and with the Second City Company.

PRINCIPAL STAGE WORK—Director: *Talley's Folly,* Whole Theatre Company, Upper Montclair, NJ, 1984; also *U.S.A., Orpheus Descending, The House of Bernarda Alba, Arms and the Man,* and *Uncle Vanya,* all Whole Theatre Company; *Six Characters in Search of an Author* and *A Touch of the Poet,* both Williamstown Theatre Festival, Williamstown, MA; *One Flew Over the Cuckoo's Nest,* Delaware Summer Festival; and *Kennedy's Children,* Commonwealth Stage.

MAJOR TOURS—With the Phoenix Theatre Company, U.S. cities, 1960.

FILM DEBUT—Woman and commentator, *Twice a Man,* Gregory J. Markopoulous, 1964. PRINCIPAL FILM APPEARANCES—Patient, *Lilith,* Columbia, 1964; John's mother, *John and Mary,* Twentieth Century-Fox, 1969; Gig's mother, *Made for Each Other,* Twentieth Century-Fox, 1971; lawyer, *Rich Kids,* United Artists, 1979; Joey's mother, *The Wanderers,* Orion, 1979; Mrs. Vacarri, *The Idolmaker,* United Artists, 1980; Mary, *Flanagan,* United Film Distributors, 1985; Rose Castorini, *Moonstruck,* Metro-Goldwyn-Mayer/United Artists, 1987. Also appeared in *Sisters* (also known as *Blood Sisters*), American International, 1973; *Death Wish,* Paramount, 1974; *National Lampoon Goes to the Movies* (also known as *National Lampoon's Movie Madness*), 1981; *Walls of Glass,* 1985; *The Rehearsal;* and *Daddy's Home.*

TELEVISION DEBUT—*CBS Workshop,* CBS. PRINCIPAL TELEVI-

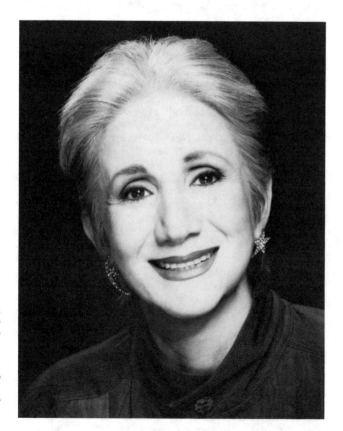

Harry Langdon Photography/Video © 1988

OLYMPIA DUKAKIS

SION APPEARANCES—Series: *Search for Tomorrow*, NBC, 1983-84. Pilots: *The Neighborhood*, NBC, 1982. Episodic: *One of the Boys*, NBC, 1982; also *The Ed Sullivan Show*, CBS; *The Nurses*, CBS; *Dr. Kildare*, NBC; "King of America," *American Playhouse*, PBS. Movies: Irene Kaminios, *Nicky's World*, CBS, 1974; also *F.D.R.—The Last Year*, NBC, 1980.

RELATED CAREER—Founding member, Charles Street Playhouse, Boston, MA, 1957-60; acting teacher, New York University, 1967-70, then 1974-83; acting teacher, Yale University, 1976; founding member, artistic director, director, and company member, Whole Theatre Company, Upper Montclair, NJ, 1976—; founding member, Edgartown Summer Theatre, Edgartown, MA; associate director, Williamstown Theatre Festival, Williamstown, MA.

WRITINGS: STAGE—All as adaptor of productions by the Whole Theatre Company, Upper Montclair, NJ: *Mother Courage and Her Children*, *The House of Bernarda Alba*, *Edith Stein*, *The Trojan Women*, and *Uncle Vanya*.

AWARDS: Obie Award from the *Village Voice*, 1963, for *A Man's a Man;* Academy Award, New York Film Critics Award, Los Angeles Film Critics Award, Golden Globe Award, and National Board of Review Award, Best Supporting Actress, and American Comedy Award, Funniest Supporting Female, all 1988, for *Moonstruck;* Obie Award for *The Marriage of Bette and Boo;* New England fencing champion.

MEMBER: Actors' Equity Association, Screen Actors Guild, American Federation of Television and Radio Artists.

SIDELIGHTS: FAVORITE ROLES—Mother Courage in *Mother Courage and Her Children*, Madame Ranevskaya in *The Cherry Orchard*, Mary Tyrone in *Long Day's Journey into Night*, Tamora in *Titus Andronicus*, and Serafina in *The Rose Tattoo*.

ADDRESSES: OFFICE—Whole Theatre Company, 544 Bloomfield Avenue, Montclair, NJ 07042.*

*   *   *

DUKES, David   1945-

PERSONAL: Born June 6, 1945, in San Francisco, CA; father, a California highway patrolman; married first wife, 1965 (divorced, 1975); married Carol Muske; children: Shawn (first marriage). EDUCATION: Attended Mann College; trained for the stage at the American Conservatory Theatre, San Francisco.

VOCATION: Actor.

CAREER: BROADWAY DEBUT—Horace, *The School for Wives*, Lyceum Theatre, 1971. PRINCIPAL STAGE APPEARANCES—Aubrey Beardsley, *The Neophyte*, Center Theatre Group, New Theatre for Now, Los Angeles, CA, 1971; Don Carlos, *Don Juan*, and committee member, *The Great God Brown*, both New Phoenix Repertory Company, Lyceum Theatre, 1972; Albert Adam, *The Play's the Thing*, Bijou Theatre, New York City, 1973; the Judge, *The Government Inspector*, New Phoenix Repertory Company, Edison Theatre, New York City, 1973; husbands number 7, 8, and 9, *The Visit*, Coustouillu, *Chemin de fer*, and Nick Potter, *Holiday*, all New Phoenix Repertory Company, Ethel Barrymore Theatre,

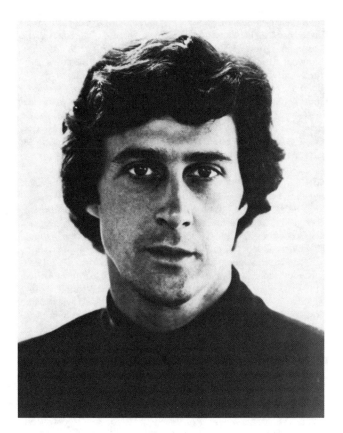

DAVID DUKES

New York City, 1973; Scandal, *Love for Love*, and Guido Venanzi, *The Rules of the Game*, both New Phoenix Repertory Company, Helen Hayes Theatre, New York City, 1974; Billy, *The Salty Dog Saga*, New Dramatists, New York City, 1975; Henry, *Travesties*, Ethel Barrymore Theatre, 1975; Harold, *The Man Who Drew Circles*, New Dramatists, 1976; General William Tecumseh Sherman, *Rebel Women*, New York Shakespeare Festival, Public Theatre, New York City, 1976; Henry, *Travesties*, Center Theatre Group, Mark Taper Forum, Los Angeles, 1977; Horst, *Bent*, New Apollo Theatre, New York City, 1979; Victor Frankenstein, *Frankenstein*, Palace Theatre, New York City, 1981; Benjamin, *Another Part of the Forest*, Center Theatre Group, Ahmanson Theatre, Los Angeles, 1982; Antonio Salieri, *Amadeus*, Broadhurst Theatre, New York City, 1982; Charles and Harold, *Light Comedies*, Center Theatre Group, Ahmanson Theatre, 1984; Rene Gallimard, *M. Butterfly*, Eugene O'Neill Theatre, New York City, 1988. Also appeared in *Murderous Angels*, Center Theatre Group, Mark Taper Forum, 1969; *In 3 Zones*, Charles Playhouse, Boston, MA, 1970; *The Death and Life of Jesse James*, New Theatre for Now, Ahmanson Theatre, 1974; *Design for Living*, Goodman Theatre, Chicago, IL, 1976; and at the National Shakespeare Festival, Old Globe Theatre, San Diego, CA, 1981.

PRINCIPAL STAGE WORK—Choreographer of sword fights, *Macbeth*, New York Shakespeare Festival, Mitzi E. Newhouse Theatre, New York City, 1974.

MAJOR TOURS—Horace, *The School for Wives*, Canadian cities, 1971-72; title role, *Dracula*, U.S. cities, 1979.

PRINCIPAL FILM APPEARANCES—Guard, *The Strawberry State-*

ment, Metro-Goldwyn-Mayer, 1970; James Morrison, *The Wild Party,* American International, 1975; George de Marco, *A Little Romance,* Orion, 1979; Daniel Blank, *The First Deadly Sin,* Filmways, 1980; David, *Only When I Laugh* (also known as *It Hurts Only When I Laugh*), Columbia, 1981; Graham Selky, *Without a Trace,* Twentieth Century-Fox, 1983; Phillip, *The Men's Club,* Atlantic, 1986; Waldo, *Catch the Heat* (also known as *Feel the Heat*), Trans World, 1987; Ed Winston, *Date with an Angel,* De Laurentiis Group, 1987; Howard Hellenbeck, *Rawhead Rex,* Empire, 1987; Myron Weston, *Deadly Intent,* Fries Distribution, 1988; Peter, *See You in the Morning,* Warner Brothers, 1989.

PRINCIPAL TELEVISION APPEARANCES—Series: Robert Lassiter, *Beacon Hill,* CBS, 1975. Mini-Series: Leslie Slote, *The Winds of War,* ABC, 1983; George William Fairfax, *George Washington,* CBS, 1984; Leopold Strabismus, *James A. Michener's "Space"* (also known as *Space*), CBS, 1985. Pilots: Dr. O'Brien, *Handle with Care,* CBS, 1977; Dr. Chase, *The Many Loves of Arthur,* NBC, 1978; Reverend Crane, *Go West, Young Girl!,* ABC, 1978. Episodic: Rapist, *All in the Family,* CBS, 1977; also *Barney Miller,* ABC, 1977; *All That Glitters,* syndicated, 1977; "Remembering Melody," *The Hitchhiker,* HBO; *Family,* ABC. Movies: Mike Koshko, *Harold Robbins' "79 Park Avenue"* (also known as *79 Park Avenue*), NBC, 1977; David Allen, *A Fire in the Sky,* NBC, 1978; Miles Standish, *Mayflower: The Pilgrim's Adventures,* CBS, 1979; Joe Dine, *Some Kind of Miracle,* CBS, 1979; Lou Ribin, *The Triangle Factory Fire Scandal,* NBC, 1979; Bill Sanger, *Portrait of a Rebel: Margaret Sanger,* CBS, 1980; Avery McPherson, *Miss All-American Beauty,* CBS, 1982; Bill Gardner, *Sentimental Journey,* CBS, 1984; David Osborne, *Kane and Abel,* CBS, 1985. Specials: Cutting, *Valley Forge,* NBC, 1975; Dr. Ned Darrell, "Strange Interlude," *American Playhouse,* PBS, 1988.

RELATED CAREER—Company member, American Conservatory Theatre, San Francisco, CA, 1966-69; company member, Alley Theatre, Houston, TX, 1969-70; company member, National Shakespeare Festival, San Diego, CA, 1970; company member, Philadelphia Drama Guild, Philadephia, PA, 1971-72; also fencing instructor, Juilliard School, New York City.

AWARDS: Los Angeles Drama Critics Award, Outstanding Actor, for *Design for Living;* Antoinette Perry Award nomination, Best Featured Actor in a Play, 1980, for *Bent.*

SIDELIGHTS: In an interview with Karen Coker of the [New York] *Daily News* (January 18, 1988), David Dukes stated, "I think I'm best onstage because the stage is an actor's milieu. No one can bring a play off without you. On film, your performance can be edited, cut or completely erased. You have no control."

ADDRESSES: AGENT—International Creative Management, 40 W. 57th Street, New York, NY 10019.*

*   *   *

DUNAWAY, Faye   1941-

PERSONAL: Full name, Dorothy Faye Dunaway; born January 14, 1941, in Bascom, FL; daughter of John (a career U.S. Army officer) and Grace Dunaway; married Peter Wolf (a singer), August 7, 1974 (divorced, 1978); married Terry O'Neill (a photographer), 1983 (divorced); children: Liam (second marriage). EDUCATION:

Graduated from Boston University, 1962; also attended Florida State University and the University of Florida.

VOCATION: Actress.

CAREER: BROADWAY DEBUT—Margaret More, *A Man for All Seasons,* American National Theatre and Academy Theatre, 1962. PRINCIPAL STAGE APPEARANCES—Nurse, then Elsie, *After the Fall,* American National Theatre and Academy (ANTA) Washington Square Theatre, New York City, 1964; Faith Prosper, *But for Whom Charlie,* ANTA Washington Square Theatre, 1964; Beatrice's maid, *The Changeling,* ANTA Washington Square Theatre, 1965; Kathleen Stanton, *Hogan's Goat,* American Place Theatre, New York City, 1965; Blanche du Bois, *A Streetcar Named Desire,* Ahmanson Theatre, Los Angeles, CA, 1973; Frances Anna Duffy Walsh, *The Curse of an Aching Heart,* Little Theatre, New York City, 1982. Also appeared in *Tartuffe,* ANTA Washington Square Theatre, 1965; in *Candida,* summer theatre production, 1971; and in *Old Times,* Mark Taper Forum, Los Angeles, 1972.

FILM DEBUT—Sandy, *The Happening,* Columbia, 1967. PRINCIPAL FILM APPEARANCES—Lou McDowell, *Hurry Sundown,* Paramount, 1967; Bonnie Parker, *Bonnie and Clyde,* Warner Brothers, 1967; Vicky Anderson, *The Thomas Crown Affair* (also known as *Thomas Crown and Company* and *The Crown Caper*), United Artists, 1968; Gwen, *The Arrangement,* Warner Brothers, 1969; Jennifer Winslow, *The Extraordinary Seaman,* Metro-Goldwyn-Mayer (MGM), 1969; Julia, *A Place for Lovers* (also known as *Amanti* and *Le Temps des amants*), MGM, 1969; Mrs. Pendrake, *Little Big Man,* National General, 1970; Lou Andrews Sand, *Puzzle of a Downfall Child,* Universal, 1970; Kate Elder, *Doc,* United Artists, 1971; Jill, *The Deadly Trap* (also known as *La Maison sous les arbres*), National General, 1972; Lena Doyle, *Oklahoma Crude,* Columbia, 1973; Evelyn Mulwray, *Chinatown,* Paramount, 1974; Susan Franklin, *The Towering Inferno,* Twentieth Century-Fox/Warner Brothers, 1974; Lady de Winter, *The Three Musketeers,* Twentieth Century-Fox, 1974; Lady de Winter, *The Four Musketeers* (also known as *The Revenge of Milady*), Twentieth Century-Fox, 1975; Kathy Hale, *Three Days of the Condor,* Paramount, 1975; Diana Christensen, *Network,* Metro-Goldwyn-Mayer/United Artists (MGM/UA), 1976; Denise Kreisler, *Voyage of the Damned,* AVCO-Embassy, 1976; title role, *The Eyes of Laura Mars,* Columbia, 1978; Annie, *The Champ,* MGM/UA, 1979; Barbara Delaney, *The First Deadly Sin,* Filmways, 1980; Joan Crawford, *Mommie Dearest,* Paramount, 1981; Lady Barbara Skelton, *The Wicked Lady,* MGM/UA, 1983; Rachel Calgary, *Ordeal by Innocence,* MGM/UA, 1984; Selena, *Supergirl,* Tri-Star, 1984; Wanda Wilcox, *Barfly,* Cannon, 1987; Helen Barton, *Midnight Crossing,* Vestron, 1988. Also appeared in *Arthur Miller: On Home Ground* (documentary), 1979; and as Sonya Tuchman, *Burning Secret,* 1989.

PRINCIPAL TELEVISION APPEARANCES—Movies: Sister Aimee McPherson, *The Disappearance of Aimee,* NBC, 1976; title role, *Evita Peron,* NBC, 1981; Maud Charteris, *Ellis Island,* CBS, 1984; Jane Wilkinson (Lady Edgeware) and Carlotta Adams, *Agatha Christie's "Thirteen at Dinner,"* CBS, 1985; Queen Isabella, *Christopher Columbus,* CBS, 1985; Lil Hutton, *Beverly Hills Madam,* NBC, 1986; Mme. D'Urfe, *Casanova,* CBS, 1987; also Wallis Simpson, *The Woman I Love,* 1971. Plays: Kathleen Stanton, *Hogan's Goat,* 1971; also *After the Fall,* 1974.

RELATED CAREER—Member, Lincoln Center Repertory Company, New York City.

AWARDS: Theatre World Award, 1966, for *Hogan's Goat;* Academy Award nomination, Best Actress, 1967, and British Academy Award, Most Promising Newcomer, 1968, both for *Bonnie and Clyde;* Academy Award nomination, Best Actress, 1974, for *Chinatown;* Academy Award, Best Actress, 1976, for *Network;* Golden Globe nomination, Best Actress in a Dramatic Film, 1988, for *Barfly.*

ADDRESSES: AGENT—Sam Cohn, International Creative Management, 40 W. 57th Street, New York, NY 10019.*

*   *   *

DUNCAN, Lindsay   1950-

PERSONAL: Born November 7, 1950, in Edinburgh, Scotland. EDUCATION: Attended the Central School for Speech and Drama, London.

VOCATION: Actress.

CAREER: OFF-BROADWAY DEBUT—Lady Nijo and Win, *Top Girls,* New York Shakespeare Festival, Public Theatre, 1982. BROADWAY DEBUT—La Marquise de Merteuil, *Les Liaisons Dangereuses,* Music Box Theatre, 1987. PRINCIPAL STAGE APPEARANCES—Charlotta/Violette, *Don Juan,* Hampstead Theatre Club, London, 1976; Margaret, *The Ordeal of Gilbert Pinfold,* Royal Exchange Theatre, Manchester, U.K., 1977, later Round House Theatre, London, 1979; Hilary, *Comings and Goings,* Hampstead Theatre Club, 1978; Dorcas Frey, *Plenty,* National Theatre Company, Lyttleton Theatre, London, 1978; Maggie, *Cat on a Hot Tin Roof,* National Theatre, London, 1988. Also appeared in *The Script,* Hampstead Theatre Club, 1976.

PRINCIPAL FILM APPEARANCES—Sally, *Loose Connections,* Twentieth Century-Fox, 1984; Anthea Lahr, *Prick Up Your Ears,* Samuel Goldwyn, 1987; Lily Sachor, *Manifesto,* Cannon, 1988.

AWARDS: Theatre World Award and Antoinette Perry Award nomination, Best Actress in a Play, both 1987, for *Les Liaisons Dangereuses.*

ADDRESSES: AGENTS—Ken McReddie Ltd., 91 Regent Street, London W1R 7TB, England; Josh Ellis Agency, 240 W. 44th Street, Suite 8, New York, NY 10036.*

*   *   *

DUNCAN, Sandy   1946-

PERSONAL: Born February 20, 1946, in Henderson, TX; daughter of Mancil Ray and Sylvia Wynne (Scott) Duncan; married Thomas C. Calcaterra (a doctor; divorced); married Don Correia (an actor and dancer); children: Jeffrey, Michael (second marriage). EDUCATION: Attended Lon Morris College; trained for the stage with Wynn Handman, Utah Ground, and Toni Beck.

VOCATION: Actress.

CAREER: STAGE DEBUT—*The King and I,* State Fair Music Hall, Dallas, TX, 1958. BROADWAY DEBUT—Zaneeta Shin, *The Music Man,* City Center Theatre, 1965. PRINCIPAL STAGE APPEARANCES—Louise, *Carousel,* City Center Theatre, New York City, 1966; Susan Mahoney, *Finian's Rainbow,* Liesl, *The Sound of Music,* and Mary Skinner, *Life with Father,* all City Center Theatre, 1967; Thulja, *The Ceremony of Innocence,* American Place Theatre, New York City, 1967; Viola, *Your Own Thing,* Orpheum Theatre, New York City, 1968; Alison, Molly, May, and Sweetheart, *Canterbury Tales,* Eugene O'Neill Theatre, New York City, 1969; April MacGregor, *Love Is a Time of Day,* Music Box Theatre, New York City, 1969; Maisie, *The Boyfriend,* Ambassador Theatre, New York City, 1970; title role, *Peter Pan,* Music Hall Theatre, Dallas, TX, 1975; Mary, *Vanities,* Mark Taper Forum, Los Angeles, CA, 1976; title role, *Peter Pan,* Opera House, John F. Kennedy Center for the Performing Arts, Washington, DC, then Lunt-Fontanne Theatre, New York City, both 1979; Irene Castle, *Parade of Stars Playing the Palace,* Palace Theatre, New York City, 1983; *5-6-7-8 . . . Dance!,* Radio City Music Hall, New York City, 1984; Edith Herbert, *My One and Only,* St. James Theatre, New York City, 1985. Also appeared in *Wonderful Town,* City Center Theatre, 1967; and in *Waitin' in the Wings,* Triplex Theatre, New York City, 1986.

MAJOR TOURS—Viola, *Your Own Thing,* U.S. and Canadian cities, 1968; title role, *Peter Pan,* U.S. cities, 1981; Edith Herbert, *My One and Only,* U.S. cities, 1985-86; and in U.S. tours of *Gypsy, The Music Man,* and *Brigadoon.*

FILM DEBUT—Katie Dooley, *The Million Dollar Duck,* Buena Vista, 1971. PRINCIPAL FILM APPEARANCES—Amy Cooper, *Star Spangled Girl,* Paramount, 1971; Liz, *The Cat from Outer Space,* Buena Vista, 1978; voice of Vixey, *The Fox and the Hound* (animated), Buena Vista, 1981.

TELEVISION DEBUT—*Bonanza,* NBC. PRINCIPAL TELEVISION APPEARANCES—Series: Sandy Stockton, *Funny Face,* CBS, 1971, renamed *The Sandy Duncan Show,* CBS, 1972; Sandy Hogan, *Valerie* (also known as *Valerie's Family*), NBC, 1987, renamed *The Hogan Family,* NBC, 1987—; also Helen, *Search for Tomorrow,* CBS. Mini-Series: Missy Anne Reynolds, *Roots,* ABC, 1977. Pilots: *The Funny World of Fred and Bunni,* CBS, 1978. Episodic: Gillian, *The Six-Million Dollar Man,* ABC; also *Laugh-In,* NBC; *The Flip Wilson Show,* NBC; *The Muppet Show,* syndicated. Specials: *Merv Griffin's St. Patrick's Day Special,* syndicated, 1968; *Keep U.S. Beautiful,* NBC, 1973; *The Burt Bacharach Special,* NBC, 1974; host, *The Sandy Duncan Show,* CBS, 1974; host, *Sandy in Disneyland,* CBS, 1974; *Bing Crosby and His Friends,* CBS, 1974; co-host, *Opryland, U.S.A.,* ABC, 1975; *The Rich Little Show,* NBC, 1975; *Celebration: The American Spirit,* ABC, 1976; *Happy Birthday, America,* NBC, 1976; tour guide, *Christmas in Disneyland,* ABC, 1976; title role, *Pinnochio,* CBS, 1976; *Bing! . . . A 50th Anniversary Gala,* CBS, 1977; *Doug Henning's World of Magic II,* NBC, 1977; *Perry Como's Music from Hollywood,* ABC, 1977; *100 Years of Golden Hits,* NBC, 1981; *Parade of Stars,* ABC, 1983.

AWARDS: Theatre World Award, 1968, for *The Ceremony of Innocence;* Antoinette Perry Award nomination, Best Supporting or Featured Actress in a Musical, 1969, for *Canterbury Tales;* Outer Critics Circle Award and New York Drama Critics Award, both 1970, and Antoinette Perry Award nomination, Best Actress in a Musical, 1971, all for *The Boyfriend;* Golden Apple Award from the Hollywood Women's Press Club, Discovery of the Year, 1971; Emmy Award nomination, Best Actress in a Comedy Series, 1972, for *Funny Face;* Emmy Award nomination, 1977, for *Roots;*

Antoinette Perry Award nomination, Best Actress in a Musical, 1980, for *Peter Pan.*

ADDRESSES: AGENT—Litke/Gale and Associates, 10390 Santa Monica Boulevard, Suite 300, Los Angeles, CA 90025.*

*   *   *

DUVALL, Robert   1931-

PERSONAL: Full name, Robert Selden Duvall; born January 5, 1931, in San Diego, CA; son of William Howard Duvall (an admiral); married Barbara Benjamin, 1964 (divorced); married Gail Youngs, 1982 (divorced, 1986). EDUCATION: Attended Principia College; studied acting with Sanford Meisner at the Neighborhood Playhouse. MILITARY: U.S. Army.

VOCATION: Actor.

CAREER: PRINCIPAL STAGE APPEARANCES—Frank Gardner, *Mrs. Warren's Profession,* Gate Theatre, New York City, 1958; Doug, *Call Me by My Rightful Name,* Sheridan Square Playhouse, New York City, 1961; Bob Smith, *The Days and Nights of Beebee Fenstermaker,* Sheridan Square Playhouse, 1962; Eddie, *A View from the Bridge,* Sheridan Square Playhouse, 1965; Walter "Teacher" Cole, *American Buffalo,* Ethel Barrymore Theatre, then Belasco Theatre, both New York City, 1977. Also appeared in "Midnight Caller" in *Two Plays by Horton Foote,* Sheridan Square Playhouse, 1958; in *Wait Until Dark,* Ethel Barrymore Theatre, 1966; and as Jackson Fentry, *Tomorrow,* 1968.

FILM DEBUT—Arthur "Boo" Radley, *To Kill a Mockingbird,* Universal, 1962. PRINCIPAL FILM APPEARANCES—Captain Paul Cabot Winston, *Captain Newman, M.D.,* Universal, 1963; motorcyclist, *Nightmare in the Sun,* Zodiac, 1964; Edwin Stewart, *The Chase,* Columbia, 1966; Weissberg, *Bullitt,* Warner Brothers, 1968; Chiz, *Countdown,* Warner Brothers, 1968; Nestor, *The Detective,* Twentieth Century-Fox, 1968; Gordon, *The Rain People,* Warner Brothers, 1969; Ned Pepper, *True Grit,* Paramount, 1969; Major Frank Burns, *M*A*S*H,* Twentieth Century-Fox, 1970; Despard, *The Revolutionary,* United Artists, 1970; Vernon Adams, *Lawman,* United Artists, 1971; title role, *THX 1138,* Warner Brothers, 1971; Tom Hagen, *The Godfather,* Paramount, 1972; Jesse James, *The Great Northfield, Minnesota Raid,* Universal, 1972; Frank Harlan, *Joe Kidd,* Universal, 1972; Jackson Fentry, *Tomorrow,* Filmgroup, 1972; Eddie Ryan, *Badge 373,* Paramount, 1973; Ford Pierce, *Lady Ice,* National General, 1973; Earl Macklin, *The Outfit* (also known as *The Good Guys Always Win*), Metro-Goldwyn-Mayer, 1973; the director, *The Conversation,* Paramount, 1974; Tom Hagen, *The Godfather, Part II,* Paramount, 1974.

Jay Wagner, *Breakout,* Columbia, 1975; George Hansen, *The Killer Elite,* United Artists, 1975; Frank Hackett, *Network,* Metro-Goldwyn-Mayer/United Artists, 1976; Bill McDonald, *The Greatest,* Columbia, 1977; Dr. Watson, *The Seven Percent Solution,*

Universal, 1977; Colonel Max Radl, *The Eagle Has Landed,* Columbia, 1977; Loren Hardeman III, *The Betsy,* Allied Artists, 1978; Lieutenant Colonel Kilgore, *Apocalypse Now,* United Artists, 1979; Bull Meechum, *The Great Santini,* Warner Brothers, 1979; Gruen, *The Pursuit of D.B. Cooper,* Universal, 1981; Tom Spellacy, *True Confessions,* United Artists, 1981; Mac Sledge, *Tender Mercies,* Universal, 1983; Joe Hillerman, *The Stone Boy,* Twentieth Century-Fox, 1984; Max Mercy, *The Natural,* Tri-Star, 1984; as himself, *Sanford Meisner—The Theatre's Best Kept Secret* (documentary), Columbia, 1984; Caspary, *The Lightship,* Warner Brothers, 1985; Preacher, *Belizaire the Cajun,* Skouras-Norstar, 1986; Carrasco, *Hotel Colonial,* Orion, 1987; Norman Shrike, *Let's Get Harry,* Tri-Star, 1987; Bob Hodges, *Colors,* Orion, 1988. Also appeared in *Aliens from Another Planet,* 1967; and *Invasion of the Body Snatchers,* United Artists, 1978.

PRINCIPAL FILM WORK—Producer (with Philip S. Hobel, Mary Ann Hobel, and Horton Foote), *Tender Mercies,* Universal, 1982; co-producer and director, *Angelo My Love,* Cinecom, 1983; also director, *We're Not the Jet Set* (documentary), 1977.

PRINCIPAL TELEVISION APPEARANCES—Mini-Series: General Dwight D. Eisenhower, *Ike* (also known as *Ike: The War Years*), ABC, 1979; Captain Augustus "Gus" McCrae, *Lonesome Dove,* CBS, 1989. Pilots: Frank Reeser, *Guilty or Not Guilty* (braodcast as an episode of *The Bob Hope Chrysler Theatre*), NBC, 1966. Episodic: Charley Parkes, "Miniature," *The Twilight Zone,* CBS, 1963; Louis Mace, "The Chameleon," *The Outer Limits,* ABC, 1964; Adam Ballard, "The Inheritors," *The Outer Limits,* 1964; also *Great Ghost Tales,* NBC, 1961; "The Invaders," *Voyage to the Bottom of the Sea,* ABC, 1964; "Chase Through Time," *The Time Tunnel,* ABC, 1966; *This Morning,* CBS, 1989; *Naked City,* ABC; *The Defenders,* CBS; *The F.B.I.,* ABC; *Route 66,* CBS. Movies: Eddie, *Fame Is the Name of the Game,* NBC, 1966; Bill Vigars, *The Terry Fox Story,* HBO, 1983; also *Cosa Nostra: An Arch Enemy of the F.B.I.,* 1968. Specials: Howard, *Flesh and Blood,* NBC, 1968.

RELATED CAREER—Singer.

WRITINGS: FILMS—*Angelo My Love,* Cinecom, 1983. Also wrote two songs in *Tender Mercies.*

AWARDS: Obie Award from the *Village Voice,* 1965, for *A View from the Bridge;* New York Film Critics Award, Best Supporting Actor, 1972, and Academy Award nomination, Best Supporting Actor, 1973, both for *The Godfather;* Academy Award nomination and British Academy Award, both Best Supporting Actor, 1979, for *Apocalypse Now;* Academy Award nomination, Best Actor, and Best Actor Award from the Montreal World Film Festival, both 1980, for *The Great Santini;* Academy Award, Best Actor, and Golden Globe Award, Best Performance by an Actor in a Motion Picture, both 1984, for *Tender Mercies;* also received a National Association of Theatre Owners Award.

ADDRESSES: MANAGER—Bill Robinson, International Creative Management, 8899 Beverly Boulevard, Los Angeles, CA 90048.

E

EASTERBROOK, Leslie

PERSONAL: Born July 29, in Los Angeles, CA.

VOCATION: Actress.

CAREER: PRINCIPAL STAGE APPEARANCES—Bunny, ''Visitor from Philadelphia,'' *California Suite*, Eugene O'Neill Theatre, New York City, 1976; Agnes, *On the Twentieth Century*, St. James Theatre, New York City, 1979; Havana McCoy, *Mike*, Walnut Street Theatre, Philadelphia, PA, 1988.

PRINCIPAL FILM APPEARANCES—Hospital nurse, *Just Tell Me What You Want*, Warner Brothers, 1980; Sergeant Callahan, *Police Academy*, Warner Brothers, 1984; Bobby Sue, *Private Resort*, Tri-Star, 1985; Lieutenant Callahan, *Police Academy 3: Back in Training*, Warner Brothers, 1986; Callahan, *Police Academy 4: Citizens on Patrol*, Warner Brothers, 1987; Callahan, *Police Academy 5: Assignment Miami Beach*, Warner Brothers, 1988; Callahan, *Police Academy 6: City Under Siege*, Warner Brothers, 1989.

PRINCIPAL TELEVISION APPEARANCES—Series: Devlin Kowalski, *Ryan's Hope*, ABC, 1975; Rhonda Lee, *Laverne and Shirley*, ABC, 1980-83. Pilots: Allison, *First and Ten*, HBO, 1984; Sharon, *His and Hers*, CBS, 1984. Episodic: Judy York, *The Law and Harry McGraw*, CBS, 1987; Glenda Morrison, *Murder, She Wrote*, CBS, 1988; Gloria, *Ohara*, ABC, 1988. Movies: Audrey, *The Taking of Flight 847: The Uli Derickson Story*, NBC, 1988.

ADDRESSES: MANAGER—Michael Mann Management, 8380 Melrose Avenue, Suite 207, Los Angeles, CA 90069.*

*   *   *

EDWARDS, Julie
See ANDREWS, Julie

*   *   *

EDWARDS, Vince   1928-

PERSONAL: Born Vincente Edwardo Zoino, July 7, 1928, in Brooklyn, NY; son of Vincente and Julia Zoino; married Kathy Kersh, June 13, 1965 (divorced, October 1965); married Linda Ann Foster, 1967 (marriage ended); married wife, Cassandra (an actress), 1980; children: one daughter (first marriage). EDUCATION: Attended Ohio State University, 1946-48, and the University of Hawaii, 1948; studied theatre at the American Academy of Dramatic Arts.

VOCATION: Actor, director, and writer.

CAREER: Also see *WRITINGS* below. BROADWAY DEBUT—Chorus, *High Button Shoes*, Century Theatre. PRINCIPAL STAGE APPEARANCES—Appeared with the Honolulu Community Theater and the University of Hawaii Players.

MAJOR TOURS—*Come Back Little Sheba*, U.S. cities.

PRINCIPAL FILM APPEARANCES—Tommy Tomkins, *Mr. Universe*, Eagle-Lion, 1951; Blayden, *Sailor Beware*, Paramount, 1951; title role, *Hiawatha*, Monogram, 1952; Langley, *Rogue Cop*, Metro-Goldwyn-Mayer (MGM), 1954; Hamilton, *Cell 2455, Death Row*, Columbia, 1955; Victor Gosset, *The Night Holds Terror*, Columbia, 1955; Val Cannon, *The Killing*, United Artists, 1956; Marco Roselli, *Serenade*, Warner Brothers, 1956; Kell Beldon, *The Hired Gun*, MGM, 1957; Frank, *Hit and Run*, United Artists, 1957; Little Wolf, *Ride Out for Revenge*, United Artists, 1957; Mike, *Island Women* (also known as *Island Woman*), United Artists, 1958; Claude, *Murder by Contract*, Columbia, 1958; Vince Ryker, *City of Fear*, Columbia, 1959; Stuart Allison, *The Scavengers* (also known as *City of Sin*), Valiant/Roach, 1959.

George, *The Outsider*, Universal, 1962; Tommy, *Too Late Blues*, Paramount, 1962; Baker, *The Victors*, Columbia, 1963; Major Cliff Bricker, *The Devil's Brigade*, United Artists, 1968; Charles Hood, *Hammerhead*, Columbia, 1969; David Galt, *The Desperados*, Columbia, 1968; Geronimo Minneli, *The Mad Bomber* (also known as *Police Connection* and *Detective Geronimo*), Cinemation, 1973; Maxwell, *The Seduction*, AVCO-Embassy, 1982; Frank Stryker, *Deal of the Century*, Warner Brothers, 1983; Hawk, *Space Raiders* (also known as *Star Child*), New World, 1983; Frank Lane, *The Fix* (also known as *The Agitators*), Reverie, 1985; Steve King, *Sno-Line* (also known as *Texas Sno-Line*), Vandom, 1986; Richard Birnbaum, *Return to Horror High*, Balcor, 1987; Meshelski, *Cellar Dweller*, Empire, 1988. Also appeared in *I Am a Camera*, Directors Corporation of America, 1955; *Three Faces of Eve*, Twentieth Century-Fox, 1957; and in *Las Vegas, Los Angeles*.

PRINCIPAL FILM WORK—Director, *Mission Galactica: The Cylon Attack*, Universal, 1979.

PRINCIPAL TELEVISION APPEARANCES—Series: Title role, *Ben Casey*, ABC, 1961-66; title role, *Matt Lincoln*, ABC, 1970-71; voice characterization, *Punky Brewster* (animated), NBC, 1985; voice characterization, *The Centurions—PowerXtreme!* (animated), syndicated, 1986. Mini-Series: General Swanson, *The Rhinemann Exchange*, NBC, 1977. Pilots: David Leopold, *Dial*

Hot Line, ABC, 1970; Spike Ryerson, *Firehouse*, ABC, 1973; Bradner, *Cover Girls*, NBC, 1977; Colonel Joe Agajanian, *The Courage and the Passion*, NBC, 1978; Inspector Frank Walker, *The Return of Mickey Spillane's Mike Hammer*, CBS, 1986; also *Knight Rider*. Episodic: *Undercurrent*, CBS; *Fireside Theatre*, NBC; *The Untouchables*, ABC; *General Electric Theatre*, CBS; *Philco Television Playhouse*, NBC; *The Deputy*, NBC; *Studio One*, CBS; *Alfred Hitchcock Presents*. Movies: Major Michael Devlin, *Sole Survivor*, CBS, 1970; Mal Weston, *Do Not Fold, Spindle, or Mutilate*, ABC, 1971; Jack Trahey, *Death Stalk*, NBC, 1975; Bret Easton, *Evening in Byzantium*, syndicated, 1978; title role, *The Return of Ben Casey*, syndicated, 1988; also *The Dirty Dozen: The Deadly Mission*, NBC, 1987. Specials: Sheriff, *Saga of Sonora*, NBC, 1973; *ABC's Silver Anniversary Celebration*, ABC, 1978; *Circus of the Stars*, CBS, 1979; *National Off-the-Wall People's Poll*, NBC, 1984; Detective Lieutenant Philip Lombardo, *You Are the Jury*, NBC, 1986; "Surviving a Heart Attack," *Lifetime Informathon*, Lifetime, 1988.

PRINCIPAL TELEVISION WORK—All as director, unless indicated. Pilots: Executive producer (with David Gerber) and creator, *The Courage and the Passion*, NBC, 1978. Episodic: *The Hardy Boys Mysteries*, ABC, 1977-79; *David Cassidy—Man Undercover*, NBC, 1978-79; *B.J. and the Bear*, NBC, 1979-80; *Battlestar Galactica*, ABC, 1978-79; *Galactica 1980*, ABC, 1980; also *Police Story*, NBC; *Ben Casey*, ABC. Movies: *Maneater*, ABC, 1973.

WRITINGS: FILM—(With Christian I. Nyby II) *Mission Galactica: The Cylon Attack*, Universal, 1979. TELEVISION—Movies: (With Marcus Demian) *Maneater*, ABC, 1973.

RECORDINGS: ALBUMS—*Vince Edwards Sings*.

ADDRESSES: AGENT—Lillian Micelli, Diamond Artists, Ltd., 9200 Sunset Boulevard, Suite 909, Los Angeles, CA 90069.*

*   *   *

EKBERG, Anita   1931-

PERSONAL: Born September 29, 1931, in Malmo, Sweden; came to the United States in 1951; married Anthony Steele, 1956 (divorced, 1959); married Rick Van Nutter, 1963.

VOCATION: Actress.

CAREER: PRINCIPAL FILM APPEARANCES—Venusian woman, *Abbott and Costello Go to Mars*, Universal, 1953; handmaiden, *The Golden Blade*, Universal, 1953; bridesmaid, *The Mississippi Gambler*, Universal, 1953; dance hall girl, *Take Me to Town*, Universal, 1953; Anita, *Artists and Models*, Paramount, 1955; Wei Long, *Blood Alley*, Warner Brothers, 1955; Rena, *Back from Eternity*, RKO, 1956; as herself, *Hollywood or Bust*, Paramount, 1956; Flo Randall, *Man in the Vault*, RKO, 1956; Helene, *War and Peace*, Paramount, 1956; Salma, *Zarak*, Columbia, 1956; Gina Broger, *Pickup Alley* (also known as *Interpol* and *International Police*), Columbia, 1957; title role, *Valerie*, United Artists, 1957; Trudie Hall, *The Man Inside*, Columbia, 1958; Zara, *Paris Holiday*, United Artists, 1958; Virginia Wilson, *Screaming Mimi*, Columbia, 1958; Zenobia, Queen of Palmyra, *Sign of the Gladiator* (also known as *Nel Segno Di Roma*), American International, 1959.

Sylvia, *La Dolce Vita*, Astor/American International, 1961; Anita, "The Temptation of Dr. Antonio," *Boccaccio '70*, Gray, 1962; Luba, *Call Me Bwana*, United Artists, 1963; Elya Carlson, *Four for Texas*, Warner Brothers, 1963; Amanda Beatrice Cross, *The Alphabet Murders* (also known as *The ABC Murders*), Metro-Goldwyn-Mayer, 1966; Huluna, *The Mongols*, Colorama, 1966; Anna Soblova, *Way . . . Way Out*, Twentieth Century-Fox, 1966; Aberchiaria, "The Unkindest Cut," *White, Red, Yellow, Pink* (also known as *Love Factory*), Seymour Borde, 1966; Lou, *The Cobra*, American International, 1968; Paulette, *The Glass Sphinx*, American International, 1968; nightclub performer, *If It's Tuesday, This Must Be Belgium*, United Artists, 1969; as herself, *I Clowns* (also known as *The Clowns* and *Les Clowns*), Levitt-Pickman, 1970; title role, *Malenka, the Vampire* (also known as *La Nipole del Vampiro* and *Fangs of the Living Dead*), Europix, 1972. Also appeared in *Northeast to Seoul*, 1974; *Cicciambomba*, 1983; *Dolce Pella Di Angela* (also known as *Angela's Sweet Skin*), Cineglobo, 1987; and in *Sheba and the Gladiator*.

PRINCIPAL TELEVISION APPEARANCES—Pilots: Dr. Else Biebling, *S*H*E*, CBS, 1980. Mini-Series: Ilsa Lund Laszlo, "Casablanca," *Warner Brothers Presents*, ABC, 1955-56. Movies: Queen Na-Eela, *Gold of the Amazon Women*, NBC, 1979. Specials: *The Bob Hope Show*, NBC, 1955, 1958, and 1966; *Intervista* (also known as *Federico Fellini's Intervista* and *The Interview*), Aljosta/RAI-TV-Cinecitta/Ferlyn, 1987.

RELATED CAREER—Model.*

*   *   *

EKLAND, Britt   1942-

PERSONAL: Born October 6, 1942, in Stockholm, Sweden; married Peter Sellers (an actor) in 1963 (divorced, 1968); married "Slim" Jim Phantom (a musician); children: three.

VOCATION: Actress.

CAREER: PRINCIPAL STAGE APPEARANCES—Olivia, *Mate!*, Comedy Theatre, London, 1978.

PRINCIPAL FILM APPEARANCES—Gina Romantica, *After the Fox*, United Artists, 1966; Olimpia Segura, *The Bobo*, Warner Brothers, 1967; Gina, *The Double Man*, Warner Brothers, 1967; Rachel Schpitendavel, *The Night They Raided Minsky's* (also known as *The Night They Invented Striptease*), United Artists, 1968; Illeana, *Stiletto*, AVCO-Embassy, 1969; Antigone, *The Cannibals*, Doria/San Marco, 1970; Irene Tucker, *Machine Gun McCann* (also known as *Gli Intoccabili*), Columbia, 1970; Anna Fletcher, *Get Carter*, Metro-Goldwyn-Mayer (MGM), 1971; Dorothy Chiltern-Barlow, *Percy*, MGM, 1971; Lucy, *Asylum* (also known as *House of Crazies*), Cinerama, 1972; Chris Bentley, *Baxter*, National General, 1973; Mary Goodnight, *The Man with the Golden Gun*, United Artists, 1974; Michelle, *The Ultimate Thrill* (also known as *The Ultimate Chase*), General Cinema, 1974; Willow MacGregor, *The Wicker Man*, British Lion/Warner Brothers, 1974; Duchess Irma, *Royal Flash*, Twentieth Century-Fox, 1975; Mrs. Anderson, *High Velocity*, First Asian Films of California, 1977; Anna Von Erken, *Slavers*, ITM, 1977; Nypeptha, *King Solomon's Treasures*, Canafox/Towers, 1978; Countess Trivulzi, *Some Like It Cool* (also known as *The Rise and Rise of Casanova* and *Casanova and Co.*), Pro International, 1979.

Lintom's mother, "The Vampire Story," *The Monster Club*, ITC, 1981; Anne-Marie, *Satan's Mistress* (also known as *Fury of the Succubus, Demon Rage,* and *Dark Eyes*), Motion Pictures Marketing, 1982; Priscilla Lancaster/Penny, *Dead Wrong*, Comworld, 1983; Annie, *Love Scenes*, Starways, 1985; Evette, *Fraternity Vacation*, New World, 1985; Linda, *Moon in Scorpio*, Trans World, 1987; Mariella Novotny, *Scandal*, Miramax, 1989. Also appeared in *Too Many Thieves*, MGM, 1968; *Endless Night* (also known as *Agatha Christie's Endless Night*), British Lion, 1971; *Night Hair Child* (also known as *Child of the Night*), Towers, 1971; *A Time for Loving* (also known as *Paris Was Made for Lovers*), London Screen Plays, 1971; and in *At Any Price* and *Tintomara.*

PRINCIPAL TELEVISION APPEARANCES—Pilots: Katrina Volana, *The Six Million Dollar Man*, ABC, 1973. Episodic: *The Trials of O'Brien*, CBS; *McCloud*, NBC. Movies: Jenny Wallenda, *The Great Wallendas*, NBC, 1978; Anny Ondra Schmelling, *Ring of Passion*, NBC, 1978; Leah, *The Hostage Tower*, CBS, 1980; Francoise, *Jacqueline Susann's "Valley of the Dolls 1981,"* CBS, 1981. Specials: Mother, *Carol for Another Christmas*, ABC, 1964; *US against the World II*, ABC, 1978; *Britt Ekland's Juke Box*, syndicated, 1979; *Circus of the Stars*, CBS, 1981 and 1986; *Women Who Rate a "10"*, NBC, 1981. Also appeared in *A Cold Peace.*

ADDRESSES: MANAGER—Paul Cohen Management, P.O. Box 241609, Los Angeles, CA 90024.*

*   *   *

ELDER, Lonne III   1931-

PERSONAL: Born December 26, 1931, in Americus, GA; son of Lonne II and Quincy Elder; married Judith Ann Johnson (an actress), February 14, 1969; children: two sons. EDUCATION: Attended New Jersey State Teachers College; also attended Yale University School of Drama, 1965-67; studied acting with Mary Welch. MILITARY: U.S. Army, 1952-54.

VOCATION: Actor, playwright, and screenwriter.

CAREER: Also see WRITINGS below. BROADWAY DEBUT—Bobo, *A Raisin in the Sun*, Ethel Barrymore Theatre, 1959. PRINCIPAL STAGE APPEARANCES—Clem, *Day of Absence*, St. Mark's Playhouse, New York City, 1965. Also appeared with Brett Warren's Actors' Mobile Theatre, during the 1950s.

MAJOR TOURS—Bobo, *A Raisin in the Sun*, U.S. cities, 1960-61.

PRINCIPAL FILM APPEARANCES—Lieutenant Daniels, *Melinda*, Metro-Goldwyn-Mayer (MGM), 1972.

RELATED CAREER—Coordinator of playwrights and directors unit, Negro Ensemble Company, New York City, 1967-69; writer, Talent Associates, New York City, 1968; writer and producer, Cinema Center Films, Hollywood, CA, 1969-70; writer, Universal Pictures, Hollywood, 1970-71; writer, Radnitz/Mattel Productions, Hollywood, 1971; writer and producer, Talent Associates, Hollywood, 1971; writer, Metro-Goldwyn-Mayer Pictures, Hollywood, 1971; writer, Columbia Pictures, Hollywood, 1972; script writer, ABC Television Network, New York City, 1972; founder (with Robert Hooks), Bannaker Productions.

NON-RELATED CAREER—Waiter, professional gambler, and dock worker.

WRITINGS: STAGE—*Ceremonies in Dark Old Men*, Wagner College, Staten Island, NY, 1965, then revised version, St. Mark's Playhouse, later Pocket Theatre, both New York City, 1969, published by Farrar, Straus & Giroux, 1969; *Charades on East Fourth Street*, Expo '67, Montreal, PQ, Canada, 1967, published in *Black Drama Anthology*, New American Library, 1971. Also wrote *A Hysterical Turtle in a Rabbit Race*, 1961; *Kissing Rattlesnakes Can be Fun*, 1966; *Seven Comes Up, Seven Comes Down*, 1966. FILM—*Melinda*, MGM, 1972; *Sounder*, Twentieth Century-Fox, 1972; *Sounder, Part 2*, Gamma III, 1976; *Bustin' Loose*, Universal, 1981. TELEVISION—Series: *Camera Three*, CBS, 1963; *N.Y.P.D.*, ABC, 1967-68; *McCloud*, NBC, 1970-71. Pilots: *Thou Shalt Not Kill*, NBC, 1982. Movies: *The Terrible Veil*, NBC, 1963; *Ceremonies in Dark Old Men*, ABC, 1975; *A Woman Called Moses*, NBC, 1978; also *Deadly Circle of Violence*, 1964. OTHER—Contributor of articles to journals, periodicals, and magazines.

AWARDS: Stanley Drama Award, 1965; John Hay Whitney Fellowship, 1965-66; ABC Television Writing Fellowship, 1965-66; Hamilton K. Bishop Award in Playwriting and American National Theatre and Academy Award, both 1967; Joseph E. Levine Fellowship in Filmmaking and John Golden Fellowship in Playwriting, both 1967; Pulitzer Prize nomination in drama, 1969, Outer Critics Circle Award, Drama Desk Award, Stella Holt Memorial Playwriting Award, and Los Angeles Drama Critics Award, 1970, all for *Ceremonies in Dark Old Men;* Award of Merit, University of Southern California Film Conference, 1971; Academy Award nomination, Best Screenplay, 1972, for *Sounder.*

MEMBER: Writers Guild of America-West, Black Academy of Arts and Letters, New Dramatists Committee, Harlem Writers Guild.

ADDRESSES: AGENT—Bart/Levy Associates, 280 S. Beverly Drive, Beverly Hills, CA 90212.*

*   *   *

ELIZONDO, Hector   1936-

PERSONAL: Born December 22, 1936, in New York, NY; son of Martin Echevarria (an accountant) and Carmen Medina (Reyes) Elizondo; married Carolee Campbell (a printer and photographer), April 13, 1969; children: Rodd. EDUCATION: Attended the High School of Music and Art and Commerce High School, both in New York City; graduated from City College of New York, 1956; trained for the stage with Mario Siletti and Frank Corsaro at the Stella Adler Studio. RELIGION: Roman Catholic.

VOCATION: Actor.

CAREER: STAGE DEBUT—Reber, *Mr. Roberts*, Equity Library Theatre, New York City, 1961. BROADWAY DEBUT—Blackface, *The Great White Hope*, Alvin Theatre, 1968. PRINCIPAL STAGE APPEARANCES—Supervisor, director, soldier, and attendant, *Kill the One-Eyed Man*, Provincetown Playhouse, New York City, 1965; Archie, *Armstrong's Last Goodnight*, Oriental manservant, *Candaules*, commissioner and Vachel Lindsay, *So Proudly We Hail*, and title role, *The Undertaker*, all Theatre Company of

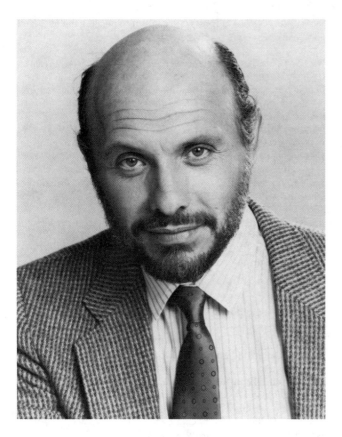

HECTOR ELIZONDO

Boston, *Boston*, MA, 1966-67; Carl Balicke, *Drums in the Night*, Circle in the Square, New York City, 1967; attendant/God, *Steambath*, Truck and Warehouse Theatre, New York City, 1970; Antony, *Antony and Cleopatra*, New York Shakespeare Festival, New York City, 1972; Mel Edison, *The Prisoner of Second Avenue*, Eugene O'Neill Theatre, New York City, 1973; Kurt, *The Dance of Death*, Vivian Beaumont Theatre, New York City, 1974; Simon Able, *Sly Fox*, Broadhurst Theatre, New York City, 1976; Mangiacavallo, *The Rose Tattoo*, Stockbridge Playhouse, Stockbridge, MA, 1980; Eddie Carbone, *A View from the Bridge*, Stockbridge Playhouse, 1983. Also appeared in *Marat/Sade*, Theatre Company of Boston, 1967; and in *Island in Infinity* and *Madonna of the Orchard*.

PRINCIPAL FILM APPEARANCES—Inspector, *The Vixens* (also known as *Friends and Lovers* and *The Women*), International Film Artists, 1969; the Geek, *Born to Win*, United Artists, 1971; Mexican rider, *Valdez Is Coming*, United Artists, 1971; Juan, *Pocket Money*, National General, 1972; Lou Kellerman, *Stand Up and Be Counted*, Columbia, 1972; Grey, *The Taking of Pelham, One, Two, Three*, United Artists, 1974; Captain D'Angelo, *Report to the Commissioner* (also known as *Operation Undercover*), United Artists, 1975; Man Below, *Thieves*, Paramount, 1977; Ramirez, *Cuba*, United Artists, 1979; Sunday, *American Gigolo*, Paramount, 1980; Inspector Raphael Andrews, *The Fan*, Paramount, 1981; Bad Character, *Deadhead Miles*, filmed in 1970, released by Paramount, 1982; Angelo and Angela Bonafetti, *Young Doctors in Love*, Twentieth Century-Fox, 1982; Arthur Willis, *The Flamingo Kid*, Twentieth Century-Fox, 1984; the Maestro, *Private Resort*, Tri-Star, 1985; Charlie Gargas, *Nothing in Common*, Tri-Star, 1986; LeHondro Tunatti, *Overboard*, Metro-Goldwyn-Mayer-

United Artists (MGM/UA), 1987; Mr. Fisk, *Astronomy* (short), Discovery Program/Chanticleer, 1988; Cobb, *Leviathan*, MGM-UA, 1989. Also appeared in *The Landlord*, United Artists, 1970; and *One Across, Two Down*.

TELEVISION DEBUT—*The Wendy Barrie Show*, 1947. PRINCIPAL TELEVISION APPEARANCES—Series: Abraham Rodriquez, *Popi*, CBS, 1976; Detective Sergeant Dan "The Bean" Delgado, *Freebie and the Bean*, CBS, 1980-81; Captain Louis Renault, *Casablanca*, NBC, 1983; Jose Sanchez/Shapiro, *a.k.a. Pablo*, ABC, 1984; District Attorney Jesse Steinberg, *Foley Square*, CBS, 1985-86; Dave Whiteman, *Down and Out in Beverly Hills*, Fox, 1987. Pilots: Abraham Rodriquez, *Popi*, CBS, 1975; Monkey Moreno, *Feel the Heat*, ABC, 1983. Episodic: Commissioner, "Medal of Honor Rag," *American Playhouse*, PBS, 1982; Joe Peters, *Matlock*, NBC, 1986; Meadows, *Amazing Stories*, NBC, 1986; Hector, *Night Heat*, CBS, 1987; Morris King, "Tales from the Hollywood Hills: Natica Jackson," *Great Performances*, PBS, 1987; Quintero, *The Equalizer*, CBS, 1989; also *All in the Family*, CBS, 1972; *Kojak*, CBS; *Columbo*, NBC; *Baretta*, ABC; *The Jackie Gleason Show*, CBS; *The Doctors*, NBC. Movies: Mr. Hernandez, *The Impatient Heart*, NBC, 1971; Pancho Villa, *Wanted: The Sundance Woman* (also known as *Mrs. Sundance Rides Again*), ABC, 1976; Ben Feeney, *The Dain Curse*, CBS, 1978; Emilio Ramirez, *Honeyboy*, NBC, 1982; Captain Mike Reyes, *Women of San Quentin*, NBC, 1983; Ben Haggerty, *Murder: By Reason of Insanity* (also known as *Death on a Day Pass*), CBS, 1985; Father George, *Out of the Darkness*, CBS, 1985; Nick Miraldo, *Courage*, CBS, 1986; Detective Currigan, *Addicted to His Love*, ABC, 1988.

PRINCIPAL TELEVISION WORK—Episodic: Director, *a.k.a Pablo*, ABC, 1984.

RELATED CAREER—Dancer, Ballet Arts Company of Carnegie Hall, New York City, 1959-61.

AWARDS: Obie Award from the *Village Voice*, 1971, for *Steambath;* Drama Desk Award nomination, 1977, for *Sly Fox.*

MEMBER: American Buddhist Academy.

SIDELIGHTS: FAVORITE ROLES—God in *Steambath*. Mel Edison in *The Prisoner of Second Avenue*, and the manservant in *Candaules*. RECREATIONS—Kendo, Zen Buddhism, chess, backpacking, classical guitar playing, and cooking.

Hector Elizondo told *CTFT* that he is an active supporter of the United Farm Workers, Amnesty International, and Oxfam America.

ADDRESSES: AGENT—Peter Kelley, William Morris Agency, 1350 Avenue of the Americas, New York, NY 10019.

*   *   *

ELWES, Cary   1962-

PERSONAL: Born October 26, 1962, in London, England; son of Dominic Elwes (a painter) and Tessa Kennedy (an interior designer). EDUCATION: Studied acting at Sarah Lawrence College with Julie Bovasso and at the London Drama Centre.

VOCATION: Actor.

CAREER: STAGE DEBUT—*Equus,* Greengate Theatre, New York City, 1981.

FILM DEBUT—Harcourt, *Another Country,* Orion Classics, 1984. PRINCIPAL FILM APPEARANCES—Lionel, *Oxford Blues,* Metro-Goldwyn-Mayer/United Artists, 1984; Josef, *The Bride,* Columbia, 1985; Guilford Dudley, *Lady Jane,* Paramount, 1986; Ganin, *Maschenka,* Goldcrest, 1987; Westley, *The Princess Bride,* Twentieth Century-Fox, 1987. Also appeared in *Glory,* Tri-Star.

RELATED CAREER—Backstage worker at the Westport Country Playhouse, Westport, CT.

ADDRESSES: AGENT—David Schiff, Creative Artists Agency, 1888 Century Park E., Suite 1400, Los Angeles, CA 90067.*

*   *   *

ENGLE, Debra   1953-

PERSONAL: Born July 4, 1953, in Baltimore, MD; daughter of Tracy R. and Mary E. (Davis) Engle; married Russ Smith (a producer), February 6, 1983. EDUCATION: Received B.F.A. from Illinois Wesleyan University.

VOCATION: Actress.

CAREER: STAGE DEBUT—Babe, *Balm in Gilead,* Steppenwolf

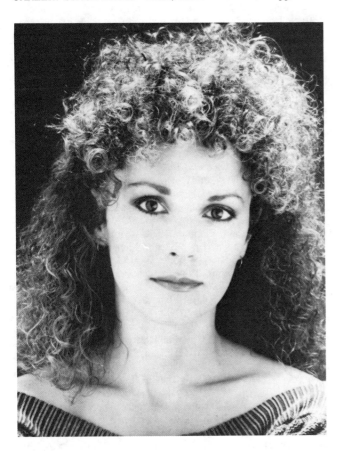

DEBRA ENGLE

Theatre, Chicago, IL, 1981, for two hundred performances. OFF-BROADWAY DEBUT—Babe, *Balm in Gilead,* Minetta Lane Theatre, New York City, 1984, for two hundred performances. PRINCIPAL STAGE APPEARANCES—Tansy, *The Nerd,* Helen Hayes Theatre, New York City, 1987; also appeared in *The Early Male Years,* North Light Repertory Theatre, Evanston, IL, 1982; *Waiting for the Parade,* Steppenwolf Theatre, Chicago, IL, 1985; *Misalliance,* Court Theatre, Chicago, 1985; *Arms and the Man,* Circle in the Square Theatre, New York City, 1985, then Court Theatre, 1986.

PRINCIPAL TELEVISION APPEARANCES—Mini-Series: Millie Preston, *Kane and Abel,* CBS, 1985. Pilots: Joanie, *Badlands 2005* (also known as *Badlands*), ABC, 1988. Episodic: Holly Dean, *Hometown,* CBS, 1985; Lissa Thomas, *Spenser: For Hire,* ABC, 1987; Jamie Carter, *Family Ties,* NBC, 1988; Gina Barrett, *Beauty and the Beast,* CBS, 1989; also *All My Children,* ABC, 1985; *Kay O'Brien,* CBS, 1986. Also appeared as Sheila, *Love Life,* Chicago television.

AWARDS: Joseph Jefferson Award, 1981, for *Balm in Gilead;* Chicago Emmy Award for *Love Life.*

ADDRESSES: AGENTS—Don Buchwald and Associates, 10 E. 44th Street, New York, NY 10150; The Agency, 10351 Santa Monica Boulevard, Suite 211, Los Angeles, CA, 90025.

*   *   *

ENRIQUEZ, Rene   1933-

PERSONAL: Born November 25, 1933, in San Francisco, CA; son of Andres (a businessman and politician) and Rosa Emilia (Castillo) Enriquez. EDUCATION: City College of San Francisco, A.A., 1955; San Francisco State University, B.A., 1958; also attended Colegio Centro America, Granada, Nicaragua; trained for the stage at the American Academy of Dramatic Art. RELIGION: Roman Catholic. MILITARY: U.S. Air Force, sergeant, 1951-55.

VOCATION: Actor.

CAREER: STAGE DEBUT—Mr. A. Ratt, *Camino Real,* Circle in the Square, New York City, 1960, for thirty-five performances. PRINCIPAL STAGE APPEARANCES—*Marco Millions,* Lincoln Center Repertory Theatre, New York City, 1963; *Diamond Orchid,* Henry Miller's Theatre, New York City, 1964; *House of Blue Leaves,* Coconut Grove Playhouse, Miami, FL, 1988; also appeared in *Truck Load,* New York City, 1975.

MAJOR TOURS—*The New Mount Olive Motel,* U.S. cities, 1973.

FILM DEBUT—*Girl in the Night,* Warner Brothers, 1960. PRINCIPAL FILM APPEARANCES—Colonel Diaz, *Bananas,* United Artists, 1971; Jesus, *Harry and Tonto,* Twentieth Century-Fox, 1974; voice, *Night Moves,* Warner Brothers, 1975; President Somoza, *Under Fire,* Orion, 1983; Max, *The Evil That Men Do,* Tri-Star, 1984; General Brogado, *Bulletproof,* Cinetel, 1987.

TELEVISION DEBUT—*The Defenders,* CBS. PRINCIPAL TELEVISION APPEARANCES—Series: Lieutenant Ray Calletano, *Hill Street Blues,* NBC, 1980-86. Mini-Series: Manolo Marquez, *Centennial,* NBC, 1978-79; General Castro, *Dream West,* CBS, 1986. Pilots: Ambassador Henriques, *High Risk,* ABC, 1976; Salvador Cruz, *The Return of Frank Cannon,* CBS, 1980; Ortiz,

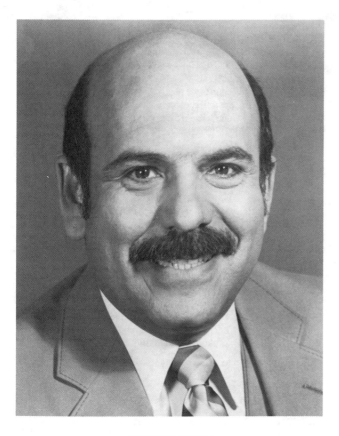

RENE ENRIQUEZ

Rosetti and Ryan: Men Who Love Women, NBC, 1977; also *Panic in Echo Park,* NBC, 1977. Episodic: *The Nurses,* CBS; *Police Story,* NBC; *Quincy, M.E.,* NBC. Movies: Mr. Torres, *Nicky's World,* CBS, 1974; Mr. Rosario, *Foster and Laurie,* CBS, 1975; Vega, *Katherine,* ABC, 1975; cook, *The Call of the Wild,* NBC, 1976; Luis, *It Happened at Lake Wood Manor* (also known as *Panic at Lake Wood Manor*), ABC, 1977; Mayor Julio Escontrerez, *Gridlock* (also known as *The Great American Traffic Jam*), NBC, 1980; Manuel, *Marathon,* CBS, 1980; Archbishop Oscar Arnulfo Romero, *Choices of the Heart,* NBC, 1983; Hector, *Hostage Flight,* NBC, 1985; Oscar Ortega, *Perry Mason: The Case of the Scandalous Scoundrel,* NBC, 1987; Ramirez, *Full Exposure: The Sex Tapes Scandal* (also known as *The Sex Tapes Scandal, The Sex Tapes,* and *Streetwise*), NBC, 1988. Specials: Father, *Santiago's America,* ABC, 1975; *The Screen Actors Guild Fiftieth Anniversary Celebration,* CBS, 1984; judge, *The 1986 Miss U.S.A. Pageant,* CBS, 1986; Sergeant Lopez, *You Are the Jury,* NBC, 1986. Also appeared in *Imagen.*

RELATED CAREER—Founder and president, National Hispanic Arts Endowment.

AWARDS: Emmy Award nomination, 1985, for *Imagen;* Lulac Theatre Award; Golden Eagle Award.

MEMBER: Screen Actors Guild (national board of directors, 1984—), Actors' Equity Association, American Federation of Television and Radio Artists.

ADDRESSES: PUBLICIST—Bollinger/Paladino Public Relations, 9200 Sunset Boulevard, Los Angeles, CA 90069.*

ESZTERHAS, Joe

PERSONAL: EDUCATION: Graduated from Ohio State University.

VOCATION: Screenwriter and producer.

CAREER: Also see *WRITINGS* below. PRINCIPAL FILM WORK—Producer, *Checking Out,* Warner Brothers, 1988; executive producer, *Betrayed,* Metro-Goldwyn-Mayer/United Artists, 1988.

RELATED CAREER—Reporter for newspapers in Dayton, OH, and Cleveland, OH; political correspondent, *Rolling Stone* magazine.

WRITINGS: FILM—(With Sylvester Stallone) *F.I.S.T.,* United Artists, 1978; (with Thomas Hedley) *Flashdance,* Paramount, 1983; *Jagged Edge,* Columbia, 1985; (with Scott Richardson) *Hearts of Fire,* Lorimar, 1987; *Big Shots,* Lorimar, 1987; *Checking Out,* Warner Brothers, 1989. TELEVISION—Movies: (Co-writer) *Pals,* CBS, 1987. OTHER—*Charlie Simpson's Apocalypse* (nonfiction), 1974.

AWARDS: National Book Award nomination, 1974, for *Charlie Simpson's Apocalypse.**

*   *   *

EVANS, Maurice   1901-1989

PERSONAL: Full name, Maurice Herbert Evans; born June 3, 1901, in Dorchester, England; naturalized American citizen, 1941; died March 12, 1989, in Rottingdean, England; son of Alfred Herbert (an analytical chemist) and Laura (Turner) Evans. EDUCATION: Attended Grocers' Company School. MILITARY: U.S. Army, major, 1941-45.

VOCATION: Actor and producer.

CAREER: STAGE DEBUT—Orestes, *The Oresteia,* Festival Theatre, Cambridge, U.K., 1926. LONDON DEBUT—P.C. Andrews, *The One-Eyed Herring,* Wyndham's Theatre, 1927. BROADWAY DEBUT—Romeo, *Romeo and Juliet,* Martin Beck Theatre, 1935. PRINCIPAL STAGE APPEARANCES—Stephani, *Listeners,* Sir Blayden Coote, *The Stranger in the House,* Hector Frome and Edward Clements, *Justice,* and Borring and Graviter, *Loyalties,* all Wyndham's Theatre, London, 1928; Jean, *The Man They Buried,* Ambassadors' Theatre, London, 1928; Wyn Hayward, *Diversion,* Little Theatre, London, 1928; Second Lieutenant Raleigh, *Journey's End,* Stage Society, Apollo Theatre, London, 1928, then Savoy Theatre, London, 1929; Young Frenchman, *The Man I Killed,* and the Sailor, *The Queen Bee,* both Savoy Theatre, 1930; Professor Agi, *The Swan,* St. James's Theatre, London, 1930; Owen Llewellyn, *To See Ourselves,* Ambassadors' Theatre, London, 1930; Marius, *Sea Fever,* New Theatre, London, 1931; Eric Masters, *Those Naughty Nineties,* Criterion Theatre, London, 1931; Nigel Chelmsford, *Avalanche,* Arts Theatre, London, 1932; Jean Jacques, *The Heart Line,* Lyric Theatre, London, 1932; Peter, *Will You Love Me Always?,* Globe Theatre, London, 1932; Reverend Peter Penlee, *Playground,* Royalty Theatre, London, 1932; Guy Daunt, *Cecilia,* Arts Theatre, 1933; Dick, *The Soldier and the Gentlewoman,* Vaudeville Theatre, London, 1933; Arnold Waite, *Other People's Lives,* Wyndham's Theatre, London, 1933; Aristide, *Ball at the Savoy,* Drury Lane Theatre, London, 1933; Edward Voysey, *The Voysey Inheritance,* Sadler's Wells Theatre, then Shaftesbury

Theatre, both London, 1934; Octavius Caesar, *Antony and Cleopatra*, title role, *Richard II*, Benedick, *Much Ado about Nothing*, and the Dauphin, *Saint Joan*, all Old Vic Company, Sadler's Wells Theatre, 1934.

Petruchio, *The Taming of the Shrew*, Iago, *Othello*, title role, *Hippolytus*, Adolphus Cusins, *Major Barbara*, Silence, *Henry IV, Part II*, and title role, *Hamlet*, all Old Vic Company, Sadler's Wells Theatre, 1935; the Dauphin, *Saint Joan*, Martin Beck Theatre, New York City, 1936; Napoleon, *St. Helena*, Lyceum Theatre, New York City, 1936; title role, *Richard II*, St. James Theatre, New York City, 1937; Sir John Falstaff, *Henry IV, Part I*, Forrest Theatre, Philadelphia, PA, 1937; title role, *Hamlet*, St. James Theatre, 1938; Sir John Falstaff, *Henry IV, Part I*, St. James Theatre, 1939; title role, *Hamlet*, 44th Street Theatre, New York City, 1939; title role, *Richard II*, and Malvolio, *Twelfth Night*, both St. James Theatre, 1940; title role, *Macbeth*, National Theatre, New York City, 1941; title role, *Hamlet* (also known as *G.I. Hamlet*), Columbus Circle Theatre, New York City, 1945, then City Center Theatre, New York City, 1946; John Tanner, *Man and Superman*, Alvin Theatre, New York City, 1947; John Tanner, *Man and Superman*, City Center Theatre, New York City, 1949; Andrew Crocker-Harris, *The Browning Version*, and Arthur Gosport, *Harlequinade* (double-bill), both Coronet Theatre, New York City, 1949.

Dick Dudgeon, *The Devil's Disciple*, City Center Theatre, then Royale Theatre, New York City, both 1950; title role, *Richard II*, and Hjalmar Ekdal, *The Wild Duck*, both City Center Theatre, 1951; Tony Wendice, *Dial M for Murder*, Plymouth Theatre, New York City, 1952; King Magnus, *The Apple Cart*, Plymouth Theatre, 1956; Captain Shotover, *Heartbreak House*, Billy Rose Theatre, New York City, 1959; Reverend Brock, *Tenderloin*, 46th Street Theatre, New York City, 1960; H.J., *The Aspern Papers*, Playhouse Theatre, New York City, 1962; *Shakespeare Revisited: A Program for Two Players* (two-person show with Helen Hayes), American Shakespeare Festival, Stratford, CT, 1962; narrator, *The Plague*, National Symphony Orchestra, Washington, DC, 1973; Oberon, Othello, Romeo, and various roles, *Shakespeare and the Performing Arts*, Festival of Shakespeare Dance and Drama, Kennedy Center for the Performing Arts, Washington, DC, 1973.

PRINCIPAL STAGE WORK—Producer: (With Joseph Verner Reed and Boris Said) *Hamlet*, St. James Theatre, New York City, 1938; *Henry IV, Part I*, St. James Theatre, 1939; *Hamlet*, 44th Street Theatre, New York City, 1939; *Richard II*, St. James Theatre, 1940; (with John Haggott) *Macbeth*, National Theatre, New York City, 1941; *Man and Superman*, Alvin Theatre, New York City, 1947; *The Linden Tree*, Music Box Theatre, New York City, 1948; *The Browning Version* and *Harlequinade* (double-bill), both Coronet Theatre, New York City, 1949; (with George Schaefer) *The Teahouse of the August Moon*, Martin Beck Theatre, New York City, 1953; (with Emmett Rogers) *No Time for Sergeants*, Alvin Theatre, New York City, 1955, then Her Majesty's Theatre, London, 1956; (with Robert L. Joseph) *Heartbreak House*, Billy Rose Theatre, New York City, 1959. Also produced *Hey Mac!* and *Shoot the Works*, both during service with U.S. Army.

MAJOR TOURS—Ralph, *After All*, U.K. cities, 1931; Romeo, *Romeo and Juliet*, U.K. cities, 1935; title role, *Richard II*, U.S. cities, 1937; Malvolio, *Twelfth Night*, U.S. cities, 1940-41; title role, *Macbeth*, U.S. cities, 1942; title role, *Hamlet* (also known as *G.I. Hamlet*), U.S. cities, 1945-47; John Tanner, *Man and Superman*, U.S. cities, 1948-49; Dick Dudgeon, *The Devil's Disciple*, U.S. cities, 1950; producer (with Schaefer), *The Teahouse of the August Moon*, U.S. cities, 1956; producer (with

Rogers), *No Time for Sergeants*, U.S. cities, 1956-58; King Magnus, *The Apple Cart*, U.S. cities, 1957; *Shakespeare Revisited: A Program for Two Players* (two-person show with Helen Hayes), U.S. cities, 1962-63. Also appeared in *The Grass Is Greener*, U.S. cities, 1965; and as title role, *Hamlet* (also known as *G.I. Hamlet*), Armed Forces tour.

FILM DEBUT—Langford, *White Cargo*, Harold Auten, 1930. PRINCIPAL FILM APPEARANCES—Rodney Langford, *Raise the Roof*, First National/Pathe, 1930; Roger Smith, *Should a Doctor Tell?*, Regal, 1931; Paul Hart, *Marry Me*, Ideal/Gaumont, 1932; Tootles, *Wedding Rehearsal*, Ideal, 1932; Didier, *The Empress and I* (also known as *Ich und die Kaiserin*, *Heart Song*, and *The Only Girl*), Twentieth Century-Fox, 1933; Robin, *Bypass to Happiness*, Twentieth Century-Fox, 1934; Anton Maroni, *The Path of Glory*, Producers Distributors, 1934; Phillip Allen, *Checkmate*, Paramount, 1935; poor man, *Scrooge*, Paramount, 1935; Henry Springer Elcott, *Kind Lady*, Metro-Goldwyn-Mayer (MGM), 1951; Caesar, *Androcles and the Lion*, RKO, 1952; Arthur Sullivan, *The Great Gilbert and Sullivan* (also known as *The Story of Gilbert and Sullivan*), United Artists, 1953; title role, *Macbeth*, Prominent, 1963; Prist, *The War Lord*, Universal, 1965; Sir Norman Swickert, *One of Our Spies Is Missing*, MGM, 1966; Nicolai, *Jack of Diamonds*, MGM, 1967; Dr. Zaius, *Planet of the Apes*, Twentieth Century-Fox, 1968; Hutch, *Rosemary's Baby*, Paramount, 1968; Dr. Matthews, *The Body Stealers* (also known as *Thin Air*), Allied Artists, 1969; Dr. Zaius, *Beneath the Planet of the Apes*, Twentieth Century-Fox, 1970; Inspector Daniels, *Terror in the Wax Museum*, Cinerama, 1973; Hobart, *The Jerk*, Universal, 1979. Also appeared in *Sam Hughes' War*, 1984.

PRINCIPAL TELEVISION APPEARANCES—Series: Maurice, *Bewitched*, ABC, 1964-72. Pilots: Dr. George Barger, *U.M.C.* (also known as *Operation Heartbeat*), CBS, 1969; Leroy Wintermore, *The Girl, the Gold Watch, and Everything*, syndicated, 1980. Episodic: The Puzzler, *Batman*, ABC, 1967; also "Caesar and Cleopatra," *General Electric Theatre*, CBS; *Tarzan*, NBC; *The Six Million Dollar Man*, ABC. Movies: Harry Masters, *Brotherhood of the Bell*, CBS, 1970; Major Geoffrey Palgrave, *Agatha Christie's "A Caribbean Mystery,"* CBS, 1983. Specials: Title role, "Hamlet," *Hallmark Hall of Fame*, NBC, 1953; title role, "Richard II," and title role, "Macbeth," both *Hallmark Hall of Fame*, NBC, 1954; Dick Dudgeon, "The Devil's Disciple," *Hallmark Hall of Fame*, NBC, 1955; host, *Hallmark Hall of Fame*, NBC, 1955-58; Petruchio, "The Taming of the Shrew," *Hallmark Hall of Fame*, NBC, 1956; John Tanner, "Man and Superman," *Hallmark Hall of Fame*, NBC, 1956; Malvolio, "Twelfth Night," *Hallmark Hall of Fame*, NBC, 1957; Tony Wendice, "Dial M for Murder," *Hallmark Hall of Fame*, NBC, 1958; Prospero, "The Tempest," and title role, "Macbeth" (color rebroadcast of 1954 production), both *Hallmark Hall of Fame*, NBC, 1960; Bishop Cauchon, "Saint Joan," *Hallmark Hall of Fame*, NBC, 1967.

PRINCIPAL TELEVISION WORK—All as producer. Specials: "The Devil's Disciple," "Dream Girl," and (with Jack Royal) "Alice in Wonderland," all *Hallmark Hall of Fame*, NBC, 1955; "The Corn Is Green," "The Good Fairy," "The Taming of the Shrew," and "The Cradle Song," all *Hallmark Hall of Fame*, NBC, 1956.

RELATED CAREER—Music publisher; in charge of Army Entertainment Section, Central Pacific Area, 1942-45; honorary artistic supervisor, City Center Theatre Company, New York City, 1949-51.

WRITINGS: STAGE—(Adaptor) *Hamlet* (also known as *G.I. Ham-*

let), Columbus Circle Theatre, New York City, 1945, then City Center Theatre, New York City, 1946, and tour of U.S. cities, 1945-47, and Armed Forces tour.

AWARDS: Drama League Medal, 1937; Legion of Merit from the U.S. Army, 1945; Antoinette Perry Award, Special Citation, 1950, for drama season at City Center Theatre; Christopher Award, 1953 and 1956; New York Drama Circle Critics Award, Best Play, 1954, for *Teahouse of the August Moon;* American Shakespeare Festival Theatre and Academy Special Award, 1956, for television production of "The Taming of the Shrew," *Hallmark Hall of Fame;* Emmy Award, Best Actor in a Single Performance, 1961, for "Macbeth," *Hallmark Hall of Fame;* Veteran's Administrative Voluntary Certificate, 1961; Salmagundi Award, 1962. Honorary degrees: University of Hawaii, Lafayette College, and Brandeis University.

OBITUARIES AND OTHER SOURCES: New York Times, March 14, 1989.*

*   *   *

EVIGAN, Greg   1953-

PERSONAL: Full name, Gregory Ralph Evigan; born October 14, 1953, in South Amboy, NJ; son of Ralph Milan and Barbara Elizabeth Evigan; married Pamela C. Serpe, June 3, 1979; children: Briana, Jason, Vanessa.

VOCATION: Actor and musician.

CAREER: PRINCIPAL STAGE APPEARANCES—Annas, then title role, *Jesus Christ Superstar,* Mark Hellinger Theatre, New York City, 1972; Danny Zuka, *Grease,* Eden Theatre, New York City, 1973.

MAJOR TOURS—*Jesus Christ Superstar,* U.S. cities, 1971-72.

PRINCIPAL FILM APPEARANCES—Alan, *Scorchy,* American International, 1976; Sergeant Heineman, *Stripped to Kill* (also known as *Strip Me Deadly*), Concorde, 1987; McBride, *Deepstar Six,* Tri-Star, 1989. Also appeared in *Echoes in Crimson,* Astral/Lorimar Home Video, 1988.

PRINCIPAL TELEVISION APPEARANCES—Series: Greg, *A Year at the Top,* CBS, 1977; B.J. McKay, *B.J. and the Bear,* NBC, 1979-81; Danny Doyle, *Masquerade,* ABC, 1983-84; Joey Harris, *My Two Dads,* NBC, 1987—. Pilots: Cliff, *Hereafter,* NBC, 1975; Billie Joe "B.J." McKay, *B.J. and the Bear,* NBC, 1978; B.J. McKay, *The Eyes of Texas,* NBC, 1980; B.J. McKay, *The Eyes of Texas II,* NBC, 1980; Craig Stone, *Scene of the Crime,* NBC, 1984;

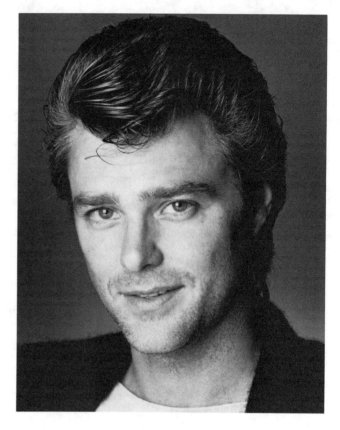

GREG EVIGAN

Major Jack North, *Northstar,* ABC, 1986; Rick, *Private Sessions,* NBC, 1985. Episodic: Trey Champion, *The Yellow Rose,* NBC, 1983; Eric Gordon, *Matlock,* NBC, 1987. Specials: *Battle of the Network Stars,* ABC, 1979 and 1980; *Debby Boone . . . The Same Old Brand New Me,* NBC, 1980; *Men Who Rate a "10",* NBC, 1980; *The Osmond Family Christmas Special,* NBC, 1980; *Circus of the Stars,* CBS, 1981; *True Confessions,* syndicated, 1986.

RELATED CAREER—Singer and songwriter; performer of theme songs for the television series *B.J. and the Bear* and *My Two Dads;* founder and musician in rock group, GhettoWay City.

MEMBER: Screen Actors Guild, American Federation of Television and Radio Artists, Actors' Equity Association, Musicians Union.

ADDRESSES: AGENT—David Westberg, Triad Artists, 10100 Santa Monica Boulevard, 16th Floor, Los Angeles, CA 90067.

F

FARENTINO, James 1938-

PERSONAL: Born James Ferrantino, February 24, 1938, in Brooklyn, NY; son of Anthony and Helen (Enrico) Ferrantino; married Michele Lee Dusick (an actress and singer; professional name, Michele Lee), February 20, 1966 (divorced); married Deborah Mullowney (an actress; professional name, Debrah Farentino), June, 1985 (separated); children: David Michael (first marriage). EDUCATION: Trained for the stage at the American Academy of Dramatic Arts.

VOCATION: Actor.

CAREER: PRINCIPAL STAGE APPEARANCES—Pedro, Night of the Iguana, Royale Theatre, New York City, 1961; Mr. Solares, In the Summer House, Little Fox Theatre, New York City, 1964; Stanley Kowalski, A Streetcar Named Desire, Vivian Beaumont Theatre, New York City, 1973; Biff Loman, Death of a Salesman, Circle in the Square, New York City, 1975. Also appeared in The Days and Nights of BeeBee Fenstermaker, Sheridan Square Playhouse, New York City, 1963; as Randall Patrick McMurphy, One Flew Over the Cuckoo's Nest, Chicago, IL, 1973; in The Best Man, Chicago, 1974; and in The Big Knife, Arlington Park Theatre, Chicago, 1976.

MAJOR TOURS—California Suite, U.S. cities, 1978.

PRINCIPAL FILM APPEARANCES—Insigna, Ensign Pulver, Warner Brothers, 1964; Charlie Perone, Psychomania (also known as Violent Midnight), Victoria-Emerson, 1964; Marc, The War Lord, Universal, 1965; Ted, The Pad . . . And How to Use It, Universal, 1966; Chris, Banning, Universal, 1967; Matt, Stone: The Ride to Hangman's Tree (also known as The Ride to Hangman's Tree), Universal, 1967; David Wheelwright, Rosie!, Universal, 1967; David Harris, Me, Natalie, National General, 1969; Bruno Cardin, Story of a Woman (also known as Storia di una donna), Universal, 1970; Commander Richard Owens, The Final Countdown, United Artists, 1980; Dan, Dead and Buried, AVCO-Embassy, 1981.

PRINCIPAL TELEVISION APPEARANCES—Series: Neil Darrell, The Lawyers, NBC, 1969-72; Jefferson Keyes, Cool Million, NBC, 1972-73; Dr. Nick Toscanni, Dynasty, ABC, 1981-82; Frank Chaney, Blue Thunder, ABC, 1984; Frank DeMarco, Mary, CBS, 1985-86; also John Dos Passos: U.S.A. Mini-Series: Simon Peter, Jesus of Nazareth, NBC, 1977; David Westfield, Sins, CBS, 1986. Pilots: Neil Darrell, The Sound of Anger, NBC, 1968; Neil Darrell, The Whole World Is Watching, NBC, 1969; Jefferson Keyes, The Mask of Marcella, NBC, 1972; Vince Rossi, Crossfire, NBC, 1975; George Bassett, My Wife Next Door, NBC, 1975; also The Singers, CBS, 1969. Episodic: Police Story, NBC, 1974 and 1975; also Naked City, ABC; The Defenders, CBS; Laredo, NBC;

Route 66, CBS; Ben Casey, ABC; Twelve O'Clock High, ABC; 77 Sunset Strip, ABC; Love Story, NBC; Alfred Hitchcock Presents.

Movies: Taff Malloy, Wings of Fire, NBC, 1967; Gene Culligan, Vanished, NBC, 1971; Gino Rico, The Family Rico, CBS, 1972; John Danbury, The Longest Night, ABC, 1972; Eddie Holcomb, The Elevator, ABC, 1974; Kevin Leahy, The Possessed, NBC, 1977; Duffy Hambleton, Silent Victory: The Kitty O'Neill Story, CBS, 1979; Barry Kaufman, Son Rise: A Miracle of Love, NBC, 1979; Juan Peron, Evita Peron, NBC, 1981; Arnie Potts, Something So Right, CBS, 1982; Dr. Edgar Highley, The Cradle Will Fall, CBS, 1983; John Peterson, License to Kill, CBS, 1984; Dan Hagan, Picking Up the Pieces, CBS, 1985; Tom Wyler, A Summer to Remember . . ., CBS, 1985; Gerald Remson, That Secret Sunday, CBS, 1986; Lieutenant Daniel Malone, The Red Spider, CBS, 1988; Buddy, Who Gets the Friends?, CBS, 1988; also Family Sins, CBS, 1987. Specials: Happy Loman, Death of a Salesman, CBS, 1966; second husband, The First Nine Months Are the Hardest, NBC, 1971; Mitzi and a Hundred Guys, CBS, 1975; Joe Crane, "Emily, Emily," Hallmark Hall of Fame, NBC, 1977; Celebrity Challenge of the Sexes, CBS, 1977.

NON-RELATED CAREER—Honorary chairor, Illinois Association of Retarded Citizens.

AWARDS: Golden Globe Award, Most Promising Newcomer, 1966, for The Pad . . . And How to Use It; Best Actor Award (Chicago), 1973; Theatre World Award, 1973, for A Streetcar Named Desire; Charles MacArthur Award from the Chicago Drama League, 1974; Emmy Award nomination, Outstanding Supporting Actor in a Drama, 1977, for Jesus of Nazareth.

ADDRESSES: AGENT—William Morris Agency, 151 El Camino Drive, Beverly Hills, CA 90212.*

*   *   *

FARER, Ronnie 1951-

PERSONAL: Full name, Rhonda Farer; born October 19, 1951, in Elizabeth, NJ; daughter of Herman (a builder) and Edith (a medical assistant; maiden name, Berman) Farer. EDUCATION: Rider College, B.F.A., 1973; trained for the stage with Stella Adler and Warren Robertson; studied voice with Marge Rivingston.

VOCATION: Actress, singer, dancer, and teacher.

CAREER: STAGE DEBUT—Chorus, Anything Goes, tour of U.S. cities, 1973. BROADWAY DEBUT—Swing, Rachael Lily Rosenbloom,

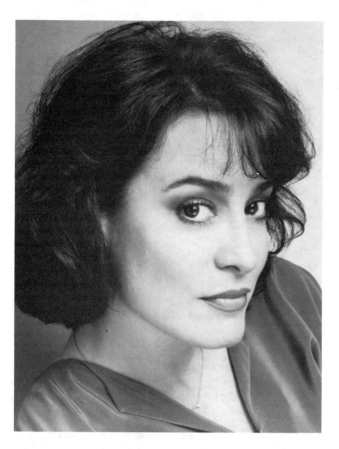

RONNIE FARER

Broadhurst Theatre, 1973. PRINCIPAL STAGE APPEARANCES—Ensemble, *Yevtushenko and Friends* (poetry concert), Felt Forum, New York City, 1972; Mildred Luce, *The Dog beneath the Skin,* Manhattan Theatre Club, New York City, 1973; Sonia Walsk, *They're Playing Our Song,* Imperial Theatre, New York City, 1980; Titania and Hippolyta, *A Midsummer Night's Dream,* University of Delaware, Newark, DE, 1984; Countess, *A Little Night Music,* Merrimack Repertory Theatre, Lowell, MA, 1985; Christine, *Room Service,* Kennedy Center for the Performing Arts, Washington, DC, 1985; Anita, *West Side Story,* Beef and Boards Dinner Theatre, Indianapolis, IN, 1985; Tzeitel, *Fiddler on the Roof,* Paper Mill Playhouse, Millburn, NJ, 1985; homecoming queen and woman two, *Is There Life after High School?,* Ford's Theatre, Washington, DC, 1986; wife, "The Deep End" in *Festival of One-Act Comedies,* Manhattan Punch Line, Judith Anderson Theatre, New York City, 1987; Penelope, *The Coconuts,* Arena Stage, Washington, DC, 1988; Barbara, *Social Security,* Indiana Repertory Theatre, Indianapolis, IN, 1988-89. Also appeared in *Sally and Marsha,* Manhattan Theatre Club, 1982; as Ruth, *We Bombed in New Haven,* Brenda, *Lovers and Other Strangers,* she, *Loveliest Afternoon of the Year,* daughter, *Bringing It All Back Home,* Edith, *Not Enough Rope,* Nun, *The House of Blue Leaves,* and ensemble, *American Hurrah,* all Merrimack Repertory Theatre; Adelaid, *Guys and Dolls,* Reno Sweeney, *Anything Goes,* and April, *Company,* all Paper Mill Playhouse.

PRINCIPAL STAGE WORK—Director, *Bringing It All Back Home,* University of Delaware, Newark, DE, 1984.

MAJOR TOURS—Maid by the fire, *Jesus Christ Superstar,* U.S.

cities, 1975; Rizzo, *Grease,* U.S. cities, 1975; also *No No Nanette,* U.S. cities, 1974.

PRINCIPAL FILM APPEARANCES—Student, *Next Stop, Greenwich Village,* Twentieth Century-Fox, 1976.

PRINCIPAL TELEVISION APPEARANCES—Episodic: Les Gifford, *Another World,* NBC, 1984; Celia Bennett, *The Guiding Light,* CBS, 1985; Dave's mom (skit), *Late Night with David Letterman,* NBC, 1985; also *Kojak,* CBS, 1975.

RELATED CAREER—Acting teacher, Contact Studios, New York City, 1984-88; acting teacher, University of Delaware, Newark, DE, 1986.

MEMBER: Amnesty International, Common Cause, American Civil Liberties Union, Greenpeace, Gay Men's Health Crisis, National Abortion Rights Action League.

ADDRESSES: AGENT—Henderson/Hogan Agency, 405 W. 44th Street, New York, NY, 10017.

*   *   *

FARLEY, Morgan   1898-1988

PERSONAL: Full name, Francis Morgan Farley; born October 3, 1898, in Mamaroneck, NY; died October 11, 1988, in San Pedro, CA; son of John Treacy (a builder) and Marie T. (Morgan) Farley. MILITARY: U.S. Army, second lieutenant, during World War II.

VOCATION: Actor.

CAREER: STAGE DEBUT—*Gammer Gurton's Needle,* Stuart Walker's Stock Company, Cleveland, OH, 1916. BROADWAY DEBUT—Joe Bullit, *Seventeen,* Booth Theatre, 1918. LONDON DEBUT—Jimmy Dugan, *The Trial of Mary Dugan,* Golder's Green Hippodrome, 1927. PRINCIPAL STAGE APPEARANCES—Joe Bullit, *Seventeen,* Portmanteau Players, Minneapolis, MN, then Murat Theatre, Indianapolis, IN, both 1917; young man, *The Laughter of the Gods,* Punch and Judy Theatre, New York City, then Murat Theatre, both 1919; Pink Youth, *A Young Man's Fancy,* Playhouse Theatre, New York City, 1919; Tim Simpkins, *The Charm School,* Bijou Theatre, New York City, 1920; Charles Deburau, *Deburau,* Belasco Theatre, New York City, 1920; Michel Alexis, *The Grand Duke,* Lyceum Theatre, New York City, 1921; Bobby, *Mary the Third,* and Tony, *Home Fires,* both 39th Street Theatre, New York City, 1923; Anthony Wescott, *The Wild Wescotts,* Frazee Theatre, New York City, 1923; George, *Fata Morgana,* Garrick Theatre, New York City, 1924; Paolo, *Paolo and Francesca,* Booth Theatre, New York City, 1924; Arthur Griswold, *Tangletoes,* 39th Street Theatre, 1925; Eugene Marchbanks, *Candida,* Comedy Theatre, New York City, 1925; Lawrence Sanbury, *The Unchastened Woman,* Princess Theatre, New York City, 1926; Benjamin, *Easter One Day Before,* Princess Theatre, 1926; Clyde Griffiths, *An American Tragedy,* Longacre Theatre, New York City, 1926; Jimmy Dugan, *The Trial of Mary Dugan,* Queen's Theatre, London, 1927; Karl Rolf, *The Comic Artist,* Strand Theatre, London, 1928.

Romeo, *Romeo and Juliet,* and Berend, *The Good Hope,* both Civic Repertory Theatre, New York City, 1930; Armand Duval, *Camille,* Civic Repertory Theatre, 1931; Lansing French, *The Passing*

Present, Ethel Barrymore Theatre, New York City, 1931; Strom Peters, *Waltz in Fire*, Masque Theatre, New York City, 1934; Raskolnikoff, *Crime and Punishment*, Biltmore Theatre, New York City, 1935; Osric, *Hamlet*, Empire Theatre, New York City, 1936; Alexander Mill, *Candida*, Empire Theatre, 1937; Randall Utterword, *Heartbreak House*, and Herault de Sechelles, *Danton's Death*, both Mercury Theatre, New York City, 1938; Scrubby, *Outward Bound*, Playhouse Theatre, 1938; the Chaplain, *The Distant City*, Longacre Theatre, 1941; Caradoc Lowell, *Portrait of a Lady*, Majestic Theatre, Boston, MA, 1941. Also appeared in *King Argimenes, The Gods of the Mountain*, and *The Very Naked Boy*, all Punch and Judy Theatre, then Murat Theatre, 1919; in *The Marquise*, El Capitan Theatre, Hollywood, CA, 1932; and as Colin Derwent, *Ten Minute Alibi*, summer theatre production, New London, CT, 1934.

PRINCIPAL STAGE WORK—Stage manager, *A Night in Avignon, Stinky, The Laughter of the Gods, The Golden Doom, King Argimenes, The Gods of the Mountain, The Very Naked Boy, The Tents of the Arabs*, and *The Book of Job*, all Punch and Judy Theatre, New York City, the Murat Theatre, Indianapolis, IN, 1919; also assistant stage manager, Stuart Walker's Stock Company, 1916.

MAJOR TOURS—Arthur Bixby, *Nobody's Fool*, U.S. cities, 1922; George, *Fata Morgana*, U.S. cities, 1932; Cassius, *Julius Caesar*, and Randall Utterword, *Heartbreak House*, both Mercury Theatre Company, U.S. cities, 1937-38; Baron Max von Alvenstor, *Margin for Error*, U.S. cities, 1940. Also appeared in *Grounds for Divorce* and *The Marquise*, California cities, 1933; *The Wind and the Rain*, U.S. cities, 1934; and with Stuart Walker's Stock Company, U.S. cities, 1916.

PRINCIPAL FILM APPEARANCES—Rex Greene, *The Greene Murder Case*, Paramount, 1929; Dick Carroll, *Half-Marriage*, RKO, 1929; Bud Woodbridge, *The Love Doctor*, Paramount, 1929; Jerry Patterson, *The Mighty*, Paramount, 1929; Monkey McConnell, *The Devil's Holiday*, Paramount, 1930; Lieutenant Lee, *A Man from Wyoming*, Paramount, 1930; Joe Fisher, *Men Are Like That*, Paramount, 1930; Tom Wendell, *Only the Brave*, Paramount, 1930; Malatroff's victim, *Slightly Scarlet*, Paramount, 1930; Eric, *Beloved*, Universal, 1934; clerk, *Gentleman's Agreement*, Twentieth Century-Fox, 1947; Topper, *Behind Locked Doors*, Eagle-Lion, 1948; Howard Anderson, *Hollow Triumph* (also known as *The Scar*), Eagle/Lion, 1948; doctor, *Macbeth*, Republic, 1948; Mitchell, *Open Secret*, Eagle/Lion, 1948; proprietor, *Walls of Jericho*, Twentieth Century-Fox, 1948; ticket taker, *You Were Meant for Me*, Twentieth Century-Fox, 1948; Gregory Milford, *Abbott and Costello Meet the Killer, Boris Karloff*, Universal, 1949; Dr. Bowen, *Special Agent*, Paramount, 1949; bookseller, *That Forsyte Woman* (also known as *The Forsythe Saga*), Metro-Goldwyn-Mayer (MGM), 1949; Edwin Livesley, *Top o' the Morning*, Paramount, 1949.

The Judge, *Barricade*, Warner Brothers, 1950; Caleb Nicholas, *Double Crossbones*, Universal, 1950; Dr. Pitt, *Goodbye, My Fancy*, Warner Brothers, 1951; Lawyer Haddon, *The Lady from Texas*, Universal, 1951; Rushton, *The Man Who Cheated Himself*, Twentieth Century-Fox, 1951; Caleb, *Sealed Cargo*, RKO, 1951; Rinville, *The Strange Door*, Universal, 1951; Minister, *High Noon*, United Artists, 1952; Dr. McCarran, *My Wife's Best Friend*, Twentieth Century-Fox, 1952; Father Simon, *The Wild North* (also known as *The Big North*), MGM, 1952; Juror, *Angel Face*, RKO, 1953; Artemidorus, *Julius Caesar*, MGM, 1953; Kyle Manning, *Remains to Be Seen*, MGM, 1953; Vinny, *Jivaro* (also known as

Lost Treasure of the Amazon), Paramount, 1954; advertising executive, *The Barefoot Executive*, Buena Vista, 1971; Book 1, *Soylent Green*, MGM, 1973; Marcus, *The Last Tycoon*, Paramount, 1976; movie fanatic, *Nickelodeon*, Columbia, 1976; Middleton, *Heaven Can Wait*, Paramount, 1978; old Lonely Hearts Club member, *Sergeant Pepper's Lonely Hearts Club Band*, Universal, 1978; old timer, *Dreamer*, Twentieth Century-Fox, 1979. Also appeared in *The Winners Circle*, Twentieth Century-Fox, 1948; *Flamingo Road*, Warner Brothers, 1949; *Hello, Dolly!*, Twentieth Century-Fox, 1969; *Scorpio*, United Artists, 1973; *At Long Last Love*, Twentieth Century-Fox, 1975; and *Sextette*, Crown International, 1978.

PRINCIPAL TELEVISION APPEARANCES—Pilots: Ben Herren, *Enigma*, CBS, 1977; Boss, *Clapper's*, NBC, 1978; Mr. Granger, *Beane's of Boston*, CBS, 1979. Episodic: Hacom, "The Return of the Archons," *Star Trek*, NBC, 1966; also *The Wild Wild West*, CBS; *The Big Valley*, ABC; *Mannix*, CBS; *The F.B.I.*, ABC; *Barnaby Jones*, CBS; *The Tony Randall Show*, CBS; *Mission: Impossible*, CBS. Movies: Bill Plog, *Eleanor and Franklin: The White House Years*, ABC, 1977; Mr. Macy, *A Killing Affair* (also known as *Behind the Badge*), CBS, 1977; Mr. McGarrity, *Orphan Train*, CBS, 1979; Mason, *Valentine*, ABC, 1979; Frazer, *Charlie and the Great Balloon Race*, NBC, 1981.

RELATED CAREER—Manager and director, Siasconset Casino Theatre and Yacht Club, Nantucket, MA, 1938-40.

OBITUARIES AND OTHER SOURCES: Variety, October 19, 1988.*

*   *   *

FARONE, Felicia   1961-

PERSONAL: Born Felicia Falzarano, March 5, 1961, in Orange, NJ; daughter of Phillip (a mechanical inspector) and Concetta (an office manager; maiden name, Nardiello) Falzarano. EDUCATION: Montclair State College, B.A., 1983; trained for the stage at Michael Shulman's British American Acting Academy.

VOCATION: Actress, dancer, and singer.

CAREER: STAGE DEBUT—Anita, *West Side Story*, Spotlight Productions, in New Jersey, 1982, for twenty-five performances. OFF-BROADWAY DEBUT—Swing, *Rabboni*, Perry Street Theatre, 1985, for sixty performances. PRINCIPAL STAGE APPEARANCES—Eva Peron, *Evita*, Darien Dinner Theatre, Darien, CT, then Carousel Dinner Theatre, Ravenna, OH, both 1985; Charlene, *The Pajama Game*, Equity Library Theatre, New York City, 1986; Dora, *Fiorello!*, Equity Library Theatre, 1988. Also appeared in *Anything Goes*, Tyrone Guthrie Theatre, Minneapolis, MN, 1985; as Carmen, *Sweet Charity*, Coachlight Dinner Theatre, Warehouse Point, CT; ensemble, *She Loves Me* (revue), Star-to-Be, *Annie*, Ellie, *Showboat*, and Ego, *They're Playing Our Song*, all Theatre by the Sea, Portsmouth, NH; Diana Morales, *A Chorus Line*, Brunswick Music Theatre, Brunswick, ME; Rosemary, *How to Succeed in Business without Really Trying*, Amy, *Where's Charley?*, Pegeen Ryan, *Mame*, and Velma, *Chicago*, all Montclair Operetta Club, Montclair, NJ.

MAJOR TOURS—Diana Morales, *A Chorus Line*, U.S. cities, 1986; Demeter, *Cats*, U.S. cities, 1987-88.

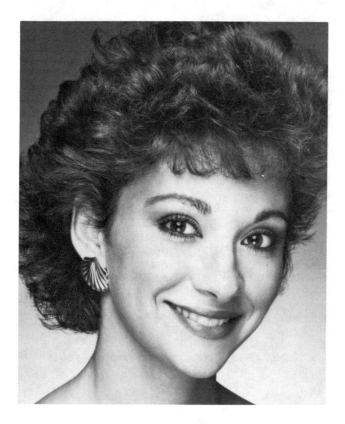

FELICIA FARONE

RELATED CAREER—Teacher, the Dance Factory, Clifton, NJ, 1983-86; featured dancer, *Canada Dry* (industrial film), SAGA Productions, New York City.

NON-RELATED CAREER—Volunteer, Belleville Friendly Visitors Organization, Belleville, NJ.

MEMBER: Actors' Equity Association.

ADDRESSES: HOME—529 W. 48th Street, New York, NY 10036.

*   *   *

FARROW, Mia   1945-

PERSONAL: Full name, Maria de Lourdes Villiers Farrow; born February 9, 1945 (some sources say 1946), in Los Angeles, CA; daughter of John Villiers Farrow (a film director) and Maureen Paula O'Sullivan (an actress); married Frank Sinatra (a singer and actor), 1966 (divorced, 1968); married Andre Previn (an orchestra conductor), September 10, 1970 (divorced, February, 1979); children: Matthew Phineas and Sascha Villiers (twins; second marriage); Satchel (with Woody Allen); Lark Song, Fletcher, Summer Song, Gigi Soon Mi, Misha (adopted).

VOCATION: Actress.

CAREER: OFF-BROADWAY DEBUT—Cecily Cardew, *The Importance of Being Earnest,* Madison Avenue Playhouse, 1966. LONDON DEBUT—Title role, *Mary Rose,* Shaw Theatre, 1972. PRINCI-

PAL STAGE APPEARANCES—Jan and Adela, *The House of Bernarda Alba,* and Irina, *The Three Sisters,* both Greenwich Theatre, London, 1973; title role, *The Marrying of Ann Leete,* Royal Shakespeare Company (RSC), Aldwych Theatre, London, 1975; Pavla Tselovnyeva, *The Zykovs,* and Sasha, *Ivanov,* both RSC, Aldwych Theatre, 1976; Phoebe Craddock, *Romantic Comedy,* Ethel Barrymore Theatre, New York City, 1979. Also appeared in *Jeanne d'Arc,* London, 1971; in the title role, *Peter Pan;* and in summer theatre productions at Warren, OH, 1963.

PRINCIPAL FILM APPEARANCES—Karen Ericksson, *Guns at Batasi,* Twentieth Century-Fox, 1964; Caroline, *A Dandy in Aspic,* Columbia, 1968; Rosemary Woodhouse, *Rosemary's Baby,* Paramount, 1968; Cenci, *Secret Ceremony,* Universal, 1968; Mary, *John and Mary,* Twentieth Century-Fox, 1969; Sarah, *See No Evil* (also known as *Blind Terror*), Columbia, 1971; Christine Dupont, *Docteur Popaul* (also known as *Scoundrel in White*), Twentieth Century-Fox/Rank/CIC, 1972; Belinda Sidley, *The Public Eye* (also known as *Follow Me*), Universal, 1972; Daisy Buchanan, *The Great Gatsby,* Paramount, 1974; Julia Lofting, *Full Circle* (also known as *The Haunting of Julia*), Fester, 1977; Caroline Brace, *Avalanche,* New World, 1978; Jacqueline de Bellefort, *Death on the Nile,* Paramount, 1978; Buffy Brenner, *A Wedding,* Twentieth Century-Fox, 1978; Charlotte Bruckner, *Hurricane* (also known as *Forbidden Paradise*), Paramount, 1979; voice of the Last Unicorn and Lady Amalthea, *The Last Unicorn* (animated), ITC, 1982; Ariel Weymouth, *A Midsummer Night's Sex Comedy,* Warner Brothers, 1982; Dr. Eudora Fletcher, *Zelig,* Warner Brothers, 1983; Tina Vitale, *Broadway Danny Rose,* Orion, 1984; Alura Zor-El, *Supergirl,* Tri-Star, 1984; Cecilia, *The Purple Rose of Cairo,* Orion, 1985; Hannah, *Hannah and Her Sisters,* Orion, 1986; Sally White, *Radio Days,* Orion, 1987; Lane, *September,* Orion, 1987; Hope, *Another Woman,* Orion, 1988; Lisa, "Oedipus Wrecks," *New York Stories,* Touchstone, 1989. Also appeared in *John Paul Jones,* Warner Brothers, 1959; in *The Age of Curiosity* (short film), 1963; and in *Sarah (animated), Yoram Gross/Sarah Enterprises-Australian Film Commission,* 1982.

PRINCIPAL TELEVISION APPEARANCES—Series: Allison Mac-Kenzie, *Peyton Place,* ABC, 1964-66. Movies: Brooke Collier, *Goodbye Raggedy Ann,* CBS, 1971; Allison MacKenzie (flashbacks only), *Murder in Peyton Place,* NBC, 1977. Specials: Belinda McDonald, *Johnny Belinda,* ABC, 1967; title role, "Peter Pan," *Hallmark Hall of Fame,* NBC, 1976.

AWARDS: Golden Globe Award, Most Promising Newcomer, 1965; French Academy Award, Best Actress, David Di Donatello Award, Rio de Janeiro Film Festival Award, and San Sebastian Film Festival Award, all 1969, for *Rosemary's Baby.*

ADDRESSES: AGENT—Lionel Larner, 130 W. 57th Street, New York, NY 10019.*

*   *   *

FEDER, Abe H.   1909-

PERSONAL: Born June 27, 1909, in Milwaukee, WI; son of Benjamin (a restaurateur) and Sane (Byfield) Feder; married Ciel Grossman (an interior decorator), March 23, 1952; children: one daughter. EDUCATION: Attended the Carnegie Institute of Technology, 1926-29. MILITARY: U.S. Army Air Forces, staff sergeant, during World War II.

VOCATION: Lighting and set designer.

CAREER: FIRST BROADWAY WORK—Lighting designer, *Trick for Trick*, Sam H. Harris Theatre, 1932. PRINCIPAL STAGE WORK—All as lighting designer, unless indicated: *One Sunday Afternoon*, Little Theatre, New York City, 1933; *Four Saints in Three Acts* (opera), 44th Street Theatre, New York City, 1934; *Calling All Stars*, Hollywood Theatre, New York City, 1934; *Gentlewoman*, Cort Theatre, New York City, 1934; *Ghosts*, Empire Theatre, New York City, 1935; *The Hook-Up*, Cort Theatre, 1935; *Walk Together Chillun, Conjurin' Man Dies, Macbeth*, and *Turpentine*, all Federal Theatre Project, Lafayette Theatre, New York City, 1936; *Triple-A Ploughed Under* and *Injunction Granted*, both Federal Theatre Project, Biltmore Theatre, New York City, 1936; *Horse Eats Hat*, Federal Theatre Project, Maxine Elliott's Theatre, New York City, 1936; *New Faces of 1936*, Vanderbilt Theatre, New York City, 1936; *Hedda Gabler*, Longacre Theatre, New York City, 1936; *The Tragical Historie of Dr. Faustus*, Federal Theatre Project, Maxine Elliott's Theatre, 1937; *Native Ground*, Al Jolson's Theatre, New York City, 1937; *How Long, Brethren*, Federal Theatre Project, Nora Bayes Theatre, New York City, 1937; *Without Warning*, National Theatre, New York City, 1937; *I'd Rather Be Right*, Alvin Theatre, New York City, 1937; *One-Third of a Nation*, Federal Theatre Project, Adelphi Theatre, New York City, 1938; *Diff'rent, Pygmalion, Coriolanus, The Big Blow*, and *Prologue to Glory*, all Federal Theatre Project, Maxine Elliott's Theatre, 1938; *The Cradle Will Rock* (opera), Living Newspaper of the Federal Theatre Project, Al Jolson's Theatre, 1938; *Immediate Comment* (ballet), Living Newspaper of the Federal Theatre Project, Adelphi Theatre, 1938; *Androcles and the Lion*, Federal Theatre Project, Lafayette Theatre, 1938; *Here Come the Clowns*, Booth Theatre, New York City, 1938; *Sing for Your Supper* (revue), Adelphi Theatre, 1939.

A Passenger to Bali, Ethel Barrymore Theatre, New York City, 1940; *Hold On to Your Hats*, Shubert Theatre, New York City, 1940; *Johnny Belinda*, Belasco Theatre, New York City, 1940; *Angel Street*, John Golden Theatre, New York City, 1941; *Autumn Hill*, Booth Theatre, 1942; *The Walking Gentleman, Magic*, and *Hello Out There*, all Belasco Theatre, 1942; *The Skin of Our Teeth*, Plymouth Theatre, New York City, 1942; *Winged Victory*, 44th Street Theatre, 1943; (also set designer) *The Gioconda Smile*, Lyceum Theatre, New York City, 1950; *The Tower Beyond Tragedy*, American National Theatre and Academy (ANTA) Theatre, New York City, 1950; *Out of This World*, New Century Theatre, New York City, 1950; *A Sleep of Prisoners*, St. James Church, New York City, 1951; *Mary Rose*, ANTA Theatre, 1951; *Dear Barbarians*, Royale Theatre, New York City, 1952; *Three Wishes for Jamie*, Mark Hellinger Theatre, New York City, 1952; *Thunderland*, Biltmore Estate, Asheville, NC, 1952; *The Immoralist*, Royale Theatre, 1953; *A Pin to See the Peep Show*, Playhouse Theatre, New York City, 1953; (also set designer) *The Boy Friend*, Royale Theatre, 1953; *What Every Woman Knows*, City Center Theatre, New York City, 1954; *The Flowering Peach*, Belasco Theatre, 1954.

The Wisteria Trees, City Center Theatre, 1955; *Inherit the Wind*, National Theatre, 1955; *Seventh Heaven*, ANTA Theatre, 1955; *The Skin of Our Teeth*, Sarah Bernhardt Theatre, Paris, France, then ANTA Theatre, both 1955; *The Young and the Beautiful*, Longacre Theatre, New York City, 1955; *My Fair Lady*, Mark Hellinger Theatre, 1956; *A Clearing in the Woods*, Belasco Theatre, 1957; *Visit to a Small Planet*, Booth Theatre, 1957; *Orpheus Descending*, Martin Beck Theatre, New York City, 1957; *Time Remembered*, Morosco Theatre, New York City, 1957; *At the Grand*, Los Angeles Civic Light Opera, Los Angeles, CA, 1958; *Goldilocks*, Lunt-Fontanne Theatre, New York City, 1958; *The Cold Wind and the Warm*, Morosco Theatre, 1958; (also set designer) *Come Play with Me*, York Playhouse, New York City, 1959; set designer, *Carmen Jones, April in Paris, Guys and Dolls, Can-Can*, and *Ballet Russe de Monte Carlo*, all Theatre-in-the-Park, New York City, 1959; *A Loss of Roses*, Eugene O'Neill Theatre, New York City, 1959.

Greenwillow, Alvin Theatre, 1960; *Camelot*, Majestic Theatre, New York City, 1960; *Tiger, Tiger Burning Bright*, Booth Theatre, 1962; (also set designer) *Once for the Asking*, Booth Theatre, 1963; (also set designer) *Blues for Mr. Charlie*, ANTA Theatre, 1964; *My Fair Lady*, City Center Theatre, 1964; *The Three Sisters*, Morosco Theatre, 1964; *On a Clear Day You Can See Forever*, Mark Hellinger Theatre, 1965; (also set designer) *Country Girl*, City Center Theatre, 1966; (also set designer) *Elizabeth the Queen*, City Center Theatre, 1966; (also set designer) *Beyond Desire*, Theatre Four, New York City, 1967; *Salute to the American Musical Theatre*, White House, Washington, DC, 1967; *The King and I, My Fair Lady*, and *Carnival!*, all City Center Theatre, 1968; *Scratch*, St. James Theatre, New York City, 1971; *Carmelina*, St. James Theatre, 1979; *A Musical Evening with Joshua Logan*, Springer Opera House, Columbus, GA, 1980; *A Musical Evening with Alan Jay Lerner*, Springer Opera House, 1982. Also *Speak of the Devil!*, 1939; (also production coordinator) *The Great American Goof* (ballet), *Peter and the Wolf* (ballet), and *Giselle* (ballet), all American Ballet Theatre, New York City, 1941; *The Sonja Henie Ice Revue*, Santa Barbara, CA, 1952; (also set designer) *Carousel*, 1966; *Goodtime Charley*, 1975; *Doctor Jazz*, 1975; and *Night of the Iguana*, Baltimore, MD, 1985.

MAJOR TOURS—Lighting designer, *Ballet Caravan, One-Third of a Nation*, and *The Father*, U.S. cities, all 1938; also lighting designer and production coordinator for the first tour of the American Ballet Theatre, U.S. cities, 1941.

PRINCIPAL FILM WORK—Lighting consultant, *Winged Victory*, Twentieth Century-Fox, 1944.

RELATED CAREER—Head of lighting, Federal Theatre Project of the WPA (Works Progress Administration, then Work Projects Administration), 1935-41; owner, Lighting by Feder (stage lighting company), New York City; lecturer and seminar conductor at universities and for lighting professionals. Also lighting designer and/or lighting consultant: New York World's Fair, Flushing, NY; Montreal Cultural Center, Montreal, PQ, Canada; Israel National Museum, Jerusalem, Israel; Gallery of Modern Art, New York City; Tulsa Civic Center, Tulsa, OK; San Francisco Civic Center, San Francisco, CA; Springer Opera House, Columbus, GA; Minskoff Theatre, New York City; Hartford Stage Company, Hartford, CT; Philharmonic Hall, New York City; the Prometheus Fountain, Rockefeller Plaza, and the RCA Building, all Rockefeller Center, New York City; Kennedy Center for the Performing Arts, Washington, DC; Special Events Center, University of Illinois; and Memorial Hall, University of South Carolina.

WRITINGS: (Contributor, chapter on lighting) *Producing the Play*, by John Gassner; also wrote articles for the *AIA Journal, Progressive Architecture, Illuminating Engineer, American City, Interior Design, Designer*, and *Contract*.

MEMBER: United Scenic Artists, U.S. Institute of Theatre Technicians, U.S. Experts Committee on Lighting Education in Architecture, Architectural League of New York, Illuminating Engineering

Society of North America (fellow), International Association of Lighting Designers (first president and fellow).

ADDRESSES: OFFICE—Lighting by Feder, 1600 Broadway, Suite 703, New York City, 10019.

*   *   *

FELLINI, Federico   1920-

PERSONAL: Born January 20, 1920, in Rimini, Italy; son of Urbano (in sales) and Ida (Barbiani) Fellini; married Giulietta Masina (an actress), October 30, 1943. EDUCATION: Attended the University of Rome.

VOCATION: Director, screenwriter, and actor.

CAREER: Also see *WRITINGS* below. PRINCIPAL FILM APPEARANCES—Stranger mistaken for St. Joseph, "Il miracolo," *L'Amore,* 1948, released in the United States as "The Miracle," *Ways of Love,* Joseph Burstyn, 1950; member of Fellini's troupe, *I Clowns* (also known as *The Clowns*), Levitt-Pickman, 1970; as himself, *Alex in Wonderland,* Metro-Goldwyn-Mayer, 1970; as himself, *Ciao, Federico!* (documentary; also known as *So Long, Federico!*), Victor Herbert, 1970; as himself, *Roma* (also known as *Fellini Roma*), United Artists, 1972; voice of interviewer, *Prova d'orchestra* (also known as *Orchestra Rehearsal*), New Yorker, 1978; as himself, *Il tassinaro* (also known as *The Cabbie*), Italian International, 1983; as himself, *Federico Fellini's Intervista* (also known as *Intervista* and *The Interview*), Aljosha/RAI-TV/Cinecitta-Fernlyn, 1987. Also appeared in *C'eravamo tanto amati,* 1974; *We All Loved Each Other So Much,* Almi/Cinema V, 1977.

PRINCIPAL FILM WORK—All as director, unless indicated: Assistant director, *Open City* (also known as *Roma, citta aperta* and *Rome, Open City*), Mayer-Burstyn, 1945; assistant director, *Paisa* (also known as *Paisan*), Mayer-Burstyn, 1946; (with Alberto Lattuada; also producer) *Luci del varieta* (also known as *Variety Lights* and *Lights of Variety*), 1950, released in the United States by Pathe, 1965; *Lo sceicco bianco* (also known as *The White Sheik*), 1951, release in the United States by Janus/API, 1956; *I Vitelloni* (also known as *Vitelloni, The Young and the Passionate,* and *Spivs*), 1953, released in the United States by Janus, 1956; *La strada* (also known as *The Road*), 1955, released in the United States by Trans-Lux, 1956; *Il bidone* (also known as *The Swindle*), 1955, released in the United States by Astor, 1962; *Le notti di Cabiria* (also known as *Nights of Cabiria* and *Cabiria*), Lopert, 1956; *La dolce vita,* 1960, released in the United States by Astor-American International, 1961; "Le tentazioni del dottor Antonio" (also known as "The Temptation of Dr. Antonio") in *Boccaccio '70,* Gray, 1962; *8 1/2* (also known as *Otte e mezzo* and *Federico Fellini's 8 1/2*), Embassy, 1963; *Giulietta degli spiriti* (also known as *Juliet of the Spirits, Juliette des esprits,* and *Julia und die Geister*), Rizzoli, 1965; (also producer) *Fellini Satyricon* (also known as *Satyricon*), United Artists, 1969; "Never Bet the Devil Your Head, or Toby Dammit," (also known as "Il ne faut jamais parier sa tete contre le diable") in *Spirits of the Dead* (also known as *Histoires extraordinaires* and *Tre passi nel delirio*), 1968, released in the United States by American International, 1969.

(Also producer) *I Clowns* (also known as *The Clowns*), Levitt-Pickman, 1970; *Roma* (also known as *Fellini Roma*), United Artists, 1972; *Amarcord,* Warner Brothers/New World, 1974;

(also production designer) *Il Casanova di Federico Fellini* (also known as *Fellini's Casanova* and *Casanova*), Universal, 1976; *Prova d'orchestra* (also known as *Orchestra Rehearsal*), New Yorker, 1978; *La citta delle donne* (also known as *City of Women*), Gaumont, 1980; *E la nave va* (also known as *And the Ship Sails On*), Vides, 1983; *Ginger et Fred* (also known as *Ginger and Fred*), Metro-Goldwyn-Mayer/United Artists, 1986; *Federico Fellini's Intervista* (also known as *Intervista* and *The Interview*), Aljosha-RAI-TV/Cinecitta/Fernlyn, 1987. Also assistant director, *Francesco, giullare di dio,* 1949; director, "Un' agenzia matrimoniale" (also known as "The Matrimonial Agency") in *Amore in citta* (also known as *Love in the City*), 1953.

PRINCIPAL TELEVISION APPEARANCES—Narrator, *Fellini: A Director's Notebook* (also known as *Block-notes di un Regista*), NBC, 1969. PRINCIPAL TELEVISION WORK—Director, *Fellini: A Director's Notebook* (also known as *Block-notes di un Regista*), NBC, 1969.

RELATED CAREER—Film gag writer, 1939-40; radio sketchwriter, 1939-42; founder (with Alberto Lattuada), Capitoleum Production Company, 1950; founder (with Angelo Rizzoli), Federiz Production Company, 1961; also comic with the Fabrizzi vaudeville troupe and circus performer.

NON-RELATED CAREER—Cartoon artist for a comic strip and various humor magazines, 1938-39; story editor, *Marc' Aurelio* (magazine), 1939.

WRITINGS: See production credits above, unless indicated. FILM—(With Sergio Amidei and Roberto Rossellini) *Open City,* 1945; (with Amidei, Rossellini, and Annalena Limentani) *Paisa,* 1946; "Il miracolo" in *L'Amore,* 1948; (with Tullio Pinelli) *Senza pieta* (also known as *Without Pity*), Lux, 1948; (with Lattuada, Pinelli, and Flaiano) *Luci del varieta,* 1950, published as "Variety Lights" (translated by Judith Green) in *Early Screenplays,* Grossman, 1971; (with Pinelli and Flaiano) *Lo sceicco bianco,* 1951, published in *Il primo Fellini,* Cappelli, 1969, and as "The White Sheik" (translated by Green) in *Early Screenplays; I Vitelloni,* 1953, published in *Il primo Fellini,* 1969, then as "The Young and the Passionate" (translated by Green) in *Three Screenplays,* Orion Press, 1970, and in *Quattro Film,* Einaudi, 1974; (with Pinelli) *La strada,* 1955, published in *Il primo Fellini,* 1969; *Il bidone,* 1955, published by Flammarion, 1956, then in *Il primo Fellini,* 1969, later as "The Swindler" (translated by Green) in *Three Screenplays,* 1970; (with Flaiano, Pinelli, and Pier Paolo Pasolini) *Le notti di Cabiria,* 1956, published by Cappelli, 1957.

(With Flaiano, Pinelli, and Brunello Rondi) *La dolce vita,* 1960, published by Cappelli, 1961, then in *Quattro Film,* 1974; (with Flaiano and Pinelli) "Le tentazioni del dottor Antonio" in *Boccaccio '70,* 1962, published in *8 1/2,* Cappelli, 1965, then as "The Temptation of Doctor Antonio" (translated by Green) in *Three Screenplays,* 1970, later in *Quattro Film,* 1974; (with Pinelli, Flaiano, and Rondi) *8 1/2,* 1963, published by Cappelli, 1965; (with Pinelli, Flaiano, and Rondi) *Juliet of the Spirits,* 1965, published by Cappelli, 1965, then Orion Press, 1965, later Ballantine, 1966, and in *Quattro Film,* 1974; (with Bernardino Zapponi and Rondi) *Fellini Satyricon,* 1969, published by Cappelli, 1969, then Ballantine, 1970; (with Zapponi and Clement Biddle Wood) "Never Bet the Devil Your Head, or Toby Dammit" in *Spirits of the Dead,* 1968, published as *Tre passi nel delirio,* Cappelli, 1968.

(With Zapponi) *I Clowns,* 1970; (with Zapponi) *Roma,* 1972, published by Cappelli, 1972; (with Tonino Guerra) *Amarcord,*

1974, published by Rizzoli, 1973; (with Zapponi) *Il Casanova di Federico Fellini,* 1976; *Prova d'orchestra,* 1978; (with Zapponi and Rondi) *La citta della donne,* 1980; (with Guerra) *E la nave va,* 1983; (with Guerra and Pinelli) *Ginger et Fred,* 1986; (with Gianfranco Angelucci) *Federico Fellini's Intervista,* 1987. Also (gag writer for Mario Mattoli) *Lo vedi come soi . . . lo vedi come sei?!,* 1939; (gag writer for Mattoli) *Non me lo dire!,* 1940; (gag writer for Mattoli) *Il pirata sono io!,* 1940; *Documento Z-3* (uncredited), 1941; *Avanti, c'e posto* (uncredited), 1942; *Chi l'ha vistro?,* 1942; *Quarta pagina,* 1942; *Apparizione* (uncredited), 1943; *Campo dei fiori* (also known as *The Path of Hope*), 1943; *Tutta la citta canta,* 1943; *L'ultima carrozzella,* 1943; co-writer, *Il delitto di Giovanni Episcopo,* 1947; co-writer, *Il passatore,* 1947; co-writer, *La fumeria d'oppio* (also known as *Ritorna Za-la-mort*), 1947; co-writer, *L'ebreo errante,* 1947; co-writer, *Il mulino del po,* 1948; co-writer, *In nome della legge* (also known as *Mafia*), 1948; co-writer, *La citta dolente,* 1948; co-writer, *Francesco, giullare di dio,* 1949; co-writer, *Il cammino della speranza,* 1950; co-writer, *Persiane chiuse,* 1950; co-writer, *La citta si difende,* 1951; co-writer, *Cameriera bella presenza offresi,* 1951; co-writer, *Il brigante di Tacca del Lupo,* 1952; co-writer, *Europa '51,* (uncredited), 1952; ''Un'agenzia matrimoniale'' in *Amore in citta,* 1953; co-writer, *Fortunella,* 1958.

TELEVISION—Specials: *Fellini: A Director's Notebook,* 1969. OTHER—(With Dominique DeLouche, *Entretiens avec Federico Fellini,* Radiodiffusion television belge, 1962; (with Francoise Sagan) *Mirror of Venus,* Random House, 1966; (contributor) *La mia Rimini,* Cappelli, 1968; *Fellini,* L'Arc, 1971; *Fellini on Fellini,* Delacorte, 1976.

AWARDS: Nastro d'Argento, 1950, for *Luci del varieta;* New York Film Critics Circle Award, 1950, for *L'Amore;* Nastra d'Argento, 1951, for *Europa '51;* Grand Prize from the Venice Film Festival, 1954, New York Film Critics Circle Award, 1956, Screen Directors Guild Award, Best Direction of Foreign Film, 1956, and Academy Award, Best Foreign Film, 1956, all for *La strada;* Academy Award, Best Foreign Film, 1957, for *Le notti di Cabiria;* Academy Award, Best Foreign Film, 1960, Golden Palm Award from the Cannes Film Festival, 1960, New York Film Critics Circle Award, 1961, all for *La dolce vita;* Academy Award, Best Foreign Film, 1963, for *8 1/2;* Golden Globe Award, 1965, for *Juliet of the Spirits;* Academy Award, Best Foreign Film, and New York Film Critics Circle Award, both 1974, for *Amarcord;* honored by the Film Society of Lincoln Center, 1985; Prix du 40th Anniversaire from the Cannes Film Festival, 1987; Moscow Film Festival Award. Honorary degrees: Columbia University, doctor of humane letters, 1970.

ADDRESSES: HOME—Corso d'Italia 356, Rome, Italy. OFFICE—141-A Via Margutta 110, Rome, Italy.*

*   *   *

FIEDLER, John   1925-

PERSONAL: Full name, John Donald Fiedler; born February 3, 1925, in Platteville, WI; son of Donald (a salesman) and Margaret (Phelan) Fiedler. EDUCATION: Trained for the stage with Sanford Meisner at the Neighborhood Playhouse, 1947, and at the Robert Lewis Workshop. MILITARY: U.S. Navy, yeoman third class, 1945-46.

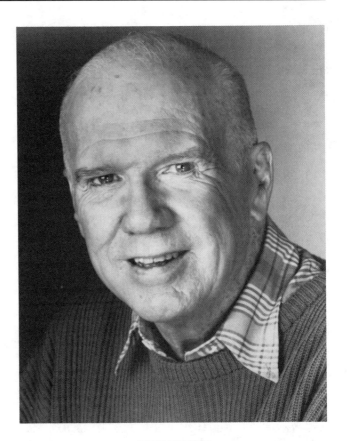

JOHN FIEDLER

VOCATION: Actor.

CAREER: PRINCIPAL STAGE APPEARANCES—Student, *Danny Larkin,* and Paw, *Cock-a-Doodle Doo,* both Experimental Theatre, Lenox Hill Playhouse, New York City, 1948; Medvedenko, *The Seagull,* and Johnny Colton Smith, *Sing Me No Lullaby,* both Phoenix Theatre, New York City, 1954; Cy Milton, *One Eye Closed,* Bijou Theatre, New York City, 1954; Squeak, *Billy Budd,* Masquers Theatre, New York City, 1955; Buckley, *The Terrible Swift Sword,* Phoenix Theatre, New York City, 1955; Karl Lindner, *A Raisin in the Sun,* Ethel Barrymore Theatre, New York City, 1959; Lew, *Harold,* Cort Theatre, New York City, 1962; Vinnie, *The Odd Couple,* Plymouth Theatre, New York City, 1965; Professor Willard, *Our Town,* American National Theatre and Academy Theatre, New York City, 1969; Father Jerome, *The Mind with the Dirty Man,* Center Theatre Group, Mark Taper Forum, Los Angeles, CA, 1972; Dr. Welch, *Rockaway,* Vineyard Theatre, New York City, 1982; servingman, ''The Frog Prince'' in *Marathon '85,* Ensemble Studio Theatre, New York City, 1985; Karl Lindner, *A Raisin in the Sun,* Roundabout Theatre, New York City, then Kennedy Center for the Performing Arts, Washington, DC, both 1986. Also appeared in *The Raspberry Picker,* American Jewish Theatre, 92nd Street YM-YWHA, New York City, 1982; *The Crate,* Ensemble Studio Theatre, 1985; and in *Neptune's Hips,* Ensemble Studio Theatre.

MAJOR TOURS—Alfred, *The Happy Time,* U.S. cities, 1950; Karl Lindner, *A Raisin in the Sun,* U.S. cities, 1987; also appeared in *The Milky Way,* U.S.O. tour of U.S. cities, 1949.

PRINCIPAL FILM APPEARANCES—Juror number two, *Twelve Angry Men,* United Artists, 1957; Adrian, *Stage Struck,* Buena Vista, 1958; Karl Lindner, *A Raisin in the Sun,* Columbia, 1961; Mr. Smith, *That Touch of Mink,* Universal, 1962; Ives, *Guns of Diablo,* Metro-Goldwyn-Mayer (MGM), 1964; Reverend Carruthers, *Kiss Me, Stupid,* Lopert, 1964; Sidney, *The World of Henry Orient,* United Artists, 1964; Mr. Penchill, *Girl Happy,* MGM, 1965; Daniel K. Papp, *A Fine Madness,* Warner Brothers, 1966; Mr. Dunne, *Fitzwilly* (also known as *Fitzwilly Strikes Back*), United Artists, 1967; Simpson, *Ballad of Josie,* Universal, 1968; Vinnie, *The Odd Couple,* Paramount, 1968; Cy Jenkins, *Rascal,* Buena Vista, 1969; J. Noble Daggett, *True Grit,* Paramount, 1969; Major Purvis, *Suppose They Gave a War and Nobody Came?* (also known as *War Games*), Cinerama, 1970; Ames, *Making It,* Twentieth Century-Fox, 1971; Pop, *The Deathmaster,* American International, 1972; Robert Grundig, *Skyjacked* (also known as *Sky Terror*), MGM, 1972; police photographer, *The Fortune,* Columbia, 1975; Howie Clemmings, *The Shaggy D.A.,* Buena Vista, 1976; voice of Owl, *The Rescuers* (animated), Disney, 1977; Bobby Taylor, *Harper Valley, P.T.A.,* April Fools, 1978; clerk, *The Cannonball Run,* Twentieth Century-Fox, 1981; voice of porcupine, *The Fox and the Hound* (animated), Buena Vista, 1981; Barrett, *Sharky's Machine,* Warner Brothers, 1982; grocery clerk, *Savannah Smiles,* Gold Coast, 1983; Arnold, *I Am the Cheese,* Almi, 1983. Also appeared in *That Kind of Woman,* Paramount, 1959; and *Honky,* Jack H. Harris, 1971.

TELEVISION DEBUT—*The Aldrich Family,* NBC, 1949. PRINCIPAL TELEVISION APPEARANCES—Series: Mr. Peterson, *The Bob Newhart Show,* CBS, 1973-78; Gordy Spangler, *Kolchak: The Night Stalker,* ABC, 1974-75; Woody Deschler, *Buffalo Bill,* NBC, 1983-84; Gilbert, *One Life to Live,* ABC, 1987-88; also voice of piglet, *Winnie the Pooh* (animated), ABC. Pilots: Jake, *Cannon,* CBS, 1971; room clerk, *Winner Take All,* CBS, 1977; Lester, *Human Feelings,* NBC, 1978; Jimmy Popadopolis, *Joe Dancer: The Monkey Mission,* NBC, 1981.

Episodic: Mr. Dundee, "Night of the Meek," *The Twilight Zone,* CBS, 1960; field representative three, "Cavender Is Coming," *The Twilight Zone,* CBS, 1962; Mr. Hengist, "Wolf in the Fold," *Star Trek,* NBC, 1967; man on boat, *Amazing Stories,* NBC, 1985; Carl, "Seize the Day," *American Playhouse,* PBS, 1986; Karl Lindner, "A Raisin in the Sun," *American Playhouse,* PBS, 1989; Eddie, *The Golden Girls,* NBC, 1989; also Alfie Higgins, *Tom Corbett, Space Cadet;* in "A Wig for Miss Devore," *Thriller,* NBC, 1961; *The Odd Couple,* ABC; *The Rockford Files,* NBC; *Police Story,* NBC; *Alice,* CBS; *Gunsmoke,* CBS; *Fantasy Island,* ABC; *Dr. Kildare,* NBC; *Bonanza,* NBC; *Alfred Hitchcock Presents,* CBS; *The Fugitive,* ABC; *Chrysler Theatre,* CBS; *The Farmer's Daughter,* ABC; *Checkmate,* NBC; *Adventures in Paradise,* ABC; *Kraft Television Theatre,* NBC; *Studio One,* CBS; *U.S. Steel Hour,* CBS; *Bewitched,* ABC; *Cannon,* CBS. Movies: Sam Jeffers, *A Tattered Web,* CBS, 1971; Jackson, *Double Indemnity,* ABC, 1973; Henry, *Hitched,* NBC, 1973; Mr. Roscoe, *Bad Ronald,* ABC, 1974; PX manager, *Who Is the Black Dahlia?,* NBC, 1975; justice of the peace, *Woman of the Year,* CBS, 1976. Specials: Taylor, "Who's Happy Now?," *Great Performances,* PBS, 1975.

RELATED CAREER—Member, Ensemble Studio Theatre, New York City.

MEMBER: Actors' Equity Association, Screen Actors Guild, American Federation of Television and Radio Artists.

SIDELIGHTS: RECREATIONS—Bridge and travel.

Concerning his long association with the role of Karl Lindner in the drama *A Raisin in the Sun,* John Fiedler told *CTFT:* "I think I'm one of the few actors who did the original Broadway version, movie, New York revival, and taped version for television of the same play."

ADDRESSES: HOME—225 Adams Street, Apartment 10-B, Brooklyn, NY 11201. AGENT—Merritt Blake, Camden Artists, 2121 Avenue of the Stars, Suite 410, Los Angeles, CA 90067.

*   *   *

FIRTH, Peter   1953-

PERSONAL: Born October 27, 1953, in Bradford, England.

VOCATION: Actor.

CAREER: STAGE DEBUT—Alan Strang, *Equus,* National Theatre Company, Olivier Theatre, London, 1973. BROADWAY DEBUT—Alan Strang, *Equus,* Plymouth Theatre, 1974. PRINCIPAL STAGE APPEARANCES—Melchior Gabor, *Spring Awakening,* Lucio and first gentleman, *Measure for Measure,* and Romeo, *Romeo and Juliet,* all National Theatre Company, Old Vic Theatre, London, 1974; Wolfgang Amadeus Mozart, *Amadeus,* Broadhurst Theatre, New York City, 1980.

PRINCIPAL FILM APPEARANCES—Alan Strang, *Equus,* United Artists, 1977; Croft, *Aces High,* EMI, 1977; title role, *Joseph Andrews,* Paramount, 1977; Stephen Ryder, *When You Comin' Back, Red Ryder?,* Columbia, 1979; Angel Clare, *Tess,* Columbia, 1980; Dinas, *Tristan und Isolde,* Von Fuerstenberg/Dobbertin, 1981; Roy, *The Aerodrome,* BBC Films, 1983; Peter Davidson, *White Elephant,* Worldoc, 1984; Inspector Caine, *Lifeforce,* Tri-Star, 1985; Peter, *A Letter to Brezhnev,* Circle, 1986; Dr. Kenneth Parrish, *A State of Emergency,* Double O Associates/Norkat, 1986; Paul Bergson, *Born of Fire,* IFEX/Vidmart, 1987; Clive Ingram, *Prisoner of Rio,* Multimedia/Palace, 1988. Also appeared in *Fire and Sword,* 1982.

PRINCIPAL TELEVISION APPEARANCES—Series: *The Flaxton Boys,* BBC, 1971-72. Episodic: Henry Tilney, "Northanger Abbey," *Masterpiece Theatre,* PBS, 1987.

AWARDS: Theatre World Award, 1974, for *Equus;* Academy Award nomination, Best Supporting Actor, 1977, for *Equus.*

MEMBER: British Actors' Equity Association, Screen Actors Guild.*

*   *   *

FISHBURNE, Larry

PERSONAL: Full name, Laurence Fishburne III.

VOCATION: Actor.

CAREER: PRINCIPAL STAGE APPEARANCES—Solomon, *Eden,* Negro Ensemble Company, St. Mark's Playhouse, New York City, 1976; Tony Pridgeon, *Section D,* New Federal Theatre, New York

City, 1975. Also appeared in *Urban Blight,* Manhattan Theatre Club, City Center Theatre, New York City, 1988.

PRINCIPAL FILM APPEARANCES—Wilford, *Cornbread, Earl, and Me,* American International, 1975; Clean, *Apocalypse Now,* United Artists, 1979; street kid, *Fast Break,* Columbia, 1979; Wilson, *Willie and Phil,* Twentieth Century-Fox, 1980; Cutter, *Death Wish II,* Columbia/EMI/Warner Brothers, 1982; Midget, *Rumble Fish,* Universal, 1983; Bumpy Rhodes, *The Cotton Club,* Orion, 1984; Swain, *The Color Purple,* Warner Brothers, 1985; Cream, *Band of the Hand,* Tri-Star, 1986; Voodoo, *Quicksilver,* Columbia, 1986; Corporal Flanagan, *Gardens of Stone,* Tri-Star, 1987; Max, *A Nightmare on Elm Street 3: Dream Warriors,* New Line Cinema, 1987; Dap Dunlap, *School Daze,* Columbia, 1988; Lieutenant Stubbs, *Red Heat,* Tri-Star, 1988.

PRINCIPAL TELEVISION APPEARANCES—Series: Corporal Don "Robby" Robinson, *The Six O'Clock Follies,* NBC, 1980; also Joshua West, *One Life to Live,* ABC. Episodic: Cowboy Curtis, *Pee-Wee's Playhouse,* CBS, 1986; Maurice Haynes, *Hill Street Blues,* NBC, 1986; Kellar, *Miami Vice,* NBC, 1986; Mukende, *Spenser: For Hire,* ABC, 1987; also "The Tooth Shall Set You Free," *M*A*S*H,* CBS, 1982; and "For Us, the Living," *American Playhouse,* PBS, 1983. Movies: Lightbulb, *A Rumor of War,* CBS, 1980; Hank Johnson, *I Take These Men,* CBS, 1983; also *The Father Clements Story,* NBC, 1987.

MEMBER: Actors' Equity Association, Screen Actors Guild, American Federation of Television and Radio Artists.*

*   *   *

FISHER, Carrie   1956-

PERSONAL: Full name, Carrie Frances Fisher; born October 21, 1956, in Beverly Hills, CA; daughter of Eddie Fisher (a singer) and Debbie Reynolds (an entertainer); married Paul Simon (a singer and songwriter), 1983 (divorced, 1984). EDUCATION: Attended the Central School of Speech and Drama.

VOCATION: Actress.

CAREER: BROADWAY DEBUT—Chorus member, *Irene,* Minskoff Theatre, 1973. PRINCIPAL STAGE APPEARANCES—Iris, *Censored Scenes from King Kong,* Princess Theatre, New York City, 1980; title role, *Agnes of God,* Music Box Theatre, New York City, 1982.

PRINCIPAL FILM APPEARANCES—Lorna Carr, *Shampoo,* Columbia, 1975; Princess Leia Organa, *Star Wars,* Twentieth Century-Fox, 1977; mystery woman, *The Blues Brothers,* Universal, 1980; Princess Leia, *The Empire Strikes Back,* Twentieth Century-Fox, 1980; Annie Clark, *Under the Rainbow,* Orion/Warner Brothers, 1981; Princess Leia, *The Return of the Jedi,* Twentieth Century-Fox, 1983; Lisa Rolfe, *Garbo Talks,* Metro-Goldwyn-Mayer-United Artists, 1984; Paula, *The Man with One Red Shoe,* Twentieth Century-Fox, 1985; April, *Hannah and Her Sisters,* Orion, 1986; Betty Melton, *Hollywood Vice Squad,* Concorde, 1986; Mary Brown, *Amazon Women on the Moon,* Universal, 1987; Petra, *The Time Guardian,* Hemdale, 1987; Nadine Boynton, *Appointment with Death,* Cannon, 1988; Carol Peterson, *The Burbs,* Universal, 1989. Also appeared in *Mr. Mike's Mondo Video,* 1979; and in *Loverboy,* Tri-Star, 1989.

TELEVISION DEBUT—Marie, *Come Back, Little Sheba,* NBC, 1977. PRINCIPAL TELEVISION APPEARANCES—Movies: Marny Clarkson, *Leave Yesterday Behind,* ABC, 1978; Emma Lazarus, *Liberty,* NBC, 1986; Franny Jessup, *Sunday Drive,* ABC, 1986. Specials: Markene, *Ringo,* NBC, 1978.

WRITINGS: *Postcards from the Edge* (novel), Simon & Schuster, 1987.

ADDRESSES: AGENT—Toni Howard, William Morris Agency, 151 El Camino Drive, Beverly Hills, CA 90212.*

*   *   *

FLETCHER, Bramwell   1904-1988

PERSONAL: Born February 20, 1904, in Bradford, England; died June 22, 1988, in Westmoreland, NH; son of Benjamin and Jean (Scott) Fletcher; married Helen Chandler, February 14, 1935 (divorced); married Diana Barrymore, July 30, 1942 (divorced); married Susan Robinson, April 12, 1950 (divorced); married Lael Tucker Wertenbaker, September 26, 1970; children: Catherine, Kent, Whitney (third marriage). EDUCATION: Studied drama with Margaret Carrington in New York City, 1935-38. MILITARY: U.S. Army, private, during World War II.

VOCATION: Actor and playwright.

CAREER: Also see *WRITINGS* below. STAGE DEBUT—Florizel, *The Winter's Tale,* Shakespeare Memorial Company, Shakespeare Memorial Theatre, Stratford-on-Avon, U.K., 1927. LONDON DEBUT—Colonel Prince Yashvil, *Paul I,* Court Theatre, 1927. BROADWAY DEBUT—Kent Heathcote, *Scotland Yard,* Sam H. Harris Theatre, 1929. PRINCIPAL STAGE APPEARANCES—Oscar Nordholm, *Sauce for the Gander,* Lyric Theatre, London, 1928; Martin, *Thunder on the Left,* Arts Theatre, then Kingsway Theatre, both London, 1928; Harold Marquess, *The Chinese Bungalow,* Duke of York's Theatre, London, 1929; Jimmie Chard, *The Devil in the Cheese,* Comedy Theatre, London, 1929; Ray Fanshawe, *Red Planet,* Cort Theatre, New York City, 1932; Colin Derwent, *Ten Minute Alibi,* Ethel Barrymore Theatre, New York City, 1933; Simon More, *These Two,* Henry Miller's Theatre, New York City, 1934; the Dreamer, *Within the Gates,* National Theatre, New York City, 1934; Dick Shale, *The Dominant Sex,* Cort Theatre, 1935; Hsieh Ping-Kuei, *Lady Precious Stream,* Booth Theatre, New York City, 1936; Rodney Bevan, *Boy Meets Girl,* Shaftesbury Theatre, London, 1936; Arnold Champion-Cheney, *The Circle,* Playhouse Theatre, New York City, 1938; title role and Don Caesar, *Ruy Blas,* Central City Opera House, Central City, CO, 1938; Mr. Prior, *Outward Bound,* Playhouse Theatre, 1938; Baron Max von Alvenstor, *Margin for Error,* Plymouth Theatre, New York City, 1939.

Jacob Wait, *Eight O'Clock Tuesday,* Henry Miller's Theatre, 1941; Louis Dubedat, *The Doctor's Dilemma,* Shubert Theatre, New York City, 1941; Captain Sutton, *Storm Operation,* Belasco Theatre, New York City, 1944; Maxim de Winter, *Rebecca,* Ethel Barrymore Theatre, 1945; newspaper reporter, *The Greatest of These,* Shubert-Lafayette Theatre, Detroit, MI, then Selwyn Theatre, Chicago, IL, 1947; Richard Brinsley Sheridan, *The Lady Maria,* Cape Playhouse, Dennis MA, 1947; George, Duke of Bristol, *The Day after Tomorrow,* Booth Theatre, 1950; Collins, *Getting Married,* American National Theatre Academy (ANTA)

Theatre, New York City, 1951; Mr. Burgess, *Candida*, National Theatre, 1952; Doolittle, *Pygmalion*, Westport Country Playhouse, Westport, CT, 1952; Alick Wylie, *Maggie*, National Theatre, 1953; Lord Summerhays, *Misalliance*, City Center Theatre, New York City, then Ethel Barrymore Theatre, both 1953; Sir Henry Harcourt-Reilly, *The Cocktail Party*, and the Duke of Altair, *Venus Observed*, Olney Theatre, Olney, MD, 1954; Gavin Leon Andree, *The Wisteria Trees*, City Center Theatre, 1955; Marechal Francois de Sevres, *The Little Glass Clock*, John Golden Theatre, New York City, 1956; Clement of Metz, *The Lovers*, Martin Beck Theatre, New York City, 1956; Aeneas Posket, *Posket's Family Skeleton*, Westport Country Playhouse, 1956.

Mephisto, *Faust*, Goodman Theatre, Chicago, 1961; Ulric Brendel, *Rosmersholm*, Fourth Street Theatre, New York City, 1962; Leonid Andreyevich Gayef, *The Cherry Orchard*, Theatre Four, New York City, 1962; *Parnassus '63* (one-man show), ANTA Theatre, 1962; title role, *The Bernard Shaw Story* (one-man show), Gate Theatre, Dublin, Ireland, 1964, then East 74th Street Theatre, New York City, 1965; Andrew Undershaft, *Major Barbara*, Doolittle, *Pygmalion*, and title role, *The Bernard Shaw Story* (one-man show), all Westport Country Playhouse, 1965; Sir Ormsby-Gore and Dr. York, *A Step Away from War*, American Place Theatre, New York City, 1965; title role, *The Miser*, Goodman Theatre, 1967; Lord Summerhays, *Misalliance*, Loeb Theatre, Boston, MA, 1974; Speaker of the House, *In the Well of the House*, Kansas City Playhouse, Kansas City, MO, 1975. Also appeared at the Ogunquit Playhouse, Ogunquit, ME, 1940; and as the understudy for the role of Henry Higgins, *My Fair Lady*, Mark Hellinger Theatre, New York City, 1956-61.

PRINCIPAL STAGE WORK—Director, *The Deadly Game* and *A Touch of the Poet*, both Washington Theatre Club, Washington, DC, 1965.

MAJOR TOURS—Various roles, *Tonight at 8:30*, U.S. cities, 1937; Maxim de Winter, *Rebecca*, U.S. cities, 1944; Sergeant Rough, *Angel Street*, U.S. cities, 1945; President Merrill, *Goodbye My Fancy*, U.S. cities, 1950; Matthew Store, *Told to the Children*, U.S. cities, 1951; Doolittle, *Pygmalion*, U.S. cities, 1953; David Slater, *The Moon Is Blue*, U.S. cities, 1954; *Love, Laughter, and Baseball* (one-man show; originally titled *Parnassus '63*), U.S. cities, 1963; title role, *The Bernard Shaw Story* (one-man show), U.S. cities, 1965, then 1976.

FILM DEBUT—*Chick*, British Lion, 1928. PRINCIPAL FILM APPEARANCES—Jim Nolan, *To What Red Hell*, Tiffany, 1929; Bunny Manders, *Raffles*, United Artists, 1930; Alfred Honeycutt, *So This Is London*, Twentieth Century-Fox, 1930; Ronald Petrie, *Daughter of the Dragon*, Paramount, 1931; Eric, *Men of the Sky*, First National/Warner Brothers, 1931; Carter Andrews, *The Millionaire*, Warner Brothers, 1931; Allen Corinth, *Once a Lady*, Paramount, 1931; Billee, *Svengali*, Warner Brothers, 1931; Bill Bronson, *The Face on the Barroom Floor*, Invincible Films, 1932; Norton, *The Mummy*, Universal, 1932; Anthony Howard, *The Silent Witness*, Twentieth Century-Fox, 1932; Herbert, *The Monkey's Paw*, RKO, 1933; Scott Hughes, *Only Yesterday*, Universal, 1933; David Morland, *Line Engaged*, British Lion, 1935; priest, *The Scarlet Pimpernel*, United Artists, 1935; Harrison, *Random Harvest*, Metro-Goldwyn-Mayer (MGM), 1942; Dr. Geoffrey Covert, *The Undying Monster* (also known as *The Hammond Mystery*), Twentieth Century-Fox, 1942; Wilbur Ashley, *White Cargo*, MGM, 1942; Symes, *The Immortal Sergeant*, Twentieth Century-Fox, 1943. Also appeared in *S.O.S.*, 1928; *Inside the Lines*, RKO, 1930; *A Bill of Divorcement*, RKO, 1932; *The Right to*

Romance, RKO, 1933; and *Nana* (also known as *Lady of the Boulevards*), United Artists, 1934.

PRINCIPAL TELEVISION APPEARANCES—Episodic: Horfield, "The Paradine Case," *Theater '62*, NBC, 1962.

RELATED CAREER—Toured the United States as a lecturer and actor for the National Endowment for the Humanities.

NON-RELATED CAREER—Clerk with an insurance company in London.

WRITINGS: See production details above. STAGE—*The Bernard Shaw Story* (one-man show), 1964; also (with Lael Wertenbaker) *Operation Gadfly*, 1970.

AWARDS: Cockefair grant from the University of Missouri, Distinguished Theatre Artist of the Year, 1975.

SIDELIGHTS: CTFT learned that as the understudy for Rex Harrison and later Edward Mulhare in the original Broadway production of *My Fair Lady*, Bramwell Fletcher appeared in the role of Henry Higgins for more than 200 performances between 1956 and 1961. According to his obituary in the *New York Times*, "During the hundreds of performances in which Mr. Fletcher stood by but did not go on, he concentrated on his lifelong passion for art, developing a second career as a portrait painter; he maintained a studio near the theatre from which he contended that he could reach the stage in 20 seconds, if necessary."

OBITUARIES AND OTHER SOURCES: New York Times, June 24, 1988; *Variety*, June 29, 1988.*

*   *   *

FO, Dario   1926-

PERSONAL: Born March 24, 1926, in San Giano, Lombardy, Italy.

VOCATION: Playwright, actor, director, and producer.

CAREER: Also see *WRITINGS* below. PRINCIPAL STAGE APPEARANCES—*Mistero Buffo*, American Repertory Theatre, Cambridge, MA, then Joyce Theatre, New York City, both 1986. PRINCIPAL STAGE WORK—Director, *Mistero Buffo*, American Repertory Theatre, Cambridge, MA, then Joyce Theatre, New York City, both 1986; director (with Franca Rame) and set and costume designer, *Archangels Don't Play Pinball*, American Repertory Theatre, 1987. PRINCIPAL FILM APPEARANCES—*Do Not Enter: The Visa War against Ideas*, New Day Films, 1986. PRINCIPAL TELEVISION APPEARANCES—Specials: *Paper Curtain* (documentary), PBS, 1986.

RELATED CAREER—Founder and director, Compagnia Dario Fo, Italy.

WRITINGS: STAGE—*We Won't Pay! We Won't Pay!*, Chelsea Theatre Center, New York City, 1980, then Actors Theatre of St. Paul, St. Paul, MN, 1985, later Whole Theatre Company, Montclair, NJ, 1987, published by Pluto Press, 1980; *Accidental Death of an Anarchist*, Center Theatre Group, Mark Taper Forum, Los Angeles, CA, 1982, then Arena Stage, Washington, DC, 1984, later

Belasco Theatre, New York City, 1984, then Denver Center Theatre Company, Denver, CO, 1985, published by Pluto Press, 1980; (with Franca Rame) *Female Parts,* Los Angeles Actors Theatre, Los Angeles, CA, 1983, published as *Female Parts: One Woman Plays,* Pluto Press, 1981; *About Face,* Yale Repertory Theatre, New Haven, CT, 1983; (with Franca Rame) *Orgasmo Adulto Escapes from the Zoo,* New York Shakespeare Festival, Public Theatre, New York City, 1983; *Mistero Buffo,* American Repertory Theatre, Cambridge, MA, then Joyce Theatre, New York City, both 1986; *Archangels Don't Play Pinball,* American Repertory Theatre, 1987; *Almost by Chance a Woman: Elizabeth,* Yale Repertory Theatre, 1987. FILM—*It Happened in Rome,* Lopert, 1959.

MEMBER: Writers Guild, Dramatists Guild.*

*   *   *

FOLEY, Ellen   1951-

PERSONAL: Born in 1951 in St. Louis, MO.

VOCATION: Actress and singer.

CAREER: PRINCIPAL STAGE APPEARANCES—Sheila, *Hair,* Biltmore Theatre, New York City, 1977; Kim Dolphin, *Eve Is Innocent,* Actors and Directors Theatre, New York City, 1983; the Witch, *Into the Woods,* Old Globe Theatre, San Diego, CA, 1987; Lisbeth, *Beautiful Bodies,* Whole Theatre Company, Montclair, NJ, 1987; Sally, *Me and My Girl,* Marquis Theatre, New York City, 1988.

PRINCIPAL FILM APPEARANCES—Sheila, *Hair,* United Artists, 1979; Jacqui, *Tootsie,* Columbia, 1982; street scum, *The King of Comedy,* Twentieth Century-Fox, 1983; Hildy, *Fatal Attraction,* Paramount, 1987; Eleanor, *Cocktail,* Buena Vista, 1988; Theresa, *Married to the Mob,* Orion, 1988.

PRINCIPAL TELEVISION APPEARANCES—Series: Regular, *3 Girls 3,* NBC, 1977; Billie Young, *Night Court,* NBC, 1984-85.

MEMBER: Actors' Equity Association, Screen Actors Guild, American Federation of Television and Radio Artists.

SIDELIGHTS: As a rock singer, Ellen Foley has performed as a background vocalist with such artists as Ian Hunter, the Clash, and Meat Loaf as well as having recorded an album of her own.

ADDRESSES: AGENT—Bob Gersh, The Gersh Agency, 222 N. Canon Drive, Suite 202, Beverly Hills, CA 90210.*

*   *   *

FOLLOWS, Megan   1968-

PERSONAL: Born March 14, 1968, in Toronto, ON, Canada; daughter of Ted Follows (an actor) and Dawn Greenhalgh (an actress).

VOCATION: Actress.

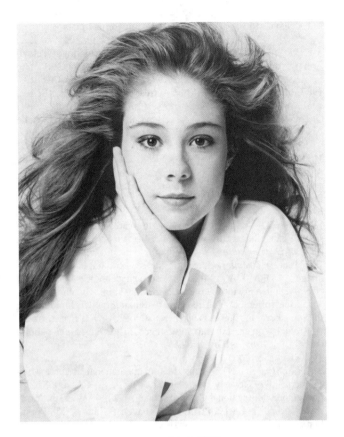

MEGAN FOLLOWS

CAREER: STAGE DEBUT—*The Effect of Gamma Rays on Man-in-the-Moon Marigolds,* Young People's Theatre, Toronto, ON, Canada, 1988. PRINCIPAL STAGE APPEARANCES—Cecile de Volanges, *Les Liaisons dangereuses,* Williamstown Theatre Festival, Williamstown, MA, 1988.

FILM DEBUT—*Claire's Wish* (short film). PRINCIPAL FILM APPEARANCES—Jane Coslaw, *Stephen King's Silver Bullet,* De Laurentiis Entertainment Group/Paramount, 1985; Anna Mae Morgan, *Stacking* (also known as *Season of Dreams*), Spectrafilm, 1987; Irene, *A Time of Destiny,* Columbia, 1988. Also appeared in *Boys and Girls,* Atlantis Films, 1982; and in *Termini Station,* 1989.

PRINCIPAL TELEVISION APPEARANCES—Series: Lucy Baxter, *The Baxters,* syndicated, 1980-81; Didi Crane, *Domestic Life,* CBS, 1984; also Jenny, *Matt and Jenny on the Wilderness Trail,* Canadian television. Mini-Series: Anne Shirley, *Anne of Green Gables,* CBC, then *Wonderworks,* PBS, 1985; Anne Shirley, *Anne of Avonlea: The Continuing Story of Anne of Green Gables,* CBC, then Disney Channel, 1987, later *Wonderworks,* PBS, 1988; Louise, *Champagne Charlie,* CTV, then syndicated in the United States, both 1989. Pilots: Tina Jackson, *The Faculty,* ABC, 1986. Episodic: *Facts of Life,* NBC, 1983. Movies: Laura McClain, *The Mating Season,* CBS, 1980; Jenny Colleran, *Sin of Innocence,* CBS, 1986; Cathy, *Hockey Night,* CBC, then *Wonderworks,* PBS, 1987; Rachel Brown, *Inherit the Wind,* NBC, 1988. Specials: *The Making of Anne of Green Gables,* PBS, 1986; Dana Sherman, "Seasonal Differences," *ABC Afterschool Special,* ABC, 1987. Also appeared in *Jen's Place,* CBC and PBS, 1982; and *The Olden Day Coat.*

RELATED CAREER—Actress in television commercials.

AWARDS: Gemini Award from the Canadian Academy of Television Arts and Sciences, Best Actress in a Drama Mini-Series, 1986, for *Anne of Green Gables;* ACE Award nomination, Best Actress, 1987, and Gemini Award, Best Actress in a Drama Mini-Series, 1988, both for *Anne of Avonlea: The Continuing Story of Anne of Green Gables;* Association of Canadian Television and Radio Artists Award nomination, Best Actress, 1988, for *Hockey Night.*

MEMBER: Actors' Equity Association, Canadian Actors' Equity Association, Screen Actors Guild, American Federation of Television and Radio Artists, Association of Canadian Television and Radio Artists.

SIDELIGHTS: Megan Follows's acting career has been building steadily since her award-winning performance as Anne Shirley in *Anne of Green Gables* for Canadian television. In the November, 1987 issue of *Premiere* magazine, she spoke about her wholesome image: "I know I've got this wholesome appearance, but it can be effective when my looks contradict the way I am. And this business is so looks-oriented. You're either a stunning model, hired for the 'he spots her—his breath is taken away' roles, or you're not. And if you're not, you can fall into any category. I've played nice people, but I'm not *Anne of Green Gables.*"

ADDRESSES: AGENTS—Brian Mann, International Creative Management, 8899 Beverly Boulevard, Los Angeles, CA 90048; Lisa Loosemore, International Creative Management, 40 W. 57th Street, New York, NY 10019. PUBLICIST—Karen Williams, 268 Poplar Plains Road, Suite 901, Toronto, ON, Canada M4V 2P2.

*   *   *

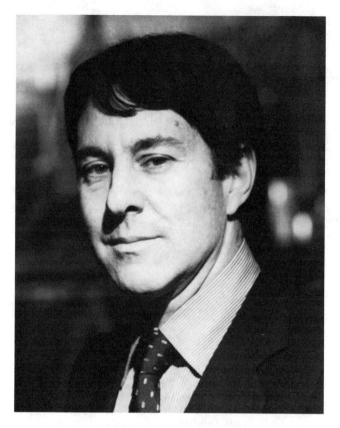

GEORGE FOLSEY, JR.

FOLSEY, George, Jr.   1939-

PERSONAL: Born January 17, 1939, in Los Angeles, CA; son of George, Sr. (a cameraman) and Angele Folsey; married Belinda Comer. EDUCATION: Pomona College, B.A., English literature, 1961.

VOCATION: Producer and film editor.

CAREER: PRINCIPAL FILM APPEARANCES—*Making Michael Jackson's Thriller,* Palace/Virgin Vision/Gold, 1983. PRINCIPAL FILM WORK—Producer and editor, *Glass Houses,* Columbia, 1972; cinematographer and editor, *Bone,* Jack H. Harris, 1972; editor, *Hammer,* United Artists, 1972; editor, *Black Caesar,* American International, 1973; executive producer and editor, *Schlock* (also known as *The Banana Monster*), Jack H. Harris Productions, 1973; editor, *Trader Horn,* Metro-Goldwyn-Mayer (MGM), 1973; editor, *Bucktown,* American International, 1975; editor, *J.D.'s Revenge,* American International, 1976; editor, *Norman . . . Is That You?,* MGM/United Artists, 1976; editor, *The Chicken Chronicles,* AVCO-Embassy, 1977; editor, *Kentucky Fried Movie,* United Film, 1977; editor, *Sourdough,* Film Saturation, 1977; editor, *Tracks,* Trio, 1977; editor, *National Lampoon's Animal House,* Universal, 1978; editorial consultant, *The Great Santini,* Orion/Warner Brothers, 1979; associate producer and editor, *The Blues Brothers,* Universal, 1980; producer, *An American Werewolf in London,* Universal, 1981; associate producer, *Twilight Zone—The Movie,* Warner Brothers, 1982; executive producer and second unit director, *Trading Places,* Paramount, 1983; producer, co-

cinematographer, and editor, *Making Michael Jackson's Thriller,* Palace/Virgin Vision/Gold, 1983; producer (with Ron Koslow) and second unit director, *Into the Night,* Universal, 1985; producer (with Brian Grazer), *Spies Like Us,* Warner Brothers, 1985; executive producer, *Clue,* Paramount, 1985; producer (with Lorne Michaels) and second unit director, *Three Amigos!,* Orion, 1986; executive producer, *Amazon Women on the Moon,* Universal, 1987; producer and editor, *Coming to America,* Paramount, 1988.

PRINCIPAL TELEVISION WORK—Movies: Editor, *It Happened at Lake Wood Manor,* ABC, 1977; editor, *Freedom Road,* NBC, 1979.

ADDRESSES: AGENT—Mike Marcus, Creative Artists Agency, 1888 Century Park E., Los Angeles, CA 90067.*

*   *   *

FONDA, Jane   1937-

PERSONAL: Full name, Jane Seymour Fonda; born December 21, 1937, in New York, NY; daughter of Henry (an actor) and Frances Seymour (Brokaw) Fonda; married Roger Vadim (a film producer and director), August 14, 1965 (divorced, 1973); married Tom Hayden (a political activist and legislator), January 20, 1973 (separated, 1989); children: Vanessa (first marriage); Troy (second marriage). EDUCATION: Attended Vassar College, 1956-60; studied acting with Lee Strasberg at the Actors Studio and with Andrea Voutsinas.

VOCATION: Actress and producer.

CAREER: STAGE DEBUT—Nancy Stoddard, *The Country Girl*, Community House, Omaha, NE, 1954. BROADWAY DEBUT—Toni Newton, *There Was a Little Girl*, Cort Theatre, 1960. PRINCIPAL STAGE APPEARANCES—Patricia Stanley, *The Male Animal*, Cape Playhouse, Dennis, MA, then Falmouth Playhouse, Falmouth, MA, both 1956; Patty O'Neill, *The Moon Is Blue*, North Jersey Playhouse, Fort Lee, NJ, 1959; Jacky Durrant, *No Concern of Mine*, Westport Country Playhouse, Westport, CT, 1960; Norma Brown, *Invitation to a March*, Music Box Theatre, New York City, 1960; Tish Stanford, *The Fun Couple*, Lyceum Theatre, New York City, 1962; Madeline Arnold, *Strange Interlude*, Hudson Theatre, New York City, 1963.

MAJOR TOURS—*Free the Army* (revue), U.S. Army bases throughout the world, 1970-71; also toured Southeast Asia with an anti-war troupe, 1971.

FILM DEBUT—June Ryder, *Tall Story*, Warner Brothers, 1960. PRINCIPAL FILM APPEARANCES—Kathleen Barclay, *The Chapman Report*, Warner Brothers, 1962; Isabel Haverstick, *Period of Adjustment*, Metro-Goldwyn-Mayer (MGM), 1962; Kitty Twist, *Walk on the Wild Side*, Columbia, 1962; Christine Bonner, *In the Cool of the Day*, MGM, 1963; Eileen Tyler, *Sunday in New York*, MGM, 1963; Melinda, *Les Felins* (also known as *Joy House* and *The Love Cage*), MGM, 1964; title role, *Cat Ballou*, Columbia, 1965; the wife, *La Ronde* (also known as *Circle of Love*), Sterling, 1965; Ellen Gordon, *Any Wednesday* (also known as *Bachelor Girl Apartment*), Warner Brothers, 1966; Anna Reeves, *The Chase*, Columbia, 1966; Corie Bratter, *Barefoot in the Park*, Paramount, 1967; Renee Saccard, *La Curee* (also known as *The Game Is Over*), Royal, 1967; Julie Ann Warren, *Hurry Sundown*, Paramount, 1967; title role, *Barbarella* (also known as *Barbarella, Queen of the Galaxy*), Paramount, 1968; Countess Frederica, "Metzengerstein" in *Histoires extraordinaires* (also known as *Spirits of the Dead* and *Tre passi nel delirio*), American International, 1969; Gloria Beatty, *They Shoot Horses, Don't They?*, ABC-Cinerama, 1969.

Bree Daniels, *Klute*, Warner Brothers, 1971; Nora, *A Doll's House*, World Film Services, 1973; Iris Caine, *Steelyard Blues* (also known as *The Final Crash*), Warner Brothers, 1973; She, *Tout va bien*, New Yorker, 1973; Night, *The Blue Bird*, Twentieth Century-Fox, 1976; Jane Harper, *Fun with Dick and Jane*, Columbia, 1977; Lillian Hellman, *Julia*, Twentieth Century-Fox, 1977; Hannah Warren, *California Suite*, Columbia, 1978; Ella Connors, *Comes a Horseman*, United Artists, 1978; Sally Hyde, *Coming Home*, United Artists, 1978; Kimberly Wells, *The China Syndrome*, Columbia, 1979; Hallie Martin, *The Electric Horseman*, Universal, 1979; Judy Bernley, *Nine to Five*, Twentieth Century-Fox, 1980; Chelsea Thayer Wayne, *On Golden Pond*, Universal, 1981; Lee Winters, *Rollover*, Warner Brothers, 1981; Dr. Martha Livingston, *Agnes of God*, Columbia, 1985; Alex Sternbergen, *The Morning After*, Twentieth Century-Fox, 1986; as herself, *Leonard Part 6*, Columbia, 1987; Harriet Winslow, *Old Gringo*, Columbia, 1989. Also appeared in *F.T.A.*, American International, 1972; *Introduction to the Enemy* (documentary), IPC, 1974; *No Nukes* (documentary), Warner Brothers, 1980; *Acting: Lee Strasberg and the Actors Studio* (documentary), Davada Enterprises, 1981; *Montgomery Clift* (documentary), Ciak Studio Productions, 1982; *We Are the World—the Video Event*, Columbia, 1985.

PRINCIPAL FILM WORK—Co-producer, *F.T.A.*, American International, 1972; co-director, *Introduction to the Enemy* (documentary), IPC, 1974; producer, *Coming Home*, United Artists, 1978;

co-producer, *The China Syndrome*, Columbia, 1979; producer, *Nine to Five*, Twentieth Century-Fox, 1980; producer, *On Golden Pond*, Universal, 1981; producer, *Rollover*, Warner Brothers, 1981; producer, *Old Gringo*, Columbia, 1989.

TELEVISION DEBUT—Gloria Winters, *A String of Beads*, ABC, 1961. PRINCIPAL TELEVISION APPEARANCES—Episodic: *Headliners with David Frost*, NBC, 1978; also O'Neal, *Nine to Five*, ABC; *Girl Talk*, ABC; *The Tonight Show*, NBC; *The Merv Griffin Show*, syndicated. Specials: *Superstunt* (documentary), NBC, 1977; *The American Film Institute Salute to Henry Fonda*, CBS, 1978; *Variety '77—The Year in Entertainment*, CBS, 1978; *The Helen Reddy Special*, ABC, 1979; *The Sensational, Shocking, Wonderful, Wacky 70s*, NBC, 1980; *Lily—Sold Out*, CBS, 1981; *I Love Liberty*, ABC, 1982; Judy Bernley, *Lily for President*, CBS, 1982; Gertie Nevels, *The Dollmaker*, ABC, 1984; *Windows on Women*, PBS, 1985; *Fit for a Lifetime* (also known as *Lifetime Health Styles*), Lifetime, 1986; host, *The American Film Institute Salute to Barbara Stanwyck*, ABC, 1987; *NBC News Report on America: Life in the Fat Lane*, NBC, 1987; *The Special Olympics Opening Ceremonies*, ABC, 1987; "Gregory Peck—His Own Man," *Crazy about the Movies*, Cinemax, 1988; *The American Film Institute Salute to Gregory Peck*, NBC, 1989.

PRINCIPAL TELEVISION WORK—Series: Executive producer, *Nine to Five*, ABC, 1982. Specials: Co-producer, *The Dollmaker*, ABC, 1984.

RELATED CAREER—As a professional model, appeared on the covers of *Esquire, Vogue, Ladies' Home Journal, Glamour*, and *McCall's*, all 1959; member, Actors Studio, New York City, 1960—; founder, Entertainment Industry for Truth and Justice (anti-war troupe), 1971; founder, IPC Films, 1976; created and performed in the fitness videos: *Jane Fonda Workout*, Lorimar, 1982; *Jane Fonda's Workout for Pregnancy, Birth, and Recovery*, Lorimar, 1983; *Jane Fonda's Workout Challenge*, Lorimar, 1983; *Jane Fonda's Easy Going Workout*, Lorimar, 1984; *Jane Fonda's New Workout*, Lorimar, 1985; *Jane Fonda's Low Impact Workout*, Lorimar, 1986; *Jane Fonda's Workout with Weights*, Lorimar, 1987; *Jane Fonda Presents SportsAid*, Lorimar, 1987; *Start Up with Jane Fonda*, Lorimar, 1988; *Jane Fonda's Complete Workout*, Lorimar, 1989; also founder, Fonda Films, Los Angeles, CA.

WRITINGS: FILMS—(With others) *F.T.A.*, American International, 1972. OTHER—All published by Simon & Schuster: *Jane Fonda's Workout Book*, 1981; (with Mignon McCarthy) *Women Coming of Age*, 1984; *Jane Fonda's Year of Fitness, Health, and Nutrition*, 1984; *Jane Fonda's New Workout and Weight-Loss Program*, 1986; *Jane Fonda's New Low Impact Workout and Weight-Loss Program*, 1988.

AWARDS: Variety New York Drama Critics Poll winner and Theatre World Award, both 1960, for *There Was a Little Girl;* Laurel Award from the Motion Picture Exhibitors of America, 1960, for *Tall Story;* Hasty Pudding Woman of the Year Award from the Harvard Hasty Pudding Theatricals, 1961; Academy Award nomination and New York Film Critics Award, both Best Actress, 1969, for *They Shoot Horses, Don't They?;* Academy Award and New York Film Critics Award, both Best Actress, 1971, for *Klute;* Golden Apple Award from the Hollywood Women's Press Club, Female Star of the Year, 1977; Academy Award nomination, Best Actress, 1977, and British Academy Award, Best Actress, 1978, both for *Julia;* Academy Award and Golden Globe Award, both Best Actress, 1978, for *Coming Home;* Academy Award nomination and British Academy Award, both Best Actress,

1979, for *The China Syndrome;* Emmy Award, Outstanding Actress in a Dramatic Special, 1984, for *The Dollmaker;* Academy Award nomination, Best Actress, 1987, for *The Morning After.*

MEMBER: Actors' Equity Association, Screen Actors Guild, American Federation of Television and Radio Artists.

ADDRESSES: OFFICE—Fonda Films, Inc., P.O. Box 491355, Los Angeles, CA 90049-9355. AGENT—Ron Meyer, Creative Artists Agency, 1888 Century Park E., 14th Floor, Los Angeles, CA 90067.

*   *   *

FOOTE, Hallie

PERSONAL: Full name, Barbarie Hallie Foote; daughter of Horton (a writer, director, and actor) and Lillian (Vallish) Foote.

VOCATION: Actress.

CAREER: PRINCIPAL STAGE APPEARANCES—Annie, *The Roads to Home,* Manhattan Punchline Theatre, New York City, 1982; Sophia, *A Little Family Business,* Center Theatre Group, Ahmanson Theatre, Los Angeles, CA, then Martin Beck Theatre, New York City, both 1982; title role, *The Widow Claire,* Circle in the Square Downtown, New York City, 1986.

PRINCIPAL FILM APPEARANCES—Waitress, *C.H.U.D.,* New World, 1984; Elizabeth Robedaux, *1918,* Cinecom International, 1984; Elizabeth Robedaux, *On Valentine's Day,* Cinecom International, 1986.

PRINCIPAL TELEVISION APPEARANCES—Mini-Series: Elizabeth Vaughn Robedaux, ''Story of a Marriage Courtship,'' *American Playhouse,* PBS, 1987. Movies: Agnes Wood, ''Roanoak,'' *American Playhouse,* PBS, 1986; Mary Margaret Dutton, *The Little Match Girl,* NBC, 1987.

MEMBER: Actors' Equity Association, Screen Actors Guild, American Federation of Television and Radio Artists.*

*   *   *

FORD, Ruth   1915-

PERSONAL: Full name, Ruth Elizabeth Ford; born July 7, 1915, in Hazelhurst, MS; daughter of Charles Lloyd (in the hotel business) and Gertrude (a painter; maiden name, Cato) Ford; married Peter Van Eyck (an actor), 1941 (divorced); married Zachary Scott (an actor), July 6, 1952 (died, 1965); children: one daughter (first marriage). EDUCATION: Attended All Saint's Episcopal Junior College and Mississippi State College for Women; received B.A. and M.A., philosophy, from the University of Mississippi.

VOCATION: Actress.

CAREER: STAGE DEBUT—Nanny, *Ways and Means,* Ivoryton Players, Ivoryton Playhouse, Ivoryton, CT, 1937. BROADWAY DEBUT—Jane, *The Shoemaker's Holiday,* Mercury Theatre, 1938. LONDON DEBUT—Mrs. Gowan Stevens (Temple Drake), *Requi-*

em for a Nun, Royal Court Theatre, 1957. PRINCIPAL STAGE APPEARANCES—Judy, *Idiot's Delight,* fourth Athenian woman, *Lysistrata,* first lady, *Dead End,* Lois Fisher, *The Children's Hour,* and Mildred, *The Jazz Age,* all Ivoryton Players, Ivoryton Playhouse, Ivoryton, CT, 1937; Rosalie, *Danton's Death,* Mercury Theatre, New York City, 1938; the Bridesmaid, *Trial by Jury,* the Lady, *The Dark Lady of the Sonnets,* Desdemona, *Othello,* Stella Cartwright, *Ways and Means,* Lady Maureen Gilpin, *Hands Across the Sea,* Mrs. Omar Dobbs, *The Best Dressed Woman in the World,* and Suzy Courtois, *Topaz,* all Green Mansions Theatre, Warrensburg, NY, 1939; Polly, *Swingin' the Dream,* City Center Theatre, New York City, 1939; Irma Szabo, *The Glass Slipper,* Barbizon-Plaza Theatre, New York City, 1940; Estelle, *No Exit,* Biltmore Theatre, New York City, 1946; Maggie, *The Man Who Came to Dinner,* Westport Country Playhouse, Westport, CT, 1947; Yolan, *This Time Tomorrow,* Ethel Barrymore Theatre, New York City, 1947; Ophelia, *Hamlet,* Kronberg Castle, Elsinore, Denmark, 1949; Deborah Pomfret, *Clutterbuck,* Elitch Gardens Theatre, Denver, CO, then Biltmore Theatre, both 1949; Estelle, *No Exit,* and the Stepdaughter, *Six Characters in Search of an Author,* both Brattle Theatre, Cambridge, MA, 1950; Martirio, *The House of Bernarda Alba,* American National Theatre and Academy Theatre, New York City, 1951; Lady Macbeth, *Macbeth,* and Dynamene, *A Phoenix Too Frequent,* both Brattle Theatre, 1951; Sally Bowles, *I Am a Camera,* Brattle Theatre, 1953; the Patient, *Too True to Be Good,* Playhouse in the Park, Philadelphia, PA, 1954; Sabina, *The Skin of Our Teeth,* Boston Commons Arts Festival, Boston, MA, 1955; Pia, *Island of Goats,* Fulton Theatre, New York City, 1955; Mrs. X, *The Stronger,* and Kristin, *Miss Julie,* both Phoenix Theatre, New York City, 1956; Mrs. Gowan Stevens (Temple Drake), *Requiem for a Nun,* John Golden Theatre, New York City, 1959.

The Nun, *The Umbrella,* and Mommy, *The American Dream,* both Festival of Two Worlds, Spoleto, Italy, 1963; Vera Ridgeway Condotti, *The Milk Train Doesn't Stop Here Anymore,* Brooks Atkinson Theatre, New York City, 1964; Virginia Varnum, *Lovey,* Cherry Lane Theatre, New York City, 1965; Hattie Loomis, *Dinner at Eight,* Alvin Theatre, New York City, 1966; Judith Hastings, *The Ninety-Day Mistress,* Biltmore Theatre, 1967; Aunt Adelaide, *Hunger and Thirst,* Berkshire Theatre Festival, Stockbridge, MA, 1969; Verena Talbo, *The Grass Harp,* Martin Beck Theatre, New York City, 1971; Comtesse de Saint-Fond, *Madame de Sade,* Theatre De Lys, New York City, 1972; Lorraine, *A Breeze from the Gulf,* Eastside Playhouse, New York City, then Bucks County Playhouse, New Hope, PA, both 1973; Clarissa Halley-Yshott, *The Charlatan,* Mark Taper Forum, Los Angeles, CA, 1974; third actress, voluptuous mistress, Irina Pavlovna Kurganova, and Countess Byelitskaya, *Poor Murderer,* Ethel Barrymore Theatre, 1976; Madame Arkadina, *The Seagull,* Goodman Theatre, Chicago, IL, 1977; Juliana Bordereau, *The Aspern Papers,* McCarter Theatre, Princeton, NJ, 1978; Mrs. Chasen, *Harold and Maude,* Martin Beck Theatre, 1980; Kathy, *Confluence,* Circle Repertory Company, New York City, 1981; Claire Zachanassian, *The Visit,* Alley Theatre, Houston, TX, 1982. Also appeared as Mrs. Billings, *Too Much Johnson,* Stoney Creek, CT, 1939; in *Interesting Experiment,* Green Mansions Theatre, 1939; as Matilda Rockley, *You Touched Me,* Mt. Kisco, NY, 1946; as Laetitia, *Children of Darkness,* summer theatre production, 1948; in *The Heiress, The Winslow Boy, Twentieth Century,* and *The Traitor,* all Elitch Gardens Theatre, 1949; in *The Failures,* Brattle Theatre, 1951; in *The Shewing Up of Blanco Posnet* and *The Apollo of Bellac,* both Westport Country Playhouse, 1954; as Dorothy Cleves, *Any Wednesday,* Coconut Grove, FL, and Miami, FL, both 1965; and in *Outward Bound,* Apple Corps Theatre, New York City, 1984.

MAJOR TOURS—Roxanne, *Cyrano de Bergerac*, U.S. cities, 1946; also in *The Button*, U.S. cities, 1970.

FILM DEBUT—*Roaring Frontiers*, Columbia, 1941. PRINCIPAL FILM APPEARANCES—Helene de Leon, *Secrets of the Lone Wolf* (also known as *Secrets*), Columbia, 1941; secretary, *Across the Pacific*, First National, 1942; Myrt, *Escape from Crime*, Warner Brothers, 1942; Janet Devon, *Gorilla Man*, Warner Brothers, 1942; Estelle, *The Hidden Hand*, Warner Brothers, 1942; young mother, *In This Our Life*, Warner Brothers, 1942; Myrtle, *The Lady Is Willing*, Columbia, 1942; Lucy Fenton, *Lady Gangster*, Warner Brothers, 1942; Beth Beebe, *The Man Who Returned to Life*, Columbia, 1942; Mrs. Gordon, *Murder in the Big House* (also known as *Human Sabotage* and *Born for Trouble*), Warner Brothers, 1942; Miss Charlton, *Secret Enemies*, Warner Brothers, 1942; Tess Torrence, *Adventures in Iraq*, Warner Brothers, 1943; nurse, *Air Force*, Warner Brothers, 1943; Lana Shane, *Murder on the Waterfront*, Warner Brothers, 1943; Claire Stillwell, *Princess O'Rourke*, Warner Brothers, 1943; Pearl, *Truck Busters*, Warner Brothers, 1943; Sister Clotilde, *The Keys of the Kingdom*, Twentieth Century-Fox, 1944; Mrs. Simms, *Circumstantial Evidence*, Twentieth Century-Fox, 1945; Ruth Gibson, *The Woman Who Came Back*, Republic, 1945; Cornelia Van Borden, *Dragonwyck*, Twentieth Century-Fox, 1946; Jane Karaski, *Strange Impersonation*, Republic, 1946; Beatrice Kaufman, *Act One*, Warner Brothers, 1964; Mrs. Gagnon, *The Tree*, Robert Guenette, 1969; Carlotta, *Play It As It Lays*, Universal, 1972; Irma, *Too Scared to Scream*, Movie Store, 1985. Also appeared in *The Devil's Trail*, Columbia, 1942; *Wilson*, Twentieth Century-Fox, 1944; *A Separate Peace*, Paramount, 1972; and *The Eyes of the Amaryllis*, 1982.

PRINCIPAL TELEVISION APPEARANCES—Episodic: *Cameo Theatre*, NBC.

RELATED CAREER—Photographer's model; consultant, Center for the Study of Southern Culture; advisory council, Circle Repertory Company, New York City.

WRITINGS: STAGE—(Adaptor) *Requiem for a Nun*, Royal Court Theatre, London, 1957.

AWARDS: London Drama Critics Award nomination, Best Actress of the Season, 1957, for *Requiem for a Nun*.

MEMBER: Actors' Equity Association, American Federation of Television and Radio Artists, Screen Actors Guild, Chi Omega (president, college chapter).

SIDELIGHTS: FAVORITE ROLES—Mrs. Gowan Stevens (Temple Drake) in *Requiem for a Nun*, Estelle in *No Exit*, and Lorraine in *A Breeze from the Gulf*. RECREATIONS—Reading, collecting art, talking, and listening to music.

ADDRESSES: HOME—1 W. 72nd Street, New York, NY, 10023.*

*   *   *

FORREST, Frederic   1936-

PERSONAL: Born December 23, 1936, in Waxahachie, TX. EDUCATION: Attended Texas Christian University and the University of Oklahoma; studied acting at the Actors Studio in New York City.

VOCATION: Actor.

CAREER: PRINCIPAL STAGE APPEARANCES—*Futz, Massachusetts Trust, Tom Paine*, and *Viet Rock*, all with the La Mama Experimental Theatre Club, New York City, 1965-69. Also appeared in *Silhouettes*, Los Angeles, CA, 1970; with the Fort Worth Community Theatre, Fort Worth, TX; the Alley Theatre, Houston, TX; and with the Center Stage, Baltimore, MD.

FILM DEBUT—*Futz*, Commonwealth United, 1969. PRINCIPAL FILM APPEARANCES—Tom Black Bull, *When the Legends Die*, Twentieth Century-Fox, 1972; Tony, *The Don Is Dead* (also known as *Beautiful but Deadly*), Universal, 1973; Rut, *The Gravy Train* (also known as *The Dion Brothers*), Columbia, 1974; Mark, *The Conversation*, Paramount, 1974; Scott Alexander, *Permission to Kill*, AVCO-Embassy, 1975; Cary, *The Missouri Breaks*, United Artists, 1976; Eugene Scott, *It Lives Again* (also known as *It's Alive II*), Warner Brothers, 1978; Hicks (the "Chef"), *Apocalypse Now*, United Artists, 1979; Dyer, *The Rose*, Twentieth Century-Fox, 1979; title role, *Hammett*, Warner Brothers, 1982; Hank, *One from the Heart*, Columbia, 1982; Steve Richman, *Valley Girl*, Atlantic Releasing, 1983; Andy Jansen, *The Stone Boy*, Twentieth Century-Fox, 1984; Brian Stoving, *Return*, Silver, 1986; Courtney Parrish, *Where Are the Children?*, Columbia, 1986; Buster McGuire, *Stacking* (also known as *Season of Dreams*), Spectrafilm, 1987; Eddie Dean, *Tucker: The Man and His Dream*, Paramount, 1988.

PRINCIPAL TELEVISION APPEARANCES—Series: Captain Jenko, *21 Jump Street*, Fox, 1987. Mini-Series: Blue Duck, *Lonesome Dove*, CBS, 1989. Movies: Larry Herman, *Larry*, CBS, 1974; Paul Hunter, *Promise Him Anything . . .*, ABC, 1975; Lee Harvey Oswald, *Ruby and Oswald*, CBS, 1978; Bob Chesneau, *Saigon—Year of the Cat*, Thames Television, 1983; Ivan Fray, *Who Will Love My Children?*, ABC, 1983; Blaise Dietz, *Best Kept Secrets*, ABC, 1984; Wild Bill Hickock, *Calamity Jane*, CBS, 1984; Richard Jahnke, Sr., *Right to Kill?*, ABC, 1985; Detective Bob Keppel, *The Deliberate Stranger*, NBC, 1986; Pap Finn, *The Adventures of Huckleberry Finn*, PBS, 1986; Tim Brady, *Little Girl Lost*, ABC, 1988; Raoul Schumacher, *Beryl Markham: A Shadow on the Sun*, CBS, 1988; Father George, *Gotham*, Showtime, 1988; Erskine Caldwell, *Margaret Bourke-White*, TNT, 1989; also *Quo Vadis*, Italian television.

AWARDS: Golden Globe Award nomination, 1972, for *When the Legends Die*; Academy Award nomination, Best Supporting Actor, 1979, for *The Rose*.

MEMBER: Actors' Equity Association, Screen Actors Guild, American Federation of Television and Radio Artists.*

*   *   *

FORREST, Steve   1925-

PERSONAL: Born William Forrest Andrews, September 29, 1925, in Huntsville, TX; wife's name, Cris; children: three sons. EDUCATION: Attended the University of California, Los Angeles, 1950.

VOCATION: Actor.

CAREER: FILM DEBUT—*The Geisha Girl*, Metro-Goldwyn-Mayer, 1951. PRINCIPAL FILM APPEARANCES—Sergeant, *Battle*

Circus, Metro-Goldwyn-Mayer (MGM), 1953; young man, *The Clown,* MGM, 1953; Louis, *Dream Wife,* MGM, 1953; Dirk DeJong, *So Big,* Warner Brothers, 1953; Lobo Naglaski, *Take the High Ground,* MGM, 1953; Professor Paul Dupin, *Phantom of the Rue Morgue,* Warner Brothers, 1954; Corporal Joseph Robert Stanton, *Prisoner of War,* MGM, 1954; Eddie Kelvaney, *Rogue Cop,* MGM, 1954; Gregory Fitzgerald, *Bedevilled,* MGM, 1955; Terry Matthews, *The Living Idol,* MGM, 1957; Larry Hall, *It Happened to Jane* (also known as *Twinkle and Shine*), Columbia, 1959; Sergeant Keller, *Five Branded Women,* Paramount, 1960; Clint Burton, *Flaming Star,* Twentieth Century-Fox, 1960; Clint Mabry, *Heller in Pink Tights,* Paramount, 1960; Dan Jones, *The Second Time Around,* Twentieth Century-Fox, 1961; Captain Harding, *The Longest Day,* Twentieth Century-Fox, 1962; Hub Wiley, *The Yellow Canary,* Twentieth Century-Fox, 1963; Willard North, *Rascal,* Buena Vista, 1969; Jim Hatch, *The Late Liz,* Gateway, 1971; Jim Tanner, *The Wild Country* (also known as *The Newcomers*), Buena Vista, 1971; Conrad Hunt, *North Dallas Forty,* Paramount, 1979; Greg Savitt, *Mommie Dearest,* Paramount, 1981; Rich Gordon, *Sahara,* Metro-Goldwyn-Mayer-United Artists, 1984; General Sline, *Spies Like Us,* Warner Brothers, 1985; Captain Nelson, *Amazon Women on the Moon,* Universal, 1987. Also appeared in *The Bad and the Beautiful,* MGM, 1952; *Man in a Looking Glass,* Twentieth Century-Fox, 1965; and *The Sagittarius Mine,* 1972.

PRINCIPAL TELEVISION APPEARANCES—Series: John "the Baron" Mannering, *The Baron,* ABC, 1966; Lieutenant Dan "Hondo" Harrelson, *S.W.A.T.,* ABC, 1975-76; Ben Stivers, *Dallas,* CBS, 1986—. Mini-Series: Martin Eaton, *Testimony of Two Men,* syndicated, 1977; James Kent, *The Manions of America,* ABC, 1981; Ross Conti, *Hollywood Wives,* ABC, 1981. Pilots: Jacks, *Honey West: Who Killed the Jackpot?,* ABC, 1965; Lou Brackett, *Captain America,* CBS, 1979; Rich Bradley, *Malibu,* ABC, 1983. Episodic: Robert Gaines, "The Parallel," *The Twilight Zone,* CBS, 1963; also *Ghost Story,* NBC, 1972; *Hec Ramsey,* NBC; *Bonanza,* NBC; *The Name of the Game,* NBC; *Gunsmoke,* CBS; *The Virginian,* NBC; *Kraft Suspense Theatre,* NBC; *Playhouse 90,* CBS; *Climax,* CBS; *Alfred Hitchcock Presents.* Movies: James Devlin, *The Hanged Man,* ABC, 1974; Randall McCoy, *The Hatfields and the McCoys,* ABC, 1975; Charlie Siringo, *Wanted: The Sundance Woman* (also known as *Mrs. Sundance Rides Again*), ABC, 1976; Hawkeye, *The Last of the Mohicans,* NBC, 1977; Hawkeye, *The Deerslayer,* NBC, 1978; David Birk, *Maneaters Are Loose,* CBS, 1978; Gus Garver, *Condominium,* syndicated, 1980; Paul Marshall, *Roughnecks,* syndicated, 1980; Colonel Atherton, *A Rumor of War,* CBS, 1980; Tom Hunter, *Hotline,* CBS, 1982; Mannon, *Gunsmoke: Return to Dodge City,* CBS, 1987. Specials: *Celebration: The American Spirit,* ABC, 1976; *ABC's Silver Anniversary Celebration—Twenty-Five and Still the One,* ABC, 1978; also *The Legend of Robin Hood,* 1968.

RELATED CAREER—Appeared on stage at the La Jolla Playhouse, La Jolla, CA, during the 1950s; also performed as a radio actor.

MEMBER: Actors' Equity Association, Screen Actors Guild, American Federation of Television and Radio Artists.

SIDELIGHTS: Steve Forrest is the brother of actor Dana Andrews.

ADDRESSES: AGENT—Michael Livingston, The Artists Agency, 10000 Santa Monica Boulevard, Suite 305, Los Angeles, CA 90067.*

FORSYTHE, John   1918-

PERSONAL: Born John Lincoln Freund, January 29, 1918, in Penn's Grove, NJ; son of Samuel Jeremiah (a stockbroker) and Blanche Materson (Blohm) Freund; married Parker McCormick (divorced); married Julie Warren (an actress), 1943; children: Dall (first marriage); Page, Brooke (second marriage). EDUCATION: Attended the University of North Carolina; trained for the stage at the Actors Studio.

VOCATION: Actor.

CAREER: STAGE DEBUT—Captain, *Dick Whittington and His Cat,* Clare Tree Major's Children's Theatre, Chappaqua, NY, 1939. BROADWAY DEBUT—Private Cootes, *Vickie,* Plymouth Theatre, 1942. PRINCIPAL STAGE APPEARANCES—Coast guardsman, *Yankee Point,* Longacre Theatre, New York City, 1942; ensemble, *Winged Victory* (revue), 44th Street Theatre, New York City, 1943; Chris Keller, *All My Sons,* Coronet Theatre, New York City, 1947; Bill Renault, *It Takes Two,* Biltmore Theatre, New York City, 1947; title role, *Mister Roberts,* Alvin Theatre, New York City, 1950; Captain Fisby, *The Teahouse of the August Moon,* Martin Beck Theatre, New York City, 1953; Detective McLeod, *Detective Story,* Westport Country Playhouse, Westport, CT, 1955; Senator MacGruder, *Weekend,* Broadhurst Theatre, New York City, 1968; Lieutenant Greenwald, *The Caine Mutiny Court Martial,* Ahmanson Theatre, Los Angeles, CA, 1971. Also appeared in *Yellowjack,* 44th Street Theatre, 1945; and *Woman Bites Dog,* Belasco Theatre, New York City, 1946.

PRINCIPAL STAGE WORK—Director, *Mister Roberts,* City Center Theatre, New York City, 1956.

MAJOR TOURS—Title role, *Mister Roberts,* U.S. cities, 1949-50.

PRINCIPAL FILM APPEARANCES—Soldier, *Northern Pursuit,* Warner Brothers, 1943; Sparks, *Destination Tokyo,* Warner Brothers, 1944; Jim Austin, *Captive City,* United Artists, 1952; Captain John Marsh, *Escape from Fort Bravo,* Metro-Goldwyn-Mayer, 1953; Don Newell, *The Glass Web,* Universal, 1953; Bob MacAvoy, *It Happens Every Thursday,* Universal, 1953; Sam Marlowe, *The Trouble with Harry,* Paramount, 1955; Danny, *The Ambassador's Daughter,* United Artists, 1956; Ernie Miller, *Everything but the Truth,* Universal, 1956; David Patton, *Kitten with a Whip,* Universal, 1964; Clay Anderson, *Madame X,* Universal, 1966; Alvin Dewey, *In Cold Blood,* Columbia, 1967; Fred Wilson, *The Happy Ending,* United Artists, 1969; Michael Nordstrom, *Topaz,* Universal, 1969; Judge Fleming, *. . . And Justice for All,* Columbia, 1979; Lew Hayward, *Scrooged,* Paramount, 1988.

PRINCIPAL TELEVISION APPEARANCES—Series: Bentley Gregg, *Bachelor Father,* CBS, 1957-58, then NBC, 1958-61, later ABC, 1961-62; Major John Foster, *The John Forsythe Show,* NBC, 1965-66; Michael Endicott, *To Rome with Love,* CBS, 1969-71; host and narrator, *The World of Survival,* syndicated, 1971-77, then 1987; voice of Charlie Townsend, *Charlie's Angels,* ABC, 1976-81; Blake Carrington, *Dynasty,* ABC, 1981-89. Pilots: Bentley Gregg, *New Girl in His Life* (broadcast as an episode of *The General Electric Theatre*), CBS, 1957; Dr. John Carter, *Belle Starr,* CBS, 1958; Andy Ballard, *Five, Six, Pick Up Sticks* (broadcast as an episode of *Alcoa Premiere*), NBC, 1963; Bill Adams, *The*

Miss and the *Missiles,* CBS, 1964; Paul Anderson, "The Andersons: Dear Elaine," *The Letters,* ABC, 1973; Dr. Robert Kier, *The Healers,* NBC, 1974; voice of Charlie Townsend, *Charlie's Angels,* ABC, 1976; E.J. Valerian, *The Feather and Father Gang: Never Con a Killer* (also known as *Never Con a Killer*), ABC, 1977; He, *The Mysterious Two,* NBC, 1982. Episodic: Blake Carrington, *The Colbys,* ABC, 1986; also *Magnavox Theatre,* CBS, 1950; *Cosmopolitan Theatre,* Dumont, 1951; *Danger,* CBS; *Curtain Call Theatre,* NBC, 1952; *Climax!,* CBS; *Light's Out,* NBC; *The Elgin Hour,* NBC; *Kraft Mystery Theatre,* NBC; *Ford Theatre Hour,* NBC; *Studio One,* CBS; *Philco Television Playhouse,* NBC; *Pulitzer Prize Playhouse,* ABC; *Schlitz Playhouse of Stars,* CBS; *Star Stage,* NBC; *Starlight Theatre,* CBS; "The Beach of Falsea," *Suspense,* CBS; *Zane Grey Theatre* (also known as *Dick Powell's Zane Grey Theatre*) CBS; *Robert Montgomery Presents,* NBC; and *Alfred Hitchcock Presents.*

Movies: General Wendell Bruce, *Shadow on the Land,* ABC, 1968; Dr. Ron Wellesley, *Murder Once Removed,* CBS, 1971; Dennis Ryder, *Cry Panic,* ABC, 1974; Daniel Overland, *Terror on the Fortieth Floor,* NBC, 1974; Lieutenant Elwood Forbes, *The Deadly Tower,* NBC, 1975; G.P. Putnam, *Amelia Earhart,* NBC, 1976; Paul Cunningham, *Tail Gunner Joe,* NBC, 1977; Reade Jamison, *The Users,* ABC, 1978; General Albert Harris, *With This Ring,* ABC, 1978; Reverend Charles Mather, *Cruise into Terror,* ABC, 1978; Postulator, *A Time for Miracles,* ABC, 1980; Mike Callahan, *Sizzle,* ABC, 1981; Joe Leary, *On Fire,* ABC, 1987; also *See How They Run,* 1964; and *Wuthering Heights.* Specials: Keith Burgess, *Stage Door,* NBC, 1948; Captain Fishby, *The Teahouse of the August Moon,* NBC, 1962; Victor Joppolo, *A Bell for Adano,* NBC, 1967; co-host, *The Light Fantastic, or How to Tell Your Past, Present, and Maybe Your Future through Social Dancing,* ABC, 1967; William Schilling, "Lisa, Bright and Dark," *Hallmark Hall of Fame,* NBC, 1973; host, *Circus of the Stars,* CBS, 1977; Niles Putnam, "Emily, Emily," *Hallmark Hall of Fame,* NBC, 1977; *ABC's Silver Anniversary Celebration—Twenty-Five and Still the One,* ABC, 1978; *Dom DeLuise and Friends,* ABC, 1983; *Bob Hope's Merry Christmas Show,* NBC, 1983; host, *George Burns Celebrates Eighty Years in Show Business,* NBC, 1983; *The Dean Martin Celebrity Roast,* NBC, 1984; *ABC All Star Spectacular,* ABC, 1985; host, *Disneyland's Thirtieth Anniversary Celebration,* NBC, 1985; host, *People's Choice Awards,* CBS, 1985; *The American Film Institute Salute to Billy Wilder,* NBC, 1986; host, *Tears of Joy, Tears of Sorrow,* ABC, 1986; *Christmas in Washington,* NBC, 1986; *Kraft Salutes George Burns' Ninetieth Birthday Special,* CBS, 1986; *The American Film Institute Salute to Barbara Stanwyck,* ABC, 1987; *America's Tribute to Bob Hope,* NBC, 1988; *Happy Birthday, Bob—Fifty Stars Salute Your Fifty Years with NBC,* NBC, 1988; *The Seventy-Fifth Anniversary of Beverly Hills* (also known as *Beverly Hills Seventy-Fifth Diamond Jubilee*), ABC, 1989.

PRINCIPAL TELEVISION WORK—Movies: Executive producer, *On Fire,* ABC, 1987.

RELATED CAREER—Public address announcer for the Brooklyn Dodgers, Ebbets Field, Brooklyn, NY; host, Hollywood Park Feature Race, 1971-74; appeared on radio soap operas.

SIDELIGHTS: RECREATIONS—Sailing, music, and painting.

ADDRESSES: OFFICE—11560 Bellagio Road, Los Angeles, CA 90049. MANAGER—Josh Baser, Charter Management, 9000 Sunset Boulevard, Suite 308, Beverly Hills, CA 90069.*

FOSTER, Jodie   1962-

PERSONAL: Born Alicia Christian Foster, November 19, 1962, in Los Angeles, CA; daughter of Lucius III (an Air Force officer) and Evelyn "Brandy" (a personal manager; maiden name, Almond) Foster. EDUCATION: Yale University, B.A., literature, 1985.

VOCATION: Actress.

CAREER: FILM DEBUT—Samantha, *Napoleon and Samantha,* Buena Vista, 1972. PRINCIPAL FILM APPEARANCES—Rita, *Kansas City Bomber,* Metro-Goldwyn-Mayer, 1972; Martha, *One Little Indian,* Buena Vista, 1973; Becky Thatcher, *Tom Sawyer,* United Artists, 1973; Audrey, *Alice Doesn't Live Here Anymore,* Warner Brothers, 1975; Tallulah, *Bugsy Malone,* Paramount, 1976; Deirdre Striden, *Echoes of a Summer* (also known as *The Last Castle*), Cine Artists, 1976; Annabel Andrews, *Freaky Friday,* Buena Vista, 1976; Iris Steensman, *Taxi Driver,* Columbia, 1976; Rynn Jacobs, *The Little Girl Who Lives Down the Lane,* American International, 1977; Fleur Bleue, *Moi, fleur bleue* (also known as *Stop Calling Me Baby!*), Megalo/CIC, 1978; Casey Brown, *Candleshoe,* Buena Vista, 1978; Donna, *Carny,* United Artists, 1980; Jeanie, *Foxes,* United Artists, 1980; Tersina, *Il cassota* (also known as *The Beach House*), Medusa Distribuzione, 1980; Barbara O'Hara, *O'Hara's Wife,* Davis-Panzer, 1983; Helene, *Les Sang des autres* (also known as *The Blood of Others*), Parafrance/Prism, 1984; Franny Berry, *The Hotel New Hampshire,* Orion, 1984; Victoria, *Mesmerized,* Thorn-EMI, 1984; Nancy, *Siesta,* Lorimar, 1987; Linda, *Five Corners,* Cineplex Odeon, 1987; Sarah Tobias, *The Accused,* Paramount, 1988; Katie Chandler, *Stealing Home,* Warner Brothers, 1988. Also appeared in *Menace on the Mountain,* Buena Vista, 1973.

PRINCIPAL FILM WORK—Co-producer, *Mesmerized,* Thorn-EMI, 1984; also director, "Hands on Time" in *Americans* (documentary), Time-Life/BBC.

TELEVISION DEBUT—*Mayberry, R.F.D.,* CBS, 1969. PRINCIPAL TELEVISION APPEARANCES—Series: Voice of Anne Chan, *The Amazing Chan and the Chan Clan* (animated), CBS, 1972; Elizabeth Henderson, *Bob and Carol and Ted and Alice,* ABC, 1973; voice of Pugsley Addams, *The Addams Family* (animated), NBC, 1973-75; Addie Pray, *Paper Moon,* ABC, 1974-75. Pilots: Henrietta "Hank" Bennett, *My Sister Hank,* CBS, 1972; Liberty Cole, *Smile Jenny, You're Dead,* ABC, 1974. Episodic: Host, *Saturday Night Live,* NBC, 1976; also Julie Lawrence, *The Partridge Family,* ABC; Joey Kelley, *The Courtship of Eddie's Father,* ABC; Priscilla, *My Three Sons,* CBS; *Ghost Story,* NBC, 1972; *Love Story,* NBC, 1973; *Who's Who,* CBS, 1977; *Sam,* CBS, 1978; *Ironside,* NBC; *Daniel Boone,* NBC; *The Wonderful World of Disney,* NBC; *Adam-12,* NBC; *Julia,* NBC; *Gunsmoke,* CBS; *Kung Fu,* ABC; *Bonanza,* NBC. Movies: Zoe Alexander, *Svengali,* CBS, 1983; Helene Bertrand, *The Blood of Others,* HBO, 1984. Specials: Sharon Lee, "Rookie of the Year," *ABC Afterschool Special,* ABC, 1973; Sue, "Alexander," *ABC Afterschool Special,* ABC, 1973; title role, "The Secret Life of T.K. Dearing," *ABC Weekend Special,* ABC, 1975.

RELATED CAREER—Actress in television commercials from the age of three; original "Coppertone Girl" character in ads for suntan lotion.

WRITINGS: FILM—"Hands on Time" in *Americans* (documentary), Time-Life/BBC. Also wrote article "Why Me?," *Esquire,* 1982.

AWARDS: Emmy Award, 1973, for "Rookie of the Year," *ABC Afterschool Special;* National Film Critics Award, Los Angeles Film Critics Award, David Di Donatello Award, Academy Award nomination, and New York Film Critics Award nomination, all Best Supporting Actress, 1976, for *Taxi Driver;* British Academy Awards, Best Supporting Actress and Most Promising Newcomer to Leading Film Roles, both 1976, for *Taxi Driver* and *Bugsy Malone;* Italian Situation Comedy Award, 1976, for *Bugsy Malone;* Golden Globe Award, Best Actress in a Motion Picture Drama, and Academy Award, Best Actress, both 1989, for *The Accused.*

ADDRESSES: AGENT—International Creative Management, 8899 Beverly Boulevard, Los Angeles, CA 90048.*

*   *   *

FOSTER, Meg   1948-

PERSONAL: Born May 10, 1948, in Connecticut. EDUCATION: Studied acting at the Neighborhood Playhouse in New York City.

VOCATION: Actress.

CAREER: PRINCIPAL STAGE APPEARANCES—Olga, *The Three Sisters,* Los Angeles Theatre Center, Los Angeles, CA, 1986. Also appeared in *Extremities,* Los Angeles Public Theatre, Los Angeles, CA, 1983.

PRINCIPAL FILM APPEARANCES—Joyce, *Adam at 6 A.M.,* National General, 1970; Chay, *Thumb Tripping,* AVCO-Embassy, 1972; Robbin Stanley, *Tender Flesh* (also known as *Welcome to Arrow Beach*), Warner Brothers, 1976; Stella, *A Different Story,* AVCO-Embassy, 1978; Gerta, *Carny,* United Artists, 1980; Ingrid, *Ticket to Heaven,* United Artists, 1981; Ali Tanner, *The Osterman Weekend,* Twentieth Century-Fox, 1983; Jean Markham, *The Emerald Forest,* Embassy, 1985; Evil Lyn, *Masters of the Universe,* Cannon, 1987; Sian Anderson, *The Wind,* Omega, 1987; Holly, *They Live,* Universal, 1988. Also appeared in *The Todd Killings* (also known as *A Dangerous Friend* and *Skipper*), National General, 1971; and *Riding Fast,* Transcontinental Pictures Industries, 1986.

PRINCIPAL TELEVISION APPEARANCES—Series: Nora, *Sunshine,* NBC, 1975; Detective Chris Cagney, *Cagney and Lacey,* CBS, 1982. Mini-Series: Jennie Jamison, *Washington: Behind Closed Doors,* ABC, 1977; Hester Prynne, *The Scarlet Letter,* PBS, 1979. Episodic: Del Scott, *Murder, She Wrote,* CBS, 1986; also "Dreams for Sale, *The Twilight Zone,* CBS, 1986; *Miami Vice,* NBC, 1987; "Blood and Roses," *Miami Vice,* NBC, 1988; and "The Martyr," *The Hitchhiker,* USA Network, 1989. Movies: Alice, *The Death of Me Yet,* ABC, 1971; Nora, *Sunshine,* CBS, 1973; Judy Pines, *Things in Their Season,* CBS, 1974; Marjorie Sherman, *Promise Him Anything . . .,* ABC, 1975; Dizzy Sheridan, *James Dean,* NBC, 1976; Nora, *Sunshine Christmas,* NBC, 1977; Katrina Van Tassel, *The Legend of Sleepy Hollow,* NBC, 1980; Jean Ritchie, *Guyana Tragedy: The Story of Jim Jones,* CBS, 1980; Joanna Walcott, *Desperate Intruder,* syndicated, 1983; Shari Mitchell, *Best Kept Secrets,* ABC, 1984; Dorymai, *Desperate,* ABC, 1987.

MEMBER: Actors' Equity Association, Screen Actors Guild, American Federation of Television and Radio Artists.

ADDRESSES: AGENT—STE Representation, Ltd., 888 Seventh Avenue, New York, NY 10019.*

*   *   *

FOX, Edward   1937-

PERSONAL: Born April 13, 1937, in London, England; son of Robin (a theatrical agent) and Angela Fox; married Tracy Pelissier (marriage ended); second wife's name, Joanna; children: one daughter (first marriage); one daughter (second marriage). EDUCATION: Attended the Royal Academy of Dramatic Art.

VOCATION: Actor.

CAREER: PRINCIPAL STAGE APPEARANCES—Faulkland, *The Rivals,* Chichester Festival Theatre, Chichester, U.K., 1971; Curly, *Knuckle,* Comedy Theatre, London, 1974; Iago, *Othello,* New Shakespeare Company, Regent's Park Open Air Theatre, London, 1976; Harry, Lord Monchensey, *The Family Reunion,* Royal Exchange Theatre, Manchester, U.K., then Round House Theatre, London, later Vaudeville Theatre, London, all 1979. Also appeared in *Anyone for Denis* and *Quartermaine's Terms,* both 1981; *Hamlet,* 1982; and *The Dance of Death,* 1983.

PRINCIPAL FILM APPEARANCES—Stewart, *The Mind Benders,* American International, 1963; prisoner number three, *The Frozen Dead,* Warner Brothers, 1967; Walter, *I'll Never Forget What's 'is Name,* Universal, 1967; Lieutenant Sprague, *The Jokers,* Universal, 1967; Hardwicke, *The Long Duel,* Rank-Lippert/Paramount, 1967; Ritchie Jackson, *The Naked Runner,* Warner Brothers, 1967; Pilot Officer Archie, *The Battle of Britain,* United Artists, 1969; aide, *Oh! What a Lovely War,* Paramount, 1969; Bruce Spofford, *Skullduggery,* Universal, 1970; Hugh Trimingham, *The Go-Between,* Metro-Goldwyn-Mayer/EMI/Columbia, 1971; "the Jackal," *The Day of the Jackal,* Universal, 1973; Krogstad, *A Doll's House,* World Film Services, 1973; Cardinal Inquisitor, *Galileo,* American Film Theatre, 1975; Lieutenant General Brian Horrocks, *A Bridge Too Far,* United Artists, 1977; Colonel Reynard, *The Duellists,* Paramount, 1977; Foreman, *The Squeeze,* Warner Brothers, 1977; Joe Brody, *The Big Sleep,* United Artists, 1978; Sergeant "Milly" Miller, *Force 10 from Navarone,* American International, 1978; Hendricks, *The Cat and the Canary,* Cinema Shares, 1979; Colonel Rafelli, *Soldier of Orange,* Rank/International Picture Show, 1979; Inspector Craddock, *The Mirror Crack'd,* Associated Film Distributors, 1980; A.T.A.C. man, *Nighthawks,* Universal, 1981; General Dyer, *Gandhi,* Columbia, 1982; Oxenby, *The Dresser,* Columbia, 1983; M, *Never Say Never Again,* Warner Brothers, 1983; Captain Greetham, *The Bounty,* Orion, 1984; Lord Gilbert Harlip, *The Shooting Party,* European Classics, 1985; Alex Faulkner, *Wild Geese II,* Universal, 1985. Also appeared in *Journey into Midnight,* Twentieth Century-Fox, 1968.

PRINCIPAL TELEVISION APPEARANCES—Mini-Series: Captain Harthouse, "Hard Times," *Great Performances,* PBS, 1977; Edward VIII, *Edward and Mrs. Simpson,* PBS, 1978; Lord Francis George Farewell, *Shaka Zulu,* Fox, 1987. Movies: Dr. Hauser, *Anastasia: The Mystery of Anna,* NBC, 1986; Lord Harry Wortham, *A Hazard of Hearts,* CBS, 1987. Plays: St. John Quartermaine, *Quartermaine's Terms,* PBS, 1987; also *A Midsummer Night's Dream,* 1971; *The School for Scandal,* 1974. Specials: "Shooting the Chandelier," *Great Performances,* PBS, 1978. Also appeared in *Portrait of a Lady,* 1958; *The Bachelors,* 1968; *The Case of the*

Rat Man, 1972; *The Darkwater Hall Mystery*, 1974; *Loyalties*, 1975; *Centre Play*, 1975; and in *Sign of the Bounty, The Voysey Inheritance, The Ragged Trousered Philanthropists,* and *The Girl of My Dreams.*

SIDELIGHTS: RECREATIONS—Piano.

ADDRESSES: AGENT—Michael Whitehall, 125 Gloucester Road, London SW7 4TE, England.*

*   *   *

FRANK, Judy   1936-

PERSONAL: Born November 26, 1936, in Cincinnati, OH; daughter of Norris Clinton (a claims manager) and Laura J. (a teacher; maiden name, Stowe) Frank; married Mike Mearian (an actor), May 28, 1970. EDUCATION: Received A.B. from Indiana University; received M.F.A. from Yale University.

VOCATION: Actress and writer.

CAREER: BROADWAY DEBUT—Mary and Tiffany, *Mary, Mary,* Helen Hayes Theatre, 1962. PRINCIPAL STAGE APPEARANCES— Madame Pace, *Six Characters in Search of an Author,* Martinique Theatre, New York City, 1963; Emily Wellspot, *Xmas in Las Vegas,* Ethel Barrymore Theatre, New York City, 1965; Eugenie Selden, *Now Is the Time for All Good Men,* Theatre De Lys, New York City, 1967; Mrs. Culver, *The Constant Wife,* Equity Library

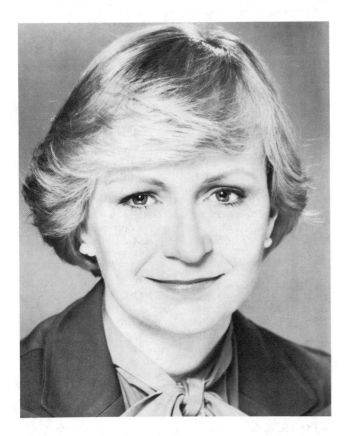

JUDY FRANK

Theatre, New York City, 1986. Also appeared as Jackie, *Find Your Way Home,* Production Company, New York City; title role, *Edie's Home,* Manhattan Theatre Club, New York City; Lady Macbeth, *Macbeth,* and Princess of Pompiona, *Knight of the Burning Pestle,* both McCarter Theatre, Princeton, NJ; Mae, *Once in a Lifetime,* Desdemona, *Othello,* and Young Queen, *Becket,* all Williamstown Theatre Festival, Williamstown, MA; Gloria, *Is the Real You Really You?,* Lambs' Theatre, New York City; Clare, *There's a Girl in My Soup,* and Smitty, *How to Succeed in Business without Really Trying,* both Playhouse on the Mall, NJ.

MAJOR TOURS—Mary and Tiffany, *Mary, Mary,* U.S. cities, 1962-63; also various roles, *Spoon River Anthology,* U.S. cities; Gloria, *Is the Real You Really You?,* U.S. cities; Smitty, *How to Succeed in Business without Really Trying,* U.S. cities.

PRINCIPAL TELEVISION APPEARANCES—Episodic: Janet Gordon and Mrs. McMartin, *Search for Tomorrow,* CBS.

RELATED CAREER—Appeared in a nightclub act in New York City.

WRITINGS: Two Ways about It, Dial Press, 1979; *Someone Slightly Different,* Dial Press, 1980.

AWARDS: Breadloaf Fellowship, 1980.

MEMBER: Actors' Equity Association, American Federation of Television and Radio Artists, Screen Actors Guild.

ADDRESSES: AGENT—Don Buchwald and Associates, 10 E. 44th Street, New York, NY 10017.

*   *   *

FRANKLIN, Bonnie   1944-

PERSONAL: Full name, Bonnie Gail Franklin; born January 6, 1944, in Santa Monica, CA; daughter of Samuel Benjamin (an investment banker) and Claire (Hersch) Franklin; married Ron Sossi, March, 1967 (divorced, 1970); married Marvin Minoff (a producer), August 31, 1980. EDUCATION: Attended Smith College, 1961-63; University of California, Los Angeles, B.A., 1966.

VOCATION: Actress and director.

CAREER: STAGE DEBUT—Viola, *Your Own Thing,* Marines Memorial Theatre, San Francisco, CA, 1968. OFF-BROADWAY DEBUT—Viola, *Your Own Thing,* Orpheum Theatre, 1968. PRINCIPAL STAGE APPEARANCES—Ruby, *Dames at Sea,* Theatre De Lys, New York City, 1969; Bonnie, *Applause,* Palace Theatre, New York City, 1970; title role, *Peter Pan,* Studio Arena Theatre, Buffalo, NY, 1972; Frankie, *Frankie and Johnny in the Clair de Lune,* Westside Arts Theatre, New York City, 1988. Also appeared in "Applause" segment, *Parade of Stars Playing the Palace,* Palace Theatre, New York City, 1983; in *Happy Birthday and Other Humiliations,* New York City, 1987; *Annie Get Your Gun,* Bucks County Playhouse, New Hope, PA, 1988; in productions of *A Thousand Clowns, George M, Carousel,* and *The Owl and the Pussycat,* and in regional theatre in Massachusetts and Ohio, 1972-74.

PRINCIPAL FILM APPEARANCES—Betty, *The Kettles in the Ozarks,*

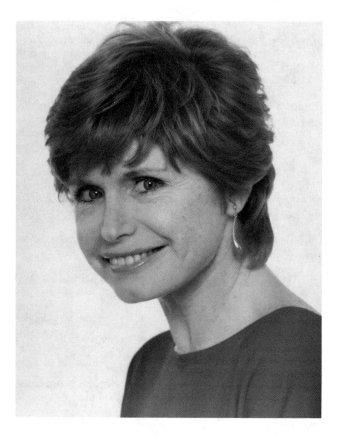

BONNIE FRANKLIN

Universal, 1956; young girl, *The Wrong Man*, Warner Brothers, 1956; young girl in dormitory, *A Summer Place*, Warner Brothers, 1959.

PRINCIPAL TELEVISION APPEARANCES—Series: Ann Romano, *One Day at a Time*, CBS, 1975-84. Episodic: Guest host, *Take Two*, Cable News Network, 1988; also *The Mary Tyler Moore Hour*, CBS, 1979; *The Comedy Zone*, CBS, 1984; as Janie Carmichael, *Gidget*, ABC; Janice, *The Munsters*, CBS; Stacey Stubing Scoggsstaad, *The Love Boat*, ABC; and in *Please Don't Eat the Daisies*, NBC. Movies: Bobbie Stone, *The Law*, NBC, 1974; Shirley, *A Guide for the Married Woman*, ABC, 1978; Gail Tobin, *Breaking Up Is Hard to Do*, ABC, 1979; title role, *Portrait of a Rebel: Margaret Sanger*, CBS, 1980; Alexandra, *Your Place or Mine*, CBS, 1983; Sister Margaret, *Sister Margaret and the Saturday Night Ladies*, CBS, 1987. Specials: A child, *A Christmas Carol*, CBS, 1954; *CBS: On the Air*, CBS, 1978; *Dean Martin Celebrity Roast: Betty White*, NBC, 1978; *Hanna-Barbera's All Star Comedy*, CBS, 1978; *National Love, Sex, and Marriage Test*, NBC, 1978; *The Bob Hope Christmas Special*, NBC, 1979; host, *Musical Comedy Tonight*, PBS, 1981; *Bob Hope's Women I Love—Beautiful But Funny*, NBC, 1982; *Bonnie and the Franklins*, CBS, 1982; *Parade of Stars*, ABC, 1983; *Happy Birthday Hollywood*, ABC, 1987; *Shalom Sesame*, PBS, 1988; *Drug Free Kids: A Parent's Guide*, PBS, 1988.

PRINCIPAL TELEVISION WORK—All as director. Episodic: *One Day at a Time*, CBS, 1983 and 1984; *Karen's Song*, Fox, 1987; also *Charles in Charge*, syndicated; *The Munsters Today*, syndicated.

RELATED CAREER—Child tap-dancer and actress; protege of

Donald O'Connor; created and appeared in *Let's Tap* (tap-dance video), Lorimar, 1985.

NON-RELATED CAREER—Spokesperson, Save the Children, for five years; honorary chair, National Committee of Arts with the Handicapped.

AWARDS: Theatre World Award, Outer Critics' Circle Award, Aegis Theatre Club Award, and Antoinette Perry Award nomination, Best Supporting or Featured Actress in a Musical, all 1970, for *Applause;* Emmy Award nomination for *One Day at a Time;* Torch of Liberty Award from the Anti-Defamation League of B'nai B'rith, 1983; Women of Achievement Award from "Women For," 1985; Women of Achievement Award from the Anti-Defamation League, 1987.

MEMBER: Actors' Equity Association, Screen Actors Guild, American Federation of Television and Radio Artists, Directors Guild of America.

ADDRESSES: AGENT—Creative Artists Agency, 1888 Century Park E., Suite 1400, Los Angeles, CA 90067. PUBLICIST—Lemack and Company Public Relations, 7060 Hollywood Boulevard, Suite 320, Los Angeles, CA 90028.

*   *   *

FRANZ, Dennis   1944-

PERSONAL: Born October 28, 1944, in Maywood, IL.

VOCATION: Actor.

CAREER: PRINCIPAL STAGE APPEARANCES—Zig, *Bleacher Bums*, Performing Garage, then American Place Theatre, both New York City, 1978; Earl MacMillan, *Brothers*, South Coast Repertory Theatre, Costa Mesa, CA, 1983.

PRINCIPAL FILM APPEARANCES—Bob, *The Fury*, Twentieth Century-Fox, 1978; Franks, *Remember My Name*, Columbia, 1978; Jerry Domino, *Stony Island* (also known as *My Main Man from Stony Island*), World-Northal, 1978; Koons, *A Wedding*, Twentieth Century-Fox, 1978; Costa, *A Perfect Couple*, Twentieth Century-Fox, 1979; Detective Marino, *Dressed to Kill*, Filmways, 1980; Spike, *Popeye*, Paramount, 1980; Manny Karp, *Blow Out*, Filmways, 1981; Toomey, *Psycho II*, Universal, 1983; Rubin, *Body Double*, Columbia, 1984; Phil, *A Fine Mess*, Columbia, 1986.

PRINCIPAL TELEVISION APPEARANCES—Series: Officer Joe Gilland, *Chicago Story*, NBC, 1982; Angelo Carbone, *Bay City Blues*, NBC, 1983; Lieutenant Norman Buntz, *Hill Street Blues*, NBC, 1985-87; Norman Buntz, *Beverly Hills Buntz*, NBC, 1987-88. Pilots: Officer Joe Gilland, *Chicago Story*, NBC, 1981; also *Scene of the Crime*, NBC, 1984. Episodic: "Bad Sal" Benedetto, *Hill Street Blues*, NBC, 1982-83. Movies: Detective Max Lucas, *Deadly Messages*, ABC, 1985. Specials: *America Talks Back*, NBC, 1986; Louie, "Tales from the Hollywood Hills: Pat Hobby Teamed with Genius," *Great Performances*, PBS, 1987.

MEMBER: Actors' Equity Association, Screen Actors Guild, American Federation of Television and Radio Artists.

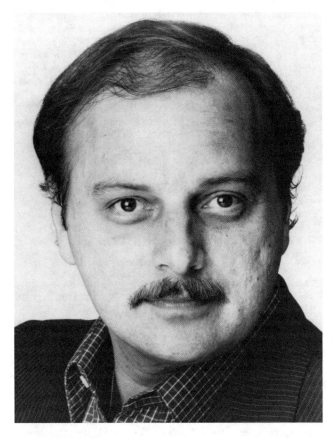

DENNIS FRANZ

ADDRESSES: AGENTS—Judith Nef Moss and Jack Fields, Gores-Fields Agency, 10100 Santa Monica Boulevard, Suite 700, Los Angeles, CA 90067. PUBLICIST—Cynthia Snyder Public Relations, 3518 Cahuenga Boulevard W., Suite 304, Los Angeles, CA 90068.

*　　*　　*

FREEMAN, Al, Jr. 1934-

PERSONAL: Full name, Albert Cornelius Freeman, Jr.; born March 21, 1934, in San Antonio, TX; son of Albert Cornelius (a jazz pianist) and Lottie Brisette (Coleman) Freeman; married Sevara E. Clemon, January 8, 1960. EDUCATION: Attended Los Angeles City College, 1951, then 1954-57; trained for the stage with Jeff Corey, Harold Clifton, and Frank Silvera. MILITARY: U.S. Air Force, 1951-54.

VOCATION: Actor, director, producer, and screenwriter.

CAREER: Also see *WRITINGS* below. STAGE DEBUT—*Detective Story,* Ebony Showcase, Los Angeles, CA, 1954. BROADWAY DEBUT—Rex "Fishbelly" Tucker, *The Long Dream,* Ambassador Theatre, 1960. LONDON DEBUT—Richard Henry, *Blues for Mister Charlie,* Actors Studio Theatre Company, World Theatre Season, Aldwych Theatre, 1965. PRINCIPAL STAGE APPEARANCES—Silky Satin, *Kicks and Co.,* Arie Crown Theatre, Chicago, IL, 1961; Dan Morris, *Tiger, Tiger, Burning Bright,* Booth Theatre,

New York City, 1962; Reverend Ridgley Washington, *Trumpets of the Lord,* Astor Place Theatre, New York City, 1963; ensemble, *The Living Premise* (revue), Premise Theatre, New York City, 1963; Richard Henry, *Blues for Mister Charlie,* American National Theatre and Academy Theatre, New York City, 1964; John, *Conversation at Midnight,* Billy Rose Theatre, New York City, 1964; Walker Vessels, *The Slave,* St. Mark's Playhouse, New York City, 1964; Eddie Satin, *Golden Boy,* Majestic Theatre, New York City, 1964; Clay, *Dutchman,* Cherry Lane Theatre, New York City, 1964, then Warner Playhouse, Los Angeles, CA, 1965; Diomedes, *Troilus and Cressida,* New York Shakespeare Festival (NYSF), Delacorte Theatre, New York City, 1965; Charles Dumaine, *All's Well That Ends Well,* and Lucio, *Measure for Measure,* both NYSF, Delacorte Theatre, 1966; Kilroy, *Camino Real,* Playhouse in the Park, Cincinnati, OH, 1968; Stanley Pollack, *The Dozens,* Booth Theatre, 1969.

Homer Smith, *Look to the Lilies,* Lunt-Fontanne Theatre, New York City, 1970; Paul Robeson, *Are You Now or Have You Ever Been . . . ?,* Yale Repertory Theatre, New Haven, CT, 1972; messenger, *Medea,* Circle in the Square, New York City, 1973; Willy Stepp, *The Poison Tree,* Westport Country Playhouse, Westport, CT, 1973; Scag, Photographer, Skull, Sheriff, Scarecrow, and Humdrum, *The Great Macdaddy,* Negro Ensemble Company, St. Mark's Playhouse, 1974; Bulldog, *One Crack Out,* Phoenix Theatre, Marymount Manhattan Theatre, New York City, 1978; Jamie Tyrone, *Long Day's Journey into Night,* Theatre at St. Peter's Church, New York City, 1981. Also appeared in *The Toilet,* St. Mark's Playhouse, 1964; *Sweet Talk,* NYSF, Other Stage Theatre, New York City, 1974; *'Tis Pity She's a Whore,* McCarter Theatre, Princeton, NJ, 1974; *Dream on Monkey Mountain,* Hartford, CT, 1976; *Kennedy's Children,* Marines Memorial Theatre, San Francisco, CA, 1976; and with the Ebony Showcase, Los Angeles, 1954-59.

PRINCIPAL STAGE WORK—Director, *Time Out of Time,* New Federal Theatre, Louis Abrons Arts for Living Center, New York City, 1986.

MAJOR TOURS—*A Raisin in the Sun,* U.S. cities, 1962.

FILM DEBUT—*Torpedo Run,* Metro-Goldwyn-Mayer, 1958. PRINCIPAL FILM APPEARANCES—Taru, *Ensign Pulver,* Warner Brothers, 1964; intern, *The Troublemaker,* Janus, 1964; Clay, *Dutchman,* Continental, 1966; Robbie, *The Detective,* Twentieth Century-Fox, 1968; Howard, *Finian's Rainbow,* Seven Arts, 1968; Private First Class Alistair Benjamin, *Castle Keep,* Columbia, 1969; Dennis Laurence, *The Lost Man,* Universal, 1969; Charles Roberts, *My Sweet Charlie,* Universal, 1970; Leader, *A Fable,* MFR, 1971; co-narrator, *Thermidor,* Altura, 1971; Danny Larwin, *Seven Hours to Judgment,* Trans World Entertainment, 1988. Also appeared in *This Rebel Breed,* Warner Brothers, 1960; *Sniper Ridge,* Twentieth Century-Fox, 1961; *Black Like Me* (also known as *No Man Walks Alone*), Continental, 1964; and *For Pete's Sake!,* World Wide, 1966.

PRINCIPAL FILM WORK—Producer and director, *A Fable,* MFR, 1971; director, *The Lost Man,* Universal, 1969.

PRINCIPAL TELEVISION APPEARANCES—Series: Captain Ed Hall, *One Life to Live,* ABC, 1972—; Charles Bingham, *Hot l Baltimore,* ABC, 1975. Mini-Series: Damon Lockwood, *King,* NBC, 1978; Malcolm X, *Roots: The Next Generations,* ABC, 1979. Episodic: *General Electric Theatre,* CBS, 1955; also *Suspicion,* NBC; *The Millionaire,* CBS; *Adventures in Paradise,* ABC; *Bourbon Street*

Beat, ABC; *The Defenders,* CBS; *Slattery's People,* CBS; *The F.B.I.,* ABC; *Judd for the Defense,* ABC; *The Mod Squad,* ABC; *Maude,* CBS; *Day in Court* (also known as *Accused*), ABC. Movies: Charles Roberts, *My Sweet Charlie,* NBC, 1970; Lieutenant Cooper, *Perry Mason Returns,* NBC, 1985. Plays: "To Be Young, Gifted and Black," *NET Playhouse,* NET, 1972. Specials: Jerry Hudson, "A Piece of Cake," *A Special Treat,* NBC, 1977.

WRITINGS: FILM—*A Fable,* MFR, 1971; (with Ossie Davis and Ladi Ladebo) *Countdown At Kusini,* Columbia, 1976.

AWARDS: Emmy Award nomination, 1970, for *My Sweet Charlie;* Emmy Award, Best Actor in a Daytime Drama Series, 1979, for *One Life to Live;* Russwurm Award; Golden Gate Award.

MEMBER: Actors' Equity Association, Screen Actors Guild, American Federation of Television and Radio Artists.

SIDELIGHTS: FAVORITE ROLES—Richard Henry in *Blues for Mister Charlie.* RECREATIONS—Golf, tennis, and woodworking.*

*   *   *

FULLER, Charles   1939-

PERSONAL: Full name, Charles Henry Fuller, Jr.; born March 5, 1939, in Philadelphia, PA; son of Charles Henry (a printer) and Lillian (Anderson) Fuller; married Miriam A. Nesbitt, August 4, 1962; children: Charles III, David. EDUCATION: Attended Villanova University, 1956-58, and LaSalle College, 1965-67. MILITARY: U.S. Army, 1959-62.

VOCATION: Writer.

CAREER: Also see *WRITINGS* below. PRINCIPAL RADIO WORK—Director, *The Black Experience,* WIP-Radio, Philadelphia, PA, 1970-71. RELATED CAREER—Co-founder and co-director, Afro-American Arts Theatre, Philadelphia, PA, 1967-71; also board member, Adolph Caesar Black Actors Memorial Fund, Theatre Communications Group.

WRITINGS: STAGE—*The Village: A Party,* McCarter Theatre, Princeton, NJ, 1968, revised as *The Perfect Party,* Tambellini's

Gate Theatre, New York City, 1969; *In My Many Names and Days* (six one-act plays), Henry Street Settlement, New York City, 1972; *The Candidate,* Henry Street Settlement, 1974; *In the Deepest Part of Sleep,* St. Mark's Playhouse, New York City, 1974; *First Love,* Billie Holiday Theatre, New York City, 1974; *The Lay Out Letter,* Freedom Theatre, Philadelphia, PA, 1975; *The Brownsville Raid,* Negro Ensemble Company, Theatre De Lys, New York City, 1976; *Sparrow in Flight,* AMAS Repertory Theatre, New York City, 1978; *Zooman and the Sign,* Negro Ensemble Company, Theatre Four, New York City, 1980, published by Samuel French, Inc., 1981; *A Soldier's Play,* Negro Ensemble Company, Theatre Four, 1981, then Center Theatre Group, Mark Taper Forum, Los Angeles, CA, 1982, later Goodman Theatre, Chicago, IL, 1983, published by Samuel French, Inc., 1982, and Hill and Wang, 1982; (contributor) *Urban Blight,* Manhattan Theatre Club, then City Center Theatre, both New York City, 1988; *Sally,* First National Black Arts Festival, Atlanta, GA, then Negro Ensemble Company, Theatre Four, both 1988; *Prince,* Negro Ensemble Company, Theatre Four, 1988.

FILM—*A Soldier's Story,* Columbia, 1984. TELEVISION—Mini-Series: *Roots, Resistance, and Renaissance,* WHYY, Philadelphia, PA, 1967. Episodic: "The Sky Is Gray," *American Short Story,* PBS, 1980. Movies: *A Gathering of Old Men,* CBS, 1987. OTHER—Short stories and nonfiction for anthologies and periodicals.

AWARDS: Creative Artist Public Service Award, 1974; Rockefeller Foundation fellowship, 1975; National Endowment for the Arts fellowship, 1976; Guggenheim fellowship, 1977-78; Obie Award from the *Village Voice* and Audelco Award for Best Writing, both 1981, for *Zooman and the Sign;* New York Drama Critics Award, Best American Play, Outer Circle Critics Award, Best Off-Broadway Play, Audelco Award, Theatre Club Award, and Pulitzer Prize in Drama, all 1982, for *A Soldier's Play;* Academy Award nomination, Best Screenplay, 1984, for *A Soldiers Story;* Hazelitt Award from the Pennsylvania State Council on the Arts, 1984. Honorary degrees: Doctor of Fine Arts, LaSalle College, 1982; Doctor of Fine Arts, Villanova Universtiy, 1983.

MEMBER: Writers Guild of America-East, Dramatists Guild (council member), P.E.N.

ADDRESSES: AGENT—Esther Sherman, William Morris Agency, 1350 Avenue of the Americas, New York City, 10019.*

G

GALARNO, Bill 1938-

PERSONAL: Full name, William S. Galarno; born March 1, 1938, in Saginaw, MI; son of Frederic William (a civil engineer) and Marie Cecelia (an office manager; maiden name, Potvin) Galarno. EDUCATION: Michigan State University, B.S., 1959; studied dance with Orest Sergievsky and voice with Ora Witte.

VOCATION: Actor, director, and playwright.

CAREER: Also see *WRITINGS* below. STAGE DEBUT—Christopher Wren, *The Mousetrap,* Pittsburgh Playhouse, Pittsburgh, PA, 1956, for thirty performances. PRINCIPAL STAGE APPEARANCES—Peter, *Plain and Fancy,* Mt. Gretna Playhouse, Gretna, PA, 1959; knight templar, *Nathan the Wise,* East 78th Street Theatre, New York City, 1962; Marchbanks, *Candida,* and Mr. Mulleady, *The*

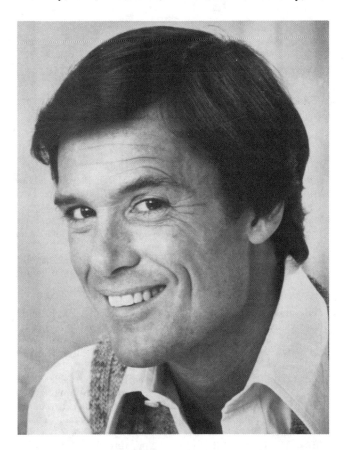

BILL GALARNO

Hostage, both Woodstock Playhouse, Woodstock, NY, 1964; Ligniere, *Cyrano de Bergerac,* and Duperret, *Marat/Sade,* both Studio Arena Theatre, Buffalo, NY, 1966-67; Rolf Gruber, *The Sound of Music,* City Center Theatre, New York City, 1967; Duke Senior and Duke Frederick, *As You Like It,* Sylvan Theatre, Washington, DC, 1968; herald, *Candide,* Avery Fisher Hall, New York City, 1968; singer, actor, and dancer, *Absurdities,* Theatre Nes, Amsterdam, Netherlands, 1976; Charley, *Where's Charley?,* Dinner Theatre of the Stars, Tidewater, VA, 1979; Herr Zeller, *The Sound of Music,* Jones Beach Amphitheatre, Long Island, NY, 1980; Andre, *Pictures at an Exhibition,* No Smoking Playhouse, New York City, 1983; Alan, *Baby,* St. Michael's Playhouse, Winooski, VT, 1985. Also appeared as Queen of Hearts, *Alice in Wonderland,* Studio Arena Theatre; Blank, *Pantagleize,* Judson Poets' Theatre, New York City; inspector, *Larry and the Gypsy,* St. Clement's Church Theatre, New York City; *Actors On and Off the Stage—A Look behind the Curtain,* American Jewish Theatre, New York City; as Aaron, *On the March to the Sea,* Hyde Park Playhouse, Hyde Park, NY; Jimmy Perry, *The Gingerbread Lady,* Piedmont Repertory Company; Sergeant Carlino, *Wait Until Dark,* Tanglewood Barn Theatre, Tanglewood, MA; Dr. Einstein, *Arsenic and Old Lace,* Winston-Salem, NC; Dussel, *The Diary of Anne Frank,* Candlewood Playhouse, New Fairfield, CT; and Beverly Carlton, *The Man Who Came to Dinner,* New Fairfield, CT.

PRINCIPAL STAGE WORK—Director: *A Christmas Carol—The Boston Broadcast of 1932,* Actors Theatre of Nantucket, Nantucket, MA, 1988; also *Your Room of Mine, Brighton Beach Memoirs, The Odd Couple,* and *The Owl and the Pussycat,* all Genetti Dinner Playhouse, Hazleton, PA; *The Owl and the Pussycat* and *Squabbles,* both Peddlers Village Dinner Theatre, New Hope, PA; *The Odd Couple,* Shepherd Hills Dinner Theatre, Allentown, PA, and Actors Theatre of Nantucket; *Angel Street,* New London Barn Players, New London, NH; *Lunch Hour* and *Blithe Spirit,* both Nantucket Theatre Workshop, Nantucket, MA; *One Touch of Venus,* Marathon Community Theatre, New York City; *Purlie Victorious, Contributions, The Ofay Watcher,* and *Happy Ending,* all African Cultural Center Theatre, Buffalo, NY; *Actors On and Off the Stage—A Look behind the Curtain,* American Jewish Theatre, New York City; *The Cretan Woman* and *The Potboiler,* both Michigan State University, East Lansing, MI; and *The Molehill,* Ohio University, Athens, OH.

MAJOR TOURS—Rolf, *The Sound of Music,* U.S. cities, 1962-63; Jim Curry, *110 in the Shade,* U.S. and Canadian cities, 1964; Alistair Spenlow, *Move Over, Mrs. Markham,* U.S. cities, 1974.

PRINCIPAL FILM APPEARANCES—Healthy kisser, *The Horror of Party Beach,* Twentieth Century-Fox, 1964; button-man, *The Godfather,* Paramount, 1972; Father Devereau, *Last Embrace,* United Artists, 1979; Ronald, *New York Nights,* Euro/London

Films, 1981; *Dave, Violated,* Cinematronics, 1987; also appeared as double and stand-in for Roy Scheider, *All That Jazz,* Twentieth Century-Fox, 1979.

TELEVISION DEBUT—Billy, *The Cold Woman,* NBC, 1961. PRINCIPAL TELEVISON APPEARANCES—Episodic: Sergeant Molina, *Serpico,* NBC; Officer York, *Somerset,* NBC; Andre, *The Edge of Night,* NBC.

RELATED CAREER—Appeared in industrial films as the prosecuting attorney in *The Trial of Clarence Birdseye* for General Foods and as Chuck Caldwell in *The Battle of the Boardroom,* for E.F. Hutton.

WRITINGS: STAGE—*Kiss, Comrades, Kiss!,* 1968; *For the Love of Suzanne,* Martinique Theatre, New York City, 1974; *A Christmas Carol—The Boston Broadcast of 1932,* Actors Theatre of Nantucket, Nantucket, MA, 1988; also (co-writer) *Actors On and Off Stage—A Look behind the Curtain,* American Jewish Theatre; *The Molehill,* Ohio University; (adaptor) *Squaring the Circle.*

AWARDS: American Society of Composers, Authors, and Publishers Award, 1968, for *Kiss, Comrades, Kiss!;* CAPS Grant in Playwriting from the Creative Artists Public Service Program, 1979, for *For the Love of Suzanne.*

MEMBER: Actors' Equity Association, Screen Actors Guild, American Federation of Television and Radio Artists, Dramatists Guild, American Society of Composers, Authors, and Publishers.

SIDELIGHTS: Bill Galarno told *CTFT:* "Theatre is my religion, my life. Pursuing it, I have traveled to the Carribbean, Europe, and throughout the U.S. and Canada."

ADDRESSES: HOME—400 W. 43rd Street, Apartment 17-0, New York, NY, 10036. AGENT—Mitch Douglas, International Creative Management, 40 W. 57th Street, New York, NY 10019.

*   *   *

GALE, Bob   1952-

PERSONAL: Born in 1952 in St. Louis, MO; father, a lawyer; mother, a violinist and art gallery owner; wife, a former publicist; children: one daughter. EDUCATION: Attended Tulane University and the University of Southern California School of Cinema.

VOCATION: Screenwriter and producer.

CAREER: Also see *WRITINGS* below. PRINCIPAL FILM WORK—Associate producer, *I Wanna Hold Your Hand,* Universal, 1978; producer, *Used Cars,* Columbia, 1980; producer (with Neil Canton), *Back to the Future,* Universal, 1985.

WRITINGS: FILM—(With Robert Zemeckis) *I Wanna Hold Your Hand,* Universal, 1978; (with Zemeckis) *1941,* Universal, 1979; (with Zemeckis) *Used Cars,* Columbia, 1980; (with Zemeckis) *Back to the Future,* Universal, 1985. TELEVISION—Pilots: *Used Cars,* CBS, 1984. Episodic: (With Zemeckis) *McCloud,* NBC; (with Zemeckis) *Kolchak: The Night Stalker,* ABC.

AWARDS: Academy Award nomination, Best Original Screenplay, 1986, for *Back to the Future.**

GALLAGHER, Megan

PERSONAL: EDUCATION: Graduated from the drama division of the Juilliard School of Music.

VOCATION: Actress.

CAREER: PRINCIPAL STAGE APPEARANCES—Elmire, *Tartuffe,* Acting Company, American Place Theatre, New York City, 1983; W2, "Play," and Ru, "Krapp's Last Tape," in *"Play" and Other Plays,* Acting Company, American Place Theatre, 1983; title role, *Miss Julie,* Theatre of the Open Eye, New York City, 1985. Also appeared in *All's Well That Ends Well,* Colorado Shakespeare Festival, Boulder, CO, 1981; *Oliver, Oliver,* Long Wharf Theatre, New Haven, CT, 1984; and in *Major Barbara,* Baltimore, MD.

MAJOR TOURS—Roxanne, *Cyrano de Bergerac,* U.S. cities, 1985-86; also *Twelfth Night* and *The Country Wife,* Acting Company, U.S. cities.

PRINCIPAL TELEVISION APPEARANCES—Series: Detective Tina Russo, *Hill Street Blues,* NBC, 1986-87; Judy Ralston, *The "Slap" Maxwell Story,* ABC, 1987; Wayloo Marie Holmes, *China Beach,* ABC, 1988—. Mini-Series: Peggy Shippen, *George Washington,* CBS, 1984. Pilots: Audrey Ritter, *At Your Service,* NBC, 1984; also *L.A. Law,* NBC, 1986. Movies: Ellen Easton, *Sins of the Past,* ABC, 1984.

ADDRESSES: AGENT—Smith-Freedman and Associates, 121 N. San Vicente Boulevard, Beverly Hills, CA 90211.*

*   *   *

GALLO, Paul

PERSONAL: Wife's name, Judith (a scenic artist); children: one daughter.

VOCATION: Lighting designer.

CAREER: PRINCIPAL STAGE WORK—Lighting designer: *The Offering,* Negro Ensemble Company, St. Mark's Playhouse, New York City, 1977; *Photograph,* Open Space in Soho Theatre, New York City, 1977; *Black Body Blues,* Negro Ensemble Company, St. Mark's Playhouse, 1978; *Conjuring an Event,* American Place Theatre, New York City, 1978; *Bonjour, la, Bonjour* and *Damn Yankees,* both Hartford Stage Company, Hartford, CT, 1979; *Absurd Person Singular,* Indiana Repertory Theatre, Indianapolis, IN, 1979; *The Winter Dancers,* Phoenix Theatre, Marymount Manhattan College, New York City, 1979.

Tintypes, American National Theatre and Academy, Theatre at St. Peter's Church, then John Golden Theatre, both New York City, 1980; *Passione,* Morosco Theatre, New York City, 1980; *John Gabriel Borkman,* Circle in the Square, New York City, 1980; *The Little Foxes,* Martin Beck Theatre, New York City, 1981, then Center Theatre Group, Ahmanson Theatre, Los Angeles, CA, 1982; *Coming Attractions,* Playwrights Horizons, New York City, 1980; *The Actor's Nightmare* and *Sister Mary Ignatius Explains It All for You,* both Playwrights Horizons, 1981; *Candida,* Circle in the Square, 1981; *Kingdoms,* Cort Theatre, New York City, 1981; *Grownups,* Lyceum Theatre, New York City, 1981, then Center Theatre Group, Mark Taper Forum, Los Angeles, 1982; *The*

Comedy of Errors and *Red River,* both Goodman Theatre, Chicago, IL, 1982; *On Borrowed Time,* Hartford Stage Company, 1982; *The Hasty Heart,* Center Theatre Group, Ahmanson Theatre, 1982; *Paper Angels,* New Federal Theatre, New York City, 1982; *Beyond Therapy,* Brooks Atkinson Theatre, New York City, 1982; *Come Back to the 5 and Dime, Jimmy Dean, Jimmy Dean,* Martin Beck Theatre, 1982; *The Lady and the Clarinet,* Long Wharf Theatre, New Haven, CT, 1983; *Heartbreak House,* Circle in the Square, 1983; *La Boheme,* New York Shakespeare Festival (NYSF), Public Theatre, New York City, 1984; *The Foreigner,* Astor Place Theatre, New York City, 1984; *The Garden of Earthly Delights,* St. Clement's Church Theatre, New York City, 1984; *Henry V* and *Cinders,* both NYSF, Delacorte Theatre, New York City, 1984; *Terra Nova,* Playwrights Horizons, American Place Theatre, New York City, 1984; *Mr. and Mrs.,* WPA Theatre, New York City, 1984.

Crossing the Bar, Playhouse 91, New York City, 1985; *Salonika* and *The Marriage of Bette and Boo,* both NYSF, Public Theatre, 1985; *South Pacific,* Dorothy Chandler Pavilion, Los Angeles, 1985; *The Mystery of Edwin Drood,* NYSF, Delacorte Theatre, then Imperial Theatre, New York City, both 1985; *Vienna: Lusthaus,* NYSF, Public Theatre, 1986; *The House of Blue Leaves,* Mitzi E. Newhouse Theatre, then Vivian Beaumont Theatre, later Plymouth Theatre, all New York City, 1986; *Orchards,* The Acting Company, Lucille Lortel Theatre, New York City, 1986; *Smile,* Lunt-Fontanne Theatre, New York City, 1986; *The Front Page,* Vivian Beaumont Theatre, 1986; *The Hunger Artist,* St. Clement's Church Theatre, 1987; *The Comedy of Errors,* Vivian Beaumont Theatre, 1987; *Anything Goes,* Vivian Beaumont Theatre, 1988; *Macbeth,* Mark Hellinger Theatre, New York City, 1988; *Wenceslas Square,* NYSF, Public Theatre, 1988; *Spoils of War,* Music Box Theatre, New York City, 1988; *Lend Me a Tenor,* Royale Theatre, 1989. Also lighting designer, *Equity Library Informals,* Bruno Walter Auditorium, Lincoln Center, New York City, 1982-83; *Miracolo D'Amore;* and with the Folger Theatre Group, Washington, DC, 1978-79, Philadelphia Drama Guild, Philadelphia, PA, 1980-81, Hartford Stage Company, 1983, and the Arena Stage, Washington, DC, 1983-86.

MAJOR TOURS—Lighting designer, *Macbeth,* U.S. cities, 1988.

AWARDS: Joseph Maharam Award, 1984, for *The Garden of Earthly Delights;* Joseph Maharam Award, 1986, for *Vienna: Lusthaus;* Antoinette Perry Award nomination, Best Lighting Design, 1986, for *The House of Blue Leaves;* Obie Award from the *Village Voice,* Sustained Excellence of Lighting Design, 1986; Obie Award, 1987, for *A Hunger Artist;* Antoinette Perry Award nomination, Best Lighting Design, 1988, for *Anything Goes.*

MEMBER: International Alliance of Theatrical Stage Employees and Moving Picture Machine Operators of the U.S. and Canada.*

*   *   *

GARDENIA, Vincent   1922-

PERSONAL: Born Vincent Scognamiglio, January 7, 1922, in Naples, Italy; came to the United States c. 1924; son of Gennaro Gardenia (an actor and singer) and Elisa (Ausiello) Scognamiglio. EDUCATION: Studied acting with Harold Clurman, 1954. MILITARY: U.S. Army, private, 1942-44.

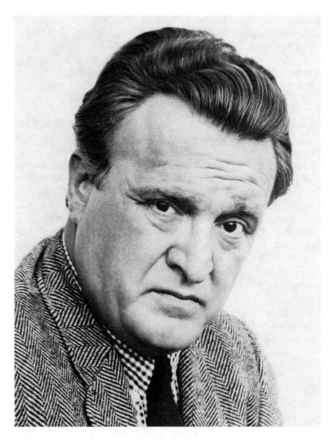

VINCENT GARDENIA

VOCATION: Actor.

CAREER: STAGE DEBUT—Shoeshine boy, *Shoe Shine,* Fifth Avenue Theatre, Brooklyn, NY, 1927. OFF-BROADWAY DEBUT—Piggy, *The Man with the Golden Arm,* Cherry Lane Theatre, 1956. BROADWAY DEBUT—Blind man, *The Visit,* Lunt-Fontanne Theatre, 1958. PRINCIPAL STAGE APPEARANCES—Stanley Kowlaski, *A Streetcar Named Desire,* Joseph, *My Three Angels,* and Stosh, *Stalag 17,* all Hampton Playhouse, Hampton, NH, 1954; Johnson, *Mister Roberts,* Sea Cliff Playhouse, Sea Cliff, NY, 1955; Hugo the Pirate, *In April Once,* Broadway Tabernacle Church, New York City, 1955; Corvino, *Volpone,* Rooftop Theatre, New York City, 1957; Fyodor, *The Brothers Karamazov,* Gate Theatre, New York City, 1957; Jim Nightingale, *The Cold Wind and the Warm,* Morosco Theatre, New York City, 1958; the Deputy, *Rashomon,* Music Box Theatre, New York City, 1959; Mittrich, *The Power of Darkness,* York Playhouse, New York City, 1959; the Chairman, *Only in America,* Cort Theatre, New York City, 1959.

George H. Jones, *Machinal,* Gate Theatre, 1960; Pavel Menkes, *The Wall,* Billy Rose Theatre, New York City, 1960; the Warden, *Gallows Humor,* Gramercy Arts Theatre, New York City, 1961; Panisse, *Fanny,* Lambertville Music Circus, Lambertville, NJ, 1961; Sergeant Manzoni, *Daughter of Silence,* Music Box Theatre, 1961; Hamm, *Endgame,* and the Warden, *Gallows Humor,* both Cherry Lane Theatre, 1962; Popoff, *The Chocolate Soldier,* Lambertville Music Circus, 1962; Wilenski, *Seidman and Son,* Belasco Theatre, New York City, 1962; Mr. Jones and workman, *The Lunatic View,* American National Theatre and Academy Matinee Series, Theatre De Lys, New York City, 1962; Eddie Carbone, *A View from the Bridge,* Charles Playhouse, Boston, MA, 1968; Carol Newquist, *Little Murders,* Circle in the Square, New York City, 1969; Charles Ferris, "The Son Who Hunted Tigers in Jakarta," and Nick Esposito, "The Burial of Esposito," in *Passing Through from Exotic Places,* Sheridan Square Playhouse, New York City, 1969.

Marty Mendelsohn, *Dr. Fish,* Ethel Barrymore Theatre, New York City, 1970; Father, *The Carpenters,* American Place Theatre, New York City, 1970; Harry Edison, *The Prisoner of Second Avenue,* Eugene O'Neill Theatre, New York City, 1971; Joe Benjamin, *God's Favorite,* Eugene O'Neill Theatre, 1974; Marvin and Mort, *California Suite,* Eugene O'Neill Theatre, 1977; Foxwell J. Sly, *Sly Fox,* Broadhurst Theatre, New York City, 1978; Alfred Rossi, *Ballroom,* Majestic Theatre, New York City, 1978; Wild Bob Culhane, *Buried Inside Extra,* Public Theatre, New York City, then Royal Court Theatre, London, both 1983; Shelly Levene, *Glengarry Glen Ross,* John Golden Theatre, New York City, 1984; Harry Edison, *The Prisoner of Second Avenue,* Burt Reynolds Theatre, Jupiter, FL, 1984. Also appeared in *Burlesque,* Clinton Theatre, Clinton, NJ, 1955; as General St. Pe, *The Waltz of the Toreadors,* Webster, MA, 1957; as Willy Loman, *Death of a Salesman,* Moorestown, NY, 1964; and as Edmund Tyrone, *Long Day's Journey into Night,* Moorestown, 1965.

MAJOR TOURS—Nat, *I'm Not Rappaport,* U.S. cities.

PRINCIPAL FILM APPEARANCES—Trainee, *The House on 92nd Street,* Twentieth Century-Fox, 1945; Lawyer Laslo, *Murder, Inc.,* Twentieth Century-Fox, 1960; bartender, *The Hustler,* Twentieth Century-Fox, 1961; Dutch Schultz, *Mad Dog Coll,* Columbia, 1961; gas station attendant, *Parrish,* Warner Brothers, 1961; Lipari, *A View from the Bridge,* Continental Distributing, 1962; Preston, *The Third Day,* Warner Brothers, 1965; Mr. Marsh, *Jenny* (also known as *And Jenny Makes Three*), Cinerama, 1969; Coach Williams, *Where's Poppa?* (also known as *Going Ape*), United Artists, 1970; Mayor Wrappler, *Cold Turkey,* United Artists, 1971; Mr. Newquist, *Little Murders,* Twentieth Century-Fox, 1971; Papadakis, *Hickey and Boggs,* United Artists, 1972; Dutch Schnell, *Bang the Drum Slowly,* Paramount, 1973; American colonel, *Re: Lucky Luciano* (also known as *A proposito Luciano* and *Lucky Luciano*), 1973, released in the United States by AVCO-Embassy, 1974; Detective Frank Ochoa, *Death Wish,* Paramount, 1974; Sheriff, *The Front Page,* Universal, 1974; Big Daddy, *The Manchu Eagle Murder Caper Mystery,* United Artists, 1975; Benny Fikus, *Fire Sale,* Twentieth Century-Fox, 1977; Sheriff Cotton, *Greased Lightning,* Warner Brothers, 1977; Lieutenant Krim, *Heaven Can Wait,* Paramount, 1978; Frank Hull, *Firepower,* Associated Film Distribution, 1979; Dr. Byrd, *Home Movies,* United Artists, 1979; Stoney, *The Last Flight of Noah's Ark,* Buena Vista, 1980; Frank Ochoa, *Death Wish II,* Columbia/EMI/Warner Brothers, 1982; Saul Gritz, *Movers and Shakers,* Metro-Goldwyn-Mayer/United Artists (MGM/UA), 1985; Mushnik, *Little Shop of Horrors,* Warner Brothers, 1986; Cosmo Castorini, *Moonstruck,* MGM-UA, 1987. Also appeared in *Cop Hater,* United Artists, 1958.

PRINCIPAL TELEVISION APPEARANCES—Series: Frank Lorenzo, *All in the Family,* CBS, 1973-74; Ray Stohler, *Breaking Away,* ABC, 1980-81. Mini-Series: J. Edgar Hoover, *Kennedy,* NBC, 1983. Pilots: Captain Sonny Miglio, *Cops,* CBS, 1973; Chef, *Dean's Place,* NBC, 1975; Chief Mike Maldonato, *Brass,* CBS, 1985. Episodic: *Voyage to the Bottom of the Sea,* ABC, 1965; *All in the Family,* CBS, 1971 and 1972; *The Mary Tyler Moore Show,* CBS, 1977; also Mr. Petri, *The Untouchables,* ABC; *Studio One,*

CBS; *Maude,* CBS. Movies: Sam Diamond, *Goldie and the Boxer,* NBC, 1979; Al Weill, *Marciano,* ABC, 1979; Peter Kessler, *The Dream Merchants,* syndicated, 1980; Traegar, *Thornwell,* CBS, 1981; Captain Maggio, *Muggable Mary: Street Cop,* CBS, 1982; Detective Al Church, *Dark Mirror,* ABC, 1984. Specials: Stephen Spettigue, *Charley's Aunt,* Entertainment Channel, 1983; *The Night of the Empty Chairs,* PBS, 1978. Also appeared as Mr. Beckerman, *Ride in Terror,* 1963.

AWARDS: Obie Award from the *Village Voice,* 1960, for *Machinal;* Obie Award, 1970, for *Passing Through from Exotic Places;* Antoinette Perry Award, Best Supporting or Featured Actor, 1972, for *The Prisoner of Second Avenue;* New York Film Critics Award, Best Supporting Actor, 1973, and Academy Award nomination, Best Supporting Actor, 1974, both for *Bang the Drum Slowly;* Academy Award nomination, Best Supporting Actor, 1988, for *Moonstruck*

MEMBER: Actors' Equity Association, American Federation of Radio and Television Artists, Screen Actors Guild.

SIDELIGHTS: FAVORITE ROLES—Willy Loman in *Death of a Salesman,* Eddie in *A View from the Bridge,* and Carol Newquist in *Little Murders.* RECREATIONS—Cooking and "mountain climbing on 12th Avenue."

ADDRESSES: AGENT—Jay Julien, 1501 Broadway, New York, NY 10036.

                    *   *   *

GARY, Lorraine

PERSONAL: Born Lorraine Gottfried in Forest Hills, NY; daughter of George Gottfried (an entertainment business manager); married Sidney J. Scheinberg (a motion picture executive); children: Jon, Billy. EDUCATION: Attended Columbia University.

VOCATION: Actress.

CAREER: FILM DEBUT—Ellen Brody, *Jaws,* Universal, 1975. PRINCIPAL FILM APPEARANCES—Hysterical lady, *Car Wash,* Universal, 1976; Mrs. Blake, *I Never Promised You a Rose Garden,* New World, 1977; Ellen Brody, *Jaws II,* Universal, 1978; Shirl, *Just You and Me, Kid,* Columbia, 1979; Joan Douglas, *1941,* Universal, 1979; Ellen Brody, *Jaws—The Revenge,* Universal, 1987.

PRINCIPAL TELEVISION APPEARANCES—Pilots: Ruthie, *The Marcus-Nelson Murders* (also known as *Kojak and the Marcus-Nelson Murders*), CBS, 1973; Myra Galen, *Lanigan's Rabbi* (also known as *Friday the Rabbi Slept Late*), NBC, 1976. Episodic: "She'll Be Company for You," *Rod Serling's Night Gallery,* NBC, 1972. Movies: Victoria Ulysses, *The City,* ABC, 1971; Margery Jordan, *Partners in Crime,* NBC, 1973; Lila Summerfield, *Pray for the Wildcats,* ABC, 1974; Nora Griffin, *Man on the Outside,* ABC, 1975; Emily Mulwray, *Crash,* ABC, 1978.

RELATED CAREER—Formerly a literary agent with Creative Artists Agency.

MEMBER: Screen Actors Guild.*

GEDRICK, Jason

PERSONAL: Born c. 1966 in Chicago, IL; attended Drake University.

VOCATION: Actor.

CAREER: PRINCIPAL STAGE APPEARANCES—George Gibbs, *Our Town*, Lyceum Theatre, New York City, 1989; also appeared in *The Miracle Worker* and *Rumplestiltskin*, both Anawim Too Players, Chicago, IL; *Mrs. Dally Has a Lover*, Westbeth Theatre, New York City; with the Second City Workshop, Chicago; and with the Philbin Theatre, Chicago.

FILM DEBUT—*Bad Boys*, EMI/Universal/Associated Film Distributors, 1983. PRINCIPAL FILM APPEARANCES—Eric Briscoe, *Massive Retaliation*, One Pass/Hammermark, 1984; Lenny Barnes, *The Heavenly Kid*, Orion, 1985; Hardin, *The Zoo Gang*, NW, 1985; Doug, *Iron Eagle*, Tri-Star, 1986; Gary Connaloe, *Stacking*, Spectrafilm, 1988; Davey Hancock, *The Promised Land*, Vestron, 1988; "T," *Rooftops*, New Century/Vista, 1989. Also appeared in *Winners Take All*, New World, 1985; *Risky Business*, Warner Brothers/Columbia, 1983; and *Dr. Detroit*, Universal, 1983.

PRINCIPAL TELEVISION APPEARANCES—Movies: *Listen to Your Heart*, CBS, 1983; also *Bozo's Circus*.

SIDELIGHTS: RECREATIONS—Motorcycling and parachuting.

ADDRESSES: AGENT—Ilene Feldman, Triad Artists, 10100 Santa Monica Boulevard, 16th Floor, Los Angeles, CA 90067.*

* * *

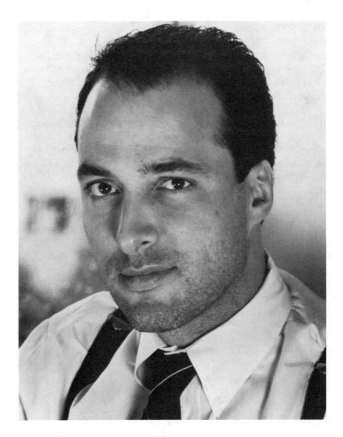

DAN GERRITY

GERRITY, Dan   1958-

PERSONAL: Born December 21, 1958, in Red Bank, NJ; son of Daniel Joseph (a construction worker) and Constance Faith (Robbins) Gerrity. EDUCATION: Attended the State University of New York, Albany, and Hofstra University; trained for the stage with Sanford Meisner at the Neighborhood Playhouse.

VOCATION: Actor, assistant director, and producer.

CAREER: OFF-BROADWAY DEBUT—Flip the Prince, *The Apple Tree*, Bert Wheeler Theatre, 1974, for forty performances. PRINCIPAL STAGE APPEARANCES—Starbuck, *110 in the Shade*, Bert Wheeler Theatre, New York City, 1978; Judd, *Bouncers*, Minetta Lane Theatre, New York City, 1987; Pierce Brennan, *Stand-Up Tragedy*, Center Theatre Group, Mark Taper Forum, Los Angeles, CA, 1988; also appeared in *A Christmas Carol*, Center Theatre Group, Mark Taper Forum, 1977; *The Impact Company*, Improvisational Theatre Project, Center Theatre Group, Mark Taper Forum, 1977; with the Improvisational Theatre Project, Mark Taper Forum, 1980-83; in *Delirious*, Los Angeles, 1985; and as Judd, *Bouncers*, Los Angeles, 1986.

PRINCIPAL STAGE WORK—Assistant director, *C'et le rossignol chantait* (French translation of *And a Nightingale Sang*), Theatre de Poche, Brussels, Belgium, 1985; *Femmes derriere les barreaux* (French translation of *Women behind Bars*), Theatre de Poche, 1986; assistant director, *Brighton Beach Memoirs* and *I'm Not Rappaport*, both Sydney Opera Playhouse, Sydney, Australia, 1987; producer, *Shakers*, Odyssey Theatre Ensemble, U.K./L.A.

Festival, Los Angeles, CA, 1987; producer, *Catwalk*, Edinburgh Festival, Edinburgh, Scotland, 1989; producer, *Hooray for Hollywood*, Mark Taper Forum, Los Angeles, 1989; also producer with the Odyssey Theatre Ensemble, 1988.

PRINCIPAL FILM APPEARANCES—Randy, *Crimes of Passion*, New World, 1984.

TELEVISION DEBUT—Arnie, *Throb*, syndicated, 1986-87. PRINCIPAL TELEVISION APPEARANCES—Episodic: Chip, *Head of the Class*, ABC, 1987; Denton, *Sidekicks*, ABC, 1987; also *Cheers*, NBC. Movies: Felix, *The Triangle Factory Fire*, NBC, 1979.

AWARDS: Los Angeles Weekly Award and *Drama-Logue* Award, both 1985, for *Delirious; Los Angeles Drama Critics Circle Award, 1986, for *Bouncers*.

MEMBER: Actors' Equity Association, Screen Actors Guild, American Federation of Television and Radio Artists, American Guild of Variety Artists.

ADDRESSES: OFFICE—1752 N. Cerrano, Los Angeles, CA 90027.

* * *

GERTZ, Jami   1965-

PERSONAL: Born October 28, 1965, in Chicago, IL; father, a builder and contractor. EDUCATION: Attended New York University.

VOCATION: Actress.

CAREER: PRINCIPAL STAGE APPEARANCES—Marie, *Come Back, Little Sheba,* Los Angeles Theatre Center, Los Angeles, CA, 1987; also appeared in *Outta Gas on Lover's Leap,* Court Playhouse, Los Angeles, CA.

PRINCIPAL FILM APPEARANCES—Big girl, *On the Right Track,* Twentieth Century-Fox, 1981; prostitute, *Alphabet City,* Atlantic Releasing, 1984; Rosalie, *Mischief,* Twentieth Century-Fox, 1985; Frances, *Crossroads,* Columbia, 1986; Terri, *Quicksilver,* Columbia, 1986; Terra, *Solarbabies,* Metro-Goldwyn-Mayer/United Artists, 1986; Blair, *Less than Zero,* Twentieth Century-Fox, 1987; Star, *The Lost Boys,* Warner Brothers, 1987.

PRINCIPAL TELEVISION APPEARANCES—Series: Muffy Tepperman, *Square Pegs,* CBS, 1982-83; Martha Spino, *Dreams,* CBS, 1984. Pilots: Monica Mitchell, *For Members Only,* CBS, 1983. Episodic: Boots St. Clair, *The Facts of Life,* NBC, 1983; also *Diff'rent Strokes,* NBC; *Family Ties,* NBC.

ADDRESSES: PUBLICIST—Susan Geller, Guttman and Pam Public Relations, 8500 Wilshire Boulevard, Suite 801, Beverly Hills, CA 90211.*

*   *   *

GIANNINI, Giancarlo   1942-

PERSONAL: Born August 1, 1942, in Spezia, Italy; children: Lorenzo, Adriano. EDUCATION: Received degree in electronics engineering; studied acting at the Rome Academy of Drama, 1963.

VOCATION: Actor, director, and screenwriter.

CAREER: STAGE DEBUT—Puck, *A Midsummer Night's Dream,* Italy, 1961. PRINCIPAL STAGE APPEARANCES—Romeo, *Romeo and Juliet,* Italy, 1964; also appeared in *Two Plus Two No Longer Make Four,* Italy, 1966.

FILM DEBUT—*Fango sulla metropoli,* 1965. PRINCIPAL FILM APPEARANCES—Cellini, *Anzio* (also known as *Lo sbarco di Anzio* and *The Battle for Anzio*), Columbia, 1968; Salverio, *Arabella,* Universal, 1969; Lieutenant Hans Ruppert, *Fraulein Doktor,* Paramount, 1969; Fabio, *The Secret of Santa Vittoria,* United Artists, 1969; Nello, *Dramma della gelosia—Tutti in particolarie in cronacal* (also known as *The Motive Was Jealousy, A Drama of Jealousy [and Other Things], Jealousy Italian Style,* and *The Pizza Triangle*), Warner Brothers, 1970; Inspector Tellini, *La tarantol dal ventre nero* (also known as *The Black Belly of the Tarantula*), Metro-Goldwyn-Mayer (MGM), 1972; Mimi, *Mimi metallurgico ferito nell' onore* (also known as *The Seduction of Mimi* and *Mimi the Metalworker*), New Line Cinema, 1972; Biagio Solise, *Sono stato io* (also known as *I Did It*), Warner Brothers, 1972; Spider, *Le Professeur* (also known as *The Professor*), Valoria, 1972; Tunin, *Film d'amore e d'anarchia* (also known as *Love and Anarchy*), Peppercorn-Wormsler, 1973; Paolo Castorini, *Paolo il caldo* (also known as *Hot-Blooded Paolo*), Medusa Distribuzione, 1973; Gennarino Carunchio, *Travolti da un insolito destino nell'azzurro mare d'Agosto* (also known as *Swept Away . . . By an Unusual Destiny in the Blue Sea of August* and *Swept Away*), Cinema V, 1974; Nino Patrovita, *Il bestione* (also known as *Beast*), Warner

Brothers, 1974; Paolo, *The Sensual Man,* Peppercorn-Wormsler, 1974.

Gino Benacio, *A mezzanotte va la ronda del piacere* (also known as *Midnight Pleasures*), Film Ventures, 1975; Tullio Murri, *Fatti di gente perbene* (also known as *Drama of the Rich*), PAC, 1975; Pasqualino Frafuso, *Pasqualino settebellezze* (also known as *Seven Beauties* and *Pasqualino: Seven Beauties*), Cinema V, 1975; Paolo, *The End of the World (in Our Usual Bed in a Night Full of Rain),* Warner Brothers, 1977; Tulio Murri, *La Grande Bourgeoise* (also known as *The Murri Affair*), Atlantic/Buckley Brothers, 1977; Tullio Hermil, *L'Innocente* (also known as *The Innocent*), Analysis Film Releasing Corporation, 1979; husband, *Buone notizie* (also known as *Good News*), Medusa Distribuzione, 1979; Nick Sammichele, *Fatto di sangue fra due uomini per causa di una Vedova. Si sospettano moventi Politici* (also known as *Blood Feud* and *Revenge*), Associated Film Distributing, 1979.

Gino Benacio, *The Immortal Bachelor,* S.J. International, 1980; Robert Mendelsson, *Lili Marleen,* United Artists, 1981; Guido, *Lovers and Liars* (also known as *A Trip with Anita* and *Travels with Anita*), Levitt-Pickman, 1981; Antonio, *La vita e bella* (also known as *Life Is Wonderful*), Cavalli Cinematographic/Mosfilm, 1982; Victor Marchand, *American Dreamer,* Warner Brothers, 1984; Charley Peru, *Fever Pitch,* Metro-Goldwyn-Mayer/United Artists, 1985; Salvatore, *Mi manda Picone* (also known as *Where's Picone?* and *Picone Sent Me*), Italtoon/Wonder Movies, 1985; Abalardi, *Saving Grace,* Embassy/Columbia, 1986; Guzman, *I Picari,* Warner Brothers, 1987; Nini, *Ternosecco,* Columbia Pictures Italia, 1987; Claudio, "Life without Zoe" in *New York Stories,* Touchstone, 1989. Also appeared in *Bello mio bellezza mia* (also known as *My Handsome My Beautiful*), PLM Film Produzione, 1982; *Rita la zansara,* 1967; *Libido,* 1967; *Non stuzzicate la Zansara,* 1967; *Stasera mi butto,* 1967; *Le sorelle,* 1969; *Una macchia rosa,* 1969; *Una prostituta al servizio del pubblico e regol con le leggi dello stato,* 1971; *Mio Padre Monsignore,* 1971; *Mazzabubu . . . quante come stanno quaggiu,?,* 1971; *Un aller simple,* 1971; *Ettore lo fusto,* 1971; *La prima notte di quiete* (also known as *The First Quiet Night*), Titanus, 1972; *Sessomatto* (also known as *Sex Crazy*), Delta, 1973; *In una notte piena di Pioggia,* 1978; as a narcotics dealer, *Indian Summer,* 1978; and as a lawyer, *Snackbar Budapest,* 1988.

PRINCIPAL FILM WORK—Producer, *Pasqualino settebellezze* (also known as *Seven Beauties* and *Pasqualino: Seven Beauties*), Cinema V, 1976; producer, *Buone notize* (also known as *Good News*), Medusa Distribuzione, 1979; director, *Ternosecco,* Columbia Pictures Italia, 1987.

PRINCIPAL TELEVISION APPEARANCES—Mini-Series: Marcello D'Itri, *Sins,* CBS, 1986.

RELATED CAREER—Partner (with Lina Wertmuller), Liberty Films; provided Italian translation of American films for the Italian film market.

WRITINGS: FILM—(With Lin Jannuzzi) *Ternosecco,* Columbia Pictures Italia, 1987.

AWARDS: Best Actor Award from the Cannes Film Festival, 1973, for *Love and Anarchy;* Academy Award nomination, Best Actor, 1976, for *Seven Beauties.*

MEMBER: Screen Actors Guild.

ADDRESSES: OFFICE—c/o C.S.C., Sr. L. Viale Mazzini 132, Rome 00195, Italy.*

*   *   *

GIELGUD, John   1904-

PERSONAL: Full name, Arthur John Gielgud; born April 14, 1904, in London, England; son of Frank (a stockbroker) and Kate (Terry-Lewis) Gielgud. EDUCATION: Trained for the stage at Lady Benson's School, 1921, and at the Royal Academy of Dramatic Art, 1922.

VOCATION: Actor, producer, and director.

CAREER: STAGE DEBUT—Herald, *Henry V*, Old Vic Theatre, London, 1921. BROADWAY DEBUT—Grand Duke Alexander, *The Patriot*, Majestic Theatre, 1928. PRINCIPAL STAGE APPEARANCES—Felix, *The Insect Play*, and aide-de-camp, *Robert E. Lee*, both Regent Theatre, London, 1923; Charles Wykeham, *Charley's Aunt*, Comedy Theatre, London, 1923; Romeo, *Romeo and Juliet*, Regent Theatre, 1924; Castalio, *The Orphan*, Aldwych Theatre, London, 1925; Nicky Lancaster, *The Vortex*, Royalty Theatre, London, 1925; Peter Trophimoff, *The Cherry Orchard*, Lyric Hammersmith Theatre, London, 1925; Konstantin Treplev, *The Seagull*, and Sir John Harington, *Gloriana*, both Little Theatre, London, 1925; Robert, *L'Ecole des cocottes*, Princes Theatre, London, 1925; Ferdinand, *The Tempest*, Savoy Theatre, London, 1926; Baron Tusenbach, *The Three Sisters*, and George Stibelev, *Katerina*, both Barnes Theatre, London, 1926; Lewis Dodd, *The Constant Nymph*, New Theatre, London, 1926; Dion Anthony, *The Great God Brown*, Strand Theatre, London, 1927; Oswald, *Ghosts*, Wyndham's Theatre, London, 1928; Dr. Gerald Marlowe, *Holding Out the Apple*, Globe Theatre, London, 1928; Captain Allenby, *The Skull*, Shaftesbury Theatre, London, 1928; Felipe Rivas, *The Lady from Albuquerque*, and Alberto, *Fortunato*, both Court Theatre, London, 1928; John Marstin, *Out of the Sea*, Strand Theatre, 1928; Fedor, *Red Dust*, Little Theatre, 1929; Henry Tremayne, *The Lady with a Lamp*, Garrick Theatre, London, 1929; Trotsky (Bronstein), *Red Sunday*, Arts Theatre, London, 1929; Romeo, *Romeo and Juliet*, Antonio, *The Merchant of Venice*, Cleante, *The Imaginary Invalid*, Oberon, *A Midsummer Night's Dream*, title role, *Richard II*, and title role, *Macbeth*, all Old Vic Company, Old Vic Theatre, London, 1929.

Title role, *Hamlet*, Queen's Theatre, London, 1930; John Worthing, *The Importance of Being Earnest*, Lyric Hammersmith Theatre, 1930; Mark Antony, *Julius Caesar*, Orlando, *As You Like It*, Emperor, *Androcles and the Lion*, title role, *Hamlet*, Hotspur, *Henry IV, Part I*, Prospero, *The Tempest*, Lord Trinket, *The Jealous Wife*, and Antony, *Antony and Cleopatra*, all Old Vic Company, Old Vic Theatre, 1930; Inigo Jollifant, *The Good Companions*, His Majesty's Theatre, London, 1931; Joseph Schindler, *Musical Chairs*, Arts Theatre, 1931; Malvolio, *Twelfth Night*, Old Vic Company, Sadler's Wells Theatre, London, 1931; Sergius Saranoff, *Arms and the Man*, Benedick, *Much Ado about Nothing*, and title role, *King Lear*, all Old Vic Company, Old Vic Theatre, 1931; Richard II, *Richard of Bordeaux*, Arts Theatre, 1932, then New Theatre, 1933; Roger Maitland, *The Maitlands*, Wyndham's Theatre, 1934; title role, *Hamlet*, New Theatre, 1934; title role, *Noah*, New Theatre, 1935; Mercutio, then Romeo, *Romeo and Juliet*, New Theatre, 1935; Boris Trigorin, *The Seagull*,

New Theatre, 1936; title role, *Hamlet*, Empire Theatre, New York City, 1936; Mason, *He Was Born Gay*, title role, *Richard II*, and Joseph Surface, *The School for Scandal*, all Queen's Theatre, 1937; Colonel Vershinin, *The Three Sisters*, Shylock, *The Merchant of Venice*, and Nicholas Randolph, *Dear Octopus*, all Queen's Theatre, 1938; John Worthing, *The Importance of Being Earnest*, Globe Theatre, 1939; title role, *Hamlet*, Lyceum Theatre, London, then Kronborg Castle, Elsinore, Denmark, both 1939.

MacHeath, *The Beggar's Opera*, Haymarket Theatre, London, 1940; title role, *King Lear*, and Prospero, *The Tempest*, both Old Vic Company, Old Vic Theatre, 1940; Will Dearth, *Dear Brutus*, Globe Theatre, 1941; title role, *Macbeth*, Piccadilly Theatre, London, 1942; John Worthing, *The Importance of Being Earnest*, Phoenix Theatre, London, 1942; Louis Dubedat, *The Doctor's Dilemma*, Haymarket Theatre, London, 1942; Valentine, *Love for Love*, Phoenix Theatre, London, 1943; Champion-Cheney, *The Circle*, Valentine, *Love for Love*, and title role, *Hamlet*, all Haymarket Theatre, 1944; Oberon, *A Midsummer Night's Dream*, and Ferdinand, *The Duchess of Malfi*, both Haymarket Theatre, 1945; Raskolnikoff, *Crime and Punishment*, New Theatre, 1946; John Worthing, *The Importance of Being Earnest*, and Valentine, *Love for Love*, both Royale Theatre, New York City, 1947; Jason, *Medea*, and Raskolnikoff, *Crime and Punishment*, both National Theatre, London, 1947; Eustace Jackson, *The Return of the Prodigal*, Globe Theatre, 1948; Thomas Mendip, *The Lady's Not for Burning*, Globe Theatre, 1949; Benedick, *Much Ado about Nothing*, Shakespeare Memorial Theatre Company, Shakespeare Memorial Theatre, Stratford-on-Avon, U.K., 1949.

Angelo, *Measure for Measure*, Cassius, *Julius Caesar*, and title role, *King Lear*, all Shakespeare Memorial Theatre Company, Shakespeare Memorial Theatre, 1950; Thomas Mendip, *The Lady's Not for Burning*, Royale Theatre, 1950; Leontes, *The Winter's Tale*, Phoenix Theatre, London, 1951; Benedick, *Much Ado about Nothing*, Phoenix Theatre, London, 1952; Mirabel, *The Way of the World*, and Jaffeir, *Venice Preserv'd*, both Lyric Hammersmith Theatre, 1953; Julian Anson, *A Day by the Sea*, Haymarket Theatre, 1953; Benedick, *Much Ado about Nothing*, and title role, *King Lear*, both Palace Theatre, London, 1955; Sebastian, *Nude with Violin*, Globe Theatre, 1956; Prospero, *The Tempest*, Shakespeare Memorial Theatre Company, Shakespeare Memorial Theatre, then Drury Lane Theatre, London, both 1957; James Callifer, *The Potting Shed*, Globe Theatre, 1958; Cardinal Wolsey, *Henry VIII*, Old Vic Theatre, 1958; *Ages of Man* (one-man show), 46th Street Theatre, New York City, 1958, then Queen's Theatre, 1959; Benedick, *Much Ado about Nothing*, Cambridge Drama Festival, Boston, MA, then Lunt-Fontanne Theatre, New York City, both 1959.

Ages of Man (one-man show), Haymarket Theatre, 1960; Prince Ferdinand Cavanati, *The Last Joke*, Phoenix Theatre, New York City, 1960; title role, *Othello*, Shakespeare Memorial Theatre Company, Shakespeare Memorial Theatre, 1961; Gaev, *The Cherry Orchard*, Shakespeare Memorial Theatre Company, Shakespeare Memorial Theatre, then Aldwych Theatre, both 1961; Joseph Surface, *The School for Scandal*, Haymarket Theatre, 1962, then Majestic Theatre, New York City, 1963; *Ages of Man* (one-man show), Lyceum Theatre, 1963; Julius Caesar, *The Ides of March*, Haymarket Theatre, 1963; voice of the Ghost, *Hamlet*, Lunt-Fontanne Theatre, 1964; Julian, *Tiny Alice*, Billy Rose Theatre, New York City, 1964; Nikolai Ivanov, *Ivanov*, Yvonne Arnaud Theatre, Guildford, U.K., then Phoenix Theatre, London, 1965, later Shubert Theatre, New York City, 1966; *Ages of Man* (one-man show), Huntington Hartford Theatre, Los Angeles, CA, 1967; Orgon, *Tartuffe,* Old Vic Theatre, 1967; *Men and Women of Shakespeare* (one-man show), Hunter College, New York City, 1967; title role, *Oedipus,* Old Vic Theatre, 1968; Headmaster, *Forty Years On,* Apollo Theatre, London, 1968.

Gideon, *The Battle of Shrivings,* Lyric Theatre, London, 1970; Harry, *Home,* Royal Court Theatre, London, then Morosco Theatre, New York City, both 1970; Julius Caesar, *Caesar and Cleopatra,* Chichester Festival Theatre, Chichester, U.K., 1971; Sir Geoffrey Kendle, *Veterans,* Royal Court Theatre, 1972; Prospero, *The Tempest,* National Theatre, 1974; William Shakespeare, *Bingo,* Royal Court Theatre, 1974; Milton, *Paradise Lost,* Royal Theatre, York, U.K., then Old Vic Theatre, both 1974; Spooner, *No Man's Land,* Old Vic Theatre, then Wyndham's Theatre, both 1975, later Kennedy Center for the Performing Arts, Washington, DC, 1976; title role, *Julius Caesar,* and Sir Politic Wouldbe, *Volpone,* both Olivier Theatre, London, 1977; Sir Noel Cunliffe, *Half-Life,* Cottesloe Theatre, London, 1977, then Duke of York's Theatre, London, 1978; Sir Sydney Cockerell, *The Best of Friends,* Apollo Theatre, 1988. Also appeared in *King Lear, Wat Tyler,* and *Peer Gynt,* all 1922; with J.B. Fagan's repertory company, Oxford Playhouse, Oxford, U.K., 1924; in *Fumed Oak, Hands Across the Sea,* and *Swan Song,* all Globe Theatre, 1940; in a revue with Beatrice Lillie and Edith Evans, military bases on Gibralter, 1942; in *Homage to Shakespeare,* Philharmonic Hall, New York City, 1964; and in *Tribute to a Lady,* Old Vic Theatre, 1976.

PRINCIPAL STAGE WORK—Director, unless indicated: *Richard of Bordeaux,* New Theatre, London, 1932; *Strange Orchestra,* St. Martin's Theatre, London, 1932; *Sheppey,* Wyndham's Theatre, London, 1933; (also producer, with Richard Clowes) *Spring 1600,* Shaftesbury Theatre, London, 1934; *Queen of Scots* and *Hamlet,* both New Theatre, 1934; *The Old Ladies* and *Romeo and Juliet,* both New Theatre, 1935; (with Emlyn Williams) *He Was Born Gay,* Queen's Theatre, London, 1937; *Richard II* and *The Merchant of Venice,* Queen's Theatre, 1938; *Spring Meeting,* Ambassadors' Theatre, London, 1938; *The Importance of Being Earnest* and *Scandal in Assyria,* both Globe Theatre, London, 1939; producer, *Rhondda Roundabout,* Globe Theatre, 1939; *The Beggar's Opera,* Haymarket Theatre, London, 1940; *Dear Brutus,* Globe Theatre, 1941; *Ducks and Drakes,* Apollo Theatre, London, 1941; *Macbeth,* Piccadilly Theatre, London, 1942; *Love for Love,* Phoenix Theatre, London, 1943; *Landslide,* Westminster Theatre, London, 1943; *The Cradle Song,* Apollo Theatre, 1944; *Crisis in Heaven,* Lyric Theatre, London, 1944; *The Last of Summer,* Phoenix Theatre, 1944; *Lady Windermere's Fan,* Haymarket Theatre, 1945; *Medea,* National Theatre, 1947; *The Importance of Being Earnest* and *Love for Love,* both Royale Theatre, New York City, 1947; *The Glass Menagerie,* Haymarket Theatre, 1948; *Medea,* Globe Theatre, 1948; *The Heiress,* Haymarket Theatre, 1949; *The Lady's Not for Burning,* Globe Theatre, 1949; *Much Ado about Nothing,* Shakespeare Memorial Theatre Company, Shakespeare Memorial Theatre, Stratford-on-Avon, U.K., 1949; *Treasure Hunt,* Apollo Theatre, 1949.

Shall We Join the Ladies? and *The Boy with a Cart* (double-bill), Lyric Hammersmith Theatre, 1950; (with Anthony Quayle) *King Lear,* Shakespeare Memorial Theatre Company, Shakespeare Memorial Theatre, 1950; *Indian Summer,* Criterion Theatre, London, 1951; *Much Ado about Nothing,* Phoenix Theatre, 1952; *Macbeth,* Shakespeare Memorial Theatre Company, Shakespeare Memorial Theatre, 1952; *Richard II,* Lyric Hammersmith Theatre, London, 1952; *The Way of the World,* Lyric Hammersmith Theatre, 1953; *A*

Day by the Sea, Haymarket Theatre, 1953; *Charley's Aunt,* New Theatre, 1954; *The Cherry Orchard,* Lyric Hammersmith Theatre, 1954; *Twelfth Night,* Shakespeare Memorial Theatre Company, Shakespeare Memorial Theatre, 1955; *Much Ado about Nothing,* Palace Theatre, London, 1955; *The Chalk Garden,* Haymarket Theatre, 1956; (with Noel Coward) *Nude with Violin,* Globe Theatre, 1956; *The Trojans* (opera), Covent Garden Theatre, London, 1957; *Variations on a Theme,* Globe Theatre, 1958; *Five Finger Exercise,* Comedy Theatre, London, 1958; *The Complaisant Lover,* Globe Theatre, 1959; *Much Ado about Nothing,* Cambridge Drama Festival, Boston, MA, then Lunt-Fontanne Theatre, New York City, both 1959; *Five Finger Exercise,* Music Box Theatre, New York City, 1959.

A Midsummer Night's Dream (opera), Covent Garden Theatre, 1961; *Big Fish, Little Fish,* American National Theatre and Academy Theatre, New York City, 1961; *Dazzling Prospect,* Globe Theatre, 1961; *The School for Scandal,* Haymarket Theatre, 1962, then Majestic Theatre, New York City, 1963; *Hamlet,* Lunt-Fontanne Theatre, 1963; *Ivanov,* Yvonne Arnaud Theatre, Guildford, U.K., then Phoenix Theatre, both 1965, later Shubert Theatre, New York City, 1966; *Halfway Up the Tree,* Queen's Theatre, 1967; *Don Giovanni* (opera), Coliseum Theatre, London, 1968; *All Over,* Martin Beck Theatre, New York City, 1971; *Private Lives,* Queen's Theatre, 1972, then 46th Street Theatre, New York City, 1975; *The Constant Wife,* Albery Theatre, London, 1973, then Shubert Theatre, 1975; *The Gay Lord Quex,* Albery Theatre, 1975.

MAJOR TOURS—Understudy and stage manager, *The Wheel,* U.K. cities, 1922; Lewis Dodd, *The Constant Nymph,* U.K. cities, 1927; John Worthing (also director), *The Importance of Being Earnest,* U.K. cities, 1939; Charles Condamine, *Blithe Spirit,* and title role, *Hamlet,* British military bases in the Far East, 1945; Raskolnikoff, *Crime and Punishment,* U.K. cities, 1946; John Worthing, *The Importance of Being Earnest,* and Valentine, *Love for Love,* Canadian and U.S. cities, 1947; title role, *Richard II,* Rhodesian cities, 1953; Benedick (also director), *Much Ado about Nothing,* and title role, *King Lear,* Shakespeare Memeorial Theatre Company, European and U.K. cities, 1955; Cardinal Wolsey, *Henry VIII,* European cities, 1958; *Ages of Man* (one-man show), U.S. and Canadian cities, 1958, Italian cities, 1959 and 1960, Israeli cities, 1962, New Zealand and Australian cities, 1963, and European cities, 1964; *Men and Women of Shakespeare* (one-man show), South American and U.S. cities, 1966; director, *Private Lives,* U.S. and Canadian cities, 1974-75; director, *The Constant Wife,* U.S. cities, 1975; also in *Fumed Oak, Hands Across the Sea,* and *Swan Song,* Entertainments National Service Association tour of British military bases, 1940.

FILM DEBUT—Daniel, *Who Is the Man?,* 1924. PRINCIPAL FILM APPEARANCES—Henri Dubois, *Insult,* Paramount, 1932; Edgar Brodie and Richard Ashenden, *The Secret Agent,* Gaumont, 1936; Benjamin Disraeli, *The Prime Minister,* Warner Brothers, 1941; voice of the Ghost, *Hamlet,* General Films Distributors, 1948; Cassius, *Julius Caesar,* Metro-Goldwyn-Mayer (MGM), 1953; chorus, *Romeo and Juliet,* United Artists, 1954; Clarence, *Richard III,* Lopert, 1956; Foster, *Around the World in 80 Days,* United Artists, 1956; Mr. Barrett, *The Barretts of Wimpole Street,* MGM, 1957; Earl of Warwick, *Saint Joan,* United Artists, 1957; voice of the Ghost, *Hamlet,* Warner Brothers, 1964; King Louis VII, *Becket,* Paramount, 1964; Sir Francis Hinsley, *The Loved One,* MGM, 1965; King Henry IV, *Chimes at Midnight* (also known as *Campanadas a medianoche* and *Falstaff*), Peppercorn/Wormser/ U-M, 1967; Curt Valayan, *Assignment to Kill,* Warner Brothers/

Seven Arts, 1968; Lord Raglan, *The Charge of the Light Brigade,* United Artists, 1968; head of Intelligence, *Sebastian,* Paramount, 1968; elder Pope, *The Shoes of the Fisherman,* MGM, 1968; Count Berchtold, *Oh! What a Lovely War,* Paramount, 1969; title role, *Julius Caesar,* American International, 1970; Lord Sissal, *Eagle in a Cage,* National General, 1971; Chang, *Lost Horizon,* Columbia, 1973; Farrell, *Gold,* Allied Artists, 1974; Beddoes, *Murder on the Orient Express,* Paramount, 1974; Meecham, *11 Harrowhouse* (also known as *Anything for Love*), Twentieth Century-Fox, 1974; old cardinal, *Galileo,* American Film Theatre, 1975; headmaster, *Aces High,* EMI, 1977; Clive Langham, *Providence,* Cinema V, 1977; doctor, *Joseph Andrews,* Paramount, 1977; Brigadier Tomlinson, *The Human Factor,* Metro-Goldwyn-Mayer/United Artists (MGM/UA), 1979; preacher, *Portrait of the Artist as a Young Man,* Howard Mahler, 1979; Lord Salisbury, *Murder by Decree,* AVCO-Embassy, 1979.

Carr Gomm, *The Elephant Man,* Paramount, 1980; Dr. Esau, *The Formula,* MGM/UA, 1980; Abdu Hamdi, *The Sphinx,* Warner Brothers, 1981; Hobson, *Arthur,* Warner Brothers, 1981; Master of Trinity, *Chariots of Fire,* Twentieth Century-Fox, 1981; title role, *The Conductor* (also known as *Dyrygent* and *The Orchestra Conductor*), Cinegate, 1981; Herbert G. Muskett, *Priest of Love,* Filmways, 1981; Sharif El Gariani, *Lion of the Desert* (also known as *Omar Mukhtar*), United Film Distribution, 1981; Lord Irwin, *Gandhi,* Columbia, 1982; Hogarth, *The Wicked Lady,* MGM/UA, 1983; Pfistermeister, *Wagner,* Alan Landsburg, 1983; Uncle Willie, *Scandalous,* Orion, 1984; Sir Leonard Darwin, *Plenty,* Twentieth Century-Fox, 1985; Reverend Clyde Ormiston, *Invitation to the Wedding,* New Realm, 1985; Cornelius Cardew, *The Shooting Party,* European Classics, 1985; as himself, *Ingrid* (documentary), Wombat Productions, 1985; Sir Adrian Chapple, *The Whistle Blower,* Hemdale, 1987; Colonel Carbury, *Appointment with Death,* Cannon, 1988; Hobson, *Arthur 2: On the Rocks,* Warner Brothers, 1988. Also appeared as Rex Trasmere, *The Clue of the New Pin,* 1929; Inigo Jollifant, *The Good Companions,* 1933; (voice only) *Full Fathom Five* (short film), 1934; in *A Diary for Timothy* (documentary), 1937; title role, *Hamlet* (documentary), 1939; (voice only) *An Airman's Letter to His Mother* (short film), 1941; in *Unfinished Journey* (short film), 1943; (voice only) *Shakespeare's Country* (short film), 1944; *The Cherry Orchard,* 1954; narrator, *The Immortal Land* (documentary), 1958; narrator, *To Die in Madrid* (also known as *Mourir a Madrid*), 1967; narrator, *October Revolution* (also known as *Revolution d'Octobre*), 1967; as Nerva, *Caligula* (also known as *Gore Vidal's Caligula*), 1978; as John Middleton Murray, *Leave All Fair,* 1985; *Barbalu Barbalu* (also known as *Bluebeard Bluebeard*), Betafilm/RAF2, 1987; and Pope Pacelli, *The Vatican Pimpernel.*

TELEVISION DEBUT—Julian Anson, *A Day by the Sea,* ITV, 1959. PRINCIPAL TELEVISION APPEARANCES—Series: Host, *The Pallisers,* BBC, 1974, then PBS, 1977; also host and narrator, *Buddenbrooks,* PBS. Mini-Series: Clinton-Meek, *QB VII,* ABC, 1974; Albert Speer, Sr., *Inside the Third Reich,* ABC, 1982; Edward Ryder, *Brideshead Revisited,* Granada, 1980, then *Masterpiece Theatre,* PBS, 1982; Doge, *Marco Polo,* NBC, 1982; Cavagnari, *The Far Pavilions,* HBO, 1984. Pilots: Harold Streeter, *Probe* (also known as *Search*), NBC, 1972. Episodic: "The Love Song of Barney Kempinski," *Stage 67,* ABC, 1966; also *Dupont Show of the Month,* CBS. Movies: Chief constable, *Frankenstein: The True Story,* NBC, 1973; Gillenormand, *Les Miserables,* CBS, 1978; Charmolue, *The Hunchback of Notre Dame,* CBS, 1982; Pope Pius XII, *The Scarlet and the Black,* CBS, 1983; Lord Durrisdeer, *The Master of Ballantrae,* CBS, 1984; Duke de Charles,

Camille, CBS, 1984; Theodore Woodward, *Romance on the Orient Express,* NBC, 1985; Jasper Swift, *Time After Time,* BBC, 1985, then Arts & Entertainment, 1987; Sir Simon de Canterville, *The Canterville Ghost,* syndicated, 1986.

Specials: Mr. Browning, *The Browning Version,* CBS, 1959; Ghost, "Hamlet," *Hallmark Hall of Fame,* NBC, 1953; *Ages of Man* (one-man show), CBS, 1966; Nikolai Ivanov, *Ivanov,* CBS, 1967; Harry, *Home,* PBS, 1970; narrator, "Peter Pan," *Hallmark Hall of Fame,* NBC, 1976; Marquis of Caterham, *The Seven Dials Mystery,* syndicated, 1981; Reverend Jones, *Why Didn't They Ask Evans?,* syndicated, 1981; Eddie Loomis, "Quartermaine's Terms," *Great Performances,* PBS, 1987; also *The Professors and the Professionals,* NET, 1966; *Alice in Wonderland,* BBC, 1966; *From Chekhov with Love,* BBC, 1967; *Saint Joan,* BBC, 1968; *In Good King Charles' Golden Days,* BBC, 1969; *Conversation at Night,* BBC, 1969; *Hassan,* BBC, 1970; *Funny You Don't Look 200,* ABC, 1987. Also appeared in *The Rehearsal,* 1963; *Edward VII,* 1974; and in *The Cherry Orchard, Heartbreak House, Great Acting, Mayfly and the Frog,* and *Deliver Us from Evil.*

RELATED CAREER—Manager, Queen's Theatre, London, 1937-38; appeared in television commercials for Paul Masson wine.

WRITINGS: STAGE—(Adaptor) *The Cherry Orchard,* Lyric Hammersmith Theatre, London, 1954, published as *The Cherry Orchard: A Comedy in Four Acts,* Heinemann, 1963; (adaptor) *Ivanov,* Yvonne Arnaud Theatre, Guildford, U.K., 1965, published as *Ivanov: A Drama in Four Acts,* Scripts Limited, 1966. TELEVISION—Specials: (Adaptor, with John Bowen) *Ivanov,* CBS, 1967. OTHER—All autobiographies. *Early Stages,* Macmillan, 1939; *Stage Directions,* Heinemann, 1963; *Distinguished Company,* Heinemann, 1972; (with John Miller and John Powell) *An Actor and His Time,* Sidgwick & Jackson, 1979.

AWARDS: British Academy Award, Best British Actor, 1953, for *Julius Caesar;* Special Antoinette Perry Award, 1959, for *Ages of Man;* Antoinette Perry Award, Best Director of a Play, 1961, for *Big Fish, Little Fish;* Academy Award nomination, Best Supporting Actor, 1964, for *Becket;* Variety poll of London critics, Best Male Performer, 1969, for *Forty Years On; Evening Standard* Award, Best Actor, 1970, Drama Desk Award and Antoinette Perry Award nomination, both Best Actor in a Play, 1971, for *Home;* British Academy Award, Best Supporting Actor, 1974, for *Murder on the Orient Express;* New York Film Critics Award, Best Actor, 1977, for *Providence;* Academy Award, Best Supporting Actor, 1981, for *Arthur;* New Standard Special Award, 1982; Emmy Award nomination, Outstanding Supporting Actor, 1985, for *The Master of Ballantrae;* Emmy Award nomination, Outstanding Supporting Actor, 1986, for *Romance on the Orient Express;* Annual Cable Excellence (ACE) Award, Best Actor in a Movie or Mini-Series, 1988, for *Time After Time;* knighted, 1953; Brandeis University Companion, 1960; Companion of Honour, 1977; Chevalier of the French Legion d'Honneur. Honorary degrees: St. Andrew's University, LL.D., 1950; Oxford University, D. Litt., 1953; Brandeis University, LL.D., 1965.

MEMBER: Actors' Equity Association, Shakespeare Reading Society (president), Royal Academy of Dramatic Art (president), Garrick Club, Players Club.

ADDRESSES: OFFICE—South Pavilion, Wotton Underwood, Aylesbury HP18 OSB, Buckinghamshire, England. AGENT—In-

ternational Creative Management, 22 Grafton Street, London, W1, England.*

*   *   *

GLEASON, Paul   1944-

PERSONAL: Born May 4, 1944, in Jersey City, NJ; son of George L. (a professional boxer, iron worker, restaurateur, and roofing manufacturer) and Eleanor (a registered nurse; maiden name, Doyle) Gleason; married Candy Moore, March 15, 1971 (divorced, 1978); children: Shannon. EDUCATION: Attended Florida State University and Yale University; trained for the stage with Lee Strasberg at the Actors Studio. RELIGION: Roman Catholic.

VOCATION: Actor and writer.

CAREER: Also see *WRITINGS* below. OFF-BROADWAY DEBUT—King McCloud, *Key Largo*, Circle Ten Theatre, 1967. BROADWAY DEBUT—*The Gingerbread Lady*, Plymouth Theatre, 1971. PRINCIPAL STAGE APPEARANCES—McMurphy, *One Flew over the Cuckoo's Nest*, Mercer Arts Theatre, New York City, 1973; Larry, *Innocent Pleasures*, Ensemble Studio Theatre, New York City, 1980; also appeared in *Bachelor Furnished*, Schoenberg Hall, University of California, Los Angeles, 1968; *Niagra Falls*, Mark Taper Forum, Los Angeles, 1969; *The Front Page*, Ethel Barrymore Theatre, New York City, then Huntington Hartford

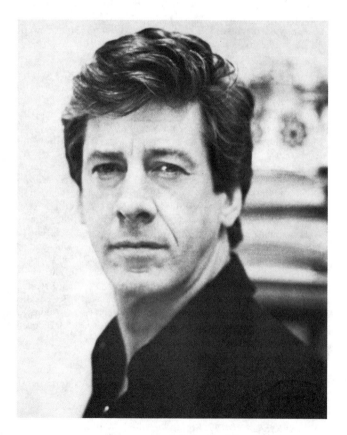

PAUL GLEASON

Theatre, Los Angeles, both 1972; *Born Yesterday*, Barn Theatre, Albuquerque, NM, 1975; *George Washington Slept Here*, Cecilwood Theatre, Fishkill, NY, 1976; *The Wakefield Trilogy*, Actors Studio, New York City, 1977; *Big John*, Carnegie Hall, New York City, 1977; *The Shanty*, Theatre at St. Clement's Church, New York City, 1978; *Valentine's Day*, Herbert Berghof Studio, New York City, 1981; *Open Admissions*, Long Wharf Theatre, New Haven, CT, 1982; *The Chain*, Hartman Theatre, Stamford, CT, 1983; and in *Economic Necessity*, New York City, 1975; *Criminal Minds*, New York City, 1978; *Violano Virtuoso*, New York City, 1979.

FILM DEBUT—*Camelot*, Warner Brothers, 1965. PRINCIPAL FILM APPEARANCES—Dr. McClintock, *Private Duty Nurses*, New World, 1972; Long Tom, *Doc Savage . . . The Man of Bronze*, Warner Brothers, 1975; (as Paul X. Gleason) Michael Loonius, *Vigilante Force*, United Artists, 1975; Lieutenant Sammy, *The Great Santini*, Orion/Warner Brothers, 1979; Daley, *He Knows You're Alone*, Metro-Goldwyn-Mayer/United Artists, 1980; detective, *Fort Apache, the Bronx*, Twentieth Century-Fox, 1980; executive, *Arthur*, Warner Brothers, 1981; Remson, *The Pursuit of D.B. Cooper*, Universal, 1981; reporter, *Tender Mercies*, EMI/ Universal, 1982; Clarence Beeks, *Trading Places*, Paramount, 1983; Richard Vernon, *The Breakfast Club*, Universal, 1985; Jay Springsteen, *Morgan Stewart's Coming Home* (also known as *Homefront*), New Century/Vista, 1987; Robert, *Forever, Lulu*, Tri-Star, 1987; Coach Wayne Hisler, *Johnny Be Good*, Orion, 1988; Dwayne T. Robinson, *Die Hard*, Twentieth Century-Fox, 1988. Also appeared in *Sergeant Deadhead*, American International, 1965; *Banning*, Universal, 1967; *Hit Man*, Metro-Goldwyn-Mayer, 1972; *Where Does It Hurt?*, Cinerama, 1972; *Little Laura and Big John*, Crown International, 1973; *She's Having a Baby*, Paramount, 1988; *Ghost Chase*, Cannon, 1989; *Night Game*, Trans World, 1989; *Miami Blues*, Orion, 1989.

TELEVISION DEBUT—*Ozzie and Harriet*, ABC, 1965. PRINCIPAL TELEVISION APPEARANCES—Series: David Thornton, *All My Children*, ABC, 1970. Mini-Series: Captain Ernest "Tex" Lee, *Ike: The War Years*, ABC, 1979. Pilots: Larry Worth, *Anything for Love*, NBC, 1985; Captain Pete McQuade, *Supercarrier*, ABC, 1988. Episodic: Harry, *The A-Team*, NBC, 1986; also Nick, *Love, American Style*, ABC; "Appalachian Spring," *CBS Playhouse*, CBS; *It's About Time*, CBS; *The Green Hornet*, ABC; *The F.B.I.*, ABC; *Then Came Bronson*, NBC; *Adam-12*, NBC; *Jigsaw*, ABC; *The Bold Ones: The Lawyers*, NBC; *The Bold Ones: The Doctors*, NBC; *Mission: Impossible*, CBS; *Columbo*, NBC; *McCloud*, NBC; *Toma*, ABC; *Banacek*, NBC; *Nurse*, CBS; *Riptide*, NBC; *Hardcastle and McCormick*, ABC; *Remington Steele*, NBC; *Scarecrow and Mrs. King*, CBS; *Cagney and Lacey*, CBS; *Call to Glory*, ABC; *Dallas*, CBS; *Magnum, P.I.*, CBS; *Hill Street Blues*, NBC; *Miami Vice*, NBC; *Gimme a Break*, NBC; *The Equalizer*, CBS; *Kate and Allie*, CBS; *Sidekicks*, ABC; *Falcoln Crest*, CBS; *Beauty and the Beast*, CBS. Movies: Major James Kirk, *Women at West Point*, CBS, 1979; John Schoonover, *Challenge of a Lifetime*, ABC, 1985; Howie Henley, *Doubletake*, CBS, 1985; also *The Ewok Adventure*, ABC, 1984. Specials: *Mother, May I?*, PBS.

WRITINGS: STAGE—*Bush*, Harold Clurman Theatre, New York City, 1982; *Crowbar*, West Bank Theatre, New York City, 1984; *Batting Practice*, Raft Theatre, New York City, 1988. OTHER— *Uleta Blues* (fiction), Creative Arts Publishers, 1988; has also had poetry published in *Paris Review, American Poetry East, Yale Review, Long Shot, Rolling Stone, National Lampoon, Home Planet News, New York Quarterly, Village Voice*, and *City Lights Journal*.

ADDRESSES: AGENT—Harris and Goldberg Agency, 2121 Avenue of the Stars, Los Angeles, CA 90067.

*   *   *

GOBEL, George   1919-

PERSONAL: Born May 20, 1919, in Chicago, IL; son of Herman and Lillian (MacDonald) Goebel; married Alice Humecke, December 13, 1942; children: Gregg, Georgia, Leslie, Alice. MILITARY: U.S. Army Air Forces, pilot instructor and first lieutenant, 1942-46.

VOCATION: Actor, singer, comedian, and producer.

CAREER: PRINCIPAL FILM APPEARANCES—Marshall "Mickey" Briggs, *I Married a Woman,* RKO/Universal, 1957; George Hamilton, *The Birds and the Bees,* Paramount, 1965; President of the U.S., *Rabbit Test,* AVCO-Embassy, 1978; preacher, *Ellie,* Film Ventures, 1984.

PRINCIPAL TELEVISION APPEARANCES—Series: Host, *The George Gobel Show,* NBC, 1954-59, then CBS, 1959-60; regular, *The Eddie Fisher Show,* NBC, 1957-59; Mayor Otis Harper, Jr., *Harper Valley P.T.A.,* NBC, 1981-82; also regular, *Hollywood Squares,* NBC, during the 1970s. Pilots: Drunk, *Benny and Barney, Las Vegas Undercover,* NBC, 1977; Dr. Farrington, *The Invisible Woman,* NBC, 1983. Episodic: *Saturday Night Revue,* NBC, 1953-54; panelist, *Who Said That?* (seven episodes), NBC, 1953; *Showtime,* CBS, 1968; *America 2-Night,* syndicated, 1978; also *My Three Sons,* ABC; *Daniel Boone,* NBC; *Love, American Style,* ABC. Movies: Hallway man, *A Guide for the Married Woman,* ABC, 1979; Captain Taylor, *Better Late than Never,* NBC, 1979; Bergman, *The Fantastic World of D.C. Collins,* NBC, 1984; Gnat, *Alice in Wonderland,* CBS, 1985. Specials: Town drunk, *Saga of Sonora,* NBC, 1973; voice of Father Mouse, *'Twas the Night before Christmas* (animated), CBS, 1974; *The John Denver Special,* ABC, 1974; *One More Time,* CBS, 1974; Nathan Terwilliger, *'Twas the Night before Christmas,* ABC, 1977; *A Country Christmas,* CBS, 1979; *NBC's Sixtieth Anniversary Celebration,* NBC, 1986; voice of ghost in shed, *The Incredible Book Escape,* 1980; *Bob Hope's Stand Up and Cheer for the National Football League's Sixtieth Year,* NBC, 1981.

PRINCIPAL TELEVISION WORK—Series: Producer, *Leave It to Beaver,* CBS, 1957-58, then ABC, 1959-1963.

PRINCIPAL RADIO APPEARANCES—(As Little Georgie Gobel) *National Barn Dance,* Chicago, IL, 1933-42.

RELATED CAREER—As a standup comedian, appeared in nightclubs, hotels, and county fairs throughout the U.S., 1946-54; dubbed "the Littlest Cowboy," sang with country music bands as a child; partner, Gomalco Enterprises (a television production company); vice-president, Gomalco, Inc.

AWARDS: Emmy Award, Outstanding New Personality, Peabody Award for Television Entertainment, Sylvania Award, Motion Picture Daily Poll, Radio-TV Daily Variety Magazine Award, *Look Magazine* Award, AP Man of the Year, TV Personality of the Year, and TV-Radio Life Award, all 1954-55, for *The George Gobel Show.*

MEMBER: Screen Actors Guild, Actors' Equity Association, Bohemian Club (San Francisco, CA), Lakeside Golf Club (North Hollywood, CA), Indian Wells Golf Club (Palm Springs, CA).

ADDRESSES: MANAGER—Roy Gerber Associates, 9046 Sunset Boulevard, Suite 208, Los Angeles, CA 90069-1819.*

*   *   *

GODARD, Jean-Luc   1930-
(Hans Lucas)

PERSONAL: Born December 3, 1930, in Paris, France; son of Paul (a physician) and Odile (Monod) Godard; married Anna Karina (an actress), March 2, 1961 (divorced, 1964); married Anne Wiasemsky (an actress), July 21, 1967 (divorced); children: one daughter. EDUCATION: Received certificate d'ethnologie from the Sorbonne, 1949.

VOCATION: Director, writer, producer, actor, and film editor.

CAREER: Also see *WRITINGS* below. PRINCIPAL FILM APPEARANCES—Man visiting a prostitute, *Une femme coquette* (short film), Jean-Luc Godard, 1955; dubbed voice, *Charlotte et son Jules* (short film), Les Films de la Pleieade, 1958; silhouette, *Paris Belongs to Us* (also known as *Paris nous appartient* and *Paris Is Ours*), 1958, released in the United States by Merlyn, 1962; informer, *Breathless* (also known as *A bout de souffle*), Georges de Beauregard/Societe Nouvelle de Cinema, 1959, released in the United States by Imperia Films, 1959; actor in comedy film, *Cleo from 5 to 7* (also known as *Cleo de 5 a 7*), Rome-Paris Films, 1961; dubbed voice, *A Woman Is a Woman* (also known as *Une femme est une femme* and *La donna e donna*), Rome-Paris Films, 1961, released in the United States by Pathe Contemporary, 1961; narrator, *My Life to Live* (also known as *Vivre sa vie* and *It's My Life*), Les Films de la Pleieade, 1962, released in the United States by Union/Pathe Contemporary, 1963; Ian's assistant director, *Contempt* (also known as *Le Mepris*), Rome-Paris Films, 1963, released in the United States by Embassy, 1963; bystander at railway station, *Le Petit soldat* (also known as *The Little Soldier*), Georges de Beauregard/Societe Nouvelle de Cinema, 1963, released in the United States by West End, 1965; narrator and man in Moroccan chechia, "Le Grand escroc" in *Les Plus belles escroqueries du monde,* Ulysse Films, 1964; narrator, *The Married Woman* (also known as *La Femme mariee, Une femme mariee,* and *A Married Woman*), Anouchka Films, 1964, released in the United States by Royal, 1965.

Orlovsky's friend, *The Defector* (also known as *Lauthose Waffen* and *L'Espion*), Warner Brothers/Seven Arts, 1966; voice on tape recorder, *Made in America* (also known as *Made in U.S.A.*), Rome-Paris Films, 1966; narrator, *Two or Three Things I Know about Her* (also known as *Deux ou trois choses que je sais d'elle*), Anouchka Films, 1966, released in the United States by New Yorker, 1970; voice, *Un film comme les autres* (also known as *A Film Like All the Others*), Leacock-Pennebaker Films, 1968; voice, *One Plus One* (also known as *Sympathy for the Devil*), Cupid Productions, 1968, released in the United States by New Line Cinema, 1969; as himself, *One P.M.* (also known as *One Parallel Movie*), Leacock-Pennebaker, 1971; narrator and policeman, *Vladimir et Rosa,* Evergreen Films, 1971; Uncle Sean, *First Name: Carmen* (also known as *Prenom: Carmen*), International Spectrafilm, 1984; the Idiot and the Prince, *Soigne tu droite,* Gaumont, 1987; professor,

King Lear, Cannon, 1988. Also appeared in *Quadrille,* 1950; *Presentation ou Charlotte et son steak,* 1951; *Le Coup du berger,* 1956; *Le Signe du lion,* 1959; *Le Soleil dans l'oeil,* 1961; "Le Nouveau Monde" in *RoGoPaG* (also known as *Laviamoci il cervello*), Lyre Cinematographique, 1962; *Scheherezade,* 1963; *The Directors,* 1963; *Paparazzi,* 1963; *Begegnung mit Fritz Lang,* 1963; *Petit jour,* 1963; "Camera-oeil" in *Loin du Vietnam,* 1967; *Wind from the East* (also known as *Vent d'est* and *East Wind*), 1969, released in the United States by New Line Cinema, 1970; narrator, *A Letter to Jane, or Investigation about a Still* (also known as *Lettre a Jane*), 1972; *Numero deux* (also known as *Number Two*), Societe Nouvelle de Cinema, 1975; and in *Grandeur et decadence d'un petit commerce de cinema,* Hamster, 1986.

PRINCIPAL FILM WORK—All as director, unless indicated: (Also producer) *Operation Beton* (short film), Actua Films, 1954; (as Hans Lucas; also producer and cinematographer) *Une femme coquette* (short film), Jean-Luc Godard, 1955; (with Francois Truffaut) *Une histoire d'eau* (short film; also known as *A History of Water*), Les Films de la Pleiade, 1958; *Charlotte et son Jules* (short film), Les Films de la Pleiade, 1958; *Breathless* (also known as *A bout de souffle*), Georges de Beauregard/Societe Nouvelle de Cinema, 1959, released in the United States by Imperia Films, 1959.

A Woman Is a Woman (also known as *Une femme est une femme* and *La donna e donna*), Rome-Paris Films, 1961, released in the United States by Pathe Contemporary, 1961; "Le Nouveau monde" in *RoGoPaG* (also known as *Laviamoci il cervello*), Lyre Cinematographique, 1962; "Laziness" in *Seven Capital Sins* (also known as *Les Sept peches capitaux* and *I sette peccati capitali*), Films Gibe, 1962, released in the United States by Embassy, 1962; *My Life to Live* (also known as *Vivre sa vie* and *It's My Life*), Les Films de la Pleiade, 1962, released in the United States by Union/Pathe Contemporary, 1963; *Contempt* (also known as *Le Mepris*), Rome-Paris Films, 1963, released in the United States by Embassy, 1963; *Le Petit soldat* (also known as *The Little Soldier*), Georges de Beauregard/Societe Nouvelle de Cinema, 1963, released in the United States by West End, 1965; *Les Carabiniers* (also known as *The Soldiers* and *The Riflemen*), Rome-Paris Films, 1963, released in the United States by New Yorker, 1968; "Montparnasse-Levallois" in *Six in Paris* (also known as *Paris vu par . . .*), Les Films du Losange, 1963, released in the United States by New Yorker, 1968; "Le Grand escroc" in *Les Plus belles escroqueries du monde,* Ulysse Films, 1964; *The Married Woman* (also known as *La Femme mariee, Une Femme mariee,* and *A Married Woman*), Anouchka Films, 1964, released in the United States by Royal, 1965; *Band of Outsiders* (also known as *Bande a part* and *The Outsiders*), Anouchka Films, 1964, released in the United States by Royal, 1966.

Alphaville, Chaumiane Productions and Filmstudio, 1965, released in the United States by Pathe, 1965; *Pierrot le fou,* Rome-Paris Films, 1965, released in the United States by Pathe/Corinth, 1968; *Masculin-feminin* (also known as *Masculin-feminin: 15 faits precis*), Anouchka Films, 1966; *Made in America* (also known as *Made in U.S.A.*), Rome-Paris Films, 1966; "Anticipation, ou L'Amour en l'an 2000" in *Le Plus vieux metier du monde* (also known as *The Oldest Profession*), Francoriz Films, 1966, released in the United States by Goldstone/VIP, 1968; *Two or Three Things I Know about Her* (also known as *Deux ou trois choses que je sais d'elle*), Anouchka Films, 1966, released in the United States by New Yorker, 1970; *La Chinoise, ou plutot a la chinoise,* Anouchka Films, 1967; "L'Enfant prodigue" in *Vangelo '70* (also known as "L'Amore" in *Amore e rabbia*), Anouchka Films, 1967; *Weekend* (also known as *Le Week-end*), Anouchka Films, 1967, released in

the United States by Ascot, 1968; *Le gai savoir* (also known as *The Joy of Learning* and *Merry Wisdom—Happy Knowledge*), Anouchka Films, 1968; *Un film comme les autres* (also known as *A Film Like All the Others*), Leacock-Pennebaker Films, 1968; *One Plus One* (also known as *Sympathy for the Devil*), Cupid Productions, 1968, released in the United States by New Line Cinema, 1969; (with Jean Pierre Gorin) *British Sounds* (also known as *See You at Mao*), Kestrel Productions, 1969; (with Gorin, Jean-Henri Roger, and Paul Burron as Groupe Dziga-Vertov) *Pravda,* Centre European Cinema Radio Television, 1969; (with Gorin) *Lotte in Italia* (also known as *Struggle in Italy* and *Luttes en Italie*), Cosmoseion, 1969; (with Gorin and Daniel Cohn-Bendit) *Wind from the East* (also known as *Vent d'est* and *East Wind*), 1969, released in the United States by New Line Cinema, 1970.

(With Gorin) *Vladimir et Rosa,* Evergreen Films, 1971; (with Gorin; also producer) *Tout va bien,* Anouchka Films, 1972, released in the United States by New Yorker, 1973; (also co-producer) *Numero deux* (also known as *Number Two*), Societe Nouvelle de Cinema, 1975; (also producer with Alain Sarde and editor with Anne Marie Mieville) *Sauve qui peut* (also known as *La Vie* and *Every Man for Himself*), New Yorker, 1980; *Passion,* 1982, released in the United States by Artificial Eye/United Artists Classics, 1983; *First Name: Carmen* (also known as *Prenom: Carmen*), International Spectrafilm, 1984; *Detective,* International Spectrafilm, 1985; *Hail, Mary* (also known as *Je vous salve Marie*), Gaumont/New Yorker, 1985; *Grandeur et decadence d'un petit commerce de cinema* (origianlly made for French television), Hamster, 1986; (also editor) "Armide" in *Aria,* Virgin Vision, 1987; (also editor) *Soigne tu droite,* Gaumont, 1987; *King Lear,* Cannon, 1988. Also as director, unless indicated: Producer, *Quadrille,* 1950; producer, *Kreutzer Sonata,* 1956; *Charlotte et Veronique ou Tous les garcons s'appellent Patrick* (short film), 1957; *Reportage sur Orly* (short film), 1964; "Camera-oeil" in *Loin du Vietnam,* 1967; *Cinetracts* (series of untitled, creditless newsreels), 1968; *One A.M.* (also known as *One American Movie;* unfinished), 1968; (with Gorin) *Jusqu'a la victoire* (also known as *Till Victory;* unfinished), 1970; (with Gorin; also producer with Gorin) *A Letter to Jane, or Investigation about a Still* (also known as *Lettre a Jane*), 1972; *Ici et ailleurs,* 1974; *Comment ca va,* 1976.

PRINCIPAL TELEVISION WORK—Series: Director, *France tour detour deux enfants,* French television, 1978. Specials: Co-director, *6 x 2: Sur et sous la communication,* French television, 1977.

RELATED CAREER—Gossip columnist, *Les Temps de Paris,* 1950; founder and film critic (as Hans Lucas), *Gazette du cinema,* 1950-51; film critic, *Cahiers du cinema,* 1952-1967; founder, Anouchka Films, 1964; assistant editor for Zurich television; publicist, Twentieth Century-Fox, Paris, France; founder, Sonimage film and video studio, Grenoble, France; contributor of articles and essays to journals and periodicals.

WRITINGS: See productions details above. FILM—*Operation Beton,* 1954; *Une Femme coquette,* 1955; *Charlotte et Veronique ou Tous les garcons s'appellent Patrick,* 1957; (with Francois Truffaut) *Une Histoire d'eau,* 1958; *Charlotte et son Jules,* 1958; *Breathless,* 1959, published by Balland, 1974, then Rutgers University Press, 1987; *A Woman Is a Woman,* 1961, published in *Godard: Three Films,* Harper, 1975; "Laziness" in *Seven Capital Sins,* 1962; *My Life to Live,* 1962; "Le Nouveau monde" in *RoGoPaG,* 1962; "Montparnasse-Levallois" in *Six in Paris,* 1963; *Contempt,* 1963; (with Jean Gruault and Roberto Rossellini) *Les Carabiniers,* 1963, published by Verlag Filmkritik, 1967; *Le Petit soldat,* 1963, published by Lorrimer Publishing, 1967, then

Simon & Schuster, 1970; "Le Grand escroc" in *Les Plus belles escroqueries du monde*, 1964; *Band of Outsiders*, 1964; *Reportage sur Orly*, 1964; *The Married Woman*, 1964, published in *Godard: Three Films*, Harper, 1975.

Alphaville, 1965, published by Lorrimer Publishing, 1966, then Simon & Schuster, 1968; *Pierrot le fou*, 1965, published by Simon & Schuster, 1969; "Anticipation, ou L'Amour en l'an 2000" in *Le Plus vieux metier du monde*, 1966; *Made in America*, 1966, published by Lorrimer Publishing, 1967; *Masculin-feminin*, 1966, published by Grove, 1969; *Two or Three Things I Know about Her*, 1966, published in *Godard: Three Films*, Harper, 1975; "L'Enfant prodigue" in *Vangelo '70*, 1967; "Camera-oeil" in *Loin du Vietnam*, 1967; *La Chinoise, ou plutot a la chinoise*, 1967, published by L'Avant-Scene, 1971; *Weekend*, 1967, published in *Weekend [and] Wind from the East*, Simon & Schuster, 1972; *Le Gai savoir*, 1968; *Un film comme les autres*, 1968; *One Plus One*, 1968; *Cinetracts*, 1968; *One A.M.*, 1968; (with Jean Pierre Gorin) *British Sounds*, 1969; (with Gorin, Jean-Henri Roger, and Paul Burron as Groupe Dziga-Vertov) *Pravda*, 1969; (with Gorin) *Lotte in Italia*, 1969; (with Daniel Cohn-Bendit) *Wind from the East*, 1969, published in *Weekend [and] Wind from the East*, Simon & Schuster, 1972; *Jusqu'a la victoire*, 1970; (with Gorin) *Vladimir et Rosa*, 1971; (with Gorin) *Tout va bien*, 1972; (with Gorin) *A Letter to Jane, or Investigation about a Still*, 1972; *Ici et ailleurs*, 1974; *Numero deux*, 1975; *Comment ca va*, 1976; *Passion*, 1982; *First Name: Carmen*, 1984; *Detective*, International Spectrafilm, 1985; *Hail, Mary*, 1985; *Grandeur et decadence d'un petit commerce de cinema*, 1986; "Armide" in *Aria*, 1987; *Soigne tu droite*, 1987; *King Lear*, 1988.

TELEVISION—Series: *France tour detour deux enfants*, 1978. Specials: Co-writer, *6 x 2: Sur et sous la communication*, 1977.

OTHER—(With Macha Meril) *Journal d'une femme mariee* (journal), Denoeel, 1965; *Jean-Luc Godard: articles, essais, entretiens*, P. Belfond, 1968; *Godard on Godard*, edited and translated by Tom Milne, Viking, 1972; also *Introduction a une veritable histoire du cinema*, 1980.

AWARDS: Prix Jean Vigo and Best Director Award, both from the Berlin Film Festival, 1960, for *Breathless;* Special Jury Prize from the Berlin Film Festival, 1961, for *A Woman Is a Woman;* Special Jury Prize and Italian Critics' Prize from the Venice Film Festival and German Critics' Prize, Best Foreign Film, all 1962, for *My Life to Live;* Special Jury Prize from the Venice Film Festival, 1967, for *La Chinoise, ou plutot a la chinoise;* Diploma of Merit from the Edinburgh Film Festival, 1968, for *Weekend;* Grand Prix National, 1982; (co-winner) Prix Delluc, 1987, for *Soigne tu droite.*

MEMBER: Directors Guild of America.

ADDRESSES: HOME—15 rue du Nord, 1180 Rouille, Switzerland.*

*   *   *

GOLDEN, Annie   1951-

PERSONAL: Born October 19, 1951, in Brooklyn, NY.

VOCATION: Actress.

CAREER: BROADWAY DEBUT—Mother, *Hair*, Biltmore Theatre,

1977. PRINCIPAL STAGE APPEARANCES—Audrey, *Little Shop of Horrors*, Orpheum Theatre, New York City, 1982; Spike, *Dementos*, The Production Company, Theatre Guinevere, New York City, 1983; as herself, *Leader of the Pack*, Ambassador Theatre, New York City, 1985; ensemble member, *National Lampoon's "Class of '86"*, Village Gate Theatre, New York City, 1986; Belle, *Ah! Wilderness*, Neil Simon Theatre, New York City, 1988. Also appeared in *Dr. Selavy's Magic Theatre*, St. Clement's Church Theatre, New York City, 1984; as Carlotta Vance, *Dinner at Eight*, in Connecticut, 1988; and in *A . . . My Name Is Alice*, in New York City.

PRINCIPAL FILM APPEARANCES—Jeannie, *Hair*, United Artists, 1979; band singer, *Desperately Seeking Susan*, Orion, 1985; Val, *Key Exchange*, Twentieth Century-Fox, 1985; Phoebe, *Streetwalkin'*, Concorde, 1985; Diana, *Forever, Lulu*, Tri-Star, 1986; nanny, *Baby Boom*, Metro-Goldwyn-Mayer/United Artists, 1987. Also appeared in *Burnin' Love* (also known as *Love at Stake*), Tri-Star, 1987.

PRINCIPAL TELEVISION APPEARANCES—Episodic: Caroline, "The House of Ramon Iglesia," *American Playhouse*, PBS, 1986. Specials: Ensemble member, *National Lampoon's Class of '86*, Showtime, 1986; Mary, "The Rec Room," *NBC Presents the American Film Institute Comedy Special*, NBC, 1987.

RELATED CAREER—Singer with the rock group, the Shirts.

RECORDINGS: ALBUMS—(With the Shirts) *The Shirts*, Capitol Records.

MEMBER: Actors' Equity Association, Screen Actors Guild.

ADDRESSES: AGENT—Kathy Rothacker, William Morris Agency, 151 El Camino Drive, Beverly Hills, CA 90212.*

*   *   *

GOLDMAN, William   1931-
(Harry Longbaugh, S. Morgenstern)

PERSONAL: Born August 12, 1931, in Chicago, IL; son of Maurice Clarence (in business) and Marion (Weil) Goldman; married Ilene Jones, April 15, 1961; children: Jenny Rebecca, Susana. EDUCATION: Oberlin College, B.A., 1952; Columbia University, M.A., 1956. MILITARY: U.S. Army, corporal, 1952-54.

VOCATION: Writer.

WRITINGS: STAGE—(With James Goldman) *Blood, Sweat, and Stanley Poole*, Morosco Theatre, New York City, 1961, published by Dramatists Play Service, 1962; (with James Goldman and John Kander) *A Family Affair*, Billy Rose Theatre, New York City, 1962. FILM—(With Michael Relph) *Masquerade*, United Artists, 1965; *Harper* (also known as *The Moving Target*), Warner Brothers, 1966; *Butch Cassidy and the Sundance Kid*, Twentieth Century-Fox, 1969; *The Hot Rock* (also known as *How to Steal a Diamond in Four Easy Lessons*), Twentieth Century-Fox, 1972; (with Bryan Forbes) *The Stepford Wives*, Columbia, 1974; *The Great Waldo Pepper*, Universal, 1975; *All the President's Men*, Warner Brothers, 1976; *Marathon Man*, Paramount, 1976; *A Bridge Too Far*, United Artists, 1977; *Magic*, Twentieth Century-Fox, 1978; *Heat*, New Century-Vista, 1987; *The Princess Bride*,

Twentieth Century-Fox, 1987. TELEVISION—Movies: *Mr. Horn,* CBS, 1979.

OTHER—Novels: *The Temple of Gold,* Knopf, 1957; *Your Turn to Curtsy, My Turn to Bow,* Doubleday, 1958; *Soldier in the Rain,* Atheneum, 1960; *Boys and Girls Together,* Atheneum, 1964; (as Harry Longbaugh) *No Way to Treat a Lady,* Gold Medal, 1964, then (as William Goldman) Harcourt, Brace & World, 1967; *The Thing of It Is . . . ,* Harcourt, Brace & World, 1964; *Butch Cassidy and the Sundance Kid,* Corgi, 1969; *Father's Day,* Harcourt Brace Jovanovich, 1970; *The Princess Bride,* Harcourt Brace Jovanovich, 1973; *Marathon Man,* Delacorte Press, 1974; *Wigger,* Harcourt Brace Jovanovich, 1974; *The Great Waldo Pepper,* Dell, 1975; *Magic,* Delacorte Press, 1976; *William Goldman's Story of "A Bridge Too Far,"* Dell, 1977; *Tinsel,* Delacorte, 1979; *Control,* Delacorte, 1982; (as S. Morgenstern) *The Silent Gondoliers,* Del Ray, 1983; *The Color of Light,* Warner Books, 1984; *Heat,* Warner Books, 1985; *Brothers,* Warner Books, 1987.

Non-Fiction: *The Season: A Candid Look at Broadway,* Harcourt, Brace & World, 1969, revised edition published by Limelight Editions, 1984; *Adventures in the Screen Trade,* Warner Books, 1983. Also writes short stories and articles for numerous periodicals.

AWARDS: Writers Guild Award and British Academy Award, both 1969, and Academy Award, Best Original Screenplay, 1970, all for *Butch Cassidy and the Sundance Kid;* Academy Award, Best Screenplay Adaptation, and Writers Guild Award, both 1976, for *All the President's Men;* Writers Guild Award nomination, Best Screenplay Based on Material from Another Medium, 1988, for *The Princess Bride.*

ADDRESSES: AGENTS—Michael Ovitz and B. Bookman, Creative Artists Agency, 1888 Century Park E., Suite 1400, Los Angeles, CA 90067.*

*   *   *

GORDON, Keith   1961-

PERSONAL: Born February 3, 1961, in New York, NY.

VOCATION: Actor, director, producer, and screenwriter.

CAREER: OFF-BROADWAY DEBUT—*Secrets of the Rich,* 1976. PRINCIPAL STAGE APPEARANCES—Kid, "Gotcha" and "Getaway" in *Gimme Shelter,* Brooklyn Academy of Music, Brooklyn, NY, 1978; Prince of Wales, *Richard III,* Cort Theatre, New York City, 1979; Boo, *Album,* Cherry Lane Theatre, New York City, 1980; Stu Fisher, *The Buddy System,* Circle in the Square Downtown, New York City, 1981; Hughes, *Back to Back,* WPA Theatre, New York City, 1982; Ron, *Third Street,* Circle Repertory Theatre, New York City, 1983. Also appeared in *A Traveling Companion, Suckers,* and *Sunday Runners.*

PRINCIPAL FILM APPEARANCES—Doug, *Jaws II,* Universal, 1978; young Joe, *All That Jazz,* Columbia/Twentieth Century-Fox, 1979; Dennis, *Home Movies,* United Artists, 1979; Peter Miller, *Dressed to Kill,* Filmways, 1980; Arnie Cunningham, *Christine,* Columbia, 1983; Lloyd Muldaur, *The Legend of Billie Jean,* Tri-Star, 1984; Jason Mellon, *Back to School,* Orion, 1986; also appeared as Ernie Blick, *Static,* 1986.

PRINCIPAL FILM WORK—Director, *The Chocolate War,* Management Company Entertainment Group, 1989; also co-producer, *Static,* 1986.

PRINCIPAL TELEVISION APPEARANCES—Mini-Series: Young Paulie, *Studs Lonigan,* NBC, 1979. Episodic: Chris, "My Palikari," *American Playhouse,* PBS, 1982. Movies: Jeff Miller, *Kent State,* NBC, 1981; Lionel, *Single Bars, Single Women,* ABC, 1984; Max Mendelsson, *Combat High,* NBC, 1986.

WRITINGS: FILM—(With Mark Romanek) *Static,* 1986; *The Chocolate War,* Management Company Entertainment Group, 1989.

AWARDS: Madrid Film Festival Award, Best Actor, 1987, for *Static.*

ADDRESSES: MANAGER—Jonathan D. Krane, M.C.E.G. Management, 11355 W. Olympic Boulevard, Los Angeles, CA 90064. AGENTS—(Directing) Steve Dontanville and Steve Rabineau, International Creative Management, 8899 Beverly Boulevard, Los Angeles, CA 90048; (acting) Nevin Dollicfiro, The Agency, 10351 Santa Monica Boulevard, Suite 211, Los Angeles, CA 90025.

*   *   *

GORMAN, Cliff

PERSONAL: Born October 13, in New York, NY; married Gayle Stevens, May 31, 1963. EDUCATION: Attended the University of New Mexico, 1954-55, and the University of California, Los Angeles, 1955-56; New York University, B.S., education, 1959; trained for the stage with Wynn Handman, 1963-64, and with Jerome Robbins' American Theatre Lab, 1965-66.

VOCATION: Actor.

CAREER: STAGE DEBUT—Peter Boyle, *Hogan's Goat,* American Place Theatre, New York City, 1965. BROADWAY DEBUT—Lenny Bruce, *Lenny,* Brooks Atkinson Theatre, 1971. PRINCIPAL STAGE APPEARANCES—Arnulf, *Ergo,* New York Shakespeare Festival, Public Theatre, New York City, 1968; Emory, *The Boys in the Band,* Theatre Four, New York City, 1968, then Huntington Hartford Theatre, Los Angeles, CA, 1969; Leo Schneider, *Chapter Two,* Ahmanson Theatre, Los Angeles, then Imperial Theatre, New York City, both 1977; Benny, *Angelo's Wedding,* Circle Repertory Company, New York City, 1985; Lennie Ganz, *Doubles,* Ritz Theatre, New York City, 1985; David Kahn, *Social Security,* Ethel Barrymore Theatre, New York City, 1986.

FILM DEBUT—Toto, *Justine,* Twentieth Century-Fox, 1969. PRINCIPAL FILM APPEARANCES—Emory, *The Boys in the Band,* National General, 1970; Tom, *Cops and Robbers,* United Artists, 1973; Hamlekh, *Rosebud,* United Artists, 1975; Charlie, *An Unmarried Woman,* Twentieth Century-Fox, 1978; Davis Newman, *All That Jazz,* Twentieth Century-Fox, 1979; Gus Soltic, *Night of the Juggler,* Columbia, 1980; Lieutenant Andrews, *Angel,* New World, 1984.

PRINCIPAL TELEVISION APPEARANCES—Pilots: Arthur McGee, *Having Babies II,* ABC, 1977; Riki Anatole, *Cocaine and Blue Eyes,* NBC, 1983. Episodic: *Hawk,* ABC; *NYPD,* ABC; *Police Story,* NBC; *Hawaii Five-O,* CBS; *The Streets of San Francisco,* ABC; *Trapper John, M.D.,* CBS; *Murder, She Wrote,* CBS;

Cagney and Lacey, CBS; *Friday the 13th—The Series,* syndicated; *Spenser: For Hire,* ABC. Movies: Mickey Swerner, *Class of '63,* ABC, 1973; Stanley Greenberg, *The Silence,* NBC, 1975; Detective Joey Gentry, *Strike Force,* NBC, 1975; Danny Conforti, *Brinks: The Great Robbery,* CBS, 1976; Joseph Goebbels, *The Bunker,* CBS, 1981; Aaron Greenberg, *Doubletake,* CBS, 1985; Aaron Greenberg, *Internal Affairs,* CBS, 1988. Specials: *The Trial of the Chicago Seven,* BBC, 1970; also *Paradise Lost,* NET.

AWARDS: Obie Award from the *Village Voice,* 1968, for *The Boys in the Band;* Drama Desk Award, Best Actor, 1971, *Show Business* (magazine) Award, 1971, Antoinette Perry Award, Best Actor in a Dramatic Play, 1972, and La Guardia Memorial Award for Cultural Achievement, 1972, all for *Lenny.*

MEMBER: Actors' Equity Association, American Federation of Television and Radio Artists, Screen Actors Guild, Honor Legion of the New York City Police Department, Friends of George Spelvin.

ADDRESSES: AGENT—STE Representation, Ltd., 888 Seventh Avenue, New York, NY 10019.

*   *   *

GRAFF, Todd

VOCATION: Actor and playwright.

CAREER: Also see *WRITINGS* below. PRINCIPAL STAGE APPEARANCES—David, *The City Suite,* Park Royal Theatre, New York City, 1979; Johnny, *American Passion,* Joyce Theatre, New York City, 1983; Danny Hooper, *Baby,* Ethel Barrymore Theatre, New York City, 1983.

PRINCIPAL FILM APPEARANCES—Rothwell T. Schwartz, *Not Quite Jerusalem,* Rank Organization, 1985; Leonard, *Sweet Lorraine,* Angelika, 1987; James, *Five Corners,* Cineplex Odeon, 1987; Larry Higgins, *Dominick and Eugene,* Orion, 1988.

PRINCIPAL TELEVISION APPEARANCES—Movies: Tough kid, *After Midnight,* ABC, 1988.

WRITINGS: STAGE—*The Grandma Plays,* Vineyard Theatre, New York City, 1988.

AWARDS: Theatre World Award, 1983, for *Baby.*

ADDRESSES: AGENT—Nancy Carson, Carson-Adler Agency, 250 W. 57th Street, Suite 808, New York, NY 10107.*

*   *   *

GRAHAM, Ronny   1919-

PERSONAL: Born August 26, 1919, in Philadelphia, PA; son of Steve (a vaudeville performer) and Florence (a vaudeville performer; maiden name, Sweeney) Graham; married Jean Spitzbarth, 1947 (divorced, 1950); married Ellen Hanley (a singer and actress), March 4, 1951 (divorced, December 4, 1963); married Sigyn Lund, 1965; children: five (one, first marriage; two, second marriage;

two, third marriage). MILITARY: U.S. Army Air Forces, sergeant, 1942-45.

VOCATION: Actor, director, composer, lyricist, and writer.

CAREER: Also see *WRITINGS* below. STAGE DEBUT—*It's about Time* (revue), Brattle Theatre, Cambridge, MA, 1951. BROADWAY DEBUT—*New Faces of 1952* (revue), Royale Theatre, 1952. PRINCIPAL STAGE APPEARANCES—Charlie Reader, *The Tender Trap,* Longacre Theatre, New York City, 1954; *Take Five* (revue), Upstairs at the Downstairs, New York City, 1957; *Graham Crackers* (revue), Upstairs at the Downstairs, 1963; Monte Checkovitch, *Something More!,* Eugene O'Neill Theatre, New York City, 1964; Weller Martin, *Jokers,* Goodspeed Opera House, East Haddam, CT, 1986. Also appeared in as Mr. Applegate, *Damn Yankees,* Camden, NJ, and Philadelphia, PA, both 1960; in *America, Be Seated,* Louisiana Pavilion, New York World's Fair, Flushing, NY, 1964; in *Room Service,* St. Louis Repertory Theatre, St. Louis, MO, 1971; and in *That Championship Season,* Seattle Repertory Theatre, Seattle, WA, 1973.

PRINCIPAL STAGE WORK—Director: *Money* (revue), Upstairs at the Downstairs, New York City, 1963; *America, Be Seated,* Louisiana Pavilion, New York World's Fair, Flushing, NY, 1964; *Mating Dance,* Eugene O'Neill Theatre, New York City, 1965; *Free Fall* (revue), Upstairs at the Downstairs, 1969; *Grin and Bare It!* and *Postcards,* both Belasco Theatre, New York City, 1970; *A Place for Polly,* Ethel Barrymore Theatre, New York City, 1970.

MAJOR TOURS—*New Faces of 1952* (revue), U.S. cities, 1952; *Luv,* U.S. cities, 1967. Also director, *Here Lies Jeremy Troy* (retitled *Jeremy Troy*), U.S. cities, 1968-69.

FILM DEBUT—*New Faces,* Twentieth Century-Fox, 1954. PRINCIPAL FILM APPEARANCES—Charlie Niles, *Dirty Little Billy,* Columbia, 1972; the Director, *The World's Greatest Lover,* Twentieth Century-Fox, 1977; Mark Bennett, *Won Ton Ton, the Dog Who Saved Hollywood,* Paramount, 1977; Oedipus, *History of the World, Part 1,* Twentieth Century-Fox, 1981; Sondheim, *To Be or Not to Be,* Twentieth Century-Fox, 1983; minister, *Spaceballs,* Metro-Goldwyn-Mayer/United Artists, 1987.

PRINCIPAL TELEVISION APPEARANCES—Series: Regular, *The New Bill Cosby Show,* CBS, 1972-73; regular, *The Wacky World of Jonathan Winters,* syndicated, 1972; regular, *The Hudson Brothers Show,* CBS, 1974; Mr. Ernest Busso, *The Bob Crane Show,* NBC, 1975; Reverend Bemis, *Chico and the Man,* NBC, 1975-76. Episodic: "Highlights of New Faces," *Play of the Week,* NTA, 1960; *M*A*S*H,* CBS, 1978; also *Toast of the Town,* CBS; *The Phil Silvers Show,* CBS; *The Colgate Comedy Hour,* NBC; *The Tonight Show,* NBC; *The Steve Allen Show,* CBS; *Omnibus,* CBS. Movies: Cap'n Andy, *The Ratings Game,* Movie Channel, 1984. Specials: *Jonathan Winters Presents 200 Years of American Humor,* NBC, 1976.

PRINCIPAL TELEVISION WORK—Series: Story consultant, *M*A*S*H,* CBS, 1977-81; comedy consultant, *Mel and Susan Together,* ABC, 1978.

RELATED CAREER—As a comedian and singer, appeared in nightclubs throughout the United States, including Punchinello's East, Chicago, IL, Ruban Bleu, Blue Angel, Plaza 9, and Brothers and Sisters, all in New York City.

WRITINGS: STAGE—Contributor of music, lyrics, and sketches,

New Faces of 1952 (revue), Royale Theatre, 1952; music, lyrics, and (with Sidney Carroll) continuity, *Mask and Gown* (revue), John Golden Theatre, New York City, 1957; *Take Five* (revue), Upstairs at the Downstairs, New York City, 1957; contributor, *Let It Ride!* (revue), Eugene O'Neill Theatre, New York City, 1961; lyrics, *Bravo, Giovanni!*, Broadhurst Theatre, New York City, 1962; contributor, *The Cat's Pajamas* (revue), Sheridan Square Playhouse, New York City, 1962; *Graham Crackers* (revue), Upstairs at the Downstairs, 1963; contributor, *Wet Paint* (revue), Renata Theatre, New York City, 1965; contributor of music, lyrics, and sketches, *New Faces of 1968* (revue), Booth Theatre, New York City, 1968.

FILM—(With Mel Brooks, Paul Lynde, Luther Davis, and John Cleveland) *New Faces*, Twentieth Century-Fox, 1954; (with Thomas Meehan) *To Be or Not to Be*, Twentieth Century-Fox, 1983; (with Terence Marsh and Charles Dennis) *Finders Keepers*, Warner Brothers, 1984; (with Brooks and Meehan) *Spaceballs*, Metro-Goldwyn-Mayer/United Artists, 1987.

TELEVISION—Series: *The New Bill Cosby Show*, CBS, 1972-73. Episodic: "Your Hit Parade," *M*A*S*H*, CBS, 1978; (with Ken Levine and David Isaacs) "Dr. Winchester and Mr. Hyde," *M*A*S*H*, CBS, 1978; "Commander Pierce," *M*A*S*H*, CBS, 1978; (with Levine, Isaacs, and Larry Balmagia) "Our Finest Hour," *M*A*S*H*, CBS, 1978; "An Eye for a Tooth," *M*A*S*H*, CBS, 1978; (with Balmagia) "C*A*V*E," *M*A*S*H*, CBS, 1979; "Mr. and Mrs. Who?," *M*A*S*H*, CBS, 1979.

AWARDS: Donaldson Award and Theatre World Award, both 1953, for *New Faces of 1952;* (with Milton Schafer) Antoinette Perry Award nomination, Best Composer and Lyricist, 1963, for *Bravo, Giovanni!*.

MEMBER: Actors' Equity Association, American Guild of Variety Artists, American Federation of Television and Radio Artists, Screen Actors Guild, American Federation of Musicians.

ADDRESSES: CONTACT—Actors' Equity Association, 165 W. 46th Street, New York, NY 10036.*

*   *   *

GRAMMER, Kelsey

PERSONAL: Born February 21, in St. Thomas, Virgin Islands; children: Spencer. EDUCATION: Trained for the stage at the Juilliard School for two years.

VOCATION: Actor.

CAREER: PRINCIPAL STAGE APPEARANCES—Aleksei Belyayev, *A Month in the Country*, Roundabout Stage One Theatre, New York City, 1980; Lennox, *Macbeth*, Vivian Beaumont Theatre, New York City, 1981; Gloucester, *Henry V*, American Shakespeare Theatre, Stratford, CT, 1981; Cassio, *Othello*, American Shakespeare Theatre, 1981, then Winter Garden Theatre, New York City, 1982; Codename Lazar, *Plenty*, New York Shakespeare Festival, Public Theatre, New York City, 1982; Mark Sackling, *Quartermaine's Terms*, Long Wharf Theatre, New Haven, CT, then Playhouse 91, New York City, both 1983; young man, soldier, and Alex Savage, *Sunday in the Park with George*, Playwrights Horizons, New York City, 1983; Demeter Stanzides and Lucio, *Measure for Measure*, Center Theatre Group, Mark Taper Forum, Los Angeles, CA,

1985. Also appeared in *The Mousetrap*, Studio Arena Theatre, Buffalo, NY, 1980; *Arms and the Man*, Studio Arena Theatre, 1984; and at the Globe Theatre, San Diego, CA, for three years.

PRINCIPAL TELEVISION APPEARANCES—Series: Frasier Crane, *Cheers*, NBC, 1984—; also Dr. Canard, *Another World*, NBC. Mini-Series: Stephen Smith, *Kennedy*, NBC, 1983; Lieutenant Stewart, *George Washington*, CBS, 1984; Craig Lawson, *Crossings*, ABC, 1986. Pilots: *Lame Duck*. Episodic: *Kate and Allie*, CBS. Movies: Ed Strull, *Dance 'til Dawn*, NBC, 1988. Specials: Stuart Cooper, *You Are the Jury*, NBC, 1987; *Paul Reiser: Out on a Whim*, HBO, 1987.

ADDRESSES: PUBLICIST—Maggie Begley, Mahoney/Wasserman Public Relations, 345 N. Maple Drive, Beverly Hills, CA 90210.*

*   *   *

GRAY, Spalding   1941-

PERSONAL: Born June 5, 1941, in Providence, RI; son of Rockwell and Elizabeth Gray. EDUCATION: Emerson College, B.A., 1965.

VOCATION: Actor, performance artist, and writer.

CAREER: Also see WRITINGS below. STAGE DEBUT—Hanibal, *The Curious Savage*, Fryeburg Academy, 1965, for two performances. OFF-BROADWAY DEBUT—King of the May, *Endicott and the Red Cross*, American Place Theatre, 1968. LONDON DEBUT—*Swimming to Cambodia* (monologue), Riverside Theatre, 1987, for

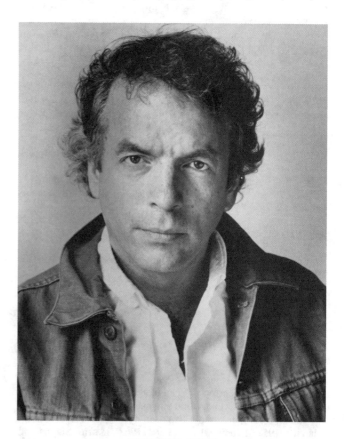

SPALDING GRAY

twenty performances. PRINCIPAL STAGE APPEARANCES—Hoss, *The Tooth of Crime*, Performing Garage, New York City, 1973; swiss cheese, *Mother Courage and Her Children,* and in *Sakonnet Point*, Performing Garage, 1975; cook, soldier, and peasant man, *Mother Courage and Her Children,* and Spud, *Rumstick Road*, both Performing Garage, 1977; Spud, *Rumstick Road,* Spalding, *Nayatt School,* and in *Sakonnet Point,* all in *Three Places in Rhode Island,* Performing Garage, 1978; Czerwicki, *Cops,* Performance Group, Envelope Theatre, New York City, 1978; bishop, *The Balcony,* Performing Garage, 1979; *Sex and Death to the Age 14, India and After (America),* and *Booze, Cars, and College Girls* (monologues), and in *Point Judith: An Epilog,* all Performing Garage, 1979.

Travels through New England (monologue), Brattle Theatre, Cambridge, MA, 1984; *Swimming to Cambodia, Parts I and II* (monologues), Performing Garage, 1984, then Center Theatre Group, Taper Too Theatre, Los Angeles, CA, 1985; *Terrors of Pleasure, Sex and Death to the Age 14,* and *Swimming to Cambodia* (monologues), all Trinity Repertory Company, Providence, RI, then Mitzi E. Newhouse Theatre, New York City, both 1986; General Lance Benders, *North Atlantic,* Kennedy Center for the Performing Arts, Washington, DC, 1986; Stage Manager, *Our Town,* Lyceum Theatre, New York City, 1988. Also appeared in *The Knack* and *Long Day's Journey into Night,* both Cape Cod, MA, 1965; *Scales,* Northampton, MA, 1966, then New York City, 1975; *Nobody Ever Wanted to Sit behind a Desk* and *A Personal History of the American Theatre* (monologues), both New York City, 1980; *Interviewing the Audience* and *47 Beds* (monologues), both New York City, 1981; *In Search of the Monkey Girl* and *8 x Gray* (monologues), both New York City, 1982; *Terrors of Pleasure: The House* (monologue), Cambridge, MA, 1985, then New York City, 1986, later London, 1987; in little theatre productions, Saratoga, NY, 1967; and in the *Carplays* series, Olympic Arts Festival.

PRINCIPAL STAGE WORK—Director (with Elizabeth LeComte), *Rumstick Road,* Performing Garage, New York City, 1977; also director, *Scales,* Northampton, MA, then Amherst, MA, both 1966.

MAJOR TOURS—Swiss Cheese, *Mother Courage and Her Children,* Performance Group, Indian cities, 1976; *Interviewing the Audience* (monologue), U.S. and European cities, 1982; also toured U.S. cities in performances of his monologues.

PRINCIPAL FILM APPEARANCES—Radical, *Cowards,* Jaylo, 1970; travel agent, *Almost You,* Twentieth Century-Fox/TLC, 1984; voice of obscene phone caller, *Variety,* Horizon, 1984; Terry Norfolk, *Hard Choices,* Screenland-Breakout, 1984; U.S. consul, *The Killing Fields,* Warner Brothers, 1984; Dr. Rodney, *Seven Minutes in Heaven,* Warner Brothers, 1986; Earl Culver, *True Stories,* Warner Brothers, 1986; as himself, *Swimming to Cambodia,* Cinecom, 1987; Reverend Cardew, *Stars and Bars,* Columbia, 1988; Peter Epstein, *Clara's Heart,* Warner Brothers, 1988; Dr. Richard Milstein, *Beaches,* Buena Vista, 1988. Also appeared in *The Communists Are Comfortable (and Three Other Stories),* 1984; *Heavy Petting* (documentary), Fossil, 1988; and in *Gray Areas* and *Spalding Gray's Map of L.A.* (videos).

PRINCIPAL TELEVISION APPEARANCES—Episodic: Gary, "Bedtime Story," *Trying Times,* PBS, 1987. Specials: *The American Dream,* NBC, 1986; "Spalding Gray: Terrors of Pleasure," *On Location,* HBO, 1987.

RELATED CAREER—Founder (with Elizabeth LeComte), Wooster Group, New York City, 1975; teacher, summer workshop in performance, University of California, Santa Cruz, 1978; teacher, New York University Experimental Theatre Wing, New York City, 1981.

WRITINGS: See production details above, unless indicated. STAGE— *Scales,* 1966; (with Elizabeth LeComte) *Sakonnet Point,* 1975, *Rumstick Road,* 1977, and *Nayatt School,* 1978, all later performed as *Three Places in Rhode Island,* 1979; (with LeComte) *Point Judith: An Epilog,* 1979; *Sex and Death to the Age 14,* 1979, published by Random House, 1986, and in *Swimming to Cambodia: The Collected Works,* Pan, 1987; *Booze, Cars, and College Girls,* 1979, published in *Sex and Death to the Age 14,* 1986; *India and After (America),* 1979; *Nobody Ever Wanted to Sit behind a Desk,* 1980, published in *Sex and Death to the Age 14,* 1986; *A Personal History of the American Theatre,* 1980; *Interviewing the Audience,* 1981; *47 Beds,* 1981, published in *Sex and Death to the Age 14,* 1986; (with Randal Levenson) *In Search of the Monkey Girl,* 1982, published by Aperture, 1982; *8 x Gray,* 1982; *Travels through New England,* 1984; *Swimming to Cambodia, Parts I and II,* 1984, published by Theatre Communications Group, 1985, and in *Swimming to Cambodia: The Collected Works,* 1987; (adaptor) *Rivkala's Ring,* first performed in Urbana, IL, 1985, then by the Acting Company, Lucille Lortel Theatre, New York City, 1986, published by Knopf, 1986; *Terrors of Pleasure: The House,* 1985, published in *Sex and Death to the Age 14,* 1986.

FILM—*Swimming to Cambodia,* 1987. TELEVISION—Episodic: (With Renee Shafransy) "Bedtime Story," *Trying Times,* 1987. Specials: "Spalding Gray: Terrors of Pleasure," *On Location,* 1987. OTHER—*Impossible Vacation* (autobiography), Knopf, 1989.

AWARDS: National Endowment for the Arts fellowship, 1977; Rockefeller Foundation fellowship, 1980; Guggenheim fellowship, 1985; Obie Award from the *Village Voice,* 1985; also Edward Albee Foundation Grant and two *Villager* Awards.

ADDRESSES: OFFICE—22 Wooster Street, New York, NY. AGENTS—Tony Martino, International Creative Management, 40 W. 57th Street, New York, NY 10019; Pat Quinn, International Creative Management, 8899 Beverly Boulevard, Los Angeles, CA 90048.

*　　*　　*

GREENBLATT, William R. 1944-

PERSONAL: Born June 11, 1944, in Brooklyn, NY; son of Jerome Milton (a salesman) and Blanche (an employment counselor; maiden name, Posner) Greenblatt; married wife, Charlotte (a potter), April 15, 1965; children: James Marshal, Kathy.

VOCATION: Producer and press representative.

CAREER: PRINCIPAL STAGE WORK—Press representative: *What Makes Sammy Run?,* 54th Street Theatre, New York City, 1954; *Oh, What a Lovely War,* Broadhurst Theatre, New York City, 1964; *The Subject Was Roses,* Royale Theatre, New York City, 1964; *The Wicked Cooks,* Orpheum Theatre, New York City, 1967.

MAJOR TOURS—Press representative, *Funny Girl,* U.S. cities.

PRINCIPAL FILM WORK—Executive producer, *Judgment in Ber-*

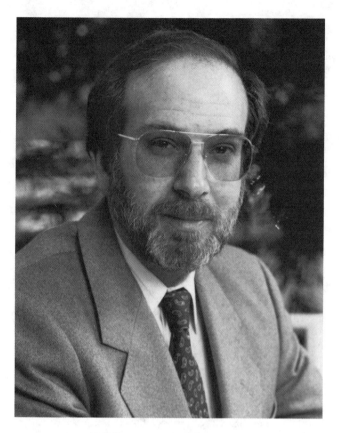

WILLIAM R. GREENBLATT

lin, New Line Cinema, 1987; executive producer, *Da,* FilmDallas, 1988.

PRINCIPAL TELEVISION WORK—Specials: Executive producer, "Babies Having Babies," *CBS Schoolbreak Special,* CBS, 1986; executive producer and producer, "No Means No," *CBS Schoolbreak Special,* CBS, 1988.

RELATED CAREER—Partner and executive vice-president, John O'Donnell Company (a public relations and financial development firm), New York City, 1967-82; founder (with Martin Sheen) and president, Sheen/Greenblatt Productions (also known as Symphony Pictures/Symphony Pictures Television), 1983—; press representative for Radio City Music Hall, New York City, Metropolitan Opera Company, New York City, and Brooklyn Academy of Music, Brooklyn, NY; past president and member of the board of directors, Los Angeles Ballet, Los Angeles, CA.

MEMBER: Academy of Television Arts and Sciences.

ADDRESSES: OFFICE—5711 W. Slauson, Suite 226, Culver City, CA 90230. AGENT—Robert Lee, Triad Artists, 10100 Santa Monica Boulevard, 16th Floor, Los Angeles, CA 90067.

*　　*　　*

GREY, Jennifer

PERSONAL: Daughter of Joel (an actor, dancer, and singer) and Jo (an actress and singer; maiden name, Wilder) Grey.

VOCATION: Actress and dancer.

CAREER: PRINCIPAL STAGE APPEARANCES—*Album,* Cherry Lane Theatre, New York City, 1980.

PRINCIPAL FILM APPEARANCES—Cathy Bennario, *Reckless,* Metro-Goldwyn-Mayer/United Artists (MGM/UA), 1984; Patsy Dwyer, *The Cotton Club,* Orion, 1984; Toni, *Red Dawn,* MGM/UA, 1984; Leslie, *American Flyers,* Warner Brothers, 1985; Jeanie Beuller, *Ferris Beuller's Day Off,* Paramount, 1986; Frances "Baby" Houseman, *Dirty Dancing,* Vestron, 1987; voice of Airelle, *Light Years* (animated), Miramax, 1988.

RELATED CAREER—Dancer in television commercials.

AWARDS: Golden Globe Award nomination, Best Actress in a Comedy or Musical, 1988, for *Dirty Dancing.*

ADDRESSES: AGENT—Smith Freedman and Associates, 121 N. San Vicente Boulevard, Beverly Hills, CA 90211.*

*　　*　　*

GRIFFIN, Lynne

PERSONAL: Born in Canada; daughter of James Joseph (a soccer player and fashion photographer) and Kay (an actress) Griffin; married Steven Poster (a cinematographer).

VOCATION: Actress.

CAREER: PRINCIPAL STAGE APPEARANCES—Cordelia, *King Lear,* Stratford Shakespearean Festival, Stratford, ON, Canada, 1980; Bianca, *The Taming of the Shrew,* and Virgilia, *Coriolanus,* both Stratford Shakespearean Festival, 1981; Kate, "Souvenir" in *Sundays at the Itchey Foot,* Center Theatre Group, Mark Taper Forum, Taper Too Theatre, Los Angeles, 1985; Louisa May Alcott, *Romance Language,* Center Theatre Group, Mark Taper Forum, 1986. Also appeared in *Thark,* Philadelphia Drama Guild, Philadelphia, PA, 1979; *There's One in Every Marriage,* Old Globe Theatre, San Diego, CA, 1987; *The Voice of the Prairie,* Old Globe Theatre, 1988; as Saint Joan, *The Lark;* Nora, *A Doll's House;* title role, *Antigone;* Ophelia, *Hamlet;* Laura, *The Glass Menagerie;* Jill, *Equus;* Cathy, *Wuthering Heights;* Violet, *Man and Superman;* Teresa, *The Hostage;* and Ellie Dunn, *Heartbreak House.*

PRINCIPAL FILM APPEARANCES—Clare Harrison, *Black Christmas,* Ambassador, 1974; Monica, *Mr. Patman,* Film Consortium of Canada, 1980; Sara Kaplan, *The Amateur,* Twentieth Century-Fox, 1982; Patti O'Connor, *Curtains,* Jensen Farley, 1983; Pam Elsinore, *Strange Brew,* Metro-Goldwyn-Mayer/United Artists, 1983; waitress, *The Heavenly Kid,* Orion, 1985; Karen Hughes, *Obsessed* (also known as *Hitting Home*), Astral/New Star, 1988. Also appeared in *A Stranger in the House.*

PRINCIPAL TELEVISION APPEARANCES—Series: Host, *Drop In,* Canadian television. Mini-Series: Candice Alexander, *I'll Take Manhattan,* CBS, 1987. Specials: *The Magic of David Copperfield,* CBS, 1983; Vicki Atkin, *The Second Time Around,* ABC, 1985; Melba, "It Takes Two," *Comedy Factory,* ABC, 1985.

RELATED CAREER—Appeared in fashion advertisements and television commercials as a child.

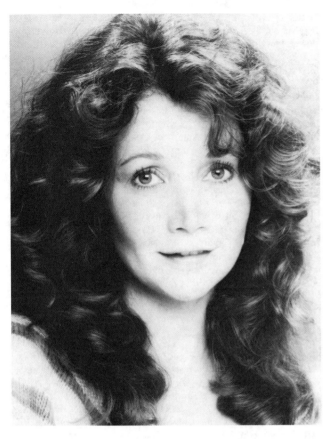

LYNNE GRIFFIN

SIDELIGHTS: FAVORITE ROLES—Cordelia in *King Lear,* Cathy in *Wuthering Heights,* Bianca in *The Taming of the Shrew,* and Virgilia in *Coriolanus.*

ADDRESSES: PUBLICIST—Lori De Waal, The Garrett Company, 6922 Hollywood Boulevard, Suite 407, Los Angeles, CA 90028.

*   *   *

GRIMES, Stephen   1927-1988

PERSONAL: Born April 18, 1927, in Weybridge, England; died of a heart attack, September 12, 1988, in Positano, Italy; children: two sons, three daughters.

VOCATION: Film production designer and art director.

CAREER: PRINCIPAL FILM APPEARANCES—Second Commissioner, *Out of Africa,* Universal, 1985. FIRST FILM WORK—Assistant art director, *Moby Dick,* Warner Brothers, 1956. PRINCIPAL FILM WORK—Art director, *Heaven Knows, Mr. Allison,* Twentieth Century-Fox, 1957; special effects (with Ivor Beddoes), *Attila,* Lux, 1958; art director (with Raymond Gabutti), *The Roots of Heaven,* Twentieth Century-Fox, 1958; art director, *The Unforgiven,* United Artists, 1960; art director (with William Newberry), *The Misfits,* United Artists, 1961; art director, *Freud* (also known as *The Secret Passion*), United Artists, 1962; associate art director, *Lawrence of Arabia,* Columbia, 1962; art director

(with Alexander Golitzen and George Webb), *The List of Adrian Messenger,* Universal, 1963; art director, *The Night of the Iguana,* Metro-Goldwyn-Mayer (MGM), 1964; production designer, *The Chalk Garden,* Universal, 1964; art director (with Hal Pereira), *This Property Is Condemned,* Paramount, 1966; produciton designer, *The Bible . . . In the Beginning,* Twentieth Century-Fox, 1966; production designer, *Reflections in a Golden Eye,* Warner Brothers, 1967; production designer, *Sinful Davey,* United Artists, 1969; production designer, *A Walk with Love and Death,* Twentieth Century-Fox, 1969.

Production designer, *Ryan's Daughter,* MGM, 1970; production designer, *The Way We Were,* Columbia, 1973; production designer, *Three Days of the Condor,* Paramount, 1975; production designer and second unit director, *The Yakuza* (also known as *Brotherhood of the Yakuza*), Warner Brothers/Toei, 1975; art director, *Independence,* Twentieth Century-Fox, 1975; production designer, *Murder by Death,* Columbia, 1976; production designer and second unit director, *Bobby Dearfield,* Columbia, 1977; production designer, *Straight Time,* Warner Brothers, 1978; production designer, *The Electric Horseman,* Universal, 1979; production designer, *Urban Cowboy,* Paramount, 1980; production designer and second unit director, *On Golden Pond,* Universal, 1981; production designer, *True Confessions,* United Artists, 1981; production designer, *The Dresser,* Columbia, 1983; production designer, *Krull,* Columbia, 1983; production designer (with Philip Harrison), *Never Say Never Again,* Warner Brothers, 1983; production designer, *Out of Africa,* Universal, 1985; production designer (with Dennis Washington), *The Dead,* Vestron/Zenith, 1988; production designer, *Haunted Summer,* Cannon Releasing, 1988.

AWARDS: Academy Award nomination, Best Art Direction and Set Decoration (black and white), 1965, for *The Night of the Iguana;* Academy Award nomination, Best Art Direction and Set Decoration, 1974, for *The Way We Were;* Academy Award, Best Production Design, 1985, for *Out of Africa.*

OBITUARIES AND OTHER SOURCES—Variety, September 21, 1988.*

*   *   *

GUEST, Christopher   1948-

PERSONAL: Born February 5, 1948, in New York, NY; married Jamie Lee Curtis (an actress); children: one daughter. EDUCATION: Attended the High School of Music and Art; also attended Bard College and New York University.

VOCATION: Actor, writer, and comedian.

CAREER: STAGE DEBUT—*Little Murders,* 1969. BROADWAY DEBUT—Bank messenger, *Room Service,* Edison Theatre, 1970. PRINCIPAL STAGE APPEARANCES—Norman, *Moonchildren,* Royale Theatre, New York City, 1972; ensemble member, *National Lampoon's Lemmings,* Village Gate Theatre, New York City, 1973; Sir Francis, *East Lynne,* Manhattan Theatre Club, New York City, 1975. Also appeared with the Arena Stage, Washington, DC, 1971-72.

PRINCIPAL FILM APPEARANCES—Resident, *The Hospital,* United Artists, 1971; policeman, *The Hot Rock* (also known as *How to Steal a Diamond in Four Easy Lessons*), Twentieth Century-Fox,

1972; Patrolman Reilly, *Death Wish,* Paramount, 1974; boy lover, *The Fortune,* Columbia, 1975; voice characterization, *La Honte de la jungle* (animated; also known as *Jungle Burger*), Entertainment Film Distributors, 1975; Eric, *Girlfriends,* Warner Brothers, 1978; Roger, *The Last Word* (also known as *Danny Travis*), International, 1979; Charlie Ford, *The Long Riders,* United Artists, 1980; voice characterization, *The Missing Link* (animated), SND, 1980; Calvin, *Heartbeeps,* Universal, 1981; Nigel Tufnel, *This Is Spinal Tap* (also known as *Spinal Tap*), Embassy, 1984; first customer, *Little Shop of Horrors,* Warner Brothers, 1986; Bob, *Beyond Therapy,* New World, 1987; Count Rugen, *The Princess Bride,* Twentieth Century-Fox, 1987; Sam, *Sticky Fingers,* Spectrafilm, 1988.

PRINCIPAL TELEVISION APPEARANCES—Series: Regular, *Saturday Night Live with Howard Cosell,* ABC, 1975; regular, *Saturday Night Live,* NBC, 1984-85. Mini-Series: Jeb Stuart Magruder, *Blind Ambition,* CBS, 1979. Pilots: *The TV Show,* ABC, 1979. Episodic: Jim, "Mike and Gloria Meet," *All in the Family,* CBS, 1977. Movies: Harry Bailey, *It Happened One Christmas,* ABC, 1977; television director, *Haywire,* CBS, 1980; Bucky Frische, *Million Dollar Infield,* CBS, 1982; Philip Ryan, *A Piano for Mrs. Cimino,* CBS, 1982. Specials: *The Lily Tomlin Special,* ABC, 1975; Al Green, *Billion Dollar Bubble,* NBC, 1977; *How to Survive the 70s and Maybe Even Bump into Happiness,* CBS, 1978; Ira, *Close Ties,* Entertainment Channel, 1983; *Martin Short Concert for the North Americas,* Showtime, 1985; Chip, *Billy Crystal—Don't Get Me Started,* HBO, 1986.

PRINCIPAL TELEVISION WORK—Director, "Johnny Appleseed," *Tall Tales and Legends,* Showtime.

RELATED CAREER—Appeared on fifty-two syndicated radio programs and six comedy albums associated with the National Lampoon; appeared in a concert tour as his *Spinal Tap* character, musician Nigel Tufnel.

WRITINGS: STAGE—Music and lyrics (with Paul Jacobs), *National Lampoon's Lemmings,* Village Gate Theatre, 1973. FILM—Screenplay, music, and lyrics (with Michael McKean, Harry Shearer, and Rob Reiner) *This Is Spinal Tap,* Embassy, 1984. TELEVISION—Specials: (With Jane Wagner, Lorne Michaels, Lily Tomlin, Earl Pomerantz, Jim Rusk, Rod Warren, and George Yanok) *The Lily Tomlin Special,* ABC, 1975; (with Bill Richmond, Gene Perret, Robert Illes, and James Stein) *Peeping Times,* NBC, 1978.

AWARDS: Emmy Award, Best Writing for a Comedy Special, 1976, for *The Lily Tomlin Special;* Obie Award from the *Village Voice,* Best Music and Lyrics, for *National Lampoon's Lemmings.*

ADDRESSES: AGENT—Hildy Gottlieb, International Creative Management, 8899 Beverly Boulevard, Los Angeles, CA 90048.*

*   *   *

GULAGER, Clu   1928-

PERSONAL: Born November 16, 1928, in Holdenville, OK; son of John Gulager (a cowboy entertainer). EDUCATION: Attended Baylor University. MILITARY: U.S. Marine Corps.

VOCATION: Actor.

CAREER: PRINCIPAL FILM APPEARANCES—Lee, *The Killers* (also known as *Ernest Hemingway's "The Killers"*), Universal, 1964; Johnny, *And Now Miguel,* Universal, 1966; Juan Clemente, *Sullivan's Empire,* Universal, 1967; Larry Morechek, *Winning,* Universal, 1969; Frank Quinn, *Company of Killers,* Universal, 1970; Abilene, *The Last Picture Show,* Columbia, 1971; deputy, *Molly and Lawless John,* Producers Distributors Corporation, 1972; Franklin Toms, *McQ,* Warner Brothers, 1974; Bill Fraser, *The Other Side of Midnight,* Twentieth Century-Fox, 1977; Sam Dunne, *A Force of One,* American Cinema, 1979; Don Fielder, *Touched by Love* (also known as *To Elvis, with Love*), Columbia, 1980; Sam, *Chattanooga Choo Choo,* April Fools, 1984; Dwight Fairchild, *The Initiation,* New World, 1984; Dr. Bartlett, *Lies,* Alpha, 1984; federal agent, *Into the Night,* Universal, 1985; Mr. Walsh, *A Nightmare on Elm Street, Part Two: Freddy's Revenge,* New Line Cinema, 1985; Paul Minsky, *Prime Risk,* Almi, 1985; Burt, *Return of the Living Dead,* Orion, 1985; Ed Flynn, *The Hidden,* New Line Cinema, 1987; Mason Rand, *Hunter's Blood,* Concorde, 1987; Stanley Burnside, *The Offspring* (also known as *From a Whisper to a Scream*), Movie Store, 1987; Will Stanton, *Summer Heat,* Atlantic, 1987; Albert, *Uninvited,* Amazing Movies, 1988; Norman Mart, *Tapeheads,* Avenue, 1989. Also appeared in *Gangsterfilmen* (also known as *The Gangster Movie*), Sandrew Film and Teater, 1974.

PRINCIPAL TELEVISION APPEARANCES—Series: Billy the Kid, *The Tall Man,* NBC, 1960-62; Sheriff Emmett Ryker, *The Virginian,* NBC, 1964-68; Senator Mark Jennings, *The Survivors,* ABC, 1969-70; Bob Hatten, *San Francisco International Airport,* NBC, 1970-71; Cuda Weber, *The Mackenzies of Paradise Cove,* ABC, 1979. Mini-Series: Lieutenant Merrick, *Once an Eagle,* NBC, 1976-77; Reuben Smith, *Black Beauty,* NBC, 1978; William Sullivan, *King,* NBC, 1978; Victor Hardesty, *James A. Michener's "Space,"* CBS, 1985; General Philip Henry Sheridan, *North and South, Book II,* ABC, 1986. Pilots: Bob Hatten, *San Francisco International,* NBC, 1970; Emmet Jergens, *Call to Danger,* CBS, 1973; Milt Bosworth, *Smile Jenny, You're Dead,* ABC, 1974; Harry Keller, *The Killer Who Wouldn't Die,* ABC, 1976; title role, *Charlie Cobb: Nice Night for a Hanging,* NBC, 1977; Cuda Weber, *Sticking Together,* ABC, 1978.

Episodic: Coker, "Bang the Drum Slowly," *The U.S. Steel Hour,* CBS, 1956; Vincent "Mad Dog" Coll, *The Untouchables,* ABC, 1959; Mike Gann, *Murder, She Wrote,* CBS, 1986; also *Magnum, P.I.,* CBS, 1986; and "A Different Drummer," *Omnibus.* Movies: Brian Courtland, *Truman Capote's "The Glass House,"* CBS, 1972; Jonas Kane, *Footsteps* (also known as *Footsteps: Nice Guys Finish Last*), CBS, 1972; Roarke, *Hit Lady,* ABC, 1974; Lou Matthews, *Houston, We've Got a Problem,* ABC, 1974; Mike Guettner, *A Question of Love,* NBC, 1978; Marv Gillman, *Ski Lift to Death,* CBS, 1978; Marvin Tayman, *This Man Stands Alone* (also known as *Lawman without a Gun*), NBC, 1979; Joe Welch, *Willa,* CBS, 1979; Steve Ward, *Skyward,* NBC, 1980; Rufe Bennett, *Kenny Rogers as "The Gambler,"* CBS, 1980; J.R. Smith, *Living Proof: The Hank Williams, Jr. Story,* NBC, 1983; Don Gregory, *Bridge across Time* (also known as *Arizona Ripper*), NBC, 1985.

RELATED CAREER—Acting teacher.

ADDRESSES: AGENT—Century Artists, Ltd., 9744 Wilshire Boulevard, Suite 308, Beverly Hills, CA 90212.*

H

HACK, Shelley 1952-

PERSONAL: Born July 6, 1952, in Greenwich, CT. EDUCATION: Attended Smith College; studied acting at the Herbert Berghof Studios.

VOCATION: Actress.

CAREER: PRINCIPAL STAGE APPEARANCES—Billie Dawn, *Born Yesterday,* Pennsylvania Stage Company, Allentown, PA, 1982.

PRINCIPAL FILM APPEARANCES—Street stranger, *Annie Hall,* United Artists, 1977; Jennifer Corly, *If Ever I See You Again,* Columbia, 1978; docent, *Time after Time,* Warner Brothers/Orion, 1979; Cathy Long, *The King of Comedy,* Twentieth Century-Fox, 1983; Anne Potter, *Troll,* Empire, 1986; Susan Blake, *The Stepfather,* New Century-Vista, 1987.

PRINCIPAL TELEVISION APPEARANCES—Series: Tiffany Welles, *Charlie's Angels,* ABC, 1979-80; Dr. Beth Gilbert, *Cutter to Houston,* CBS, 1983; Jackie Shea, *Jack and Mike,* ABC, 1986-87. Movies: Janette Clausen, *Death Car on the Freeway,* CBS, 1979; Leslie Phillips, *Found Money* (also known as *My Secret Angel*), NBC, 1983; Logan Gay, *Trackdown: Finding the Goodbar Killer,* CBS, 1983; Frankie, *Singles Bars, Single Women,* ABC, 1984; Maggie, *Kicks,* ABC, 1985. Specials: Mary, *Vanities,* HBO, 1981; Anna, *Close Ties,* Entertainment Channel, 1983.

RELATED CAREER—Model; appeared in television commercials as Revlon's Charlie Girl.

ADDRESSES: AGENT—Joe Funicello, International Creative Management, 8899 Beverly Boulevard, Los Angeles, CA 90048.*

* * *

HAID, Charles 1943-

PERSONAL: Born June 2, 1943, in Palo Alto, CA; son of Charles Maurice and Grace Marian (Folger) Haid; married Penelope Windust (an actress; divorced, 1983); married Deborah Richter, February 17, 1985; children: Arcadia Elizabeth, Brittany Catherine (first marriage). EDUCATION: Received B.F.A. from Carnegie Institute of Technology.

VOCATION: Actor, producer, and director.

CAREER: BROADWAY DEBUT—Various roles, *Elizabeth I,* Lyceum Theatre, New York City, 1972. PRINCIPAL STAGE APPEAR-

ANCES—*The Merchant of Venice,* National Shakespeare Festival, Old Globe Theatre, San Diego, CA, 1973; also appeared with the Purdue Professional Theatre, Lafayette, IN, 1969-70; and with the Arena Stage, Washington, DC, 1973-74.

PRINCIPAL STAGE WORK—Associate producer, *Godspell,* Cherry Lane Theatre, New York City, 1971, then Plymouth Theatre, New York City, 1976; assistant director, *The Sign in Sidney Brustein's Window,* Longacre Theatre, New York City, 1972.

PRINCIPAL FILM APPEARANCES—Sergeant Nick Yanov, *The Choirboys,* Universal, 1977; Stephen Simpson, *Oliver's Story,* Paramount, 1978; Eddy, *Who'll Stop the Rain?,* United Artists, 1978; Mason Parrish, *Altered States,* Warner Brothers, 1980; Fats, *The House of God,* United Artists, 1984; Whitey Haines, *Cop* (also known as *Blood on the Moon*), Atlantic Releasing, 1987; Commander Howard, *The Rescue,* Buena Vista, 1988.

PRINCIPAL FILM WORK—Executive producer (with Michael Nesmith and Jane Alexander), *Square Dance* (also known as *Home Is Where the Heart Is*), Island, 1987.

PRINCIPAL TELEVISION APPEARANCES—Series: Ed McShane, *Kate McShane,* CBS, 1975; Sergeant Paul Shonski, *Delvecchio,* CBS, 1976-77; Officer Andy Renko, *Hill Street Blues,* NBC, 1981-87. Mini-Series: George Lumden, *The Bastard* (also known as *Kent Family Chronicles*), syndicated, 1978. Pilots: Ed McShane, *Kate McShane,* CBS, 1975; Dr. Lawrence "Red" Hacker, *Scalpels,* NBC, 1980; Jim Blanton, *Code of Vengeance,* NBC, 1985; Dwight Perry, *Fort Figueroa,* CBS, 1988. Episodic: *Barney Miller,* ABC. Movies: Brockmeyer, *The Execution of Private Slovik,* NBC, 1974; Jimmy, *Remember When,* NBC, 1974; Dr. Willie McCreevy, *Things in Their Season,* CBS, 1974; Sergeant Bray, *Foster and Laurie,* CBS, 1975; Sergeant Case, *A Death in Canaan,* CBS, 1978; Earl Wheelie, *Deathmoon,* CBS, 1978; Matt Jordan, *Twirl,* NBC, 1981; Fred Bemous, *Divorce Wars,* ABC, 1982; Fred Chandler, *Children in the Crossfire,* NBC, 1984; "Crazy" Sam Shockley, *Six against the Rock,* NBC, 1987; Sergeant Kupjack, *Weekend War,* ABC, 1988; Sergeant MacKenzie, *The Great Escape II: The Untold Story,* NBC, 1988; James Pierson, *A Deadly Silence,* ABC, 1989. Specials: *Working,* PBS, 1982; *Battle of the Network Stars,* ABC, 1983 and 1984; *The Best of Farm Aid: An American Event,* HBO, 1986; *The Academy of Country Music's Twentieth Anniversary Reunion,* NBC, 1986; *A Program for Vietnam Veterans . . . And Everyone Else Who Should Care,* PBS, 1986; *Willie Nelson's Picnic,* syndicated, 1987.

PRINCIPAL TELEVISION WORK—Producer (with Frank Prendergast and George Schaefer), *Children in the Crossfire,* NBC, 1984; associate producer, *Who Are the Debolts and Where Did They Get Nineteen Kids?* (documentary).

RELATED CAREER—Assistant director, American Shakespeare Festival, Stratford, CT, 1971; director, Repertory Theatre of St. Louis, St. Louis, MO, 1972; member, California Arts Council, 1982-84.

AWARDS: Emmy Award nominations, both Best Supporting Actor, 1981 and 1982, for *Hill Street Blues*.

MEMBER: Screen Actors Guild, Actors' Equity Association, Academy of Television Arts and Sciences.

ADDRESSES: AGENT—Writers and Artists Agency, 11726 San Vicente Boulevard, Suite 300, Los Angeles, CA 90049.*

*   *   *

HALE, Barbara   1922-

PERSONAL: Born April 18, 1922, in DeKalb, IL; married Bill Williams (an actor); children: William Katt. EDUCATION: Attended the Chicago Academy of Fine Arts.

VOCATION: Actress.

CAREER: PRINCIPAL FILM APPEARANCES—Young lover, *The Seventh Victim*, RKO, 1943; Barbara, *Around the World*, RKO, 1943; Catherine Keating, *Higher and Higher*, RKO, 1943; Sarah Cavanaugh, *The Iron Major*, RKO, 1943; Angie, *Heavenly Days*, RKO, 1944; Peggy Callahan, *The Falcon in Hollywood*, RKO, 1944; Marion, *The Falcon Out West*, RKO, 1944; Patty, *Goin' to Town*, RKO, 1944; Abby Drake, *First Yank into Toyko* (also known as *Mask of Fury*), RKO, 1945; Rill Lambeth, *West of the Pecos*, RKO, 1945; Mary Audrey, *Lady Luck*, RKO, 1946; Vickie North, *A Likely Story*, RKO, 1947; Mrs. Woodry, *The Window*, RKO, 1949; Jacqueline Walsh, *And Baby Makes Three*, Columbia, 1949; Miss Brand, *The Boy with the Green Hair*, RKO, 1949; Martha Gregory, *The Clay Pigeon*, RKO, 1949; Ellen Clark, *Jolson Sings Again*, Columbia, 1949.

Helen Hunt, *Emergency Wedding*, Columbia, 1950; Amy Lawrence, *The Jackpot*, Twentieth Century-Fox, 1950; title role, *Lorna Doone*, Columbia, 1951; Betsey Bennet, *The First Time*, Columbia, 1952; Julia Lanning, *Last of the Commanches* (also known as *The Sabre and the Arrow*), Columbia, 1952; Verity Wade, *A Lion Is in the Streets*, Warner Brothers, 1953; Sarah Jane Skaggs, *The Lone Hand*, Universal, 1953; Revere Muldoon, *Seminole*, Universal, 1953; Julia Hancock, *The Far Horizons* (also known as *The Untamed West*), Paramount, 1955; Mary Davitt, *Unchained*, Warner Brothers, 1955; Zoe Crane, *The Houston Story*, Columbia, 1956; Martha Kellogg, *Seventh Cavalry*, Columbia, 1956; Anne Barnes, *The Oklahoman*, Allied Artists, 1957; Allie Hanneman, *Slim Carter*, Universal, 1957; Celie Edwards, *Desert Hell*, Twentieth Century-Fox, 1958.

Sarah Cody, *Buckskin*, Paramount, 1968; Sarah Demerest, *Airport*, Universal, 1970; Mrs. Grierson, *The Red, White, and Black* (also known as *Soul Soldiers* and *Men of the Tenth*), Hirschman-Northern, 1970; Jenny, *The Giant Spider Invasion*, Group I, 1975; Mrs. Barlow, *Big Wednesday*, Warner Brothers, 1978. Also appeared in *Mexican Spitfire's Blessed Event*, RKO, 1943; *Gildersleeve's Bad Day*, RKO, 1943; *Government Girl*, RKO, 1943; and *Belle of the Yukon*, RKO, 1944.

PRINCIPAL TELEVISION APPEARANCES—Series: Della Street, *Perry Mason*, CBS, 1957-66. Pilots: June Waters, *Meet the Governor*, NBC, 1955; also *Whatever Became of . . . ?*, ABC, 1981. Episodic: *Footlights Theatre*, CBS; *Crossroads*, ABC; *The Loretta Young Theatre*, NBC; *Playhouse 90*, CBS; *Schlitz Playhouse of Stars*, CBS; *The Greatest American Hero*, ABC; also *Ford Theatre* and *Screen Director's Playhouse*. Movies: Della Street, *Perry Mason Returns*, NBC, 1985; Della Street, *Perry Mason: The Case of the Notorious Nun*, NBC, 1986; Della Street, *Perry Mason: The Case of the Shooting Star*, NBC, 1986; Della Street, *Perry Mason: The Case of the Lost Love*, NBC, 1987; Della Street, *Perry Mason: The Case of the Murdered Madam*, NBC, 1987; Della Street, *Perry Mason: The Case of the Scandalous Scoundrel*, NBC, 1987; Della Street, *Perry Mason: The Case of the Avenging Ace*, NBC, 1988; Della Street, *Perry Mason: The Case of the Lady in the Lake*, NBC, 1988.

RELATED CAREER—Appeared in television commercials as spokesperson for Amana appliances for twelve years.

AWARDS: Emmy Award, Best Supporting Actress in a Drama, 1959, for *Perry Mason*.

ADDRESSES: AGENT—Bob Edmiston, Associated Talent International, 1930 Central Park W., Suite 303, Los Angeles, CA 90067.*

*   *   *

HALL, Anthony Michael   1968-

PERSONAL: Full name, Michael Anthony Thomas Charles Hall; born April 14, 1968, in Boston, MA; son of Mercedes Hall (an actress and singer); stepson of Thomas Chestaro (a show business manager and producer). EDUCATION: Attended the Professional Children's School, New York, NY.

VOCATION: Actor.

CAREER: STAGE DEBUT—*The Wake*, Philadelphia, PA, 1977. PRINCIPAL STAGE APPEARANCES—*St. Joan of the Microphone*, Lincoln Center Festival, New York City; *Segments of a Contemporary Morning*, Griffin Repertory Theater.

FILM DEBUT—Doc, *Six Pack*, Twentieth Century-Fox, 1982. PRINCIPAL FILM APPEARANCES—Rusty Griswold, *National Lampoon's Vacation*, Warner Brothers, 1983; Brian Johnson, *The Breakfast Club*, Universal, 1984; Ted the Geek, *Sixteen Candles*, Universal, 1984; Gary, *Weird Science*, Universal, 1985; Daryl Cage, *Out of Bounds*, Columbia, 1986; Johnny Walker, *Johnny Be Good*, Orion, 1988.

PRINCIPAL TELEVISION APPEARANCES—Series: Regular, *Saturday Night Live*, NBC, 1985-86. Movies: Huck Finn, *Rascals and Robbers—The Secret Adventures of Tom Sawyer and Huck Finn*, CBS, 1982; Kylie, *Running Out*, CBS, 1983. Also appeared in *Jennifer's Journey*, 1979; *Gold Bug*, ABC; *The Body Human;* and *Orphans, Waifs, and Wards*.

RELATED CAREER—Appeared in television commercials from age eight to thirteen.

SIDELIGHTS: Anthony Michael Hall told *CTFT* that he became an

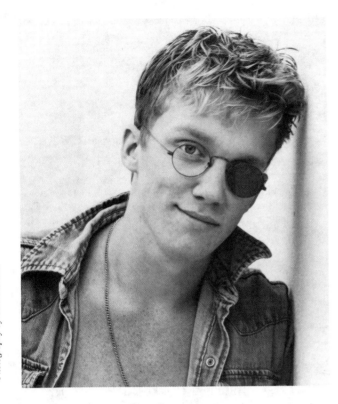

Photography by Ciro Barbaro

ANTHONY MICHAEL HALL

actor "to express my talents and share them with the audience—it's fun."

ADDRESSES: AGENT—Martin Bauer, Bauer/Benedek Agency, 9255 Sunset Boulevard, Suite 710, Los Angeles, CA, 90069. PUBLICIST—G. Freeman, P/M/K Public Relations, 8436 W. Third Street, Suite 650, Los Angeles, CA 90048.

*   *   *

HALL, Arsenio   1957-

PERSONAL: Born February 12, 1957, in Cleveland, OH. EDUCATION: Graduated from Kent State University.

VOCATION: Actor, comedian, and talk show host.

CAREER: Also see *WRITINGS* below. FILM DEBUT—Apartment victim, "Mondo Condo" segment, *Amazon Women on the Moon,* Universal, 1987. PRINCIPAL FILM APPEARANCES—Semmi, Morris, extremely ugly girl, and Reverend Brown, *Coming to America,* Paramount, 1988.

PRINCIPAL TELEVISION APPEARANCES—Series: Host, *The Half Hour Comedy Hour,* ABC, 1983; regular, *Thicke of the Night,* syndicated, 1984; regular, *The New Love, American Style,* ABC, 1985; regular, *Motown Revue,* NBC, 1985; voice characterization, *The Real Ghostbusters* (also known as *Slimer and the Real Ghostbusters;* animated), ABC, 1986; regular, *Solid Gold,* syndicated, 1987; host, *The Late Show,* Fox, 1987; host, *The Arsenio*

Hall Show, syndicated, 1989—. Episodic: Cleavon, *Alfred Hitchcock Presents,* NBC, 1986. Specials: "Uptown Comedy Express," *On Location,* HBO, 1987; host, *MTV's 1988 Video Music Awards Show,* MTV, 1988; *The Comedy Store 15th Year Class Reunion* (also known as *The Comedy Store Reunion*), NBC, 1989; *The Twenty-First Annual NAACP Image Awards,* NBC, 1989; also host, *The Magic of Christmas,* broadcast on a local station in Cleveland, OH.

PRINCIPAL TELEVISION WORK—Series: Executive producer, *The Arsenio Hall Show,* syndicated, 1989—.

RELATED CAREER—As a stand-up comedian, has appeared in comedy clubs throughout the United States, 1979—; magician; drum player with a pop music band.

NON-RELATED CAREER—In advertising.

WRITINGS: TELEVISION—Series: *Motown Revue,* NBC, 1985; *The Arsenio Hall Show,* syndicated, 1989—.*

*   *   *

HAMEL, Veronica   1945-

PERSONAL: Born November 20, 1945 (some sources say 1943), in Philadelphia, PA; father, a carpenter. EDUCATION: Attended Temple University.

VOCATION: Actress.

CAREER: STAGE DEBUT—*The Big Knife,* Off Off-Broadway production, New York City. PRINCIPAL STAGE APPEARANCES—Annie Sullivan, *The Miracle Worker,* St. Louis, MO, 1982.

MAJOR TOURS—*Cactus Flower,* U.S. cities.

PRINCIPAL FILM APPEARANCES—Linda, *Cannonball* (also known as *Carquake*), New World, 1976; Suzanne Constantine, *Beyond the Poseidon Adventure,* Warner Brothers, 1979; Nikki, *When Time Ran Out,* Warner Brothers, 1980; Kay Hutton, *A New Life,* Paramount, 1988.

PRINCIPAL TELEVISION APPEARANCES—Series: Joyce Davenport, *Hill Street Blues,* NBC, 1981-87. Mini-Series: Laura DeWitt Koshko, *Harold Robbins' "79 Park Avenue,"* NBC, 1977; Kate Kane, *Kane and Abel,* CBS, 1985. Episodic: "Peeper-Two," *The Bob Newhart Show,* CBS, 1976; Thelma, *City of Angels,* NBC, 1976; also *Starsky and Hutch,* ABC. Movies: Helen Thornton, *The Gathering,* ABC, 1977; Andrea Mason, *Ski Lift to Death,* CBS, 1978; Helen Thornton, *The Gathering, Part II,* NBC, 1979; Sheila Dodge, *The Hustler of Muscle Beach,* ABC, 1980; Jennifer North, *Jacqueline Susann's "Valley of the Dolls 1981,"* CBS, 1981; Leigh Churchill, *Sessions,* ABC, 1983; Deborah, *Twist of Fate,* NBC, 1989.

RELATED CAREER—Model.

AWARDS: Emmy Award nominations, 1981, 1982, and 1983, all for *Hill Street Blues.*

ADDRESSES: AGENT—Agency for Performing Arts, 9000 Sunset Boulevard, Suite 1200, Los Angeles, CA 90059.*

HAMER, Joseph 1932-

PERSONAL: Born July 29, 1932, in Dayton, OH; son of Gail B. and Amelie A. (Blot) Hamer; married Susan Lynn Martin (deceased); married Patricia Field Morthland (divorced, 1973); children: Christopher Gordon, Michael Grant, Vanessa Helen. EDUCATION: Miami University, B.A., 1956; University of California, Los Angeles, M.A., 1957; post-graduate work at Ohio State University, 1957-59. MILITARY: U.S. Army, 1953-55.

VOCATION: Actor, designer, and announcer.

CAREER: BROADWAY DEBUT—Bratby and Hewlett, *The Great White Hope,* Alvin Theatre, 1968. PRINCIPAL STAGE APPEARANCES—Fred Ashley, *White Cargo,* Players Theatre, New York City, 1960; Caelius, *Cicero,* St. Mark's Theatre, New York City, 1961; Shpigelski and Schaff, *A Month in the Country,* Maidman Playhouse, New York City, 1963; Somerset, *The White Rose and the Red,* Stage 73, New York City, 1964; Devery, *Born Yesterday,* Manhattan Theatre Club, New York City, 1974. Also appeared in *Henry IV, Part II,* Phoenix Theatre, New York City, 1960; as Thom Khoury, *Something That Matters,* American Theatre, New York City; Thomas Mendip, *The Lady's Not for Burning,* Center Stage, Baltimore, MD; Falstaff, *The Merry Wives of Windsor,* New Jersey Shakespeare Festival, Madison, NJ; Julien Berniers, *Toys in the Attic,* and Michael Starkwedder, *The Unexpected Guest,* both Hyde Park Playhouse, Hyde Park, NY; Father Riccardo, *The Deputy,* Circle Theatre, Kansas City; Rubin, *Dark at the Top of the Stairs,* Robin Hood Theatre; Murry, *A Thousand Clowns,* Mt. Cathalia Playhouse.

PRINCIPAL STAGE WORK—Director and designer of more than twenty summer theatre and regional theatre productions; also produced plays at Hyde Park Playhouse, Hyde Park, NY.

PRINCIPAL FILM APPEARANCES—Detective Stern, *The Sentinel,* Universal, 1977; Joey (the fan), *It's My Turn,* Columbia, 1980; garden ticketman, *Paternity,* Paramount, 1981; Officer Pollack, **batteries not included,* Universal, 1987.

PRINCIPAL TELEVISION APPEARANCES—Series: Detective Lieutenant Quinn, *The Corner Bar,* ABC, 1972-73; also Police Captain Craig, *The Guiding Light,* CBS; Joe, *I Am Joe's Body,* syndicated; Ralph, *Living Together,* syndicated. Pilots: Detective Brody, *People Versus.* Episodic: *Saturday Night Live,* NBC. Specials: Dad, "Nags," *Young People's Specials,* syndicated, 1987; Barry Sennett, "Seasonal Differences," *ABC Afterschool Special,* ABC, 1987; also as Dr. Roskovik, *The Silent Countdown.*

RELATED CAREER—Partner, Hamer and Herd Management Associates; appeared in films for the U.S. Armed Forces and in industrial films; actor in more than 250 radio commercials, 150 television commercials, and more than twenty-five radio shows; guest lecturer, U.S. universities.

NON-RELATED CAREER—Authors' representative.

MEMBER: Actors' Equity Association, Screen Actors Guild, American Federation of Television and Radio Artists, Players Club, Dutch Treat Club, Miami University Alumni of New York.

SIDELIGHTS: RECREATIONS—Farming, flower gardening, painting, photography, sketching, miniature building, jogging, golf, tennis, ping-pong, swimming, archery, softball, and bowling.

ADDRESSES: AGENT—Don Buchwald and Associates, 10 E. 44th Street, New York, NY 10017.

*   *   *

HAMILTON, Linda

PERSONAL: Born September 26, in Salisbury, MD.

VOCATION: Actress.

CAREER: PRINCIPAL STAGE APPEARANCES—Reporter, *Looice,* New York Shakespeare Festival, Public Theatre, New York City, 1975; Young Elizabeth, *Richard III,* Actors' Studio Theatre, New York City, 1977.

PRINCIPAL FILM APPEARANCES—Susan, *T.A.G.: The Assassination Game,* New World, 1982; Vicky Baxter, *Children of the Corn,* New World, 1984; Eva Crescent moon lady, *The Stone Boy,* Twentieth Century-Fox, 1984; Sarah Conner, *The Terminator,* Orion, 1984; Nina, *Black Moon Rising,* New World, 1986; Amy Franklin, *King Kong Lives,* De Laurentiis Entertainment Group, 1986.

PRINCIPAL TELEVISION APPEARANCES—Series: Lisa Rogers, *The Secrets of Midland Heights,* CBS, 1980-81; Lauren Hollister, *King's Crossing,* ABC, 1982; Catherine Chandler, *Beauty and the Beast,* CBS, 1987—. Episodic: Carol McDermott, *Murder, She Wrote,* CBS, 1986; also Sandy Velpriso, *Hill Street Blues,* NBC.

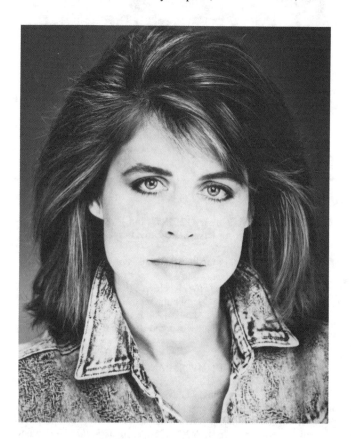

LINDA HAMILTON

Movies: Greta Rideout, *Rape and Marriage—The Rideout Case*, CBS, 1980; Anne Samoorian, *Reunion*, CBS, 1980; Josie Greenwood, *Country Gold*, CBS, 1982; Susan Becker, *Secrets of a Mother and Daughter*, CBS, 1983; Elena Koslov, *Secret Weapons*, NBC, 1985; Kate, *Club Med*, ABC, 1986; Claire Madison, *Go Toward the Light*, CBS, 1988.

AWARDS: Golden Globe Award nomination, Best Performance by an Actress in a Television Series—Drama, 1988 and 1989, for *Beauty and the Beast.*

ADDRESSES: AGENT—John Kimble, Triad Artists, 10100 Santa Monica Boulevard, 16th Floor, Los Angeles, CA 90067. MANAGER—Bobbie Edrick, Artist Circle Entertainment, 8957 Norma Place, Los Angeles, CA 90069.

*   *   *

HAMPTON, Christopher   1946-

PERSONAL: Full name, Christopher James Hampton; born January 26, 1946, in Fayal, Azores; son of Bernard Patrick (a marine telecommunications engineer) and Dorothy Patience (Herrington) Hampton; married Laura Margaret de Holesch (a social worker), 1971; children: two daughters. EDUCATION: Attended Lancing College, 1956-63; Oxford University, B.A., French and German, 1968; also received M.A. from Oxford University.

VOCATION: Playwright.

CAREER: See *WRITINGS* below. RELATED CAREER—Report writer, Schauspielhaus, Hamburg, West Germany, 1967; translator of lectures on James Joyce, Paris, France, 1967; resident dramatist, Royal Court Theatre, London, 1968-70; fellow, Royal Society of Literature, 1976, then council member, 1984—.

WRITINGS: STAGE—*When Did You Last See My Mother?*, Royal Court Theatre, then Comedy Theatre, both London, 1966, later Young People's Repertory Theatre, Sheridan Square Playhouse, New York City, 1967, published by Faber and Faber, 1967, then Grove Press, 1967; (adaptor) *Marya*, Royal Court Theatre, 1967, then Jewish Repertory Theatre, New York City, 1981, published in *Plays of the Year 35*, Elek, 1969; *Total Eclipse*, Royal Court Theatre, 1968, then in Washington, DC, 1972, later in New York City, 1974, published by Faber and Faber, 1969, then Samuel French, Inc., 1972, revised version produced in London, 1981, published by Faber and Faber, 1981; (adaptor) *Uncle Vanya*, Royal Court Theatre, 1970, published in *Plays of the Year 39*, Elek, 1971; (adaptor) *Hedda Gabler*, National Theatre, Stratford, ON, Canada, 1970, then Roundabout Theatre, New York City, 1981, later Center Theatre Group, Mark Taper Forum, Los Angeles, 1985, published by Samuel French, Inc., 1971; *The Philanthropist: A Bourgeois Comedy*, Royal Court Theatre, then May Fair Theatre, London, both 1970, later Ethel Barrymore Theatre, New York City, 1972, published by Faber and Faber, 1970, then Samuel French, Inc., 1971, revised version published by Faber and Faber, 1985; (adaptor) *Don Juan*, Theatre Royal, Bristol, U.K., 1972, published by Faber and Faber, 1974; (adaptor) *A Doll's House*, Playhouse Theatre, New York City, 1971, then Criterion Theatre, London, 1973, published by Samuel French, Inc., 1972; *Savages*, Royal Court Theatre, then Comedy Theatre, both 1973, later Mark Taper Forum, 1974, then Hudson Guild Theatre, New York City, 1977,

published by Faber and Faber, 1974, revised version published by Samuel French, Inc., 1977.

Treats, Royal Court Theatre, then May Fair Theatre, both 1976, later Indiana Repertory Theatre, Indianapolis, IN, 1980, published by Faber and Faber, 1976, then Samuel French, Inc., 1976; (adaptor) *Signed and Sealed*, Comedy Theatre, 1976; (adaptor and translator) *Tales from the Vienna Woods*, National Theatre Company, Olivier Theatre, London, 1977, then Arena Stage, Washington, DC, 1978, published by Faber and Faber, 1977; (translator) *Don Juan Comes Back from the War*, National Theatre Company, Cottesloe Theatre, London, 1978, then Manhattan Theatre Club, New York City, 1979, published by Faber and Faber, 1978; (adaptor) *Ghosts*, Key Theatre, Peterborough, U.K., 1978, published by Samuel French, Inc., 1983; (adaptor) *The Wild Duck*, National Theatre Company, Olivier Theatre, 1979, published by Faber and Faber, 1980, then Samuel French, Inc., 1981; *After Mercer*, first produced in London, 1980; *The Prague Trial*, first produced in Paris, France, 1980; (with Ronald Harwood) *A Night of the Day of the Imprisoned Writer*, first produced in London, 1981; (adaptor) *The Portage to San Cristobal of A.H.*, Mermaid Theatre, London, 1982, then Hartford Stage Company, Hartford, CT, 1982, published by Faber and Faber, 1983; *Tales from Hollywood*, Mark Taper Forum, 1982, then in London, 1983, published by Faber and Faber, 1983; (adaptor) *Tartuffe, or The Imposter*, first produced in London, 1983, published by Faber and Faber, 1984; *Les Liaisons Dangereuses*, Royal Shakespeare Company, Other Place Theatre, Stratford-on-Avon, U.K., 1985, then London, 1986, later Music Box Theatre, New York City, 1987, published by Faber and Faber, 1985.

FILM—*A Doll's House*, Paramount, 1973; *Beyond the Limit* (also known as *The Honorary Consul*), Paramount, 1983; *The Good Father*, Skouras, 1986; *The Wolf at the Door*, Manson, 1986; (with Maximilian Schell) *Geschichten aus dem Wiener-Wald* (also known as *Tales from the Vienna Woods*), Constantin, 1979, published by Suhrkamp, 1979; *Dangerous Liaisons*, Warner Brothers, 1988. Also wrote the unproduced screenplays: *When Did You Last See My Mother?*, 1966; *The Tenant*, 1972; *A Temporary Life*, 1974; *The Moon and Sixpence*, 1975; *Carrington*, 1978; and *The Last Secret*, 1979.

TELEVISION—Plays: *Able's Will*, 1977, published by Faber and Faber, 1979; (adaptor) *The History Man*, BBC, 1981; *Hotel du Lac*, BBC, then Arts and Entertainment, 1986; also *Total Eclipse, The Philanthropist, Savages, Treats*, and *Marya.*

RADIO—Plays: *Don Juan*, BBC Radio 3, 1970; *The Prague Trial*, 1980. Also *2 Children Free to Wander* (documentary), 1969.

AWARDS: Plays and Players London Critics Award, Best Play, and *Evening Standard* Award, Best Comedy, both 1970, for *The Philanthropist; Variety* New York Drama Critics Poll, Most Promising Playwright, 1971; (co-winner) *Plays and Players* London Critics Award, Best Play, 1973, for *Savages;* Los Angeles Drama Critics Circle Playwriting Award, Distinguished Theatrical Productions and Performances, 1975, for *Savages; Evening Standard* Award, Best Comedy, 1984; *Evening Standard* Award and Olivier Award both 1986, and Antoinette Perry Award nomination, Best Play, 1988, all for *Les Liaisons Dangereuses;* Academy Award nomination, Best Screenplay (Adaptation), 1989, for *Dangerous Liaisons.*

MEMBER: Dramatists Club.

SIDELIGHTS: RECREATIONS—Travel and cinema.

ADDRESSES: HOME—2 Kensington Park Gardens, London W11, England. AGENT—Margaret Ramsay, Ltd., 14-A Goodwin's Court, St. Martin's Lane, London WC2N 4LL, England.*

*   *   *

HAMPTON, James   1936-

PERSONAL: Born July 9, 1936, in Oklahoma City, OK.

VOCATION: Actor.

CAREER: PRINCIPAL FILM APPEARANCES—Private Menzies, *Soldier Blue,* AVCO-Embassy, 1970; Cotton, *Mackintosh and T.J.,* Penland, 1975; bus driver, *Hustle,* Paramount, 1975; Junior, *W.W. and the Dixie Dancekings,* Twentieth Century-Fox, 1975; Howard Clemmons, *Hawmps!,* Mulberry Square, 1976; Captain Anderson, *The Cat from Outer Space,* Buena Vista, 1978; Bill Gibson, *The China Syndrome,* Columbia, 1979; Lew Price, *Hangar 18* (also known as *Invasion Force*), Sunn Classic, 1980; Harry Oslo, *Condorman,* Buena Vista, 1981; Harold Howard, *Teen Wolf,* Atlantic, 1985; Uncle Howard, *Teen Wolf Too,* Atlantic, 1987; Mayor of Miami, *Police Academy 5: Assignment Miami,* Warner Brothers, 1988. Also appeared in *The Longest Yard,* Paramount, 1974.

PRINCIPAL TELEVISION APPEARANCES—Series: Bugler Hannibal Dobbs, *F Troop,* ABC, 1965-67; Leroy B. Simpson, *The Doris Day Show,* CBS, 1968-69; regular, *Love, American Style,* ABC, 1971-74; regular, *Mary,* CBS, 1978; Len Weston, *Maggie,* ABC, 1981-82. Mini-Series: Defense attorney Prescott, *Centennial,* NBC, 1978-79. Pilots: Lester White, *Force Five,* CBS, 1975; Lieutenant O'Brien, *Bravo Two,* CBS, 1977; Sam Tuttle, *Through the Magic Pyramid,* NBC, 1981; Dub Dennible, *Kudzu,* CBS, 1983. Episodic: Odell Mitchell, *Simon and Simon,* CBS, 1986; Sheriff Buster Moon, *The Dukes of Hazzard,* CBS. Movies: Harry Dudley, *Attack on Terror: The FBI Versus the Ku Klux Klan,* CBS, 1975; Wilbur Peterson, *The Amazing Howard Hughes,* CBS, 1977; Alvin Karl, *Thaddeus Rose and Eddie,* CBS, 1978; Ernest, *Three on a Date,* ABC, 1978; Billy Sherrill, *Stand by Your Man,* CBS, 1981; Richard Hickman, *World War III,* NBC, 1982; police witness, *The Burning Bed,* NBC, 1984.

WRITINGS: TELEVISION—Specials: *A Whole Lotta Fun,* NBC, 1988.*

*   *   *

HAREWOOD, Dorian   1950-

PERSONAL: Born August 6, 1950, in Dayton, OH; married Ann McCurry, February 14, 1979; children: Olivia Ruth. EDUCATION: Graduated from the University of Cincinnati Conservatory of Music.

VOCATION: Actor.

CAREER: PRINCIPAL STAGE APPEARANCES—Understudy for Valentine, *The Two Gentlemen of Verona,* New York Shakespeare

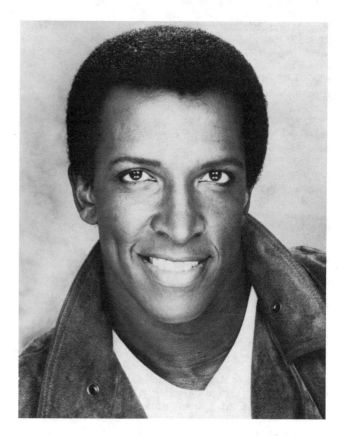

DORIAN HAREWOOD

Festival (NYSF), St. James Theatre, New York City, 1972; father, Raymond, and rock singer, *Brainchild,* Forrest Theatre, Philadelphia, PA, 1974; *Over Here!,* Shubert Theatre, New York City, 1974; Morgan Evans, *Miss Moffat,* Shubert Theatre, Philadelphia, PA, 1974; Clarence, *Don't Call Back,* Helen Hayes Theatre, New York City, 1975; Carlyle, *Streamers,* NYSF, Mitzi E. Newhouse Theatre, New York City, 1976; Frankie, *The Mighty Gents,* Ambassador Theatre, New York City, 1978. Also appeared in *A Gala Tribute to Joshua Logan,* Imperial Theatre, New York City, 1975; *Bloodshot Wine,* Manhattan Theatre Club, New York City, 1975; *To Sir with Love,* Broadway production, 1989; and in the chorus, *A Tribute to Oscar Hammerstein,* Philharmonic Hall, New York City.

MAJOR TOURS—Judas, *Jesus Christ, Superstar,* U.S. cities.

FILM DEBUT—Levi, *Sparkle,* Warner Brothers, 1976. PRINCIPAL FILM APPEARANCES—Fowler, *Gray Lady Down,* Universal, 1978; Lieutenant Masters, *Looker,* Warner Brothers, 1981; Tommy, *Against All Odds,* Columbia, 1984; Sergeant Tippet, *Tank,* Universal, 1984; Gene, *The Falcon and the Snowman,* Orion, 1985; Eightball, *Full Metal Jacket,* Warner Brothers, 1987.

TELEVISION DEBUT—Gregory Foster, *Foster and Laurie,* CBS, 1975. PRINCIPAL TELEVISION APPEARANCES—Series: Detective Paul Strobber, *Strike Force,* ABC, 1981-82; Dr. Nate "Skate" Baylor, *Trauma Center,* ABC, 1983; Earl Tobin, *Glitter,* ABC, 1984-85; voice characterization, *The New Adventures of Jonny Quest* (animated), syndicated, 1987; voice characterization, *Sky Commanders* (animated), syndicated, 1987. Mini-Series: Simon Haley, *Roots: The Next Generations,* ABC, 1979; Floyd, *Beulah*

Land, NBC, 1980; Jeffrey Wyman, *Amerika* (also known as *Topeka, Kansas . . . U.S.S.R.*), ABC, 1987. Pilots: Dr. Michael Stoner, *Panic in Echo Park*, NBC, 1977; Lieutenant Jack Hill, *Dirty Work*, CBS, 1985; Hank Whittaker, *Kingpins*, CBS, 1987; James Reynolds, *Hope Division*, ABC, 1987; Ben Colter, *Half 'n' Half* (also known as *Momma's Boys* and *Black and White*), ABC, 1988; also *We Are Vivian Dawn*, ABC, 1989. Episodic: Sheriff Cox, *Murder, She Wrote*, CBS, 1986; also Jake, *Kojak*, CBS. Movies: Simon, *Siege*, CBS, 1978; Matt Reeves, *An American Christmas Carol*, ABC, 1979; Lieutenant Zack Hawkins, *High Ice*, NBC, 1980; Detective Jerry van Ness, *I, Desire*, ABC, 1982; Ray Ellsworth, *The Ambush Murders*, CBS, 1982; title role, *The Jesse Owens Story*, syndicated, 1984; title role, *Guilty of Innocence: The Lenell Geter Story*, CBS, 1987; Calvin, *God Bless the Child*, ABC, 1988; also *Kiss Shot*, CBS, 1989. Specials: *We the People 200: The Constitutional Gala*, CBS, 1987.

PRINCIPAL TELEVISION WORK—Series: Creator, *Half 'n' Half* (also known as *Momma's Boys* and *Black and White*), ABC, 1988.

WRITINGS: Seven songs for *Dorian Harewood: Love Will Stop Calling*, Emeric Records, 1989.

RECORDINGS: ALBUMS—*Dorian Harewood: Love Will Stop Calling*, Emeric Records, 1989.

AWARDS: Theatre World Award, 1975, for *Don't Call Back;* Image Award nomination from the National Association for the Advancement of Colored Peopl for *Guilty of Innocence: The Lenell Geter Story.*

MEMBER: Actors' Equity Association, Screen Actors Guild, American Federation of Television and Radio Artists.

ADDRESSES: AGENT—Bob Schwartz, Paul Kohner Agency, 9169 Sunset Boulevard, Los Angeles, CA 90024. PUBLICISTS—Phil Paladino and John Blanchette, Paladino Public Relations, 9200 Sunset Boulevard, Suite 418, Los Angeles, CA 90069.

*   *   *

HARMON, Mark   1951-

PERSONAL: Born September 2, 1951, in Burbank, CA; son of Tom Harmon (a football player and sportscaster) and Elyse Knox (an actress and artist); married Pam Dawber (an actress), March 21, 1987; children: one son. EDUCATION: University of California, Los Angeles, B.A., communications, 1974.

VOCATION: Actor.

CAREER: PRINCIPAL FILM APPEARANCES—Billy Joe Meynert, *Comes a Horseman*, United Artists, 1978; Larry Simpson, *Beyond the Poseidon Adventure*, Warner Brothers, 1979; Harry Burck, *Let's Get Harry*, Tri-Star, 1987; Freddy Shoop, *Summer School*, Paramount, 1987; narrator, *Dear America: Letters Home from Vietnam*, HBO Films, 1987; Jay Austin, *The Presidio*, Paramount, 1988; Billy Wyatt, *Stealing Home*, Warner Brothers, 1988.

TELEVISION DEBUT—*Adam-12*, NBC, 1975. PRINCIPAL TELE-VISION APPEARANCES—Series: Officer Mike Breen, *Sam*, CBS, 1978; Deputy Dwayne Thibideaux, *240-Robert*, ABC, 1979-80; Fielding Carlyle, *Flamingo Road*, NBC, 1981-82; Dr. Robert

Caldwell, *St. Elsewhere*, NBC, 1983-85. Pilots: Officer Mike Breen, *Sam*, CBS, 1977; Fielding Carlyle, *Flamingo Road*, NBC, 1980. Episodic: *Ozzie's Girls*, ABC; *Adam-12*, NBC; *Police Story*, NBC; *Laverne and Shirley*, ABC; *The Nancy Drew Mysteries*, ABC; *Moonlighting*, ABC. Mini-Series: John McIntosh, *Centennial*, NBC, 1978-79. Movies: Robert Dunlap, *Eleanor and Franklin: The White House Years*, ABC, 1977; Howie Lesser, *Getting Married*, CBS, 1978; Norman Brinker, *Little Mo*, NBC, 1978; Johnny Edge, *The Dream Merchants*, syndicated, 1980; Peter Cabot, *Goliath Awaits*, syndicated, 1981; Tommy, *Intimate Agony*, ABC, 1983; Robin Prince, *Prince of Belair*, ABC, 1986; Ted Bundy, *The Deliberate Stranger*, NBC, 1986; Elmer Jackson, *After the Promise*, CBS, 1987. Specials: *The New and Spectacular Guinness Book of World Records*, ABC, 1980; *Battle of the Network Stars*, ABC, 1981, 1982, and 1984.

RELATED CAREER—Commercial spokesman for Coors beer.

NON-RELATED CAREER—Sales representative for sports shoe company, lifeguard, and bartender.

AWARDS: Emmy Award nomination, Best Supporting Actor, 1977, for *Eleanor and Franklin: The White House Years.*

MEMBER: American Federation of Television and Radio Artists, Screen Actors Guild.

SIDELIGHTS: RECREATIONS—T'ai chi ch'uan, running, and carpentry.

ADDRESSES: MANAGER—Neal Koenigsberg Management, 1022 Gayley, Suite 201, Los Angeles, CA 90024.*

*   *   *

HARPER, Tess   1950-

PERSONAL: Born Tessie Jean Washam, 1950, in Mammoth Spring, AR. EDUCATION: Received B.S. in education and theatre from Southwest Missouri State College.

VOCATION: Actress.

CAREER: FILM DEBUT—Rosa Lee, *Tender Mercies*, EMI, 1982. PRINCIPAL FILM APPEARANCES—Nancy Baxter, *Amityville 3-D*, Orion, 1983; Linda Dawson, *Silkwood*, Twentieth Century-Fox, 1983; Ellen, *Flashpoint*, Tri-Star, 1984; Chick Boyle, *Crimes of the Heart*, De Laurentiis Entertainment Group, 1986; Willa, *Ishtar*, Columbia, 1987; Rita, *Far North*, Alive, 1988; Detective Stillwell, *Criminal Law*, Tri-Star, 1989.

PRINCIPAL TELEVISION APPEARANCES—Mini-Series: Carrie Lee, *Chiefs*, CBS, 1983; Susan French, *Celebrity*, NBC, 1984. Episodic: Sarah, "Welcome to Winfield," *The Twilight Zone*, CBS, 1985. Movies: Lorna Whateley, *Kentucky Woman*, CBS, 1983; Janet Briggs, *Starflight: The Plane That Couldn't Land*, ABC, 1983; Gwen Palmer, *Promises to Keep*, CBS, 1985; Meredith Craig, *Reckless Disregard*, Showtime, 1985; Jeannie Wyler, *A Summer to Remember*, CBS, 1985; Ann Burnette, *Daddy*, ABC, 1987; Clara Brady, *Little Girl Lost*, ABC, 1988; Mary Flowers, *Unconquered*, CBS, 1989.

RELATED CAREER—Performed in dinner theatre and children's

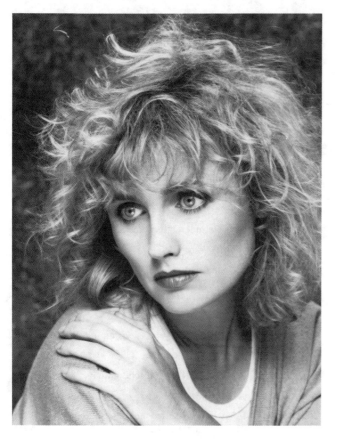

TESS HARPER

theatre for eight years; also appeared in local television commercials in Texas.

AWARDS: Academy Award nomination, Best Supporting Actress, 1987, for *Crimes of the Heart.*

MEMBER: Screen Actors Guild, American Federation of Television and Radio Artists.

ADDRESSES: AGENTS—Scott Zimmerman and Ames Cushing, William Morris Agency, 151 El Camino Drive, Beverly Hills, CA 90212. PUBLICIST—Susan Geller, 420 Spaulding Drive, Beverly Hills, CA 90212.

*   *   *

HARROLD, Kathryn   1950-

PERSONAL: Born August 2, 1950, in Tazewell, VA. EDUCATION: Attended Mills College; studied acting at the Neighborhood Playhouse and with Uta Hagan in New York City.

VOCATION: Actress.

CAREER: PRINCIPAL STAGE APPEARANCES—Rebecca West, *Rosmersholm,* Classic Theatre, New York City, 1977.

FILM DEBUT—Anne Dillon, *Nightwing,* Columbia, 1979. PRINCI-

PAL FILM APPEARANCES—Dotty, *The Hunter,* Paramount, 1980; Hannah, *The Pursuit of D.B. Cooper,* Universal, 1981; Mary Harvard, *Modern Romance,* Columbia, 1981; Pamela Taylor, *Yes, Giorgio,* Metro-Goldwyn-Mayer/United Artists, 1982; Gail Farmer, *The Sender,* Paramount, 1982; Cyd Mills, *Heartbreakers,* Orion, 1984; Christie, *Into the Night,* Universal, 1985; Monique, *Raw Deal,* De Laurentiis, 1986. Also appeared in *Someone to Love,* International Rainbow, 1987.

PRINCIPAL TELEVISION APPEARANCES—Series: Detective Jenny Loud, *MacGruder and Loud,* NBC, 1985; Sara Newhouse, *The Bronx Zoo,* NBC, 1987-88; also Nora Aldrich, *The Doctors,* NBC. Episodic: Megan Dougherty, *The Rockford Files,* NBC; also *Starsky and Hutch,* ABC. Movies: Leslie Rawlins, *Vampire,* ABC, 1979; Dr. Jill Bates, *Women in White,* NBC, 1979; Suzie Kaufman, *Son-Rise: A Miracle of Love,* NBC, 1979; Bliss, *The Women's Room,* ABC, 1980; Lauren Bacall, *Bogie,* CBS, 1980; Cynthia Malcolm, *An Uncommon Love,* CBS, 1983; Marilyn Butler, *Man against the Mob,* NBC, 1988; also *Dead Solid Perfect,* HBO, 1988. Specials: Leslie Applegate, *The Best Legs in the Eighth Grade,* HBO, 1984.

RELATED CAREER—As a member of Section Ten (experimental theatre group), taught and performed at Connecticut College and New York University.

MEMBER: Actors' Equity Association, Screen Actors Guild, American Federation of Television and Radio Artists.

ADDRESSES: AGENT—Bob Gersh, The Gersh Agency, 222 N. Canon Drive, Suite 202, Beverly Hills, CA 90210.*

*   *   *

HARTMAN, Phil   1948-

PERSONAL: Born Philip Edward Hartmann, September 24, 1948, in Brantford, ON, Canada; son of Rupert L. (in sales) and Doris M. Hartmann; married Vicki Jo Omdahl (an actress and writer), November 25, 1987; children: Sean Edward. EDUCATION: Attended Santa Monica College, 1967-68, and San Fernando Valley State College, 1972-73.

VOCATION: Actor, comedian, and screenwriter.

CAREER: Also see *WRITINGS* below. PRINCIPAL STAGE APPEARANCES—*Olympic Trials,* Olympic Arts Festival, Los Angeles, CA, 1984.

PRINCIPAL FILM APPEARANCES—Chick Hazard, *Cheech and Chong's Next Movie,* Universal, 1980; Joe Chicago, *Weekend Pass,* Crown, 1984; reporter, *Pee-Wee's Big Adventure,* Warner Brothers, 1985; Jean-Michel, *The Last Resort,* Trinity, 1985; Ted Davis, *Blind Date,* Tri-Star, 1986; voice of Air Conditioner and Hanging Lamp, *The Brave Little Toaster* (animated), Hyperion Kushner/Lockec, 1987; baseball announcer, "Murray in Videoland," *Amazon Women on the Moon,* Universal, 1987; Bly manager, *Fletch Lives,* Universal, 1989; also appeared in *The Three Amigos,* Universal, 1986.

TELEVISION DEBUT—Sergeant Rubin, *Six O'Clock Follies,* NBC, 1979. PRINCIPAL TELEVISION APPEARANCES—Series: Voice characterization, *Pink Panther and Sons* (animated), NBC, 1984-85; regular, *Our Time,* NBC, 1985; voice of Mr. Wilson, *Dennis*

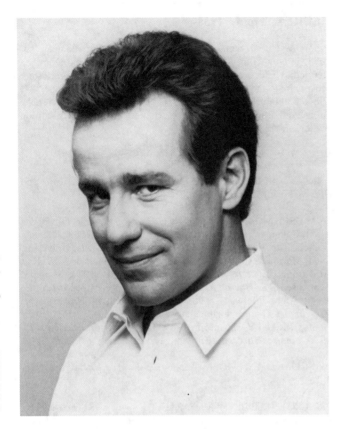

PHIL HARTMAN

the Menace (animated), syndicated, 1986; Kapt'n Karl, *Pee-Wee's Playhouse*, CBS, 1987; regular, *Saturday Night Live*, NBC, 1986—. Pilots: Regular, *Top Ten*, NBC, 1980; co-anchor, *The Natural Snoop*, NBC, 1983.

PRINCIPAL TELEVISION WORK—Series: Associate producer, *Our Time*, NBC, 1985.

RELATED CAREER—Member of the Groundlings (an improvisational comedy troupe), 1975-86.

WRITINGS: FILM—(With Paul Reubens and Michael Varhol) *Pee-Wee's Big Adventure*, Warner Brothers, 1985. TELEVISION—Series: Co-writer, *Saturday Night Live*, NBC, 1986—. Specials: Co-writer, *The Pee-Wee Herman Show*, HBO, 1982.

AWARDS: Emmy Award nomination (writing), 1987, for *Saturday Night Live*.

MEMBER: Cousteau Society.

ADDRESSES: AGENT—J.J. Harris, William Morris Agency, 151 El Camino Drive, Beverly Hills, CA, 90212.

*   *   *

HASSELHOFF, David   1952-

PERSONAL: Born July 17, 1952, in Baltimore, MD; married Catherine Hickland (an actress; divorced).

VOCATION: Actor.

CAREER: PRINCIPAL FILM APPEARANCES—Simon, *Starcrash* (also known as *Stella Star* and *Star Crash*), New World, 1979. Also appeared in *Starke Zeiten*, 1988; *W.B. Blue and the Bean*, 1989; and *The Final Alliance*, 1989. PRINCIPAL FILM WORK—Producer (with Max Kleven), *W.B. Blue and the Bean*, 1989.

PRINCIPAL TELEVISION APPEARANCES—Series: Snapper Foster, *The Young and the Restless*, CBS, 1975-82; Shake Tiller, *Semi-Tough*, ABC, 1980; Michael Knight, *Knight Rider*, NBC, 1982-86. Pilots: *Star Search*, syndicated, 1983. Episodic: Detective, *Scene of the Crime*, NBC, 1985; also *Police Story*, CBS; *The Love Boat*, ABC. Movies: Scott, *Pleasure Cove*, NBC, 1979; Curt Taylor, *The Cartier Affair*, NBC, 1984; Don Gregory, *Bridge across Time* (also known as *Arizona Ripper*), NBC, 1985; Billy Travis, *Perry Mason: The Case of the Lady in the Lake*, NBC, 1988; also *Griffin and Phoenix: A Love Story*, ABC, 1976; *Baywatch*, NBC, 1989. Specials: *After Hours: Getting to Know Us*, CBS, 1977; *Disneyland's Thirtieth Anniversary Celebration*, NBC, 1985; *The NBC All-Star Hour*, NBC, 1985; *On Top All over the World*, syndicated, 1985; *Fame, Fortune, and Romance*, syndicated, 1986; *NBC's Sixtieth Anniversary Celebration*, NBC, 1986; *The Noel Edmonds Show*, ABC, 1986; *A Crystal Christmas* (also known as *A Crystal Christmas in Sweden*), syndicated, 1987; *AIDS: The Global Explosion*, syndicated, 1988.

RELATED CAREER—As a singer, has released two albums in Europe.

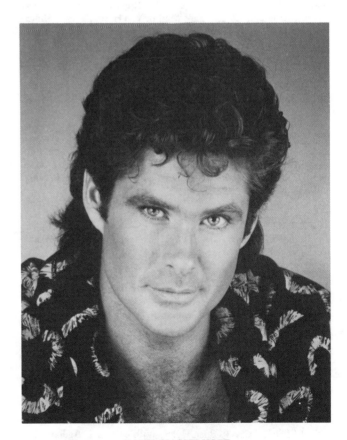

DAVID HASSELHOFF

MEMBER: Screen Actors Guild, American Federation of Television and Radio Artists.

ADDRESSES: AGENT—Merritt Blake, Camden Artists, 2121 Avenue of the Stars, Suite 410, Los Angeles, CA 90067. PUBLICIST—Jonni Hartman, Slade, Grant, Hartman, and Hartman, 9145 Sunset Boulevard, Suite 218, Los Angeles, CA 90069.

*   *   *

HAUER, Rutger   1944-

PERSONAL: Born January 23, 1944, in Breukelen, Netherlands. MILITARY: Served in the Dutch Army and Navy.

VOCATION: Actor.

CAREER: FILM DEBUT—*Turkish Delight* (also known as *Turks Fruit*), Nederland, 1972. PRINCIPAL FILM APPEARANCES—Rik Van de Loo, *Pusteblume* (also known as *Hard to Remember*), Cinecenta, 1974; Blaine Van Niekirk, *The Wilby Conspiracy,* United Artists, 1975; Johan Nagel, *Mysteries,* Cine-Vog, 1979; Erik, *Soldier of Orange,* International Picture Show, 1979; Etienne De Balsan, *Chanel Solitaire,* United Film Distribution, 1981; Wulfgar, *Nighthawks,* Universal, 1981; Roy Batty, *Blade Runner,* Warner Brothers, 1982; Claude Maillot Van Horn, *Eureka,* United Artists, 1983; John Tanner, *The Osterman Weekend,* Twentieth Century-Fox, 1983; Brigadier Rinus de Gier, *Outsider in Amsterdam* (also know as *Grijpstra and De Gier*), Verenigade Nederland, 1983; Gerrit Witkamp, *Spetters,* Embassy, 1983; Jim Malden, *A Breed Apart,* Orion, 1984; Martin, *Flesh and Blood,* Riverside, 1985; Navarre, *Ladyhawke,* Warner Brothers, 1985; John Ryder, *The Hitcher,* Tri-Star, 1986; Nick Randall, *Wanted: Dead or Alive,* New World, 1987. Also appeared in *Keetje Tippl'e* (also known as *Keetje Tippel*), Tuschinski Film Distribution, 1975; *Max Havelaar,* Netherlands Fox Film Corporation, 1976; Driann, *A Woman between Dog and Wolf* (also known as *Een Vrouw Tussen Hond en Wolf*), Gaumont International, 1979; and as Andreas, *La Legenda del Santo Bevitore,* 1988.

PRINCIPAL TELEVISION APPEARANCES—Movies: Albert Speer, *Inside the Third Reich,* ABC, 1982; Lieutenant Alexander "Sasha" Pechersky, *Escape from Sobibor,* CBS, 1987.

RELATED CAREER—Stage actor in Amsterdam for six years prior to film debut.

AWARDS: Golden Globe Award, Best Performance by an Actor in a Supporting Role in a Mini-Series or Motion Picture Made for Television, 1987, for *Escape from Sobibor.*

MEMBER: Screen Actors Guild.

ADDRESSES: AGENT—Joan Hyler, William Morris Agency, 151 El Camino Drive, Beverly Hills, CA 90212.*

HEDREN, Tippi   1935-

PERSONAL: Full name, Nathalie Kay Hedren; born January 19, 1935, in New Ulm, MN; daughter of Bernard Carl and Dorothea Henrietta (Eckhardt) Hedren; married Peter Griffith (a real estate broker; marriage ended); married Noel Marshall, September 27, 1964; children: Melanie Griffith (first marriage). EDUCATION: Attended Pasadena City College; studied acting with Gertrude Fogler and Claudia Franck.

VOCATION: Actress.

CAREER: PRINCIPAL STAGE APPEARANCES—*Hatful of Rain* and *Black Comedy,* both summer theatre productions.

FILM DEBUT—Ice Box, *The Petty Girl* (also known as *Girl of the Year*), Columbia, 1950. PRINCIPAL FILM APPEARANCES—Melanie Daniels, *The Birds,* Universal, 1963; title role, *Marnie,* Universal, 1964; Martha, *A Countess from Hong Kong,* Universal, 1969; Rita Armstrong, *Tiger by the Tail,* Commonwealth, 1970; Margaret Tenhausen, *The Harrad Experiment,* Cinerama, 1973; Madeleine, *Roar,* Alpha-Filmways, 1981. Also appeared in *Hitchcock, Il Brivido del Genio* (documentary; also known as *The Thrill of Genius*), RAI-TV/Channel 1, 1985; *The Man with the Albatross,* 1970; *Satan's Harvest,* 1970; and *Adonde muere el Viento.*

PRINCIPAL FILM WORK—Producer, *Roar,* Alpha-Filmways, 1981.

PRINCIPAL TELEVISION APPEARANCES—Series: Host, *New Yorkers.* Episodic: Casey Drummond, *The Courtship of Eddie's Father,* ABC. Movies: Waitress, "Man from the South," *Alfred Hitchcock Presents,* NBC, 1985. Also appeared in *Mr. Kingstreet's War,* 1973.

RELATED CAREER—Professional model, 1952-60; actress in television commercials; toured with the U.S.O. in Vietnam.

NON-RELATED CAREER—Director of the Women's Council, Channel 28-TV; spokesperson for the March of Dimes.

MEMBER: Screen Actors Guild, Food for the Hungry, Multiple Sclerosis Foundation, International Orphans.*

*   *   *

HELM, Levon   1943-

PERSONAL: Born May 26, 1943, in Marvel, AR; father, a cotton farmer; children: Amy.

VOCATION: Actor, musician, and singer.

CAREER: PRINCIPAL FILM APPEARANCES—As himself, *The Last Waltz* (documentary), United Artists, 1978; Ted Webb, *Coal Miner's Daughter,* Universal, 1980; Jack Ridley and narrator, *The Right Stuff,* Warner Brothers, 1983; Bo, *Best Revenge,* Black Cat/RKR Releasing, 1984; Harry, *Smooth Talk,* Spectrafilm, 1985; Sheriff Leland Laughlin, *Man Outside,* Virgin Vision, 1987; Led Pickett, *End of the Line,* Orion, 1988.

PRINCIPAL TELEVISION APPEARANCES—Movies: Clovis Nevels, *The Dollmaker,* ABC, 1984. Specials: *Live from the Lone Star,* syndicated, 1982; *Folk/Rock Crossroads* (also known as *A 60's Folk/Rock Reunion*), PBS, 1986; narrator, "Elvis '56," *Crazy about the Movies,* Cinemax, 1987.

RELATED CAREER—Rock musician (with Rick Danko, Garth Hudson, Richard Manuel, and Robbie Robertson) in the Hawks (backing group for rockabilly performer Ronnie Hawkins), then as Levon and the Hawks, the Canadian Squires, and the Crackers; renamed the Band, 1967-76.

RECORDINGS: ALBUMS—*Levon Helm and the RCO All-Stars,* ABC, 1977; *Levon Helm,* ABC, 1978; *American Son,* MCA, 1978; (contributor) *The Legend of Jesse James,* A&M, 1980; *Levon Helm,* Capitol, 1982.

With the Band: *Music from Big Pink,* Capitol, 1968; *The Band,* Capitol, 1969; *Stage Fright,* Capitol, 1970; *Cahoots,* Capitol, 1971; *Rock of Ages,* Capitol, 1972; *Moondog Matinee,* Capitol, 1973; (also with Bob Dylan) *Before the Flood,* Asylum, 1974; *Northern Lights, Southern Cross,* Capitol, 1975; (also with Dylan) *The Basement Tapes,* Columbia, 1975; *Best of the Band,* Capitol, 1976; *Islands,* Capitol, 1977; *The Last Waltz* (original soundtrack), Warner Brothers, 1978; *Anthology, Volume I,* Capitol, 1978; *Anthology, Volume II,* Capitol, 1980.

ADDRESSES: HOME—Springdale, AR.*

*   *   *

HEMMINGS, David   1941-

PERSONAL: Full name, David Leslie Edward Hemmings; born November 18, 1941, in Guildford, England; married Genista Ouvry, 1960 (marriage ended); married Gayle Hunnicutt (an actress), 1969 (divorced, 1975); married Prudence J. de Casembroot, 1976; children: one daughter (first marriage); one son (second marriage); two sons (third marriage). EDUCATION: Attended Glyn College.

VOCATION: Actor, director, producer, and screenwriter.

CAREER: Also see *WRITINGS* below. PRINCIPAL STAGE APPEARANCES—Bertie Wooster, *Jeeves,* Her Majesty's Theatre, London, 1975. Also appeared in *The Turn of the Screw,* English Opera Group, 1954; and *Adventures in the Skin Trade.*

PRINCIPAL FILM APPEARANCES—Danny Willard, *The Heart Within,* Rank, 1957; schoolboy, *In the Wake of a Stranger,* Paramount, 1960; Ginger, *The Wind of Change,* Bryanston, 1961; Roy, *Murder Can Be Deadly* (also known as *The Painted Smile*), Colorama/Schoenfeld, 1963; Dave Martin, *Sing and Swing* (also known as *Live It Up*), Universal, 1964; Bert, *Some People,* American International, 1964; Kenny, *No Tree in the Street,* Seven Arts, 1964; Brian, *Two Left Feet,* British Lion, 1965; Dave, *Be My Guest,* Three Kings, 1965; Thomas, *Blow-Up,* Premier, 1966; David, *The Girl Getters* (also known as *The System*), American International, 1966; Mordred, *Camelot,* Warner Brothers/Seven Arts, 1967; Christian de Caray, *Eye of the Devil* (also known as *Thirteen*), Metro-Goldwyn-Mayer (MGM), 1967; Dildano, *Barbarella* (also known as *Barbarella, Queen of the Galaxy*), Paramount, 1968; Captain Nolan, *The Charge of the Light Brigade,* United Artists, 1968; Bob, *Only When I Larf,* Paramount, 1968; John, *The Long Day's Dying,* Paramount, 1968; title role, *Alfred*

the Great, MGM, 1969; Benjamin Oakes, *The Best House in London,* MGM, 1969.

Leigh Hartley, *The Walking Stick,* MGM, 1970; Tom Brett, *Fragment of Fear,* Columbia, 1971; Jerry Nelson, *The Love Machine,* Columbia, 1971; John Ebony, *Unman, Wittering, and Zigo,* Paramount, 1971; Charlie Braddock, *Juggernaut,* United Artists, 1974; Richard Swiveller, *Mr. Quilp* (also known as *The Old Curiosity Shop*), AVCO-Embassy, 1975; Marcus Daly, *Profondo Rosso* (also known as *Deep Red, The Hatchet Murders, Dripping Deep Red,* and *The Deep Red Hatchet Murders*), Seda Spettacoli Mahler/ Fletcher Video, 1976; Eddy, *Islands in the Stream,* Paramount, 1977; Keith, *The Squeeze,* Warner Brothers, 1977; Jack Armstrong, *Les Liens de sang* (also known as *Blood Relatives*), SNS, 1978; Hugh Hendon, *Crossed Swords* (also known as *The Prince and the Pauper*), Warner Brothers, 1978; Colonel Anthony Narriman, *Power Play,* Robert Cooper, 1978; Captain Hermann Kraft, *Just a Gigolo* (also known as *Schoner Gigolo—Armer Gigolo*), United Artists, 1979; Inspector Foxborough, *Murder by Decree,* AVCO-Embassy, 1979; Dr. Fraser, *Thirst,* New Line Cinema, 1979; Inspector Bruce Hutton, *Beyond Reasonable Doubt,* Endeavour, 1980; Senator Nick Rast, *Harlequin,* New Image, 1980; Edward, *The Disappearance,* World Northal, 1981; Gavin Wilson, *Man, Woman, and Child,* Paramount, 1983. Also appeared in *The Rainbow Jacket,* General Films Distributors, 1954; *Saint Joan,* United Artists, 1957; *Voices,* Hemdale, 1973; *Prisoners,* Endeavor, 1983; and in *Five Clues to Fortune,* 1957; *Men of Tomorrow,* 1958; *Don't Worry Momma,* 1973; and *Disappearance,* 1977.

PRINCIPAL FILM WORK—Director, *Running Scared,* Paramount, 1972; director, *The Fourteen,* Anglo/EMI, 1973; co-producer, *Power Play,* Robert Cooper, 1978; director, *Just a Gigolo* (also known as *Schoner Gigolo—Amer Gigolo*), United Artists, 1979; director, *The Survivor,* Greater Union Organization, 1980; executive producer, *Turkey Shoot,* Hemdale, 1981; executive producer, *Dead Kids,* Hemdale, 1981; executive producer, *Prisoners,* Endeavor, 1983; producer (with Anthony I. Ginnane and John Barnett) and director, *Treasure of the Yankee Zephyr* (also known as *Race for the Yankee Zephyr*), Film Ventures, 1984. Also produced *Disappearance,* 1977; and *Strange Behaviour,* 1981.

PRINCIPAL TELEVISION APPEARANCES—Episodic: Dr. Moffett, *Airwolf,* CBS, 1984. Movies: Title role, *Scott Fitzgerald,* BBC, 1975; Ian Blaize, *Beverly Hills Cowgirl Blues,* CBS, 1985; Captain James O'Neill, *Calamity Jane,* syndicated, 1985; Major Sanford Smith, *The Key to Rebecca,* syndicated, 1985; Maxwell "Newt" Newton, *Three on a Match,* NBC, 1987; Jack Roarke, *Harry's Hong Kong,* ABC, 1987. Also appeared in *The Rime of the Ancient Mariner,* ITV, 1978; *Charlie Muffin,* ITV, 1979; *Auto Stop, The Big Toe,* and *Out of the Unknown.*

PRINCIPAL TELEVISION WORK—All as director. Pilots: *In the Heat of the Night,* NBC, 1988; *Down Delaware Road,* NBC, 1988. Episodic: *Hawaiian Heat,* ABC, 1984; *Airwolf,* CBS, 1984; *Mickey Spillane's Mike Hammer* (also known as *The New Mike Hammer*), CBS, 1984; *The Last Precinct,* NBC, 1986; *Werewolf,* Fox, 1987. Movies: *The Key to Rebecca,* syndicated, 1985.

WRITINGS: FILM—(With Clive Exton) *Running Scared,* Paramount, 1972. TELEVISION—Episodic: *Airwolf,* CBS, 1984; *The Last Precinct,* NBC, 1986.

AWARDS: Silver Bear Award from the Berlin Film Festival, 1973, for *The Fourteen.*

MEMBER: Screen Actors Guild, American Federation of Television and Radio Artists, British Actors' Equity Association.

ADDRESSES: HOME—94 Onslow Gardens, London SW 7, England.*

*   *   *

HENNER, Marilu   1952-

PERSONAL: Born April 6, 1952, in Chicago, IL; married Frederic Forrest (an actor), September 28, 1980 (divorced). EDUCATION: Attended the University of Chicago.

VOCATION: Actress.

CAREER: PRINCIPAL STAGE APPEARANCES—Marty, *Grease,* Royale Theatre, New York City, 1972; Donna, *Over Here!,* Shubert Theatre, New York City, 1974; Sonia Walsk, *They're Playing Our Song,* Burt Reynolds' Dinner Theatre, Jupiter, FL, 1984; Marilu, *Pal Joey,* Circle in the Square, New York City, 1976; Barbara Kahn, *Social Security,* Ethel Barrymore Theatre, New York City, 1987. Also appeared in *Carnal Knowledge,* in Los Angeles, CA; and in productions of *Once Upon a Mattress* and *The Roar of the Greasepaint, the Smell of the Crowd.*

MAJOR TOURS—*Grease,* U.S. cities, 1971.

PRINCIPAL FILM APPEARANCES—Danielle, *Between the Lines,* Midwest Film, 1977; Annette, *Blood Brothers,* Warner Brothers, 1978; Kit Conger and Sue Alabama, *Hammett,* Warner Brothers, 1982; Agnes, *The Man Who Loved Women,* Columbia, 1983; Betty, *Cannonball Run II,* Warner Brothers, 1984; Lil, *Johnny Dangerously,* Twentieth Century-Fox, 1984; Sally, *Perfect,* Columbia, 1985; Miss Tracy, *Rustler's Rhapsody,* Paramount, 1985.

PRINCIPAL TELEVISION APPEARANCES—Series: Elaine Nardo, *Taxi,* ABC, 1978-82, then NBC, 1982-83. Pilots: Ashley Walters, *Stark,* CBS, 1985; also *Channel 99,* NBC, 1988. Movies: Laura Griffith, *Dream House,* CBS, 1981; Victoria Ducane, *Love with a Perfect Stranger,* Showtime, 1986.

ADDRESSES: AGENT—International Creative Management, 8899 Beverly Boulevard, Los Angeles, CA 90048. PUBLICISTS—Doug Taylor and Neil Koenigsberg, P/M/K Public Relations, 8436 W. Third Street, Suite 650, Los Angeles, CA 90048.*

*   *   *

HEPBURN, Audrey   1929-

PERSONAL: Born Edda van Heemstra Hepburn-Ruston, May 4, 1929, in Brussels, Belgium; daughter of Joseph Anthony and Baroness Ella (van Heemstra) Hepburn-Ruston; married Mel Ferrer (an actor), 1954 (divorced, 1968); married Andrea Dotti (a psychiatrist), 1969 (divorced); children: Sean (first marriage), Luca (second marriage). EDUCATION: Studied ballet at the Arnheim Conservatory of Music, with Sonia Gaskel in Amsterdam, and with Marie Rambert in London; studied acting with Felix Aylmer.

VOCATION: Actress.

CAREER: STAGE DEBUT—Chorus, *High Button Shoes,* London production, 1949. BROADWAY DEBUT—Title role, *Gigi,* Fulton Theatre, 1951. PRINCIPAL STAGE APPEARANCES—Title role, *Ondine,* 46th Street Theatre, New York City, 1954. Also appeared with Sauce Tartare and Sauce Piquante, both in London.

FILM DEBUT—(As Edda Hepburn) Stewardess, *Nederland in 7 Lessen* (a semi-travelogue; also known as *Dutch at the Double*), 1948. PRINCIPAL FILM APPEARANCES—Extra, *One Wild Oat,* Eros, 1951; cigarette girl, *Laughter in Paradise,* Associated British Films/Pathe, 1951; Chiquita, *The Lavender Hill Mob,* Universal, 1951; Nora Brentano, *Secret People,* Lippert, 1952; Linda Farrel, *Monte Carlo Baby,* Favorite, 1953; Princess Anne, *Roman Holiday,* Paramount, 1953; title role, *Sabrina* (also known as *Sabrina Fair*), Paramount, 1954; Eve Lester, *Young Wives' Tales,* Allied Artists, 1954; Natasha Rostov, *War and Peace,* Paramount, 1956; Jo Stockton, *Funny Face,* Paramount, 1957; Ariane Chavasse, *Love in the Afternoon,* Allied Artists, 1957; Rima, *Green Mansions,* Metro-Goldwyn-Mayer, 1959; Sister Luke/Gabrielle Van Der Mal, *The Nun's Story,* Warner Brothers, 1959.

Rachel Zachery, *The Unforgiven,* United Artists, 1960; Holly Golightly, *Breakfast at Tiffany's,* Paramount, 1961; Karen Wright, *The Children's Hour* (also known as *The Loudest Whisper*), United Artists, 1961; Reggie Lampert, *Charade,* Universal, 1963; Eliza Doolitle, *My Fair Lady,* Warner Brothers, 1964; Gabrielle Simpson, *Paris When It Sizzles,* Paramount, 1964; Nicole Bonnet, *How to Steal a Million,* Twentieth Century-Fox, 1966; Joanna Wallace, *Two for the Road,* Twentieth Century-Fox, 1967; Susy Hendrix, *Wait until Dark,* Warner Brothers, 1967; Maid Marian, *Robin and Marian,* Columbia, 1976; Elizabeth Roffe, *Bloodline* (also known as *Sidney Sheldon's ''Bloodline''*), Paramount, 1979; Angela Niotes, *They All Laughed,* Twentieth Century-Fox/United Artists Classics, 1981. Also appeared as Melissa Walter, *Nous irons a Monte Carlo,* 1951; and *Introducing Audrey Hepburn,* 1953.

PRINCIPAL TELEVISION APPEARANCES—Episodic: ''Mayerling,'' *Producers Showcase,* NBC, 1957; ''Directed by William Wyler,'' *American Masters,* PBS, 1987; ''Gregory Peck—His Own Man,'' *Crazy about the Movies,* Cinemax, 1988. Movies: Baroness Caroline DuLac, *Love among Thieves,* ABC, 1987. Specials: *A World of Love,* CBS, 1970; *The American Film Institute Salute to Fred Astaire,* CBS, 1981; *The American Film Institute Salute to Billy Wilder,* NBC, 1986; *Lerner and Loewe: Broadway's Last Romantics,* PBS, 1988.

RELATED CAREER—Ballet dancer in London; acted as courier and performed in underground concerts to raise funds for the Dutch Resistance during World War II.

AWARDS: Theatre World Award, 1952, for *Gigi;* Academy Award, New York Film Critics Award, and British Academy Award, all Best Actress, 1953, for *Roman Holiday;* Antoinette Perry Award, Best Actress (Dramatic), 1954, for *Ondine;* Star of Tomorrow, 1954; Academy Award nomination, Best Actress, 1954, for *Sabrina;* Academy Award nomination, British Academy Award, both Best Actress, 1959, for *The Nun's Story;* Academy Award nomination, Best Actress, 1961, for *Breakfast at Tiffany's;* British Academy Award, Best Actress, 1964, for *Charade;* Academy Award nomination, Best Actress, 1967, for *Wait until Dark;* Special Antoinette Perry Award, 1968.

MEMBER: Actors' Equity Association, Screen Actors Guild, American Federation of Television and Radio Artists.*

HERZOG, Werner   1942-

PERSONAL: Born Werner H. Stipetic, September 5, 1942, in Munich, Germany; married Martje Grohmann (a journalist), 1966; children: Rudolph Amos Achmed. EDUCATION: Attended the University of Munich, the University of Pittsburgh, and Duquesne University.

VOCATION: Director, producer, writer, and actor.

CAREER: Also see *WRITINGS* below. PRINCIPAL FILM APPEARANCES—Glass carrier, *Herz aus Glas* (also known as *Heart of Glass*), Cine International Filmvertrieb, 1976; narrator, *La Soufriere* (documentary short film), New Yorker, 1977; monk, *Nosferatu—Phantom der Nacht* (also known as *Nosferatu the Vampire* and *Nosferatu, Phantom of the Night*), Twentieth Century-Fox, 1979; father, *Man of Flowers*, International Spectrafilm, 1984; narrator, *Ballade vom kleinen Soldaten* (also known as *Ballad of the Little Soldier*), New Yorker, 1984. Also appeared in *Was Ich Bin, Sind Meine Filme* (also known as *I Am My Films: A Portrait of Werner Herzog, I Am My Films*, and *I Am What My Films Are;* documentary), Filmwelt verleib/New Yorker, 1978; *Garlic Is as Good as Ten Mothers*, Les Blank, 1980; *Werner Herzog Eats His Shoe* (short), Les Blank, 1980; *Burden of Dreams* (also known as *Die Last der Traume;* documentary about the making of *Fitzcarraldo*), Contemporary Films, Ltd., 1982; *Werner Herzog in Peru* (short), Les Blank, 1982; *Chambre 666* (also known as *Chambre 666 n' importe quand . . .* and *Room 666;* documentary), Gray City, 1982; *Tokyo-Ga* (documentary), Filmverlag der Autoren, 1984.

PRINCIPAL FILM WORK—All as producer and director, unless indicated: *Die beispiellose Verteidigung der Festung Deutschkreuz* (also known as *The Unparalleled Defense of the Fortress of Deutschkreuz*), Werner Herzog Filmproduktion, 1966; *Lebenszeichen*, Werner Herzog Filmproduktion, 1968, released in the United States as *Signs of Life*, New Yorker, 1981; *Letzte Worte* (also known as *Last Words;* short film), Werner Herzog Fillmproduktion, 1968; *Massnahmen gegen Fanatiker* (also known as *Measures against Fanatics*), Werner Herzog Filmproduktion, 1969; *Die fliegenden Arzte von Ostafrika* (also known as *The Flying Doctors of East Africa;* documentary short film), Werner Herzog Filmproduktion, 1970; *Auch Zwerge haben klein angefangen* (also known as *Even Dwarfs Started Small*), New Line Cinema, 1970; *Behinderte Zukunft* (also known as *Frustrated Future* and *Impeded Future;* documentary), Werner Herzog Filmproduktion, 1970; *Fata Morgana*, Werner Herzog Filmproduktion, 1970; *Land des Schweigens und der Dunkelheit* (also known as *Land of Silence and Darkness;* documentary), New Yorker, 1971; *Aguirre, der Zorn Gottes* (also known as *Aguirre, the Wrath of God*), New Yorker, 1972; *Die grosse Ekstase des Bildschnitzers Steiner* (also known as *The Great Ecstasy of the Sculptor Steiner;* documentary short film), New Yorker, 1974; *Jeder fur sich und Gott gegen alle* (also known as *Every Man for Himself and God against All* and *The Mystery of Kaspar Hauser*), Cine International/Cinema V, 1974.

How Much Wood Would a Woodchuck Chuck? (documentary short film), Werner Herzog Filmproduktion, 1976; *Mit mir will keiner spielen* (also known as *No One Will Play with Me;* short film), Werner Herzog Filmproduktion, 1976; *Herz aus Glas* (also known as *Heart of Glass*), Cine International Filmvertrieb, 1976; (director only) *La Soufriere* (documentary short film), New Yorker, 1977; *Stroszek*, Werner Herzog Filmproduktion, 1977; *Nosferatu—Phantom der Nacht* (also known as *Nosferatu, the Vampire* and *Nosferatu, Phantom of the Night*), Twentieth Century-Fox, 1979; *Woyzeck*, Werner Herzog Filmproduktion, 1979; *Huie's Predigt* (also known

as *Huie's Sermon;* documentary short film), New Yorker, 1980; (director only) *Glaube und Wahrung* (also known as *God's Angry Man*), New Yorker, 1980; *Fitzcarraldo*, New World, 1982; *Ballade vom kleinen Soldaten* (also known as *Ballad of the Little Soldier*), New Yorker, 1984; *Gasherbrum—Der leuchtende Berg* (also known as *The Dark Glow of the Mountains;* documentary), New Yorker, 1984; (director only) *Wo die grunen Ameisen traumen* (also known as *Where the Green Ants Dream*), Orion Classics, 1985; (director only) *Cobra Verde*, De Laurentiis Entertainment Group, 1988. Also producer and director, *Herakles* (short film), 1962; *Spiel im Sand* (also known as *Playing in the Sand* and *Game in the Sand;* incomplete), 1964.

RELATED CAREER—Founder, Werner Herzog Filmproduktion.

NON-RELATED CAREER—Worked for the National Aeronautics and Space Administration (NASA), 1966; also dockworker, Manchester, U.K.; steel factory worker, parking lot attendant, and rodeo hand, Pittsburgh, PA.

WRITINGS: FILM—See production details above, unless indicated. *Herakles* (short film), 1962; *Spiel im Sand* (incomplete), 1964; *Die beispiellose Verteidigung der festung Deutschkreuz*, 1966; *Lebenszeichen*, 1968; *Letzte Worte*, 1968; *Massnahmen gegen Fanatiker*, 1969; *Die fliegenden Arzte von Ostafrika*, 1970; *Auch Zwerge haben klein angefangen*, 1970; *Behinderte Zukunft* (documentary), 1970; *Fata Morgana*, 1970; *Land des Schweigens und der Dunkelheit* (documentary), 1971; *Aguirre, der Zorn Gottes*, 1972, dialogue and cutting continuity published as ''Aguirre, la colere de Dieu'' in *Avant-Scene du cinema*, June 15, 1978; *Die grosse Ekstase des Bildschnitzers Steiner* (documentary short film), 1974; *Jeder fur sich und Gott gegen alle*, 1974, dialogue and cutting continuity published as ''L'enigme de Kaspar Hauser'' in *Avant-Scene du cinema*, June, 1976; (co-writer) *Herz aus Glas*, 1976; *How Much Wood Would a Woodchuck Chuck?* (documentary short film), 1976; (with Herbert Achternbusch) *Mit mir will keiner spielen* (short film), 1976; *La Soufriere*, 1977; *Stroszek*, 1977, published in *2 Filmerzahlungen*, 1979; *Nosferatu—Phantom der Nacht*, 1979, published in *2 Filmerzahlungen*, 1979; *Woyzeck*, 1979; *Huie's Predigt*, 1980; *Glaube und Wahrung*, 1980; *Fitzcarraldo*, 1982, published as *Fitzcarraldo: The Original Story*, translated by Martje Herzog and Alan Greenberg, Fjord Press, 1982; *Ballade vom kleinen Soldaten*, 1984; *Gasherbrum—Der leuchtende Berg* (documentary), 1984; (with Bob Ellis) *Wo die grunen Ameisen traumen*, 1985; *Cobra Verde*, 1988; also *Screenplays* (a collection), translated by Alan Greenberg, published by Tanan Press, 1980.

OTHER—*Werner Herzog: Drehbucher I*, 1977; *Werner Herzog: Drehbucher II*, 1977; *Vom Gehen im Eis*, 1978, translated by Alan Greenberg, published as *Walking on Ice*, Tanan Press, 1980; *Sur la chemin des glaces: Munich-Paris 23.11 au 14.12 1974*, 1979. Also contributor of articles to film magazines and journals.

AWARDS: Prize from Oberhausen Film Festival, 1967, for *Letze Worte;* Bundesfilmpreis and Silver Bear Award, Best First Film, both from the Berlin Film Festival, 1968, for *Lebenszeichen;* Bundesfilmpreis and Special Jury Prize from the Cannes Film Festival, both 1975, for *Jeder fur sich und Gott gegen alle;* (with Bruno S.) German Film Critics Prize, 1977, for *Stroszek;* Rauriser Literaturpreis, 1978, for *Vom Gehen im Eis;* Best Director Award from the Cannes Film Festival, 1982, for *Fitzcarraldo.*

ADDRESSES: OFFICE—Neureutherstrasse 20, D-8000 Munchen 13, West Germany.*

HICKEY, William 1928-

PERSONAL: Full name, William Edward Hickey; born in 1928 in Brooklyn, NY; son of Edward and Nora Hickey. EDUCATION: Studied acting with Herbert Berghof and Uta Hagen.

VOCATION: Actor, director, and teacher.

CAREER: BROADWAY DEBUT—*Saint Joan,* Cort Theatre, 1951. PRINCIPAL STAGE APPEARANCES—Francisco, *Hamlet,* New York Repertory Group, Cherry Lane Theatre, New York City, 1948; concierge, *Tovarich,* City Center Theatre, New York City, 1952; Jimmy, *Mardi Gras,* Locust Theatre, Philadelphia, PA, 1954; title role, *Amedee,* Tempo Playhouse, New York City, 1955; Pierrot, *Don Juan, or the Feast with the Statue,* Downtown Theatre, New York City, 1956; Chandra, *The Lesser Comores,* Bucks County Playhouse, New Hope, PA, 1956; Fats Goldsmith, *Miss Lonelyhearts,* Music Box Theatre, New York City, 1957; Albert, *The Body Beautiful,* Broadway Theatre, New York City, 1958; second gravedigger, *Hamlet,* Flute, *A Midsummer Night's Dream,* and the young shepherd, *The Winter's Tale,* all American Shakespeare Festival, Stratford, CT, 1958; Bernie Leeds, *Make a Million,* Playhouse Theatre, New York City, 1958; Ozzie, *On the Town,* Carnegie Hall Playhouse, New York City, 1959; Scaltivo, *The Queen and the Rebels,* Bucks County Playhouse, 1959; Etienne Perisson, *Moonbirds,* Cort Theatre, New York City, 1959.

Fabian, *Twelfth Night,* and Trinculo, *The Tempest,* both American Shakespeare Festival, 1960; Sir Andrew Aguecheek, *Twelfth Night,* American Shakespeare Festival, 1961; Boats, *The Undercover Lover,* Adelphi College Summer Theatre Workshop, Garden City, NY, 1961; neighbor, "Not Enough Rope" in *3 x 3,* Maidman Playhouse, New York City, 1962; Bagdad, *Step on a Crack,* Ethel Barrymore Theatre, New York City, 1962; *Diary of a Madman* (one-man show), Gramercy Arts Theatre, New York City, 1964; ensemble, *The Decline and Fall of the Entire World As Seen through the Eyes of Cole Porter, Revisited* (revue), Square East Theatre, New York City, 1965; Arnold, *This Winter's Hobby,* Shubert Theatre, New Haven, CT, then Walnut Street Theatre, Philadelphia, 1966; Adam, *The Devils,* Mark Taper Forum, Los Angeles, CA, 1967; the Centurion, *Androcles and the Lion,* and Costard, *Love's Labour's Lost,* both American Shakespeare Festival, 1968; second watch, *Much Ado about Nothing,* and second gravedigger, *Hamlet,* both American Shakespeare Festival, 1969; Marion Cheever, *Next,* Greenwich Mews Theatre, New York City, 1969.

Looseleaf Harper, *Happy Birthday, Wanda June,* Theatre de Lys, New York City, 1970; Steve, *Small Craft Warnings,* Truck and Warehouse Theatre, New York City, 1972; Seth Beckwith, *Mourning Becomes Electra,* Circle in the Square, New York City, 1972; "Grandmother Kroner," *Siamese Connections,* New York Shakespeare Festival (NYSF), Public Theatre, New York City, 1973; Pandarus and Calchas, *Troilus and Cressida,* NYSF, Mitzi E. Newhouse Theatre, New York City, 1973; Johnny MacDonald, *Thieves,* Broadhurst Theatre, New York City, 1974; Ralph Waldo Emerson and Mitch Bouyer, *Romance Language,* Playwrights Horizons, New York City, 1984; Uncle Salvatore, *Angelo's Wedding,* Circle Repertory Theatre, New York City, 1985; title role, *Lippe,* Quaigh Theatre, New York City, 1985; Dr. Einstein, *Arsenic and Old Lace,* 46th Street Theatre, New York City, 1986. Also appeared as Cash, *As I Lay Dying,* 1955; and in *Sunday Runners.*

PRINCIPAL STAGE WORK—Assistant stage manager, *Tovarich,*

City Center Theatre, New York City, 1952; director, *All You Need Is One Good Break,* Phoenicia Playhouse, Phoenicia, NY, 1961; associate director, *Do You Know the Milky Way?,* Billy Rose Theatre, New York City, 1961; director, "Not Enough Rope" in *3 x 3,* Maidman Playhouse, New York City, 1962; director, *Name of a Soup,* HB Studio, New York City, 1963; director, *Diary of a Madman,* Gramercy Arts Theatre, New York City, 1964; consultant, *On the Necessity of Being Polygamous,* Gramercy Arts Theatre, 1964.

MAJOR TOURS—Concierge, *Tovarich,* U.S. cities, 1952; Flute, *A Midsummer Night's Dream,* American Shakespeare Festival, U.S. cities, 1960; also *The Play's the Thing,* U.S. cities, 1952. Director, *The Lady's Not for Burning,* U.S. cities, 1954.

PRINCIPAL FILM APPEARANCES—Apples, *A Hatful of Rain,* Twentieth Century-Fox, 1957; Jo-Jo, *Invitation to a Gunfighter,* United Artists, 1964; drunk in theatre bar, *The Producers,* Embassy, 1967; Eugene T. Rourke, *The Boston Strangler,* Twentieth Century-Fox, 1968; historian, *Little Big Man,* National General, 1970; Looseleaf Harper, *Happy Birthday, Wanda June,* Columbia, 1971; Mr. Skelton, *92 in the Shade,* United Artists, 1975; Sid Fine, *Mikey and Nicky,* Paramount, 1976; Perry, *The Sentinel,* Universal, 1977; Papa, *Flanagan,* United Film, 1985; Don Corrado Prizzi, *Prizzi's Honor,* Twentieth Century-Fox, 1985; Coney Island barker, *Remo Williams: The Adventure Begins,* Orion, 1985; Ubertino de Casale, *The Name of The Rose,* Twentieth Century-Fox, 1986; Old Man Beckersted, *One Crazy Summer,* Warner Brothers, 1986; ferret man, *Bright Lights, Big City,* United Artists, 1988; Drumm, *Da,* Film Dallas, 1988. Also appeared in *Operation Madball,* Columbia, 1957; *Something Wild,* United Artists, 1961; *The Telephone Book,* Rosebud, 1971; *Wise Blood,* New Line, 1979; *Walls of Glass,* 1985; and *Seize the Day,* 1986.

PRINCIPAL TELEVISION APPEARANCES—Episodic: Artful Dodger, "Oliver Twist," *Dupont Show of the Month,* CBS, 1959; also *Studio One,* CBS; *Camera Three,* CBS; *Philco Playhouse,* NBC; *The Reporter,* CBS; *The Phil Silvers Show,* CBS; *Mr. Broadway,* CBS; *Hawk,* ABC. Movies: Hotel desk clerk, *Izzy and Moe,* CBS, 1985; Mr. Pierson, *Stranded,* NBC, 1986. Specials: Menagerie keeper, *Androcles and the Lion,* NBC, 1967.

RELATED CAREER—Acting teacher.

AWARDS: Academy Award nomination, Best Supporting Actor, 1986, for *Prizzi's Honor.*

MEMBER: Actors' Equity Association, Screen Actors Guild, American Federation of Television and Radio Artists.

ADDRESSES: OFFICE—HB Studio, 120 Bank Street, New York, NY 10014. AGENT—Bob Waters Agency, 1501 Broadway, New York, NY 10036.*

*   *   *

HICKS, Catherine 1951-

PERSONAL: Born August 6, 1951, in Scottsdale, AZ. EDUCATION: Attended Notre Dame University.

VOCATION: Actress.

CAREER: PRINCIPAL STAGE APPEARANCES—Sally Haines, *Tribute*, Brooks Atkinson Theatre, New York City, 1978.

PRINCIPAL FILM APPEARANCES—Sally, *Death Valley*, Universal, 1982; Sable, *Better Late Than Never*, Warner Brothers, 1983; Jane Mortimer, *Garbo Talks*, Metro-Goldwyn-Mayer/United Artists (MGM/UA), 1984; Isabel, *The Razor's Edge*, Columbia, 1984; Flo, *Fever Pitch*, MGM/UA, 1985; Carol Heath, *Peggy Sue Got Married*, Tri-Star, 1986; Dr. Gillian Taylor, *Star Trek IV: The Voyage Home*, Paramount, 1986; Dr. Amy Larkin, *Like Father, Like Son*, Tri-Star, 1987; Tina Boyer, *Souvenir*, Palisades Entertainment, 1988; Karen Barclay, *Child's Play*, MGM/UA, 1988.

PRINCIPAL TELEVISION APPEARANCES—Series: Dr. Emily Rappant, *The Bad News Bears*, CBS, 1979-80; Amanda Tucker, *Tucker's Witch*, CBS, 1982-83; also Faith Coleridge, *Ryan's Hope*, ABC. Pilots: (As Cathy Hicks) Valerie, *Sparrow*, CBS, 1978. Movies: Annie, *Love for Rent*, ABC, 1979; Marilyn Monroe, *Marilyn: The Untold Story*, ABC, 1980; Beth, *To Race the Wind*, CBS, 1980; Ann Welles, *Jacqueline Susann's "Valley of the Dolls 1981"* CBS, 1981; Lisa Sage, *Happy Endings*, CBS, 1983; Jane Algernon, *Laguna Heat*, HBO, 1987.

AWARDS: Emmy Award nomination, Outstanding Actress, 1980, for *Marilyn: The Untold Story*.

ADDRESSES: AGENT—Nicole David, Triad Artists, 10100 Santa Monica Boulevard, 16th Floor, Los Angeles, CA 90067.*

*   *   *

HIGGINS, Anthony

VOCATION: Actor.

CAREER: PRINCIPAL STAGE APPEARANCES—Mick, *The Caretaker*, Greenwich Theatre, London, 1977; Eddie, German soldier, and Angelo, *Piaf*, and Corporal Moat, *Captain Swing*, both Royal Shakespeare Company (RSC), Other Place Theatre, Stratford-on-Avon, U.K., 1978, then Warehouse Theatre, London, 1979; Ron, *Men's Beano*, and Andy, *The Innocent*, both RSC, Warehouse Theatre, 1979.

PRINCIPAL FILM APPEARANCES—Heinz Berg, *Voyage of the Damned*, AVCO-Embassy, 1976; Stephen Zelli, *Quartet*, New World, 1981; Gobler, *Raiders of the Lost Ark*, Paramount, 1981; Mr. Neville, *The Draughtsman's Contract*, United Artists, 1983; Clerval, *The Bride*, Columbia, 1985; Tom, *She'll Be Wearing Pink Pyjamas*, Film Four International, 1985; Rathe, *Young Sherlock Holmes*, Paramount, 1985; Peter, *Max Mon Amour* (also known as *Max My Love*), Allied Artists, 1986. Also appeared in *Gossip*, Boyd's Company, 1983.

PRINCIPAL TELEVISION APPEARANCES—Mini-Series: Tallyrand, *Napoleon and Josephine: A Love Story*, ABC, 1987. Movies: Erich, *The Cold Room*, HBO, 1984; Abdullah, *Lace*, ABC, 1984; Abdullah, *Lace II*, ABC, 1985.*

HIKEN, Gerald   1927-

PERSONAL: Born May 23, 1927, in Milwaukee, WI; son of Nathan (a merchant) and Marian (Shapiro) Hiken; married Barbara Lerner (a make-up artist), September 23, 1961; children: one daughter. EDUCATION: University of Wisconsin, B.A., 1949; trained for the stage with Uta Hagen, 1955-56, and at the Actors Studio, 1959.

VOCATION: Actor, director, and producer.

CAREER: OFF-BROADWAY DEBUT—Trofimoff, *The Cherry Orchard*, Fourth Street Theatre, 1955. LONDON DEBUT—Andrei, *The Three Sisters*, Actors Studio, World Theatre Season, Aldwych Theatre, 1965. PRINCIPAL STAGE APPEARANCES—Richard, *Hay Fever*, Linden Circle Theatre, Milwaukee, WI, 1949; Eddie Brock, *Born Yesterday*, Erie Playhouse, Erie, PA, 1951; Telegin, then title role, *Uncle Vanya*, Fourth Street Theatre, New York City, 1956; Don Parritt, *The Iceman Cometh*, Circle in the Square, New York City, 1956; Blaise, *The Lovers*, Martin Beck Theatre, New York City, 1956; Semyon Semyonovitch, Medvedenko, *The Seagull*, Fourth Street Theatre, 1956; Wong, *The Good Woman of Setzuan*, Phoenix Theatre, New York City, 1956; Alceste, *The Misanthrope*, Theatre East, New York City, 1956; the Father, *The Cave Dwellers*, Bijou Theatre, New York City, 1957; Clov, *Endgame*, Cherry Lane Theatre, New York City, 1958; the Supervisor, *The Enchanted*, Renata Theatre, New York City, 1958; Hovstad, *An Enemy of the People*, Actors Playhouse, New York City, 1959; Max the Millionaire, *The Nervous Set*, Henry Miller's Theatre, New York City, 1959; Andrei Prozoroff, *The Three Sisters*, Fourth Street Theatre, 1959; Michepain, *The Fighting Cock*, American National Theatre and Academy Theatre, New York City, 1959.

Morris "Moishe" Golub, *The 49th Cousin*, Ambassador Theatre, New York City, 1960; the Condemned Man and the Hangman, *Gallows Humor*, Gramercy Arts Theatre, New York City, 1961; Arthur Groomkirby, *One Way Pendulum*, East 74th Street Theatre, New York City, 1961; title role, *Gideon*, Plymouth Theatre, New York City, 1961; Shortcut, *Foxy*, Ziegfeld Theatre, New York City, 1964; Andrei, *The Three Sisters*, Actors Studio, Morosco Theatre, New York City, 1964; Stanley, *The Birthday Party*, University of California at Los Angeles Theatre Group, Los Angeles, CA, 1965; title role, *Scapin*, Stanford University Repertory Theatre, Stanford, CA, 1965; Lafeu, *All's Well That Ends Well*, Wong, *The Good Woman of Setzuan*, and Caesar, *Antony and Cleopatra*, all Stanford University Repertory Theatre, 1966; Gaev, *The Cherry Orchard*, Bill Maitland, *Inadmissable Evidence*, the Playwright, *Once in a Lifetime*, and the Author, *The Cavern*, all Stanford University Repertory Theatre, 1967; Mathern, *Cock-a-Doodle Dandy*, Ossip, *The Inspector General*, and Sidney, *The Sign in Sidney Brustein's Window*, all Stanford University Repertory Theatre, 1968.

Morris Meyerson, *Golda*, Morosco Theatre, 1977; Ed Lemon, *Mackerel*, Hartford Stage Company, Hartford, CT, 1978; Steve Miller, *Gracious Living*, Eisenhower Theatre, Kennedy Center for the Performing Arts, Washington, DC, 1978; the Common Man, *A Man for All Seasons*, Ahmanson Theatre, Los Angeles, 1979; title role and Actor, *Strider: The Story of a Horse*, Chelsea Theatre Center, Westside Theatre, then Helen Hayes Theatre, both New York City, 1979; Snetsky, *Fools*, Eugene O'Neill Theatre, New York City, 1981; David Malter, *The Chosen*, Second Avenue Theatre, New York City, 1988. Also appeared in *Twelfth Night* and *The Physician in Spite of Himself*, both Little Theatre, Houston, TX, 1949; in *Dig We Must*, John Drew Theatre, East Hampton,

NY, 1959; as Stockman, *An Enemy of the People,* and in *Major Barbara,* both Princeton, NJ, 1960; in *Brecht on Brecht,* Theatre De Lys, New York City, 1962; *An Enemy of the People,* Los Angeles Actor's Theatre, Los Angeles, 1984; *The Quartered Man,* Los Angeles Actor's Theatre, 1986; *Barabbas,* Los Angeles Theatre Center, Los Angeles, 1987; and in various productions at Lake Geneva, WI, 1950; at the Erie Playhouse, 1951-53; Brattle Theatre, Cambridge, MA, 1952; with the Port Players, in Wisconsin, 1953; at the Arena Stage, Washington, DC, 1953-55; and with the New Theatre, in Los Angeles, 1968-77.

PRINCIPAL STAGE WORK—Producer and director, *Hay Fever,* Linden Circle Theatre, Milwaukee, WI, 1949; director, *Beautiful People* and *Earnest,* both Rice Institute, Houston, TX, 1951; assistant director, *Mother Courage and Her Children,* Martin Beck Theatre, New York City, 1963.

MAJOR TOURS—Moishe, *Sweet and Sour,* U.S. cities, 1958; also with the New Theatre, U.S. cities, 1968-77.

FILM DEBUT—Ilya Ilyich Telegin ("Waffles"), *Uncle Vanya,* Continental Distributing, 1958. PRINCIPAL FILM APPEARANCES— Uncle, *The Goddess,* Columbia, 1958; Gully, *Invitation to a Gunfighter,* United Artists, 1964; Mahlon, *Funnyman,* New Yorker, 1967; Chick, *Company of Killers,* Universal, 1970; station master, *The Candidate,* Warner Brothers, 1972; painter, *Fuzz,* United Artists, 1972; Andrei, *The Three Sisters,* NTA, 1977; Dr. Lorber, *Reds,* Paramount, 1981; Reb Shulem, *War and Love,* Cannon, 1985.

TELEVISION DEBUT—Title role, "Uncle Vanya," *Camera Three,* CBS, 1956. PRINCIPAL TELEVISION APPEARANCES—Mini-Series: Urquhart, *Sandburg's Lincoln,* NBC, 1974; Professor Anderson, *James A. Michener's "Space"* (also known as *Space*), CBS, 1985; Erdheim, *Nutcracker: Money, Madness, and Murder,* CBS, 1987. Pilots: Etienne Jacoby, *Once Upon a Dead Man,* NBC, 1971; Father Heller, *Spencer's Pilots,* CBS, 1976; Kokotchka, *Circus,* ABC, 1987. Episodic: St. Ignatius, *Lamp Unto My Feet,* CBS, 1956; Dr. Bernie Applebaum, *The Partridge Family,* ABC, 1970; Squire Hacker, "A Message from Charity," *The Twilight Zone,* CBS, 1985; Alexandrov Dimitri, *Newhart,* CBS, 1986; Robin Baskins, *St. Elsewhere* (two episodes), NBC, 1987; Mr. Crebbin, *Who's the Boss?,* ABC, 1987; Denis, *Cheers* (two episodes), NBC, 1988; Dr. Redding, *Matlock,* NBC, 1988; Horowitz, *Something Is Out There,* NBC, 1988; also *All in the Family,* CBS, 1976; as Private Lester Mendelsohn, *The Phil Silvers Show,* CBS; in *Armstrong Circle Theatre,* CBS; *U.S. Steel Hour,* CBS; *Car 54, Where Are You?,* NBC; *The Untouchables,* ABC; *You'll Never Get Rich,* CBS; *Studio One,* CBS; *The Defenders,* CBS; *Eleventh Hour,* NBC; *Dupont Show of the Month,* NBC; *The Farmer's Daughter,* ABC; *Naked City,* ABC; *Occasional Wife,* NBC; *Judd for the Defense,* ABC; *Mission Impossible,* CBS; *Play of the Week,* NTA; *Omnibus.*

Movies: Judge Arnold Lerner, *The Law,* NBC, 1974; Fischel Shpunt, *The Wall,* CBS, 1982; Jack, *Love Leads the Way,* Disney Channel, 1984; Theo Grant, *Blackout,* HBO, 1985; Mr. Freilich, *Crossings,* ABC, 1986; John, *Liberace,* ABC, 1988; Dix, *Street of Dreams,* NBC, 1988; also *A Case of Rape,* NBC, 1974; *Strange Voices,* CBS, 1987. Specials: Frank Olmstead, "There Shall Be No Night," *Hallmark Hall of Fame,* NBC, 1957; also *The Ballad of Louie the Louse,* CBS, 1959; *The Whirlwind,* CBS, 1974. Also appeared *The Lady's Not for Burning, Eternal Light,* and *Cain's Hundred.*

RELATED CAREER—Assistant director, Little Theatre, Houston, TX, 1949-50; company member, Stanford University Repertory Theatre, Stanford, CA, 1965-68, and artistic director, 1966-68; acting lecturer, Stanford University, 1966-68; founder (with Paul E. Richards), the New Theatre (a two-man repertory theatre performing original works), Los Angeles, CA, 1968-77; National Humanities Faculty, 1970-72; member, Actors Studio, New York City.

AWARDS: Obie Award from the *Village Voice* and Clarence Derwent Award, both 1955, for *Uncle Vanya;* Outer Critics Circle Award, Outstanding Performance by an Actor, 1980, for *Strider: The Story of a Horse.*

MEMBER: Actors' Equity Association (council member, 1961-67), Screen Actors Guild, American Federation of Television and Radio Artists.

SIDELIGHTS: FAVORITE ROLES—All Chekhov roles.

ADDRESSES: HOME—910 Moreno Avenue, Palo Alto, CA 94303.*

                 *   *   *

HILL, Dana   1964-

PERSONAL: Born May 6, 1964, in Encino, CA.

VOCATION: Actress.

CAREER: PRINCIPAL STAGE APPEARANCES—Millie Owens, *Picnic,* Ahmanson Theatre, Los Angeles, CA, 1986; Annelle Dupuy-Desoto, *Steel Magnolias,* Pasadena Playhouse, Pasadena, CA, 1988.

FILM DEBUT—Sherry, *Shoot the Moon,* Metro-Goldwyn-Mayer, 1982. PRINCIPAL FILM APPEARANCES—Ellie Turner, *Cross Creek,* Universal, 1983; Audrey Griswald, *National Lampoon's European Vacation,* Warner Brothers, 1985.

TELEVISION DEBUT—Deborah, *The Paul Williams Show,* NBC, 1978. PRINCIPAL TELEVISION APPEARANCES—Series: Gabrielle "Gabby" Gallagher, *The Two of Us,* CBS, 1981-82; voice characterization, *Mighty Mouse: The New Adventures* (animated), CBS, 1987. Mini-Series: Maggie Joy, *The French Atlantic Affair,* ABC, 1979. Pilots: Courteney Featherstone, *Featherstone's Nest,* CBS, 1979; Gussie Mapes, *Branagan and Mapes,* CBS, 1983. Episodic: Cassie Farraday, *The Fall Guy,* ABC, 1981; also *Magnum, P.I.,* CBS; *The Tonight Show,* NBC; and *The Merv Griffin Show,* syndicated. Movies: Kim Lissik, *The $5.20 an Hour Dream,* CBS, 1980; Jennifer Phillips, *Fallen Angel,* CBS, 1981; Cindy Lewis, *Silence of the Heart,* CBS, 1984; Andrea, *Combat High,* NBC, 1986; Millie Owens, *Picnic,* Showtime, 1986; also *The Kids Who Knew Too Much.* Specials: Michelle Mudd, "What Are Friends For?," *ABC Afterschool Special,* ABC, 1980; Frankie Addams, *The Member of the Wedding,* NBC, 1982; Geraldine Oxley, "Welcome Home, Jellybean," *CBS Schoolbreak Special,* CBS, 1984; voice of Stoney, *The Flintstone Kids "Just Say No" Special* (animated), ABC, 1988.

RELATED CAREER—Actress in television commercials.

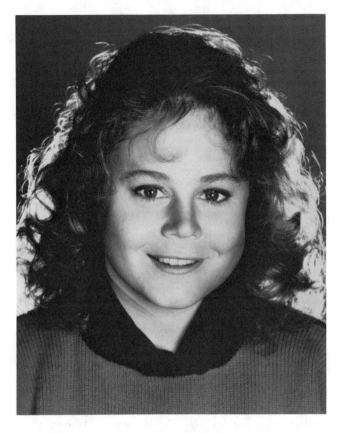

DANA HILL

ADDRESSES: PUBLICIST—Paul Shefrin, The Shefrin Company, 800 S. Robertson Boulevard, Suite 5, Los Angeles, CA 90035.

*   *   *

HOFFMAN, Dustin   1937-

PERSONAL: Full name, Dustin Lee Hoffman; born August 8, 1937, in Los Angeles, CA; son of Harry (a set decorator) and Lillia (a jazz pianist; maiden name, Gold) Hoffman; married Anne Byrne (a ballet dancer), May 4, 1969 (divorced, 1980); married Lisa Gottsegen (a lawyer), September, 1980; children: Karina, Jenna (first marriage); two sons and one daughter (second marriage). EDUCATION: Trained for the stage at the Pasadena Playhouse, 1958, and with Barney Brown, Lonny Chapman, and Lee Strasberg; also studied music at the Los Angeles Conservatory of Music and attended Santa Monica City College.

VOCATION: Actor and director.

CAREER: BROADWAY DEBUT—Ridzinski, *A Cook for Mr. General,* Playhouse Theatre, 1961. PRINCIPAL STAGE APPEARANCES—Clov, *Endgame,* Dunlavin, *The Quare Fellow,* C. Couch (Babboon), *In the Jungle of Cities,* Nicholas Trilestski, *A Country Scandal,* Ben, *The Dumbwaiter,* Bert Hudd, *The Room,* Pozzo, *Waiting for Godot,* Zapo, *Picnic on the Battlefield,* Hugo, *Dirty Hands,* and Peter, *The Cocktail Party,* all Theatre Company of Boston, Boston, MA, 1964; Frankie, *Three Men on a Horse,* McCarter Theatre, Princeton, NJ, 1964; Immanuel, *Harry, Noon and Night,* American

Place Theatre, New York City, 1965; Zoditch, *The Journey of the Fifth Horse,* American Place Theatre, 1966; title role, ''The Old Jew,'' Max, ''Reverberations,'' and Jax, ''Fragments,'' in *Fragments* (triple-bill), Berkshire Theatre Festival, Stockbridge, MA, 1966; Valentine Bross, *Eh?,* Circle in the Square, New York City, 1966; title role, *Jimmy Shine,* Brooks Atkinson Theatre, New York City, 1968; Willy Loman, *Death of a Salesman,* Broadhurst Theatre, New York City, 1984; Shylock, *The Merchant of Venice,* Phoenix Theatre, London, 1989. Also appeared in productions of *Star Wagon,* 1966; *The Subject Was Roses* and *A View from the Bridge.*

PRINCIPAL STAGE WORK—Assistant to director, *A View from the Bridge,* Sheridan Square Playhouse, New York City, 1965; director, *Jimmy Shine,* Brooks Atkinson Theatre, New York City, 1968; director, *All over Town,* Booth Theatre, New York City, 1974; co-producer, *Death of a Salesman,* Broadhurst Theatre, New York City, 1984.

FILM DEBUT—Hap, *The Tiger Makes Out,* Columbia, 1967. PRINCIPAL FILM APPEARANCES—Ben Braddock, *The Graduate,* Embassy, 1967; John, *John and Mary,* Twentieth Century-Fox, 1969; Enrico ''Ratso'' Rizzo, *Midnight Cowboy,* United Artists, 1969; Jack Crabb, *Little Big Man,* National General, 1970; Jack Fisher, *Madigan's Millions,* American International, 1970; Georgie Soloway, *Who Is Harry Kellerman, and Why Is He Saying Those Terrible Things about Me?,* National General, 1971; David Sumner, *Straw Dogs,* Cinerama, 1971; title role, *Alfredo, Alfredo,* Paramount, 1973; Louis Dega, *Papillon,* Allied Artists, 1973; Lenny Bruce, *Lenny,* United Artists, 1974; Carl Bernstein, *All the President's Men,* Warner Brothers, 1976; Babe Levy, *Marathon Man,* Paramount, 1976; Max Dembo, *Straight Time,* Cinerama, 1978; Wally Stanton, *Agatha,* Warner Brothers, 1979; Ted Kramer, *Kramer vs. Kramer,* Columbia, 1979; Michael Dorsey/Dorothy Michaels, *Tootsie,* Columbia, 1982; Chuck Clark, *Ishtar,* Columbia, 1987; Raymond, *Rain Man,* Metro-Goldwyn-Mayer/United Artists, 1988. Also appeared in *Private Conversations* (documentary), Teleculture, 1985.

PRINCIPAL FILM WORK—Director, *Straight Time,* Cinerama, 1978.

TELEVISION DEBUT—*The Naked City,* ABC, 1961. PRINCIPAL TELEVISION APPEARANCES—Specials: Willy Loman, *Death of a Salesman,* CBS, 1985. Also appeared in *The Star Wagon,* 1975; *The Trap of Solid Gold* and *The Journey of the Fifth Horse.* PRINCIPAL TELEVISION WORK—Executive producer, *Death of a Salesman,* CBS, 1985.

RECORDINGS: Young Ben, *Death of a Salesman,* Caedmon, 1968.

AWARDS: Obie Award from the *Village Voice,* 1966, for *The Journey of the Fifth Horse;* Drama Desk Award, Vernon Rice Award, and Theatre World Award, all 1967, for *Eh?;* Academy Award nomination, Best Actor, 1968, for *The Graduate;* Academy Award nomination, Best Actor, 1970, for *Midnight Cowboy;* Academy Award nomination, Best Actor, 1975, for *Lenny;* Academy Award and New York Film Critics Circle Award, both Best Actor, 1980, for *Kramer vs. Kramer;* New York Film Critics Circle Award, National Society of Film Critics Award, Golden Globe, and Academy Award nomination, all Best Actor, 1983, for *Tootsie;* Drama Desk Award, 1985, for *Death of a Salesman;* Emmy Award nomination, Outstanding Actor, 1986, for *Death of a Salesman;*

Academy Award and Golden Bear from the Berlin Film Festival, both Best Actor, 1989, for *Rain Man.*

SIDELIGHTS: Recognized for the breadth of his performances as well as the depth and believability with which he imbues them, ''Dustin Hoffman has played them all in a career of dazzling virtuosity,'' remarks Gerald Clarke (*Time,* December 3, 1979). Hoffman believes that ''one of the things you can do as an actor is compensate for the things you can't do in life,'' states Peter Travers (*People,* January 17, 1983). And since his theatrical debut as Tiny Tim in a junior high school production of *A Christmas Carol,* he has compensated by definitively portraying a wide spectrum of memorable and critically acclaimed roles. From the theatre to the television screen, ''Hoffman's signature as an actor has been to appear in roles far outside his experience,'' says Tony Schwartz (*New York Times,* December 16, 1979), adding that ''perhaps no other actor has played so daring and disparate a range of parts.''

An actor of boundless versatility, Hoffman possesses a keen talent for observation and mimicry. Calling him ''a sponge for mannerisms and dialects, an instinctive prober, a clown and a mimic,'' Schwartz suggests that ''acting has legitimized his curiosity.'' Hoffman approaches roles with tenacity and thoroughness; his ''method is to exhaustively research the characters he plays,'' says Schwartz, who offers Hoffman's own explanation: ''My job is to do you, and the only way that's possible is if I've got you inside me. I've got to find out what you're doing. Nobody simply *is,* except infants. Once we gets self-conscious, we act—all the way to the grave. So an actor shows you how people act. That's what Diane Arbus was doing in her pictures: showing you what the person was, plus the image the person had of himself.''

Hoffman's performance of the young and bewildered Benjamin Braddock in *The Graduate* earned him the first of several Academy Award nominations, plus star status. Mel Gussow (*New York Times Magazine,* March 18, 1984) recalls: ''As he said to me about his sudden success, 'I plummeted to stardom,' a statement that he cherishes . . . as a total summary of that eventful period in his life. Soon he was a household name and a role model for future actors.'' Striving relentlessly for perfection in his work, Hoffman has the reputation, especially among directors, as ''the archetypical difficult actor,'' observes Clarke. ''Getting it right—his character, a scene, the film itself—is Mr. Hoffman's obsession, and it is not always an endearing one,'' says Schwartz. ''Being difficult comes quite naturally to him.'' Gussow quotes one director's experience: ''He's one of the most inventive actors I've ever known. He's so full of ideas that he almost gives you too much. I loved working with him, but I'm not sure I'd want to do it again soon.'' Hoffman is sensitive about the reluctance of some directors to work with him ''because of his insistence on rehearsal time and frequent script revisions,'' notes Travers; but as Schwartz suggests, ''For Mr. Hoffman, personal instinct is the key to quality. 'A director will say, ''Just trust me.'' Well I can't work that way. I either agree with you or I don't. I go by my own gut. In a film, it's a fine line, a half beat. It's meant to look effortless, but it's all worked out with such hair-splitting scrutiny. The game is to give goosebumps, then you're home.'''

According to Gussow, playwright Arthur Miller thinks that Hoffman ''has to know with his brain and his belly what the center of the dramatic issue is. He peels it off like an onion, getting to the middle of the middle.'' And while Hoffman's working relationship with directors may be tense, his fellow actors seem to understand his intent. For instance, Schwartz relates a comment by Hoffman's *Kramer vs. Kramer* co-star, Meryl Streep: ''Dustin has a techni-

cian's thoroughness and he is very demanding, but it isn't the star temperament I'd been led to expect. It isn't vanity. He is a perfectionist about the craft and about the structuring of the film, and his own ego is subjugated to that.'' Hoffman's peers also recognize that he is as concerned about their performances as he is about his own. Gussow reports that John Malkovich, who appeared with Hoffman in the television production of *Death of a Salesman,* considers him ''as relentless a performer as I've ever encountered,'' adding that ''a lot of stars cast mediocre people around them and put them in a dim light, but he wants everybody around him to be very good.''

Although he is widely regarded as a character actor, Hoffman expressed to Leslie Bennetts (*New York Times,* December 21, 1982) that his portrayal of the scavenging pimp, Ratso Rizzo, in *Midnight Cowboy,* for example, was not character acting: ''That was just an autobiography of subjective feelings about oneself.'' Gussow indicates that Hoffman ''models his look, manner and voice on people he knows. *The Graduate* was based on his brother; Ratso was the super of a building he lived in; Tootsie was patterned after his mother.'' Similarly, Hoffman infused his portrayal of Willy Loman in *Death of a Salesman* with recollections of his own father who had been a furniture salesman; and during the filming of *Kramer vs. Kramer,* for which Hoffman won the Academy Award for his performance of what he describes to Travers as ''a bad father who tried to be a good mother,'' Hoffman's own first marriage was dissolved. Clarke believes, though, that in *Kramer vs. Kramer,* Hoffman ''assumed perhaps the most difficult persona of all: Dustin Hoffman.''

While Hoffman draws frequently on personal observations or experience for his performances, his roles are also marked by a capacity for change; and the role that has apparently affected him most profoundly is that of the indomitable Dorothy Michaels in *Tootsie,* a film that explores issues of what is inherently male or female. Travers reports that one of Hoffman's deepest disappointments was that Hollywood, with all of its cosmetic artistry, was unable to make Dorothy ''beautiful.'' ''The discovery that he might portray a woman convincingly but that he could never turn himself into a pretty one was shattering,'' observes Bennetts. ''The next step was outrage over how he was treated by men.'' And Travers reports that if the film ''deepened Hoffman's regard for women, it lowered his estimation of his own sex. . . . 'It hit me when I realized I wouldn't take myself out or go to bed with me.''' The character, which ''was born out of [Hoffman's] frustrations,'' says Travers, was a ''powerful personal experience,'' observes Bennetts, and plunged ''him into an intensive self-examination that has changed him in many ways.''

''Hoffman began to build a local reputation as a wild-eyed perfectionist unafraid to walk the gangplank of any role—he seemed to harbor an insatiable need to reach out and scrape his knuckles against his limits in order to convince himself that they hadn't closed around his throat,'' states Gary Smith (*Rolling Stone,* February 3, 1983), who finds that ''there is, nonetheless, a deepened humanness that Hoffman is discovering. 'He has seen that change is the only thing that is absolute, that is immortal,' says Marvin Belsky, a close friend. 'That is why the kind of roles he takes will keep changing dramatically, and why there must be so much arc within those roles.'''

OTHER SOURCES: New York Times, December 16, 1979, December 21, 1982; *New York Times Magazine,* March 18, 1984; *People,* January 17, 1983, May 25, 1987; *Rolling Stone,* February 3, 1983;

Saturday Review, January/February, 1986; *Time,* December 3, 1979.

ADDRESSES: OFFICE—Punch Productions, 75 Rockefeller Plaza, New York, NY 10019.*

*   *   *

HOGAN, Paul   1942-

PERSONAL: Born in 1942 in Lightning Ridge, New South Wales, Australia; wife's name, Noelene; children: Loren, Scott, Clay, Todd, Brett.

VOCATION: Actor, producer, and screenwriter.

CAREER: Also see *WRITINGS* below. FILM DEBUT—Title role, *"Crocodile" Dundee,* Paramount, 1986. PRINCIPAL FILM APPEARANCES—Title role, *"Crocodile" Dundee II,* Paramount, 1988. PRINCIPAL FILM WORK—Executive producer, *"Crocodile" Dundee II,* Paramount, 1988.

TELEVISION DEBUT—Contestant, *New Faces,* Australian television. PRINCIPAL TELEVISION APPEARANCES—Series: Host, *The Paul Hogan Show,* syndicated, 1981; commentator, *A Current Affair,* Australian television. Movies: Pat Cleary, *Anzacs: The War Down Under,* syndicated, 1987. Specials: Co-host, *The Fifty-Ninth Annual Academy Awards Presentation,* ABC, 1987; *Australia Live: Celebration of a Nation,* Nine Network (Australia), 1988; *The Barbara Walters Special,* ABC, 1988. PRINCIPAL TELEVISION WORK—Producer, *The Paul Hogan Show,* syndicated, 1981.

RELATED CAREER—Founder (with John Cornell), JP Productions, 1972—; appeared in and (with John Cornell) contributed to scripts of television commercials for the Australian Tourist Commission, Foster's beer, and Winfield cigarettes (in Australia).

NON-RELATED CAREER—Bridge rigger, prizefighter, salesman, and construction worker.

WRITINGS: See above for production details. FILM—(With Ken Shade and John Cornell) *"Crocodile" Dundee,* Paramount, 1986; (with Brett Hogan) *"Crocodile" Dundee II,* Paramount, 1988. TELEVISION—*The Paul Hogan Show,* syndicated, 1981.

AWARDS: Golden Globe Award, Best Actor in a Comedy or Musical, and Academy Award nomination, Best Screenplay, both 1987, for *"Crocodile" Dundee.**

*   *   *

HOLBROOK, Hal   1925-

PERSONAL: Full name, Harold Rowe Holbrook, Jr.; born February 17, 1925, in Cleveland, OH; son of Harold Rowe, Sr. and Aileen (a vaudeville dancer; maiden name, Davenport) Holbrook; married Ruby Elaine Johnston, September 22, 1945 (divorced); married Carol Rossen (an actress), December 28, 1966 (divorced); married Dixie Carter (an actress), 1984; children: Victoria, David (first marriage); Eve (second marriage). EDUCATION: Denison University, B.A. 1948; trained for the stage with Uta Hagen at the

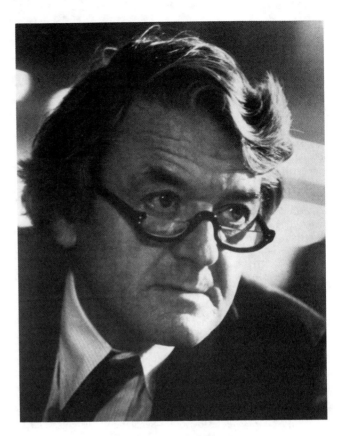

HAL HOLBROOK

the Herbert Berghof Studios, 1953. MILITARY: U.S. Army, Corps of Engineers, private, 1943-46.

VOCATION: Actor.

CAREER: STAGE DEBUT—Richard, *The Man Who Came to Dinner,* Cain Park Theatre, Cleveland, OH, 1942. OFF-BROADWAY DEBUT—Title role, *Mark Twain Tonight!* (one-man show), 41st Street Theatre, 1959. BROADWAY DEBUT—Young man, *Do You Know the Milky Way?,* Billy Rose Theatre, 1961. PRINCIPAL STAGE APPEARANCES—Title role, *Mark Twain Tonight!* (one-man show), Lock Haven State Teachers College, Lock Haven, PA, 1954; *Mark Twain Tonight!* (one-man show), Purple Onion, San Francisco, CA, then Upstairs at the Duplex, New York City, both 1955; John of Gaunt, *Richard II,* and Hotspur, *Henry IV, Part I,* both American Shakespeare Festival, Stratford, CT, 1962; title role, *Abe Lincoln in Illinois,* Phoenix Theatre Company, Anderson Theatre, New York City, 1963; Reverend Harley Barnes, then Quentin, *After the Fall,* major, *Incident at Vichy,* and Marco Polo, *Marco Millions,* all Repertory Theatre of Lincoln Center, American National Theatre and Academy (ANTA) Washington Square Theatre, New York City, 1964; M. Loyal and prologue, *Tartuffe,* Repertory Theatre of Lincoln Center, ANTA Washington Square Theatre, 1965; Jim O'Connor, *The Glass Menagerie,* Brooks Atkinson Theatre, New York City, 1965; title role, *Mark Twain Tonight!* (one-man show), Longacre Theatre, New York City, 1966; Adam, Captain Sanjar, and Prince Charming, *The Apple Tree,* Shubert Theatre, New York City, 1966; Gene Garrison, *I Never Sang for My Father,* Longacre Theatre, 1968; Cervantes and Don Quixote, *Man of La Mancha,* Martin Beck Theatre, New York

City, 1968; Mr. Winters, *Does a Tiger Wear a Necktie?*, Belasco Theatre, New York City, 1969.

Winnebago, *Lake of the Woods*, American Place Theatre, New York City, 1971; title role, *Mark Twain Tonight!* (one-man show), Ford's Theatre, Washington, DC, 1972; title role, *Mark Twain Tonight!* (one-man show), Imperial Theatre, New York City, 1977, then Theatre Three, Dallas, TX, 1981; Jake K. Bowsky, *Buried Inside Extra*, New York Shakespeare Festival, Public Theatre, New York City, then in London, both 1983; Frank Elgin, *The Country Girl*, Chelsea Playhouse, New York City, 1984. Also appeared in *The Vagabond King* and *In Time to Come*, both Cain Park Theatre, Cleveland, OH, 1942; *Three Men on a Horse*, *The Male Animal*, *George Washington Slept Here*, *Our Town*, *The Guardsman*, and *The Constant Wife*, all Denison University, Granville, OH, 1947-50; and in *The Doctor in Spite of Himself*, Westport Country Playhouse, Westport, CT, 1958.

PRINCIPAL STAGE WORK—Director, *The Winslow Boy*, Denison University, Granville, OH.

MAJOR TOURS—Title role, *Mark Twain Tonight!* (one-man show), U.S. cities, 1954-59, then U.S., European, and Saudi Arabian cities, 1959-61, later U.S. cities, 1962 and 1963; Andrew Mackerel, *The Mackerel Plaza*, U.S. cities, 1963; King Arthur, *Camelot*, U.S. cities, 1969; title role, *Mark Twain Tonight!* (one-man show), U.S. cities, 1975-77; also appeared (with Ruby Johnston) in scenes from classic plays, U.S. cities, 1948-53.

FILM DEBUT—Gus Leroy, *The Group*, United Artists, 1966. PRINCIPAL FILM APPEARANCES—Senator John Fergus, *Wild in the Streets*, American International, 1968; Cameron, *The Great White Hope*, Twentieth Century-Fox, 1970; David Hoffman, *The People Next Door*, AVCO-Embassy, 1970; Dr. Watkins, *They Only Kill Their Masters*, Metro-Goldwyn-Mayer, 1972; voice of Elder, *Jonathan Livingston Seagull*, Paramount, 1973; Lieutenant Briggs, *Magnum Force*, Warner Brothers, 1973; Joe, *The Girl from Petrovka*, Universal, 1974; Deep Throat, *All the President's Men*, Warner Brothers, 1976; Commander Joseph J. Rochefort, Jr., *Midway* (also known as *The Battle of Midway*), Universal, 1976; Alan Campbell, *Julia*, Twentieth Century-Fox, 1977; Dr. James Kelloway, *Capricorn One*, Warner Brothers, 1978; Paul Steward, *Natural Enemies*, Cinema V, 1979; Father Malone, *The Fog*, AVCO-Embassy, 1980; President Adam Scott, *The Kidnapping of the President*, Crown International, 1980; Harry, *Rituals* (also known as *The Creeper*), Coast, 1980; Henry Northrup, "The Crate" in *Creepshow*, Warner Brothers, 1982; Benjamin Caulfield, *The Star Chamber*, Twentieth Century-Fox, 1983; Lou Mannheim, *Wall Street*, Twentieth Century-Fox, 1987; Archbishop Mosely, *The Unholy*, Vestron, 1988; Ham Johnson, *Fletch Lives*, Universal, 1989. Also appeared in *Girls Night Out* (also known as *The Scaremaker*), Aries, 1984; and *Final Clue*.

TELEVISION DEBUT—Grayling Dennis, *Hollywood Screen Test*, ABC, 1953. PRINCIPAL TELEVISION APPEARANCES— Series: Grayling Dennis, *The Brighter Day*, CBS, 1954-59; Senator Hayes Stowe, *The Senator*, NBC, 1970-71; host, *Portrait of America*, WTBS (Atlanta, GA), 1983-88. Mini-Series: Abraham Lincoln, *Sandburg's Lincoln*, NBC, 1974-76; Portius Wheeler, *The Awakening Land*, NBC, 1978; District Attorney Calvin Sledge, *Celebrity*, NBC, 1984; John Adams, *George Washington*, CBS, 1984; Abraham Lincoln, *North and South*, ABC, 1985; Abraham Lincoln, *North and South, Book II*, ABC, 1986; Jonas Coe, *Emma: Queen of the South Seas*, syndicated, 1988; Dr. Andrew McKaig, *Mario Puzo's Fortunate Pilgrim*, NBC, 1988. Pilots: Jonathan

Murray, "The Cliff Dwellers," *Preview Tonight*, ABC, 1966; Chancellor Graham, *The Whole World Is Watching*, NBC, 1969; Matthew Sand, *Travis Logan, D.A.*, CBS, 1971; Hays Stowe, *A Clear and Present Danger*, NBC, 1970; Dr. Simon Abbott, *The Oath: 33 Hours in the Life of God*, ABC, 1976; John Hammer/ J.R. Swackhamer, *The Legend of the Golden Gun*, NBC, 1979; Colonel Calvin Turner, *Behind Enemy Lines*, NBC, 1985.

Episodic: Mark Twain, *The Tonight Show*, NBC, 1956; Mark Twain, *The Ed Sullivan Show*, CBS, 1956; Mark Twain, *The Sound of Laughter*, NBC, 1958; Abraham Lincoln, *Exploring*, NBC, 1963; Abraham Lincoln in scenes from "Abe Lincoln in Illinois," *The Ed Sullivan Show*, CBS, 1963; Reese Watson, *Designing Women* (recurring role), CBS, 1986—; also *I Remember Mama*, CBS, 1958; *The New Love, American Style*, ABC, 1985; *Coronet Blue*, CBS; *The F.B.I.*, ABC. Movies: Harlan Webb, *Goodbye Raggedy Ann*, CBS, 1971; Larry Hackett, *Suddenly Single*, ABC, 1971; Doug Salter, *That Certain Summer*, ABC, 1972; Jeremiah Denton, Jr., *When Hell Was in Session*, NBC, 1979; Arthur Sinclair, *Murder by Natural Causes*, CBS, 1979; Budd Johansen, *Off the Minnesota Strip*, ABC, 1980; John Webster, *The Killing of Randy Webster*, CBS, 1981; Grandpa, *The Three Wishes of Billy Grier*, ABC, 1984; President Maxwell Monroe, *Under Siege*, NBC, 1986; General Charles Hedges, *Dress Gray*, NBC, 1986; Sam Nash, "Act I," *Plaza Suite*, ABC, 1987; Joseph Bundy, *I'll Be Home for Christmas* (also known as *A Rockport Christmas*), NBC, 1988; General George C. Marshall, *Day One*, CBS, 1989.

Specials: Tom Wingfield, *The Glass Menagerie*, CBS, 1966; title role, *Mark Twain Tonight!* (one-man show), CBS, 1967; Commander Lloyd M. Boucher, "Pueblo," *ABC Theatre*, ABC, 1974; host, "Cyrano de Bergerac," "Enemies," "June Moon," "King Lear," "Monkey, Monkey Bottle of Beer, How Many Monkeys Have We Here?" "A Touch of the Poet," and "The Widowing of Mrs. Holroyd," all *Great Performances: Theatre in America*, PBS, 1974; host, "Brother to Dragons," "Forget-Me-Not-Lane," "Rules of the Game," "The School for Scandal," "The Seagull," "Who's Happy Now?," "The Year of the Dragon," and "Zalmen, or the Madness of God," all *Great Performances: Theatre in America*, PBS, 1975; host, "The Time of Your Life," "All Over," "Beyond the Horizon," "The Christmas Chester Mystery Plays," "Eccentricities of a Nightingale," "The First Breeze of Summer," "The Mound Builders," "The Patriots," and "Sea Marks," all *Great Performances: Theatre in America*, PBS, 1976; narrator, *The Animals Nobody Loved*, PBS, 1976; Stage Manager, *Our Town*, NBC, 1977; host, "The Prince of Homburg," *Great Performances*, PBS, 1977; narrator, *Willa Cather's America*, PBS, 1978; host, *Omnibus*, ABC, 1980 and 1981; narrator, "Four Americans in China," *National Geographic Special*, PBS, 1985; *All Star Party for Clint Eastwood*, CBS, 1986; narrator, *Adolph Hitler: Portrait of a Tyrant*, HBO, 1987; *Superman's Fiftieth Anniversary: A Celebration of the Man of Steel*, CBS, 1988; *The Kennedy Center Honors: A Celebration of the Performing Arts*, CBS, 1988; host and narrator, *An American Image*, syndicated, 1989.

PRINCIPAL TELEVISION WORK—Episodic: Director, *Designing Women*, CBS, 1988 and 1989.

RELATED CAREER—Appeared in *Army Engineer Show*, ABC, 1946, and other Army Special Services radio programs; singer, 1956-58.

WRITINGS: STAGE—*Mark Twain Tonight!* (one-man show), first performed in 1954.

AWARDS: Vernon Rice Award, Obie Award from the *Village Voice,* and Outer Critics Circle Award, all 1959, for *Mark Twain Tonight!;* New York Drama Critics Circle special citation and Antoinette Perry Award, Best Actor (Dramatic), both 1966, for *Mark Twain Tonight!;* Emmy Award nomination, 1970, for *A Clear and Present Danger;* Emmy Award, Outstanding Continued Performance by an Actor in a Leading Role in a Dramatic Series, 1971, for *The Senator;* Emmy Award nomination, Outstanding Actor, 1972, for *That Certain Summer;* Torch of Liberty Award from the Anti-Defamation League of B'nai B'rith, 1972; Emmy Awards, Outstanding Lead Actor in a Special, and Actor of the Year in a Special, both 1974, for "Pueblo," *ABC Theatre;* Emmy Award, Outstanding Lead Actor in a Limited Series, 1976, for *Sandburg's Lincoln;* Emmy Award nomination, Outstanding Lead Actor in a Drama or Comedy Special, 1977, for *Our Town;* Emmy Award nomination, Outstanding Lead Actor in a Limited Series, 1978, for *The Awakening Land;* ACE (Annual Cable Excellence) Award, Best Informational or Documentary Host, 1988, for *Portrait of America.* Honorary degrees: Kenyon College, doctor of arts, 1979; Denison University, doctor of arts, 1979; Ohio State University, doctor of humane letters, 1979.

MEMBER: Actors' Equity Association, American Federation of Television and Radio Artists, Screen Actors Guild, Commission on International Cultural Exchange, National Council on Arts and Government, International Platform Association, Mark Twain Memorial Association, Players Club, Lambs Club.

ADDRESSES: AGENT—William Morris Agency, 151 El Camino Boulevard, Beverly Hills, CA 90212.*

*   *   *

HOLLIDAY, Polly   1937-

PERSONAL: Full name, Polly Dean Holliday; born July 2, 1937, in Jasper, AL; daughter of Ernest Sullivan (a truck driver) and Velma Mabell (Cain) Holliday. EDUCATION: Alabama State Women's College, B. Mus Ed., 1959; postgraduate work at Florida State University, 1960.

VOCATION: Actress.

CAREER: OFF-BROADWAY DEBUT—*Orphee,* 1964. BROADWAY DEBUT—Philomena Hopkins, *All Over Town,* Booth Theatre, 1974. PRINCIPAL STAGE APPEARANCES—Bananas Shaughnessy, *The House of Blue Leaves,* Asolo Theatre Festival, Sarasota, FL, 1971; Annabelle, *Wedding Band,* New York Shakespeare Festival, Public Theatre, New York City, 1972; Dolly, *The Red Blue-Grass Western Flyer Show,* New Dramatists, New York City, 1972; Lee, *The Girls Most Likely to Succeed,* Playwrights Horizons, New York City, 1973; Jean Manning, *A Sense of Humor,* Center Theatre Group, Ahmanson Theatre, Los Angeles, CA, 1983; Julie Cavendish, *The Royal Family,* GeVa Theatre, Rochester, NY, 1985; Martha Brewster, *Arsenic and Old Lace,* 46th Street Theatre, New York City, 1986. Also appeared in *Major Barbara* and *As You Like It,* both Asolo Theatre Festival, 1967; *Servant of Two Masters* and *Look Back in Anger,* both Asolo Theatre Festival, 1968; *Joe Egg,* Asolo Theatre Festival, 1970; *Candida* and *The Subject Was Roses,* both Asolo Theatre Festival, 1971; *Black Coffee,* GeVa Theatre, 1985; *Dinner on the Ground,* New York City; and with the Asolo State Theatre, Sarasota, FL, 1962-73.

MAJOR TOURS—Jean Manning, *A Sense of Humor,* U.S. cities, 1983.

PRINCIPAL FILM APPEARANCES—Miss Pearson, *The Catamount Killings,* Hallmark, 1975; secretary, *All the President's Men,* Warner Brothers, 1976; Mrs. Crawford, *The One and Only,* Paramount, 1978; Mrs. Deagle, *Gremlins,* Warner Brothers, 1984; Midge, *Moon over Parador,* Universal, 1988.

PRINCIPAL TELEVISION APPEARANCES—Series: Florence Jean "Flo" Castleberry, *Alice,* CBS, 1976-80; Flo Castleberry, *Flo,* CBS, 1980-81; Captain Betty, *Stir Crazy,* CBS, 1985-86. Mini-Series: Bertie Bartolotti, "Konrad," *Wonderworks,* PBS, 1985. Pilots: Flo Castleberry, *Alice,* CBS, 1976. Episodic: Mrs. Harvey, "Bernice Bobs Her Hair," *American Short Story,* PBS, 1977; Major Amanda Allen, *Private Benjamin,* CBS, 1983. Movies: Mrs. Watson, *The Silence,* NBC, 1975; Mary Gertrude, *Missing Children: A Mother's Story,* CBS, 1982; Aunt Min, *The Gift of Love: A Christmas Story,* CBS, 1983; Lucille, *Lots of Luck,* Disney Channel, 1985. Specials: Mrs. Lucas, "Eliza," *Our Story,* PBS, 1975; Mrs. Cronkite, "Luke Was There," *Special Treat,* NBC, 1976; Mrs. Kirby, *You Can't Take It with You,* CBS, 1979; Aunt Hannah, *All the Way Home,* NBC, 1981; Mrs. Wooster, "The Shady Hill Kidnapping," *American Playhouse,* PBS, 1981.

NON-RELATED CAREER—Music teacher, public school system, Sarasota, FL, 1961.

AWARDS: Golden Globe Award, Best Supporting Actress on a Television Series, 1978 and 1979, and five Emmy Award nominations, all for *Alice;* honorary degrees: D.H.L. from Mount St. Mary's College, 1982.

ADDRESSES: AGENT—The Lantz Office, 9255 Sunset Boulevard, Suite 505, Los Angeles, CA 90069.*

*   *   *

HOOPER, Tobe

PERSONAL: Born in Texas.

VOCATION: Director, producer, and screenwriter.

CAREER: Also see *WRITINGS* below. PRINCIPAL FILM APPEARANCES—*The Windsplitter,* Pop Films, 1971; *The Texas Chainsaw Massacre, Part II,* Cannon, 1986. FIRST FILM WORK—Director, *Eggshells.* PRINCIPAL FILM WORK—Director: (Also producer) *The Texas Chainsaw Massacre,* Bryanston, 1974; *Eaten Alive* (also known as *Death Trap, Starlight Slaughter, Horror Hotel Massacre,* and *Legend of the Bayou*), Virgo International, 1976; *The Funhouse,* Universal, 1981; *Poltergeist,* Metro-Goldwyn-Mayer/ United Artists, 1982; *Lifeforce,* Tri-Star, 1985; *Invaders from Mars,* Cannon, 1986; (also producer and model maker) *The Texas Chainsaw Massacre, Part II,* Cannon, 1986.

PRINCIPAL TELEVISION WORK—All as director. Episodic: *Amazing Stories,* NBC, 1987; *The Equalizer,* CBS, 1988. Movies: *Salem's Lot,* CBS, 1979.

RELATED CAREER—Documentary and industrial filmmaker; director of television commercials; former assistant director, University of Texas film program.

WRITINGS: FILM—Screenplay (With Kim Henkel) and music (with Wayne Bell), *The Texas Chainsaw Massacre,* Bryanston, 1974; music (with Jerry Lambert), *The Texas Chainsaw Massacre, Part II,* Cannon, 1986.

ADDRESSES: AGENT—Audrey Caan, Triad Artists, 10100 Santa Monica Boulevard, Los Angeles, CA 90067.*

*   *   *

HOTCHKIS, Joan   1927-

PERSONAL: Born September 21, 1927, in Los Angeles, CA; daughter of Preston (in the insurance and investment business) and Katharine (Bixby) Hotchkis; married Robert Foster (a film director and writer), June, 1958 (divorced, 1966); children: Paula Lee. EDUCATION: Smith College, B.A., 1949; Bank Street College of Education, M.S., 1952; studied acting with Lee Strasberg, Sanford Meisner, Kristen Linklater, Eric Morris and dialects with Robert Easton.

VOCATION: Actress and writer.

CAREER: STAGE DEBUT—Lizzie, *The Rainmaker,* Players Ring Theatre, Hollywood, CA, 1954, for six months. BROADWAY DEBUT—Liz, *Advise and Consent,* Cort Theatre, 1960, for seven months. PRINCIPAL STAGE APPEARANCES—Stella, *A Streetcar Named Desire,* Northland Theatre, Detroit, MI, 1956; understudy for Julie, *Write Me a Murder,* Belasco Theatre, New York City, 1961; Lois Lane, *Superman,* Walnut Street Theatre, Philadelphia, PA, 1962; Jackie, *O Boy,* Goodspeed Opera House, East Haddam, CT, 1964; Fluffy Mother, *Cowboy Jack Street,* Taper Too Theatre, Los Angeles, CA, 1976; Amanda Wingfield, *The Glass Menagerie,* Callboard Theatre, Los Angeles, 1981, then James Polk Theatre, Nashville, TN, 1982; Madame Irma, *The Balcony,* Odyssey Theatre Ensemble, Santa Monica, CA, 1983; Paulina, *The Winter's Tale,* Judith Bliss, *Hay Fever,* and Lady Gay Spanker, *London Assurance,* all Oregon Shakespearean Festival, Ashland, OR, 1984; Isabella, Louise, and Mrs. Kidd, *Top Girls,* and Mrs. Sutphen, *A Woman without Means,* both Milwaukee Repertory Theatre, Milwaukee, WI, 1985; Amanda Wingfield, *The Glass Menagerie,* Playhouse in the Park, Cincinnati, OH, 1985; Amanda Wingfield, *The Glass Menagerie,* and Lydia Ptitsyna, *Sarcophagus,* both Los Angeles Theatre Center, Los Angeles, 1987; Mrs. Temptwell, *The Grace of Mary Traverse,* Los Angeles Theatre Works, Los Angeles, 1988. Also appeared in *O Lady Lady,* Goodspeed Opera House, 1963; and in more than twenty summer theatre productions.

PRINCIPAL FILM APPEARANCES—Sally Pearson, *The Late Liz,* Gateway, 1971; Paula Harmon, *Breezy,* Universal, 1973; Bissie Hapgood, *Legacy,* Kino, 1976; Mama Hartley, *Ode to Billy Joe,* Warner Brothers, 1976; Pamela Shaw, *Old Boyfriends,* AVCO-Embassy, 1979.

PRINCIPAL TELEVISION APPEARANCES—Series: Ellen Monroe, *My World and Welcome to It,* NBC, 1969-70; Dr. Nancy Cunningham, *The Odd Couple,* ABC, 1970-72; Lydia Knitzer, *The Life and Times of Eddie Roberts,* syndicated, 1980; also *L.A.T.E.R.* Pilots: Iris Michaels, *The 416th,* CBS, 1979; Cissie Vanderplas, "Meet the Munceys," *Disney Sunday Movie,* NBC, 1988. Episodic: *St. Elsewhere,* NBC; *Lou Grant,* CBS; *Charlie's Angels,* ABC; *General Hospital,* ABC; *The F.B.I.,* ABC; *The Dick Van Dyke Show,* CBS; *Bewitched,* ABC; *Mannix,* CBS; *Medical Center,* CBS; *Marcus Welby, M.D.,* ABC; *Barnaby Jones,* CBS; *Owen Marshall, Counselor at Law,* ABC. Also appeared in *Once a Daughter.*

RELATED CAREER—Member, Actors Studio, New York City.

WRITINGS: STAGE—*Legacy,* Actors Studio West, Los Angeles, CA, 1974. FILM—*Legacy,* Kino, 1976. OTHER—(With Eric Morris) *No Acting Please* (acting manual), 1979.

AWARDS: Odyssey Theatre Award, 1983, for *The Balcony; Los Angeles Weekly* Award nomination, Best Ensemble Acting, 1988, for *The Grace of Mary Traverse;* Independent Filmmakers Grant from the American Film Institute for *Legacy.*

MEMBER: Dramatists Guild, American Civil Liberties Union, National Organization for Women, California Abortion Rights Action League, National Abortion Rights Action League, National Women's Political Caucus, Nature Conservancy, California Historical Society.

ADDRESSES: OFFICE—201 Ocean Avenue, Apartment 509-P, Santa Monica, CA 90402. AGENTS—Bret Adams, Ltd., 448 W. 44th Street, New York, NY 10036; Henderson/Hogan Agency, 247 S. Beverly Drive, Suite 102, Beverly Hills, CA 90212.

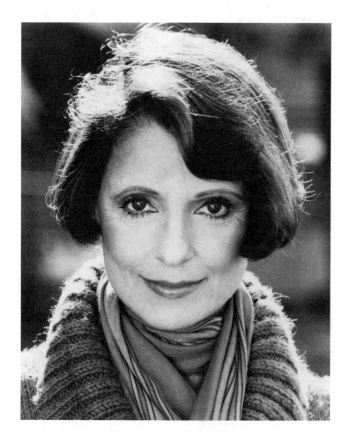

JOAN HOTCHKIS

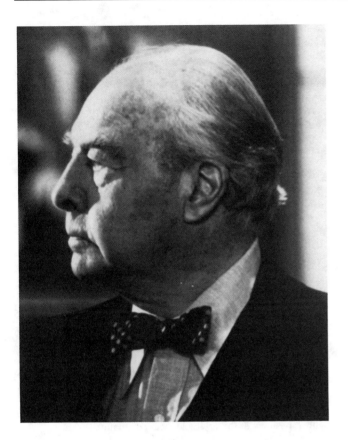

JOHN HOUSEMAN

HOUSEMAN, John   1902-1988

OBITUARY NOTICE: See index for *CTFT* sketch. Born Jacques Haussmann, September 22, 1902, in Bucharest, Rumania; died of spinal cancer, October 31, 1988, in Malibu, CA. Although he spent most of his career as an innovative stage and screen producer and director, John Houseman first attracted the attention of mass audiences as Professor Kingsfield, the imperious law school instructor in the 1973 film *The Paper Chase.* With his haughty demeanor and a voice described by Harry Haun in the [New York] *Daily News* as ''a measured, thought-filled, erudite rumble,'' Houseman's portrayal earned him an Academy Award as Best Supporting Actor. Through subsequent film and television appearances, he gained even greater recognition, especially with a series of popular television commercials in which he promoted a brokerage house by claiming, ''They make money the old fashioned way. They *earn* it.''

Prior to his success as an actor, Houseman was widely regarded as one of the most influential and respected innovators of the American stage. His theatrical affiliations included the Mercury Theatre, which he co-founded with Orson Welles in 1937; the American Shakespeare Festival, of which he was artistic director between 1956-59; the Professional Theatre Group of the University of California, Los Angeles, which later became part of the Mark Taper Forum; and the Acting Company, a New York City-based repertory group whose members have included Kevin Kline, Patti LuPone, and William Hurt. The John Houseman Theatre was established in 1986 as a permanent home for the Acting Company. His association with Welles produced such noteworthy events in American culture as a 1935 production of *Macbeth* set in Haiti with an all-black cast,

the staging of the proletarian musical *The Cradle Will Rock* that was closed by the police in 1936, and the radio broadcast of *The War of the Worlds* that panicked audiences who believed it was real. Their partnership ended in a disagreement over script credits for the film *Citizen Kane.* As a movie producer, Houseman was responsible for such films as *The Blue Dahlia,* 1946, *Letter from an Unknown Woman,* 1948, *They Live by Night,* 1949, *Julius Caesar,* 1953, and *Lust for Life,* 1956. His final acting credits included roles in Woody Allen's *Another Woman, Bright Lights, Big City,* and *Scrooged,* all released in 1988.

OBITUARIES AND OTHER SOURCES: [New York] *Daily News,* November 1, 1988; *New York Times,* November 1, 1988; *Variety,* November 2, 1988.*

*   *   *

HOWARD, Clint   1959-

PERSONAL: Born April 20, 1959, in Burbank, CA; son of Rance (an actor and writer) and Jean (Speegle) Howard.

VOCATION: Actor.

CAREER: PRINCIPAL FILM APPEARANCES—Jo-Hi, *An Eye for an Eye,* Embassy, 1966; Mark Wedloe, *Gentle Giant,* Paramount, 1967; voice of an elephant, *The Jungle Book* (animated), Buena Vista, 1967; Andrew Tanner, *The Wild Country* (also known as *The Newcomers*), Buena Vista, 1971; Tim, *Salty,* Saltwater, 1975; Georgie, *Eat My Dust!,* New World, 1976; Ace, *Grand Theft Auto,* New World, 1977; Corley, *Harper Valley P.T.A.,* April Fools, 1978; Eaglebauer, *Rock 'n' Roll High School,* New World, 1979; Coopersmith, *Evilspeak,* Moreno, 1982; Jefferey, *Night Shift,* Warner Brothers, 1982; wedding guest, *Splash,* Buena Vista, 1984; John Dexter, *Cocoon,* Twentieth Century-Fox, 1985; Paul, *Gung Ho,* Paramount, 1986; Rughead, *The Wraith,* New Century/Vista, 1986; Les Sullivan, *End of the Line,* Orion Classics, 1987; Ronnie, *Freeway,* New World, 1988.

TELEVISION DEBUT—Leon, *The Andy Griffith Show,* CBS, 1962. PRINCIPAL TELEVISION APPEARANCES—Series: Stanley, *The Baileys of Balboa,* CBS, 1964-65; Mark Wedloe, *Gentle Ben,* CBS, 1967-69; Steve, *The Cowboys,* ABC, 1974; Googie, *Gung Ho,* ABC, 1986-87. Episodic: Leon, ''The Bank Job'' and ''One Ranch Opie,'' *The Andy Griffith Show,* CBS, 1962; Leon, ''A Black Day for Mayberry'' and ''The Shoplifters,'' *The Andy Griffith Show,* CBS, 1964; Baalok, ''The Corbomite Maneuver,'' *Star Trek,* NBC, 1966; Randy Granger, *The Odd Couple,* ABC, 1970; also ''The Boy Who Predicted Earthquakes,'' *Rod Serling's Night Gallery,* NBC, 1971. Movies: Jody Tifflin, *The Red Pony,* NBC, 1973; Arch, *Huckleberry Finn,* ABC, 1975; Peanuts, *The Death of Richie,* NBC, 1977; Corky MacFearson, *Cotton Candy,* NBC, 1978; also *Skyward,* NBC, 1980. Specials: Voice of Roo, *Winnie the Pooh and the Honey Tree* (animated), NBC, 1970.

WRITINGS: TELEVISION—Movies: (With Ron Howard) *Cotton Candy,* NBC, 1978.*

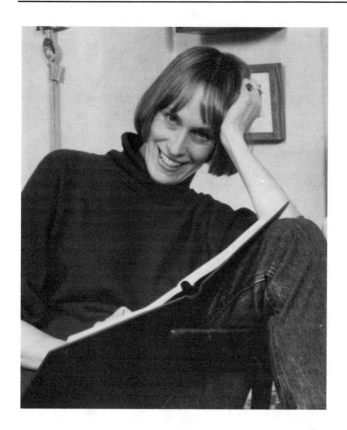

Photography by J.P. Laffont/Sygma

TINA HOWE

HOWE, Tina   1937-

PERSONAL: Born November 21, 1937, in New York, NY; daughter of Quincy (a broadcaster and writer) and Mary (an artist; maiden name, Post) Howe; married Norman Levy (a writer), 1961; children: Eben, Dara. EDUCATION: Sarah Lawrence College, B.A., 1959; graduate work, Chicago Teachers College, 1963-64, and Columbia University.

VOCATION: Playwright.

CAREER: See *WRITINGS* below. RELATED CAREER—Adjunct professor in playwriting, New York University, 1983—; also high school English teacher in Bath, ME; Chicago, IL; and Madison, WI.

WRITINGS: STAGE—*Closing Time,* Sarah Lawrence College, Bronxville, NY, 1959; *The Nest,* Act IV Theatre, Provincetown, MA, 1969, then Mercury Theatre, New York City, 1970; *Museum,* Los Angeles Actors Theatre, Los Angeles, CA, 1976, then New York Shakespeare Festival (NYSF), Public Theatre, New York City, 1977, published by Samuel French, Inc., 1979, and in *Three Plays,* Avon, 1984; *The Art of Dining,* NYSF, Public Theatre, 1979, then Kennedy Center for the Performing Arts, Washington, DC, 1980, published by Samuel French, Inc., 1980, and in *Three Plays,* 1984; *Appearances,* Ensemble Studio Theatre, New York City, 1982; *Painting Churches,* Second Stage, then Lamb's Theatre, both New York City, 1983, published in *Three Plays,* 1984; *Coastal Disturbances,* Second Stage, 1986, then Circle in the Square, New York City, 1987, published by Samuel French, Inc., 1987, and in *Coastal Disturbances: Four Plays by Tina Howe,* Theatre Communications Group, 1989; *Approaching Zanzibar,*

Second Stage, 1989. Also *Birth and After Birth,* published in *The New Women's Theatre,* Vintage Books, 1977.

AWARDS: Rosamond Gilder Award, 1983; Obie Award from the *Village Voice,* Distinguished Playwriting, 1983; Outer Critics Circle awards, 1983 and 1984; John Gassner Award, 1984; Antoinette Perry Award nomination, Best Play, 1987, for *Coastal Disturbances;* also Rockefeller grant, 1983; National Endowment for the Arts grant, 1984. Honorary degrees: Bowdoin College, Doctor of Letters, 1988.

SIDELIGHTS: Tina Howe told *CTFT:* "I feel passionate about giving credit to the courageous off-Broadway theatres that produce new work. If it weren't for them, new voices would never be discovered."

ADDRESSES: AGENT—Flora Roberts, Inc., 157 W. 57th Street, New York, NY 10019.

*   *   *

HUBER, Kathleen   1947-

PERSONAL: Born March 3, 1947, in New York, NY; daughter of Henry Hans (a photographer) and Mary Catherine (a speech therapist; maiden name, Wehe) Huber. EDUCATION: University of California, Santa Barbara, B.A., drama, 1968; trained for the stage with John Ingle at the Idyllwild Arts Foundation.

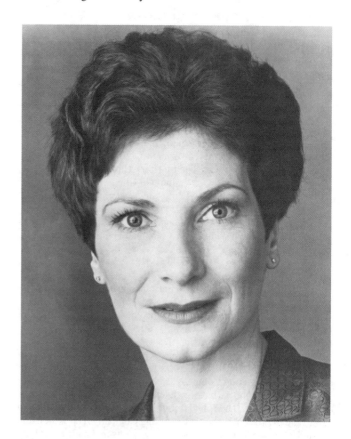

KATHLEEN HUBER

VOCATION: Actress and writer.

CAREER: Also see *WRITINGS* below. STAGE DEBUT—Louison, *The Imaginary Invalid,* California State College, Los Angeles, 1957, for four performances. OFF-BROADWAY DEBUT—Zoe, *A Scent of Flowers,* Martinique Theatre, 1969. PRINCIPAL STAGE APPEARANCES—Mrs. Sullen, *The Beaux' Stratagem,* Pasadena Playhouse, Pasadena, CA, 1968; Volumnia, *Coriolanus,* Jean Cocteau Theatre, New York City, 1972; Hannah Adler, *Throne of Straw,* St. Clement's Church Theatre, New York City, 1978; Barbara Fawcett, *The Constant Wife,* Equity Library Theatre, New York City, 1986; Mavis Kelly, *The Tronzini Ristorante Murders,* Meat and Potatoes Company, Alvina Kraus Theatre, New York City, 1987; Luisa Baccara and Aelis Mazoyer, *Tamara,* Park Avenue Armory, New York City, 1988. Also appeared in *The Virgin and the Unicorn.*

FILM DEBUT—Kathleen, *The Molders of Troy,* Bowling Green, 1978.

WRITINGS: STAGE—*A Song for Tomorrow,* Santa Barbara Children's Opera, Santa Barbara, CA, 1969; *Two on the Isles,* Edinburgh Festival Fringe, Edinburgh, Scotland, 1979, revised as *Song of the Sea* New Shandol Theatre, New York City, 1981; *The Hallowed Halls,* Sargent Theatre, New York City, 1983; *Dark Wings,* Sargent Theatre, 1985; *Conquistador Aisle,* Sargent Theatre, 1988. OTHER—Short stories published in *Prize Stories from "Seventeen,"* Macmillan, 1968; also contributor of short stories to *Seventeen, Homes and Gardens, Highlights for Children, Jack and Jill, Young World,* and *Child Life.*

RELATED CAREER—Partner (with Jerome Martin) in a repertory duet performing in and directing plays aboard cruise ships, 1974-75; founder, Actors' Holiday Theatre Company, 1981—.

MEMBER: Dramatists Guild.

SIDELIGHTS: FAVORITE ROLES—Luisa Baccara in *Tamara,* Phoebe Merryl in *The Yeomen of the Guard,* Nettie Cleary in *The Subject Was Roses,* and Gertrude Rhead in *Milestones.*

ADDRESSES: OFFICE—P.O. Box 367, Gracie Station, New York, NY 10028.

*   *   *

HUDDLESTON, David   1930-

PERSONAL: Born September 17, 1930, in Vinton, VA; son of Lewis Melvin and Ismay Hope (Dooley) Huddleston; children: David Michael. EDUCATION: Trained for the stage at the American Academy of Dramatic Arts, 1957. MILITARY: U.S. Air Force, 1950-54.

VOCATION: Actor, producer, and songwriter.

CAREER: PRINCIPAL STAGE APPEARANCES—Soldier, *Harry, Noon, and Night,* Pocket Theatre, New York City, 1965; Boscombe, *Woman Is My Idea,* Belasco Theatre, New York City, 1968; Denver Cody, *The Roast,* Winter Garden Theatre, New York City, 1980; Branch Rickey, *The First,* Martin Beck Theatre, New York City, 1981; Byrne, *Big Maggie,* Douglas Fairbanks Theatre, New York City, 1983; Charley, *Death of a Salesman,* Broadhurst Theatre,

New York City, 1984. Also appeared with the Center Stage, Baltimore, MD, 1968-69; and in productions of *A Man for All Seasons, The Front Page, Ten Little Indians, Silk Stockings, Fanny,* and *Guys and Dolls.*

MAJOR TOURS—Charlie Cowell, *The Music Man,* U.S. cities, 1961-62; Mr. Upson, *Mame,* U.S. cities, 1968; also in *A Funny Thing Happened on the Way to the Forum,* U.S. cities, 1963-64.

PRINCIPAL FILM APPEARANCES—Holland, *Slaves,* Continental, 1969; Uncle Lonnie, *Norwood,* Paramount, 1970; Dr. Jones, *Rio Lobo,* National General, 1970; heavy man, *WUSA,* Paramount, 1970; Homer Grindstaff, *Fools' Parade* (also known as *Dynamite Man from Glory Jail*), Columbia, 1971; Malachi Morton, *Something Big,* National General, 1971; Big Joe, *Bad Company,* Paramount, 1972; Mr. Carroll, *Nightmare Honeymoon* (also known as *Deadly Honeymoon*), Metro-Goldwyn-Mayer, 1972; Copeland, *Billy Two Hats* (also known as *The Lady and the Outlaw*), United Artists, 1973; Olson Johnson, *Blazing Saddles,* Warner Brothers, 1974; Mayor Hardy, *The Klansman,* Paramount, 1974; Edward M. "Pinky" Farrow, *McQ,* Warner Brothers, 1974; Dr. Edward Molyneux, *Breakheart Pass,* United Artists, 1976; barber, *The World's Greatest Lover,* Twentieth Century-Fox, 1977; Cruikshank, *The Greatest,* Columbia, 1977; Hollis Peaker, *Capricorn One,* Warner Brothers, 1978; Captain McBride, *Due superpiedi quasi piatti* (also known as *Crime Busters*), Columbia/Warner Brothers, 1979; Walrus Wallman, *Gorp,* Filmways, 1980; John Conn, *Smokey and the Bandit II* (also known as *Smokey and the Bandit Ride Again*), Universal, 1980; Corky, *The Act* (also known as *Bless 'em All*), Film Ventures, 1984; title role, *Santa Claus: The Movie,* Tri-Star, 1985; Peter, *Frantic,* Warner Brothers, 1988. Also appeared in *Country Blue,* General Film, 1975.

PRINCIPAL TELEVISION APPEARANCES—Series: Lieutenant Sam Church, *Tenafly,* NBC, 1973-74; Lieutenant John Ponce, *Petrocelli,* NBC, 1974-76; Jasper T. Kallikak, *The Kallikaks,* NBC, 1977; Christy Judson, *How the West Was Won,* ABC, 1977; Mayor Michael Cooper, *Hizzoner,* NBC, 1979. Mini-Series: Earl Preis, *Once an Eagle,* NBC, 1976-77. Pilots: Sheriff Bridges, *The Homecoming—A Christmas Story,* CBS, 1971; Harrison Davis, *The Priest Killer,* NBC, 1971; Tyler, *Sarge: The Badge or the Cross,* NBC, 1971; Jack Dawson, *Brock's Last Case,* NBC, 1973; Lieutenant Sam Church, *Tenafly,* NBC, 1973; Joseph Harrelson, *Hawkins on Murder,* CBS, 1973; Mr. Ross, *The Gun and the Pulpit,* ABC, 1974; Painted Face Kelly, *Oregon Trail,* NBC, 1976; Hiram Yerby, *Winner Take All,* CBS, 1977; Chief Sorrenson, *Computercide,* NBC, 1982.

Episodic: District Attorney Harrelson, *Hawkins,* CBS, 1974; Frank Petersen, *Magnum P.I.,* CBS, 1985; Edgar Sheridan, *Blacke's Magic,* CBS, 1986; J.J. Moon, *Our House,* NBC, 1986 and 1987; Charlie Bullets, *J.J. Starbuck,* NBC, 1987. Movies: Ed McCaskey, *Brian's Song,* ABC, 1971; Bennie, *Suddenly Single,* ABC, 1971; Arnold Brady, *Heatwave!,* ABC, 1974; Bearde, *Shark Kill,* NBC, 1976; Inspector Lafferty, *Sherlock Holmes in New York,* NBC, 1976; sheriff, *Kate Bliss and the Ticker Tape Kid,* ABC, 1978; Senator Chester Winfield, *Family Reunion,* NBC, 1981; J.D. Hines, *The Oklahoma City Dolls,* ABC, 1981; Steve Blankenship, *M.A.D.D.: Mothers Against Drunk Drivers,* NBC, 1983; Jack Archer, *Finnegan Begin Again,* HBO, 1985; Reverend August McCaffrey, *When the Bough Breaks,* NBC, 1986; Marshall Lane Crawford, *The Tracker,* HBO, 1988; Bemis, *Margaret Bourke-White,* TNT, 1989; also *Spot Marks the X,* Disney Channel, 1986. Specials: *Plimpton! Showdown at Rio Lobo,* ABC, 1970; *Super*

Comedy Bowl II, CBS, 1972; Edgar Watson, "Amy and the Angel," *ABC Afterschool Special,* ABC, 1982.

PRINCIPAL TELEVISION WORK—Series: Creator and executive producer (with Sheldon Keller), *Hizzoner,* NBC, 1979. Episodic: Director, *Our House,* NBC, 1988.

RELATED CAREER—President and owner: Shama Productions Inc., the Huddleston Company, and Huddleston Music Company.

WRITINGS: Songwriter, "Home Town Blues," 1978; also wrote theme songs for various television series.

MEMBER: Screen Actors Guild, American Federation of Television and Radio Artists, Actors' Equity Association, Players Club, California Yacht Club.*

* * *

HUFFMAN, Felicity

PERSONAL: Daughter of Moore Peters (a banker) and Grace Valle (an actress; maiden name, Ewing) Huffman. EDUCATION: Received B.F.A. from New York University.

VOCATION: Actress.

CAREER: STAGE DEBUT—Joe, *A Taste of Honey,* Stage Theatre, New York City, 1982, for twenty performances. BROADWAY

DEBUT—Karen, *Speed-the-Plow,* Royale Theatre, 1988. PRINCIPAL STAGE APPEARANCES—Jill, *Been Taken,* 18th Street Playhouse, New York City, 1986; Maggie, *Boys' Life,* Mitzi E. Newhouse Theatre, New York City, 1988.

FILM DEBUT—Wheel of fortune girl, *Things Change,* Columbia, 1988.

TELEVISION DEBUT—Pam, "A Home Run for Love," *After School Special,* 1978. PRINCIPAL TELEVISION APPEARANCES—Specials: "Lip Service," *HBO Showcase,* HBO, 1988.

RELATED CAREER—Founding member, Atlantic Theatre Company.

ADDRESSES: AGENT—c/o Richard Shmenner, STE Representation, 888 Seventh Avenue, New York, 10019.

* * *

HUGHES, Barnard   1915-

PERSONAL: First name is pronounced "Bar-nid"; born July 16, 1915, in Bedford Hills, NY; son of Owen and Madge (Kiernan) Hughes; married Helen Stenborg (an actress), April 19, 1950; children: Douglas, Laura. EDUCATION: Attended Manhattan College. MILITARY: U.S. Army.

VOCATION: Actor.

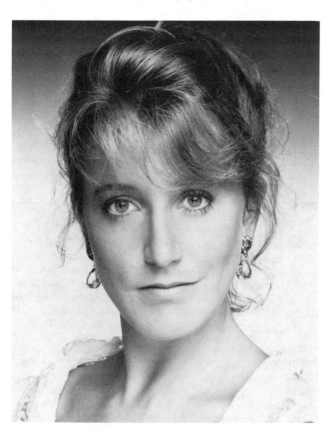

FELICITY HUFFMAN

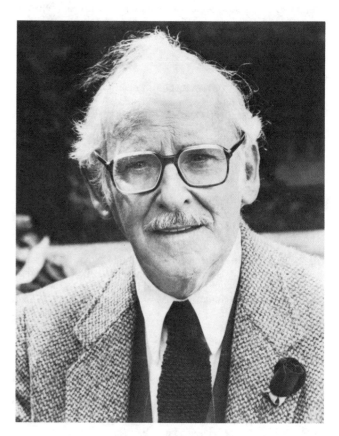

BARNARD HUGHES

CAREER: STAGE DEBUT—Haberdasher, *The Taming of the Shrew,* Shakespeare Fellowship Company, New York City, 1934. BROADWAY DEBUT—*The Cat and the Canary,* Majestic Theatre, 1937. PRINCIPAL STAGE APPEARANCES—Joe, *Please, Mrs. Garibaldi,* Belmont Theatre, New York City, 1939; Martin, *The Ivy Green,* Lyceum Theatre, New York City, 1949; Clancy, *Dinosaur Wharf,* National Theatre, New York City, 1951; Captain McLean, *The Teahouse of the August Moon,* City Center Theatre, New York City, 1956; Major Joppolo, *A Bell for Adano,* and T.J., *Home of the Brave,* both Equity Library Theatre, Lennox Hall Playhouse, New York City, 1957; Lantry, *The Will and the Way,* Theatre East, New York City, 1957; Dr. Genoni, *Enrico IV,* Erlanger Theatre, Philadelphia, PA, 1958; Inspector Norcross, *A Majority of One,* Shubert Theatre, New York City, 1959; Senator Tom August, *Advise and Consent,* Cort Theatre, New York City, 1960; Peter Mortensgaard, *Rosmersholm,* Fourth Street Theatre, New York City, 1962; Nils Krogstad, *A Doll's House,* Theatre Four, New York City, 1963; the Governor, *The Advocate,* American National Theatre and Academy Theatre, New York City, 1963; Bert Howell, *Nobody Loves an Albatross,* Lyceum Theatre, 1963; Marcellus and priest, *Hamlet,* Lunt-Fontanne Theatre, New York City, 1964; Father Frank Feeley, *I Was Dancing,* Lyceum Theatre, 1964; Jim Bolton, *Generation,* Morosco Theatre, New York City, 1965; Father Stanislas Coyne, *Hogan's Goat,* American Place Theatre, New York City, 1965; Senator McFetridge, *How Now, Dow Jones,* Lunt-Fontanne Theatre, 1967; Judge Belknap, *The Wrong-Way Light Bulb,* John Golden Theatre, New York City, 1969.

General Fitzhugh, *Sheep on the Runway,* Helen Hayes Theatre, New York City, 1970; Arnall, *Line,* Theatre De Lys, New York City, 1971; Fulbert, *Abelard and Heloise,* Brooks Atkinson Theatre, New York City, 1971; various roles, *Older People,* New York Shakespeare Festival (NYSF), Public Theatre, New York City, 1972; Polonius, *Hamlet,* NYSF, Delacorte Theatre, New York City, 1972; Dogberry, *Much Ado about Nothing,* NYSF, Delacorte Theatre, then Winter Garden Theatre, New York City, both 1972; Alexander Serebryakov, *Uncle Vanya,* Circle in the Square/Joseph E. Levine Theatre, New York City, 1973; the Voice (recorded), *Edgar Allan Poe,* Alice Tully Hall, New York City, 1973; various roles, *The Good Doctor,* Eugene O'Neill Theatre, New York City, 1973; Sir John Falstaff, *The Merry Wives of Windsor,* and Gower, *Pericles, Prince of Tyre,* both NYSF, Delacorte Theatre, 1974; Dr. Lionel Morris, *All Over Town,* Booth Theatre, New York City, 1974; voice of newspaper (recorded), *Edgar Allan Poe: A Condition of Shadow with Jerry Rockwood,* URGENT Theatre, New York City, 1975; Tchebutykin, *The Three Sisters,* Brooklyn Academy of Music Playhouse, Brooklyn, NY, 1977; Reverend Anthony Anderson, *The Devil's Disciple,* Center Theatre Group, Ahmanson Theatre, Los Angeles, CA, 1977, then Brooklyn Academy of Music Opera House, Brooklyn, NY, 1978; title role, *Da,* Hudson Guild Theatre, New York City, then Morosco Theatre, both 1978.

Hugh, *Translations,* Manhattan Theatre Club, New York City, 1981; Orgon, *Tartuffe,* Kennedy Center for the Performing Arts, Washington, DC, 1982; Father William Doherty, *Angels Fall,* Circle Repertory Theatre, New York City, 1982, then Longacre Theatre, New York City, 1983; Philip Stone, *End of the World,* Music Box Theatre, New York City, 1984; Harry Hope, *The Iceman Cometh,* Lunt-Fontanne Theatre, 1985. Also appeared in *Herself, Mrs. Patrick Crowley,* Wilmington, DE, 1939; *Homeward Bound,* 1980; *The Sky Is No Limit,* 1984; with the Tenthouse Theatre, Highland Park, IL; Shelton-Amos Players, Richmond, VA; Palm Springs Playhouse, Palm Spring, CA; and companies in Surrey, ME, and Middletown, NY.

MAJOR TOURS—Captain McLean, *The Teahouse of the August Moon,* U.S. cities, 1954-56; Jim Bolton, *Generation,* U.S. cities, 1966; title role, *Da,* U.S. cities, 1979-80.

PRINCIPAL FILM APPEARANCES—Dr. Kent O'Donnell, *The Young Doctors,* United Artists, 1961; Marcellus, *Hamlet,* Warner Brothers, 1964; Towny, *Midnight Cowboy,* United Artists, 1969; Colonel Hendriks, *Where's Poppa?* (also known as *Going Ape*), United Artists, 1970; Dr. Proctor, *Cold Turkey,* United Artists, 1971; Drummond, *The Hospital,* United Artists, 1971; Judge Vogel, *The Pursuit of Happiness,* Columbia, 1971; Dr. Spencer, *Rage,* Warner Brothers, 1972; Mr. McLennen, *Sisters* (also known as *Blood Sisters*), American International, 1973; Judge Baker, *Oh, God!,* Warner Brothers, 1977; Chief Justice Crawford, *First Monday in October,* Paramount, 1981; Tim McCullen, *Best Friends,* Warner Brothers, 1982; old man, *Deadhead Miles,* filmed in 1970, released by Paramount, 1982; Dr. Walter Gibbs and Dumont, *Tron,* Buena Vista, 1982; Bishop Campbell, *Maxie,* Orion, 1985; Jonathan Knowles, *Where Are the Children?,* Columbia, 1986; Grandpa, *The Lost Boys,* Warner Brothers, 1987; title role, *Da,* FilmDallas, 1988.

TELEVISION DEBUT—Bob Cratchit, *A Christmas Carol,* 1946. PRINCIPAL TELEVISION APPEARANCES—Series: "Doc" Joe Bogert, *Doc,* CBS, 1975-76; title role, *Mr. Merlin,* CBS, 1981-82; Francis "Pop" Cavanaugh, *The Cavanaughs,* CBS, 1986-87; also Dr. Bruce Banning, *The Guiding Light,* CBS. Pilots: Mr. Rhenquist, *The Thanksgiving Treasure,* CBS, 1973; Marion Weston, *Another April,* CBS, 1974; "Doc" Joe Bogert, *Doc,* CBS, 1975; Jess Halliday, *Ransom for Alice!,* NBC, 1977; Andy Borchard, *The World Beyond,* CBS, 1978; Father John Brown, *Sanctuary of Fear* (also known as *Girl in the Park*), NBC, 1979; Gordon Hackles, *Tales from the Darkside,* syndicated, 1983. Episodic: Priest, *All in the Family,* CBS, 1971-73; Herb Hartley, *The Bob Newhart Show,* CBS, 1974-78; judge, *Lou Grant,* CBS, 1977; the King, "The Adventures of Huckleberry Finn," *American Playhouse,* PBS, 1986; Lester Simmons, *The Days and Nights of Molly Dodd,* NBC, 1988; also *Robert Montgomery Presents,* NBC; *Hawkins Falls, Pop. 6,200,* NBC; *Hollywood Screen Test,* ABC; *The Defenders,* CBS; *Naked City,* ABC; *Kraft Theatre,* NBC; *Car 54, Where Are You?,* NBC; *U.S. Steel Hour,* ABC; *Nova,* PBS; *Armstrong Circle Theatre,* NBC; *The Nurses,* CBS; *Dupont Show of the Week,* CBS.

Movies: Dr. Helm, *The Borgia Stick,* NBC, 1967; Elias Hart, *Dr. Cook's Garden,* ABC, 1971; Dr. Benjamin Simon, *The UFO Incident,* NBC, 1975; Philip J. Madden, *Guilty or Innocent: The Sam Sheppard Murder Case,* NBC, 1975; Judge Fricke, *Kill Me if You Can,* NBC, 1977; Uncle Tyler, *Tell Me My Name,* CBS, 1977; John Matusak, *See How She Runs,* CBS, 1978; Harry Seaton, *Homeward Bound,* CBS, 1980; Justice John Francis Carew, *Little Gloria . . . Happy at Last,* NBC, 1982; Mr. Rafiel, *Agatha Christie's "A Caribbean Mystery,"* CBS, 1983; Arthur Bennett, *The Sky's No Limit,* CBS, 1984; Chance Carson, *A Hobo's Christmas,* CBS, 1987; Abner Ableson, *Night of Courage,* ABC, 1987; Colonel Henry L. Stimson, *Day One,* CBS, 1989; CIA Director William Casey, *Guts and Glory: The Rise and Fall of Oliver North* (also known as *The Rise and Fall of Oliver North*), CBS, 1989. Specials: Mr. Wallace, *The Million Dollar Incident,* CBS, 1961; Secretary of the Navy, "Pueblo," *ABC Theatre,* ABC, 1973; Mr. Crampfurl, "The Borrowers," *Hallmark Hall of Fame,* NBC, 1973; Jim, "A Memory of Two Mondays," *Great Performances,* PBS, 1974; "The 75th," *The Booth,* PBS, 1985; *The Magic of David Copperfield,* CBS, 1981; Jake Tibbits, "Home Fires Burning," *Hallmark Hall of Fame,* CBS, 1989; also *Much Ado about Nothing* and *Look Homeward Angel.*

RELATED CAREER—Member, Circle Repertory Theatre.

NON-RELATED CAREER—Wall Street runner.

AWARDS: Antoinette Perry Award nomination, Best Supporting or Featured Actor, 1973, for *Much Ado about Nothing;* St. Clair Bayfield Award, 1973; Antoinette Perry Award, Drama Desk Award, and Outer Critics Circle Award, all Best Actor in a Play, 1978, for *Da;* Emmy Award, Outstanding Lead Actor for a Single Appearance in a Drama or Comedy Series, 1978, for *Lou Grant;* Theatre Father of the Year Award from the Eire Society of Boston, 1983.

MEMBER: Actors' Equity Association, Screen Actors Guild, American Federation of Television and Radio Artists, Players Club.

SIDELIGHTS: FAVORITE ROLES—Dogberry in *Much Ado about Nothing,* Polonius in *Hamlet,* Serebryakov in *Uncle Vanya,* and Da.

ADDRESSES: AGENT—Milton Goldman, International Creative Management, 40 W. 57th Street, New York, NY 10019.*

*   *   *

HUGHES, Wendy

PERSONAL: Born in Australia.

VOCATION: Actress.

CAREER: PRINCIPAL FILM APPEARANCES—Patricia Kent, *Petersen* (also known as *Jock Petersen*), AVCO-Embassy, 1974; Lynn Carson, *Sidecar Racers,* Universal, 1975; Barbie, *High Rolling* (also known as *High Rolling in a Hot Corvette*), Hexagon Roadshow, 1977; Amy McKenzie, *Newsfront,* Roadshow, 1979; Cathy, *Kostas,* Kostas Film Productions/Victorian Film Corporation, 1979; Eva Gilmour, *Touch and Go,* Great Union, 1980; Aunt Helen, *My Brilliant Career,* New South Wales, 1980; Lucy, *Hoodwink,* New South Wales, 1981; Sophie, *A Dangerous Summer* (also known as *A Burning Man*), Virgin Vision, 1981; Barbara Dunstan, *Duet for Four* (also known as *Partners*), Burstall Releasing, 1982; Patricia Curnov, *Lonely Hearts,* Samuel Goldwyn, 1983; Vanessa Scott, *Careful, He Might Hear You,* TLC/Twentieth Century-Fox, 1984; Honour Langtry, *An Indecent Obsession,* PBL, 1985; Margaret, *I Can't Get Started,* David Evans Enterprises, 1985; Helen, *My First Wife,* Spectrafilm, 1985; Carolyn Benedict, *Happy New Year,* Columbia, 1987; Maria McEvory, *Shadows of the Peacock* (also known as *Promises to Keep*), Laughing Kookaburra/Australian European Finance Corporation, 1987; art teacher, *Warm Nights on a Slow Moving Train,* Filmpac Holdings, 1987; Stella Marsden, *Boundaries of the Heart,* International Film Management, 1988; Maria, *Echoes of Paradise,* Quartet, 1989. Also appeared in *The Spiral Bureau.*

PRINCIPAL FILM WORK—Associate producer, *Boundaries of the Heart,* International Film Management, 1988.

PRINCIPAL TELEVISION APPEARANCES—Mini-Series: Jilly Stewart, *Return to Eden,* syndicated, 1984; Marion, *Amerika* (also known as *Topeka, Kansas . . . U.S.S.R.*), ABC, 1987. Also appeared in *The Alternative, Power without Glory, Lucinda Brayford,*

Coralie Lansdown Says No, Women of the House, and *The Company of Men,* all for Australian television.

AWARDS: Australian Film Institute Award, Best Actress, 1984, for *Careful, He Might Hear You;* Penguin Award, Best Actress in a Television Drama, for *The Alternative;* Australian Film and Television Award, Best Actress, and Logie Award, Best Actress in a Supporting Role, both for *Power without Glory.*

ADDRESSES: AGENT—Ed Limato, William Morris Agency, 151 El Camino Drive, Beverly Hills, CA 90212.*

*   *   *

HUPPERT, Isabelle   1955-

PERSONAL: Full name, Isabelle Anne Huppert; born March 16, 1955, in Paris, France; daughter of Raymond and Annick Beau Huppert. EDUCATION: Attended Versailles Conservatory and Faculte de Clichy; studied acting at the Conservatoire National d'Art Dramatique.

VOCATION: Actress.

CAREER: STAGE DEBUT—*Viendra-t-il un autre ete?,* 1973.

FILM DEBUT—*Faustine et le bel ete,* 1971. PRINCIPAL FILM APPEARANCES—Marite, *Cesar and Rosalie,* Orion/Cinema V, 1972; Annie, *Le Bar de la fourche* (also known as *The Bar at the Crossing*), Societe Nouvelle de Cinema, 1972; woman, *L'Ampelopede,* Nanou Film, 1973; Jacqueline, *Les Valseuses* (also known as *Going Places*), Cinema V, 1974; Brigitte, *Dupont lajoie* (also known as *The Common Man*), Planfilm/Sirius, 1974; Yvette, *Le Petit Marcel* (also known as *Little Marcel*), Gaumont International, 1975; maid, *Le Grand delire* (also known as *The Big Delirium*), Lugo Films, 1975; Helene, *Rosebud,* United Artists, 1975; sister, *Je suis Pierre Riviere* (also known as *I Am Pierre Riviere*), UZ Diffusion, 1975; title role, *Aloise,* Framo Diffusion, 1976; Pomme, *La Dentelliere* (also known as *The Lacemaker*), Janus, 1977; Jenny Kern, *Les indiens sont encore loin* (also known as *The Indians Are Still Far Away*), Films 2001/Filmkollektiv Zurich, 1977; Elisabeth Gailland, *Docteur Francoise Gailland* (also known as *No Time for Breakfast*), Daniel Bourla, 1978; title role, *Violette Noziere* (also known as *Violette*), New Yorker, 1978; Jeanne, *Retour a la bien-aimee* (also known as *Return to the Beloved*), Societe Nouvelle Prodis/World Marketing, 1978; Anne Bronte, *Les Soeurs Bronte* (also known as *The Bronte Sisters*), Gaumont, 1979; Rose, *Le Juge et l'assassin* (also known as *The Judge and the Assassin*), Libra, 1979.

Isabelle Aiviere, *Sauve que peut la vie* (also known as *Every Man for Himself* and *Slow Motion*), New Yorker, 1980; Ella Watson, *Heaven's Gate,* United Artists, 1980; Nelly, *Loulou,* New Yorker, 1980; Rose Mercaillou, *Coup de torchon,* (also known as *Clean Slate*), Parafrance, 1981; Frederique, *La Truite* (also known as *The Trout*), Triumph, 1982; Piera as an adult, *Storia di Piera* (also known as *Story of Piera*), CIDFFilmexport ᴳroup, 1982; Lena, *Entre nous* (also known as *Coup de foudre*), Metro-Goldwyn-Mayer/United Artists, 1983; Isabelle, *Passion* (also known as *Passion, travail et amour*), United Artists Classics, 1983; Viviane Arthaud, *La Femme de mon pote* (also known as *My Best Friend's Girl*), European International, 1984; Rose Marie, *Sac du noeuds* (also known as *All Mixed Up*), Columbia-Warner Distributors/

World Marketing, 1985; title role, *Signe Charlotte* (also known as *Sincerely Charlotte* and *Signed Charlotte*), New Line Cinema, 1986; Colo, *Cactus,* International Spectrafilm, 1986; Sylvia Wentworth, *The Bedroom Window,* De Laurentiis Entertainment Group, 1987; Maria Shatov, *Les Possedes* (also known as *The Possessed*), Gaumont, 1988; Sarah, *Milan Noir,* Capital Cinema-World Marketing, 1988; Marie, *Une Affaire de femmes* (also known as *Women's Affair* and *Women's Business*), Marin Karmitz, 1988.

Also appeared in *Glissements progressifs du plaisir* (also known as *Successive Slidings of Pleasure*), Fox-Lira, 1973; *Serieux comme le plaisir* (also known as *Serious Is as Pleasure*), Lugo Films, 1974; *Des Enfants gates* (also known as *Spoiled Children*), Roissy-Gaumont International, 1977; *La Garce,* Sara Films, 1984; *Flash Back,* 1975; *Orokseg* (also known as *Les Heritieres* and *The Heiresses*), 1980; *La vera storia della signora delle camelie* (also known as *The Story of Camille* and *Dame aux camelias*), 1981; *Les Ailes de la colombe,* 1981; *Eaux profondes* (also known as *Deep Water*), 1981.

TELEVISION DEBUT—*Proust.*

AWARDS: Prix Susanne Blanchetti and Prix Bistingo, both 1976; British Academy Award, Most Promising Newcomer, 1977, for *La Dentelliere;* Best Actress Award from the Cannes International Film Festival, 1978, for *Violette Noziere;* Prix Cesar, Golden Palm Award, and Prix d'interpretation, all from the Cannes International Film Festival, 1978.

ADDRESSES: OFFICE—c/o Art Media, 10 Avenue George V, 75008 Paris, France.*

*   *   *

HUSSEY, Olivia   1951-

PERSONAL: Born Olivia Osuna, April 17, 1951, in Buenos Aires, Argentina; daughter of Andreas (an opera singer) and Joy Alma (Hussey) Osuna; married Dean Paul Martin (an actor; divorced); married Akira Fuse (a composer; divorced); children: Alexander (first marriage); one son (second marriage). EDUCATION: Studied acting at the Italia Conti Stage School.

VOCATION: Actress.

CAREER: PRINCIPAL STAGE APPEARANCES—*The Prime of Miss Jean Brodie,* London production.

FILM DEBUT—Donna, *The Battle of the Villa Fiorita* (also known as *Affair at the Villa Fiorita*), Warner Brothers, 1965. PRINCIPAL FILM APPEARANCES—Juliet, *Romeo and Juliet,* Paramount, 1968; Val, *All the Right Noises,* Twentieth Century-Fox, 1973; Maria, *Lost Horizon,* Columbia, 1973; Tonia Alfredi, *Summertime Killer,* AVCO-Embassy, 1973; Jess, *Black Christmas,* Ambassador, 1974; Rosalie Otter-Bourne, *Death on the Nile,* Paramount, 1978; Cicily Young, *The Cat and the Canary,* Cinema Shares, 1979; Elsa Borsht, *The Man with Bogart's Face* (also known as *Sam Marlow, Private Eye*), Twentieth Century-Fox, 1980; Marit, *Virus* (also known as *Fukkatsu Nohi*), Media, 1980; Chris Walters, *Escape 2000* (also known as *Turkey Shoot*), New World, 1983; Amy,

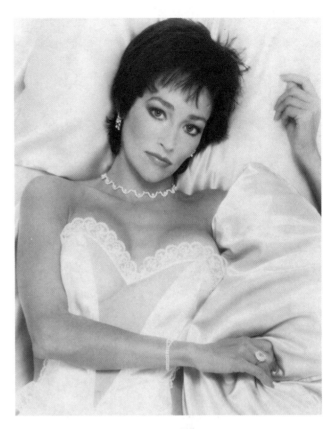

OLIVIA HUSSEY

Distortions, Cori, 1987. Also appeared in *Cup Fever,* CFF, 1965; *The Jeweler's Shop,* 1989; and *Good Friday.*

PRINCIPAL TELEVISION APPEARANCES—Mini-Series: Virgin Mary, *Jesus of Nazareth,* NBC, 1977; Ione, *The Last Days of Pompeii,* ABC, 1984. Pilots: Title role, *The Thirteenth Day: The Story of Esther,* ABC, 1979. Episodic: Kitty Trumbull, *Murder, She Wrote,* CBS, 1986. Movies: Alicia, *The Bastard* (also known as *Kent Family Chronicles*), syndicated, 1978; Leila, *Harold Robbins' "The Pirate,"* CBS, 1978; Rebecca, *Ivanhoe,* CBS, 1982; Annamaria de Guidice, *The Corsican Brothers,* CBS, 1985. Specials: Judge, *Miss Hollywood, 1986,* CBS, 1986.

RELATED CAREER—Appeared in television commercials in Japan.

NON-RELATED CAREER—Photographer.

WRITINGS: Lyricist for nine songs published in Japan.

AWARDS: David DiDonatello Awards, Most Promising Actress and Best Actress, New York Film Critics Award, and Golden Globe Award, both Best Actress, all for *Romeo and Juliet.*

ADDRESSES: OFFICE—10350 Santa Monica Boulevard, Suite 200, Los Angeles, CA 90025. AGENT—Agency for the Performing Arts, 9000 Sunset Boulevard, Suite 1200, Los Angeles, CA 90069. MANAGER—Kendal Kaldwell Concepts Management, 8605 Santa Monica Boulevard, Suite 276, Los Angeles, CA 90069.

IRONS, Jeremy 1948-

PERSONAL: Full name, Jeremy John Irons; born September 19, 1948, in Cowes, England; son of Paul Dugan and Barbara Anne (Sharpe) Irons; married Sinead Moira Cusack (an actress; professional name, Sinead Cusack), March 28, 1978; children: Samuel James, Maximilian Paul. EDUCATION: Trained for the stage at the Bristol Old Vic Theatre School.

VOCATION: Actor.

CAREER: BROADWAY DEBUT—Henry Boot, *The Real Thing,* Plymouth Theatre, 1984. PRINCIPAL STAGE APPEARANCES—Simon, *Hay Fever,* Nick, *What the Butler Saw,* and Florizel, *The Winter's Tale,* all Bristol Old Vic Theatre, Bristol, U.K., 1971; John the Baptist, *Godspell,* Round House Theatre, London, 1972, then Wyndham's Theatre, London, 1973; Don Pedro, *Much Ado*

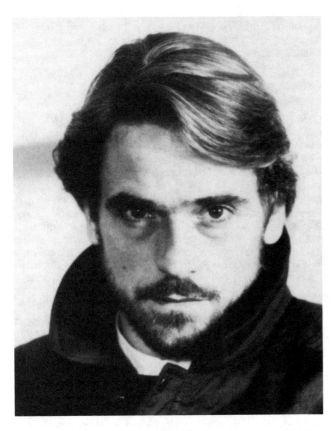

JEREMY IRONS

about Nothing, and Mick, *The Caretaker,* both Young Vic Theatre, London, 1974; Petruchio, *The Taming of the Shrew,* New Shakespeare Company, Round House Theatre, 1975; Harry Thunder, *Wild Oats,* Royal Shakespeare Company (RSC), Aldwych Theatre, London, 1976, then Piccadilly Theatre, London, 1977; James Jameson, *The Rear Column,* Globe Theatre, London, 1978; Gustav Manet, *An Audience Called Edouard,* Greenwich Theatre, London, 1978. Also appeared in *Diary of a Madman,* Act Inn Lunchtime Theatre, London, 1973; *An Inspector Calls,* Key Theatre, Peterborough, U.K., 1975; *The Rover,* Mermaid Theatre, London, 1987; as Leontes, *The Winter's Tale,* and in *Richard II,* both RSC, Royal Shakespeare Theatre, Stratford-on-Avon, U.K.

FILM DEBUT—Mikhail Fokine, *Nijinsky,* Paramount, 1980. PRINCIPAL FILM APPEARANCES—Charles Smithson/Mike, *The French Lieutenant's Woman,* United Artists, 1981; Nowak, *Moonlighting,* Universal, 1982; Jerry, *Betrayal,* Twentieth Century-Fox, 1983; Harold Ackland, *The Wild Duck,* Orion, 1983; Charles Swann, *Swann in Love* (also known as *Un Amour de Swann*), Orion, 1984; Father Gabriel, *The Mission,* Warner Brothers, 1986; Beverly and Elliot Mantle, *Dead Ringers,* Twentieth Century-Fox, 1988.

PRINCIPAL TELEVISION APPEARANCES—Mini-Series: Franz Liszt, *Notorious Woman,* BBC, then *Masterpiece Theatre,* PBS, 1975; Frank Tregear, *The Pallisers,* PBS, 1977; Charles Ryder, *Brideshead Revisited,* Granada, 1980-81, then *Great Performances,* PBS, 1982; also Alex Sanderson, *Love for Lydia,* London Weekend Television, then *Masterpiece Theatre,* PBS. Episodic: *The Talk Show,* HBO, 1986. Movies: William Smith, *Danny, The Champion of the World,* Disney Channel, 1989. Specials: Voice, *Statue of Liberty,* PBS, 1985; *The Bugs Bunny/Looney Tunes Fiftieth Anniversary Special,* CBS, 1986; *Sesame Street Special,* PBS, 1988. Also appeared as Alex Hepburn, *The Captain's Doll,* BBC, 1982; Otto Beck, *Langrishe Go Down,* BBC; Edward Voysey, *The Voysey Inheritance,* BBC.

AWARDS: Clarence Derwent Award from British Actors' Equity Association, Best Actor, 1978, for *The Rear Column;* Variety Artists of Great Britain Award and British Academy of Film and Television Arts Award nomination, both Best Actor, 1981, for *The French Lieutenant's Woman;* Antoinette Perry Award, Best Actor in a Play, and Drama League Distinguished Performance Award, both 1984, for *The Real Thing;* New York Film Critics Circle Award and Genie Award, both Best Actor, 1988, for *Dead Ringers;* also British Academy of Film and Television Arts Award nomination, Golden Globe nomination, and Emmy Award nomination, all for *Brideshead Revisited.*

ADDRESSES: AGENTS—Creative Artists Agency, 1888 Century Park E., 14th Floor, Los Angeles, CA 90067; Hutton Management, 200 Fulham Road, London SW10 9PN, England.

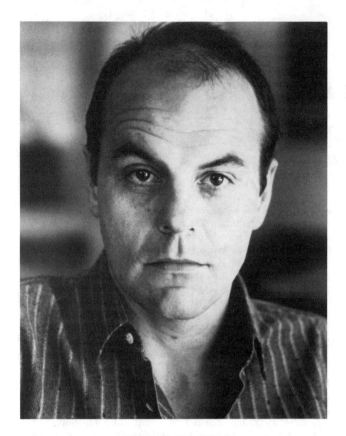

MICHAEL IRONSIDE

IRONSIDE, Michael   1950-

PERSONAL: Born February 12, 1950, in Toronto, ON, Canada; son of Robert Walter and Patricia June (Passmore) Ironside; wife's name, Karen Virginia (an actress); children: Adrienne Katrina. EDUCATION: Graduated from the Ontario College of Art.

VOCATION: Actor.

CAREER: PRINCIPAL FILM APPEARANCES—Drunk, *Outrageous!,* Almi Cinema V, 1977; Dr. Paul Johnson, *I, Maureen,* New Cinema, 1978; Butch, *High Ballin',* American International, 1978; Jimmy, *Suzanne,* Ambassador, 1980; Darryl Revok, *Scanners,* AVCO-Embassy, 1981; Wayne, *Surfacing,* Pan-Canadian Film Distributors, 1981; Colt Hawker, *Visiting Hours* (also known as *The Fright* and *Get Well Soon*), Twentieth Century-Fox, 1982; Detective Sergeant Ed Roersch, *Cross Country,* Metro-Goldwyn-Mayer/United Artists, 1983; Overdog McNabb, *Spacehunter: Adventures in the Forbidden Zone* (also known as *Road Gangs* and *Adventures in the Creep Zone*), Columbia, 1983; Skylar, *American Nightmare,* Mano, 1984; George Kiber, *The Surrogate,* Cinepix, 1984; dealer, *Best Revenge,* RKR Releasing, 1984; FBI agent, *The Falcon and the Snowman,* Orion, 1985; Detective Lawrence, *Jo Jo Dancer, Your Life Is Calling,* Columbia, 1986; Dick Wetherly ("Jester"), *Top Gun,* Paramount, 1986; Major Paul Hackett, *Extreme Prejudice,* Tri-Star, 1987; Ben, *Nowhere to Hide,* New Century-Vista, 1987; Principal Bill Nordham, *Hello Mary Lou: Prom Night II* (also known as *The Haunting of Hamilton High*), Norstar, 1987; Lem Johnston, *Watchers,* Caralco, 1988; Larry Gaylord, *Office Party,* SC Films, 1988; Kendrick, *Destiny to*

Order, Atlantis, 1988; Rick Fender, *Deadly Surveillance,* Shapiro Glickenhaus, 1988; Kellen O'Reilly, *Mindfield,* Allegro, 1988.

PRINCIPAL TELEVISION APPEARANCES—Series: Ham Tyler, *V,* NBC, 1984-85. Mini-Series: Ham Tyler, *V: The Final Battle,* NBC, 1984. Movies: Bartender, *The Family Man,* CBS, 1979; Alan Campbell, *The Sins of Dorian Gray,* ABC, 1983; Captain Neal Braddock, *Murder in Space,* Showtime, 1985; Harry Bennett, *Ford: The Man and the Machine,* syndicated, 1987. Specials: "The Fruit at the Bottom of the Bowl," *Ray Bradbury Theatre III,* First Choice, 1988.

MEMBER: Association of Canadian Television and Radio Artists, Screen Actors Guild.

ADDRESSES: OFFICE—321 S. Beverly Drive, Suite M, Beverly Hills, CA 90212. AGENT—Triad Artists, 10100 Santa Monica Boulevard, 16th Floor, Los Angeles, CA 90067.

*   *   *

IRWIN, Bill   1950-

PERSONAL: Full name, William Mills Irwin; born April 11, 1950, in Santa Monica, CA; son of Horace G. (an aerospace engineer) and Elizabeth (a teacher; maiden name, Mills) Irwin; married Kimi Okada (a dancer and choreographer), April 19, 1977 (divorced). EDUCATION: Oberlin College, B.A., 1974; also attended the University of California, Los Angeles, 1968-70; California Institute of the Arts, 1970-71; and Ringling Brothers and Barnum & Bailey's Clown College, 1974; trained for the stage with Herbert Blau.

VOCATION: Actor, dancer, clown, and writer.

CAREER: Also see *WRITINGS* below. OFF-BROADWAY DEBUT—*The Regard of Flight,* American Place Theatre, 1982. BROADWAY DEBUT—Sergeant, *Accidental Death of an Anarchist,* Belasco Theatre, 1984. PRINCIPAL STAGE APPEARANCES—Galy Gay, *A Man's a Man,* and Medvedenko, *The Sea Gull,* both La Jolla Playhouse, La Jolla, CA, 1985; the Post-Modern Hoofer, *Largely/New York (The Further Adventures of a Post-Modern Hoofer),* City Center Theatre, New York City, 1988; Lucky, *Waiting for Godot,* Mitzi E. Newhouse Theatre, New York City, 1988; the Post-Modern Hoofer, *Largely/New York,* St. James Theatre, New York City, 1989. Also appeared in *The Seeds of Atreus* and *The Donner Party, It's Crossing,* both Kraken Theatre Ensemble, Oberlin, OH, 1971; *Circa* and *Murdoch and the Regard of Flight,* both Oberlin Dance Collective, San Francisco, CA, 1977; *Not Quite/New York,* New York City, 1980; *5-6-7-8 . . . Dance!,* Radio City Music Hall, New York City, 1983; *The Regard of Flight,* Center Theatre Group, Mark Taper Forum, Los Angeles, CA, 1983, then Arena Stage, Washington, DC, 1985; *The Garden of Earthly Delights* (dance work), New York City, 1984; *The Courtroom,* Theatre at St. Clement's Church, New York City, 1985; *The Regard of Flight* and *The Clown Bagatelles,* both Vivian Beaumont Theatre, New York City, 1987; *Strike Up the Band,* Philadelphia, PA; with the Oberlin Dance Collective, Dance Theatre Workshop, New York City, 1979; and in a post-modern mime show, New York City, 1979.

PRINCIPAL STAGE WORK—Choreographer, *Circa* and *Murdoch and the Regard of Flight,* both Oberlin Dance Collective, San Francisco, CA, 1977; choreographer, *The Courtroom,* Theatre at St. Clement's, New York City, 1985; circus/clown consultant, *Times and Appetites of Toulouse-Lautrec,* American Place Theatre, New York City, 1985; producer, *Largely/New York (The Further Adventures of a Post-Modern Hoofer),* City Center Theatre, New York City, 1988.

PRINCIPAL FILM APPEARANCES—Ham Gravy, *Popeye,* Paramount, 1980; Eric, *A New Life,* Paramount, 1988; Eddie Collins, *Eight Men Out,* Orion, 1988.

PRINCIPAL TELEVISION APPEARANCES—Episodic: Santa Claus, *Who's the Boss?,* ABC, 1985; Senator Platt, *Silver Spoons,* NBC, 1985; Eddie Bartholomew, *The Cosby Show,* NBC, 1987; Gus, *Boys Will Be Boys,* Fox, 1988; also *Alive from Off Center,* PBS; *Saturday Night Live,* NBC. Mini-Series: "Katherine Anne Porter: The Eye of Memory," *American Masters,* PBS, 1986. Specials: *New Vaudevillians III,* Disney Channel, 1988; *Bette Midler's Mondo Beyondo,* HBO, 1988; also "The Regard of Flight," *Great Performances,* PBS; and *The Paul Daniels Magic Show.*

RELATED CAREER—Teaching assistant in theatre, Oberlin College, Oberlin, OH, 1974-75; original member, Kraken Theatre Ensemble, 1971-75; teacher and performer, San Francisco Public Schools, San Francisco, CA, 1975-78; Willy the Clown, Pickle Family Circus, San Francisco, 1975-79; teacher of professional workshops in physical comedy, Dance Theatre Workshop, New York City, 1982—; member, Arts Advisory Committee, New York Festival of the Arts, New York City, 1988; advisory board member, National Theatre of the Deaf; street performer as mime and (as Carno the Magnificent Salamander) fire-eater, San Francisco.

WRITINGS: See production details above. STAGE— *Circa* and (with Doug Skinner) *Murdoch and the Regard of Flight,* both 1977; *Not Quite/New York,* 1980; *The Regard of Flight,* 1982, then 1987; *The Courtroom,* 1985; (also video designer with Skip Sweeney) *Largely/New York (The Further Adventures of a Post-Modern Hoofer,* 1988. TELEVISION—Episodic: *Alive from Off Center,* PBS. Specials: "The Regard of Flight," *Great Performances,* PBS.

AWARDS: Obie Award from the *Village Voice,* Special Citation, 1981, for "inspired clowning"; Choreographers Fellowship from the National Endowment for the Arts, 1983; Guggenheim fellowship and MacArthur Foundation fellowship, both 1984.

MEMBER: Actors' Equity Association, Screen Actors Guild, American Federation of Radio and Television Artists.

ADDRESSES: OFFICE—56 Seventh Avenue, Suite 4-E, New York, NY 10011. AGENT—Bridget Aschenberg, International Creative Management, 40 W. 57th Street, New York, NY 10019.*

ITALIANO, Anne
See BANCROFT, Anne

*   *   *

ITO, Robert   1931-

PERSONAL: Born July 2, 1931, in Vancouver, BC, Canada.

VOCATION: Actor.

CAREER: PRINCIPAL STAGE APPEARANCES—*Flower Drum Song,* St. James Theatre, New York City, 1958; *Our Town,* Circle in the Square, New York City, 1959.

PRINCIPAL FILM APPEARANCES—Sato, *Dimension 5,* Feature Films, 1966; Tang, *Women of the Prehistoric Planet,* Real Art, 1966; George Toyota, *Some Kind of a Nut,* United Artists, 1969; anaesthetist, *The Terminal Man,* Warner Brothers, 1974; Oriental instructor, *Rollerball,* United Artists, 1975; butler, *Peeper* (also known as *Fat Chance*), Twentieth Century-Fox, 1975; Mr. Chu, *Special Delivery,* American International, 1976; Professor Hikita, *The Adventures of Buckaroo Banzai: Across the Eighth Dimension,* Twentieth Century-Fox, 1984; Koga, *Pray for Death,* Transworld Entertainment/American Distribution Group, 1986; Kim, *P.I. Private Investigations,* Metro-Goldwyn-Mayer/United Artists, 1987. Also appeared in *The Naked Ape,* Universal, 1973; and *Midway* (also known as *Battle of Midway*), Universal, 1976.

PRINCIPAL TELEVISION APPEARANCES—Series: Regular, *The Burns and Schreiber Comedy Hour,* ABC, 1973; voice of Henry Chan, *The Amazing Chan and the Chan Clan* (animated), CBS, 1974; Sam Fujiyama, *Quincy, M.E.,* NBC, 1976-83; voice characterization, *Rambo* (animated), syndicated, 1986. Pilots: Fong, *Kung Fu,* ABC, 1972; Li-Teh, *Men of the Dragon,* ABC, 1974; Dr. Sam Fujiyama, *The Eyes of Texas II,* NBC, 1980. Episodic: Sato, "WGOD," *The Hitchhiker,* HBO, 1985; Tran Van Hieu, *Airwolf,* CBS, 1986; Yoshio Shinno, *Knots Landing,* CBS, 1986; Vang Pau, *Supercarrier,* ABC, 1988; Kazu, *Ohara,* ABC, 1988; Joe Matsumuro, *Tour of Duty,* CBS, 1988; Lawrence Mishima, *Falcon Crest,* CBS, 1988; Tac Officer Chang, "Coming of Age," *Star Trek: The Next Generation,* syndicated, 1988. Movies: Masai Ikeda, *Fer de Lance* (also known as *Death Dive*), CBS, 1974; Arnold, *Aloha Means Goodbye,* CBS, 1974; intern, *Death Scream* (also known as *The Woman Who Cried Murder*), ABC, 1975; Drees Darrin, *Helter Skelter,* CBS, 1976; Roy Nakamura, *SST—Death Flight* (also known as *SST: Disaster in the Sky*), ABC, 1977; Mr. Hashimoto, *American Geisha,* CBS, 1986. Specials: North Korean negotiator, "Pueblo," *ABC Theatre,* ABC, 1973; Mr. Sumida, "The War between the Classes," *CBS Schoolbreak Special,* CBS, 1985.

RELATED CAREER—Member of the National Ballet of Canada for ten years.

ADDRESSES: AGENT—Diamond Artists Ltd., 9200 Sunset Boulevard, Suite 909, Los Angeles, CA 90069.*

J

JACKSON, Anne 1926-

PERSONAL: Full name, Anna June Jackson; born September 3, 1926, in Allegheny, PA; daughter of John Ivan (a beautician) and Stella Germaine (Murray) Jackson; married Eli Wallach (an actor), March 5, 1948; children: Peter, Roberta, Katherine. EDUCATION: Attended the New School for Social Research, 1943; trained for the stage with Sanford Meisner at the Neighborhood Playhouse, 1943-44, and with Herbert Berghof and Lee Strasberg at the Actors Studio, 1948.

VOCATION: Actress.

CAREER: STAGE DEBUT—Anya, *The Cherry Orchard,* Wilmington, DE, 1944. BROADWAY DEBUT—Guest, *The Cherry Orchard,* City Center Theatre, 1945. LONDON DEBUT—Sylvia, "The Typists," and Gloria, "The Tiger," in *"The Typists" and*

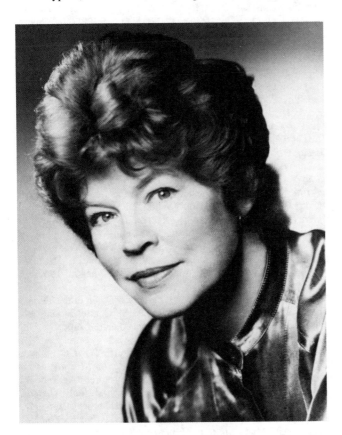

ANNE JACKSON

"The Tiger" (double-bill), Globe Theatre, 1964. PRINCIPAL STAGE APPEARANCES—Alice Stewart, *Signature,* Forrest Theatre, Philadelphia, PA, 1945; Frida Foldal, *John Gabriel Borkman,* and a Christian, *Androcles and the Lion,* both American Repertory Company, International Theatre, New York City, 1946; Miss Blake, *Yellow Jack,* American Repertory Company, International Theatre, 1947; Judith, *The Last Dance,* Belasco Theatre, New York City, 1948; Pat, *The Young and Fair,* Falmouth Playhouse, Falmouth, MA, 1948; Nellie Ewell, *Summer and Smoke,* Music Box Theatre, New York City, 1948; Nita, *Magnolia Alley,* Mansfield Theatre, New York City, 1949; Margaret Anderson, *Love Me Long,* 48th Street Theatre, New York City, 1949; Hilda, *The Lady from the Sea,* Fulton Theatre, New York City, 1950; Louka, *Arms and the Man,* Hotel Edison Theatre, New York City, 1950; Coralie Jones, *Never Say Never,* Booth Theatre, New York City, 1951; Mildred Turner, *Oh Men! Oh Women!,* Henry Miller's Theatre, New York City, 1953; the Daughter, *The Middle of the Night,* American National Theatre and Academy Theatre, New York City, 1956; title role, *Major Barbara,* Martin Beck Theatre, New York City, 1956; Laura, *The Glass Menagerie,* Westport Country Playhouse, Westport, CT, then John Drew Theatre, Easthampton, NY, both 1959; Daisy, *Rhinoceros,* Longacre Theatre, New York City, 1961; Sylvia, "The Typists," and Gloria, "The Tiger," in *"The Typists" and "The Tiger"* (double-bill), Orpheum Theatre, New York City, 1963; Ellen Manville, *Luv,* Booth Theatre, New York City, 1964; the Actress, *The Exercise,* Berkshire Festival, Stockbridge, MA, 1967, then John Golden Theatre, New York City, 1968; Molly Malloy, *The Front Page,* Ethel Barrymore Theatre, New York City, 1969.

Ethel Rosenberg, *The Inquest,* Music Box Theatre, 1970; Mother H., Doris, and Joan J., *Promenade, All!,* Alvin Theatre, New York City, 1972; Madame St. Pe, *Waltz of the Toreadors,* Eisenhower Theatre, Kennedy Center for the Performing Arts, Washington, DC, then Circle in the Square, New York City, both 1973; Madame Ranevskaya, *The Cherry Orchard,* Hartford Stage Company, Hartford, CT, 1974; Mrs. McBride, *Marco Polo Sings a Solo,* New York Shakespeare Festival (NYSF), Public Theatre, New York City, 1977; Diana, *Absent Friends,* Long Wharf Theatre, New Haven, CT, 1977; Mrs. Frank, *The Diary of Anne Frank,* Theatre Four, New York City, 1978; Margaret Heinz, "A Need for Brussels Sprouts," and Edie Frazier, "A Need for Less Expertise," *Twice Around the Park* (double-bill), Syracuse Stage Theatre, Syracuse, NY, 1981, then Cort Theatre, New York City, 1982, later Edinburgh Theatre Festival, Edinburgh, Scotland, 1984; Natalya Gavrilovna, *The Nest of the Wood Grouse,* NYSF, Public Theatre, 1984; title role, *The Madwoman of Chaillot,* Mirror Repertory Company, New York City, 1985; Odile, *Opera Comique,* Eisenhower Theatre, Kennedy Center for the Performing Arts, 1987; Anna Cole, *Cafe Crown,* NYSF, Public Theatre, 1988, then Brooks Atkinson Theatre, New York City, 1989. Also appeared in *What*

Every Woman Knows and *Henry VIII*, both American Repertory Company, International Theatre, 1946; in a poetry reading at the John Drew Playhouse, 1960; in *Brecht on Brecht* (staged reading), Theatre De Lys, New York City, 1962; in *Just an Evening with Anne Jackson and Eli Wallach;* with the Arena Stage, Washington, DC, 1977-78; Bucks County Playhouse, New Hope, PA; Clinton Playhouse, Clinton, NJ; Equity Library Theatre, New York City; and the Actors Studio, New York City.

MAJOR TOURS—Zelda Rainier, *Donnigan's Daughter*, U.S. cities, 1945; Bella, *The Barretts of Wimpole Street*, U.S. cities, 1947; Mildred, *Oh Men! Oh Women!*, U.S. cities, 1955; Ellen Manville, *Luv*, U.S. cities, 1964; Sylvia, "The Typists," and Gloria, "The Tiger," in *"The Typists" and "The Tiger"* (double-bill), U.S. cities, 1966; Mother H., Doris, and Joan J., *Promenade, All!*, U.S. cities, 1971; Madame St. Pe, *Waltz of the Toreadors*, U.S. cities, 1973; Diana, *Absent Friends*, U.S. and Canadian cities, 1977.

FILM DEBUT—Jackie, *So Young, So Bad*, United Artists, 1950. PRINCIPAL FILM APPEARANCES—Mrs. Margie Rhinelander, *The Journey*, Metro-Goldwyn-Mayer (MGM), 1959; Myra Sullivan, *Tall Story*, Warner Brothers, 1960; Gloria Fiske, *The Tiger Makes Out*, Columbia, 1967; Muriel Laszlo, *How to Save a Marriage—and Ruin Your Life* (also known as *Band of Gold*), Columbia, 1968; Victoria Layton, *The Secret Life of an American Wife*, Twentieth Century-Fox, 1968; Belle, *Dirty Dingus Magee*, MGM, 1970; lady in the store, *The Angel Levine*, United Artists, 1970; Cathy, *Lovers and Other Strangers*, Cinerama, 1970; Jean Cameron, *Zigzag* (also known as *False Witness*), MGM, 1970; Abigail Adams, *Independence*, Twentieth Century-Fox, 1975; Sub-Prioress Mildred, *Nasty Habits*, Brut, 1976; Dr. Nolan, *The Bell Jar*, AVCO-Embassy, 1979; doctor, *The Shining*, Warner Brothers, 1980; as herself, *Sanford Meisner—The Theatre's Best Kept Secret* (documentary), Columbia, 1984; Harriet Orowitz, *Sam's Son*, Invictus, 1984; narrator, *Are We Winning, Mommy? America and the Cold War* (documentary), Cine Information/National Film Board of Canada/Channel Four/Svenges TV2, 1986. Also appeared in *A View to a Kill*, Metro-Goldwyn-Mayer/United Artists, 1984.

PRINCIPAL TELEVISION APPEARANCES—Series: Rae Matthews, *Everything's Relative*, CBS, 1987; also *Love of Life*, CBS. Pilots: Jenny Dutton, *Acres and Pains*, CBS, 1965. Episodic: Gwen Schaeffer, *The Facts of Life*, NBC, 1985; Mrs. Fields, *The Equalizer*, CBS, 1985; Marge Malloy, *Highway to Heaven*, NBC, 1987; also *Academy Theatre*, NBC, 1949; "Johnny Pickup," *The Armstrong Circle Theatre*, NBC, 1951; *The Vanished Hours*, CBS, 1952; *The Doctor* (also known as *The Visitor*), NBC, 1952-53; "The Big Deal," *Philco Playhouse*, NBC, 1953; "Statute of Limitations," *Philco Playhouse*, NBC, 1954; "The Merry-Go-Round," *Goodyear Playhouse*, NBC, 1955; "O'Hoolihan and the Leprechaun," *General Electric Theatre*, CBS, 1956; "Lullaby," *Play of the Week*, WNTA, 1960; "Cooker in the Sky," *The Untouchables*, ABC, 1962; "Moment of Truth," *The Defenders*, CBS, 1964; "Dear Friends," *CBS Playhouse*, CBS, 1967; "The Typists," *Hollywood Television Theatre*, 1971; *Gunsmoke*, CBS, 1972; *Marcus Welby, M.D.*, ABC, 1972; *Robert Montgomery Presents Your Lucky Strike Theatre*, NBC; *Danger*, CBS; *Suspense*, CBS; *The Web*, CBS. Movies: Maggie Madden, *The Family Man*, CBS, 1979; Frances Bowers, *Blinded by the Light*, CBS, 1980; Kathryn Morgan Ryan, *A Private Battle*, CBS, 1980; Shirlee Thum, *Leave 'em Laughing*, CBS, 1981; Lou Kaddar and narrator, *A Woman Called Golda*, syndicated, 1982; Bella Abzug, *Out on a Limb*, ABC, 1987; Lorraine Abraham, *Baby M*, ABC, 1988. Plays: *Sticks and Bones*, CBS, 1973; *Come into My Parlour*, Anglia

Television, 1974. Also appeared in *84 Charing Cross Road*, British television.

WRITINGS: *Early Stages* (autobiography), Little, Brown, 1979.

AWARDS: Obie Award from the *Village Voice*, 1962, for *"The Typists" and "The Tiger;"* Lions of the Performing Arts Award from the New York Public Library, 1987.

MEMBER: Actors' Equity Association, American Federation of Television and Radio Artists, Screen Actors Guild.

SIDELIGHTS: FAVORITE ROLES—Hilde in *The Master Builder* and *The Madwoman of Chaillot*. RECREATIONS—Writing.

ADDRESSES: AGENT—International Creative Management, 8899 Beverly Boulevard, Los Angeles, CA 90048.

*   *   *

JACOBI, Derek 1938-

PERSONAL: Born October 22, 1938, in London, England; son of Alfred George (a store manager) and Daisy Gertrude (a secretary; maiden name, Masters) Jacobi. EDUCATION: Received M.A. from Cambridge University.

VOCATION: Actor.

CAREER: LONDON DEBUT—Laertes, *Hamlet*, National Theatre Company, Old Vic Theatre, 1963. BROADWAY DEBUT—Semyon Semyonovich Podsekalnikov (Senya), *The Suicide*, American National Theatre and Academy Theatre, 1980. PRINCIPAL STAGE APPEARANCES—Title role, *Hamlet*, English National Youth Theatre, Edinburgh Festival, Edinburgh, Scotland, 1955; title role, *Edward II*, Marlowe Society, Cambridge, U.K., 1959; Stanley Honeybone, *One Way Pendulum*, Birmingham Repertory Theatre, Birmingham, U.K., 1961; Brother Martin, *Saint Joan*, and P.C. Liversedge, *The Workinghouse Donkey*, both Chichester Festival Theatre, Chichester, U.K., 1963; Fellipillo, *The Royal Hunt of the Sun*, Cassio, *Othello*, and Simon Bliss, *Hay Fever*, all National Theatre Company, Old Vic Theatre, London, 1964; Don John, *Much Ado about Nothing*, Chichester Festival Theatre, 1965; Brindsley Miller, *Black Comedy*, Chichester Festival Theatre, then Old Vic Theatre, later Queen's Theatre, London, all 1966; Tusenbach, *The Three Sisters*, and Touchstone, *As You Like It*, both National Theatre Company, Old Vic Theatre, 1967; King of Navarre, *Love's Labour's Lost*, National Theatre Company, Old Vic Theatre, 1968; Edward Hotel, *Macrune's Guevara*, and Adam, *Back to Methuselah*, both National Theatre Company, Old Vic Theatre, 1969.

Myshkin, *The Idiot*, and Lodovico, *The White Devil*, both National Theatre Company, Old Vic Theatre, 1970; Sir Charles Mountford, *A Woman Killed with Kindness*, National Theatre Company, Old Vic Theatre, 1971; Orestes, *Electra*, Greenwich Theatre, London, 1971; title role, *Oedipus Rex*, and Mr. Puff, *The Critic*, both Birmingham Repertory Company, 1972; title role, *Ivanov*, Prospect Theatre Company, London, 1972; Sir Andrew Aguecheek, *Twelfth Night*, Prospect Theatre Company, Round House Theatre, London, 1973; title role, *Pericles*, Prospect Theatre Company, Round House Theatre, 1973, then Her Majesty's Theatre, London, 1974; Rakitin, *A Month in the Country*, Chichester Festival Theatre, 1974; Will Mossop, *Hobson's Choice*, Yvonne Arnaud Theatre, Guildford, U.K., 1975; Rakitin, *A Month in the Country*, and Cecil Vyse, *A Room with a View*, both Prospect Theatre Company, Albery Theatre, London, 1975; title role, *Hamlet*, and Octavius Caesar, *Antony and Cleopatra*, Prospect Theatre Company, Old Vic Theatre, 1977; Thomas Mendip, *The Lady's Not for Burning*, and title role, *Ivanov*, both Prospect Theatre Company, Old Vic Theatre, 1978; title role, *Hamlet*, Prospect Theatre Company, Old Vic Theatre, 1979.

Benedick, *Much Ado about Nothing*, Royal Shakespeare Company (RSC), Aldwych Theatre, London, 1982, then Gershwin Theatre, New York City, 1984; title role, *Peer Gynt*, RSC, Aldwych Theatre, 1982; Prospero, *The Tempest*, RSC, Aldwych Theatre, 1983; title role, *Cyrano de Bergerac*, RSC, Aldwych Theatre, 1983, then Gershwin Theatre, 1984; Alan Turing, *Breaking the Code*, Haymarket Theatre, London, 1986, then Eisenhower Theatre, Kennedy Center for the Performing Arts, Washington, DC, 1986, later Neil Simon Theatre, New York City, 1987; title role, *Richard II*, Phoenix Theatre, London, 1988; title role, *Richard III*, Phoenix Theatre, 1989. Also appeared in *Henry VIII*, Birmingham Repertory Theatre, 1960; as Buckingham, *Richard III*, 1972; in *The Grand Tour*, Goldsmith's Hall, London, 1973; *The Lunatic, the Lover, and the Poet* and *The Grand Tour*, both Old Vic Theatre, 1978.

MAJOR TOURS—Sir Andrew Aguecheek, *Twelfth Night*, and title role, *Pericles*, both Prospect Theatre Company, European and Middle Eastern cities, 1973; also appeared in *The Hollow Crown* and *Pleasure and Repentance*, both 1975; and in *The Grand Tour* and *Hamlet*, both Scandinavian, Australian, Japanese, and Chinese cities.

FILM DEBUT—Cassio, *Othello*, Warner Brothers, 1965. PRINCIPAL FILM APPEARANCES—Paul, *Interlude*, Columbia, 1968; Caron, *The Day of the Jackal*, Universal, 1973; Klaus Wenzer, *The Odessa File*, Columbia, 1974; Andrei, *The Three Sisters*, American Film Theatre, 1974; Townley, *The Medusa Touch*, Warner Brothers, 1978; Arthur Davis, *The Human Factor*, Metro-Goldwyn-Mayer/United Artists (MGM/UA), 1979; Martin Beck, *Mannen som gick upp i rök* (also known as *The Man Who Went Up in Smoke*), Svenska Filminstitet/Europafilm, 1980; voice of Nicodemus, *The Secret of NIMH* (animated), MGM/UA, 1982; Kurt Limmer, *Enigma*, Embassy, 1983; Arthur Clennam, *Little Dorrit*, Sands Films/Cannon, 1987. Also appeared in *Blue Blood*, Mallard/Impact Quadrant, 1973; *Charlotte*, 1980.

PRINCIPAL TELEVISION APPEARANCES—Mini-Series: Josef Lanner, *The Strauss Family*, ABC, 1973; Lord Fawn, *The Pallisers*, PBS, 1977; title role, *I, Claudius*, BBC, 1976, then *Masterpiece Theatre*, PBS, 1977; Adolf Hitler, *Inside the Third Reich*, ABC, 1982. Episodic: "Angela's Skin," *Tales of the Unexpected*, syndicated. Movies: Dom Claude Frollo, *The Hunchback of Notre Dame*, CBS, 1982; Archibald Craven, "The Secret Garden," *Hallmark Hall of Fame*, CBS, 1987; the Imposter, "Graham Greene's The Tenth Man," *Hallmark Hall of Fame*, CBS, 1988. Specials: Narrator, *Statue of Liberty* (documentary), PBS, 1985; narrator of animated sequences, *Cathedral* (documentary), PBS, 1986; host, *Jessye Norman's Christmas Symphony*, PBS, 1987; narrator, *Pyramid* (documentary), PBS, 1988; voice, *The Congress* (documentary), PBS, 1989. Plays: Title role, *Richard II*, BBC, then *The Shakespeare Plays*, PBS, 1979; title role, *Hamlet*, BBC, then *The Shakespeare Plays*, PBS, 1980; also *She Stoops to Conquer*. Also appeared in *Man of Straw*, 1971-72; *Budgie*, 1972; *Markheim*, 1973; *Affairs of the Heart*, 1973; *Paths of the Future*,

1978; *Skin*, 1979; as Burgess, *Philby, Burgess, and MacLean*, 1979-80; in *A Stranger in Town*, 1982; and in *Mr. Pye*.

RELATED CAREER—Artistic associate, Old Vic Company (formerly Prospect Theatre Company), London, 1976-81; vice president, National Youth Theatre, London, 1982—.

RECORDINGS: *1984* (taped reading), Listen for Pleasure; *A Severed Head* (taped reading), G.K. Hall.

AWARDS: Variety Club of Great Britain Award, Television Personality the Year, Royal Television Society Award, and Press Guild Award, all 1976, and British Academy of Film and Television Arts Award, Best Actor, 1977, all for *I, Claudius*; Antoinette Perry Award nomination, Best Actor in a Play, 1980, for *The Suicide*; Emmy Award nomination, Outstanding Supporting Actor in a Limited Series or Special, 1982, for *Inside the Third Reich*; Antoinette Perry Award, Best Actor in a Play, 1985, for *Much Ado about Nothing*; Antoinette Perry Award nomination and Drama Desk Award nomination, both Best Actor in a Play, 1988, for *Breaking the Code*; Commander of the British Empire.

SIDELIGHTS: RECREATIONS—Music, gardening, and reading.

OTHER SOURCES: *New York Times*, November 26, 1987, November 29, 1987.

ADDRESSES: AGENT—International Creative Management, 388 Oxford Street, London W1, England.*

* * *

JACOBI, Lou   1913-

PERSONAL: Full name, Louis Harold Jacobi; born December 28, 1913, in Toronto, ON, Canada; son of Joseph and Fay Jacobi; married Ruth Ludwin, July 15, 1957.

VOCATION: Actor.

CAREER: STAGE DEBUT—Young Hero, *The Rabbi and the Priest*, Princess Theatre, Toronto, ON, Canada, 1924. BROADWAY DEBUT—Mr. Van Daan, *The Diary of Anne Frank*, Cort Theatre, 1955. LONDON DEBUT—Morris Rosenberg, *Remains to Be Seen*, Her Majesty's Theatre, 1952. PRINCIPAL STAGE APPEARANCES—Ensemble, *Spring Thaw* (revue), Museum Theatre, Toronto, ON, Canada, 1949; Liver Lips Louie, *Guys and Dolls*, Coliseum Theatre, London, 1953; Ludlow Lowell, *Pal Joey*, Prince's Theatre, London, 1954; Father Abraham, "Bontche Schweig," Rabbi David, "A Tale of Chelm," and Russian tutor, "The High School," in *The World of Sholom Aleichem*, Embassy Theatre, London, 1955; Miller, *Into Thin Air*, Streatham Hill Theatre, London, 1955; Schlissel, *The Tenth Man*, Booth Theatre, New York City, 1959; Mr. Baker, *Come Blow Your Horn*, Brooks Atkinson Theatre, New York City, 1961; Lionel Z. Governor, *Fade Out—Fade In*, Mark Hellinger Theatre, New York City, 1964, reopened 1965; Walter Hollander, *Don't Drink the Water*, Morosco Theatre, New York City, 1966; Max Krieger, *A Way of Life*, American National Theatre and Academy Theatre, New York City, 1969; Ben Chambers, *Norman, Is That You?*, Lyceum Theatre, New York City, 1970; title role, "Epstein" and Tzuref "Eli, the Fanatic," in *Unlikely Heroes*, Plymouth Theatre, New York City, 1971; ensemble, *Milliken Breakfast Show*, Waldorf-Astoria Hotel, New York

City, 1972; Al Lewis, *The Sunshine Boys,* Shubert Theatre, New York City, 1973; Howard, *Cheaters,* Biltmore Theatre, New York City, 1978.

MAJOR TOURS—Mr. Van Daan, *The Diary of Anne Frank,* U.S. cities, 1957-58; Al Lewis, *The Sunshine Boys,* U.S. cities, 1974.

PRINCIPAL FILM APPEARANCES—Captain Noakes, *Is Your Honeymoon Really Necessary?,* Adelphi, 1953; theatre manager, *Charley Moon,* British Lion, 1956; Blackie Isaacs, *A Kid for Two Farthings,* Independent Film Distributors/Lopert, 1956; Mr. Van Daan, *The Diary of Anne Frank,* Twentieth Century-Fox, 1959; Potin, *Song Without End,* Columbia, 1960; Moustache, *Irma la Douce,* United Artists, 1963; Papa Leo, *The Last of the Secret Agents?,* Paramount, 1966; Ducky, *Penelope,* Metro-Goldwyn-Mayer, 1966; Goodman, *Cotton Comes to Harlem,* United Artists, 1970; judge, *Little Murders,* Twentieth Century-Fox, 1971; Sam, *Everything You Always Wanted to Know About Sex* (*but were afraid to ask),* United Artists, 1972; Herb, *Next Stop, Greenwich Village,* Twentieth Century-Fox, 1976; Stan, "The Waltz," in *Roseland,* Cinema Shares, 1977; Wolsky, *The Magician of Lublin,* Cannon, 1979; Elia Goldberg, *The Lucky Star,* Telemetropole Internationale, 1980; plant store owner, *Arthur,* Warner Brothers, 1981; landlord, *Chu Chu and the Philly Flash,* Twentieth Century-Fox, 1981; Uncle Morty, *My Favorite Year,* Metro-Goldwyn-Mayer/United Artists, 1982; Abe Kapp, *Isaac Littlefeathers,* Lauron, 1984; Harry Taphorn, *The Boss' Wife,* Tri-Star, 1986; Murray, "Murray in Videoland," in *Amazon Women on the Moon,* Universal, 1987. Also appeared in *The Good Beginning,* Associated British/Pathe, 1953; and *Off Your Rocker,* 1980.

TELEVISION DEBUT—*The Rheingold Theatre,* BBC, 1954. PRINCIPAL TELEVISION APPEARANCES—Series: Regular, *The Dean Martin Show,* NBC, 1971-73; title role, *Ivan the Terrible,* CBS, 1976; Jack, *Melba,* CBS, 1986. Pilots: Lieutenant Lou Finch, *Kibbe Hates Finch,* CBS, 1965; proprietor, *The Happeners,* syndicated, 1967; Harold Fisher, *Allan,* NBC, 1971; Lieutenant Wolfson, *The Judge and Jake Wyler,* NBC, 1972; Raskin, *Rear Guard,* ABC, 1976; Max, *Saint Peter,* NBC, 1981; Rosenthal, *Joanna,* ABC, 1985; "Stormtrooper" Bernie Sagowitz, "The Arena," *ABC Comedy Specials,* ABC, 1986. Episodic: "Volpone," *Play of the Week,* NTA, 1960; *The Dick Van Dyke Show,* CBS, 1965; *Barney Miller,* ABC, 1975; *Somerset,* NBC, 1976; *Douglas Fairbanks, Jr. Presents the Rheingold Theatre,* NBC; *The Milton Berle Show,* NBC; *The Defenders,* CBS; *Alfred Hitchcock Presents,* CBS; *Playhouse 90,* CBS; *The Texan,* CBS; *Trials of O'Brien,* CBS; *Sam Benedict,* CBS; *The Nurses,* CBS; *That's Life,* ABC; *That Girl,* ABC; *Love, American Style,* ABC; *Man from U.N.C.L.E.,* NBC; *Make Room for Granddaddy,* ABC; *The Judge and Jake Wyler,* NBC; Paul, *Too Close for Comfort.* Movies: Waiter, *Coffee, Tea or Me?,* CBS, 1973; Milton Cohen, *Better Late Than Never,* NBC, 1979; Ed Blye, *If It's Tuesday It Still Must Be Belgium,* NBC, 1987. Specials: *Ed Sullivan's Broadway,* CBS, 1973; Mayor R. Van Winkle, "The Day the Kids Took Over," *ABC Weekend Special,* ABC, 1986; also "Tales from the Hollywood Hills: The Old Reliable," *Great Performances,* PBS, 1988.

PRINCIPAL RADIO APPEARANCES—Series: Regular, *Mid-Day Music Hall,* BBC, 1953-54.

RELATED CAREER—Drama director, Young Men's Hebrew Association, Toronto, ON, Canada, 1940; also appeared in cabaret at Ciro's, London, 1951, and in a Command Performance at the London Palladium, 1952.

MEMBER: Actors' Equity Association, Screen Actors Guild, American Federation of Television and Radio Artists.

ADDRESSES: AGENT—William Morris Agency, 1350 Avenue of the Americas, New York, NY 10019.*

*   *   *

JAMES, Dorothy Dorian   1930-

PERSONAL: Born August 24, 1930, in Connecticut. EDUCATION: Trained for the stage with Alvina Krause at Northwestern University's School of Speech, with Sanford Meisner at the Neighborhood Playhouse, at Circle in the Square Shakespeare Seminar, at Roger Rees's Royal Shakespeare Company Workshop, and at the Royal Court Theatre Writers' Workshop.

VOCATION: Actress.

CAREER: PRINCIPAL STAGE APPEARANCES—Pat Nixon, *An Evening with Richard Nixon,* Shubert Theatre, New York City, 1972; Catherine Lynch, *All the Way Home,* South Coast Repertory Theatre, Costa Mesa, CA, 1986. Also appeared as Alma, *Summer and Smoke,* 1970; in *Sarcophagus,* Los Angeles Theatre Center, Los Angeles Festival, Los Angeles, CA, 1987; as Mary Tyrone, *Long Day's Journey into Night,* PCPA Theaterfest, Los Angeles; Giza, *Catsplay,* American Theatre Arts, Los Angeles; in *The Glass Menagerie,* Los Angeles Theatre Center, Los Angeles; *Mercy*

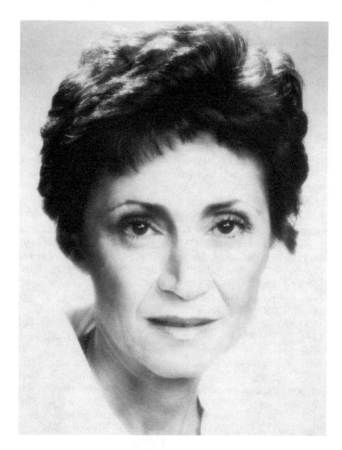

DOROTHY DORIAN JAMES

Street, American Place Theatre, New York City; *All's Well That Ends Well,* Globe Theatre, San Diego, CA; as Alice Russell, *The Best Man;* Jennet, *The Lady's Not for Burning;* Ruth Gordon, *Years Ago;* in productions of *The Prisoner of Second Avenue, Forty Carats, Hostile Witness, A Man for All Seasons, The Prime of Miss Jean Brodie,* and *O Men! O Women!,* with the New York Shakespeare Festival, New York City, and at the Stratford Shakespearean Festival, Stratford, ON, Canada.

PRINCIPAL FILM APPEARANCES—Mrs. Gomez, *The Cross and the Switchblade,* Ross, 1970; tourist, *Bobby Deerfield,* Columbia, 1977; Jean MacArthur, *Inchon,* Metro-Goldwyn-Mayer/United Artists, 1982; Mom, *Alone in the Dark,* New Line Cinema, 1982. Also appeared in *A Matter of Time,* American International, 1976; *The Cassandra Crossing,* AVCO-Embassy, 1977; *Radioactive Dreams,* De Laurentiis Entertainment Group, 1986; and *The Garden Party,* De Laurentiis Entertainment Group, 1986.

PRINCIPAL TELEVISION APPEARANCES—Series: Esther Kensington, *Days of Our Lives,* NBC; Frances Quinton, *General Hospital,* ABC; Mrs. Jablonsky, *Capitol,* CBS. Episodic: *Half Nelson,* NBC, 1985; also Rose, *Coverup,* CBS; *Cagney and Lacey,* CBS; "Zola versus Zola," *Divorce Court; The Judge.* Movies: Edna Elias, *Mrs. Delafield Wants to Marry,* CBS, 1986; Irene McNally, *Addicted to His Love* (also known as *Sisterhood*), ABC, 1988. Specials: *A Place at the Table* (also known as *The Best Kept Secret*), NBC, 1988; also as Mary, *Three Days,* NBC. Also appeared as Elizabeth Reilly, *A New Day in Eden;* in *A World Apart;* and in *Best of Everything.*

AWARDS: Connecticut Council for the Arts Award, Best Actress, 1970, for *Summer and Smoke* and *The Lady's Not for Burning.*

MEMBER: Screen Actors Guild, American Federation of Television and Radio Artists, Actors' Equity Association.

ADDRESSES: HOME—237 S. Elm Drive, Beverly Hills, CA 90212. AGENT—Brooke, Dunn, Oliver, 9165 Sunset Boulevard, Suite 202, Los Angeles, CA 90069.

*   *   *

JAMES, Roderick
See COEN, Ethan and Joel

*   *   *

JONES, Eddie

PERSONAL: Born in Washington, PA.

VOCATION: Actor.

CAREER: OFF-BROADWAY DEBUT—*Dead End,* 1960. PRINCIPAL STAGE APPEARANCES—Ellis, *Curse of the Starving Class,* New York Shakespeare Festival, Public Theatre, New York City, 1978; Mike, *The Ruffian on the Stair,* South Street Theatre, New York City, 1978; Sheriff George McKinstry, *Devour the Snow,* John Golden Theatre, New York City, 1979; Ellis, *Curse of the Starving Class,* Studio Arena Theatre, Buffalo, NY, 1980; Hal, *Big Apple Messenger,* WPA Theatre, New York City, 1981; Tarsh,

Maiden Stakes, Theatre at St. Clement's Church, New York City, 1982; Dr. Joe Quigly, *The Freak,* Douglas Fairbanks Theatre, New York City, 1982; Whitaker Chambers, *Knights Errant,* INTAR Theatre, New York City, 1982; Edwin, "Slacks and Tops," on a bill as *Triple Feature,* Manhattan Theatre Club, New York City, 1983; Ed Burke, *Burkie,* Hudson Guild Theatre, New York City, 1984; Weston, *Curse of the Starving Class,* INTAR Theatre, then Promenade Theatre, both New York City, 1985; Dee, "Pilgrim," on a bill as *Sorrows and Sons,* Vineyard Theatre, New York City, 1986; Leonard Christofferson, "The Tablecloth of Turin," on a bill as *Bigfoot Stole My Wife,* Manhattan Punch Line, New York City, 1987; Alan, *The Downside,* Long Wharf Theatre, New Haven, CT, 1987. Also appeared in *That Championship Season,* Booth Theatre, New York City, 1974; *An Act of Kindness,* Harold Clurman Theatre, New York City, 1980; *Jass,* New Dramatists, New York City, 1981; *A Touch of the Poet,* Whole Theatre Company, Montclair, NJ, 1982; and in *The Skirmishers.*

PRINCIPAL FILM APPEARANCES—Blackie, *Bloodbrothers,* Warner Brothers, 1978; Lieutenant Olson, *On the Yard,* Midwest, 1978; Ned Chippy, *Prince of the City,* Warner Brothers, 1981; watchman, *Q* (also known as *The Winged Serpent*), United Film Distribution, 1982; cop, *Trading Places,* Paramount, 1983; Jack Peurifoy, *When the Mountains Tremble* (documentary), New Yorker, 1983; Chief O'Brien, *C.H.U.D.,* New World, 1984; Cassidy, *Invasion U.S.A.,* Cannon, 1985; Charlie, *The New Kids,* Columbia, 1985; William McKenna, *Year of the Dragon,* Metro-Goldwyn-Mayer/United Artists, 1985; police patient, *The Believers,* Orion, 1987; Tom Kelly, *Apprentice to Murder,* New World, 1988.

PRINCIPAL TELEVISION APPEARANCES—Mini-Series: Barney Coster, *I'll Take Manhattan,* CBS, 1987. Pilots: Victor Muldoon, *Tales from the Darkside,* syndicated, 1983. Episodic: Howard Winslow, *The Equalizer,* CBS, 1986; J.D., *Spenser: For Hire,* ABC, 1988. Movies: Sweeney, *Doubletake,* CBS, 1985; captain, *Case Closed,* CBS, 1988.

ADDRESSES: AGENT—The Gage Group, 1650 Broadway, New York, NY 10019.*

*   *   *

JONES, Freddie   1927-

PERSONAL: Born in 1927 in London, England.

VOCATION: Actor.

CAREER: PRINCIPAL STAGE APPEARANCES—Tom, *Mister,* Duchess Theatre, London, 1971; Creon, *Antigone,* Greenwich Theatre, London, 1971; Edgar, *Play Strindberg,* Hampstead Theatre Club, London, 1973; Alec Kooning, *Dear Janet Rosenberg, Dear Mr. Kooning,* Hampstead Theatre Club, 1975; Mathias, *The Bells,* Greenwich Theatre, 1979; Robert, *A Life in the Theatre,* Open Space Theatre, London, 1979.

PRINCIPAL FILM APPEARANCES—Frantic man, *Accident,* Lippert, 1967; Cainy Ball, *Far from the Madding Crowd,* Metro-Goldwyn-Mayer (MGM), 1967; Cucurucu, *The Persecution and Assassination of Jean-Paul Marat as Performed by the Inmates of the Asylum of Charenton under the Direction of the Marquis de Sade* (also known as *Marat/Sade*), United Artists, 1967; Detective Sergeant Dylan, *The Bliss of Mrs. Blossom,* Paramount, 1968; Professor

Richter, *Frankenstein Must Be Destroyed!*, Warner Brothers, 1969; master-at-arms, *Doctor in Trouble*, Rank, 1970; David Curry, *Goodbye Gemini*, Cinerama, 1970; Dr. Harris, *The Man Who Haunted Himself*, Levitt-Pickman, 1970; reporter, *Assault* (also known as *In the Devil's Garden*), Rank, 1971; Cluny Macpherson, *Kidnapped*, American International, 1971; MacNeil, *Sitting Target*, MGM, 1972; Pompey, *Antony and Cleopatra*, Rank, 1973; Mr. Buckland, *Juggernaut*, United Artists, 1974; Dr. Frankenstein, *Son of Dracula* (also known as *Young Dracula*), Apple, 1974; Gilmore, *Old Dracula* (also known as *Vampira* and *Old Drac*), American International, 1975; Professor Keeley, *Count Dracula and His Vampire Bride* (also known as *Satanic Rites of Dracula*), Dynamic Entertainment, 1978.

Bytes, *The Elephant Man*, Paramount, 1980; Bishop Colenso, *Zulu Dawn*, Warner Brothers, 1980; Kenneth Aubrey, *Firefox*, Warner Brothers, 1982; Orlando, *And the Ship Sails On* (also known as *La Nave Va*), RAI/Vides, 1983; Ynyr, *Krull*, Columbia, 1983; Thufir Hawat, *Dune*, Dino De Laurentiis/Universal, 1984; Dr. Joseph Wanless, *Firestarter*, Dino De Laurentiis/Universal, 1984; voice of Dallben, *The Black Cauldron* (animated), Buena Vista, 1985; Cragwitch, *Young Sherlock Holmes*, Paramount, 1985; vicar, *Comrades*, Film Four International/Curzon, 1987; Podtaygin, *Maschenka*, Goldcrest, 1987; Graham Chumly, *Consuming Passions*, Samuel Goldwyn, 1988.

PRINCIPAL TELEVISION APPEARANCES—Mini-Series: Mr. Fall, *The Mayor of Casterbridge*, BBC, then *Masterpiece Theatre*, PBS, 1978; Squire Cass, "Silas Marner," *Masterpiece Theatre*, PBS, 1987; also *Vanity Fair*, Arts and Entertainment, 1988. Episodic: Arnold Tully, "Appointment with a Killer" (also known as "A Midsummer Nightmare"), *Thriller*, ABC, 1975; also "Journey to Where," *Space: 1999*, syndicated, 1976. Movies: Cranford, *All Creatures Great and Small*, NBC, 1975; Diomedes, *The Nativity*, ABC, 1978; Constable Reed, *Agatha Christie's "Murder Is Easy,"* CBS, 1982; Dr. Pavlov, *Eleanor, First Lady of the World*, CBS, 1982; Leo Porter, *Lost in London*, CBS, 1985; Ulick Uniake, *Time after Time*, BBC, then Arts and Entertainment, later Australian Broadcasting Corporation, all 1985. Also appeared as in *Never Too Young to Rock*, 1976; as Mr. Leach, *Captain Starrick*, 1982; and in *Nana*, *Treasure Island*, and *The Caesars*.

AWARDS: Monte Carlo Festival Award, Best Television Actor, 1969, for *The Caesars*.*

*   *   *

JONES, Grace   1952-

PERSONAL: Born May 19, 1952, in Spanishtown, Jamaica; father, a clergyman; children: Paulo. EDUCATION: Attended Syracuse University.

VOCATION: Actress, singer, and model.

CAREER: PRINCIPAL FILM APPEARANCES—Mary, *Gordon's War*, Twentieth Century-Fox, 1973; Zula, *Conan the Destroyer*, Universal, 1984; May Day, *A View to a Kill*, Metro-Goldwyn-Mayer/United Artists, 1985; Katrina, *Vamp*, NW Films, 1986; Conchita, *Siesta*, Lorimar, 1987; Sonya, *Straight to Hell*, Island, 1987. Also appeared in *Army of Lovers*, 1978.

RELATED CAREER—Model, nightclub performer, and appeared in and directed the music video, *I'm Not Perfect*.

RECORDINGS: ALBUMS—*Living My Life*, Island, 1982; also *No Compromise*, Capitol; *Inside Story*, Manhattan; *Warm Leatherette*, Island; *Fame*, Island; *Portfolio*, Island; *Nightclubbing*, Island; and *Island Life*, Island. SINGLES—"On Your Knees" and "I Need a Man."

MEMBER: Screen Actors Guild.*

*   *   *

JONES, LeRoi
See BARAKA, Amiri

*   *   *

JONES, Sam   1954-

PERSONAL: Full name, Sam Jerald Jones; born August 12, 1954, in Chicago, IL; father, a traveling salesman; married Lynn Eriks (a singer, dancer, and actress); children: one son. MILITARY: U.S. Marines.

VOCATION: Actor.

CAREER: PRINCIPAL STAGE APPEARANCES—*SPQR*, Cast Theatre, Los Angeles, CA, 1978.

PRINCIPAL FILM APPEARANCES—David, *10*, Warner Brothers, 1979; title role, *Flash Gordon*, Universal, 1980; Battle Witherspoon, *My Chauffeur*, Crown International, 1985; Jungle Jack Buck, *Jane and the Lost City*, Marcel/Robinson, 1987; Sam, *Silent Assassins*, Action, 1988; also appeared in *Nightshift*, Warner Brothers, 1982.

PRINCIPAL TELEVISION APPEARANCES—Series: Chris Rorchek, *Code Red*, ABC, 1981-82; title role, *The Highwayman*, NBC, 1988. Pilots: Bo Carlson, *Stunts Unlimited*, ABC, 1980; Chris Rorchek, *Code Red*, ABC, 1981; Eli Howe, *No Man's Land*, NBC, 1984; title role, *The Highwayman*, NBC, 1987; Denny Colt/title role, *The Spirit*, ABC, 1987. Episodic: *The Dating Game*, 1978. Movies: Roy, *The Incredible Journey of Doctor Meg Laurel*, CBS, 1979; Tommy Sellers, *This Wife for Hire*, ABC, 1985. Specials: *Battle of the Network Stars*, ABC, 1981.

RELATED CAREER—Model.

NON-RELATED CAREER—National spokesperson for the John Rossi Youth Foundation Movement; also worked as a cook and a bouncer.

SIDELIGHTS: RECREATIONS—Tae kwon do.

ADDRESSES: AGENT—Triad Artists, 10100 Santa Monica Boulevard, 16th Floor, Los Angeles, CA 90067.*

*   *   *

JONES, Terry   1942-

PERSONAL: Born February 1, 1942, in Colwyn Bay, North Wales; son of Alick George Parry (a bank clerk) and Dilys Louisa (Newnes) Jones; married Alison Telfer (a botanist); children: Sally, Bill. EDUCATION: Attended Oxford University, 1961-64.

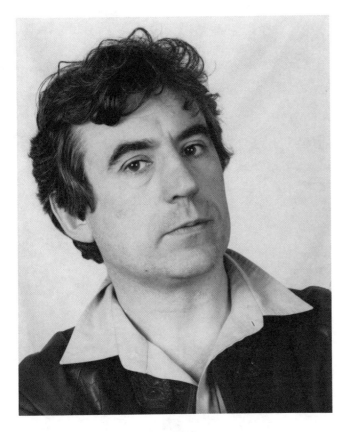

TERRY JONES

VOCATION: Actor, director, and writer.

CAREER: Also see *WRITINGS* below. PRINCIPAL STAGE APPEARANCES—Various roles, *Monty Python's First Farewell Tour,* Drury Lane Theatre, London, 1974; various roles, *Monty Python Live!,* City Center Theatre, New York City, 1976; various roles, *Monty Python Live at the Hollywood Bowl,* Hollywood Bowl, Los Angeles, CA, 1980.

MAJOR TOURS—As a member of the comedy troupe Monty Python (with Graham Chapman, John Cleese, Terry Gilliam, Eric Idle, and Michael Palin) in concert tours of U.S., U.K., and Canadian cities, during the 1970s.

PRINCIPAL FILM APPEARANCES—Various roles, *And Now for Something Completely Different,* Columbia, 1972; Sir Bedevere, not-quite-dead corpse, Dennis' wife, head of the Three-Headed Knight, Knight Who Says ''Ni'', and Herbert, *Monty Python and the Holy Grail,* Cinema V, 1975; poacher, *Jabberwocky,* Cinema V, 1977; mother of Brian, Colin, Simon the Holy Man, Bob Hoskins, and saintly passerby, *Monty Python's Life of Brian* (also known as *The Life of Brian*), Warner Brothers/Orion, 1979; various roles, *Monty Python Live at the Hollywood Bowl,* Columbia, 1982; various roles, *Monty Python's The Meaning of Life,* Celandine-Monty Python Partnership/Universal, 1983; King Arnulf, *Erik the Viking,* Orion, 1989. Also appeared in *Pleasure at Her Majesty's,* Roger Graef, 1976; and in *The Secret Policeman's Ball,* Tigon-Amnesty International, 1979.

PRINCIPAL FILM WORK—Director: (With Terry Gilliam) *Monty Python and the Holy Grail,* Cinema V, 1975; *Monty Python's Life*

of Brian (also known as *The Life of Brian*), Warner Brothers/Orion, 1979; *Monty Python's The Meaning of Life,* Celandine/Monty Python Partnership/Universal, 1983; *Personal Services,* VIP-Vestron, 1987; *Erik the Viking,* Orion, 1989.

PRINCIPAL TELEVISION APPEARANCES—Series: *Do Not Adjust Your Set,* BBC, 1968; *Complete and Utter History of Britain,* BBC, 1969; *Monty Python's Flying Circus,* BBC, 1969-74, then PBS, 1974-82; *Ripping Yarns,* BBC, 1976-77, then PBS, 1979. Movies: *Pythons in Deutschland,* Bavaria Atelier, 1971.

RELATED CAREER—Member, Monty Python (a comedy troupe), 1969—.

WRITINGS: See production details above, unless indicated. FILM—(With Monty Python [Graham Chapman, John Cleese, Terry Gilliam, Michael Palin, and Eric Idle]) *And Now for Something Completely Different,* 1972; (with Monty Python) *Monty Python and the Holy Grail,* 1975, published by Methuen, 1977, and as *Monty Python's Second Film: A First Draft,* Methuen, 1977; (with Monty Python) *Monty Python's Life of Brian,* 1979, published in *Monty Python's Life of Brian (of Nazareth) [and] Montypythonscrapbook,* Grosset, 1979; (with Monty Python) *Monty Python Live at the Hollywood Bowl,* 1982; (with Monty Python; also songwriter) *Monty Python's The Meaning of Life,* 1983, published by Methuen, 1983; (with Laura Phillips) *Labyrinth,* Tri-Star, 1986; *Erik the Viking,* 1989. TELEVISION—Series: *The Frost Report,* BBC, 1965-67; *Do Not Adjust Your Sets,* 1968; *Complete and Utter History of Britain,* 1969; (with Monty Python) *Monty Python's Flying Circus,* 1969-74; (with Michael Palin) *Ripping Yarns,* PBS, 1979. Movies: (With Monty Python) *Pythons in Deutschland,* 1971. Plays: *Secrets,* BBC, 1973.

OTHER—(With Monty Python) *Monty Python's Big Red Book,* edited by Eric Idle, published by Methuen, 1972, then Warner Books, 1975, and in *The Complete Works of Shakespeare and Monty Python,* Methuen, 1981; (with Monty Python) *The Brand New Monty Python Book,* edited by Idle, published by Eyre Methuen, 1973, then as *The Brand New Monty Python Papperbok,* Methuen, 1974, and in *The Complete Works of Shakespeare and Monty Python,* 1981; (with Monty Python) *Monty Python's Life of Brian (of Nazareth) [and] Montypythonscrapbook,* Grosset, 1979; (with Michael Palin) *Bert Fegg's Nasty Book for Boys and Girls,* Methuen, 1974, then as *Dr. Fegg's Nasty Book of Knowledge,* Peter Bedrick Books, 1985; (with Palin) *Ripping Yarns,* Methuen, 1978, then Pantheon, 1979; (with Palin) *More Ripping Yarns,* Methuen, 1980; *Chaucer's Knight: The Portrait of a Medieval Mercenary* (nonfiction), Louisiana State University Press, 1980; *Fairy Tales* (juvenile), Schocken, 1981; *The Saga of Erik the Viking* (juvenile), Schocken, 1983; (with Palin) *Dr. Fegg's Encyclopaedia of All World Knowledge,* Peter Bedrick Books, 1985; *Nicobobinus,* Peter Bedrick Books, 1986; *Goblins of the Labyrinth,* Holt & Company, 1986; *Attacks of Opinion,* Penguin, 1988; *The Curse of the Vampire's Socks,* Pavilion, 1989.

RECORDINGS: ALBUMS—All with Monty Python: *Monty Python's Flying Circus,* BBC Records, 1969; *Another Monty Python Record,* Charisma, 1970; *Monty Python's Previous Record,* Charisma, 1972; *Monty Python's Matching Tie and Handkerchief,* Charisma, 1973, then Arista, 1975; *Monty Python Live at Drury Lane,* Charisma, 1974; *The Album of the Soundtrack of the Trailer of the Film ''Monty Python and the Holy Grail,''* Arista, 1975; *Monty Python Live at City Center,* Arista, 1976; *Monty Python's Instant Record Collection,* Charisma, 1977; *Monty Python's Life of Brian,* Warner Brothers, 1979; *Monty Python's Contractual Obli-*

gation Album, Arista, 1980; *Monty Python's The Meaning of Life,* Columbia Records, 1983.

AWARDS: Press Critics of Great Britain Award, Best Comedy Show, 1977, for *Ripping Yarns;* (co-winner) Golden Palm Award from the Cannes International Film Festival, 1983, for *Monty Python's The Meaning of Life.*

OTHER SOURCES: Contemporary Authors, Vol. 116, Gale, 1986.

ADDRESSES: OFFICE—Fegg Features, Ltd., 68-A Delancey Street, London NW1 7RY, England.

K

KACZMAREK, Jane

PERSONAL: Born December 21, in Milwaukee, WI.

VOCATION: Actress.

CAREER: PRINCIPAL STAGE APPEARANCES—Lizzy Bennet, *Pride and Prejudice,* Long Wharf Theatre, New Haven, CT, 1985; Diane Newbury, *The Hands of Its Enemy,* Manhattan Theatre Club, City Center Theatre, New York City, 1986. Also appeared in *Timon of Athens* and *The Suicide,* both Yale Repertory Theatre, New Haven, CT, 1980; *Rip Van Winkle or "The Works," The Man Who Could See through Time,* and *Love's Labour's Lost,* all Yale Repertory Theatre, 1981-82.

PRINCIPAL FILM APPEARANCES—Mrs. Wilkes, *Uncommon Valor,* Paramount, 1983; Katherine Holloway, *Door to Door,* Shapiro, 1984; Ann Raftis, *Falling in Love,* Paramount, 1984; Emily, *The Heavenly Kid,* Orion, 1985; Gail Cornell, *D.O.A.,* Touchstone, 1988; Robyn, *Vice Versa,* Columbia, 1988; Linda, *All's Fair* (also known as *Skirmish*), New Century/Vista, 1988.

PRINCIPAL TELEVISION APPEARANCES—Series: Connie Lehman, *The Paper Chase: The Second Year,* Showtime, 1983-84; Mary Newell Abbott, *Hometown,* CBS, 1985. Mini-Series: Nina Stern, *I'll Take Manhattan,* CBS, 1987. Pilots: Margie Spoleto, *For Lovers Only,* ABC, 1982. Episodic: Officer Clara Tilsky, *Hill Street Blues,* NBC, 1981; Nurse Sandy Burns, *St. Elsewhere,* NBC, 1982; Susan Glaspell, "Journey into Genius," *American Playhouse,* PBS, 1988. Movies: Mrs. Hall, *Something about Amelia,* ABC, 1984; Donna Olian, *Flight 90: Disaster on the Potomac,* NBC, 1984; Alicia Frost, *The Right of the People,* ABC, 1986; Susan, *The Christmas Gift,* CBS, 1986; Dr. Paula Bolet, *The Three Kings,* ABC, 1987. Specials: Joanna Brady, *The Last Leaf,* syndicated, 1984.*

*   *   *

KAIN, Amber   1975-

PERSONAL: Full name, Amber Peyote Khykhan Kain; born November 2, 1975, in New York, NY; daughter of Gylan (an actor, writer, and poet) and Karen O. (a costume designer; maiden name, Perry) Kain. EDUCATION: Attended the Jose Feliciano School of Performing Arts.

VOCATION: Actress.

CAREER: PRINCIPAL STAGE APPEARANCES—Little girl, *Col-*

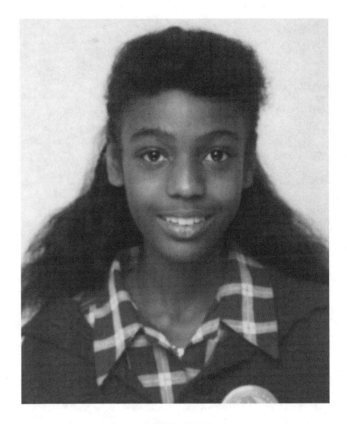

AMBER KAIN

ored Museum, New York Shakespeare Festival, Public Theatre, New York City, 1986; Janet Harris, *Good Black . . .,* Harry DeJur Playhouse, New York City, 1988. Also appeared as Annie, *Alice in Wonderland,* Jose Feliciano Theatre, New York City; in *Ebony,* Playwrights Horizons, New York City; and in *P.S. We Love You,* Riverside Theatre, New York City.

FILM DEBUT—Little girl, *The Brother from Another Planet,* Cinecom International, 1983. PRINCIPAL FILM APPEARANCES—*Angel Heart,* Tri-Star, 1987; also appeared in *Frederick Douglass: American Life,* and *Hot Shot.*

TELEVISON DEBUT—Maggie, *Fast Forward Future,* PBS, 1988. PRINCIPAL TELEVISION APPEARANCES—Episodic: Homeless girl, "Slake's Limbo," *Wonderworks,* PBS, 1988.

PRINCIPAL RADIO APPEARANCES—Series: Storyteller, *Pinkney's*

Place, WBAI, New York City, 1987-88; host, *Summer in the City,* WNYE, New York City, 1988.

WRITINGS: Thank You for Being a Friend, Erza Jeats Foundation.

MEMBER: Screen Actors Guild, Actors' Equity Association, American Federation of Television and Radio Artists.

SIDELIGHTS: RECREATIONS—Ice skating, music, writing, horseback riding, and video games.

ADDRESSES: HOME—1505 Park Avenue, New York, NY 10029. AGENT—Terrific Talent, 419 Park Avenue, New York, NY 10016.

*　　*　　*

KAPOOR, Shashi 1938-

PERSONAL: Born March 18, 1938, in Calcutta, India; son of Prithviraj Kapoor (an actor and theatre company manager); married Jennifer Kendal (an actress; died, 1985); children: Kunal and Karan (sons), Sanjana (a daughter).

VOCATION: Actor.

CAREER: FILM DEBUT—*Aag,* 1950. PRINCIPAL FILM APPEARANCES—Prem Sagar, *The Householder* (also known as *Gharbar*), Royal, 1963; Sanju, *Shakespeare Wallah,* Continental Distributing, 1966; Amaz, *A Matter of Innocence* (also known as *Pretty Polly*), Universal, 1968; Vikram, *Bombay Talkie,* Merchant-Ivory, 1970; title role, *Siddhartha,* Columbia, 1972; Javed Khan, *Junoon* (also known *Obsession*), Film-Valas/Glanard Wood, 1978; the Nawab, *Heat and Dust,* Curzon/Universal, 1983; Samsthanaka, *Utsav* (also known as *Festival*), Film Valas, 1984; Rafi Rahman, *Sammy and Rosie Get Laid,* Cinecom, 1987; Chandra Singh, *The Deceivers,* Cinecom International, 1988. Also appeared in *Char Diwari,* 1960; *Kalyug,* 1980; *Vijeta* (also known as *Conquest*), Film Valas, 1983; *New Delhi Times,* PK Communication Private, 1987; *Anjaam,* 1987; and in more than two hundred films in India.

PRINCIPAL FILM WORK—Producer: *Junoon,* Film-Valas/Glanard Wood, 1978; *Vijeta,* Film Valas, 1983; (with Dharampriya Das) *Utsav,* Film Valas, 1984. Also producer (with Dharampriya Das), *36 Chowringee Lane.*

RELATED CAREER—Assistant stage manager, prop boy, and actor with the Prithvi Theatre Company, 1957—; actor with Jennifer Kendal's troupe, Shakespeariana; founder, Prithvi Theatre, Juhu Beach, Bombay, India; owner, Film-Valas Production Company.

AWARDS: Best Actor Award (India), 1986, for *New Delhi Times.* *

*　　*　　*

KAUFMAN, Lloyd 1945-
(Louis Su, Samuel Weil)

PERSONAL: Born December 30, 1945, in New York, NY; son of Stanley Lloyd (a lawyer) and Ruth (Fried) Kaufman; married Patricia Swinney (a film buyer), July 13, 1974; children: Lily-

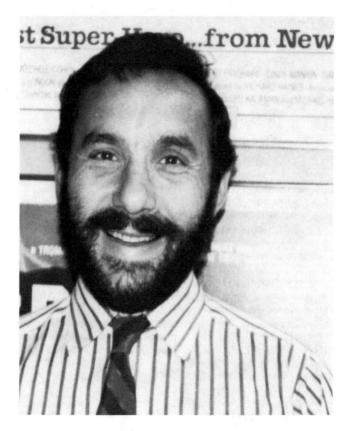

LLOYD KAUFMAN

Hayes, Lisbeth, Charlotte. EDUCATION: Yale University, B.A., 1969.

VOCATION: Director, producer, cinematographer, and screenwriter.

CAREER: Also see *WRITINGS* below. FILM DEBUT—Abacrombie, *The Battle of Love's Return,* Standard Films, 1971. PRINCIPAL FILM APPEARANCES—Drunk, *Rocky,* United Artists, 1976; usher, *Slow Dancing in the Big City,* United Artists, 1978; Lieutenant Commander Kaufman, *The Final Countdown,* United Artists, 1980.

FIRST FILM WORK—Producer (with Garrard Glen and Frank Vitale), director, and editor, *The Battle of Love's Return,* Standard Films, 1971. PRINCIPAL FILM WORK—(As Louis Su) Producer (with David Wynn) and editor, *The Divine Obsession,* Oppidan, 1975; location executive, *Saturday Night Fever,* Paramount, 1977; producer (with Charles Kaufman and David Stitt) and cinematographer, *The Secret Dreams of Mona Q.,* Troma, 1977; (as Louis Su) cinematographer, *My Sex Rated Wife,* Melody, 1977; cinematographer, *Lustful Desires,* Tigon, 1978; production supervisor, *Slow Dancing in the Big City,* United Artists, 1978; associate producer, *Mother's Day,* United Film Distribution, 1980; associate producer and unit production manager, *The Final Countdown,* United Artists, 1980; production manager, *My Dinner with Andre,* New Yorker, 1981; (as Samuel Weil) producer (with Michael Herz), director, and cinematographer, *Squeeze Play,* Troma, 1981; executive producer (with Herz), *Adventure of the Action Hunters* (also known as *Two for the Money*), Troma, 1982; (as Samuel Weil) producer (with Herz), director (with Herz), and cinematographer, *Waitress* (also known as *Soup to Nuts*), Troma, 1982; (as Samuel Weil) producer (with Herz), director (with Herz), and cinematographer, *Stuck on You!*, Troma, 1983; (as Samuel Weil) producer (with Herz), director (with Herz), and cinematographer, *The First Turn-On!!*, Troma, 1984; executive producer (with Herz), *When Nature Calls*, Troma, 1984; executive producer (with Herz), *Screamplay*, Troma, 1984; producer (with Herz, Richard W. Haines, and John Michaels) and creative consultant, *Splatter University*, Troma, 1984; executive producer (with Herz), *Girls School Screamer*, Troma, 1984; executive producer (with Herz), *The Dark Side of Midnight*, Troma, 1984.

(As Samuel Weil) Executive producer (with Herz), director (with Herz), and cinematographer (with James London), *The Toxic Avenger*, Troma, 1985; executive producer (with Herz), *The G.I. Executioner*, Troma, 1985; (as Samuel Weil) producer (with Herz), director (with Richard W. Haines), and camera operator, *Class of Nuke 'em High* (also known as *Nuke 'em High*), Troma, 1986; executive producer (with Herz), *Combat Shock*, Troma, 1986; executive producer (with Herz), *Lust for Freedom* (also known as *Georgia County Lock-Up*), Troma, 1987; producer (with Herz), *Surf Nazis Must Die*, Troma, 1987; executive producer (with Herz), *Monster in the Closet*, Troma, 1987; executive producer (with Herz), *Blood Hook*, Troma, 1987; producer (with Herz) and (as Samuel Weil) director, *War* (also known as *Troma's War*), Troma, 1988; executive producer (with Herz), *Redneck Zombies*, Trans World Entertainment, 1988; executive producer (with Herz), *War Cat*, Trans World Entertainment, 1988; (as Samuel Weil) producer (with Herz) director (with Herz), *The Toxic Avenger, Part II*, Troma, 1989.

RELATED CAREER—Founder and president, Troma, Inc., 1971—.

WRITINGS: See production details above, unless indicated. FILM—(Also composer with Andre Golino) *The Battle of Love's Return*, 1971; (with Theodore Gershuny) *Sugar Cookies*, General, 1973; (as Louis Su; with David Wynn and Robert Kalen) *The Divine Obsession*, 1975; (as Samuel Weil; with others) *Stuck on You!*, 1983; (as Samuel Weil; additional material) *The First Turn-On!!*, 1984; (with Joe Ritter, Gay Terry, and Stuart Strutin) *The Toxic Avenger*, 1985; (as Samuel Weil; with Haines, Strutin, and Mark Rudnitsky) *Class of Nuke 'em High*, 1986; (with Michael Dana, Eric Hattler, and Thomas Martinek) *War*, 1988; (as Samuel Weil; with Terry) *The Toxic Avenger, Part II*, 1989.

ADDRESSES: OFFICE—Troma Building, 733 Ninth Avenue, New York, NY 10019.

*   *   *

KELLEY, William   1929-

PERSONAL: Born May 27, 1929, in Staten Island, NY; son of Edward Thomas (a lawyer) and Alethea (a lawyer; maiden name, Waldegrave) Kelley; married Cornelia Ann Chamberlin (an artist), September 18, 1954; children: Maura, Shaun. EDUCATION: Brown University, B.A., 1955; Harvard University, M.A., 1957. MILITARY: U.S. Air Force, sergeant, 1947-50.

VOCATION: Screenwriter and producer.

CAREER: Also see *WRITINGS* below. PRINCIPAL TELEVISION APPEARANCES—Pilots: Kelly, *Key Tortuga*, CBS, 1981. PRINCIPAL TELEVISION WORK—Pilots: Producer, *Key Tortuga*, CBS,

1981. Movies: Co-producer, *The Blue Lightning*, CBS, 1986. RELATED CAREER—Editor, Doubleday & Company, New York City, 1957-58, then West Coast editor, San Francisco, CA, 1958-61; editor, McGraw-Hill Book Company, New York City, 1961-62.

WRITINGS: FILM—(With Earl W. Wallace) *Witness*, Paramount, 1985, published by Pocket Books, 1985; also *Sitka*. TELEVISION—Pilots: (With Michael Bendix) *Key Tortuga*, CBS, 1981. Episodic: *Three for the Road*, CBS, 1975; also *Route 66*, CBS; *How the West Was Won*, ABC; *Gunsmoke*, CBS; *Kung Fu*, ABC; *Judd for the Defense*, ABC. Movies: (With Jeb Rosebrook) *The Winds of Kitty Hawk*, NBC, 1978; *The Demon Murder Case*, NBC, 1983; *The Blue Lightning*, CBS, 1986. Specials: *True Believer*, HBO, 1986. OTHER—All novels, unless indicated. *Gemini*, Doubleday, 1959; *Miracle in the Evening* (biography), Doubleday, 1961; *The God Hunters*, Doubleday, 1964; *The Tyree Legend*, Simon & Schuster, 1979.

AWARDS: Spur Award from the Western Writers of America, Best Western Television Script, 1975, for *Gunsmoke*, and 1978, for *How the West Was Won*; Academy Award, Best Original Screenplay, 1986, for *Witness*.

MEMBER: Phi Beta Kappa, E Clampus Vitus, Harvard Club, Brown Club, California Yacht Club, Mammoth Bucket Brigade, Riviera Country Club (Los Angeles), Los Angeles Athletic Club.

ADDRESSES: HOME—P.O. Box 18, Mammoth Lakes, CA 93546. OFFICE—501 S. Fuller Avenue, Los Angeles, CA 90036. AGENT—Ned Brown, 407 N. Maple Drive, Suite 228, Beverly Hills, CA 90210.*

*   *   *

KELLY, Marguerite   1959-

PERSONAL: Born December 7, 1959, in Washington, DC; daughter of Thomas Vincent (a writer) and Marguerite Alice (a writer; maiden name, Lelong) Kelly; married Tony Rizzoli (an actor), December 19, 1981. EDUCATION: Attended Catholic University; trained for the stage at Circle in the Square and with Gene Bua.

VOCATION: Actress.

CAREER: STAGE DEBUT—Rebecca Gibbs, *Our Town*, Arena Stage, Washington, DC, 1972. OFF-BROADWAY DEBUT—Kitty, *Taking Steps*, York Theatre Company, Church of the Heavenly Rest, 1986, for sixteen performances. BROADWAY DEBUT—Essie, *The Devil's Disciple*, Circle in the Square, New York City, 1988. PRINCIPAL STAGE APPEARANCES—Time, *The Winter's Tale*, Folger Theatre, Washington, DC, 1973; Melinda, *Inherit the Wind*, Arena Stage, Washington, DC, 1973; Pamela, *Five Finger Exercise*, Studio Theatre, Washington, DC, 1979; Yellow Peril, *Da*, and Babe, *Crimes of the Heart*, both ACE-Charlotte's Repertory Theatre, Charlotte, NC, 1984; Ella Delahay, *Charley's Aunt*, GeVa Theatre, Rochester, NY, 1987.

MAJOR TOURS—Rebecca Gibbs, *Our Town*, and Melinda, *Inherit the Wind*, with Arena Stage, Soviet cities, both 1973.

TELEVISION DEBUT—Shauna, *Kate and Allie*, NBC, 1988.

also *The Mary Tyler Moore Show,* CBS, 1974; Sharon Cleary, *St. Elsewhere,* NBC, 1986; *Murder, She Wrote,* CBS, 1986; *Barnaby Jones,* CBS; *Emergency,* NBC; *The Rookies,* ABC; *Harry O,* ABC; *The Rockford Files,* NBC. Movies: Beatrice Hallward, *The Picture of Dorian Gray,* ABC, 1973; Lucy Mercer, *Eleanor and Franklin,* ABC, 1976; Lucy Mercer, *Eleanor and Franklin: The White House Years,* ABC, 1977; Joyce Cappelletti, *Something for Joey,* CBS, 1977; Miranda McLloyd, *A Perfect Match,* CBS, 1980; Kathy Mitchell, *Attack on Fear,* CBS, 1984; Katherine Beck, *His Mistress,* NBC, 1984; Jean Gelson, *Baby Girl Scott,* CBS, 1987; Elaine Bradshaw Dropman, *Nutcracker: Money, Madness, and Murder,* NBC, 1987. Specials: Susan Palmer, "Home Sweet Homeless," *CBS Schoolbreak,* CBS, 1988; also *The Last of Mrs. Lincoln,* PBS.

AWARDS: Five Emmy Award nominations for *Lou Grant.*

ADDRESSES: AGENT—Smith-Freedman and Associates, 850 Seventh Avenue, New York, NY 10019.*

*   *   *

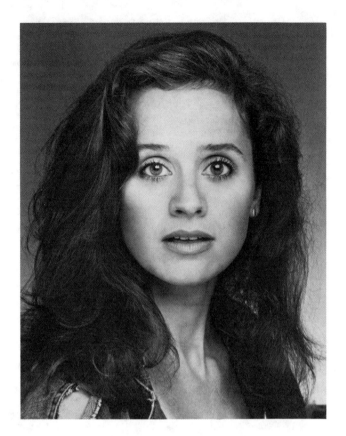

MARGUERITE KELLY

MEMBER: American Federation of Television and Radio Artists.

ADDRESSES: AGENT—Monty Silver Agency, 145 W. 45th Street, Suite 1204, New York, NY 10036.

*   *   *

KELSEY, Linda   1946-

PERSONAL: Born July 28, 1946, in Minneapolis, MN; married Glenn Strand; children: Sophia Nellist, Margit Isabella. EDUCATION: Received B.F.A. from the University of Minnesota.

VOCATION: Actress.

CAREER: PRINCIPAL STAGE APPEARANCES—Miranda, *The Tempest,* Teresa, *The Hostage,* and Maggie, *The Winners,* all Tyrone Guthrie Theatre, Minneapolis, MN; also appeared in productions of *The Crucible, Summer and Smoke,* and *Duet for One,* all in Los Angeles, CA.

PRINCIPAL FILM APPEARANCES—Betty, *The Midnight Man,* Universal, 1974.

PRINCIPAL TELEVISION APPEARANCES—Series: Gwen Bogert, *Doc,* CBS, 1975-76; Billie Newman, *Lou Grant,* CBS, 1977-82; Kate Harper, *Day by Day,* NBC, 1988—. Mini-Series: Peg, *Captains and the Kings,* NBC, 1976. Episodic: Cynthia McGrew, *Spencer's Pilots,* CBS, 1976; Nurse Baker, *M*A*S*H,* CBS, 1974;

KEMPSON, Rachel   1910-

PERSONAL: Born May 28, 1910, in Dartmouth, England; daughter of Eric William Edward (a headmaster) and Beatrice Hamilton (Ashwell) Kempson; married Michael Redgrave (an actor), July 18, 1935 (died, March 21, 1985); children: Vanessa, Lynn, Corin. EDUCATION: Trained for the stage at the Royal Academy of Dramatic Art.

VOCATION: Actress.

CAREER: STAGE DEBUT—Hero, *Much Ado about Nothing,* Shakespeare Memorial Theatre, Stratford-on-Avon, U.K., 1933. LONDON DEBUT—Blanca, *The Lady from Alfaqueque,* Westminster Theatre, 1933. PRINCIPAL STAGE APPEARANCES—Juliet, *Romeo and Juliet,* and Ophelia, *Hamlet,* both Shakespeare Memorial Theatre, Stratford-on-Avon, U.K., 1933; Ariel, *The Tempest,* Olivia, *Twelfth Night,* Princess, *Love's Labour's Lost,* and Titania, *Hero and Juliet,* all Shakespeare Memorial Theatre, 1934; Christina, *Two Kingdoms,* Savoy Theatre, London, 1934; Anne, *The Witch,* and Stella, *The Sacred Flame,* both Oxford Playhouse, Oxford, U.K., 1935; Naomi, *Flowers of the Forest,* Liverpool Repertory Company, Liverpool Playhouse, Liverpool, U.K., 1935; Yvonne, *Youth at the Helm,* Eulalia, *A Hundred Years Old,* Anne of Bohemia, *Richard of Bordeaux,* Anne, *The Wind and the Rain,* Viola, *Twelfth Night,* Agnes Boyd, *Boyd's Shop,* and Victoria, *A Storm in a Teacup,* all Liverpool Repertory Company, Liverpool Playhouse, 1935-36; Princess of France, *Love's Labour's Lost,* Old Vic Theatre, London, 1936; Celia, *Volpone,* Westminster Theatre, London 1937; Viola, *Twelfth Night,* Oxford University Dramatic Society, Oxford, U.K., 1937; Maria, *The School for Scandal,* Queen's Theatre, London, 1937; Jane, *The Shoemaker's Holiday,* Playhouse Theatre, 1938; Faith Ingalls, *Wingless Victory,* Phoenix Theatre, London, 1943; Lucy Forrest, *Uncle Harry,* Garrick Theatre, London, 1944; Marianne, *Jacobowsky and the Colonel,* Piccadilly Theatre, London, 1945; Charlotte, *Fatal Curiosity,* Arts Theatre, London, 1946; Chris Forbes, *Happy as Kings,* and Councillor Dr. Rosamond Long, *The Sparks Fly Upward,* both Q Theatre, London, 1947; Joan, *The Paragon,* Fortune Theatre, London, 1948; Violet Jackson, *The Return of the Prodigal,* Globe Theatre, London, 1948; title role, *Candida,* Oxford Playhouse, 1949.

Hilda Taylor-Snell, *Venus Observed,* and Katie, *Top of the Ladder,* both St. James's Theatre, London, 1950; Maman, *The Happy Time,* St. James's Theatre, 1952; Queen Elizabeth, *Richard III,* and Regan, *King Lear,* both Shakespeare Memorial Theatre Company, Shakespeare Memorial Theatre, 1953; Octavia, *Antony and Cleopatra,* Shakespeare Memorial Theatre Company, Shakespeare Memorial Theatre, then Princes Theatre, London, both 1953; Mrs. Thea Elvsted, *Hedda Gabler,* Lyric Hammersmith Theatre, London, then Westminster Theatre, both 1954; Theodora, *Not for Children,* Gate Theatre Company, Belfast, Ireland, 1955; Cora Fellowes, *The Mulberry Bush,* Mrs. Ann Putnam, *The Crucible,* Evelyn, *The Death of Satan,* Miss Black Panorbis, *Cards of Identity,* and Mrs. Mi Tzu, *The Good Woman of Setzuan,* all English Stage Company, Royal Court Theatre, London, 1956; Lady Capulet, *Romeo and Juliet,* Dionyza, *Pericles,* and Ursula, *Much Ado about Nothing,* all Shakespeare Memorial Theatre Company, Shakespeare Memorial Theatre, Stratford-on-Avon, 1958; Mary, *Teresa of Avila,* Dublin Theatre Festival, Dublin, Ireland, then Vaudeville Theatre, London, both 1961; Polina Andreyevna, *The Seagull,* and Martha, *Saint Joan of the Stockyards,* both Queen's Theatre, 1964; Chorus, *Samson Agonistes,* and Lady Mary, *Lionel and Clarissa,* both Yvonne Arnaud Theatre, Guildford, U.K., 1965; older lady, *A Sense of Detachment,* Royal Court Theatre, 1972; Lady Childress, *Gomes,* Queen's Theatre, 1973; Nancy, *The Freeway,* National Theatre Company, Old Vic Theatre, 1974; Blanche, *A Family and a Fortune,* Apollo Theatre, London, 1975; Bron, *The Old Country,* Queen's Theatre, 1977. Also appeared as Jean Howard, *Under One Roof,* Richmond, U.K., 1940; and Queen Margaret, *The Saxon Saint,* Dunfermline Abbey, U.K., 1949.

MAJOR TOURS—Naomi, *Family Portrait,* U.K. cities, 1941; Naomi, *Noah,* U.K. cities, 1942; Mrs. Bradman, *Blithe Spirit,* U.K. cities, 1942; Octavia, *Antony and Cleopatra,* European cities, 1953; Mrs. Thea Elvsted, *Hedda Gabler,* European cities, 1955; Lady Capulet, *Romeo and Juliet,* Soviet cities, 1958.

PRINCIPAL FILM APPEARANCES—Emily Maurier, *A Woman's Vengeance,* Universal, 1947; Celia Mitchell, *The Captive Heart,* Ealing Studios, 1948; Mrs. Waltby, *The Sea Shall Not Have Them,* United Artists, 1955; Bridget Allworthy, *Tom Jones,* Lopert, 1963; Mildred Hoving, *The Third Secret,* Twentieth Century-Fox, 1964; Madame Fournier, *Curse of the Fly,* Twentieth Century-Fox, 1965; Ellen, *Georgy Girl,* Columbia, 1966; Mrs. Stoddard, *Grand Prix,* Metro-Goldwyn-Mayer, 1966; Mrs. Tremayne, *The Jokers,* Universal, 1967; Mrs. Codrington, *The Charge of the Light Brigade,* United Artists, 1968; Sister Harvey, *Thank You All Very Much* (also known as *A Touch of Love*), Columbia, 1969; Mrs. Ashby-Kydd, *Two Gentlemen Sharing,* American International, 1969; Mrs. Raskin, *The Virgin Soldiers,* Columbia, 1970; Mrs. Fairfax, *Jane Eyre,* British Lion, 1971; Lady Belfield, *Out of Africa,* Universal, 1985; prioress, *Stealing Heaven,* Scotti Brothers Pictures, 1989. Also appeared in *Girl in Distress* (also known as *Jeannie*), General Films Distributors, 1941.

PRINCIPAL TELEVISION APPEARANCES—Mini-Series: Duchess of Marlborough, *Jennie: Lady Randolph Churchill,* PBS, 1975; Lady Manners, "The Jewel in the Crown," *Masterpiece Theatre,* PBS, 1984; Grace Willison, "The Black Tower," *Mystery!,* PBS, 1988; also "Love for Lydia" *Masterpiece Theatre,* PBS. Movies: Lady Lorradaile, *Little Lord Fauntleroy,* CBS, 1980; Hortense, *Camille,* CBS, 1984. Specials: Mrs. Fairfax, "Jane Eyre," *Hallmark Hall of Fame,* NBC, 1971. Also appeared in *Sweet Wine of Youth* and *Kate the Good Neighbour.*

WRITINGS: *Life among the Redgraves* (autobiography), Dalton, 1988.

ADDRESSES: OFFICE—42 Ebury Mews, London SW1, England.*

*   *   *

KENNY, Jack   1958-

PERSONAL: Born March 9, 1958, in Chicago, IL; son of John Joseph, Jr. (a business manager) and Sally (Cheviak) Kenny. EDUCATION: Attended the University of North Carolina, Greensboro, 1976-78; Juilliard Theatre Center, B.F.A. drama, 1982. POLITICS: Democrat.

VOCATION: Actor and screenwriter.

CAREER: STAGE DEBUT—Ronnie, *All the Girls Came Out to Play,* Barn Dinner Theatre, Greensboro, NC, 1978, for thirty performances. LONDON DEBUT—Junior Mister and President Prexy, *The Cradle Will Rock,* Old Vic Theatre, 1985, for forty performances. PRINCIPAL STAGE APPEARANCES—Fisherman and Pandar, *Pericles,* Loyal, *Tartuffe,* and M, "Play" in *Play and Other Plays,* all Acting Company, American Place Theatre, New York City, 1983; Tranio, *The Taming of the Shrew,* Huntington Theatre Company, Boston, MA, 1983; President Prexy, *The Cradle Will Rock,* Plaza Theatre, Dallas, TX, 1984; various roles, *Pieces of 8,* Acting Company, Public Theatre, New York City, 1984; Alphonse, Grover, Troll, Yeti, Mr. Coffee, Mme. Nhu, Gus,

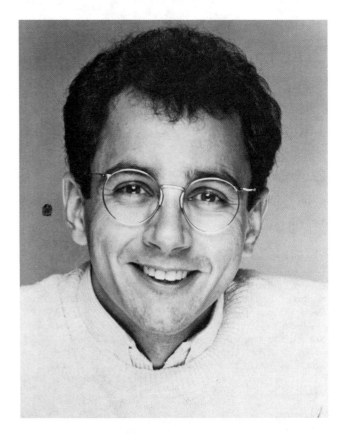

JACK KENNY

and Nicky, *On the Verge,* Syracuse Stage, Syracuse, NY, 1986; Rubin, *Cafe Crown,* Public Theatre, 1988, then Brooks Atkinson Theatre, New York City, 1989. Also appeared as Naphtali and Chaikin, *The Rise of David Levinsky,* George Street Playhouse, New Brunswick, NJ, then in New York City; James Taxi, *In a Pig's Valise,* Center Stage, Baltimore, MD; Max, *A Quiet End,* St. Louis Repertory Theatre, St. Louis, MO; La Fleche and Jacques, *The Miser,* Lincoln Center Insitiute, New York City; Shishkin, *Philistines,* Perry Street Theatre, New York City; Craig and Grady, *The Normal Heart,* and Jake Seward, *Rum and Coke,* both Public Theatre; Fields, *Emily,* Manhattan Theatre Club, New York City; Silas Slick, *Naughty Marietta,* New York City Opera, New York City; Sir Jaspar Fidget, *The Country Wife,* Acting Company, New York City; the Pope, *Issue? I Don't Even Know You!,* Prince Alf, *Cinderella Waltz,* and Tranio, *The Taming of the Shrew,* all in New York City.

TELEVISION DEBUT—Jerry Lee Lutin, *Miami Vice,* NBC, 1987. PRINCIPAL TELEVISION APPEARANCES—Episodic: Stevens, *The Guiding Light,* CBS. Specials: *Daytime Emmy Awards,* CBS.

RELATED CAREER—Actor in television commercials and industrial films.

WRITINGS: TELEVISION—*Square One,* PBS, 1987.

MEMBER: Actors' Equity Association, Screen Actors Guild, American Federation of Television and Radio Artists.

ADDRESSES: AGENT—Select Artists Representatives, 337 W. 43rd Street, New York, NY 10036.

*   *   *

KENTON, Maxwell
See SOUTHERN, Terry

*   *   *

KILMER, Val

PERSONAL: Born in Los Angeles, CA; married Joanna Whalley (an actress), March, 1988. EDUCATION: Trained for the stage at the Juilliard School.

VOCATION: Actor and playwright.

CAREER: Also see *WRITINGS* below. STAGE DEBUT—Michael Baumann, *How It All Began,* New York Shakespeare Festival, Public Theatre, New York City, 1981. PRINCIPAL STAGE APPEARANCES—Servant to Hotspur, *Henry IV, Part I,* New York Shakespeare Festival, Delacorte Theatre, New York City, 1981; Orlando, *As You Like It,* Tyrone Guthrie Theatre, Minneapolis, MN, 1982; Alan Downie, *Slab Boys,* Playhouse Theatre, New York City, 1983; title role, *Hamlet,* Colorado Shakespeare Festival, Boulder, CO, 1988.

FILM DEBUT—Nick Rivers, *Top Secret!,* Paramount, 1984. PRINCIPAL FILM APPEARANCES—Chris Knight, *Real Genius,* TriStar, 1985; Tom "Iceman" Kasanzky, *Top Gun,* Paramount, 1986;

Madmartigan, *Willow,* Metro-Goldwyn-Mayer/United Artists, 1988.

PRINCIPAL TELEVISION APPEARANCES—Movies: Philippe Huron, *The Murders in the Rue Morgue,* CBS, 1986; Robert Eliot Burns, *The Man Who Broke 1,000 Chains,* HBO, 1987. Specials: Eric, *One Too Many,* ABC, 1985.

WRITINGS: STAGE—Co-author, *How It All Began,* New York Shakespeare Festival, Public Theatre, New York City, 1981.

ADDRESSES: AGENT—Creative Artists Agency, 1888 Century Park E., Suite 1400, Los Angeles, CA 90067.*

*   *   *

KINBERG, Judy   1948-

PERSONAL: Born September 15, 1948, in Freeport, NY; daughter of Jack and Rose (Schwartz) Kinberg. EDUCATION: Hofstra University, B.A., theatre, 1970.

VOCATION: Producer.

CAREER: PRINCIPAL TELEVISION WORK—Series: Producer (with Merrill Brockway), *Camera Three,* CBS, 1970-75. Specials: Co-producer, "Pilobolus Dance Theatre" and "Trailblazers of Modern Dance," both *Dance in America,* PBS, 1977; co-producer, "San Francisco Ballet: Romeo and Juliet" and "Choreography by Balanchine, Part III," both *Dance in America,* PBS, 1978; producer, "Out of Our Fathers' House," *Great Performances,* PBS, 1978; co-producer, "Choreography by Balanchine, Part IV," co-producer, "The Martha Graham Dance Company: Clytemnestra," and producer, "The Feld Ballet," all *Dance in America,* PBS, 1979; co-producer, "When Hell Freezes Over I'll Skate," *Theatre in America,* PBS, 1979.

Co-producer, "Two Duets with Choreography by Jerome Robbins and Peter Martins," *Dance in America,* PBS, 1980; co-producer, "The Spellbound Child," "Nureyev and the Joffrey Ballet: In Tribute to Nijinsky," and "The Tempest: Live with the San Francisco Ballet," all *Dance in America,* PBS, 1981; producer, "The Green Table, with the Joffrey Ballet," producer, "Paul Taylor: Two Landmark Dances," co-producer, "Paul Taylor: Three Modern Classics," and co-producer, "Bournonville Dances, with Members of the New York City Ballet," all *Dance in America,* PBS, 1982; "The Magic Flute, with the New York City Ballet," *Dance in America,* PBS, 1983; producer, "San Francisco Ballet: A Song for Dead Warriors," "A Choreographer's Notebook: Stravinsky Piano Ballets by Peter Martins," and "Balanchine, Parts I and II," all *Dance in America,* PBS, 1984; producer (with Emile Ardolino), *He Makes Me Feel Like Dancin',* NBC, 1984; producer, "San Francisco Ballet in Cinderella," *Dance in America,* PBS, 1985; producer, "Mark Morris," "Choreography by Jerome Robbins," and "Dance Theatre of Harlem in A Streetcar Named Desire," all *Dance in America,* PBS, 1986; producer, "In Memory of . . . A Ballet by Jerome Robbins," and "Agnes, the Indomitable de Mille," both *Dance in America,* PBS, 1987; producer, "Paul Taylor: Roses [and] Last Look," "Balanchine and Cunningham: An Evening at American Ballet Theatre," and "Baryshnikov Dances Balanchine," all *Dance in America,* PBS, 1988; producer and director (with Thomas Grimm), "A Night at the Joffrey: Monotones II, Love Songs, [and] Round of Angels," all *Dance in America*, PBS, 1989.

RELATED CAREER—Production secretary for a sports program featuring Frank Gifford, WCBS-TV, New York City, 1970.

AWARDS: First Place Award from the Ninth Annual Dance and Film Video Festival, 1977, for "Trailblazers of Modern Dance," *Dance in America;* Silver Plaque from the Chicago International Film Festival, 1978, for "Choreography by Balanchine, Part III," *Dance in America;* Emmy Award, 1979, for "Choreography by Balanchine, Part IV," *Dance in America;* Golden Hugo Award from the Chicago International Film Festival, 1979, for "The Martha Graham Dance Company: Clytemnestra," *Dance in America;* Peabody Award, 1981, for "Nureyev and the Joffrey Ballet: In Tribute to Nijinsky," *Dance in America;* Monitor Award, Silver Plaque from the Chicago International Film Festival, and Gold Medal from the International Film and Television Festival of New York, all 1984, for "Balanchine, Parts I and II," *Dance in America;* Academy Award, Best Documentary Feature, Emmy Award, Silver Hugo Award from the Chicago International Film Festival, and CINE Golden Eagle Award, all 1984, for *He Makes Me Feel Like Dancin'*.

Parent's Choice Award, CINE Golden Eagle Award, and Gold Medal from the International Film and Television Festival of New York, all 1985, for "San Francisco Ballet in Cinderella," *Dance in America;* Red Ribbon Award from the American Film and Video Festival and CINE Golden Eagle Award, both 1986, for "Mark Morris," *Dance in America;* CINE Golden Eagle Award and Silver Hugo Award from the Chicago International Film Festival, both 1986, for "Choreography by Jerome Robbins," *Dance in America;* Silver Hugo Award from the Chicago International Film Festival, 1986, for "Dance Theatre of Harlem in A Streetcar Named Desire," *Dance in America;* CINE Golden Eagle Award and Silver Hugo Award from the Chicago International Film Festival, both 1987, for "In Memory of . . . A Ballet by Jerome Robbins," *Dance in America;* Emmy Award, Silver Hugo Award from the Chicago International Film Festival, and CINE Golden Eagle Award, all 1987, for "Agnes, the Indomitable de Mille," *Dance in America*.

MEMBER: Directors Guild of America, Academy of Television Arts and Sciences.

SIDELIGHTS: Judy Kinberg explained to John Gruen in the *New York Times* (April 23, 1989), "One of the founding precepts of *Dance in America* was that it would be a collaborative effort between the choreographer and the television team. This means that we would not violate the choreographer's intention and that his or her involvement would be an essential aspect of filming. Not only would the choreographer's presence and input be vital during taping but he'd be called back during editing, perhaps the most crucial factor of any dance show." She continued, ". . . dance on television can do things that can't be done in a theatre—close-ups for example, which provide a new focus and place the viewer in the midst of a dance. And we can give audiences supportive information, through archival material and interviews with the choreographers."

ADDRESSES: OFFICE—c/o *Dance in America*, WNET, 356 W. 58th Street, New York, NY 10019.

KINNEAR, Roy   1934-1988

PERSONAL: Full name, Roy Mitchell Kinnear; born January 8, 1934, in Wigan, England; died as the result of a fall from a horse, September 20, 1988, in Madrid, Spain; son of Roy Muir and Annie Smith (Durie) Kinnear; married Carmel Cryan (an actress); children: four. EDUCATION: Trained for the stage at the Royal Academy of Dramatic Art.

VOCATION: Actor.

CAREER: STAGE DEBUT—Albert, *The Young in Heart*, Newquay Theatre, Newquay, U.K., 1955. LONDON DEBUT—Fred, *Make Me an Offer*, Royal Stratford Theatre, 1959. PRINCIPAL STAGE APPEARANCES—Fred, *Make Me an Offer*, New Theatre, London, 1959; Master Mathew, *Every Man in His Humour*, R.O. man and Sid, *Sparrers Can't Sing*, and Charlie Modryb, *Progress to the Park*, all Royal Stratford Theatre, London, 1960; R.O. man and Sid, *Sparrers Can't Sing*, Wyndham's Theatre, London, 1961; Blevins Playfair, *They Might Be Giants*, and Mr. Marris, *Big Soft Nellie*, both Royal Stratford Theatre, 1961; Father Matthew, *On a Clear Day You Can See Canterbury*, Royal Stratford Theatre, 1962; ensemble, *England, Our England* (revue), Prince's Theatre, London, 1962; Sid Hotson, *The Affliction*, Oxford Playhouse, Oxford, U.K., 1963; Leo Herman, *A Thousand Clowns*, Comedy Theatre, London, 1964; John P. Jones, *Meals on Wheels*, Royal Court Theatre, London, 1965; Nicholas, *Babes in the Wood*, London Palladium, London, 1965; the Baron, *The Thwarting of Baron Bolligrew*, Royal Shakespeare Company (RSC), Aldwych Theatre, London, 1966; Bull, *The Relapse*, RSC, Aldwych Theatre, 1967; Baptista, *The Taming of the Shrew*, and Touchstone, *As You Like It*, both RSC, Aldwych Theatre, then Royal Shakespeare Theatre, Stratford-on-Avon, U.K., 1967, later Ahmanson Theatre, Los Angeles, 1968; title role, *The Travails of Sancho Panza*, National Theatre Company, Old Vic Theatre, London, 1969; Ligurio, *Mandrake*, Criterion Theatre, London, 1970; Superintendent Baxter, *Dead Easy*, St. Martin's Theatre, London, 1974; Ben, *The Can Opener*, RSC, Place Theatre, London, 1974; Valeria, *Cinderella*, Casino Theatre, London, 1974; Fred, *Roger's Last Stand*, Duke of York's Theatre, London, 1975; Gepetto, *Pinocchio*, Yvonne Arnaud Theatre, Guildford, U.K., 1977; Mayor Enrico, *Beyond the Rainbow*, Adelphi Theatre, London, 1978. Also appeared as the Common Man, *A Man for All Seasons*, West End production.

FILM DEBUT—*The Millionairess*, Twentieth Century-Fox, 1960. PRINCIPAL FILM APPEARANCES—Charles Salmon, *The Boys*, Gala, 1962; Captain Tom Enderby, *Tiara Tahiti*, Zenith, 1962; Fred Smith, *Heavens Above!*, British Lion/Romulus/Janus, 1963; Lucky Dave, *The Small World of Sammy Lee*, Seven Arts, 1963; Fred Gooding, *Sparrows Can't Sing*, Janus, 1963; Henry, *French Dressing*, Warner Brothers, 1964; Bunting, *A Place to Go*, British Lion, 1964; Algernon, *Help!*, United Artists, 1965; Monty Bartlett, *The Hill*, Metro-Goldwyn-Mayer, 1965; Shorty, *Underworld Informers* (also known as *The Informers* and *The Snout*), Continental Distributing, 1965; instructor, *A Funny Thing Happened on the Way to the Forum*, United Artists, 1966; Adam Scarr, *The Deadly Affair*, Columbia, 1967; Clapper, *How I Won the War*, United Artists, 1967; fire extinguisher salesman, *The Mini-Affair*, United Screen Arts, 1968; plastic mac man, *The Bed Sitting Room*, United Artists, 1969; Sir Tunbelly Clumsey, *Lock Up Your Daughters*, Columbia, 1969.

Park keeper, *Egghead's Robot*, Film Producer's Guild, 1970; Roscoe, *The Firechasers*, R.F.D. Productions, 1970; Prince Regent, *On a Clear Day You Can See Forever*, Paramount, 1970;

portly gentleman, *Scrooge,* National General, 1970; Weller, *Taste the Blood of Dracula,* Warner Brothers, 1970; Mr. Perkins, *Melody* (also known as *S.W.A.L.K.*), Levitt-Pickman, 1971; Mr. Salt, *Willy Wonka and the Chocolate Factory,* Paramount, 1971; Burgermeister, *The Pied Piper,* Paramount, 1972; Social Director Curain, *Juggernaut,* United Artists, 1974; Planchet, *The Three Musketeers,* Twentieth Century-Fox, 1974; Moriarty's aide, *The Adventures of Sherlock Holmes' Smarter Brother,* Twentieth Century-Fox, 1975; Bishop of Paris, *Barry McKenzie Holds His Own,* Roadshow, 1975; Planchet, *The Four Musketeers* (also known as *The Revenge of Milady*), Twentieth Century-Fox, 1975; Superintendent Grubbs, *One of Our Dinosaurs Is Missing,* Buena Vista, 1975; Old Roue, *Royal Flash,* Twentieth Century-Fox, 1975; Hoskins, *Not Now, Comrade,* EMI Film Distributors, 1976; Quincey, *Herbie Goes to Monte Carlo,* Buena Vista, 1977; Corporal Boldini, *The Last Remake of Beau Geste,* Universal, 1977; voice of Pipkin, *Watership Down* (animated), AVCO-Embassy, 1978; Bidley, *The Omega Connection* (also known as *The London Connection*), Buena Vista, 1979.

Innkeeper, *Hawk the Slayer,* ITC, 1980; Seldon, *The Hound of the Baskervilles,* Atlantic, 1980; Mr. Garnett, *High Rise Donkey,* Children's Film Foundation, 1980; English Eddie Hagedorn, *Hammett,* Warner Brothers, 1982; Hector Lloyd, *The Boys in Blue,* Rank, 1983; Gardener, *Pavlova—A Woman for All Time,* Poseidon, 1985; Dutch, *Pirates,* Cannon, 1986; Vormieter, *Unusual Ground Floor Conversation* (short film), Film Four International, 1987; Jack Splendide, *Just Ask for Diamond* (also known as *The Falcon's Malteser*), Twentieth Century-Fox/King's Road Entertainment, 1988. Also appeared in *Alice's Adventures in Wonderland,* American National Enterprises, 1972; *Rentadick,* Virgin, 1972; *Candleshoe,* Buena Vista, 1978; and in *Raising the Roof, The Garnett Saga, That's Your Funeral, Eskimo Nell, Three for All, The Amorous Milkman,* and *Dick Turpin.*

PRINCIPAL TELEVISION APPEARANCES—Series: Jerry, *George and Mildred,* syndicated, 1984; also *Shades of Greene,* PBS; *That Was the Week That Was; Inside George Webley;* and *Andy Robson.* Movies: Holidaymaker, *Madame Sin,* ABC, 1972; Friar Tuck, *The Zany Adventures of Robin Hood,* CBS, 1984; Balbi, *Casanova,* ABC, 1987; the Common Man, *A Man for All Seasons,* TNT, 1988. Specials: *Squaring the Circle* (documentary), TVS, 1983. Also appeared in *The Princess and the Pea* and *A Slight Case of. . . .**

OBITUARIES AND OTHER SOURCES: *Variety,* September 28, 1988.*

*   *   *

KIRKLAND, Sally 1944-

PERSONAL: Born October 31, 1944, in New York, NY; daughter of Sally Kirkland (a fashion editor); father, in the scrap metal business; married Michael Jarrett (marriage ended). EDUCATION: Studied at the Actors Studio.

VOCATION: Actress.

CAREER: BROADWAY DEBUT—*Step on a Crack,* Ethel Barrymore Theatre, 1962. PRINCIPAL STAGE APPEARANCES—Cindy Sweetspent, *The Love Nest,* Writers' Stage, New York City, 1963; title role, *Fitz,* Circle in the Square, New York City, 1966; various roles, *Tom Paine,* Stage 73, New York City, 1968; narrator, *Futz!,* Theatre de

Lys, New York City, 1968; the Girl, *Sweet Eros,* and Miss Presson, *Witness,* both Gramercy Arts Theatre, New York City, 1968; Young Girl, "The Noisy Passenger" in *One Night Stands of a Noisy Passenger,* Actors Playhouse, New York City, 1970; Delphine, *The Justice Box,* Theatre de Lys, 1971; Avis Honor, *Delicate Champion,* Forum Theatre, New York City, 1971; Nedda Lemon, *Where Has Tommy Flowers Gone?,* Eastside Playhouse, New York City, 1971; Marcia, *Felix,* Actors Studio, New York City, 1972; Lee, *The Chickencoop Chinaman,* American Place Theatre, New York City, 1972; Zuzana, *Largo Desolato,* New York Shakespeare Festival, Public Theatre, New York City, 1986. Also appeared in *Bicycle Ride to Nevada,* Cort Theatre, New York City, 1963; *Marathon '33,* American National Theatre Academy Theatre, New York City, 1963; *A Midsummer Night's Dream,* Delacorte Mobile Theatre, 1964; *The Bitch of Waverly Place,* Bridge Theatre, New York City, 1965; *Women Beware Women,* City Center Acting Company, Good Faith-Shepherd Church, New York City, 1972; *Canadian Gothic,* Mark Taper Forum Lab, Los Angeles, CA, 1974; as Rona, *Kennedy's Children,* San Francisco, CA, 1976; in *In the Boom Boom Room,* Los Angeles, 1981; and in *These Men,* Los Angeles Actors Theatre, Los Angeles, 1982.

PRINCIPAL FILM APPEARANCES—Ann Graham, *Going Home,* Metro-Goldwyn-Mayer, 1971; Pony Dunbar, *The Way We Were,* Columbia, 1973; fleet chick, *Cinderella Liberty,* Twentieth Century-Fox, 1973; Crystal, *The Sting,* Universal, 1973; patient, *The Young Nurses* (also known as *Nightingale*), New World, 1973; Barney's woman, *Big Bad Mama,* New World, 1974; Honey, *Bite the Bullet,* Columbia, 1975; Ella Mae, *Crazy Mama,* New World, 1975; Two Street Betty, *Pipe Dreams,* AVCO-Embassy, 1976; photographer, *A Star Is Born,* Warner Brothers, 1976; Helga, *Private Benjamin,* Warner Brothers, 1980; Katherine, *Human Highway,* Shakey, 1982; Sally, *Love Letters* (also known as *My Love Letters*), New World, 1983; title role, *Anna,* Vestron, 1987; hooker, *Talking Walls* (also known as *Motel Vacancy*), New World, 1987. Also appeared in *Coming Apart,* 1969; *Brand X,* 1970; *Hometown U.S.A.,* Film Ventures International, 1979; *Fatal Games,* 1983; *The Killing Touch,* 1983; *Paint It Black,* 1989; and *Cold Feet,* 1989.

PRINCIPAL TELEVISION APPEARANCES—Series: *Falcon Crest,* CBS. Mini-Series: Aggie, *Captains and the Kings,* NBC, 1976. Pilots: Mona Phillips, *Shaughnessey,* NBC, 1976; Della Bianco, *Stonestreet: Who Killed the Centerfold Model?,* NBC, 1977; Vivian Stark, *The Georgia Peaches,* CBS, 1980; Kate Stewart, *Willow B: Women in Prison,* ABC, 1980; mother, *Summer,* CBS, 1984. Episodic: Officer Joan Harley, *Bronk,* CBS. Movies: Mary, *Death Scream* (also known as *The Woman Who Cried Murder*), ABC, 1975; Wilma Floyd, *The Kansas City Massacre,* ABC, 1975; also *Griffin and Phoenix: A Love Story,* ABC, 1976.

RELATED CAREER—Partner (with Daniel and Mark Buntzman), Artists Alliance Productions (a film production company), 1988—. In addition to the credits listed above, Sally Kirkland appeared in a number of Pop artist Andy Warhol's underground films and worked with the La Mama Experimental Theatre Club in New York City during the 1960s.

AWARDS: Drama-Logue Award, Best Actress, 1981, for *In the Boom Boom Room;* Los Angeles Film Critics Award, Best Actress, 1987, Golden Globe Award, Best Actress in a Motion Picture Drama, 1988, and Academy Award nomination, Best Actress, 1988, all for *Anna.*

SIDELIGHTS: RECREATIONS—Painting.

ADDRESSES: AGENT—William Morris Agency, 151 El Camino Drive, Beverly Hills, CA 90210.*

*   *   *

KNOX, Terence

PERSONAL: Born December 16, in Richland, WA.

VOCATION: Actor.

CAREER: PRINCIPAL STAGE APPEARANCES—Brick, *Cat on a Hot Tin Roof,* and Teddy, *When You Comin' Back, Red Ryder?,* both Coconut Grove Playhouse, Coconut Grove, FL, 1985.

PRINCIPAL FILM APPEARANCES—Reese, *Used Cars,* Columbia, 1980; Jack's friend, *Heart Like a Wheel,* Twentieth Century-Fox, 1983; Eric Macklin, *Lies,* Alpha, 1984; Buddy, *Truckin' Buddy McCoy,* Bedford Entertainment, 1984; Hightower and McHugh, *Rebel Love,* Troma, 1986. Also appeared in *Distortions,* Cori, 1988.

PRINCIPAL TELEVISION APPEARANCES—Series: Dr. Peter White, *St. Elsewhere,* NBC, 1982-85; Matt Russell, *All Is Forgiven,* NBC, 1986; Sergeant Zeke Anderson, *Tour of Duty,* CBS, 1987. Pilots: Dr. Michael Rourke, *J.O.E. and the Colonel,* ABC, 1985. Episodic: Steve Grenowski, "Mighty Pawns," *Wonderworks,* PBS, 1987. Movies: Leo Kalb, *City Killer,* NBC, 1984; Craig Phelan, *Chase,* CBS, 1985; Martin Anderson, *Murder Ordained,* CBS, 1987.

ADDRESSES: AGENT—Artists Agency, 10000 Santa Monica Boulevard, Suite 305, Los Angeles, CA 90067. PUBLICIST—Freeman and Sutton Public Relations, 8961 Sunset Boulevard, Suite 2-A, Los Angeles, CA 90069.*

*   *   *

KOMACK, James   1930-

PERSONAL: Born August 3, 1930, in New York, NY; married Marilyn "Cluny" Cohen; children: Maxx (a daughter). MILITARY: U.S. Army Air Corps, flight gunner.

VOCATION: Producer, director, actor, and screenwriter.

CAREER: Also see *WRITINGS* below. PRINCIPAL STAGE AP-PEARANCES—Rocky, *Damn Yankees,* New York City, 46th Street Theatre, New York City, 1955; Matt Holly, *Sixth Finger in a Five Finger Glove,* Plymouth Theatre, Boston, MA, then Longacre Theatre, New York City, both 1956. Also appeared in *New Faces,* Royale Theatre, New York City, 1952.

PRINCIPAL FILM APPEARANCES—(As Jimmie Komack) Rocky, *Damn Yankees* (also known as *What Lola Wants*), Warner Brothers, 1958; Dog, *Senior Prom,* Columbia, 1958; Julius Manetta, *A Hole in the Head,* United Artists, 1959. PRINCIPAL FILM WORK—Director, *Porky's Revenge,* Twentieth Century-Fox, 1985.

PRINCIPAL TELEVISION APPEARANCES—Series: Harvey Spencer Blair III, *Hennessey,* CBS, 1959-62; Norman Tinker, *The Court-*

ship of Eddie's Father, ABC, 1969-72; voice of principal John Lazarus, *Welcome Back, Kotter,* ABC, 1975-79; Dag Larson, *9 to 5,* ABC, 1982-83. Pilots: Angel First Class Charlie, *Charlie Angelo,* CBS, 1962. Episodic: Horshack's uncle, *Welcome Back Kotter,* ABC; also *The June Allyson Show,* CBS. Specials: Hunk, *Best Foot Forward,* NBC, 1954.

PRINCIPAL TELEVISION WORK—Series: Producer, *Get Smart,* NBC, 1965-69, then CBS, 1969-70; producer, *Mr. Roberts,* NBC, 1965-66; creator and executive producer, *The Courtship of Eddie's Father,* ABC, 1969-72; creator and executive producer, *Chico and the Man,* NBC, 1974-78; creator and executive producer, *Welcome Back Kotter,* ABC, 1975-79; executive producer, *Mr. T. and Tina,* ABC, 1976; executive producer, *Another Day,* CBS, 1978; executive producer, *Sugar Time,* ABC, 1977-78; creator and executive producer, *The Rollergirls,* NBC, 1978; executive producer, *Me and Maxx,* NBC, 1980; producer, *9 to 5,* ABC, 1982-83. Pilots: Producer and director, *Lady Luck,* NBC, 1973; executive producer and director, *Whatever Happened to Dobie Gillis?,* CBS, 1977; executive producer, *The Archie Situation Comedy Musical Variety Show,* ABC, 1978; executive producer and director, *Shipshape,* CBS, 1978. Episodic: All as director, unless indicated. "Empress Carlotta's Necklace," *The Dick Van Dyke Show,* CBS, 1961; *Ensign O'Toole,* NBC, 1962-63; *My Favorite Martian,* CBS, 1963-66; *Mr. Roberts,* NBC, 1965-66; "A Piece of the Action," *Star Trek,* NBC, 1967; *The Courtship of Eddie's Father,* ABC, 1969-72; *Chico and the Man,* NBC, 1974-78; *Welcome Back Kotter,* ABC, 1975-79; *Mr. T. and Tina,* ABC, 1976; *Another Day,* CBS, 1978; *The Rollergirls,* NBC, 1978; *Me and Maxx,* NBC, 1980; executive producer, "King of the Building," *CBS Summer Playhouse,* CBS, 1987; also *77 Sunset Strip,* ABC.

RELATED CAREER—As a comedian, appeared in nightclubs through-out the United States, including the Blue Angel, Bon Soir, One Fifth Avenue, and the Village Vanguard, all New York City, Mr. Kelly's, in Chicago, and in resorts in the Catskill Mountains in New York; bandleader, Jimmie Komack and His Orchestra; comedy writer for Art Carney and Red Buttons; songwriter for Eartha Kitt, Coral Records, and RCA Victor; singer.

WRITINGS: TELEVISION—Episodic: *Hennessey,* CBS, 1959-62; *My Favorite Martian,* CBS, 1963-66; *The Courtship of Eddie's Father,* ABC, 1969-72; *Chico and the Man,* NBC, 1974-78; *Welcome Back Kotter,* ABC, 1975-79; *The Rollergirls,* NBC, 1978; *Me and Maxx,* NBC, 1980. OTHER—"Nic-Name Song" (song).*

*   *   *

KRASNER, Milton   1904-1988

PERSONAL: Born February 17, 1904 (some sources say 1898 or 1901), in Philadelphia, PA; died of a heart attack, July 16, 1988, in Woodland Hills, CA; children: one son.

VOCATION: Cinematographer.

CAREER: PRINCIPAL FILM WORK—All as cinematographer, unless indicated: Cameraman, *A Woman Commands,* RKO, 1932; cameraman, *Is My Face Red?,* RKO, 1932; cameraman, *Ride Him, Cowboy* (also known as *The Hawk*), Warner Brothers, 1932; cameraman, *70,000 Witnesses,* Paramount, 1932; *Golden Harvest,* Paramount, 1933; *I Love That Man,* Paramount, 1933; *Sitting*

Pretty, Paramount, 1933; *Strictly Personal*, Paramount, 1933; *Death of the Diamond*, Metro, 1934; *The Great Flirtation*, Paramount, 1934; *Paris Interlude*, Metro-Goldwyn-Mayer (MGM), 1934; *Private Scandal*, Paramount, 1934; *She Made Her Bed*, Paramount, 1934.

Great God Gold, Monogram, 1935; *The Great Impersonation*, Universal, 1935; *Make a Million*, Republic, 1935; *Murder in the Fleet*, MGM, 1935; *The Virginia Judge*, Paramount, 1935; *Women Must Dress*, Monogram, 1935; (with Harry Neumann) *Cheers of the Crowd*, Monogram, 1936; *Forbidden Heaven*, Republic, 1936; *The Girl on the Front Page*, Universal, 1936; *Honeymoon Limited*, Monogram, 1936; (with Reggie Lanning) *Laughing Irish Eyes*, Republic, 1936; *Love Letters of a Star*, Universal, 1936; *Mister Cinderella*, MGM, 1936; *Yellowstone*, Universal, 1936; *Crash Donovan*, Universal, 1936; *A Girl with Ideas*, Universal, 1937; *Lady Fights Back*, Universal, 1937; *Love in a Bungalow*, Universal, 1937; *Mysterious Crossing*, Universal, 1937; *Oh, Doctor*, Universal, 1937; *Prescription for Romance*, Universal, 1937; *She's Dangerous*, Universal, 1937; *There Goes the Groom*, RKO, 1937; *We Have Our Moments*, Universal, 1937; *The Crime of Dr. Hallet*, Universal, 1938; *The Devil's Party*, Universal, 1938; *The Jury's Secret*, Universal, 1938; *Midnight Intruder*, Universal, 1938; *The Missing Guest*, Universal, 1938; *Nurse from Brooklyn*, Universal, 1938; *The Storm*, Universal, 1938; *The Family Next Door*, Universal, 1939; *The House of Fear*, Universal, 1939; *I Stole a Million*, Universal, 1939; *Little Accident*, Universal, 1939; *Missing Evidence*, Universal, 1939; *Newsboy's Home*, Universal, 1939; *You Can't Cheat an Honest Man*, Universal, 1939.

The Bank Dick (also known as *The Bank Detective*), Universal, 1940; *Diamond Frontier*, Universal, 1940; *Hired Wife*, Universal, 1940; *The House of the Seven Gables*, Universal, 1940; *The Invisible Man Returns*, Universal, 1940; *The Man from Montreal*, Universal, 1940; *Oh Johnny, How You Can Love!*, Universal, 1940; *Private Affairs*, Universal, 1940; *Sandy Is a Lady*, Universal, 1940; *Ski Patrol*, Universal, 1940; (with Joseph Valentine) *Trail of the Vigilantes*, Universal, 1940; *Zanzibar*, Universal, 1940; *Bachelor Daddy*, Universal, 1941; *Buck Privates* (also known as *Rookies*), Universal, 1941; *Lady from Cheyenne*, Universal, 1941; *Paris Calling*, Universal, 1941; *Too Many Blondes*, Universal, 1941; *This Woman Is Mine*, Universal, 1942; *Arabian Nights*, Universal, 1942; *A Gentleman After Dark*, United Artists, 1942; (with Elwood Bredell) *The Ghost of Frankenstein*, Universal, 1942; *Men of Texas* (also known as *Men of Destiny*), Universal, 1942; *Pardon My Sarong*, Universal, 1942; *The Spoilers*, Universal, 1942; *Gung Ho!*, Universal, 1943; *The Mad Ghoul*, Universal, 1943; (with Bredell) *So's Your Uncle*, Universal, 1943; *Two Tickets to London*, Universal, 1943; *We've Never Been Licked* (also known as *Fighting Command* and *Texas to Tokyo*), Universal, 1943; *Hat Check Honey*, Universal, 1944; *The Invisible Man's Revenge*, Universal, 1944.

Along Came Jones, RKO, 1945; *Delightfully Dangerous*, United Artists, 1945; *Scarlet Street*, Universal, 1945; *The Woman in the Window*, RKO, 1945; *The Dark Mirror*, Universal, 1946; *Without Reservations*, RKO, 1946; *A Double Life*, Universal, 1947; *The Egg and I*, Universal, 1947; *The Farmer's Daughter*, RKO, 1947; *Something in the Wind*, Universal, 1947; *The Saxon Charm*, Universal, 1948; *Up in Central Park*, Univeral, 1948; *The Accused* (also known as *Strange Deception*), Paramount, 1949; *Holiday Affair*, RKO, 1949; *House of Strangers*, Twentieth Century-Fox, 1949; *The Set-Up*, RKO, 1949.

All About Eve, Twentieth Century-Fox, 1950; *No Way Out*, Twentieth Century-Fox, 1950; *Three Came Home*, Twentieth Century-Fox, 1950; *Half Angel*, Twentieth Century-Fox, 1951; *I Can Get It for You Wholesale* (also known as *Only the Best* and *This Is My Affair*), Twentieth Century-Fox, 1951; *The Model and the Marriage Broker*, Twentieth Century-Fox, 1951; *People Will Talk*, Twentieth Century-Fox, 1951; *Rawhide* (also known as *Desperate Siege*), Twentieth Century-Fox, 1951; *Deadline—U.S.A.* (also known as *Deadline*), Twentieth Century-Fox, 1952; *Dreamboat*, Twentieth Century-Fox, 1952; *Monkey Business*, Twentieth Century-Fox, 1952; "The Ransom of Red Chief" in *O. Henry's Full House* (also known as *Full House*), Twentieth Century-Fox, 1952; *Phone Call from a Stranger*, Twentieth Century-Fox, 1952; *Dream Wife*, MGM, 1953; *Taxi*, Twentieth Century-Fox, 1953; *Vicki*, Twentieth Century-Fox, 1953; *Demetrius and the Gladiators*, Twentieth Century-Fox, 1954; *Desiree*, Twentieth Century-Fox, 1954; *Garden of Evil*, Twentieth Century-Fox, 1954; *Three Coins in the Fountain*, Twentieth Century-Fox, 1954.

The Girl in the Red Velvet Swing, Twentieth Century-Fox, 1955; *How to Be Very, Very Popular*, Twentieth Century-Fox, 1955; *The Rains of Ranchipur*, Twentieth Century-Fox, 1955; *The Seven Year Itch*, Twentieth Century-Fox, 1955; *Bus Stop* (also known as *The Wrong Kind of Girl*), Twentieth Century-Fox, 1956; *23 Paces to Baker Street*, Twentieth Century-Fox, 1956; *An Affair to Remember*, Twentieth Century-Fox, 1957; *Boy on a Dolphin*, Twentieth Century-Fox, 1957; *Kiss Them for Me*, Twentieth Century-Fox, 1957; *A Certain Smile*, Twentieth Century-Fox, 1958; *The Gift of Love*, Twentieth Century-Fox, 1958; (with George Folsey) *Count Your Blessings*, MGM, 1959; *The Man Who Understood Women*, Twentieth Century-Fox, 1959; *The Remarkable Mr. Pennypacker*, Twentieth Century-Fox, 1959.

Bells Are Ringing, MGM, 1960; *Home from the Hill*, MGM, 1960; *Go Naked in the World*, MGM, 1961; (with Franz F. Planer and Manuel Berenguer) *King of Kings*, MGM, 1961; *The Four Horsemen of the Apocalypse*, MGM, 1962; (with Joseph La Shelle, Charles Lang, Jr., William Daniels, and Harold Wellman) *How the West Was Won*, MGM, 1962; *Sweet Bird of Youth*, MGM, 1962; *Two Weeks in Another Town*, MGM, 1962; *The Courtship of Eddie's Father*, MGM, 1963; *Love with the Proper Stranger*, Paramount, 1963; *A Ticklish Affair*, MGM, 1963; *Advance to the Rear* (also known as *Company of Cowards?*), MGM, 1964; *Fate Is the Hunter*, Twentieth Century-Fox, 1964; *Goodbye Charlie*, Twentieth Century-Fox, 1964; *Looking for Love*, MGM, 1964.

(With Haskell Boggs) *Red Line 7000*, Paramount, 1965; *The Sandpiper*, MGM, 1965; *Made in Paris*, MGM, 1966; *The Singing Nun*, MGM, 1966; (with Loyal Griggs) *Hurry Sundown*, Paramount, 1967; *The St. Valentine's Day Massacre*, Twentieth Century-Fox, 1967; (with Enzo Serafin) *The Venetian Affair*, MGM, 1967; *The Ballad of Josie*, Universal, 1968; *Don't Just Stand There*, Universal, 1968; *The Sterile Cuckoo* (also known as *Pookie*), Paramount, 1969; *Beneath the Planet of the Apes*, Twentieth Century-Fox, 1970; *Zachariah*, Cinerama, 1971. Also cinematographer for short films, including *Arbor Day*, 1936; *Beat Me Daddy, Eight to the Bar!*, 1940; *Swing Frolic*, 1942; and *The Roger Wagner Chorale*, 1954.

PRINCIPAL TELEVISION WORK—Series: Cinematographer, *MacMillan and Wife*, NBC, 1971-76, renamed *MacMillan*, NBC, 1976-77.

RELATED CAREER—Laboratory worker and assistant editor, Vitagraph, New York City; camera assistant and second cameraman for various Hollywood studios during the 1920s, including work on the Bronco Billy Anderson westerns and the Johnny Hines comedies for First National, the Harry Carey westerns for Pathe, and the Ken Maynard westerns for Universal.

AWARDS: Academy Award nomination, Best Cinematography (Color), 1943, for *Arabian Nights;* Academy Award nomination, Best Cinematography (Black and White), 1951, for *All About Eve;* Academy Award, Best Cinematography (Color), 1955, for *Three Coins in the Fountain;* Academy Award nomination, Best Cinematography, 1958, for *An Affair to Remember;* Academy Award nomination, Best Cinematography (Black and White), 1964, for *Love with the Proper Stranger;* Academy Award nomination, Best Cinematography (Color), 1964, for *How the West Was Won;* Academy Award nomination, Best Cinematography (Black and White), 1965, for *Fate Is the Hunter.*

MEMBER: American Society of Cinematographers.

OBITUARIES AND OTHER SOURCES: Variety, July 20, 1988.*

*   *   *

KRIGE, Alice   1954-

PERSONAL: Born June 28, 1954, in South Africa.

VOCATION: Actress.

CAREER: PRINCIPAL STAGE APPEARANCES—With the Royal Shakespeare Company in England, 1984-85.

FILM DEBUT—Sybil Gordon, *Chariots of Fire,* Twentieth Century-Fox, 1981. PRINCIPAL FILM APPEARANCES—Alma Mobley/Eva Galli, *Ghost Story,* Universal, 1981; Bathsheba, *King David,* Paramount, 1985; Tully Sorenson, *Barfly,* Cannon, 1987; Mary Shelley, *Haunted Summer,* Cannon, 1988; Beth, *See You in the Morning,* Warner Brothers, 1989.

PRINCIPAL TELEVISION APPEARANCES—Mini-Series: Bridget O'Donnell, *Ellis Island,* CBS, 1984; Baroness Lisl Kemery, *Wallenberg: A Hero's Story,* NBC, 1985; Jessie Benton Fremont, *Dream West,* CBS, 1986. Episodic: Nita, *Murder, She Wrote,* CBS, 1985. Movies: Lucie Manette, *A Tale of Two Cities,* CBS, 1980; Gwen, *Second Serve,* CBS, 1986; Patsy Cline, *Baja Oklahoma,* HBO, 1988.

ADDRESSES: AGENTS—Al Parker Agency, 55 Park Lane, London W1, England; Marion Rosenberg, The Lantz Office, 9255 Sunset Boulevard, Suite 505, Los Angeles, CA 90069. PUBLICIST—N. Koenigsberg, P/M/K Public Relations, 8436 W. Third Street, Suite 650, Los Angeles, CA 90048.*

*   *   *

KUBRICK, Stanley   1928-

PERSONAL: Born July 26, 1928, in Bronx, NY; son of Jacques L. (a doctor) and Gertrude (Perveler) Kubrick; married Toba Metz, 1947 (divorced, 1952); married Ruth Sobotka (a dancer), 1952 (marriage ended); married Suzanne Christiane Harlan (an actress and painter), April, 1958; children: Katherine (second marriage);

Anya, Vivian (third marriage). EDUCATION: Attended City College (now known as City University of New York).

VOCATION: Director, producer, screenwriter, film editor, and cinematographer.

CAREER: Also see *WRITINGS* below. PRINCIPAL FILM WORK—Director: (Also producer, editor, and cinematographer) *Day of the Fight* (documentary short film), RKO, 1952; (also producer and cinematographer) *Flying Padre* (documentary short film), RKO/Pathe, 1952; (also cinematographer) *The Seafarers,* Seafarers International Union, 1953; (also producer, cinematographer, and editor) *Fear and Desire,* Joseph Burstyn, 1953; (also producer with Morris Bousel, cinematographer, and editor) *Killer's Kiss,* United Artists, 1955; (also producer with James B. Harris) *The Killing,* United Artists, 1956; (also producer with Harris) *Paths of Glory,* United Artists, 1957; *Spartacus,* Universal, 1960; *Lolita,* Metro-Goldwyn-Mayer (MGM), 1962; (also producer) *Dr. Strangelove: Or How I Learned to Stop Worrying and Love the Bomb,* Columbia, 1964; (also producer and special photographic effects designer) *2001: A Space Odyssey,* MGM, 1968; (also producer) *A Clockwork Orange,* Warner Brothers, 1971; (also producer) *Barry Lyndon,* Warner Brothers, 1975; (also producer) *The Shining,* Warner Brothers, 1980; (also producer) *Full Metal Jacket,* Warner Brothers, 1987.

RELATED CAREER—Freelance photographer, 1945-46; staff photographer, *Look* magazine, 1946-50; founder (with James B. Harris), Harris-Kubrick Productions, 1955-62.

WRITINGS: FILM—See production details above. *Day of the Fight,* 1952; *Flying Padre,* 1952; (with Howard O. Sackler) *Fear and Desire,* 1953; (with Sackler) *Killer's Kiss,* 1955; *The Killing* (based on the novel *Clean Break* by Lionel White), 1956; (with Calder Willingham and Jim Thompson) *Paths of Glory* (based on the novel by Humphrey Cobb), 1957; (with Peter George and Terry Southern) *Dr. Strangelove: Or How I Learned to Stop Worrying and Love the Bomb* (based on the novel *Red Alert* by George), 1964; (with Arthur C. Clarke) *2001: A Space Odyssey* (based on the short story ''The Sentinel'' by Clarke), 1968; *A Clockwork Orange* (based on the novel by Anthony Burgess), 1971, published in *Stanley Kubrick's A Clockwork Orange: Based on the Novel by Anthony Burgess,* Ballantine, 1972; *Barry Lyndon* (based on the novel by William Makepeace Thackeray), 1975; (with Diane Johnson) *The Shining* (based on the novel by Stephen King), 1980; (with Michael Herr and Gustav Hasford) *Full Metal Jacket* (based on the novel *The Short-Timers* by Hasford), 1987, published by Knopf, 1987.

AWARDS: New York Film Critics Award, Best Director, and (with Peter George and Terry Southern) Writers Guild Award, Best Written American Comedy (screenplay), both 1964, for *Dr. Strangelove: Or How I Learned to Stop Worrying and Love the Bomb;* Academy Award, Best Special Visual Effects, and Academy Award nomination, Best Screenplay, both 1968, for *2001: A Space Odyssey;* New York Film Critics Awards, Best Director and Best Film, and Academy Award nominations, Best Director and Best Film, all 1971, for *A Clockwork Orange;* National Board of Review of Motion Pictures Awards, Best Director and Best English Language Film, and Academy Award nominations, Best Director and Best Film, all 1975, for *Barry Lyndon;* Academy Award nomination, Best Screenplay, and Writers Guild Award nomination, Best Screenplay Based on Material from Another Medium, both 1988, for *Full Metal Jacket.*

SIDELIGHTS: RECREATIONS—Reading and listening to classical music.

ADDRESSES: HOME—P.O. Box 123, Boreham Wood, Hertfordshire, England. OFFICE—c/o Louis C. Blau, Loeb and Loeb, 10100 Santa Monica Boulevard, Suite 2200, Los Angeles, CA 90067.*

*   *   *

KWAN, Nancy   1939-

PERSONAL: Full name, Nancy Kashen Kwan; born May 19, 1939, in Hong Kong.

VOCATION: Actress.

CAREER: PRINCIPAL STAGE APPEARANCES—Mai O'Connor, *The Quartered Man,* Los Angeles Theatre Center, Los Angeles, CA, 1986.

PRINCIPAL FILM APPEARANCES—Suzie Wong, *The World of Suzie Wong,* Paramount, 1960; Linda Low, *Flower Drum Song,* Universal, 1961; Tessa, *The Main Attraction,* Metro-Goldwyn-Mayer (MGM), 1962; Sally Fraser, *Fate Is the Hunter,* Twentieth Century-Fox, 1964; Lynn Hope, *Honeymoon Hotel,* MGM, 1964; title role, *Tamahine,* ABF/MGM, 1964; Baby, *Arriverderci, Baby!,* Paramount, 1966; Wednesday, *Lt. Robin Crusoe, U.S.N.,* Buena Vista, 1966; Marjorie Lee, *The Wild Affair,* Goldstone, 1966; Tina, *The Corrupt Ones* (also known as *Il Sigillo de Pechino, Die Holle Von Macao, Les Corrompus, The Peking Medallion,* and *Hell to Macao*), Warner Brothers, 1967; Tomiko Momoyama, *Nobody's Perfect,* Universal, 1968; Yu-Rang, *The Wrecking Crew,* Columbia, 1968; Revel, *The Girl Who Knew Too Much,* Commonwealth, 1969; Robin, *The McMasters* (also known as *The Blood Crowd* and *The McMasters . . . Tougher than the West Itself*), Chevron, 1970; Dr. Tsu, *Wonder Women,* General, 1973; Leslie, *Night Creature* (also known as *Out of the Darkness* and *Fear*), Dimension, 1979; Christine, *Walking the Edge,* Empire, 1985; Sue, *Angkor-Cambodia Express,* Monarex, 1986. Also appeared in *Project Kill,* Stirling Gold, 1976; *Supercock,* 1975; *Fortress in the Sun,* 1978; and *Streets of Hong Kong,* 1979.

PRINCIPAL TELEVISION APPEARANCES—Pilots: Rosemary Quong, *Hawaii Five-O,* CBS, 1968; Lily, *Blade in Hong Kong,* CBS, 1985. Mini-Series: Claudia Chen, *James Clavell's "Noble House,"* NBC, 1988. Movies: Noriko, *The Last Ninja,* ABC, 1983. Specials: *The Bob Hope Show,* NBC, 1961.*

L

LADD, Diane 1939-

PERSONAL: Born Diane Ladner, November 29, 1939, in Meridian, MS; daughter of Preston P. (a poulterer) and Mary Bernadette (Anderson) Ladner; married Bruce Dern (an actor; divorced); children: Laura Elizabeth. EDUCATION: Trained for the stage with Frank Corsaro at the Actors Studio.

VOCATION: Actress.

CAREER: STAGE DEBUT—*The Verdict*, Meridian, MS. PRINCIPAL STAGE APPEARANCES—Carol Cutrere, *Orpheus Descending*, Gramercy Arts Theatre, New York City, 1959; Alma Sue Bates, *Carry Me Back to Morningside Heights*, John Golden Theatre, New York City, 1968; Woman, "Last Stand" in *One Night Stands of a Noisy Passenger*, Actors Playhouse, New York City, 1970; Lu Ann Hampton, "Lu Ann Hampton Laverty

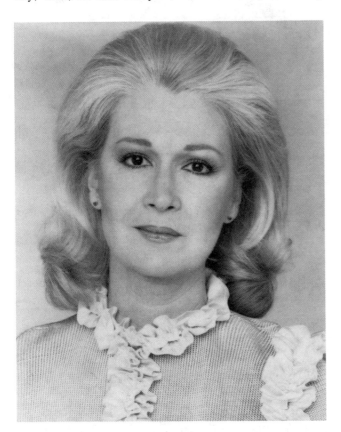

DIANE LADD

Oberlander" in *A Texas Trilogy*, Broadhurst Theatre, New York City, then Kennedy Center for the Performing Arts, Washington, DC, both 1976. Also appeared in regional theatre and summer theatre productions of *Women Speak, The Fantasticks, The Wall, The Goddess, Toys in the Attic, The Deadly Game,* and *Hamlet.*

MAJOR TOURS—*Medium Rare* (revue), U.S. cities, 1960-61; also *A Hatful of Rain,* U.S. cities.

PRINCIPAL FILM APPEARANCES—Gaysh, *The Wild Angels*, American International, 1966; Phoebe, *The Reivers*, National General, 1969; girl, *Macho Callahan*, AVCO-Embassy, 1970; Karen, *Rebel Rousers* (also known as *Limbo*), Four Star Excelsior, 1970; Mrs. Forbes, *The Steagle*, AVCO-Embassy, 1971; Maggie, *White Lightning* (also known as *McKlusky*), United Artists, 1973; Ida Sessions, *Chinatown*, Paramount, 1974; Flo, *Alice Doesn't Live Here Anymore*, Warner Brothers, 1975; Martha, *Embryo*, Cine Artists, 1976; Laura Taylor, *The November Plan*, CIC, 1976; Helen Dupler, *All Night Long*, Universal, 1981; Mrs. Nightshade, *Something Wicked This Way Comes*, Buena Vista, 1983; Etta, *Black Widow*, Twentieth Century-Fox, 1987; Jane Melway, *Plain Clothes*, Paramount, 1988. Also appeared in *Something Wild*, United Artists, 1961; and in *WUSA*, Paramount, 1970.

PRINCIPAL TELEVISION APPEARANCES—Series: Belle Dupree, *Alice*, CBS, 1980-81; also Kitty Styles, *The Secret Storm*, CBS; Kitty Styles, *Search for Tomorrow*, CBS. Mini-Series: Amelia Gordon, *Black Beauty*, NBC, 1978; Verna Howland, *Bluegrass*, CBS, 1988. Pilots: Irene Davis, *Addie and the King of Hearts*, CBS, 1976. Episodic: Christa Johansson, *Love Boat*, ABC, 1985; also *Father Dowling Mysteries*, NBC, 1989. Movies: Alice Shaw, *The Devil's Daughter*, ABC, 1973; Mae, *Willa*, CBS, 1979; Lynetta Jones, *Guyana Tragedy: The Story of Jim Jones*, CBS, 1980; Carol Cameron, *Desperate Lives*, CBS, 1982; Margaret Kelly, *Grace Kelly*, ABC, 1983; Jeannette Bryan, *I Married a Centerfold*, NBC, 1984; Carlotta, *Thaddeus Rose and Eddie*, CBS, 1984; Rose Hayward, *Crime of Innocence*, NBC, 1985; Mrs. Heflin, *Celebration Family*, ABC, 1987. Specials: *Battle of the Network Stars*, ABC, 1980.

WRITINGS: God, Give Me One More Minute (autobiography), 1982.

AWARDS: Academy Award nomination, Golden Globe Award nomination, and British Academy Award, all Best Supporting Actress, 1974, for *Alice Doesn't Live Here Anymore;* Golden Globe Award, Best Supporting Actress, for *Alice;* Broadway Tour Award and UCLA Favorite Actress Award, both for *A Texas Trilogy;* Eleanore Duse Mask Award.*

LANDAU, Martin

PERSONAL: Born June 20, in Brooklyn, NY; son of Morris (a machinist) and Selma (Buchman) Landau; married Barbara Bain (an actress), January 31, 1957 (separated); children: Susan Meredith, Juliet Rose. EDUCATION: Attended the Pratt Institute; trained for the stage at the Actors Studio with Lee Strasberg, Harold Clurman, and Elia Kazan.

VOCATION: Actor and director.

CAREER: STAGE DEBUT—Charley Gemini, *Detective Story,* Peaks Island Playhouse, Peaks Island, ME, 1951. OFF-BROADWAY DEBUT—Nick, *First Love,* Provincetown Playhouse, 1951, for eighteen performances. PRINCIPAL STAGE APPEARANCES—Lally, *The Penguin,* Current Stages Theatre, New York City, 1952; Juvan, *Goat Song,* Equity Library Theatre, New York City, 1953; Husband, *Middle of the Night,* American National Theatre and Academy Theatre, New York City, 1957. Also appeared in productions of *Uncle Vanya, Wedding Breakfast,* and *Dracula.*

MAJOR TOURS—Husband, *Middle of the Night,* U.S. and Canadian cities, 1957-58; also *Stalag 17,* U.S. cities, 1952.

FILM DEBUT—Leonard, *North by Northwest,* Metro-Goldwyn-Mayer, 1959. PRINCIPAL FILM APPEARANCES—The Duke, *The Gazebo,* Metro-Goldwyn-Mayer (MGM), 1959; Marshall, *Pork Chop Hill,* United Artists, 1959; Dade Coleman, *Stagecoach to Dancer's Park,* Universal, 1962; Rufio, *Cleopatra,* Twentieth Century-Fox, 1963; Caiaphas, *The Greatest Story Ever Told,* United Artists, 1965; Chief Walks-Stooped-Over, *The Hallelujah Trail,* United Artists, 1965; Jesse Coe, *Nevada Smith,* Paramount, 1966; Reverend Logan Sharpe, *They Call Me Mister Tibbs,* United Artists, 1970; Colonel, *A Town Called Hell* (also known as *A Town Called Bastard*), Scotia International, 1971; Capelli, *Black Gunn,* Columbia, 1972; Dr. George Tracer, *Strange Shadows in an Empty Room* (also known as *Shadows in an Empty Room* and *Blazing Magnum*), American International, 1977; Captain Garrity, *The Last Word* (also known as *Danny Travis*), International, 1979; General Barry Adlon, *Meteor,* American International, 1979; Roderick Usher, *The Fall of the House of Usher,* Sunn Classic, 1980; Marshal, *The Return,* Greydon Clark, 1980; Fred, *Without Warning* (also known as *It Came . . . Without Warning*), Filmways, 1980; Bryon "Preacher" Sutcliff, *Alone in the Dark,* New Line Cinema, 1982; Garson Jones, *The Being,* BFV, 1983; the Captain, *L'Ile au Tresor* (also known as *Treasure Island*), Films du Passage/Cannon Releasing, 1985; Bosarian, *Cyclone,* Cinetel, 1987; Chuck, *Empire State,* Virgin/Miracle, 1987; Cicero, *Sweet Revenge,* Concorde, 1987; Abe Karatz, *Tucker: The Man and His Dream,* Paramount, 1988. Also appeared in *Operation SNAFU,* 1970; *Under the Sign of Capricorn,* 1971; *Operation Moonbase Alpha,* 1980; *The Alien's Return,* 1980; *Beauty and the Beast,* 1981; *Trial by Terror,* 1983; *Access Code,* 1984; and *Delta Fever,* New World Video/Image Organization, 1988.

PRINCIPAL FILM WORK—Director, *Meteor,* American International, 1979.

PRINCIPAL TELEVISION APPEARANCES—Series: Rollin Hand, *Mission: Impossible,* CBS, 1966-69; Commander John Koenig, *Space 1999,* syndicated, 1975-77. Pilots: Paul Savage, *Savage,* NBC, 1973; Lyle Stenning, *The Return of the Six Million Dollar Man and the Bionic Woman,* NBC, 1987; also *The Ghost of Sierra de Cobra,* CBS, 1966. Episodic: Hotaling, "Mr. Denton on Doomsday," *The Twilight Zone,* CBS, 1959; Andro, "The Man Who Was

Never Born," *The Outer Limits,* ABC, 1963; Richard Bellero, Jr., *The Bellero Shield,* ABC, 1964; Major Ivan Kuchenko, "The Jeopardy Room," *The Twilight Zone,* CBS, 1964; Cooper-Janes, "The Beacon," *The Twilight Zone,* CBS, 1985; Miles Broderick, *Blacke's Magic,* NBC, 1986; also Hayden Stone, *Buffalo Bill,* NBC; *Playhouse 90,* CBS; *Omnibus,* CBS; *Studio One,* CBS; *Philco Playhouse,* NBC; *I Spy,* NBC; *Goodyear Playhouse,* NBC; *The Wild Wild West,* CBS; *Bonanza,* NBC; *General Electric Theatre,* CBS; *Gunsmoke,* CBS; *Kraft Theatre.* Movies: Title role, *Welcome Home, Johnny Bristol,* CBS, 1972; Tom Flood, *The Death of Ocean View Park,* ABC, 1979; J.J. Pierson, *The Harlem Globetrotters on Gilligan's Island,* NBC, 1981; Roderick Usher, *The Fall of the House of Usher,* NBC, 1982; John Martin Perkins III, *Kung Fu: The Movie,* CBS, 1986. Specials: *The Screen Actors Guild Fiftieth Anniversary Celebration,* CBS, 1984.

RELATED CAREER—Member of board of directors, Actors Studio, 1955—; executive director, Actors Studio West; acting teacher.

NON-RELATED CAREER—Editorial artist and staff cartoonist, *[New York] Daily News;* illustrator, Billy Rose's "Pitching Horseshoes" newspaper column; cartoonist for "The Gumps" comic strip.

AWARDS: Emmy Award nominations, Outstanding Supporting Actor in a Television Series, 1967, 1968, and 1969, and Golden Globe Award, Best Television Star—Male, 1968, all for *Mission: Impossible;* Golden Globe Award nomination, Best Supporting Actor in a Motion Picture, and Academy Award nomination, Best Supporting Actor, both 1989, for *Tucker: The Man and His Dream;* also Bravo Award (Germany), Viewers Award (Belgium), and SACI Award (Brazil).

MEMBER: Actors' Equity Association, Screen Actors Guild, American Federation of Television and Radio Artists, Academy of Motion Picture Arts and Sciences, Academy of Television Arts and Sciences.

SIDELIGHTS: RECREATIONS—Painting, photography, and writing.

ADDRESSES: AGENT—Allen Goldstein and Associates, 15010 Ventura Boulevard, Suite 234, Sherman Oaks, CA 91403.*

*   *   *

LANDIS, John   1950-

PERSONAL: Born August 30, 1950, in Chicago, IL; son of Marshall David and Shirley (Magaziner) Landis; married Deborah Nadoolman (a costume designer), July 27, 1980; children: Rachel.

VOCATION: Director, producer, screenwriter, actor, and stuntman.

CAREER: Also see WRITINGS below. PRINCIPAL FILM APPEARANCES—Jake's friend, *Battle for the Planet of the Apes,* Twentieth Century-Fox, 1973; Schlockthropus, *Schlock* (also known as *The Banana Monster*), Jack Harris, 1973; mechanic, *Death Race 2000,* New World, 1975; Mizerany, *1941,* Universal, 1979; Trooper La Fong, *The Blues Brothers,* Universal, 1980; Savak, *Into the Night,* Universal, 1985; also appeared in *Making Michael Jackson's "Thriller"* (documentary), Palace/Virgin Vision/Gold, 1983; and in *The Muppets Take Manhattan,* Tri-Star, 1984.

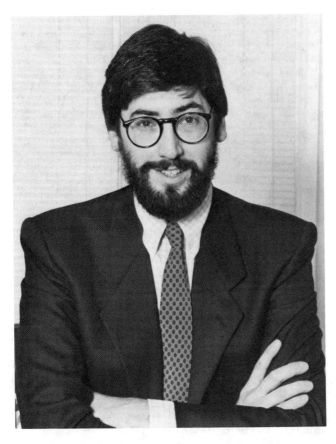

JOHN LANDIS

PRINCIPAL FILM WORK—Director and stuntman, *Schlock* (also known as *The Banana Monster*), Jack Harris, 1973; director, *Kentucky Fried Movie*, United, 1977; director, *National Lampoon's Animal House*, Universal, 1977; director, *The Blues Brothers*, Universal, 1980; director and stuntman, *An American Werewolf in London*, Universal, 1981; director, "Prologue" and "Back There" segments, and producer (with Steven Spielberg), *Twilight Zone—The Movie*, Warner Brothers, 1983; producer and director, *Making Michael Jackson's "Thriller"* (documentary), Palace/Virgin Vision/Gold, 1983; director, *Trading Places*, Paramount, 1983; director, *Into the Night*, Universal, 1985; director, *Spies Like Us*, Warner Brothers, 1985; executive producer, *Clue*, Paramount, 1985; director, *Three Amigos!*, Orion, 1986; executive producer and director (with Joe Dante, Carl Gottlieb, Peter Horton, and Robert K. Weiss), *Amazon Women on the Moon*, Universal, 1987; director, *Coming to America*, Paramount, 1988.

PRINCIPAL TELEVISION WORK—Episodic: Director, *George Burns Comedy Week*, CBS, 1985; executive producer, "Fuzzbucket," *Disney Sunday Movie*, ABC, 1986.

RELATED CAREER—Crew member, *Kelly's Heroes*, Metro-Goldwyn-Mayer, 1970; stuntman "spaghetti westerns" in Europe, 1971; co-producer and director of the Michael Jackson music video *Thriller*, 1983.

WRITINGS: FILM—See production details above. *Schlock*, 1973; (with Dan Aykroyd) *The Blues Brothers*, 1980; *An American Werewolf in London*, 1981; "Prologue" and "Back There" segments, *Twilight Zone—The Movie*, 1983; part one, *Making Mi-*

chael Jackson's "Thriller" (documentary), 1983; *Into the Night*, 1985; (story only, with Jonathan Lynn) *Clue*, 1985. OTHER—Co-writer, *Thriller* (music video), 1983.

MEMBER: Writers Guild of America, Directors Guild of America, Screen Actors Guild, Academy of Motion Pictures Arts and Sciences.

OTHER SOURCES: *Contemporary Authors*, Vol. 122, Gale, 1988.

ADDRESSES: OFFICE—Universal Studios, 100 Universal City Plaza, Building 423, Universal City, CA 91608. AGENT—Mike Marcus, Creative Artists Agency, 1888 Century Park E., Suite 1400, Los Angeles, CA 90067.*

*   *   *

LANDON, Michael   1936-

PERSONAL: Born Eugene Maurice Orowitz, October 31, 1936, in Forest Hills, NY; son of Eli Maurice (a film studio publicist) and Peggy (an actress and comedienne; maiden name, O'Neill) Orowitz; married second wife, Lynn Noe (a model), 1963 (divorced, 1982); married Cindy Clerico (a make-up artist); children: Mark, Josh, Cheryl, Michael, Leslie Ann, Shawna Leigh, Christopher Beau, Jennifer, Sean. EDUCATION: Attended the University of Southern California.

VOCATION: Actor, director, producer, and screenwriter.

CAREER: Also see WRITINGS below. PRINCIPAL FILM APPEARANCES—Boy in poolroom, *These Wilder Years*, Metro-Goldwyn-Mayer (MGM), 1956; Tony, *I Was a Teenage Werewolf*, American International, 1957; Steve Bentley, *High School Confidential* (also known as *The Young Hellions*), MGM, 1958; Dave Dawson, *God's Little Acre*, United Artists, 1958; Lago Orlando, *Maracaibo*, Paramount, 1958; title role, *The Legend of Tom Dooley*, Columbia, 1959; as himself, *The Errand Boy*, Paramount, 1961; Gene Orman, *Sam's Son*, Invictus, 1984; John Everingham, *Comeback*, Twentieth Century-Fox, 1982. PRINCIPAL FILM WORK—Director, *Sam's Son*, Invictus, 1984.

PRINCIPAL TELEVISION APPEARANCES—Series: Little Joe Cartwright, *Bonanza*, NBC, 1959-73; Charles Ingalls, *Little House on the Prairie*, NBC, 1974-82; Jonathan Smith, *Highway to Heaven*, NBC, 1984-88. Pilots: Sandy, *The Restless Gun*, CBS, 1957; Don Burns, *Belle Starr*, CBS, 1958; title role, *Johnny Risk*, NBC, 1958; Little Joe Cartwright, *Sam Hill*, NBC, 1961; Tough, *Luke and the Tenderfoot*, CBS, 1965; Charles Ingalls, *Little House on the Prairie*, NBC, 1974; also *A Country Happening*, NBC, 1969; and *The Amateur's Guide to Love*, CBS, 1971. Episodic: *The Adventures of Jim Bowie*, ABC, 1956; "Too Good with a Gun," *General Electric Theatre*, CBS, 1974; *The Wil Shriner Show*, syndicated, 1987; also *The Sheriff of Cochise*, syndicated; *Tales of Wells Fargo*, NBC; *Wanted: Dead or Alive*, CBS; *Wire Service*, ABC; *Cavalcade of America* (also known as *DuPont Cavalcade Theatre*) ABC; *Telephone Time*, ABC; *Playhouse 90*, CBS; *The Texan*, CBS; *The Tonight Show*, NBC.

Movies: John Curtis as an adult, *The Loneliest Runner*, NBC, 1976; John Everingham, *Love Is Forever*, NBC, 1983; Charles Ingalls, *Little House: Look Back to Yesterday*, NBC, 1983; Charles Ingalls, *Little House: The Last Farewell*, NBC, 1984. Specials: *Swing Out, Sweet Land*, NBC, 1971; *Monsanto Presents Mancini*, syndicated,

1971; *Mitzi and a Hundred Guys*, CBS, 1975; *Doug Henning's World of Magic*, NBC, 1976; *General Electric's All-Star Anniversary*, ABC, 1978; *The Dean Martin Celebrity Roast*, NBC, 1984; *Bob Hope Buys NBC*, NBC, 1985; *NBC's Sixtieth Birthday Celebration*, NBC, 1986; *NBC Investigates Bob Hope*, NBC, 1987; *Happy Birthday, Bob—Fifty Stars Salute Your Fifty Years with NBC*, NBC, 1988; also *Surviving a Heart Attack*, 1988.

PRINCIPAL TELEVISION WORK—Series: Creator and executive producer, *Little House on the Prairie*, NBC, 1974-82, renamed *Little House: A New Beginning*, NBC, 1982-83; creator and executive producer, *Father Murphy*, NBC, 1981-84; creator and executive producer, *Highway to Heaven*, NBC, 1984-88. Pilots: Producer and director, *Little House on the Prairie*, NBC, 1974. Episodic: Director, *Little House on the Prairie*, NBC, 1974-82, renamed *Little House: A New Beginning*, NBC, 1982-83; director, *Father Murphy*, NBC, 1981-84; director, *Highway to Heaven*, NBC, 1984-88; also director, *Bonanza*, NBC. Movies: Director, *It's Good to Be Alive*, CBS, 1974; producer and director, *The Loneliest Runner*, NBC, 1976; producer and director, *Killing Stone*, NBC, 1978; executive producer, *Love Is Forever*, NBC, 1983; executive producer, *Little House: Look Back to Yesterday*, NBC, 1983; executive producer, *Little House: Bless All the Dear Children*, NBC, 1984; executive producer and director, *Little House: The Last Farewell*, NBC, 1984; also director, *The Roy Campanella Story*.

WRITINGS: FILM—*Sam's Son*, Invictus, 1984. TELEVISION—Episodic: *Little House on the Prairie*, NBC, 1974-82, renamed *Little House: A New Beginning*, NBC, 1982-83; *Highway to Heaven*, NBC, 1984-88; also *Bonanza*, NBC. Movies: *The Loneliest Runner*, NBC, 1976; *Killing Stone*, NBC, 1978; *Little House: The Last Farewell*, NBC, 1984. Also *Love Came Laughing*.

AWARDS: Academy Founders Award from the National Academy of Television Arts and Sciences, 1982.

MEMBER: Screen Actors Guild, American Federation of Television and Radio Artists, Writers Guild-West, Directors Guild of America, National Academy of Television Arts and Sciences.

ADDRESSES: OFFICE—Michael Landon Productions, Box 951, Malibu, CA 90265.

*   *   *

LANSBURY, Angela   1925-

PERSONAL: Full name, Angela Brigid Lansbury; born October 16, 1925, in London, England; came to the United States in 1940; naturalized U.S. citizen, 1951; daughter of Edgar Isaac (a lumber merchant) and Moyna (an actress; maiden name, Macgill) Lansbury; married Richard Cromwell (an actor), 1945 (divorced, 1946); married Peter Pullen Shaw (an agent), August, 12, 1949; children: Anthony Peter, Deirdre Angela (second marriage); David (stepson). EDUCATION: Trained for the stage at the Webber-Douglas School for Dramatic Arts, 1939-40, and at the the Feagin School of Drama, 1940-42.

VOCATION: Actress.

CAREER: BROADWAY DEBUT—Marcelle, *Hotel Paradiso*, Henry Miller's Theatre, 1957. LONDON DEBUT—Mistress, *All Over*,

Royal Shakespeare Company, Aldwych Theatre, 1972. PRINCIPAL STAGE APPEARANCES—Helen, *A Taste of Honey*, Lyceum Theatre, New York City, 1960; Cora Hoover Hooper, *Anyone Can Whistle*, Majestic Theatre, New York City, 1964; title role, *Mame*, Winter Garden Theatre, New York City, 1966; Countess Aurelia, *Dear World*, Mark Hellinger Theatre, New York City, 1969; Prettybelle Sweet, *Prettybelle*, Shubert Theatre, Boston, MA, 1971; title role, *Mame*, Westbury Music Fair, Long Island, NY, 1972; ensemble, *Sondheim: A Musical Tribute* (revue), Shubert Theatre, New York City, 1973; Mama Rose, *Gypsy*, Piccadilly Theatre, London, 1973, then Shubert Theatre, Los Angeles, CA, later Winter Garden Theatre, New York City, both 1974; Gertrude, *Hamlet*, National Theatre Company, Old Vic Theatre, London, 1975, then Lyttelton Theatre, London, 1976; Anna, *The King and I*, Uris Theatre, New York City, 1978; Mrs. Lovett, *Sweeney Todd*, Uris Theatre, 1979; Lillian, *A Little Family Business*, Center Theatre Group, Ahmanson Theatre, Los Angeles, then Martin Beck Theatre, New York City, both 1982; title role, *Mame*, Gershwin Theatre, New York City, 1983. Also appeared in *Counting the Ways* and *Listening*, both Hartford Stage Company, Hartford, CT, 1976-77.

MAJOR TOURS—Mrs. Lovett, *Sweeney Todd*, U.S. cities, 1980.

FILM DEBUT—Nancy Oliver, *Gaslight* (also known as *The Murder in Thornton Square*), Metro-Goldwyn-Mayer, 1944. PRINCIPAL FILM APPEARANCES—Edwina Brown, *National Velvet*, Metro-Goldwyn-Mayer (MGM), 1944; Sybil Vane, *The Picture of Dorian Gray*, MGM, 1945; Dusty Millard, *The Hoodlum Saint*, MGM, 1946; guest performer, *Till the Clouds Roll By*, MGM, 1946; Em, *The Harvey Girls*, MGM, 1946; Mabel Sabre, *If Winter Comes*, MGM, 1947; Clottide de Marelle, *The Private Affairs of Bel Ami*, United Artists, 1947; Kay Thorndyke, *State of the Union* (also known as *The World and His Wife*), MGM, 1948; Susan Bratten, *Tenth Avenue Angel*, MGM, 1948; Queen Anne, *The Three Musketeers*, MGM, 1948; Audrey Quail, *The Red Danube*, MGM, 1949; Semador, *Samson and Delilah*, Paramount, 1949; Mrs. Edwards, *Kind Lady*, MGM, 1951; Leslie, *Mutiny*, United Artists, 1952; Valeska Chauvel, *Remains to Be Seen*, MGM, 1953; Doris Hillman, *Key Man* (also known as *A Life at Stake*), Anglo-Amalgamated, 1954; Tally Dickinson, *A Lawless Street*, Columbia, 1955; Madame Valentine, *The Purple Mask*, Universal, 1955; Princess Gwendolyn, *The Court Jester*, Paramount, 1956; Myra Leeds, *Please Murder Me*, Distributors Corporation of America, 1956; Minnie Littlejohn, *The Long, Hot Summer*, Twentieth Century-Fox, 1958; Mabel Claremont, *The Reluctant Debutante*, MGM, 1958.

Countess Lina, *A Breath of Scandal*, Paramount, 1960; Mavis Pruitt, *The Dark at the Top of the Stairs*, Warner Brothers, 1960; Sarah Lee Gates, *Blue Hawaii*, Paramount, 1961; Pearl, *Season of Passion* (also known as *Summer of the Seventeenth Doll*), United Artists, 1961; Annabel Willart, *All Fall Down*, MGM, 1962; voice of Marguerite Laurier, *The Four Horsemen of the Apocalypse*, MGM, 1962; Mrs. Iselin, *The Manchurian Candidate*, United Artists, 1962; Sibyl Logan, *In the Cool of the Day*, MGM, 1963; Phyllis, *Dear Heart*, Warner Brothers, 1964; Isabel Boyd, *The World of Henry Orient*, United Artists, 1964; Lady Blystone, *The Amorous Adventures of Moll Flanders*, Paramount, 1965; Claudia, *The Greatest Story Ever Told*, United Artists, 1965; Mama Jean Bello, *Harlow*, Paramount, 1965; Gloria, *Mister Buddwing* (also known as *Woman without a Face*), MGM, 1966; Countess Herthe von Ornstein, *Something for Everyone* (also known as *The Rook* and *Black Flowers for the Bride*), National General, 1970; Eglantine Price, *Bedknobs and Broomsticks*, Buena Vista, 1971; Mrs. Salome

Otterbourne, *Death on the Nile,* Paramount, 1978; Miss Froy, *The Lady Vanishes,* Rank/Group 1, 1980; Miss Jane Marple, *The Mirror Crack'd,* Associated Film Distribution, 1980; voice of Mommy Fortuna, *The Last Unicorn* (animated), ITC, 1982; Ruth, *The Pirates of Penzance,* Universal, 1983; Granny, *The Company of Wolves,* Cannon, 1985; as herself, *Ingrid* (documentary), Wombat Productions, 1985.

PRINCIPAL TELEVISION APPEARANCES—Series: Jessica Beatrice Fletcher, *Murder, She Wrote,* CBS, 1984—. Mini-Series: Aunt Hortense Boutin, *Lace,* ABC, 1984. Pilots: *Scene of the Crime,* NBC, 1984. Episodic: *Revlon Mirror Theater,* CBS, 1953; *Henry Fonda Presents the Star and the Story* (also known as *The Star and the Story*), syndicated, 1955; *Rheingold Theatre,* syndicated, 1955; *Stage 7,* CBS, 1955; *Star Time Playhouse,* CBS, 1955; also *Climax!,* CBS; *Fireside Theatre,* NBC; *Four Star Playhouse,* CBS; *Front Row Center,* CBS; *Playhouse 90,* CBS; *Schlitz Playhouse of Stars,* CBS; *Ford Television Theatre,* NBC; *Robert Montgomery Presents Your Lucky Strike Theatre,* NBC; *The Danny Kaye Show,* CBS; *Alcoa Preview,* ABC; *The Eleventh Hour,* NBC; *The Man from U.N.C.L.E.,* NBC; *The Trials of O'Brien,* CBS; *The Merv Griffin Show,* syndicated; *The Today Show,* NBC; *Suspense Theatre,* syndicated; *The Perry Como Show,* NBC; *Four Star Playhouse,* CBS; *General Electric Theatre,* CBS; *The Art of Film,* NET; *Studio One,* CBS; *Kraft Theatre; The Lux Video Theatre;* and *Pantomine Quiz.*

Movies: Gertrude Vanderbilt Whitney, *Little Gloria . . . Happy at Last,* NBC, 1982; Amanda Fenwick, *The Gift of Love: A Christmas Story,* CBS, 1983; Alice Garrett, *The First Olympics—Athens, 1896,* NBC, 1984; Marchesa Allabrandi, *Rage of Angels: The Story Continues,* NBC, 1986; Nan Moore, *Shootdown,* NBC, 1988. Specials: *The Perry Como Christmas Show,* NBC, 1964; *The Perry Como Thanksgiving Special,* NBC, 1966; voice of Sister Theresa, *The First Christmas Snow* (animated), NBC, 1975; *Circus of the Stars,* CBS, 1980; Mrs. Lovett, *Sweeney Todd,* Entertainment Channel, 1982; *The Barbara Walters Special,* ABC, 1985; *Clue: Movies, Murder, and Mystery,* CBS, 1986; *The Spencer Tracy Legacy: A Tribute by Katherine Hepburn,* PBS, 1986; *Liberty Weekend,* ABC, 1986; host, *The Forty-First Annual Tony Awards,* CBS, 1987; *Kennedy Center Honors: A Celebration of the Performing Arts,* CBS, 1987; *People Magazine on TV,* CBS, 1988; host, *The Forty-Second Annual Tony Awards,* CBS, 1988.

RELATED CAREER—Singer, Samovar Club, Montreal, PQ, Canada, 1942.

NON-RELATED CAREER—Sales clerk, Bullocks (department store), Wilshire, CA.

RECORDINGS: ALBUMS—*Anyone Can Whistle* (original cast recording), CBS Special Products, 1964; *Mame* (original cast recording), Columbia, 1966; *Dear World* (original cast recording), CBS Special Products, 1969; *Sweeney Todd* (original cast recording), RCA, 1979; also *The Beggar's Opera,* 1982.

AWARDS: Academy Award nomination, Best Supporting Actress, 1945, for *Gaslight;* Golden Globe Award and Academy Award nomination, both Best Supporting Actress, 1946, for *The Picture of Dorian Gray;* Golden Globe Award and Academy Award nomination, both Best Supporting Actress, 1963, for *The Manchurian Candidate;* Antoinette Perry Award, Best Actress in a Musical, 1966, for *Mame;* Hasty Pudding Woman of the Year Award from the Harvard Hasty Pudding Theatricals, 1968; Antoinette Perry Award, Best Actress in a Musical, 1969, for *Dear World;* Antoi-

nette Perry Award, Best Actress in a Musical, and Sarah Siddons Award, both 1975, for *Gypsy;* Antoinette Perry Award, Best Actress in a Musical, Drama Desk Award, Outstanding Actress in a Musical, and *After Dark*'s Ruby Award, Performer of the Year, all 1979, for *Sweeney Todd;* Sarah Siddons Award, 1980, for *Mame;* inducted into the Theatre Hall of Fame, 1982; Golden Globe Award, Best Performance by an Actress in a Television Series—Drama, 1984 and 1987, both for *Murder, She Wrote;* Golden Globe Award nomination, Best Performance by an Actress in a Television Series—Drama, 1988, for *Murder, She Wrote.*

MEMBER: Actors' Equity Association, Screen Actors Guild, American Federation of Television and Radio Artists, Players Club.

ADDRESSES: AGENT—William Morris Agency, 151 El Camino Drive, Beverly Hills, CA 90212.*

*   *   *

LAPINE, James   1949-

PERSONAL: Full name, James Elliot Lapine; born January 10, 1949, in Mansfield, OH; son of David Sanford and Lillian (Feld) Lapine; married Sarah Marshall Kernochan, February 24, 1985; children: Phoebe. EDUCATION: Received B.A. from Franklin and Marshall College; received M.F.A. from California Institute of the Arts.

VOCATION: Director and playwright.

CAREER: Also see *WRITINGS* below. PRINCIPAL STAGE WORK—Director: *Photograph,* Open Space in Soho Theatre, New York City, 1977; *Table Settings,* Playwrights Horizons, New York City, 1980; *March of the Falsettos,* Playwrights Horizons, then Cheryl Crawford Theatre, Westside Arts Center, both New York City, 1981; *Twelve Dreams,* New York Shakespeare Festival (NYSF), Public Theatre, New York City, 1981; *A Midsummer Night's Dream,* NYSF, Delacorte Theatre, New York City, 1982; *Sunday in the Park with George,* Playwrights Horizons, 1983, then Booth Theatre, New York City, 1984; *Into the Woods,* Old Globe Theatre, San Diego, CA, then Martin Beck Theatre, New York City, both 1987; *The Winter's Tale,* NYSF, Public Theatre, 1989. Also served as advisor, "A Fool's Errand," *The New Directors Project,* Perry Street Theatre, New York City, 1984.

RELATED CAREER—Teacher, Yale School of Drama, New Haven, CT.

NON-RELATED CAREER—Freelance photographer and graphic designer.

WRITINGS: See production details above. STAGE—(Adaptor) *Photograph,* 1977; *Table Settings,* 1980, published by Samuel French, 1980; *Twelve Dreams,* 1981, published by Doubleday, 1982; (book for musical) *Sunday in the Park with George,* 1983, published by Dodd Mead, 1986; (book for musical) *Into the Woods,* 1987.

AWARDS: Obie Award from the *Village Voice,* 1977, for *Photograph;* New York Drama Critics Circle Award, Best Musical, 1984, Antoinette Perry Award nominations, Best Director of a Musical and Best Book of a Musical, 1984, and Pulitzer Prize for Drama, 1985, all for *Sunday in the Park with George;* Antoinette

Perry Award, Best Book of a Musical, 1987, for *Into the Woods;* also received Drama Desk Award, George Oppenheimer Playwrighting Award, and a Guggenheim fellowship.

MEMBER: Dramatists Guild, Society of Stage Directors and Choreographers.

ADDRESSES: AGENTS—George Lane, William Morris Agency, 1350 Avenue of the Americas, New York, NY 10019; Sam Cohn, International Creative Management, 40 W. 57th Street, New York, NY 10036.*

*   *   *

LARSON, Glen A.

PERSONAL: Born c. 1937; first wife's name, Carol (marriage ended); married second wife, Janet Curtis; children: six (first marriage); two (second marriage).

VOCATION: Producer, director, writer, and composer.

CAREER: Also see *WRITINGS* below. PRINCIPAL FILM WORK—Producer, *Buck Rogers in the Twenty-Fifth Century,* Universal, 1979; producer, *Conquest of the Earth,* Glen A. Larson, 1980.

PRINCIPAL TELEVISION WORK—All as executive producer, unless indicated. Series: (With Leslie Stevens) *McCloud,* NBC, 1970-77; (also creator) *Alias Smith and Jones,* ABC, 1971-73; *The Six Million Dollar Man,* ABC, 1973-78; *Get Christie Love!,* ABC, 1974-75; (with Matthew Rapf) *Switch,* CBS, 1975-78; *Quincy, M.E.,* NBC, 1976-83; *The Nancy Drew Mysteries,* ABC, 1977-78; *The Hardy Boys Mysteries,* ABC, 1977-79; (also creator) *Sword of Justice,* NBC, 1978-79; *Battlestar Galactica,* ABC, 1978-79, renamed *Galactica 1980,* ABC, 1980; *Buck Rogers in the Twenty-Fifth Century,* NBC, 1979-80; (with Michael Sloan and John Peyser) *B.J. and the Bear,* NBC, 1979-81; *The Misadventures of Sheriff Lobo,* NBC, 1979-80, renamed *Lobo,* NBC, 1980-81; (with Donald P. Bellisario) *Magnum, P.I.,* CBS, 1980-88; *Fitz and Bones,* NBC, 1981; *The Fall Guy,* ABC, 1981-86; (with Robert A. Cinader and Robert Foster) *Knight Rider,* NBC, 1982-86; (with Paul Mason) *Manimal,* NBC, 1983; *Trauma Center,* ABC, 1983; (with Renee Valente) *Masquerade,* ABC, 1983-84; (with Larry Brody) *Automan,* ABC, 1983-84; *Cover Up,* CBS, 1984-85; *Half-Nelson,* NBC, 1985; (also creator) *The Highwayman,* NBC, 1988.

Pilots: Producer, *Alias Smith and Jones,* ABC, 1971; *Fools, Females, and Fun: I've Gotta Be Me,* NBC, 1974; *Fools, Females, and Fun: What about That One?,* NBC, 1974; *Fools, Females, and Fun: Is There a Doctor in the House?,* NBC, 1974; producer, *Switch* (also known as *Las Vegas Roundabout*), CBS, 1975; producer, *Benny and Barney: Las Vegas Undercover,* NBC, 1977; *B.J. and the Bear,* NBC, 1978; producer, *The Islander,* CBS, 1978; *The Misadventures of Sheriff Lobo,* NBC, 1979; *The Murder That Wouldn't Die* (also known as *Battles: The Murder That Wouldn't Die*), NBC, 1980; (with Sloan) *The Eyes of Texas,* NBC, 1980; (with Sloan) *The Eyes of Texas II,* NBC, 1980; (with Stephen J. Cannell) *Nightside,* ABC, 1980; (also creator) *How Do I Kill a Thief—Let Me Count the Ways,* ABC, 1982; (with Lou Shaw) *Terror at Alcatraz,* NBC, 1982; *Rooster,* ABC, 1982; (with Foster) *All That Glitters,* NBC, 1984; *In Like Flynn,* ABC, 1985; *Crazy Dan,* NBC, 1986; *The Highwayman,* NBC, 1987. Episodic: Producer and director, *McCloud,* NBC, 1970-77; producer and direc-

tor, *Alias Smith and Jones,* ABC, 1971-73; producer and director, *The Six Million Dollar Man,* ABC, 1973-78; producer and director, *Get Christie Love!,* ABC, 1974-75. Movies: Producer (with Sloan), *Evening in Byzantium,* syndicated, 1978; *The Road Raiders,* CBS, 1989.

RELATED CAREER—Member of the Four Preps singing group, during the 1950s; founder, Glen A. Larson Productions, Inc.

WRITINGS: FILM—*Battlestar Galactica,* Universal, 1979; *Mission Galactica: The Cylon Attack,* Universal, 1979; *Buck Rogers in the Twenty-Fifth Century,* Universal, 1979; *Conquest of the Earth,* Glen A. Larson, 1980.

TELEVISION—Series: All as composer. *Switch,* CBS, 1975-78; (with Stu Phillips) *The Nancy Drew Mysteries,* ABC, 1977-78; *The Hardy Boys Mysteries,* ABC, 1977-79; *Battlestar Galactica,* ABC, 1978-79, renamed *Galactica 1980,* ABC, 1980; *Buck Rogers in the Twenty-Fifth Century,* NBC, 1979-80; *B.J. and the Bear,* NBC, 1979-81; (with Gail Jensoen and David Sommerville) *The Fall Guy,* ABC, 1981-86; (with Michael Sloan) *Knight Rider,* NBC, 1982-86. Pilots: (With Matthew Howard) *Alias Smith and Jones,* ABC, 1971; (with Michael Gleason; also composer) *Fools, Females, and Fun: I've Gotta Be Me,* NBC, 1974; (with Gleason; also composer) *Fools, Females, and Fun: What about That One?,* NBC, 1974; (with Gleason; also composer) *Fools, Females, and Fun: Is There a Doctor in the House?* NBC, 1974; *Switch* (also known as *Las Vegas Roundabout*), CBS, 1975; *Benny and Barney: Las Vegas Undercover,* NBC, 1977; (with Christopher Crowe; also composer) *B.J. and the Bear,* NBC, 1978; *The Islander,* CBS, 1978; (with Sloan; also composer with Stu Phillips and Joe Harnell) *The Murder That Wouldn't Die,* NBC, 1980; *The Eyes of Texas,* NBC, 1980; *The Eyes of Texas II,* NBC, 1980; (with Stephen J. Cannell) *Nightside,* ABC, 1980; *How Do I Kill a Thief—Let Me Count the Ways,* ABC, 1982; (with Lou Shaw) *Terror at Alcatraz,* NBC, 1982; (with Paul Williams) *Rooster,* ABC, 1982; (also composer) *In Like Flynn,* ABC, 1985; (with Kim Weiskopf and Michael S. Baser) *Crazy Dan,* NBC, 1986; *The Highwayman,* NBC, 1987.

Episodic: All as co-writer. *It Takes a Thief,* ABC, 1968-70; *McCloud,* NBC, 1970-77; *Alias Smith and Jones,* ABC, 1971-73; *The Six Million Dollar Man,* ABC, 1973-78; *Switch,* CBS, 1975-78; *The Nancy Drew Mysteries,* ABC, 1977-78; *The Hardy Boys Mysteries,* ABC, 1977-79; *Battlestar Galactica,* ABC, 1978-79, renamed *Galactica 1980,* ABC, 1980; *Buck Rogers in the Twenty-Fifth Century,* NBC, 1979-80; *B.J. and the Bear,* NBC, 1979-81; *The Misadventures of Sheriff Lobo,* 1979-80, renamed *Lobo,* NBC, 1980-81; *Magnum, P.I.,* CBS, 1980-88; *Fitz and Bones,* NBC, 1981; *The Fall Guy,* ABC, 1981-86; *Knight Rider,* NBC, 1982-86; *Simon and Simon,* CBS, 1982-83; *Manimal,* NBC, 1983; *Trauma Center,* ABC, 1983; *Masquerade,* ABC, 1983-84; *Automan,* ABC, 1983-84; *Cover Up,* CBS, 1984-85; *The Highwayman,* NBC, 1988. Movies: (With Sloan) *Evening in Byzantium,* syndicated, 1978; (with Mark Jones) *The Road Raiders,* CBS, 1989.

OTHER—Novels: (With Robert Thurston) *Battlestar Galactica,* Berkley, 1978; (with Leslie Stevens) *Buck Rogers in the Twenty-Fifth Century,* Fotonovel, 1979; also wrote novelizations based on *The Nancy Drew Mysteries* and *The Hardy Boys Mysteries* television series.

RECORDINGS: All with the Four Preps. SINGLES—''26 Miles,'' ''Big Man,'' and ''Down by the Station.''

AWARDS: Academy of Science Fiction Television Awards, Best

Series, 1979 and 1980, for *Buck Rogers in the Twenty-Fifth Century;* Media Access Award of Excellence, 1985, for *The Fall Guy;* Television Showmanship Award from the Publicists Guild of America, 1986; also received gold records for "26 Miles," "Big Man," and "Down by the Station."

ADDRESSES: OFFICE—c/o Twentieth Century-Fox Television, P.O. Box 900, Los Angeles, CA 90213.*

*   *   *

LAURIA, Dan   1947-

PERSONAL: Born April 12, 1947, in Brooklyn, NY. EDUCATION: Received B.A. in history and philosophy from Southern Connecticut University, M.A. from Yale University, and M.F.A. in playwriting from the University of Connecticut. MILITARY: U.S. Marine Corps, captain, 1970-73.

VOCATION: Actor and playwright.

CAREER: Also see *WRITINGS* below. PRINCIPAL STAGE APPEARANCES—Johnny Ryan, *Game Plan*, Theatre Four, New York City, 1978; Vinnie Ventura, "The Shangri-La Motor Inn," *Niagara Falls*, Urban Arts Theatre, New York City, 1981; Top, *Dustoff*, Westside Mainstage Theatre, New York City, 1982; Donny Dukes, *Punchy*, Westside Mainstage Theatre, 1983. Also appeared in *These Days the Watchmen Sleep* and *La Visionaria*, both New

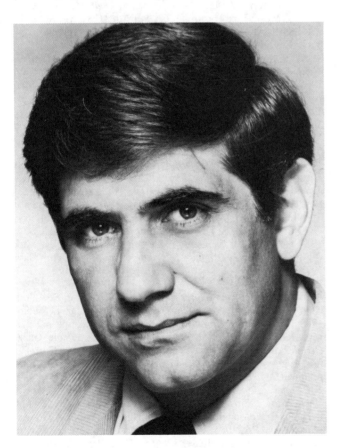

DAN LAURIA

Dramatists, New York City, 1980-81; in productions of *All My Sons, Marlon Brando Sat Here, Collective Portraits*, and *Home of the Brave*, all in New York City; and with the Washington Theatre Club, Washington, DC.

PRINCIPAL FILM APPEARANCES—Baker, *Without a Trace*, Twentieth Century-Fox, 1983; janitor, *9 1/2 Weeks*, Metro-Goldwyn-Mayer/United Artists, 1986; Phil Coldshank, *Stakeout*, Buena Vista, 1987. Also appeared in *South Bronx Heroes* (also known as *The Runaways* and *Revenge of the Innocents*), Continental, 1985.

TELEVISION DEBUT—*Love of Life*, CBS. PRINCIPAL TELEVISION APPEARANCES—Series: Jack Arnold, *The Wonder Years*, ABC, 1988—; also *One Life to Live*, ABC, for two years. Pilots: Detective Navarro, *Brass*, CBS, 1985. Episodic: Artie Karnovsky, *Simon and Simon*, CBS, 1986; Daroca, *Moonlighting*, ABC, 1986; Jacoby, *Cagney and Lacey*, CBS, 1986; Rogan, *Scarecrow and Mrs. King*, CBS, 1986; Broder, *Hunter*, NBC, 1986; also *Growing Pains*, ABC; *Spenser: For Hire*, ABC; *Hill Street Blues*, NBC; *L.A. Law*, ABC; *Hooperman*, ABC. Movies: Vince Palucci, *Muggable Mary: Street Cop*, CBS, 1982; Captain Lubway, *Doing Life*, NBC, 1986; Skuska, *Johnny Bull*, ABC, 1986; John Cirillo, *David*, ABC, 1988; also Sergeant Len Taggart, *Cop Killer*, 1988.

RELATED CAREER—Director, Raft Theatre, New York City.

WRITINGS: STAGE—*Game Plan*, Theatre Four, New York City, 1978; *'Til Jason Comes*, Raft Theatre, New York City, 1985. Also *The Setup*, Raft Theatre.

MEMBER: Actors' Equity Association, Screen Actors Guild, American Federation of Television and Radio Artists.

ADDRESSES: AGENTS—Barry Douglas, 1650 Broadway, Suite 806, New York, NY 10019; Diana Davis, Twentieth Century Artists, 3800 Barham Boulevard, Suite 303, Burbank, CA 90068.

*   *   *

LAW, John Phillip   1937-

PERSONAL: Born September 7, 1937, in Hollywood, CA. EDUCATION: Attended the University of Hawaii; studied acting with Elia Kazan at the Repertory Theatre of Lincoln Center.

VOCATION: Actor.

CAREER: PRINCIPAL FILM APPEARANCES—Ronald, "The Infidelity," in *High Infidelity* (also known as *Alta Infidelta* and *Haute Infidelite*), Magna, 1965; Alexei Kolchin, *The Russians Are Coming, the Russians Are Coming*, United Artists, 1966; Rad McDowell, *Hurry Sundown*, Paramount, 1967; Pygar, *Barbarella* (also known as *Barbarella, Queen of the Galaxy*), Paramount, 1968; Diabolik, *Danger: Diabolik* (also know as *Diabolik* and *Danger Diabolik*), Paramount, 1968; Private First Class Tom Swanson, *The Sergeant*, Warner Brothers, 1968; Stash, *Skidoo*, Paramount, 1968; Bill, *Death Rides a Horse*, United Artists, 1969; Fra Felice, "Fate benefratelli," in *Three Nights of Love* (also known as *Tre notti d'amore*), Magna, 1969; Crispino, *Certain, Very Certain, As a Matter of Fact . . . Probable*, Clesi/San Marco, 1970; Noel Hoxworth, *The Hawaiians* (also known as *Master of the Islands*), United Artists, 1970; Baron Manfred Von Richthofen, *Von Richthofen and Brown* (also known as *The Red Baron*), United Artists, 1970;

little brother, *The Last Movie* (also known as *Chinchero*), Universal/CIC, 1971; Robin Stone, *The Love Machine*, Columbia, 1971; sailor, *Polvere di Stelle* (also known as *Star Dust*), Fida Cinematografica, 1973; Sinbad, *The Golden Voyage of Sinbad*, Columbia, 1974; Greg, *Open Season*, Columbia, 1974.

Steven, *The Spiral Staircase*, Warner Brothers, 1975; Major Stack, *The Cassandra Crossing*, AVCO-Embassy, 1977; Holt, *Tarzan, the Ape Man*, Metro-Goldwyn-Mayer/United Artists, 1981; Lieutenant Jan Vietch, *Attack Force Z* (also known as *Z Men*), Virgin Vision, 1981; Harry Billings, *Night Train to Terror*, Vista International, 1985; Stephen Kendricks, *Rainy Day Friends* (also known as *L.A. Bad*), Prism Entertainment, 1985; Kelly, *American Commandos* (also known as *Hitman*), Panorama/Ader-Spiegelman, 1986; Ted Barner, *No Time to Die*, Rapid-Lisa-Rapi, 1986; Maximilian Steiner, *Johann Strauss le roi sans couronne* (also known as *Johann Strauss: The King without a Crown*), Metro-Goldwyn-Mayer, 1987; Allen, *Moon in Scorpio*, Trans World Entertainment, 1988. Also appeared in *Target of an Assassin*, 1978; and in *Tin Man*, Goldfarb Distributors, 1983.

PRINCIPAL TELEVISION APPEARANCES—Episodic: Hank, *It's a Living*, syndicated. Movies: Dr. Gary Mancini, *The Best Place to Be*, NBC, 1979.

MEMBER: Screen Actors Guild.

ADDRESSES: AGENT—Contemporary Artists, 132 Lasky Drive, Beverly Hills, CA 90212.*

*   *   *

LeGAULT, Lance

VOCATION: Actor.

CAREER: PRINCIPAL STAGE APPEARANCES—Iago, *Catch My Soul*, Round House Theatre, London, 1970.

PRINCIPAL FILM APPEARANCES—Barker, *Roustabout*, Paramount, 1964; Warren, *The Swinger*, Paramount, 1966; Curly, *The Young Runaways*, Metro-Goldwyn-Mayer, 1968; dancer, *Sweet Charity*, Universal, 1969; Iago, *Catch My Soul* (also known as *To Catch a Spy* and *Santa Fe Satan*), Metromedia Producers Corporation, 1974; Tom/Burt, *French Quarter*, Crown International, 1978; Vince, *Coma*, United Artists, 1978; Edgar Wamback, *Amy*, Buena Vista, 1981; Colonel Glass, *Stripes*, Columbia, 1981; Lieutenant Barnes, *Fast-Walking*, Pickman, 1982; general, *Iron Eagle*, Tri-Star, 1985; Victor Nardi, *Kidnapped*, Hickman, 1987.

PRINCIPAL TELEVISION APPEARANCES—Series: Colonel Roderick Decker, *The A-Team*, NBC, 1983-87; narrator, *Airwolf*, CBS, 1984-86; voice characterization, *Super Sunday* (animated), syndicated, 1987. Mini-Series: Lester Foyles, *The French Atlantic Affair*, ABC, 1979. Pilots: Mel Drew, *The Busters*, CBS, 1978; Harley, *Captain America*, CBS, 1979; Van Dyke, *Reward*, ABC, 1980; also *Constantinople*, ABC, 1977. Episodic: Noble Flowers, *Airwolf*, CBS, 1986; Colonel Green, *Magnum, P.I.*, CBS, 1986; Alamo Joe, *Werewolf*, Fox, 1987; also "Underground," *Land of the Giants*, ABC, 1968; "Showdown in Saskatchewan," *Murder, She Wrote*, CBS, 1988; "Jack in the Box," *MacGyver*, ABC, 1988; "Unfinished Business," *Magnum P.I.*, CBS, 1988; Ray Bonning, *Dynasty*, ABC. Movies: Joe Wormsler, *Pioneer Woman*,

ABC, 1973; Charles Stanton, *Donner Pass: The Road to Survival*, NBC, 1978; Kaufman, *Nowhere to Run*, NBC, 1978; Weasel, *Undercover with the KKK*, NBC, 1979; Stevens, *Power*, NBC, 1980; Doc Palmer, *Kenny Rogers as "The Gambler,"* CBS, 1980. Specials: Hamilton, *Year of the Gentle Tiger*, CBS, 1979.

MEMBER: Screen Actors Guild, American Federation of Television and Radio Artists.

ADDRESSES: AGENT—Contemporary Artists, 132 Lasky Drive, Beverly Hills, CA 90212.*

*   *   *

LEIBMAN, Ron   1937-

PERSONAL: Born October 11, 1937, in New York, NY; son of Murray and Grace (Marks) Leibman; married Linda Lavin (an actress), September 7, 1969 (divorced); married Jessica Walter (an actress), June 26, 1983. EDUCATION: Attended Ohio Wesleyan University; trained for the stage at the American Academy of Dramatic Arts and the Actors Studio.

VOCATION: Actor.

CAREER: STAGE DEBUT—Rudolfo, *A View from the Bridge*, Barnard Summer Theatre, New York City, 1959. OFF-BROADWAY DEBUT—Orpheus, *Legend of Lovers*, 41st Street Theatre, 1959. BROADWAY DEBUT—Peter Nemo, *Dear Me, the Sky Is Falling*, Music Box Theatre, 1963. PRINCIPAL STAGE APPEARANCES—Kilroy, *Camino Real*, Barnard Summer Theatre, New York City, 1959; Rip Calabria, *Bicycle Ride to Nevada*, Cort Theatre, New York City, 1963; Captain Salzer, *The Deputy*, Theatre of Living Arts, Brooks Atkinson Theatre, New York City, 1964; Gordon Miller, *Room Service*, Mineola Playhouse, Mineola, NY, 1967; Teddy, *The Poker Session*, Martinique Theatre, New York City, 1967; Hermes, *Prometheus Bound*, Solyony, *The Three Sisters*, Mosca, *Volpone*, and Sergeant Henderson, *We Bombed in New Haven*, all Yale Repertory Theatre, New Haven, CT, 1967-68; Sergeant Henderson, *We Bombed in New Haven*, Ambassador Theatre, New York City, 1968; various roles, *Cop-Out*, Cort Theatre, 1969; Starr, "Transfers," Bob, "The Rooming House," and title role, "Dr. Galley," in *Transfers*, Village South Theatre, New York City, 1970; Gordon Miller, *Room Service*, Edison Theatre, New York City, 1970; Richard, "The Lover," and Harry, "The Score," in *Love Two*, Billy Munk Theatre, New York City, 1975; various roles, *Rich and Famous*, Public Theatre, New York City, 1976; title role, *Richard III*, Actors Studio, New York City, 1977.

Herb, *I Ought to Be in Pictures* Eugene O'Neill Theatre, New York City, 1980; Count LaRuse, *Children of Darkness*, Actors Studio, 1982; Don Pasquale, *Non Pasquale*, New York Shakespeare Festival, Delacorte Theatre, New York City, 1983; Lennie Ganz, *Doubles*, Ritz Theatre, New York City, 1985; title role, *Tartuffe*, Los Angeles Theatre Center, Los Angeles, CA, 1986. Also appeared in *Dead End*, Equity Library Theatre, New York City, 1960; *The Premise*, Premise Theatre, New York City, 1960; as Astrov, *Uncle Vanya*, Clov, *Endgame*, Alceste, *The Misanthrope*, Mr. Puff, *The Critic*, and in *Galileo*, all with the Theatre of Living Arts, Philadelphia, PA, 1965; as Gordon Miller, *Room Service*, Theatre of Living Arts, Philadelphia, 1966; in *Long Day's Journey into Night*, Springfield Theatre Company, Springfield, MA, 1968; at the Eugene O'Neill Theatre Center, Waterford, CT, 1968; in *Julius Caesar*, Yale Repertory Theatre, 1976; and in *Rumors*, Broadhurst Theatre, New York City, 1988.

FILM DEBUT—Sidney Hocheiser, *Where's Poppa?* (also known as *Going Ape*), United Artists, 1970. PRINCIPAL FILM APPEARANCES—Murch, *The Hot Rock* (also known as *How to Steal a Diamond in Four Easy Lessons*), Twentieth Century-Fox, 1972; Paul Lazzaro, *Slaughterhouse-Five*, Universal, 1972; Mike, *Your Three Minutes Are Up*, Cinerama, 1973; Dave Greenberg, *The Super Cops*, Metro-Goldwyn-Mayer, 1974; Rudy Montague, *Won Ton Ton, the Dog Who Saved Hollywood*, Paramount, 1976; Reuben, *Norma Rae*, Twentieth Century-Fox, 1979; Major, *Up the Academy* (also known as *Mad Magazine's Up the Academy* and *The Brave Young Men of Weinberg*), Warner Brothers, 1980; Esteban, *Zorro, the Gay Blade*, Twentieth Century-Fox, 1981; Leo, *Romantic Comedy*, Metro-Goldwyn-Mayer/United Artists, 1983; Freddie, *Rhinestone*, Twentieth Century-Fox, 1984; Larry Price, *Door to Door*, Shapiro, 1984; Dave Davis, *Phar Lap* (also known as *Phar Lap—Heart of a Nation*), Twentieth Century-Fox, 1985; David Reardon, *Seven Hours to Judgment*, Trans World Entertainment, 1988.

PRINCIPAL TELEVISION APPEARANCES—Series: Martin "Kaz" Kazinsky, *Kaz*, CBS, 1978-79. Pilots: Roman Grey, *The Art of Crime*, NBC, 1975; Richie Martinelli, *The Outside Man*, CBS, 1977; Stan Rivkin, *Rivkin: Bounty Hunter*, CBS, 1981; *Twilight Theatre II*, NBC, 1982; Joey Caruso, *Side by Side*, ABC, 1984. Movies: Detective Louis Kazinsky, *A Question of Guilt*, CBS, 1978; Huffner, *Christmas Eve*, NBC, 1986; Jerry Brenner, *Many Happy Returns*, CBS, 1986; Simon Resnik, *Terrorists on Trial: The United States vs. Salim Ajami*, CBS, 1988. Specials: *Linda in Wonderland*, CBS, 1980; *Steve Martin's The Winds of Whoopie*, NBC, 1983.

RELATED CAREER—Acting teacher, Yale Drama School, New Haven, CT, 1967-68.

AWARDS: Drama Desk Award, 1968, and Theatre World Award, 1969, both for *We Bombed in New Haven;* Obie Award from the *Village Voice* and Drama Desk Award, both 1970, for *Transfers;* Emmy Award, Outstanding Lead Actor in a Drama Series, 1979, for *Kaz;* Golden Globe nomination, 1987, for *Christmas Eve.*

MEMBER: Actors' Equity Association, Screen Actors Guild.

ADDRESSES: OFFICE—27 W. 87th Street, New York, NY 10024. AGENT—Agency for the Performing Arts, 9000 Sunset Boulevard, Suite 1200, Los Angeles, CA 90069.*

*   *   *

LEISURE, David

BRIEF ENTRY: Born c. 1950, in San Diego, CA. David Leisure suddenly became a sensation in 1986 as Joe Isuzu, the spokesman for Isuzu cars and trucks who boasted that his cars come with such "standard" features as a breakfast nook and a frozen yogurt machine. Joe Isuzu has gone on to make even more outlandish claims in a series of award-winning television commercials. Leisure summed up the success of his character to Marty Goldensohn of *New York Newsday:* "It's because I am lying, I know I am lying,

and you know I am lying. . . . Their commercials have stated what everybody's always known: that car dealers lie to you."

Prior to his stint for Isuzu, Leisure struggled for thirteen years to make a career as an actor, at one point even shaving his head for the role of a Hare Krishna in the 1980 movie *Airplane!* Leisure recalled his lowest point for Alan Carter of the [New York] *Daily News:* "I lost my job, my marriage broke up, I moved into my car. All at the same time." These circumstances forced Leisure in a new direction, as he remembered: "I . . . figured the people who were making money from acting were doing commercials, so I signed up for a commercial acting class." He began working again and scored a minor success as a Joe Friday clone in a number of commercials for Atlantic Bell Yellow Pages that parodied the *Dragnet* television series.

As Leisure explained to Carter, "I'm getting all the jobs now I used to never be able to even audition for. Joe Isuzu broke the ice, he made me famous, and it's the reason I'm working in other areas." Leisure has appeared in the television movie *If It's Tuesday, It Still Must Be Belgium*, on episodes of *Alf, 227*, and *Sledge Hammer!*, and in the feature film *You Can't Hurry Love* (Vestron, 1987). Recently, he has appeared in the recurring role of Charley on the NBC-TV series *Empty Nest*.

OTHER SOURCES: [New York] *Daily News*, January 28, 1988; *New York Newsday*, October 31, 1988.

ADDRESSES: AGENT—J. Carter Gibson Agency, 9000 Sunset Boulevard, Suite 801, Los Angeles, CA 90069.*

*   *   *

Le MAT, Paul

PERSONAL: Born in New Jersey. EDUCATION: Studied acting with Milton Katselas and Herbert Berghof. MILITARY: U.S. Armed Forces (served in Vietnam).

VOCATION: Actor.

CAREER: PRINCIPAL STAGE APPEARANCES—In productions with the Actors Studio, New York City.

MAJOR TOURS—*Tobacco Road*, U.S. cities.

FILM DEBUT—John Milner, *American Graffiti*, Universal, 1973. PRINCIPAL FILM APPEARANCES—Bobby, *Aloha, Bobby and Rose*, Columbia, 1975; Blaine "Spider" Lovejoy, *Citizens Band* (also known as *Handle with Care*), Paramount, 1977; John Milner, *More American Graffiti*, Universal, 1979; Melvin Dummar, *Melvin and Howard*, Universal, 1980; John, *Jimmy the Kid*, New World, 1982; Mike, *Death Valley*, Universal, 1982; Kid Kane, *P.K. and the Kid*, Castle Hill, 1982; Charles Bigelow, *Strange Invaders*, EMI/Orion, 1983; Hubman, *The Hanoi Hilton*, Cannon, 1987; Lieutenant Wexler, *Private Investigations*, Metro-Goldwyn-Mayer/United Artists (MGM/UA), 1987. Also appeared in *Rock and Rule*, MGM/UA, 1982; and *Annabelle Lee* (short film).

PRINCIPAL TELEVISION APPEARANCES—Pilots: Bill Dalzell, *Firehouse*, ABC, 1973; Nick Sandusky, *Long Time Gone*, ABC, 1986. Episodic: *Murder, She Wrote*, CBS. Movies: Dwayne Sutton, *The Gift of Love*, CBS, 1982; Michael Baldwin, *The Night They*

Saved Christmas, ABC, 1984; Mickey Hughes, *The Burning Bed,* NBC, 1984; Jay Coburn, *On Wings of Eagles,* NBC, 1986; Derrick Winston, *Into the Homeland,* HBO, 1987; Kurt Blackburn, *Secret Witness* (also known as *No Secrets*), CBS, 1988.

NON-RELATED CAREER—Boxer.

AWARDS: Golden Globe Award, Best Supporting Actor in a Mini-Series or Made for Television Movie, 1984, for *The Burning Bed.*

MEMBER: Actors' Equity Association, Screen Actors Guild, American Federation of Television and Radio Artists.

SIDELIGHTS: CTFT learned that Paul Le Mat trained for the 1972 U.S. Olympic boxing team.

ADDRESSES: AGENT—Kevin Dul, The Gersh Agency, 222 N. Canon Drive, Suite 202, Beverly Hills, CA, 90210. PUBLICIST—Michael Levine Public Relations, 8730 Sunset Boulevard, 6th Floor, Los Angeles, CA 90069.*

*   *   *

LEMMON, Chris   1954-

PERSONAL: Born January 22, 1954, in Los Angeles, CA; son of Jack (an actor) and Cynthia Boyd (Stone) Lemmon; married Gina Raymond (a model), April 23, 1988.

VOCATION: Actor.

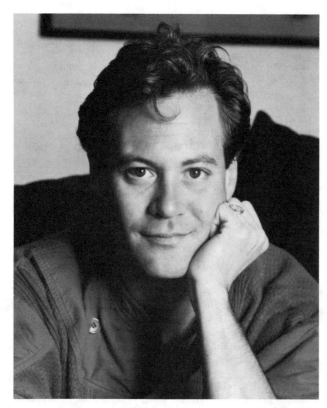

Daniel Adams Photography © 1988

CHRIS LEMMON

CAREER: PRINCIPAL FILM APPEARANCES—Radioman, *Airport '77,* Universal, 1977; Jonathan, *Just before Dawn,* Oakland, 1980; policeman, *Seems Like Old Times,* Columbia, 1980; Albert, *C.O.D.* (also known as *Snap!*), Lone Star, 1983; young cop, *Cannonball Run II,* Warner Brothers, 1984; Lieutenant O'Connor, *Swing Shift,* Warner Brothers, 1984; Josh Fairchild, *That's Life,* Columbia, 1986; Vince Tucker, *Weekend Warriors,* Movie Store, 1986; Henry Brilliant, *Going Undercover* (also known as *Yellow Pages*), Miramax, 1988. Also appeared in *The Happy Hooker Goes to Hollywood,* Cannon, 1980.

PRINCIPAL TELEVISION APPEARANCES—Series: Milos "Checko" Sabolcik, *Brothers and Sisters,* NBC, 1979; Richard Phillips, *Duet,* Fox, 1987—. Pilots: Reggie, *Uncommon Valor,* CBS, 1983; Eugene Griswold, *The Outlaws,* ABC, 1984. Movies: Jonathan Shelton, *Mirror, Mirror,* NBC, 1979. Specials: *The American Film Institute Salute to Jack Lemmon,* CBS, 1988.

MEMBER: Screen Actors Guild, American Federation of Television and Radio Artists.

ADDRESSES: AGENT—Bob Gersh, The Gersh Agency, 222 N. Canon Drive, Suite 202, Beverly Hills, CA 90210. PUBLICIST—Skip Heinecke, Hanson and Schwam Public Relations, 9200 Sunset Boulevard, Suite 307, Los Angeles, CA 90069.

*   *   *

LEMMON, Jack   1925-

PERSONAL: Full name, John Uhler Lemmon III; born February 8, 1925, in Boston, MA; son of John Uhler, Jr. and Mildred LaRue (Noel) Lemmon; married Cynthia Boyd Stone (an actress), May 7, 1950 (divorced, 1956); married Felicia Farr (an actress), August 17, 1962; children: Christopher (first marriage); Courtney (second marriage). EDUCATION: Harvard University, B.A. and B.S., 1947. MILITARY: U.S. Naval Reserve, communications officer, 1945-46.

VOCATION: Actor, director, and producer.

CAREER: BROADWAY DEBUT—Leo Davis, *Room Service,* Playhouse Theatre, 1953. PRINCIPAL STAGE APPEARANCES—David Poole, *Face of a Hero!,* Eugene O'Neill Theatre, New York City, 1960; Scottie Templeton, *Tribute,* Brooks Atkinson Theatre, New York City, 1978; Richard Dale, *A Sense of Humor,* Center Theatre Group, Ahmanson Theatre, Los Angeles, CA, 1983; James Tyrone, *Long Day's Journey into Night,* Broadhurst Theatre, New York City, 1986. Also appeared in *Idiot's Delight,* Los Angeles Music Center, Los Angeles, 1970; *Juno and the Paycock,* Los Angeles Music Center, 1975; and in summer theatre productions, 1940-48.

MAJOR TOURS—Scottie Templeton, *Tribute,* U.S. and Israeli cities, 1978-79; Richard Dale, *A Sense of Humor,* U.S. cities, 1983-84.

FILM DEBUT—Pete Sheppard, *It Should Happen to You,* Columbia, 1954. PRINCIPAL FILM APPEARANCES—Robert Tracy, *Phffft!,* Columbia, 1954; Ensign Frank Thurlowe Pulver, *Mister Roberts,* Warner Brothers, 1955; Bob Baker, *My Sister Eileen,* Columbia, 1955; Marty Stewart, *Three for the Show,* Columbia, 1955; Peter Warne, *You Can't Run Away from It,* Columbia, 1956; Tony, *Fire Down Below,* Columbia, 1957; Private Hogan, *Operation Mad*

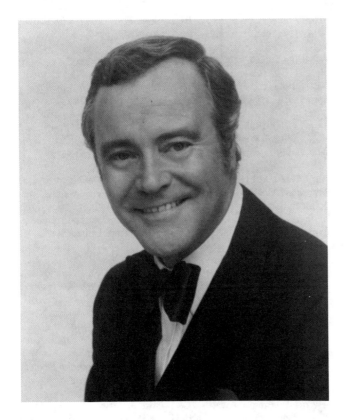

JACK LEMMON

Ball, Columbia, 1957; Nicky Holroyd, *Bell, Book, and Candle*, Columbia, 1958; Frank Harris, *Cowboy*, Columbia, 1958; George Denham, *It Happened to Jane* (also known as *Twinkle and Shine*), Columbia, 1959; Jerry/Daphne, *Some Like It Hot*, United Artists, 1959; C.C. Baxter, *The Apartment*, United Artists, 1960; as himself, *Pepe*, Columbia, 1960; Lieutenant Rip Crandall, *The Wackiest Ship in the Army*, Columbia, 1961; Joe, *Days of Wine and Roses*, Warner Brothers, 1962; William Gridley, *The Notorious Landlady*, Columbia, 1962; narrator, *Stowaway in the Sky* (also known as *Le Voyage en ballon* and *Voyage in a Balloon*), Lopert, 1962; Nestor, *Irma La Douce*, United Artists, 1963; Hogan, *Under the Yum-Yum Tree*, Columbia, 1963; Sam Bissel, *Good Neighbor Sam*, Columbia, 1964; Professor Fate, *The Great Race*, Warner Brothers, 1965; Stanley Ford, *How to Murder Your Wife*, United Artists, 1965; Harry Hinkle, *The Fortune Cookie* (also known as *Meet Whiplash Willie*), United Artists, 1966; Harry Berlin, *Luv*, Columbia, 1967; Felix Ungar, *The Odd Couple*, Paramount, 1968; Howard Brubaker, *The April Fools*, National General, 1969.

George Kellerman, *The Out of Towners*, Paramount, 1970; stranger on bus, *Kotch*, Cinerama, 1971; Wendell Armbruster, *Avanti!*, United Artists, 1972; Peter Wilson, *The War between Men and Women*, National General, 1972; Harry Stoner, *Save the Tiger*, Paramount, 1973; Hildy Johnson, *The Front Page*, Universal, 1974; Archie Rice, *The Entertainer*, Seven Keys, 1975; Mel Edison, *The Prisoner of Second Avenue*, Warner Brothers, 1975; Alexander Main, *Alex and the Gypsy*, Twentieth Century-Fox, 1976; Don Gallagher, *Airport '77*, Universal, 1977; Jack Godell, *The China Syndrome*, Columbia, 1979; Scottie Templeton, *Tribute*, Twentieth Century-Fox, 1980; Victor Clooney, *Buddy Buddy*, Metro-Goldwyn-Mayer/United Artists, 1981; Ed Horman, *Missing*, Universal, 1982; Father Tim Farley, *Mass Appeal*, Universal,

1984; Robert Traven, *Macaroni* (also known as *Maccheroni*), Paramount, 1985; Harvey Fairchild, *That's Life*, Columbia, 1986; narrator, *Debonair Dancers* (documentary), Filmmakers Library, 1986. Also appeared in *The Gentleman Tramp* (documentary), Fox-Rank, 1974; *Wednesday*, 1974; and *Portrait of a Sixty Percent Perfect Man* (documentary), Janus, 1980.

PRINCIPAL FILM WORK—Executive producer, *Cool Hand Luke*, Warner Brothers, 1967; director, *Kotch*, Cinerama, 1971; producer (with Keith Gordon and Harry Sutherland), *Track Two*, DEC, 1981.

PRINCIPAL TELEVISION APPEARANCES—Series: Harold, *That Wonderful Guy*, ABC, 1949-50; host, *Toni Twin Time* (also known as *Twin Time*), CBS, 1950; regular, *Ad Libbers*, CBS, 1951; Pete Bell, *Heaven for Betsy*, CBS, 1952; regular, *Turn of Fate* (also known as *Alcoa Theatre*), NBC, 1957-58; also *Road of Life*, CBS; *The Brighter Day*, CBS. Pilots: "The Times Square Story," *Old Knickerbocker Music Hall*, CBS, 1948; *Tom Snyder's Celebrity Spotlight*, NBC, 1980; *War of the Stars*, syndicated, 1985. Episodic: Pete Bell, "The Couple Next Door," *The Frances Langford-Don Ameche Show*, ABC, 1951; host, *Goodyear Television Playhouse*, NBC, 1951; "Size 12 Tantrum," *News Stand Theatre*, ABC, 1952; also *Zane Grey Theatre* (also known as *Dick Powell's Zane Grey Theatre*), CBS; "The Day Lincoln Was Shot," *Ford Star Jubilee*, CBS; as Nel's friend, *I Remember Mama*, CBS; in *Kraft Television Theatre*, NBC; *Chrysler Medallion Theatre* (also known as *Medallion Theatre*), CBS; *The Campbell Television Sound Stage* (also known as *TV Sound Stage*), NBC; *Danger*, CBS; *Playhouse 90*, CBS; *Pulitzer Prize Playhouse*, ABC; *The Web*, CBS; *The Dick Cavett Show*, ABC.

Movies: Governor John M. Slaton, *The Murder of Mary Phagan*, NBC, 1988. Specials: *Super Comedy Bowl*, CBS, 1971; host, *Super Comedy Bowl II*, CBS, 1972; host, *Jack Lemmon in 'S Wonderful, 'S Marvelous, 'S Gershwin*, NBC, 1972; host, *Jack Lemmon—Get Happy*, NBC, 1973; *Show Business Salute to Milton Berle*, NBC, 1973; *American Film Institute Salute to James Cagney*, CBS, 1974; Archie Rice, *The Entertainer*, NBC, 1976; *Celebration: The American Spirit*, ABC, 1976; host, *The Best of Ernie Kovacs*, PBS, 1977; *The American Film Institute Salute to Henry Fonda*, CBS, 1978; *Musical Comedy Tonight*, PBS, 1981; *Bob Hope's Stars over Texas*, NBC, 1982; *The American Film Institute Salute to Frank Capra*, CBS, 1982; co-host, *Hollywood: The Gift of Laughter*, ABC, 1982; *The Funniest Joke I Ever Heard*, ABC, 1984; *Screen Actors Guild Fiftieth Anniversary Celebration*, CBS, 1984; host, *Academy Awards*, ABC, 1985; *Liberty Weekend*, ABC, 1986; *American Film Institute Salute to Billy Wilder*, NBC, 1986; James Tyrone, *Long Day's Journey into Night*, PBS, 1987; *Television Academy Hall of Fame*, Fox, 1987; *American Film Institute Salute to Jack Lemmon*, CBS, 1988; "Gregory Peck—His Own Man," *Crazy about the Movies*, Cinemax, 1988; *Smothers Brothers Comedy Hour*, CBS, 1988. Also appeared in more than four hundred productions on live television during the 1950s.

PRINCIPAL TELEVISION WORK—Series: All as producer. *That Wonderful Guy*, ABC, 1949-50; *Ad Libbers*, CBS, 1951; *Heaven for Betsy*, CBS, 1952.

RELATED CAREER—Piano player, Old Nick Saloon, New York City, 1947; actor in radio soap operas, 1948; founder and president, Jalem Production Company, 1952—.

WRITINGS: FILM—*Track Two*, DEC, 1981.

AWARDS: Academy Award, Best Supporting Actor, 1955, for *Mister Roberts;* Academy Award nomination, Best Actor, and British Academy Award, Best Foreign Actor, both 1959, for *Some Like It Hot;* Academy Award nomination, Best Actor, and British Academy Award, Best Foreign Actor, both 1960, for *The Apartment;* Academy Award nomination, Best Actor, 1962, for *Days of Wine and Roses;* Emmy Award, Outstanding Single Program (Variety and Popular Music), 1972, for *Jack Lemmon in 'S Wonderful, 'S Marvelous, 'S Gershwin;* Academy Award, Best Actor, 1973, for *Save the Tiger;* Emmy Award nomination, 1975, for *The Entertainer;* Academy Award nomination, British Academy Award, and Cannes Film Festival Award, all Best Actor, 1979, for *The China Syndrome;* Drama Guild Award, 1979, for stage production of *Tribute;* Academy Award nomination, Best Actor, 1980, and Berlin Film Festival Award, Best Actor, 1981, for film of *Tribute;* Cannes Film Festival Award, Best Actor, 1982, for *Missing;* inducted into the Television Academy Hall of Fame, 1987; Emmy Award, 1988, for *The Murder of Mary Phagan;* Golden Globe Award, Best Performance by an Actor in a Mini-Series or Motion Picture Made for Television, 1988, for *Long Day's Journey into Night;* American Film Institute Lifetime Achievement Award, 1988.

MEMBER: Players Club.

SIDELIGHTS: RECREATIONS—Composing at the piano, golf, fishing, and photography.

ADDRESSES: OFFICE—Jalem Productions, 141 El Camino Drive, Suite 201, Beverly Hills, CA 90212. AGENT—Leonard Hirshan, William Morris Agency, 151 El Camino Drive, Beverly Hills, CA 90212. PUBLICIST—Mahoney/Wasserman Public Relations, 345 N. Maple Drive, Suite 185, Beverly Hills, CA 90210.*

*   *   *

LETTERMAN, David   1947-

PERSONAL: Born April 12, 1947, in Indianapolis, IN; son of Joseph Letterman (a florist) and his wife (a church secretary); married Michelle Cook, 1969 (divorced, 1977). EDUCATION: Received a degree in radio and television broadcasting from Ball State University, 1970.

VOCATION: Television host, writer, and comedian.

CAREER: PRINCIPAL TELEVISION APPEARANCES—Series: Announcer and regular, *The Starland Vocal Band,* CBS, 1977; regular, *Mary,* CBS, 1978; host, *The David Letterman Show,* NBC, 1980; host, *Late Night with David Letterman,* NBC, 1982—. Episodic: Interviewer, *TV's Bloopers and Practical Jokes,* NBC, 1984; also guest host, *Tonight Show* (fifty-one episodes), NBC; *The Gong Show,* syndicated; *Mork and Mindy,* ABC; *Rock Concert;* and *Good Friends.* Movies: Matt Morgan, *Fast Friends,* NBC, 1979. Specials: *Battle of the Network Stars,* ABC, 1976; Dan Cochran, *Peeping Times,* NBC, 1978; *The NBC All-Star Hour,* NBC, 1985; *Late Night Film Festival,* NBC, 1985; *The Jay Leno Show,* NBC, 1986; *David Letterman's Second Annual Holiday Film Festival,* NBC, 1986; *Television Academy Hall of Fame,* NBC, 1986; *Late Night with David Letterman Fifth Anniversary Show,* NBC, 1987; host, *David Letterman's Old-Fashioned Christmas,* NBC, 1987; *Paul Shaffer: Viva Shaf Vegas,* Cinemax, 1987; *Action Family,* Cinemax, 1987; *Late Night with David Letterman*

Sixth Anniversary Show, NBC, 1988; *Late Night with David Letterman Seventh Anniversary Show,* NBC, 1989.

PRINCIPAL TELEVISION WORK—All as executive producer. Specials: *David Letterman's Second Annual Holiday Film Festival,* NBC, 1986; *Late Night with David Letterman Fifth Anniversary Show,* NBC, 1987; *David Letterman's Old-Fashioned Christmas,* NBC, 1987; *Late Night with David Letterman Sixth Anniversary Show,* NBC, 1988; *Carol Doesn't Leifer Anymore* (also known as *I Was a Woman Who Loved Too Much*), Cinemax, 1988; *Late Night with David Letterman Seventh Anniversary Show,* NBC, 1989.

RELATED CAREER—Announcer for late-night movie program, *Freeze Dried Movies,* moderator for 4-H television show, announcer, and weatherman, all for ABC affiliate in Indianapolis, IN; radio talk show host, Indianapolis; as a comedian, has performed in comedy clubs and concert halls throughout the United States.

WRITINGS: TELEVISION—Series: *The Starland Vocal Band,* CBS, 1977; *Mary,* CBS, 1978; *The David Letterman Show,* NBC, 1980; *Late Night with David Letterman,* NBC, 1982—. Episodic: *Good Times,* CBS. Specials: *The Paul Lynde Comedy Hour,* ABC, 1977; *Bob Hope's All-Star Comedy Special from Australia,* NBC, 1978; *David Letterman's Second Annual Holiday Film Festival,* NBC, 1986; *Late Night with David Letterman Fifth Anniversary Show,* NBC, 1987; *Late Night with David Letterman Sixth Anniversary Show,* NBC, 1988; *Late Night with David Letterman Seventh Anniversary Show,* NBC, 1989; also *The John Denver Special.*

AWARDS: Emmy Awards, Best Host and Best Writing for a Daytime Variety Series, both 1981, for *The David Letterman Show;* Emmy Awards, Best Writing for a Variety Show, 1984, 1985, 1986, and 1987, all for *Late Night with David Letterman;* Jack Benny Award from the University of California, Los Angeles, 1984.

MEMBER: Sigma Chi.

SIDELIGHTS: David Letterman hosts NBC's *Late Night* program, a mix of celebrity interviews and comedy that "may be the hippest show on network television," as Jane Hall told readers of *People* (June 14, 1986). He spoofs both show business and popular culture, delighting audiences with such regular features as "Stupid Pet Tricks" and ten-point lists of useless advice. Known for his "patented platypus grin," in the words of *Time*'s Richard Corliss (March 22, 1982), Letterman addresses his fans "in a voice as gracefully modulated and wickedly bland as that of a hip, small town disk jockey reading a mortuary commercial."

A native of Indianapolis, Indiana, Letterman attended Ball State University in nearby Muncie and then spent several years in local television and radio. He reported the weekend weather, hosted a children's show and a late night movie, and talked with callers on a radio phone-in program. "For five hours each day," Letterman later said in *Newsweek* (July 7, 1980), "I handled calls from people who were certain the Commies were behind the rain." He began spiking his broadcasts with unconventional humor that management didn't always appreciate—on the movie show he exploded a model of the television station where he worked. Finally, in 1975, he left for Los Angeles and tried to establish himself as a television writer and comic.

Working the city's stand-up comedy circuit, Letterman sharpened his performance style by observing Jay Leno, who later became one of America's top comedians. Leno's act, Letterman recalled (*News-*

week, February 3, 1986), "was all smart, shrewd observations, and it could be anything—politics, television, education. The dynamic of it was, you and I both understand that this is stupid. We're Jay's hip friends." Letterman became a regular performer at the Comedy Store, a major Los Angeles club, wrote for television, and in 1978 joined the cast of Mary Tyler Moore's variety hour. Before Moore's show finished its short run, he was spotted by talent scouts for the *Tonight Show*, Johnny Carson's highly popular late-night talk program. Letterman quickly became one of Carson's favorite guest comedians and often served as host in Carson's absence.

In 1980 *The David Letterman Show* debuted on NBC's mid-morning television schedule. The program format departed from the usual lineup of celebrities and household advisers familiar to daytime broadcasting, featuring instead much of the quirky irreverence that would characterize *Late Night*. Though the show received favorable reviews and won two Emmy awards, it was largely ignored by daytime viewers and left the air after only a few months. But reviewers suggested that the daytime program simply presented Letterman to the wrong audience, and NBC was so impressed with his potential that they offered him a one-year holding contract, paying him an estimated $625,000 so that he would not switch to a rival network.

Late Night with David Letterman premiered on NBC in 1982. Generally broadcast after midnight, the show gradually built a following until it had become a major ratings success by 1984. Advertisers soon recognized Letterman's popularity with young adults, making his program more valued among some sponsors than the long-established Carson show. Television critics suggested that Letterman's humorous skepticism is well suited to an emerging generation of viewers who grew up familiar with television, its limitations, and its pretensions. Traditionally, for instance, talk shows adulate show business—celebrities arrive to promote products, movies, or television shows. But Letterman is known to poke fun at guests who are so business-like. As *Late Night* producer Barry Sand told Jane Hall, the most successful guests "understand the show and come ready to play." Cybill Shepherd, the glamorous star of television's *Moonlighting*, was well received when she appeared on stage wearing nothing but a designer towel. "Sometimes," *Newsweek*'s Bill Barol observed (February 3, 1986), *Late Night* "peel[s] back the video facade in unexpected ways," going backstage with handheld cameras or using the "Late Night Thrill-Cam," an overhead camera mounted on rollers that careens toward the stage as the audience screams in mock terror.

As Carson entered his sixties, Letterman was often mentioned as likely successor to the veteran *Tonight Show* host. But Letterman, whose show is associated with Carson's own production company, was quick to distance himself from such talk, merely noting that he considered Carson a role model and an inspiration. In *Time* Letterman recalled the 1950s, when he saw Carson hosting a wacky television show called *Who Do You Trust?* "There was one guy who balanced a lawnmower on his chin—quite a booking coup," Letterman said, "and Carson just made fun of him. I thought, 'What a great way to make a living!'"

OTHER SOURCES: [New York] *Daily News*, January 31, 1988; *Esquire*, December, 1981, November, 1986; *New York Times*, July 27, 1986; *Newsweek*, July 7, 1980, February 3, 1986; *People*, July 14, 1986; *Rolling Stone*, June 20, 1985; *Time*, March 22, 1982.

ADDRESSES: OFFICE—c/o NBC, 30 Rockefeller Plaza, New York, NY 10038. AGENT—William Morris Agency, 151 El Camino Drive, Beverly Hills, CA 90212. MANAGER—Jack Rollins,

Rollins, Joffe, Morra, and Brezner, 801 Westmount, Los Angeles, CA 90069.*

*   *   *

LEVY, Eugene   1946-

PERSONAL: Born December 17, 1946, in Hamilton, ON, Canada.

VOCATION: Actor, comedian, and writer.

CAREER: Also see *WRITINGS* below. PRINCIPAL FILM APPEARANCES—Clifford Sturges, *Cannibal Girls*, American International, 1973; Richard Rosenberg, *Running*, Universal, 1979; voice of Edsel and male reporter, *Heavy Metal* (animated), Columbia, 1981; Sal di Pasquale, *Going Berserk*, Universal, 1983; car salesman, *National Lampoon's Vacation*, Warner Brothers, 1983; Walter Kornbluth, *Splash*, Buena Vista, 1984; Norman Kane, *Armed and Dangerous*, Columbia, 1986; Barry Steinberg, *Club Paradise*, Warner Brothers, 1986. Also appeared in *Nothing Personal*, American International/Filmways, 1980; and *The Canadian Conspiracy*, HBO Pictures/Canadian Broadcasting/Schtick, 1986; *Speed Zone*, Orion, 1989.

PRINCIPAL TELEVISION APPEARANCES—Series: Earl Camembert and various roles, *Second City TV*, syndicated, 1977-81; various roles, *SCTV Network 90*, NBC, 1981-83. Pilots: Fred Wexelblatt, *The Lovebirds*, CBS, 1979; regular, *From Cleveland*, CBS, 1980; Bobby Bittman, *Autobiographies: The Enigma of Bobby Bittman*, Cinemax, 1988. Episodic: As himself, *George Burns Comedy Week*, CBS, 1985; Tom Lynch, "Bride of Boogedy," *Disney Sunday Movie*, ABC, 1987. Specials: *The Magic of David Copperfield*, CBS, 1983; Stan Schmenge, *The Last Polka*, HBO, 1985; first soldier, *Dave Thomas: The Incredible Time Travels of Henry Osgood*, Showtime, 1986; *Comic Relief*, HBO, 1986; Mort Arnold, *Billy Crystal—Don't Get Me Started*, HBO, 1986; *Second City's Fifteenth Anniversary Special* (also known as *The Second City Anniversary Reunion*), Showtime, 1988; "Skeleton," *Ray Bradbury Theatre III*, First Choice, 1988.

PRINCIPAL TELEVISION WORK—Pilots: Executive producer and director, *Autobiographies: The Enigma of Bobby Bittman*, Cinemax, 1988. Specials: Producer and director, *Second City's Fifteenth Anniversary Special*, (also known as *The Second City Anniversary Reunion*), Showtime, 1988.

RELATED CAREER—Member, Second City (improvisational comedy troupe), Toronto, ON, Canada.

WRITINGS: See production details above. TELEVISION—Series: *Second City TV*, 1977-81; *SCTV Network 90*, 1981-83. Pilots: *From Cleveland*, 1980; *Autobiographies: The Enigma of Bobby Bittman*, 1988. Specials: *The Last Polka*, 1985.

AWARDS: Emmy awards, Best Writing for a Comedy Program, 1982 and 1983, for *SCTV Network 90*.

MEMBER: Screen Actors Guild, American Federation of Television and Radio Artists.

ADDRESSES: AGENT—John Gaines, Agency for the Performing Arts, 9000 Sunset Boulevard, Suite 1200, Los Angeles, CA 90069.*

LEVY, Jonathan 1935-

PERSONAL: Born February 20, 1935, in New York, NY; son of Milton Jerome (an attorney) and Sylvia (a teacher and writer; maiden name, Narins) Levy; married Geraldine Carro (a journalist), November 24, 1968 (died, 1984); children: Catherine Sylvia. EDUCATION: Harvard University, A.B., 1956; graduate work, University of Rome, 1956-57; Columbia University, M.A., 1959, Ph.D., 1966. MILITARY: U.S. Army, staff sergeant.

VOCATION: Writer.

CAREER: See *WRITINGS* below. RELATED CAREER—Humanities instructor, Juilliard School of Music, 1960-61; lecturer, Columbia University, New York City, 1960-62; speech lecturer, University of California, Berkeley, 1964-65; member, Theatre Playwrights Unit, 1966-67; member, Bar-Albee Playwrights Unit, 1970; co-founder and president, Playwrights for Children's Theatre, 1971-75; playwright-in-residence, Manhattan Theatre Club, New York City, 1973-78; senior fellow, Lincoln Center Institute, New York City, 1975-77; professor of theatre arts, State University of New York, Stonybrook, 1978—, chairman of the department, 1980—; Fannie Hurst Visiting Professor of Theatre Arts, Brandeis University, Waltham, MA, 1979; co-chair of theatre for youth panel, National Endowment for the Arts, 1979-81, and member of theatre policy panel, 1980-81; visiting scholar, Harvard University, Cambridge, MA, 1985—.

WRITINGS: STAGE—*Sabbatai Zevi* (staged reading), Theatre Company of Boston, Boston, MA, 1966; (narration) *The Mystery of Elche*, Trinity College, Hartford, CT, 1967; (adaptor) *Turandot*, New Paltz Players, New Paltz, NY, 1967, then Cafe LaMama, New York City, and Brigham Young University, Provo, UT, published in *The Genius of the Italian Theatre*, New American Library, 1964; *The Play of Innocence and Change*, 92nd Street Young Men's Hebrew Association, New York City, 1967, published in *New Plays for Children*, 1970; *An Exploratory Operation*, New Jewish Theatre Workshop, New York City, 1968; *Jack N's Awful Demands*, Playbox Theatre, New York City, 1968; *The War between the Amazons and the Baboons*, 92nd Street Young Men's Hebrew Association, 1968; (adaptor) *The Little Green Bird*, Young Hampton Players, Bridgehampton, NY, 1968; *Ziskin's Revels*, New Theatre Workshop, New York City, 1968; *The Cushman Touch*, New York University Graduate School of Theatre, New York City, 1969.

The Master of the Blue Mineral Mines, Bar-Albee Playwrights Unit, New York City, 1970; *The Shrinking Bride*, Mercury Theatre, New York City, 1971; *The Marvelous Adventures of Tyl*, Triangle Theatre, New York City, 1971, published in *Contemporary Children's Theatre*, Avon, 1974; *Boswell's Journal*, Alice Tully Hall, New York City, 1972, published in *Ricordi*, Milan, Italy, 1972; *Monkey Play*, Clark Center for the Performing Arts, New York City, 1972; *Charlie the Chicken*, American Shakespeare Festival, Stratford, CT, 1972, then Manhattan Theatre Club, New York City, 1983, published in *Best Short Plays 1983*, Chilton, 1984, produced as an opera at the Toronto Free Theatre, Toronto, ON, Canada, 1975; *Master Class*, Manhattan Theatre Club, 1973; *Marco Polo: A Fantasy for Children*, Manhattan Theatre Club, 1973, then Phoenix Theatre, New York City, 1976, published by Dramatists Play Service, 1977; *Theatre Games*, Theatre Calgary, Calgary, AB, Canada, 1973; *Inner Voices* (staged reading), *The Pornographer's Daughter*, and *Near Fall* (staged reading), all Manhattan Theatre Club, 1975; *Old Blues* and *Pansy*, both Impossible Ragtime Theatre, New York City, 1978; (adaptor) *Wild Rose*,

Brooklyn Academy of Music, Brooklyn, NY, 1978; *Arts and Letters*, New York Stageworks, New York City, 1981.

TELEVISION—Pilots: (With John Pleshette) *Review Material*, PBS, 1969.

OTHER—*The TV Book* (nonfiction), Workman, 1977; contributor to *The Poem Itself* (nonfiction), Holt, 1962; and has contributed fiction, poems, and reviews to the *Village Voice*, *Harper's Bookletter*, *Cricket*, and the *New York Times*.

AWARDS: Charlotte B. Chorpenning Cup from the Children's Theatre Association of America, Outstanding Play for Children, 1979, for *Charlie the Chicken;* also Fulbright research grant, 1963-64; New York State Council for the Arts grant, 1973; and Creative Arts Public Service grant in playwrighting, 1975.

MEMBER: Dramatists Guild, American Society of Composers, Authors, and Publishers.

ADDRESSES: HOME—P.O. Box 295, Patterson, NY 12563. OFFICE—Department of Theatre Arts, State University of New York, Stonybrook, Stonybrook, NY 11794.

*   *   *

LEWIS, Emmanuel 1971-

PERSONAL: Born March 9, 1971, in Brooklyn, NY; son of Margaret Lewis (a computer programmer and personal manager).

VOCATION: Actor.

CAREER: STAGE DEBUT—Attendant to the Duke, *A Midsummer Night's Dream*, New York Shakespeare Festival, Delacorte Theatre, New York City, 1982.

MAJOR TOURS—Singer and dancer, Japanese cities.

PRINCIPAL TELEVISION APPEARANCES—Series: Title role, *Webster*, ABC, 1983-87, then syndicated, 1987-89. Movies: Davey Williams, *Lost in London*, CBS, 1985. Episodic: *The Tonight Show*, NBC; *The Phil Donahue Show*, NBC. Specials: Host, *The World's Funniest Commercial Goofs*, ABC, 1983, 1984, and 1985; *Salute to Lady Liberty*, CBS, 1984; *Mr. T and Emmanuel Lewis in a Christmas Dream*, 1984; *Circus of the Stars*, CBS, 1984; *The Screen Actors Guild Fiftieth Anniversary Celebration*, CBS, 1984; *Secret World of the Very Young*, CBS, 1984; *The Bob Hope Christmas Show*, NBC, 1985; *The Fiftieth Presidential Inaugural Gala*, ABC, 1985; *The ABC All-Star Spectacular*, ABC, 1985; *Christmas in Washington*, NBC, 1985; *All Star Party for "Dutch" Reagan*, CBS, 1985; *Bob Hope's Royal Command Performance from Sweden*, NBC, 1986; *Life's Most Embarrassing Moments*, ABC, 1986; *Walt Disney World Fifteenth Birthday Celebration*, ABC, 1986; *Candid Camera: The First Forty Years*, CBS, 1987; *Emmanuel Lewis: My Very Own Show*, ABC, 1987; *King Orange Jamboree Parade*, NBC, 1987; *Bob Hope's High Flying Birthday Extravaganza*, NBC, 1987.

RELATED CAREER—Owner, Emmanuel Lewis Entertainment Enterprises, Inc.; actor in over fifty television commercials.

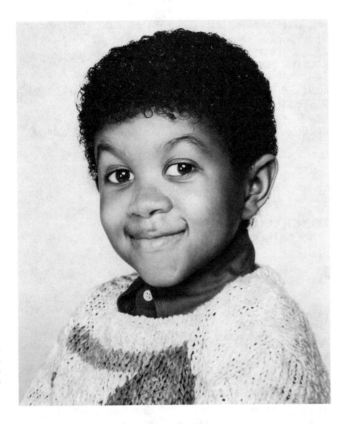

EMMANUEL LEWIS

MEMBER: American Federation of Television and Radio Artists, Screen Actors Guild, Actors' Equity Association.

ADDRESSES: AGENT—Monica Stuart, Schuller Talent/New York Kids, 276 Fifth Avenue, New York, NY 10001.

* * *

LIOTTA, Ray

PERSONAL: Born December 18, c. 1954, in Newark, NJ; son of Alfred (an auto parts store owner, politician, and personnel director) and Mary Liotta. EDUCATION: Graduated from the University of Miami.

VOCATION: Actor.

CAREER: FILM DEBUT—Joe Heron, *The Lonely Lady,* Universal, 1983. PRINCIPAL FILM APPEARANCES—Ray Sinclair, *Something Wild,* Orion, 1986; Eugene Luciano, *Dominick and Eugene,* Orion, 1988; Shoeless Joe Jackson, *Field of Dreams,* Universal, 1989. Also appeared as the Artist, *Arena Brains,* 1987.

PRINCIPAL TELEVISION APPEARANCES—Series: Joey Perrini, *Another World,* NBC, 1978-80; Sacha, *Casablanca,* NBC, 1983; Officer Ed Santini, *Our Family Honor,* NBC, 1985-86. Pilots: Johnny "Wizard" Lazarra, *Crazy Times,* ABC, 1981. Movies: Family, *Hardhat and Legs,* CBS, 1980.

AWARDS: Boston Critics Award and Golden Globe Award nomination, Best Supporting Actor, both for *Something Wild.*

MEMBER: Screen Actors Guild, American Federation of Television and Radio Artists.

SIDELIGHTS: Although he had been working steadily as an actor since 1978, Ray Liotta first received widespread critical acclaim in 1986 for his portrayal of Ray Sinclair, an obsessive ex-convict in director Jonathan Demme's *Something Wild.* Bob Strauss in *Premiere* magazine described his performance as "the cinematic equivalent of a Silkworm missle strike: all speed, danger, and high impact," while J. Hoberman in the *Village Voice* claimed that the role was "played to wired perfection."

Liotta's professional career began when he landed a role in a television commercial within three days of his arrival in New York City after college. Six months later he was cast as Joey Perrini on the soap opera *Another World* and stayed with the show for more than two years. Recurring roles on two prime-time series preceded his auditioning for the role of Ray Sinclair. Surprisingly, he was initially rejected, but was so convinced that he was right for the part that he lobbied with *Something Wild* co-star Melanie Griffith for another chance. Called back to audition on a Wednesday, Liotta so impressed director Demme that the role—for which he would win a Golden Globe nomination—was given to him that Sunday.

OTHER SOURCES: American Film, April, 1988; [New York] *Daily News,* March 20, 1988; *New York Native,* April 18, 1988; *New York Times,* January 2, 1987; [Newark] *Sunday Star-Ledger,* April 17, 1988; *Premiere,* March, 1988; *Village Voice,* November 11, 1986.

ADDRESSES: AGENTS—Nicole David, Triad Artists, 10100 Santa Monica Boulevard, Suite 300, Los Angeles, CA 90049; Rick Nicita, Creative Artists Agency, 1888 Century Park E., Suite 1400, Los Angeles, CA 90067. PUBLICIST—Monique Moss, Michael Levine Public Relations, 8730 Sunset Boulevard, 6th Floor, Los Angeles, CA 90069.*

* * *

LLOYD, Emily

BRIEF ENTRY: Born Emily Lloyd Pack, c. 1971; daughter of Roger Lloyd Pack (an actor); mother, a secretary. With her very first role, British actress Emily Lloyd commanded the attention of critics and film producers around the world. Lloyd starred as Lynda, an uninhibited teenager growing up in a stodgy English seacoast town during the 1950s in *Wish You Were Here* (Atlantic, 1987). Lynda provokes the disapproval of her neighbors by openly flaunting her sexuality. Her escapades get her fired from a number of jobs and an affair with a friend of her father results in her pregnancy. Lynda decides to leave town but, once again defying the conventional thinking of the townspeople and the times, she returns months later with her child. Of her character, Lloyd told Susan Linfield of *American Film,* "I thought Lynda was a brilliant character. I admired her because of her amazing guts. She refused to conform, despite everyone's trying to break her spirit."

Raised in a show business family (both her father and grandfather are well-known British stage actors and her mother was secretary to dramatist Harold Pinter), Lloyd, according to Jamie Diamond in

Premiere, attended "schools without rules, where her dramatic instincts were encouraged." Nevertheless, with only limited professional experience, she was passed over for the role of Lynda in her first audition but returned a second time and eventually convinced director-screenwriter David Leland that she was the right actress for the role. Although *Wish You Were Here* received only mixed reviews, Lloyd's performance was hailed by many critics as an astonishing debut and resulted in her being cast in two major Hollywood films of 1989. In *Cookie,* directed by Susan Seidelman, she stars opposite Peter Falk and Dianne Wiest as the Brooklyn-born daughter of a Mafia don, while her leading role in Norman Jewison's adaptation of Bobbie Ann Mason's acclaimed novel *In Country* casts her as Samantha, a Kentucky teenager coming to terms with her father's death in the Vietnam War.

OTHER SOURCES: American Film, September, 1987; *The 1988 Motion Picture Guide Annual,* by Jay Robert Nash and Stanley Ralph Ross, Cinebooks, Inc., 1988; *Premiere,* March, 1989.*

*   *   *

LOCKWOOD, Gary   1937-

PERSONAL: Born John Gary Yusolfsky, February 21, 1937, in Van Nuys, CA.

VOCATION: Actor.

CAREER: PRINCIPAL FILM APPEARANCES—Artist, *Call Me Genius* (also known as *The Rebel*), ABF, 1961; Toots, *Splendor in the Grass,* Warner Brothers, 1961; Cliff Macy, *Wild in the Country,* Twentieth Century-Fox, 1961; St. George, *The Magic Sword,* United Artists, 1962; Danny Burke, *It Happened at the World's Fair,* Metro-Goldwyn-Mayer (MGM), 1963; Earl, *Firecreek,* Warner Brothers, 1968; Frank Poole, *2001: A Space Odyssey,* MGM, 1968; George Matthews, *The Model Shop,* Columbia, 1969; Tony Vincenzo, *They Came to Rob Las Vegas,* Warner Brothers/Seven Arts, 1969; Rossiter, *R.P.M.* (also known as *R.P.M. [Revolutions Per Minute]*), Columbia, 1970; Eliot Travis, *Stand Up and Be Counted,* Columbia, 1972; Captain Kramer, *The Wild Pair* (also known as *Devil's Odds*), Transworld Entertainment, 1987. Also appeared in *Manhunt in Space,* 1954; *Kitten with a Whip,* Universal, 1964; *Project: Kill,* Stirling Gold, 1976; and *Bad Georgia Road,* Dimension, 1977.

PRINCIPAL TELEVISION APPEARANCES—Series: Eric Jason, *Follow the Sun,* ABC, 1961-62; Lieutenant William "Bill" Rice, *The Lieutenant,* NBC, 1963-64. Pilots: Eric, *Chalk One Up for Johnny,* ABC, 1962; Sam Cody, *Sally and Sam,* CBS, 1965; Lieutenant Commander Gary Mitchell, "Where No Man Has Gone Before," *Star Trek,* NBC, 1966. Episodic: "The Ring with the Red Velvet Ropes," *Rod Serling's Night Gallery,* NBC, 1972; also Edward St. John, *Vega$,* ABC; Dr. Matthew Ashfield, *Trapper John, M.D.,* CBS; *Barnaby Jones,* CBS; *Police Story,* NBC; *Simon and Simon,* CBS. Movies: David Seville, *Earth II,* ABC, 1971; Frank Clinger, *Manhunter,* CBS, 1974; Fred Barker, *The FBI Story: The FBI Versus Alvin Karpis, Public Enemy Number One* (also known as *The FBI Story—Alvin Karpis*), CBS, 1974; Jordan Evanhower, *The Ghost of Flight 401,* NBC, 1978; Harley Moon, *The Incredible Journey of Doctor Meg Laurel,* CBS, 1979; Dave Cully, *The Top of the Hill,* syndicated, 1980; Sheriff Earl Baker, *The Girl, the Gold Watch, and Dynamite,* syndicated, 1981; Dr. David Becker, *Emergency Room,* syndicated, 1983; John Praiser, *The Return of the Six*

Million Dollar Man and the Bionic Woman, NBC, 1987. Specials: *Nashville Remember Elvis on His Birthday,* NBC, 1978.

RELATED CAREER—Motion picture stuntman.

MEMBER: Screen Actors Guild, American Federation of Television and Radio Artists.

ADDRESSES: OFFICE—3083 1/2 Rambla Pacifica, Malibu, CA 90265.*

*   *   *

LONGBAUGH, Harry
See GOLDMAN, William

*   *   *

LOVITZ, Jon   1957-

PERSONAL: Born July 21, 1957, in Tarzana, CA.

VOCATION: Comedian and actor.

CAREER: PRINCIPAL FILM APPEARANCES—Doug, *Jumpin' Jack Flash,* Twentieth Century-Fox, 1986; bartender, *The Last Resort,* Concorde/Cinema Group/Trinity, 1986; party guest, *Ratboy,* Warner Brothers, 1986; Morty, *Three Amigos,* Orion, 1986; voice of the Radio, *The Brave Little Toaster* (animated), Hyperion/Kushner/Lockec, 1987; Scotty Brennen, *Big,* Twentieth Century-Fox, 1988; Ron Mills, *My Stepmother Is an Alien,* Weintraub Entertainment Group, 1988.

PRINCIPAL TELEVISION APPEARANCES—Series: Mole, *Foley Square,* CBS, 1985-86; regular, *Saturday Night Live,* NBC, 1985—. Specials: *Comic Relief,* HBO, 1987; Injun Larry, "I'll Do It Guy's Way," *Cinemax Comedy Experiment,* Cinemax, 1987; *Comic Relief 2,* HBO, 1987; host, *Coca-Cola Presents Live: The Hard Rock* (also known as *Live: The Hard Rock*), NBC, 1988.

SIDELIGHTS: Jon Lovitz has achieved acclaim for his work on *Saturday Night Live,* especially for his characterization of a pathological liar whose refrain "Yeah, that's the ticket" became a popular catchphrase.

ADDRESSES: AGENT—David Schiff, Creative Artists Agency, 1888 Century Park E., Suite 1400, Los Angeles, CA 90067.*

*   *   *

LOWE, Chad   1968-

PERSONAL: Born January 15, 1968, in Dayton, OH.

VOCATION: Actor.

CAREER: PRINCIPAL FILM APPEARANCES—Billy Kelly, *Apprentice to Murder* (also known as *The Long Lost Friends* and *The Long Lost Friend*), New World, 1988.

PRINCIPAL TELEVISION APPEARANCES—Series: Spencer Winger, *Spencer*, NBC, 1984-85. Movies: Al Hamilton, *Flight 90: Disaster on the Potomac*, NBC, 1984; Skip Lewis, *Silence of the Heart*, CBS, 1984; Josh Sydney, *There Must Be a Pony*, ABC, 1986. Specials: Michael Wells, "No Means No," *CBS Schoolbreak Special*, CBS, 1988; Adam Cooper, "April Morning," *Hallmark Hall of Fame*, CBS, 1988.

ADDRESSES: AGENT—Scott Zimmerman, William Morris Agency, 151 El Camino Drive, Beverly Hills, CA 90212.*

*   *   *

LUCAS, Hans
  See GODARD, Jean-Luc

*   *   *

LUCAS, J. Frank   1920-

PERSONAL: Born March 15, 1920, in Houston, TX; son of Frank Clarence and Mattie Velera (Yarbrough) Lucas. EDUCATION: Graduated from Texas Christian University, 1941; trained for the stage at the Leland Powers School of the Theatre, 1942.

VOCATION: Actor.

CAREER: OFF-BROADWAY DEBUT—*A Man's House*, 1943.

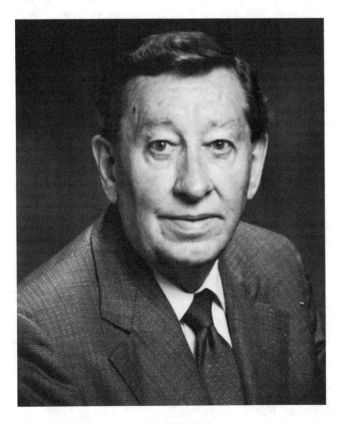

J. FRANK LUCAS

PRINCIPAL STAGE APPEARANCES—Francis Tear, "Ravenswood," and Dr. Toynbee, "Dunelawan," in *Bad Habits*, Astor Place Theatre, then Booth Theatre, both New York City, 1974; Geronte, *Scapino*, Circle in the Square, then Ambassador Theatre, both New York City, 1974; Mayor Rufus Poindexter and Senator Wingwoah, *The Best Little Whorehouse in Texas*, Entermedia Theatre, then 46th Street Theatre, both New York City, 1978, later Eugene O'Neill Theatre, New York City, 1982. Also appeared in *Othello*, Shakespearewrights, New York City, 1953; *Coriolanus*, Phoenix Theatre, New York City, 1954; *Inherit the Wind*, Margo Jones Theatre, Dallas, TX, 1955; *Edward II*, American National Theatre and Academy (ANTA) Matinee Series, Theatre De Lys, New York City, 1958; *The Long Gallery*, RNA Theatre, New York City, 1958; *The Trip to Bountiful*, Theatre East, New York City, 1959; *Guitar*, Jan Hus Theatre, New York City, 1959; *Orpheus Descending*, Gramercy Arts Theatre, New York City, 1959; *O'Casey and Carrol Twin Bill*, ANTA Matinee Series, Theatre De Lys, 1960; *Marcus in the High Grass*, Greenwich Mews Theatre, New York City, 1960; *To Bury a Cousin*, Bouwerie Lane Theatre, New York City, 1967; *Chocolates*, Gramercy Arts Theatre, 1967; *Geese*, Players Theatre, New York City, 1969; *One World at a Time*, Lamb's Club, New York City, 1972; *40 Carats*, Meadowbrook, NJ, 1972; *Gypsy*, Chateau de Ville Theatre, MA, 1972; *Twentieth Anniversary Gala*, ANTA Matinee Series, Theatre De Lys, 1975; *The Long Valley*, Theatre De Lys, 1975; *Home*, Long Wharf Theatre, New Haven, CT, 1976; *My Daughter's Rated X*, Canal-Fulton Dinner Playhouse, Canal-Fulton, OH, 1976; *The Torch-Bearers*, McCarter Theatre Company, Princeton, NJ, 1978; and in summer theatre productions at North Conway, NH, Hampton, NH, Virginia Beach, VA, Ocean City, NJ, Pompton Lakes, NJ, Sayville, NY, Clinton, CT, and Fayetteville, PA.

MAJOR TOURS—Geronte, *Scapino*, U.S. cities, 1975; Abner Dillon, *42nd Street*, U.S. cities, 1983; also in *Mr. Roberts*, U.S. cities, 1953; *Time for Elizabeth*, U.S. cities, 1958; *Once More, with Feeling*, U.S. cities, 1959; *Crazy October*, U.S. cities, 1959; *Goodbye Again*, U.S. cities, 1960; *God Bless Our Bank*, U.S. cities, 1963; *Breakfast at Tiffany's*, U.S. cities, 1966; *Don't Drink the Water*, U.S. cities, 1968; *Hadrian VII*, U.S. cities, 1970; *Charley's Aunt*, U.S. cities, 1976; *Make a Million*, U.S. cities, 1977; *Heaven Can Wait*, U.S. cities, 1977; *The Best Little Whorehouse in Texas*, U.S. cities, 1982.

PRINCIPAL FILM APPEARANCES—Seth Lucas, *Curse of the Living Corpse*, Twentieth Century-Fox, 1964; Flasher, *Law and Disorder*, Columbia, 1974; television psychologist, *Simon*, Warner Brothers, 1979. Also appeared in *A Little Sex*, Universal, 1981; *Arthur II*, Warner Brothers, 1988.

PRINCIPAL TELEVISION APPEARANCES—Series: *Texas*, NBC, 1981; *Another World*, NBC, 1982; *One Life to Live*, ABC, 1983. Pilots: *Sparrow*, CBS, 1978. Episodic: *Day in Court*, ABC, 1964. Movies: *The Life and Assassination of the Kingfish*, NBC, 1977. Specials: *Time for Elizabeth*, NBC, 1964.

RELATED CAREER—Appeared in industrial films for New Jersey Bell, 1978, and AT&T, 1982.

MEMBER: Actors' Equity Association, American Federation of Television and Radio Artists, Screen Actors Guild, American Guild of Variety Artists.

ADDRESSES: HOME—400 W. 43rd Street, Apartment 40-G, New York, NY 10036. AGENT—Sanders Agency, 156 Fifth Avenue, New York, NY 10010.

LUCCI, Susan   1950-

PERSONAL: Born December 23, 1950, in Westchester, NY; father, a building contractor; married Helmut Huber (a restaurateur); children: Liza Victoria, Andreas Martin.

VOCATION: Actress.

CAREER: PRINCIPAL TELEVISION APPEARANCES—Series: Erica Kane, *All My Children,* ABC, 1970—. Episodic: *Fame, Fortune, and Romance,* syndicated, 1986; also *Fantasy Island,* ABC; *The Love Boat,* ABC. Movies: Jessica Jones, *Invitation to Hell,* ABC, 1984; Darya Romanoff, *Anastasia: The Mystery of Anna,* NBC, 1986; Antoinette Giancana, *Mafia Princess,* NBC, 1986; Karen Beckett, *Haunted by Her Past,* NBC, 1987; Laurel March, *Lady Mobster,* ABC, 1988. Specials: Host, *Ninety-Nine Ways to Attract the Right Man,* ABC, 1985; host, *Working Women's Survival Hour,* Lifetime, 1987; host, *Soap Opera Awards* (also known as *Soap Opera Digest Awards*), NBC, 1988.

AWARDS: Eight Daytime Emmy Award nominations, all Best Actress, for *All My Children.*

ADDRESSES: AGENTS—Sylvia Gold, International Creative Management, 8899 Beverly Boulevard, Los Angeles, CA 90048; Abrams Artists and Associates, 420 Madison Avenue, New York, NY 10017. PUBLICIST—Alan Nierob, Rogers and Cowan Public Relations, 10000 Santa Monica Boulevard, Suite 1400, Los Angeles, CA 90067.*

*   *   *

LUMBLY, Carl

PERSONAL: Born in Jamaica; married Vonetta McGee (an actress); children: one son.

VOCATION: Actor.

CAREER: PRINCIPAL STAGE APPEARANCES—Hugh, *Meetings,* Phoenix Theatre Company, Marymount Manhattan Theatre, New York City, 1981; Francisco, *The Tempest,* New York Shakespeare Festival (NYSF), Delacorte Theatre, New York City, 1981; Theseus, *The Gospel at Colonus,* Carey Playhouse, Brooklyn Academy of Music, Brooklyn, NY, 1983; Oberon, *A Midsummer Night's Dream,* NYSF, Public Theatre, New York City, 1988. Also appeared in *Nevis Mountain Dew,* Los Angeles Actors' Theatre, Los Angeles, CA, 1981; *Sus,* Los Angeles Actors' Theatre, 1983; "The Damned Thing" and "The Facts in the Case of M. Valdemar and Berenice" in *Sundays at the Itchey Foot,* Center Theatre Group, Mark Taper Forum, Los Angeles, 1986; *Eyes of the American,* Los Angeles Theatre Center, Los Angeles, 1986; *Sizwe Banzi Is Dead* and *The Island,* both San Francisco, CA; and with the Arena Stage, Washington, DC, 1984-85.

MAJOR TOURS—*Sizwe Banzi Is Dead* and *The Island,* California cities.

PRINCIPAL FILM APPEARANCES—Inmate, *Escape from Alcatraz,* Paramount, 1979; Bork, *Caveman,* United Artists, 1981; John Parker, *The Adventures of Buckaroo Banzai: Across the Eighth Dimension,* Twentieth Century-Fox, 1984; Detective Quirk, *The Bedroom Window,* De Laurentiis Entertainment Group, 1987; Ed-

win Palmer, *Judgment in Berlin,* New Line Cinema, 1988; Marvel Blue, *Everybody's All-American,* Warner Brothers, 1988.

PRINCIPAL TELEVISION APPEARANCES—Series: Detective Marcus Petrie, *Cagney and Lacey,* CBS, 1982-88. Pilots: Petrie, *Cagney and Lacey,* CBS, 1981. Episodic: Theseus, "The Gospel at Colonus," *Great Performances,* PBS, 1985. Movies: Reverend Howell, *Undercover with the KKK,* NBC, 1979; Bobby Seale, *Conspiracy: The Trial of the Chicago Eight,* HBO, 1987. Specials: *Destined to Live: One Hundred Roads to Recovery,* NBC, 1988.

NON-RELATED CAREER—Writer for the Associated Press and the 3M Company.

ADDRESSES: AGENT—Susie Schwartz, Century Artists, 9744 Wilshire Boulevard, Suite 308, Beverly Hills, CA 90212.*

*   *   *

LuPONE, Robert   1946-

PERSONAL: Born July 29, 1946, in Brooklyn, NY; son of Orlando Joseph and Angela Louise LuPone. EDUCATION: Graduated from Juilliard School of Music.

VOCATION: Actor.

CAREER: BROADWAY DEBUT—*Minnie's Boys,* Imperial Theatre, 1970. PRINCIPAL STAGE APPEARANCES—Dancer, *Arabian Nights,* Jones Beach Theatre, Long Island, NY, 1967; A-Rab, *West Side Story,* State Theatre, New York City, 1968; sailor, *Charlie Was Here and Now He's Gone,* Eastside Playhouse, New York City, 1971; Manny, *The Magic Show,* Cort Theatre, New York City, 1974; Zach, *A Chorus Line,* Shubert Theatre, New York City, 1975; the Dauphin, *Saint Joan,* Circle in the Square, New York City, 1977; Antonio, *Twelfth Night,* Circle Repertory Theatre, New York City, 1980; Andrew Call, *In Connecticut,* GeVa Theatre, Rochester, NY, 1980, then Circle Repertory Theatre, 1981; older John Lennon, Stuart Sutcliffe, Les Chadwick, and Brian Epstein, *Lennon,* Entermedia Theatre, New York City, 1982; Bob Hawkins, M.P., and third hooded man, *Black Angel,* and Sebbie, *Snow Orchid,* both Circle Repertory Theatre, 1982; Reverend Prue Dimmes, *The Quilling of Prue,* AMDA Studio One, New York Theatre Studio, New York City, 1983; Zach, *A Chorus Line,* Shubert Theatre, 1989. Also appeared in *Noel Coward's Sweet Potato,* Ethel Barrymore Theatre, then Booth Theatre, both New York City, 1968; *The Rothschilds,* Lunt-Fontanne Theatre, New York City, 1970; *Jesus Christ Superstar,* Mark Hellinger Theatre, New York City, 1971; *The Tooth of Crime,* Goodman Theatre Center, Chicago, IL, 1973; *Boccaccio,* Arena Stage, Washington, DC, 1974; *Daddy's Duet,* Center Theatre Group, Mark Taper Forum, Los Angeles, CA, 1976; *Swing,* Kennedy Center for the Performing Arts, Washington, DC, 1980; *Late Night Comic,* Ritz Theatre, New York City, 1987; *Time Framed;* and *Class I Acts.*

PRINCIPAL STAGE WORK—Director (with Myra Turley), *It's Me Marie,* Actors Studio, New York City, 1980.

MAJOR TOURS—Zach, *A Chorus Line,* U.S. cities, 1976.

PRINCIPAL FILM APPEARANCES—Apostle, *Jesus Christ Superstar,* Universal, 1973.

PRINCIPAL TELEVISION APPEARANCES—Series: Zack Grayson, *All My Children,* ABC; Neil Cory, *Another World,* NBC. Pilots: Jeffrey Sinclair, "The Saint," *CBS Summer Playhouse,* CBS, 1987.

RELATED CAREER—Acting teacher, New York University, New York City, 1981; executive director (with Bernard Telsey), Manhattan Class Company, New York City, 1984—.*

*   *   *

LYMAN, Will   1948-

PERSONAL: Full name, William Lyman; born May 20, 1948, in Burlington, VT; son of Edward Phelps (an educator) and Mabry (an educator and editor; maiden name, Remington) Lyman; married Anastasia Sylvester (in human relations), January 8, 1972; children: Georgia. EDUCATION: Boston University, B.F.A., 1971; studied mime with Kenyon Martin; studied singing with Floria Mari.

VOCATION: Actor.

CAREER: OFF-BROADWAY DEBUT—Title role, *The Passion of Dracula,* Cherry Lane Theatre, 1978, for one hundred eighty-two performances. PRINCIPAL STAGE APPEARANCES—Dolek Berson, *The Wall,* National Jewish Theatre, Boston, MA, 1973; Randall Patrick McMurphy and Chief Bromden, *One Flew over the Cuckoo's Nest,* Charles Playhouse, Boston, MA, 1973; Ian, *The Grind-*

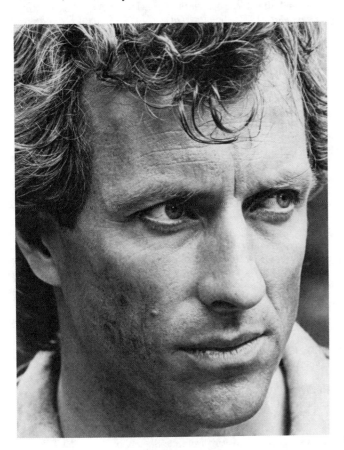

WILL LYMAN

ing Machine, American Place Theatre, New York City, 1978; Theseus and Oberon, *A Midsummer Night's Dream,* Trissotin, *The Learned Ladies,* and the Storyteller, *Caucasian Chalk Circle,* all Denver Center Theatre Company, Denver, CO, 1980; Jerry, *Betrayal,* George Street Playhouse, New Brunswick, NJ, 1981; Tom, *The Seven Year Itch,* Merrimack Regional Theatre, Lowell, MA, 1982; Oronte, *The Misanthrope,* Hartford Stage Company, Hartford, CT, 1983; Robert, *Betrayal,* Theatre by the Sea, Portsmouth, NH, 1984; John Proctor, *The Crucible,* Pennsylvania Stage Company, Allentown, PA, 1985.

FILM DEBUT—Coast guard ensign, *Jaws,* Universal, 1975; Greg Smolen, *Office Party,* SC Entertainment, 1988.

TELEVISION DEBUT—Ken Palmer, *Another World,* NBC, 1976. PRINCIPAL TELEVISION APPEARANCES—Series: Detective Nate Burroughs, *The Doctors,* NBC, 1980; narrator, *Frontline,* PBS, 1984-85; William Tell, *Crossbow,* syndicated, 1986-88. Mini-Series: Narrator, *Vietnam: A Television History,* PBS, 1981; Lawrence Washington, *George Washington,* CBS, 1984; narrator, *Crisis in Central America,* PBS, 1987; narrator, *Apartheid,* PBS, 1987; narrator, *The History of Surgery,* PBS, 1988; narrator, *China in Revolution,* PBS, 1989; narrator, *The AIDS Quarterly,* PBS, 1989. Episodic: Captain Morrison, *Spenser: For Hire,* ABC, 1985; narrator, "My Husband Is Going to Kill Me," *Frontline,* PBS, 1988; narrator, "The Race for the Superconductor," *Nova,* PBS, 1988; Lieutenant Commander Grant, *Spenser: For Hire,* ABC, 1988. Specials: John Corbin, *The Fight to Be Remembered,* PBS, 1973; title role, *Kosciuszko: An American Portrait,* PBS, 1976; Reverend Mr. Parris, *Three Sovereigns for Sarah,* PBS, 1984; Gabriel Javsicas, *Concealed Enemies,* PBS, 1983; narrator, *Einstein on the Beach: The Changing Image of Opera,* PBS, 1986; also Alex, *The Knock on the Door,* NBC.

MEMBER: Actors' Equity Association, Screen Actors Guild, American Federation of Television and Radio Artists.

ADDRESSES: AGENT—Abrams Artists and Associates, Inc., 420 Madison Avenue, Suite 1400, New York, NY 10017.

*   *   *

LYNE, Adrian

PERSONAL: Born c. 1941 in England; children: three (first marriage); one daughter (second marriage).

VOCATION: Director.

CAREER: PRINCIPAL FILM WORK—Director: *Foxes,* United Artists, 1980; *Flashdance,* Paramount, 1983; *9 1/2 Weeks,* Metro-Goldwyn-Mayer/United Artists, 1986; *Fatal Attraction,* Paramount, 1987. Also director of the short films *The Table* and *Mr. Smith.*

RELATED CAREER—Director of television commercials and short films.

AWARDS: Golden Globe Award nomination, Directors Guild of America Award nomination, and Academy Award nomination, all Best Director, 1988, for *Fatal Attraction;* Palme d'Or, Cannes Commercial Film Festival, for television commercials; also received numerous awards for television commercial work.

SIDELIGHTS: Between film projects, Adrian Lyne and his family live in a village in Provence in southern France. As he told *CTFT,* life in this region gives him "another take on things."

ADDRESSES: AGENT—Jeff Berg/Jim Wiatt, International Creative Management, 8899 Beverly Boulevard, Los Angeles, CA 90048.

*   *   *

LYNNE, Gillian   1926-

PERSONAL: Born February 20, 1926, in Bromley, England; daughter of Leslie Pyrke (in business) and Barbara (a dancer; maiden name, Hart) Lynne; married Patrick St. John Back (a lawyer; divorced); married Peter Land (a theatrical agent and actor), 1980. EDUCATION: Attended the Arts Educational School; studied ballet at the Royal Ballet School; studied jazz dance with Matt Mattocks.

VOCATION: Dancer, choreographer, and director.

CAREER: STAGE DEBUT—Dancer, Sadler's Wells Ballet Company, London, 1944. PRINCIPAL STAGE APPEARANCES—Claudine, *Can-Can,* Coliseum Theatre, London, 1954; narrator, *Peter and the Wolf,* London Philharmonic Orchestra, London, 1958. Also appeared in *Becky Sharp,* Windsor, U.K., 1959; *New Cranks,* Lyric Hammersmith Theatre, London, 1960; as the Queen of the Wilis, *Giselle* (ballet), and the Lilac Fairy, *Sleeping Beauty* (ballet), both Sadler's Wells Ballet Company, London; and in repertory

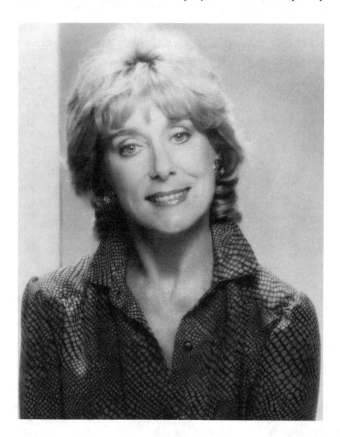

GILLIAN LYNNE

at Hythe, U.K., Windsor, U.K., and at the Devon Theatre Festival, Devon, U.K., all 1953.

PRINCIPAL STAGE WORK—All as choreographer, unless indicated: (Also director) *Round Leicester Square* and *Collages,* both Edinburgh Festival, Edinburgh, Scotland, 1963; *Pickwick,* 46th Street Theatre, New York City, 1965; *The Roar of the Greasepaint—The Smell of the Crowd,* Shubert Theatre, New York City, 1965; *A Comedy of Errors,* Royal Shakespeare Company (RSC), Royal Shakespeare Theatre, Stratford-on-Avon, U.K., 1976, then Aldwych Theatre, London, 1977; *The Trojans* (opera) and *Parsifal* (opera), both Covent Garden Opera House, London, 1977; director (with John Barton) *A Midsummer Night's Dream,* RSC, Royal Shakespeare Theatre, then Aldwych Theatre, both 1977; *As You Like It,* RSC, Royal Shakespeare Theatre, 1977; *The Yeoman of the Guard,* Tower of London, London, 1978; *Once in a Lifetime,* RSC, Aldwych Theatre, 1979; *My Fair Lady,* Adelphi Theatre, London, 1979; *Songbook,* Globe Theatre, London, 1979; (also associate director) *Cats,* New London Theatre, London, 1981, then Winter Garden Theatre, New York City, 1982; (also director) *Cats,* Vienna, Austria, 1983; director, *Jeeves Takes Charge,* Space at City Center, then Roundabout Theatre, both New York City, 1983, later Ford's Theatre, Washington, DC, 1986; (also director) *Cafe Soir* (ballet), Houston Ballet Company, Houston, TX, 1985; (also director) *Cabaret,* Strand Theatre, London, 1986; *The Phantom of the Opera,* Her Majesty's Theatre, London, 1986, then Majestic Theatre, New York City, 1988. Also choreographer, unless indicated: *The Owl and the Pussycat* (ballet), Western Theatre Ballet, 1961; *England, Our England,* 1962; director, *The Matchgirls,* 1966; director, *Bluebeard,* Sadler's Wells Opera Company, London, 1969; director, *Love on the Dole,* Nottingham, U.K., 1971; *Ambassador,* 1971; director, *Once Upon a Time,* 1972; *Liberty Ranch,* 1972; *The Papertown Chase,* 1973; *The Card,* 1973; *Hans Anderson,* 1974; director, *Home Is Best,* Amsterdam, Netherlands, 1978; *The Way of the World,* RSC, 1979.

MAJOR TOURS—Associate director and choreographer, *Cats,* U.S. cities, 1983—, and of various productions throughout the world.

PRINCIPAL FILM APPEARANCES—Marianne, *The Master of Ballantrae,* Warner Brothers, 1953; Gaskin's girl, *The Last Man to Hang,* Columbia, 1956; also appeared in *Make Mine a Million* (also known as *Look before You Laugh*), Schoenfeld, 1965.

PRINCIPAL FILM WORK—Choreographer: *Seaside Swingers* (also known as *Every Day's a Holiday*), Embassy, 1965; *Swingers' Paradise* (also known as *Wonderful Life*), American International, 1965; *Three Hats for Lisa,* Warner Brothers/Pathe, 1965; *Half a Sixpence,* Paramount, 1967; *Two Hundred Motels,* United Artists, 1971; *Man of La Mancha,* United Artists, 1972; *Mr. Quilp* (also known as *The Old Curiosity Shop*), AVCO-Embassy, 1975; *Yentl,* Metro-Goldwyn-Mayer/United Artists, 1983; *National Lampoon's European Vacation,* Warner Brothers, 1985.

PRINCIPAL TELEVISION WORK—Specials: Director and choreographer, *A Simple Man,* BBC. Also choreographer: *Morte d'Arthur,* BBC; *Easy Money,* BBC; *Mrs. F.'s Friends,* BBC; *Fool on the Hill,* Australian television.

RELATED CAREER—Dancer, Sadler's Wells Ballet Company, London; principal dancer in revues, Palladium Theatre, London, 1951-52.

AWARDS: Olivier Award from the Society of West End Theatre, Outstanding Achievement in a Musical, 1981, Antoinette Perry

Award, Best Choreography, 1983, and Silver Order of Merit from the Austrian government, 1984, all for *Cats;* Samuel G. Engel International TV Drama Award, 1985, for *Morte d'Arthur;* British Academy of Film and Television Arts Award, 1988, for *A Simple Man;* Antoinette Perry Award nomination, Best Choreography, 1988, for *The Phantom of the Opera*.

SIDELIGHTS: RECREATIONS—Cooking and rehearsing.

ADDRESSES: OFFICE—18 Rutland Street, Knightsbridge, London SW7 1EF, England.

M

MACNEE, Patrick 1922-

PERSONAL: Full name, Daniel Patrick Macnee; born February 6, 1922, in London, England; son of Daniel (a race horse trainer) and Dorothea Mary (Henry) Macnee; married Barbara Douglas, November, 1942 (divorced, 1956); married Kate Woodville (an actress), 1965 (divorced, 1969); married Baba Majos de Nagyzsenye, February 25, 1988; children: Rupert, Jenny (first marriage). EDUCATION: Trained for the stage at the Webber Douglas Academy of Dramatic Art, 1940. MILITARY: Royal Navy, first lieutenant, 1942-46.

VOCATION: Actor.

CAREER: STAGE DEBUT—Gerald Forbes, *When We Are Married,* Forbes Russell's Repertory Company, St. Francis Theatre, Letchworth, U.K., 1940, for five days. LONDON DEBUT—Laurie, *Little Women,* Westminster Theatre, 1941, for three months. BROAD-

WAY DEBUT—Andrew Wyke, *Sleuth,* Music Box Theatre, 1972. PRINCIPAL STAGE APPEARANCES—Demetrius, *A Midsummer Night's Dream,* Old Vic Theatre Company, Edinburgh Festival, Edinburgh, Scotland, then Metropolitan Opera House, New York City, both 1954; the Odd Man, *Made in Heaven,* Chichester Festival Theatre, Chichester, U.K., 1975; Andrew Wyke, *Sleuth,* Coconut Grove Playhouse, Miami, FL, 1984; Andrew Wyke, *Sleuth,* New Century Theatre, Toronto, ON, Canada, 1987. Also in *The Grass Is Greener,* Yvonne Arnaud Theatre, Guildford, U.K., 1979; as Lucifer, *Don Juan in Hell* (staged reading), Dallas, TX, 1983; in *Killing Jessica,* Savoy Theatre, London, 1986; and appeared in numerous productions in the U.K., 1939-42 and 1946-52, and in Canadian and U.S. productions, 1952-60.

MAJOR TOURS—Laurie, *Little Women,* U.K. cities, 1941; Demetrius, *A Midsummer Night's Dream,* Old Vic Theatre Company, U.S. cities, 1954; Andrew Wyke, *Sleuth,* U.S. cities, 1973-75. Also in *Secretary Bird,* Australian and New Zealand cities, 1970, later Canadian cities, 1973; *Absurd Person Singular,* U.S. cities, 1975; *The Grass Is Greener,* U.K., Middle Eastern, and Canadian cities, 1979-80; and *House Guest,* Australian cities, 1982.

FILM DEBUT—*Colonel Blimp* (also known as *The Life and Death of Colonel Blimp*), General Films Distributors, 1945. PRINCIPAL FILM APPEARANCES—Tony, *The Fatal Night,* Columbia, 1948; Honorable John Bristow, *The Fighting Pimpernel* (also known as *The Elusive Pimpernel*), British Lion, 1950; Hugh Hurcombe, *The Girl Is Mine,* British Lion, 1950; young Marley, *A Christmas Carol* (also known as *Scrooge*), United Artists, 1951; Private Duff, *Until They Sail,* Metro-Goldwyn-Mayer (MGM), 1957; Sir Percy, *Les Girls,* MGM, 1957; Lieutenant Commander Medley, *Pursuit of the Graf Spee* (also known as *The Battle of the River Plate*), Rank, 1957; Major Derek Longbow, *Incense for the Damned* (also known as *Doctors Wear Scarlet* and *The Bloodsuckers*), Lucinda/Titan International, 1970; Captain Good, *King Solomon's Treasure.*

Stark, *The Creature Wasn't Nice* (also known as *Spaceship*), Creature Features, 1981; Dr. George Waggner, *The Howling,* AVCO-Embassy, 1981; Major Yogi Crossley, *The Sea Wolves,* Paramount, 1981; Dr. Jacobs, *Young Doctors in Love,* Twentieth Century-Fox, 1982; John Morgan, *Sweet Sixteen,* Century International, 1983; Sir Denis Eton-Hogg, *This Is Spinal Tap* (also known as *Spinal Tap*), Embassy, 1984; Sir Cyril Landau, *Shadey,* Film Four International/Skouras, 1985; Tibbett, *A View to a Kill,* Metro-Goldwyn-Mayer/United Artists, 1985; Major Vickers, *For the Term of His Natural Life,* Filmco, 1985; host, *Tales from the Darkside,* International Video Entertainment, 1985; Sir Wilfred, *Waxwork,* Vestron, 1988. Also appeared in *Dead of Night,* Rank/Universal, 1946; *Hamlet,* General Films Distributors, 1948; *All Over the Town,* Rank/General Films Distributors, 1949; *Hour of Glory* (also known as *The Small Back Room*), British Lion, 1949;

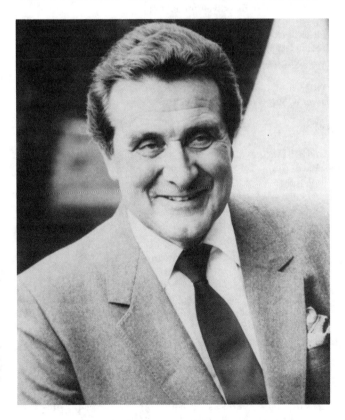

PATRICK MACNEE

239

Dick Barton at Bay, Marylebone/Hammer, 1950; *Flesh and Blood,* British Lion, 1951; *Three Cases of Murder,* Wessex Associated Artists, 1955; *Mission of Danger,* MGM, 1959; *Dick Turpin,* 1980; *The Hot Touch,* 1981; *Transformations,* 1987; *The Chill Factor,* 1988; *Lobster Man from Mars,* 1989; and *A Stroke of Luck.*

TELEVISION DEBUT—Laertes, *Hamlet,* BBC, 1947. PRINCIPAL TELEVISION APPEARANCES—Series: John Steed, *The Avengers,* British television, 1960-69, and ABC, 1966-69; John Steed, *The New Avengers,* CBS, 1978-80; Milo Bentley, *Gavilan,* NBC, 1982-83; regular, *Vintage Quiz,* TVS, 1983; Calvin Cromwell, *Empire,* CBS, 1984; Sir Geoffrey Rimbatten, *Lime Street,* ABC, 1985; also *For the Term of His Natural Life,* Australian television, 1981-82; host, *Patrick Macnee Presents Sherlock Holmes,* 1987. Mini-Series: *Around the World in Eighty Days,* 1989. Pilots: Shawcross, *Matt Helm,* ABC, 1975; Horatio Black, *The Billion Dollar Threat,* ABC, 1979; Maximilian Boudreau, *Stunt Seven,* CBS, 1979; host, *Comedy of Horrors,* CBS, 1981; also *Where There's a Will,* TSW, 1987.

Episodic: First officer, "Judgement Night," *The Twilight Zone,* CBS, 1959; voice of Imperious Cylon Leader and narrator, *Battlestar Galactica,* ABC, 1978; subject, *This Is Your Life,* Thames, 1984; Oliver Trumbull, *Murder, She Wrote,* CBS, 1985; Beechum, *Blacke's Magic,* NBC, 1986; also *Suspicion,* NBC, 1957; "Night of April 14," *One Step Beyond,* ABC, 1959; "Logoda's Heads," *Night Gallery,* NBC, 1971; *Khan,* CBS, 1975; *Caribe,* ABC, 1975; *Sweepstakes,* NBC, 1979; *Matinee Theater,* NBC, 1957; *Magnum P.I.,* CBS, 1984; *Hart to Hart,* ABC, 1984; *The Love Boat,* ABC, 1984; *Hotel,* ABC, 1985; *Mary,* CBS, 1986; *Alfred Hitchcock Presents,* NBC, 1986; *Murphy's Law,* ABC, 1988; *War of the Worlds,* syndicated, 1988; *Playhouse 90* (three episodes), CBS; *Diana,* NBC; *Columbo,* NBC; *Automan,* ABC; *First Class* (two episodes), 1983; *Ultra Quiz,* 1984; *Alfred Hitchcock Presents* (two episodes of the original series); *Kraft Television Theatre; Great Mysteries; Dial M for Murder;* and *Thriller.*

Movies: Dudley Jerico, *Mister Jerico,* ABC, 1970; Dr. John Watson, *Sherlock Holmes in New York,* NBC, 1976; Ian Wadleigh, *Evening in Byzantium,* syndicated, 1978; David Matthews, *Rehearsal for Murder,* CBS, 1982; Sir John Raleigh, *The Return of the Man from U.N.C.L.E.,* CBS, 1983; Gilbert Anthony Paige, *Club Med,* ABC, 1986. Specials: Lucius, *Caesar and Cleopatra,* NBC, 1956; also *The Miss Universe Pageant,* syndicated, 1986. Also appeared in *Beyond Reasonable Doubt,* and in more than thirty plays on Canadian television, 1952-58.

WRITINGS: (With Marie Cameron) *Blind in One Ear* (autobiography), Harrap, 1988.

AWARDS: Variety Club of Great Britain Award, Joint Television Personalities of the Year (with Honor Blackman), 1963, for *The Avengers;* Straw Hat Award, Best Performance in a Long-Running Play, 1974, for *Sleuth;* Golden Camera Award (Germany), Popular Television Personality, 1983, for *The Avengers;* Freedom of the Town of Filey, U.K., 1962; Freedom of the City of Macon, GA, 1984.

MEMBER: Actors' Equity Association, American Federation of Television and Radio Artists, Screen Actors Guild, British Actors' Equity Association, Association of Canadian Television and Radio Artists.

SIDELIGHTS: RECREATIONS—Reading, walking, tennis, and swimming.

ADDRESSES: AGENTS—Russ Lyster, The Agency, 10351 Santa Monica Boulevard, Suite 211, Los Angeles, CA 90025; Kenneth Earle, London Management, 235-241 Regent Street, London W1A 2JT, England.

*   *   *

MacNICOL, Peter   1954-

PERSONAL: Born April 10, 1954, in Dallas, TX. EDUCATION: Attended the University of Minnesota.

VOCATION: Actor.

CAREER: BROADWAY DEBUT—Barnette Lloyd, *Crimes of the Heart,* John Golden Theatre, 1981. PRINCIPAL STAGE APPEARANCES—Barnette Lloyd, *Crimes of the Heart,* Manhattan Theatre Club Upstage, New York City, 1980, then Center Theatre Group, Ahmanson Theatre, Los Angeles, CA, 1982; Little Earl 5, *Found a Peanut,* New York Shakespeare Festival (NYSF), Public Theatre, New York City, 1984; Jake Seward, *Rum and Coke,* NYSF, Susan Stein Shiva Theatre, New York City, 1986; Sir Andrew Aguecheek, *Twelfth Night,* NYSF, Delacorte Theatre, New York City, 1986; Romeo, *Romeo and Juliet,* NYSF, Public Theatre, New York City, 1988. Also appeared in *Another Country,* Long Wharf Theatre, New Haven, CT, 1982; *Tartuffe,* Alaska Repertory Theatre, Anchorage and Fairbanks, AK, 1984; *Execution of Justice,* Tyrone Guthrie Theatre, Minneapolis, MN, 1985; *All the King's Men,* Trinity Repertory Company, Providence, RI, 1987; with the Tyrone Guthrie Theatre, Minneapolis, MN, 1978-80 and 1985-86; and in *Richard II,* Off-Broadway production.

PRINCIPAL FILM APPEARANCES—Galen, *Dragonslayer,* Paramount, 1981; Stingo, *Sophie's Choice,* Universal, 1982; Cyrus Kinnick, *Heat,* New Century-Vista, 1987.

PRINCIPAL TELEVISION APPEARANCES—Movies: Joe Kovacs, *Johnny Bull,* ABC, 1986.

AWARDS: Theatre World Award, 1982, for *Crimes of the Heart.*

ADDRESSES: AGENT—Katy Rothacker and Chris Black, William Morris Agency, 1350 Avenue of the Americas, New York, NY 10019.*

*   *   *

MADSEN, Virginia   1961-

PERSONAL: Born September 11, 1961, in Chicago, IL; daughter of Cal (a fireman) and Elaine (a writer of documentaries) Madsen. EDUCATION: Studied drama at Northwestern University with Ted Liss for three years.

VOCATION: Actress.

CAREER: PRINCIPAL FILM APPEARANCES—Lisa, *Class,* Orion, 1983; Madeline, *Electric Dreams,* Metro-Goldwyn-Mayer/United Artists, 1984; Princess Irulan, *Dune,* De Laurentiis Entertainment Group/Universal, 1984; Barbara Spencer, *Creator,* Universal, 1985; Lisa Taylor, *Fire with Fire,* Paramount, 1986; Kelly,

Modern Girls, Atlantic, 1986; Yolanda Carlyle, *Slamdance,* Island, 1987; Andrea Miller, *Zombie High,* Cinema Group, 1987; Sally Boffin, *Mr. North,* Samuel Goldwyn, 1988; Allison Rowe, *Hot to Trot,* Warner Brothers, 1988.

PRINCIPAL TELEVISION APPEARANCES—Mini-Series: Claretta Petacci, *Mussolini: The Untold Story,* NBC, 1985. Movies: Lou Ellen Purdy, *A Matter of Principal,* PBS, 1984; Marion Davies, *The Hearst and Davies Affair,* ABC, 1985; Dixie Lee Boxx, *Long Gone,* HBO, 1987; Rachel Carlyle, *Gotham,* Showtime, 1988; Anne Scholes, *Third Degree Burn,* HBO, 1989.

RELATED CAREER—Appeared in television commercials.

ADDRESSES: MANAGER—Loree Rodkin, Rodkin Company, 8600 Melrose Avenue, Los Angeles, CA 90069.*

*   *   *

MAGNUSON, Ann   1956-

PERSONAL: Born in 1956 in Charleston, WV; father, a lawyer; mother, a journalist. EDUCATION: Studied theatre at Dennison University and at the British and European Studies Group; interned at the Ensemble Studio Theatre, New York City, 1978.

VOCATION: Actress, comedienne, and writer.

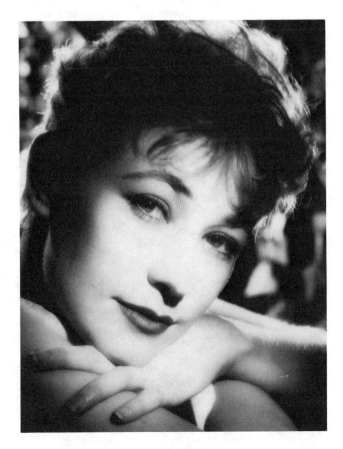

Photography by Ricky Schenck

ANN MAGNUSON

CAREER: PRINCIPAL STAGE APPEARANCES—Lavinia, *Titus Andronicus,* Pyramid Club, New York City, 1985; Sister Alice Tully Hall, "Alice Tully Hall and the Family: Transmissions" for the *Serious Fun!* series, Alice Tully Hall, Lincoln Center, New York City, 1987. Also appeared at the Festival Della Donna, Bologna, Italy, 1982; in the Art in Action show, Segetsu Hall, Tokyo, Japan, 1985; in *Occupational Hazards,* Brattle Theatre, Boston, MA; *After Dark,* Walker Arts Center, Minneapolis, MN; *Tammy's Nightmare,* L.A.C.E., Los Angeles, CA; *Art on the Beach,* Creative Time, Inc., Battery Park Landfill, New York City; *Somewhere Outside of Orlando,* Pittsburgh Center for the Arts, Pittsburgh, PA, then Lhasa Club, Los Angeles; and in *A Christmas Special,* The Kitchen (Club), New York City.

PRINCIPAL FILM APPEARANCES—Pamela Fleming, *Vortex,* B Movies, 1982; woman in disco, *The Hunger,* Metro-Goldwyn-Mayer/United Artists, 1983; feminist, *Perfect Strangers* (also known as *Blind Alley*), New Line Cinema, 1984; cigarette girl, *Desperately Seeking Susan,* Orion, 1985; Isabelle, *Sleepwalk* (also known as *Year of the Dog*), New Cinema Cinema, 1986; Frankie Stone, *Making Mr. Right,* Orion, 1987; Arzt, *The Critical Years* (also known as *Les Annees critiques*), Dexter, 1987; Joyce Fickett, *A Night in the Life of Jimmy Reardon,* Twentieth Century-Fox, 1988; Shaleen, *Tequila Sunrise,* Warner Brothers, 1988; Connie, *Checking Out,* Warner Brothers, 1989. Also appeared in *Mondo New York,* Island, 1988; *Heavy Petting* (documentary), International Film Exchange/Filmpac Holdings/Fossil Films, Inc., 1988; and in *Love at Large,* 1989.

PRINCIPAL TELEVISION APPEARANCES—Series: Co-host, *Alive from Off-Center,* PBS, 1988. Episodic: "Made for TV," *Alive from Off-Center,* PBS, 1984; "Love Comics," *New Television,* WNYC (New York), 1985; "Fallopia," *Night Flight,* USA, 1985. Specials: Sweet Pea and various roles, "Ann Magnuson's Vandemonium," *Cinemax Comedy Experiment,* Cinemax, 1987; Darlene, "Tales from the Hollywood Hills: A Table at Ciro's," *Great Performances,* PBS, 1987.

RELATED CAREER—Co-founder and manager, Club 57, New York City, 1979; devised *Upwardly Mobile,* a tribute to Muzak which was held in an elevator of the Whitney Museum, New York City, 1982; performed in the cabaret production *No Entiendes,* Palladium (dance club), New York City; in *Pagan Place,* Palladium; has appeared in nightclubs with Joey Arias in *Salvador Dali and His Wife Gala, Andy Warhol and Edie Sedgwick, Charles Manson and Squeaky Fromme,* etc., in "Duets" with Eric Bogosian, in art spaces in New York City, and in colleges throughout the northeastern United States; producer and director of such performance pieces as *A Tribute to Lawrence Welk, Putt-Putt Reggae,* and *The Stay-Free Mini Prom,* all at Club 57, *Festival de San de Niro,* at Danceteria, New York City, and productions at the Pyramid Club and Folk City, both in New York City and at the Lhasa Club, Los Angeles; performer in the music groups Pulsallama, Bleaker Street Incident, Vulcan Death Grip, and Bongwater at clubs in Los Angeles, San Francisco, Hoboken, Washington, DC, and New York City.

NON-RELATED CAREER—Lady wrestler, Club 57 and Fashion Moda, both in New York City.

WRITINGS: STAGE—*Tammy's Nightmare,* L.A.C.E., Los Angeles, CA, published in *Drama Review;* also creator of the characters Sister Alice Tully Hall, Fallopia, Raven, Tammy Jan, Kimberly Crump, Ms. Rambo, Anoushka, and others for theatre and club performances.

TELEVISION—Episodic: (With Barry Shills, Steve Brown, and Andy Rees) "Love Comics," *New Television,* WNYC (New York City), 1985. Specials: "Ann Magnuson's Vandemonium," *Cinemax Comedy Experiment,* Cinemax, 1987. OTHER—Contributor of fiction and travel articles to *Soho Weekly News, High Times, Vogue, The Paper, Interview, L.A. Weekly,* and *Conde Nast Traveler.*

RECORDINGS: SINGLES—(With Bongwater) "You Don't Love Me Yet," Shimmy Disc, 1989. ALBUMS—(With Pulsallama) *The Devil Lives in My Husband's Body,* Y Records, 1982; (with Bongwater) *Breaking No New Ground,* Shimmy Disc, 1987; (with Bongwater) *Double Bummer,* Shimmy Disc, 1988; also (with Bongwater) *Bongwater Plus* (compact disc), Shimmy Disk Europe/Semaphore Productions; (with Vulcan Death Grip) song on *Tellus: The Audio Cassette Magazine #18,* "Experimental Theatre"; "Made for Radio" segments, *The Uproar Tapes, Volume I,* Antilles Records.

ADDRESSES: AGENTS—Cary Woods, William Morris Agency, 151 El Camino Drive, Beverly Hills, CA 90210; George Lane, William Morris Agency, 1350 Avenue of the Americas, New York, NY 10019. MANAGER—Buddy Morra, Rollins, Rollins, Joffe, Morra, and Brezner, 801 Westmount Drive, Los Angeles, CA 90069.

*   *   *

MALIK, Art   1952-
(Athar Malik)

PERSONAL: Born Athar Ul-Haque Malik, November 13, 1952, in Bahawalpur, Pakistan; immigrated to England in 1956; son of Mazhar Ul-Haque (an eye surgeon) and Zaibunisa Malik; married Gina Rowe (an actress, artist, and writer), August 19, 1988; children: Jessica, Keira. EDUCATION: Graduated from Guildhall School of Music and Drama, 1977. POLITICS: Labor.

VOCATION: Actor and writer.

CAREER: PRINCIPAL STAGE APPEARANCES—Page to Tybalt, *Romeo and Juliet,* and nappi and sentry, *The 88,* both Old Vic Company, Old Vic Theatre, London, 1979; also appeared in *The Government Inspector,* Old Vic Company, Old Vic Theatre, 1979; as John, *Whose Life Is It Anyway?,* Mercury Theatre, Colchester, U.K.; Ahmed, *Aliens,* Soho Poly Theatre, London; Iachimo, *Cymbeline,* and Herbert Pocket, *Great Expectations,* both Royal Exchange Theatre, Manchester, U.K.; in *A Man for All Seasons* and *Equus,* both Leeds Playhouse, Leeds, U.K.; *Destiny* and *Timon of Athens,* both Bristol Old Vic Theatre, Bristol, U.K.; *Trial Run,* Oxford Playhouse, Oxford, U.K., and Young Vic Theatre, London; *Othello,* Royal Shakespeare Company.

PRINCIPAL FILM APPEARANCES—(As Athar Malik) Monk, *Meetings with Remarkable Men,* Enterprise, 1979; (as Athar Malik) Mahmoud, *An Arabian Adventure,* Columbia/EMI/Warner, 1979; Mahmoud Ali, *A Passage to India,* Columbia, 1984; Fluke, *Underworld,* Limehouse Pictures/Green Man, 1985; Kamran Shah, *The Living Daylights,* Metro-Goldwyn-Mayer/United Artists, 1987. Also appeared in *Richard's Things,* Southern, 1980; *Telephone Behavior: The Power and the Perils,* 1986.

PRINCIPAL TELEVISION APPEARANCES—Series: Dr. Ved Lahari,

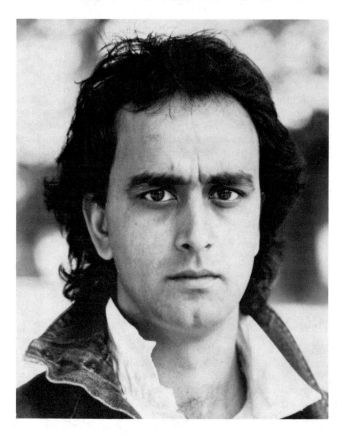

ART MALIK

Hothouse, ABC, 1988. Mini-Series: Hari Kumar, *The Jewel in the Crown,* Granada, then *Masterpiece Theatre,* PBS, 1984; Zarin, *The Far Pavilions,* HBO, 1984; Julius Court, *The Black Tower,* Anglia, then *Mystery,* PBS, 1988; also *Shadow of the Cobra,* BBC, 1989; *Stolen,* London Weekend Television (LWT), 1989. Episodic: Ravi Chavan, *Bergerac,* BBC, then Entertainment Channel, 1982; also in "The Reaper," *ITV Playhouse,* ITV. Movies: Pasha, *Harem,* ABC, 1986. Also appeared in *Death Is Part of the Process,* BBC, 1986; *West of Paradise,* Yorkshire Television, 1986; as Aziz, *Chessgame,* Granada, then PBS, 1987; Aziz Ul Haque, *Crown Court,* Granada; Turk, *The Gentle Touch,* LWT; Jerome Leblanc, *After the War,* Granada; in *Mixed Blessings,* LWT; and *The Professionals,* Euston.

WRITINGS: "Karachi," "Another Day," and "Rise Kingston and Explain," (short stories).

AWARDS: British Academy of Film and Television Arts Award nomination, Best Actor, 1985, and Milano Television Internationale Award, Best Actor, 1988, both for *The Jewel in the Crown.*

MEMBER: Groucho Club, Browns Club.

SIDELIGHTS: CTFT learned that Art Malik is currently writing a four-part television series and a film script.

ADDRESSES: AGENTS—Caroline Dawson, Caroline Dawson Associates, Apartment 20, 47 Courtfield Road, London SW7 4DB, England; Bob Duva, Gersh Agency, 130 W. 42nd Street, New York, NY 10036.

MANCUSO, Nick   1956-

PERSONAL: Born in 1956 in Italy.

VOCATION: Actor.

CAREER: PRINCIPAL STAGE APPEARANCES—Bassanio, *Merchant of Venice*, Diomedes, *Antony and Cleopatra*, and Lysander, *A Midsummer Night's Dream*, all Stratford Shakespeare Festival, Stratford, ON, Canada, 1976. Also appeared in *Tiger Tail*, Alliance Theatre Company, Atlanta, GA, 1977.

PRINCIPAL FILM APPEARANCES—Youngman Duran, *Nightwing*, Columbia, 1979; Nick, *Death Ship*, AVCO-Embassy, 1980; David Kappell, *Ticket to Heaven*, United Artists, 1981; Jean Dupre, *Mother Lode* (also known as *Search for the Mother Lode* and *The Last Great Treasure*), Agamemnon, 1982; Francois Paradis, *Maria Chapdelaine*, Movie Store, 1982; Chris Dalton, *Blame It on the Night*, Tri-Star, 1984; Eli Kahn, *Heartbreakers*, Orion, 1984; Michael, *La Nuit Magique* (also known as *Night Magic*), RSL/Fildbroc/TFI, 1985; Father Angel, *Death of an Angel*, Twentieth Century-Fox/TLC, 1985; Spallner, "The Crowd" in *The Bradbury Trilogy*, Atlantic, 1985; Peter Marker, *Paroles et Musiques* (also known as *Love Songs*), Spectrafilm, 1986; reunion friend, *Tiger Warsaw*, Sony, 1988. Also appeared in *Tell Me That You Love Me*, 1980.

PRINCIPAL TELEVISION APPEARANCES—Series: Title role, *Stingray*, NBC, 1986-87. Mini-Series: Vito Orsini, *Scruples*, CBS, 1980. Pilots: John Shackelford, *Dr. Scorpion*, ABC, 1978; Max Catlin, *Unit 4*, CBS, 1981; Andy Thorn and narrator, *Feel the Heat*, ABC, 1983; title role, *Stingray*, NBC, 1985; Harry Brackett, *Embassy*, ABC, 1985. Movies: Ari, *The House on Garibaldi Street*, ABC, 1979; Horses Ghost, *The Legend of Walks Far Woman*, NBC, 1982; Mike, *Desperate Intruder*, syndicated, 1983; William Hall/Worthington Hawkes, *H—The King of Love*, ABC, 1987. Specials: Toby, "Half a Lifetime," *HBO Showcase*, HBO, 1986.

ADDRESSES: PUBLICIST—Michael Levine Public Relations, 8730 Sunset Boulevard, 6th Floor, Los Angeles, CA 90069.*

*   *   *

MARCHAND, Nancy   1928-

PERSONAL: Born June 19, 1928, in Buffalo, NY; daughter of Raymond L. (a physician) and Marjorie (a pianist; maiden name, Freeman) Marchand; married Paul Sparer (an actor, writer, and director), July 7, 1951; children: David, Kathryn, Rachel. EDUCATION: Carnegie Institute of Technology, B.F.A., 1949.

VOCATION: Actress.

CAREER: STAGE DEBUT—*The Late George Apley*, Ogunquit, ME, 1946. PRINCIPAL STAGE APPEARANCES—Reporter, *The Winslow Boy*, Falmouth Theatre, Falmouth, MA, 1949; Princess of France, *Love's Labour's Lost*, Mrs. Dudgeon, *The Devil's Disciple*, Tibueina, *The Critic*, first witch, *Macbeth*, and Regan, *King Lear*, all Brattle Theatre, Cambridge, MA, 1950-52; hostess of the tavern, *The Taming of the Shrew*, City Center Theatre, New York City, 1951; Princess of France, *Love's Labour's Lost*, and Nerissa, *The Merchant of Venice*, both City Center Theatre, 1953; Kate, *The*

Taming of the Shrew, Nurse, *Romeo and Juliet*, and Amelia, *Othello*, all Antioch Shakespeare Festival, Antioch, OH, 1954; Mrs. Grant, *Teach Me How to Cry*, Theatre De Lys, New York City, 1955; Mrs. Mi Tzu, *The Good Woman of Setzuan*, Phoenix Theatre, New York City, 1956; Miriam Ackroyd, *Miss Isobel*, Royale Theatre, New York City, 1957; Paulina, *The Winter's Tale*, American Shakespeare Festival, Stratford, CT, 1958; Lady Capulet, *Romeo and Juliet*, and Mistress Page, *The Merry Wives of Windsor*, both American Shakespeare Festival, 1959; Ursula, *Much Ado about Nothing*, Lunt-Fontanne Theatre, New York City, 1959.

Madame Irma, *The Balcony*, Circle in the Square, New York City, 1960; Jane Peyton, *Laurette*, Shubert Theatre, New Haven, CT, 1960; Lady Sneerwell, *The School for Scandal*, and Madame Irina Arkadina, *The Seagull*, both American Producing Artists (APA), Folksbiene Playhouse, New York City, 1962; Beatrice, *Much Ado about Nothing*, APA, Ann Arbor, MI, 1963; Amalia Agazzi, *Right You Are If You Think You Are*, and Vasilissa Karpovna Kostilyova, *The Lower Depths*, both APA, Ann Arbor, 1963, then Phoenix Theatre, New York City, 1964; the Woman, *The Tavern*, APA, Phoenix Theatre, 1964; prostitute, *Judith*, and Ann Whitefield, *Man and Superman*, both APA, Ann Arbor, MI, 1964, then Phoenix Theatre, 1965; the Old Lady, *Good Day*, Cherry Lane Theatre, New York City, 1965; Genevieve, *Three Bags Full*, Henry Miller's Theatre, New York City, 1966; woman of Canterbury, *Murder in the Cathedral*, American Shakespeare Festival, 1966; Dol Common, *The Alchemist*, and Dolores, *Yerma*, both Lincoln Center Repertory Theatre, Vivian Beaumont Theatre, New York City, 1966; Gertrude Forbes-Cooper, *After the Rain*, John Golden Theatre, New York City, 1967; Duenna (Sister Clare), *Cyrano de Bergerac*, Vivian Beaumont Theatre, then Center Theatre Group, Los Angeles, CA, both 1968; Mrs. Latham, *Forty Carats*, Morosco Theatre, New York City, 1968.

Queen Elizabeth, *Christmas Dinner*, Berkshire Theatre Festival, Stockbridge, MA, 1971; Ceil Adams, *And Miss Reardon Drinks a Little*, Morosco Theatre, 1971; Queen Elizabeth, *Mary Stuart*, Vivian Beaumont Theatre, 1971; Tatiana, *Enemies*, Vivian Beaumont Theatre, 1972; Mrs. Gogon, *The Plough and the Stars*, Vivian Beaumont Theatre, 1973; Myra Power, *Patrick's Day*, Long Wharf Theatre, New Haven, CT, 1973; Vera Simpson, *Pal Joey*, and Madame Ranevskaya, *The Cherry Orchard*, both Goodman Theatre, Chicago, IL, 1974; Mother, *Children*, Manhattan Theatre Club, New York City, 1976; Esther, *The Song of Solomon*, New Dramatists, New York City, 1976; Ruth Chandler, *Taken in Marriage*, New York Shakespeare Festival, Public Theatre, New York City, 1979; Ida Bolton, *Morning's at Seven*, Lyceum Theatre, New York City, 1980; title role, *Sister Mary Ignatius Explains It All for You*, Westside Arts Center, New York City, 1982; Agnes, *A Delicate Balance*, McCarter Theatre, Princeton, NJ, 1983; Bessie Berger, *Awake and Sing!*, Circle in the Square, 1984; Connie (Mrs. David Emerson), *The Octette Bridge Club*, Music Box Theatre, New York City, 1985; Judith Tiverton, *Oliver Oliver*, Long Wharf Theatre, 1984, then Manhattan Theatre Club, City Center Theatre, 1985; Stella Livingston, *Light Up the Sky*, Center Theatre Group, Ahmanson Theatre, 1987; Ann, *The Cocktail Hour*, Old Globe Theatre, San Diego, CA, then Promenade Theatre, New York City, both 1988; Melissa Gardner, *Love Letters*, Promenade Theatre, 1989. Also appeared in *Antigone*, Carnegie Hall Playhouse, New York City, 1956; *Tchin-Tchin*, Plymouth Theatre, New York City, 1962; *Strange Interlude*, Hudson Theatre, New York City, 1963; *The Sorrows of Frederick*, Mark Taper Forum, Los Angeles, 1967; *Veronica's Room*, Music Box Theatre, 1973; *Awake and Sing!*, Playwrights Horizons, New York City, 1978; as Clytemnestra,

Elektra, New York City, 1987; and in productions of *On the Town, The Duel, Parent's Day,* and *Playboy of the Western World.*

PRINCIPAL FILM APPEARANCES—Julie, *The Bachelor Party,* United Artists, 1957; Mrs. Andrews, *Ladybug, Ladybug,* United Artists, 1963; Mrs. Miller, *Me, Natalie,* National General, 1969; Nurse Oxford, *Tell Me That You Love Me, Junie Moon,* Paramount, 1970; Mrs. Christie, *The Hospital,* United Artists, 1971; Mrs. Burrage, *The Bostonians,* Almi, 1984; Roberta Winnaker, *From the Hip,* De Laurentiis Entertainment Group, 1987; Mayor, *The Naked Gun—From the Files of Police Squad!,* Paramount, 1988. Also appeared in *Goodbye Mr. Chips,* Metro-Goldwyn-Mayer, 1969; *The Rise and Rise of Michael Rimmer,* Warner Brothers, 1970; and *Promise at Dawn* (also known as *La Promesse de l'aube*), AVCO-Embassy, 1970.

PRINCIPAL TELEVISION APPEARANCES—Series: Mary Lassiter, *Beacon Hill,* CBS, 1975; Edith Cushing, *Lovers and Friends,* NBC, 1977; Margaret Pynchon, *Lou Grant,* CBS, 1977-82; also Mrs. McCrea, *Another World,* NBC; Vinnie Phillips, *Love of Life,* CBS; and in *Search for Tomorrow,* CBS. Mini-Series: Mrs. Smith, *The Adams Chronicles,* PBS, 1976; Claudine Roux, *Spearfield's Daughter,* syndicated, 1986; Dorothea Dix, *North and South, Book II,* ABC, 1986.

Episodic: Jo March, "Little Women," *Studio One,* CBS, 1950; Clara Davis, "Marty," *The Goodyear Television Playhouse,* NBC, 1953; judge, *The Edge of Night,* CBS, 1970; Frasier's mother, "Diane Meets Mom," *Cheers,* NBC, 1984; Emily Garden, *Spenser: For Hire,* ABC, 1986; also "Of Famous Memory," *Kraft Television Theatre,* NBC, 1951; "The Hospital," *Studio One,* CBS, 1952; "The Peaceful Warrior," *Kraft Television Theatre,* NBC, 1952; "The Office Dance," "Career," "A Child Is Born," and "The Old Maid," all *Kraft Television Theatre,* NBC, 1954; "The Renaissance," *Omnibus,* CBS, 1955; "The Trial of Captain Kidd," *Omnibus,* CBS, 1957; "Mayerling," *Producer's Showcase,* NBC, 1957; "Rudy," *Studio One,* CBS, 1957; "Material Witness," *Kraft Television Theatre,* NBC, 1958; "The Sleeping Beauty," *Shirley Temple's Story Book,* ABC, 1958; "The Miracle at Spring Hill," *Armstrong Circle Theatre,* CBS, 1958; "Free Weekend" and "The Hidden Image," both *Playhouse 90,* CBS, 1959; "The Long Echo," *The Law and Mr. Jones,* ABC, 1960; "The Attack," *The Defenders,* CBS, 1960; "What's a Nice Girl Like You . . .?," *N.Y.P.D.,* ABC, 1968; *The DuPont Show of the Week,* NBC; *Philco Television Playhouse,* NBC; *Naked City,* ABC; *Southern Baptist Hour,* NBC; *Directions '66,* ABC.

Movies: Mrs. Stanch, *Willa,* CBS, 1979; Ruth Nicoff, *Some Kind of Miracle,* CBS, 1979; Mrs. Demerjian, *Once upon a Family,* CBS, 1980; Dr. Martha Trenton, *Killjoy,* CBS, 1981; Lucilla Drake, *Agatha Christie's "Sparkling Cyanide,"* CBS, 1983; also *The Golden Moment: An Olympic Love Story,* NBC, 1980. Specials: Sister Michael, *The Bells of Saint Mary's,* CBS, 1959; Ana, *Don Juan in Hell,* NET, 1965; Vassilissa, *The Lower Depths,* NET, 1966; Elizabeth the Queen, *Dark Lady of the Sonnets,* NET, 1966; Nora Melody, "A Touch of the Poet," *Great Performances,* PBS, 1974; Mother, *After the Fall,* NBC, 1974; Auntie, "Valley Forge," *Hallmark Hall of Fame,* NBC, 1975; Grandpa, *Will You Run with Me?,* NBC, 1983. Also appeared in *The Catered Affair,* 1954; *The Indestructable Mr. Gore,* 1959; as Angustias, *The House of Bernarda Alba,* 1960; *A Piece of Blue Sky,* 1960; and *The Statesman,* 1966.

AWARDS: Obie Award from the *Village Voice,* 1960, for *The Balcony;* Emmy Awards, Outstanding Supporting Actress in a Drama Series, 1979, 1980, 1981, and 1982, all for *Lou Grant;*

Drama Desk Award and Outer Critics Circle Award, both 1980, for *Morning's at Seven;* Obie Award, 1989, for *The Cocktail Hour.*

MEMBER: Actors' Equity Association, American Federation of Television and Radio Artists, Screen Actors Guild.

SIDELIGHTS: RECREATIONS—Needlework and reading.

ADDRESSES: HOME—205 W. 89th Street, New York, NY 10025. AGENT—Biff Liff, William Morris Agency, 1350 Avenue of the Americas, New York, NY 10019.*

*　　*　　*

MARGULIES, Stan   1920-

PERSONAL: Born December 14, 1920, in New York, NY. EDUCATION: New York University, B.S., 1940. MILITARY: U.S. Army Air Corps.

VOCATION: Producer.

CAREER: PRINCIPAL FILM WORK—Producer: *Forty Pounds of Trouble,* Universal, 1962; *Those Magnificent Men in Their Flying Machines, or How I Flew from London to Paris in 25 Hours and 11 Minutes* (also known as *Those Magnificent Men in Their Flying Machines*), Twentieth Century-Fox, 1965; *Don't Just Stand There,* Universal, 1968; *The Pink Jungle,* Universal, 1968; *If It's Tuesday, This Must Be Belgium,* United Artists, 1969; *I Love My Wife,* Universal, 1970; (with David L. Wolper) *Willy Wonka and the Chocolate Factory,* Paramount, 1971; *One Is a Lonely Number* (also known as *Two Is a Happy Number*), Metro-Goldwyn-Mayer, 1972. Also *Visions of Eight,* 1973.

PRINCIPAL TELEVISION WORK—All as producer, unless indicated. Series: *Tales of the Vikings,* ABC. Pilots: Executive producer, *Men of the Dragon,* ABC, 1974; *Embassy,* ABC, 1985. Mini-Series: *Roots,* ABC, 1977; *Roots: The Next Generations,* ABC, 1979; *The Thorn Birds,* ABC, 1983; executive producer (with David L. Wolper), *The Mystic Warrior,* ABC, 1984. Movies: *The 500-Pound Jerk,* CBS, 1973; *She Lives,* ABC, 1973; *The Morning After,* ABC, 1974; *Unwed Father,* ABC, 1974; *I Will Fight No More Forever,* ABC, 1975; *Moviola: This Year's Blonde,* (also known as *The Secret Love of Marilyn Monroe*), NBC, 1980; *Moviola: The Silent Lovers,* NBC, 1980; *Moviola: The Scarlett O'Hara War,* NBC, 1980; *Agatha Christie's "Murder Is Easy,"* CBS, 1982; *A Killer in the Family,* ABC, 1983; *Agatha Christie's "Sparkling Cyanide,"* CBS, 1983; *Agatha Christie's "A Caribbean Mystery,"* CBS, 1983; *A Bunny's Tale,* ABC, 1985; *Out on a Limb,* ABC, 1987; executive producer, *Broken Angel* (also known as *Best Intentions*), ABC, 1988.

RELATED CAREER—Feature article writer and assistant Sunday editor, *Salt Lake City Tribune,* Salt Lake City, UT; publicist, RKO Film Studios, Hollywood, CA, 1947, then CBS-Radio, Twentieth Century-Fox, and Walt Disney; publicist, Bryna Films, 1955, then vice-president, 1958; also held executive positions with ABC Circle Films and Telecom Entertainment, Inc.

AWARDS: Emmy Award, Outstanding Limited Series, 1977, for *Roots;* Emmy Award, Outstanding Limited Series, 1979, for *Roots: The Next Generations.**

MARINARO, Ed   1951-

PERSONAL: Full name, Edward Francis Marinaro; born March 31, 1951, in New York, NY; son of Louis John and Rose Marie (Errico) Marinaro. EDUCATION: Received B.S. from Cornell University.

VOCATION: Actor.

CAREER: PRINCIPAL FILM APPEARANCES—Gino, *Fingers*, Brut, 1978; Malcolm ''Mace'' Douglas, *Mace*, Double Helix, 1987. Also appeared in *The Gong Show Movie*, Universal, 1980.

PRINCIPAL TELEVISION APPEARANCES—Series: Sonny St. Jacques, *Laverne and Shirley*, ABC, 1980-81; Officer Joe Coffey, *Hill Street Blues*, NBC, 1981-86. Pilots: Tony Rossi, *Three Eyes*, NBC, 1982. Episodic: John Remick, *Falcon Crest*, CBS, 1987. Movies: Doug Trainer, *Born Beautiful*, NBC, 1982; Nick Velano, *Policewoman Centerfold*, NBC, 1983; Mr. Powell, *What If I'm Gay?*, CBS, 1987; Hayden Fox, *Tonight's the Night* (also known as *Single Men*), ABC, 1987; Dr. Richard Bronowski, *Sharing Richard*, CBS, 1988; Detective Brendan Thomas, *The Diamond Trap*, CBS, 1988. Specials: *Crystal Light National Aerobic Championship*, syndicated, 1986.

NON-RELATED CAREER—Professonal football player with the Minnesota Vikings, New York Jets, and the Seattle Seahawks.

MEMBER: Screen Actors Guild, American Federation of Television and Radio Artists.

ADDRESSES: AGENT—Steve Glick, William Morris Agency, 151 El Camino Drive, Beverly Hills, CA 90212.*

*   *   *

MARKHAM, Monte   1935-

PERSONAL: Born June 21, 1935, in Manatee, FL; son of Jesse Edward (a merchant) and Millie Content (Willbur) Markham; married Klaire Keevil Hester, June 1, 1961; children: Keevil Lee (a daughter), Jason Morgan. EDUCATION: University of Georgia, M.F.A., 1960. MILITARY: U.S. Coast Guard Reserve, 1958-67.

VOCATION: Actor, director, and producer.

CAREER: STAGE DEBUT—Morris, *The Heiress*, Priscilla Beach Theatre, White House Beach, MA, 1954. BROADWAY DEBUT—Donald Marshall, *Irene*, Minskoff Theatre, 1973, for two hundred performances. PRINCIPAL STAGE APPEARANCES—George, *Same Time Next Year*, Brooks Atkinson Theatre, then Ambassador Theatre, both New York City, 1978; Lord Arthur Dilling, *The Last of Mrs. Cheyney*, Kennedy Center for the Performing Arts, Washington, DC, 1978; Starbuck, *110 in the Shade*, Pittsburgh Civic Light Opera, Pittsburgh, PA, 1986. Also appeared in the title role, *Hamlet*, University of California; in *Sleuth*, Hyde Park Festival Theatre, Hyde Park, NY, 1986; with the Burt Reynolds Jupiter Theatre, Jupiter, FL, 1985-86; Old Globe Shakespeare Festival, San Diego, CA; Ashland Shakespeare Festival, Ashland, OR; resident theatre company, Stephens College, Columbia, MO; and with the Actors' Workshop, San Francisco, CA.

PRINCIPAL STAGE WORK—Producer and director, *Dinner and*

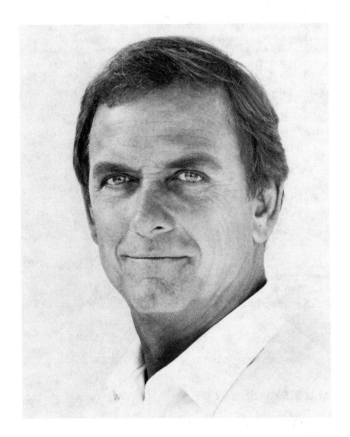

MONTE MARKHAM

Drinks, Tiffany Theatre, Los Angeles, CA, 1986; also participated in the Directors Unit of the Actors Studio, Los Angeles, CA.

MAJOR TOURS—Aaron Burr, *Together Tonight: Jefferson, Hamilton, and Burr*, U.S. cities, 1976; Lord Arthur Dilling, *The Last of Mrs. Cheyney*, U.S. cities, 1978-79.

PRINCIPAL FILM APPEARANCES—Sherman McMasters, *Hour of the Gun*, United Artists, 1967; Gregory Gallea, *Project X*, Paramount, 1968; Keno, *Guns of the Magnificent Seven*, United Artists, 1969; Howard Carpenter, *One Is a Lonely Number* (also known as *Two Is a Happy Number*), Metro-Goldwyn-Mayer, 1972; Joe, *Ginger in the Morning*, National, 1973; Commander Max Leslie, *Midway* (also known as *The Battle of Midway*), Universal, 1976; Banker, *Airport '77*, Universal, 1977; Governor, *Off the Wall*, Jensen Farley, 1983; Mr. Winston, *Jake Speed*, New World, 1986; Bill Cronenberg, *Hot Pursuit*, Paramount, 1987; Colonel Mark Denton, *Defense Play*, Trans World Entertainment, 1988. Also appeared in *Separate Ways*, Crown International, 1981.

PRINCIPAL FILM WORK—Director, *Defense Play*, Trans World Entertainment, 1988.

TELEVISION DEBUT—*Mission: Impossible*, CBS, 1966. PRINCIPAL TELEVISION APPEARANCES—Series: Luke Carpenter and Ken Carpenter, *The Second Hundred Years*, ABC, 1967-68; Longfellow Deeds, *Mr. Deeds Goes to Town*, ABC, 1969-70; title role, *Perry Mason* (also known as *The New Perry Mason*), CBS, 1973; Clint Ogden, *Dallas*, CBS, 1981; host, *Breakaway*, syndicated, 1983; Carter Robinson, *Rituals*, syndicated, 1984-85. Pilots: Tom McKell, *Ellery Queen: Too Many Suspects*, NBC, 1975; also

Baywatch, NBC, 1989; *Nikki and Alexander*, NBC, 1989. Episodic: Douglas Shayne, *Blacke's Magic*, NBC, 1986; Ned Olson, *Murder, She Wrote*, CBS, 1986; Inspector Matheney, *Murder, She Wrote*, CBS, 1987; Clayton, *The Golden Girls*, NBC, 1988; also *The Mary Tyler Moore Show*, CBS, 1971; *Hotel*, ABC, 1987; Barney Hillver, *The Six Million Dollar Man*, ABC. Movies: David Smith, *Death Takes a Holiday*, ABC, 1971; Eddie Reese and Colonel Brice Randolph, *The Astronaut*, ABC, 1972; Professor Mark Lowell, *Visions*, CBS, 1972; Orin Dietrich, *Hustling*, ABC, 1975; Paul Vickers, *Relentless*, CBS, 1977; Tony Malgrado, *Drop-Out Father*, CBS, 1982; Kyle Durham, *Hotline*, CBS, 1982. Specials: *Mitzi and a Hundred Guys*, CBS, 1975.

RELATED CAREER—Acting teacher, Stephens College, Columbia, MO, 1960-62.

AWARDS: Theatre World Award, 1973, for *Irene.*

ADDRESSES: AGENTS—David Shapira and Associates, 15301 Ventura Boulevard, Sherman Oaks, CA 91403; Lionel Larner, Ltd., 130 W. 57th Street, New York, NY 10019; (commercials) Arlene Thornton and Associates, 5757 Wilshire Boulevard, Los Angeles, CA 90036.

*   *   *

MARKS, Arthur   1927-

PERSONAL: Full name, Arthur Ronald Marks; born August 2, 1927, in Los Angeles, CA; son of Dave (a film production manager and assistant director) and Marion (Freibrun) Marks; married Phyllis Marie Lehman, May 14, 1948; children: Kathleen, Beau, Elizabeth, Paul. EDUCATION: Attended Santa Monica College and the University of Southern California. MILITARY: U.S. Navy, 1948-54.

VOCATION: Director, producer, and screenwriter.

CAREER: Also see *WRITINGS* below. PRINCIPAL FILM WORK—Producer and director, *Detroit 9000*, General Film, 1973; director, *The Roommates*, General Film, 1973; director, *Bonnie's Kids*, General Film, 1973; executive producer, *The Centerfold Girls*, General Film, 1974; director, *Bucktown*, American International, 1975; producer and director, *Friday Foster*, American International, 1975; director, *A Woman for All Men*, General Film, 1975; producer and director, *J.D.'s Revenge*, American International, 1976; producer and director, *The Monkey Hustle*, American International, 1976. Also producer and director, *Togetherness*, 1970; director, *Class of '74*, 1972; executive in charge of production, *Wonder Women*, 1972; executive producer, *The Candy Snatchers*, 1972; producer and director, *Times Like These*, 1985; producer and director, *Moongames*, 1977.

PRINCIPAL TELEVISION WORK—All as director. Series: *Perry Mason*, CBS, 1957-66 (also producer, 1960-66). Episodic: *I Spy*, NBC, 1967; *My Friend Tony*, NBC, 1969; *Mannix*, CBS, 1972; *The New Perry Mason*, CBS, 1973; *Young Dan'l Boone*, CBS, 1977; also *Starsky and Hutch*, ABC; *The Dukes of Hazzard*, CBS; *Steve Canyon*, NBC; *Casablanca*, ABC; *The Man behind the Badge*, CBS; *CHiPs*, NBC; *The Eddie Capra Mysteries*, NBC.

RELATED CAREER—Production department, Metro-Goldwyn-Mayer, 1949-51; assistant director, Columbia Studios, 1951-53;

assistant director and production manager, Columbia, Warner Brothers, Twentieth Century-Fox, CBS television, and Revue-MCA, all 1953-56; president, Arthur Productions, Inc., 1976—; president, ARMS Service Company, 1980—; executive head of production, Henry Plitt Productions, Inc., 1981-83; executive producer, Plitt Theatres, 1981-83; executive, Century Entertainment, Inc., 1984; vice-president and executive producer, New Concepts Entertainment, 1985-86; executive producer and director, Cineventure Group-Lionshead, Ltd., London, 1987-88; served on Television Academy Blue Ribbon Award panels for selection of producers and directors.

WRITINGS: FILM—(With John Durren) *The Roommates*, General Film, 1973; *Bonnie's Kids*, General Film, 1973; also *Togetherness*, 1970; *Class of '74*, 1972; *Times Like These*, 1985; *Something to Shoot For*, 1986; *Empress of the China Seas*, 1986; *Streets*, 1986; *The Stone Kingdom*, 1986; *Tiger Boy (The Mario Lanza Story)*, 1986; *Hot Times*, 1987; *Gold Stars*, 1988; and *Mean Intentions*, 1988.

TELEVISION—Pilots: *Rainbow Bend*, CBS; *Kops*, CBS; also *Cheyenne Crossing*. Episodic: *Murder, She Wrote*, CBS, 1987; also *Perry Mason*, CBS; *I Spy*, NBC; *Mannix*, CBS; *Starsky and Hutch*, ABC; *The Dukes of Hazzard*, CBS; *CHiPs*, NBC; *The Eddie Capra Mysteries*, NBC; *Young Dan'l Boone*, CBS.

AWARDS: Television Academy Award nominations, Best Produced Drama Series, 1961-64, and Producers Guild Award nomination, Best Television Program of the Year, 1964-65, both for *Perry Mason;* National Association of Theatre Owners Award, Best Independently Produced Film of the Year, 1973, for *Detroit 9000;* Edgar Allan Poe Award; Limelight Award; Television Today Award; *Radio/TV Daily* Best Mystery Program Award; Newspapers Nationwide Award.

MEMBER: Directors Guild of America, Writers Guild of America.

ADDRESSES: OFFICE—Arthur Productions, Inc., 20010 Wells Drive, Woodland Hills, CA 91634.

*   *   *

MARS, Kenneth   1936-

PERSONAL: Born in 1936 in Chicago, IL.

VOCATION: Actor.

CAREER: PRINCIPAL STAGE APPEARANCES—Martin Eliot, *The Affair*, Henry Miller's Theatre, New York City, 1962; Baron Stockmar, *The Crown, the Ring, and the Roses*, American National Theatre and Academy, Theatre De Lys, New York City, 1963; Cass Henderson, *Any Wednesday*, Music Box Theatre, New York City, 1965; Dr. Ralph Brodie, *The Best Laid Plans*, Brooks Atkinson Theatre, New York City, 1966. Also appeared in *Help*, Center Theatre Group, New Theatre for Now, Los Angeles Music Center, Los Angeles, CA, 1972; and *Flint*, Studio Arena Theatre, Buffalo, NY, 1974.

MAJOR TOURS—Baron Elberfeld, *The Sound of Music*, U.S. cities, 1961.

PRINCIPAL FILM APPEARANCES—Franz Liebkind, *The Produc-*

ers, Embassy, 1967; Don Hopkins, *The April Fools*, National General, 1969; marshall, *Butch Cassidy and the Sundance Kid*, Twentieth Century-Fox, 1969; Dr. Sam Gillison, *Viva Max!*, Commonwealth United, 1969; Otto, *Desperate Characters*, Paramount, 1971; Hugh Simon, *What's Up, Doc?*, Warner Brothers, 1972; former F.B.I. Agent Turner, *The Parallax View*, Paramount, 1974; Inspector Kemp, *Young Frankenstein*, Twentieth Century-Fox, 1974; Nick, *Night Moves*, Warner Brothers, 1975; Kruse, *Goin' Coconuts*, Osmond, 1978; Marshall, *The Apple Dumpling Gang Rides Again*, Buena Vista, 1979; Crisp/Verdugo, *Yellowbeard*, Orion, 1983; Stanton Boyd, *Fletch*, Universal, 1984; Lou, *Protocol*, Warner Brothers, 1984; Lyndon B. Johnson, *Prince Jack*, Castle Hill, 1985; voice of Vultor and Buzzard, *Adventures of the American Rabbit* (animated), Atlantic Releasing, 1985; A.J. Norbecker, *Beer*, Orion, 1986; Rabbi Baumel, *Radio Days*, Orion, 1987; Mr. Bobrucz, *For Keeps*, Tri-Star, 1988; Reverend Farrell, *Rented Lips*, Cineworld, 1988; Hal Keeler, *Illegally Yours* (also known as *Double Duty*), Metro-Goldwyn-Mayer/United Artists, 1988; mayor, *Police Academy 6: City under Siege*, Warner Brothers, 1989. Also appeared in *Full Moon High*, Filmways, 1982.

PRINCIPAL TELEVISION APPEARANCES—Series: Harry Zarakardos, *He and She*, CBS, 1967-68; regular, *The Don Knotts Show*, NBC, 1970-71; regular, *Sha Na Na*, syndicated, 1977-78; regular, *Carol Burnett and Company*, CBS, 1979; voice of Lou Granite, *Flintstone Family Adventures* (animated), NBC, 1981; voice of Sergeant Turnbuckle, *Laverne and Shirley in the Army* (animated), ABC, 1981-82, then *Laverne and Shirley with the Fonz* (animated), ABC, 1982-83; voice characterization, *Saturday Supercade* (animated), CBS, 1983-85; voice characterization, *The Biskitts* (animated), CBS, 1983-85; voice characterization, *The New Jetsons* (animated), ABC, 1985; voice characterization, *The Thirteen Ghosts of Scooby-Doo* (animated), ABC, 1985-86; voice characterization, *The Flintstone Kids* (also known as *Captain Caveman and Son*; animated), ABC, 1986; voice characterization, *Foofur* (animated), NBC, 1986-88; voice characterization, *My Little Pony and Friends* (animated), syndicated, 1986—.

Pilots: Jack Shepherd, *Shepherd's Flock*, CBS, 1971; reporter, *Comedy News II*, ABC, 1973; Eddie, *The Karen Valentine Show*, ABC, 1973; Colonel Von Balasko, *The New, Original Wonder Woman*, ABC, 1975; Frank Campbell, *Full House*, NBC, 1976; bank manager, *Bunco*, NBC, 1977; Colonel H. Jonas Boyette, *The Fighting Nightingales*, CBS, 1978; William Tarkington IV, *The Killin' Cousin*, CBS, 1980; Arthur Krantz, *Full House*, CBS, 1983. Episodic: William W.B. "Bud" Prize, *America 2-Night*, syndicated, 1978; Donner, *Misfits of Science*, NBC, 1985; photographer, *Remington Steele*, NBC, 1985; Paul Brubaker, *The Last Precinct*, NBC, 1986; Tooth Fairy, "Tooth or Consequences," *The Twilight Zone*, CBS, 1986; Gerald Hardcastle, *Hardcastle and McCormick*, ABC, 1986; Fritz Markham, *Simon and Simon*, CBS, 1986; Ned Bartlett/Don Diablo, *Simon and Simon*, CBS, 1986; Mr. Harris, *The Facts of Life*, NBC; ghost of Charlie's uncle, *Head of the Class*, ABC, 1988; also Dr. Cobb, *Hart to Hart*, ABC.

Movies: Dr. Julius Roth, *Second Chance*, ABC, 1972; Mitchell Bernard, *Guess Who's Sleeping in My Bed*, ABC, 1973; Paul Wrightwood, *Someone I Touched*, ABC, 1975; Ben Fryer, *Before and After*, ABC, 1979; Red Hewitt, *The Rules of Marriage*, CBS, 1982; Commander Douglas Drury, *Get Smart, Again!*, ABC, 1989. Specials: *The Alan King Show*, NBC, 1968; Max Mencken, *It's a Bird, It's a Plane, It's Superman*, ABC, 1975; *Van Dyke and Company*, NBC, 1975; Kolenkov, *You Can't Take It with You*, CBS, 1979; voice of the bald man, "Hugh Pine" (animated), *CBS*

Storybreak, CBS, 1985; voice of Sugar Cane, "Chocolate Fever" (animated), *CBS Storybreak*, CBS, 1985.

MEMBER: Screen Actors Guild, American Federation of Television and Radio Artists.*

*   *   *

MARSDEN, Roy   1941-

PERSONAL: Born June 25, 1941, in London, England; married Polly Hemingway; children: Joseph. EDUCATION: Attended the Royal Academy of Dramatic Art.

VOCATION: Actor.

CAREER: PRINCIPAL STAGE APPEARANCES—Crispen, *The Friends*, Round House Theatre, London, 1970; Casca and Lucilius, *Julius Caesar*, Young Vic Theatre, London, 1972; Paul Schippel, *Schippel*, Open Space Theatre, London, 1974; Heinrich Krey, *The Plumber's Progress*, Prince of Wales Theatre, London, 1975. Also appeared in *Breman Coffee*, Hampstead Theatre Club, London, 1974.

PRINCIPAL FILM APPEARANCES—Alpha, *Toomorrow*, Rank, 1970; Barry, *The Squeeze*, Warner Brothers, 1976.

PRINCIPAL TELEVISION APPEARANCES—Series: Neil Bernside, *The Sandbaggers*, 1978-79, then PBS, 1986. Mini-Series: George Osborne, "Vanity Fair," *Masterpiece Theatre*, PBS, 1972; Adam Dalgliesh, "Death of an Expert Witness," *Mystery*, PBS, 1985; Chief Superintendent Adam Dalgliesh, "Shroud for a Nightingale," *Mystery*, PBS, 1986; Arthur Chipping, "Goodbye Mr. Chips," *Masterpiece Theatre*, PBS, 1987; Chief Superintendent Adam Dalgliesh, "Cover Her Face," *Mystery*, PBS, 1987; Inspector Adam Dalgliesh, "The Black Tower," *Mystery*, PBS, 1988; John Bennet, *Inside Story*, ABC, 1988. Also appeared in *Airline*.

ADDRESSES: AGENT—Caroline Dawson Associates, 31 Kings Road, London SW3 4RP, England.*

*   *   *

MARSHALL, Frank

PERSONAL: EDUCATION: Attended the University of California, Los Angeles.

VOCATION: Actor and producer.

CAREER: PRINCIPAL FILM APPEARANCES—Tommy Logan, *The Last Picture Show*, Columbia, 1971; Dinsdale's assistant, *Nickelodeon*, Columbia, 1976; pilot, *Raiders of the Lost Ark*, Paramount, 1981.

PRINCIPAL FILM WORK—Associate producer, *Paper Moon*, Paramount, 1973; associate producer, *Daisy Miller*, Paramount, 1974; associate producer, *Nickelodeon*, Columbia, 1976; line producer, *The Last Waltz*, United Artists, 1978; associate producer, *The Driver*, Twentieth Century-Fox, 1978; executive producer, *The Warriors*, Paramount, 1979; producer (with Steven Spielberg),

Raiders of the Lost Ark, Paramount, 1981; producer (with Spielberg), *Poltergeist,* Metro-Goldwyn-Mayer/United Artists, 1982; production supervisior, *E.T.: The Extra-Terrestrial,* Universal, 1982; executive producer, *Twilight Zone—The Movie,* Warner Brothers, 1983; executive producer and second unit director, *Indiana Jones and the Temple of Doom,* Paramount, 1984; executive producer, *Gremlins,* Warner Brothers, 1984; executive producer, *The Goonies,* Warner Brothers, 1985; producer (with Spielberg, Kathleen Kennedy, Quincy Jones, Jon Peters, and Peter Guber) and second unit director, *The Color Purple,* Warner Brothers, 1985; executive producer and second unit director, *Back to the Future,* Universal, 1985; executive producer, *Young Sherlock Holmes,* Paramount, 1985; executive producer, *Fandango,* Warner Brothers, 1985; producer (with Kennedy and Art Levinson), *The Money Pit,* Universal, 1986; executive producer, *An American Tail,* Universal, 1986; producer (with Spielberg and Kennedy) and second unit director, *Empire of the Sun,* Warner Brothers, 1987; executive producer (with Spielberg and Kennedy), *Innerspace,* Warner Brothers, 1987; executive producer, **batteries not included,* Universal, 1987; producer and second unit director, *Who Framed Roger Rabbit?,* Buena Vista, 1988; executive producer (with Spielberg), *The Land before Time,* Universal, 1988; producer (with Spielberg), *Indiana Jones and the Lost Crusade,* Paramount, 1989. Also line producer, *Orson Welles' The Other Side of the Wind* (unreleased).

PRINCIPAL TELEVISION WORK—Specials: Executive producer (with Sid Ganis), *Heroes and Sidekicks—Indiana Jones and the Temple of Doom* (documentary), CBS, 1984; also executive producer, *China Odyssey: Empire of the Sun* (documentary), 1987; executive producer, *Roger Rabbit and the Secrets of Toontown* (documentary), 1988. Also creator, *The Bretts,* 1987.

ADDRESSES: OFFICE—Amblin Entertainment, 100 Universal Plaza, Universal City, CA 91608.*

*   *   *

MARTIN, Andrea   1947-

PERSONAL: Born January 15, 1947, in Portland, ME. EDUCATION: Graduated from Emerson College.

VOCATION: Actress, comedienne, and writer.

CAREER: Also see *WRITINGS* below. OFF-BROADWAY DEBUT—*Hard Sell,* New York Shakespeare Festival, Public Theatre, 1980. PRINCIPAL STAGE APPEARANCES—Liz, *Sorrows of Stephen,* New York Shakespeare Festival, Public Theatre, New York City, 1980; also appeared in *What's a Nice Country Like You Doing in a State Like This?,* Theatre in the Dell, Toronto, ON, Canada, 1974; and in *She Loves Me,* Playwrights Horizons, New York City.

PRINCIPAL FILM APPEARANCES—Gloria Wellaby, *Cannibal Girls,* American International, 1973; Phyl, *Black Christmas,* Ambassador, 1974; Zipporah, *Wholly Moses!,* Columbia, 1980; Concord seductress, *Soup for One,* Warner Brothers, 1982; Linda White, *Club Paradise,* Warner Brothers, 1986; waiting room patient, *Innerspace,* Warner Brothers, 1987; Ruth, *Martha, Ruth, and Edie,* Norstar Releasing/Simcom International, 1988; Claire, *Worth Winning,* Twentieth Century-Fox, 1989; Toots, *Boris and Natasha,* MCEG, 1989; April, *Rude Awakening,* Aaron Russo Productions, 1989.

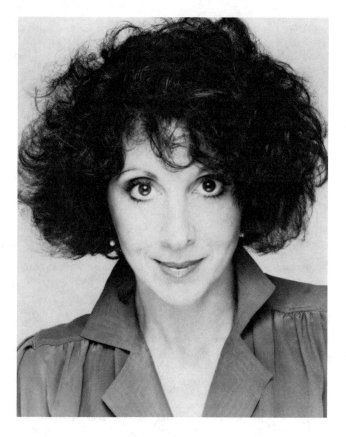

ANDREA MARTIN

PRINCIPAL TELEVISION APPEARANCES—Series: Edith Prickly and various other roles, *Second City TV,* syndicated, 1977-81; regular, *SCTV Network 90,* NBC, 1981-83; title role, *Roxie,* CBS, 1987; voice of Mr. Freebus, *The Completely Mental Misadventures of Ed Grimley* (animated), NBC, 1988—; Melissa, *Poison,* Showtime, 1988. Pilots: Regular, *From Cleveland,* CBS, 1980. Episodic: Eddie, *Kate and Allie* (two episodes), CBS, 1982; also *The Comedy Zone,* CBS, 1984; *The Smothers Brothers Comedy Hour,* CBS, 1988. Movies: Steffie Conti, *Torn between Two Lovers,* CBS, 1979. Specials: *That Thing on ABC,* ABC, 1978; *That Second Thing on ABC,* ABC, 1978; *The Robert Klein Show,* NBC, 1981; *Late Night Film Festival,* NBC, 1985; *Second City (Chicago) Twenty-Fifth Anniversary,* ABC, 1985; *Martin Short Concert for the North Americas,* Showtime, 1985; *Comic Relief,* HBO, 1986; *Comic Relief* (also known as *Comic Relief II*), HBO, 1987; host, *Just for Laughs,* Showtime, 1987; *The Best of SCTV,* ABC, 1988; *Sesame Street Special,* PBS, 1988; *Merrill Markoe's Guide to Glamorous Living,* Cinemax, 1988; host, *Women of the Night II,* HBO, 1988; *Second City [Toronto] Fifteenth Anniversary Special* (also known as *The Second City Anniversary Reunion*), Showtime, 1988; *Andrea Martin: Together Again,* Showtime, 1989.

WRITINGS: TELEVISION—Series: *SCTV Network 90,* NBC, 1981-83. Pilots: *From Cleveland,* CBS, 1980.

AWARDS: Emmy Awards, Best Writing for a Comedy Program, 1982 and 1983, for *SCTV Network 90;* Emmy Award nomination, Best Supporting Actress, 1982, for *SCTV Network 90.*

ADDRESSES: AGENT—Nancy Geller, International Creative Management, 8899 Beverly Boulevard, Los Angeles, CA 90048.

*　　*　　*

MARTIN, Kiel 1945-

PERSONAL: Born July 26, 1945, in Pittsburgh, PA; children: Jesse. EDUCATION: Attended Trinity University and University of Miami. MILITARY: U.S. Army, 1962-64.

VOCATION: Actor.

CAREER: PRINCIPAL STAGE APPEARANCES—*Bent*, University of Alabama, 1984. Also appeared with the National Shakespeare Company, Old Globe Theatre, San Diego, CA, 1966; and in repertory in Miami, FL, New Orleans, LA, and New York City.

PRINCIPAL FILM APPEARANCES—Union runner, *The Undefeated*, Twentieth Century-Fox, 1969; Chico, *Panic in Needle Park*, Twentieth Century-Fox, 1971; Ludie Gutshall, *Lolly-Madonna XXX* (also known as *The Lolly-Madonna War*), Metro-Goldwyn-Mayer, 1973; White Folks, *Trick Baby* (also known as *The Double Con*), Universal, 1973; Bobby Lee, *Moonrunners*, United Artists, 1975.

PRINCIPAL TELEVISION APPEARANCES—Series: Raney Cooper, *The Edge of Night*, ABC, 1977-78; Detective John "J.D." LaRue, *Hill Street Blues*, NBC, 1981-86; Charles Russell, *Second Chance*, Fox, 1987. Pilots: Wes Watkins, *The Catcher*, NBC, 1972. Episodic: *Delvecchio*, CBS; *Harry-O*, ABC; *The Bold Ones*, NBC; *Ironside*, NBC; *Kung Fu*, ABC. Movies: Christopher Sand, *The Log of the Black Pearl*, NBC, 1975; Bob Kalish, *Child Bride of Short Creek*, NBC, 1981; Van, *Convicted: A Mother's Story*, CBS, 1987; Zane Drinkwater, *If It's Tuesday, It Still Must Be Belgium*, NBC, 1987.

NON-RELATED CAREER—Partner, Mt. Jackson Cellars, Sonoma County, CA, 1982—.

SIDELIGHTS: RECREATIONS—Jogging, racquetball, softball, golf, and fishing.

ADDRESSES: AGENT—The Artists Agency, 10000 Santa Monica Boulevard, Suite 305, Los Angeles, CA 90067.*

*　　*　　*

MARTIN, Millicent 1934-

PERSONAL: Born June 8, 1934, in Romford, England; daughter of William Andrew and Violet Eileen (Bedford) Martin; married Ronnie Carroll (divorced); married Norman Eshley (divorced); married Marc Alexander. EDUCATION: Trained for the stage at the Italia Conti Stage School.

VOCATION: Actress and singer.

CAREER: STAGE DEBUT—Children's chorus, *The Magic Flute*, Royal Opera House, London, 1948. BROADWAY DEBUT—Nancy, *The Boy Friend*, Royale Theatre, 1954. PRINCIPAL STAGE

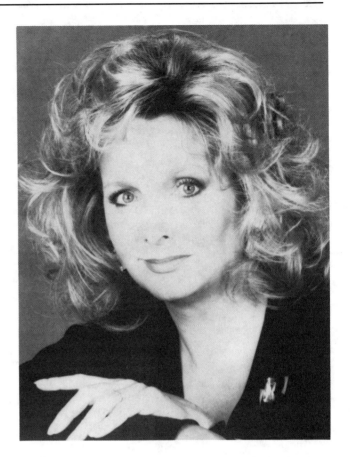

MILLICENT MARTIN

APPEARANCES—Handmaiden, *The Lute Song*, Winter Garden Theatre, London, 1948; Dejanira, *Mistress of the Inn*, Bucks County Playhouse, New Hope, PA, 1957; Polly Brown, *The Boy Friend*, Coconut Grove Playhouse, Miami, FL, 1957; Maisie, *Expresso Bongo*, Saville Theatre, London, 1958; Cora, *The Crooked Mile*, Cambridge Theatre, London, 1959; Marion Laverne, *The Dancing Heiress*, Lyric Hammersmith Theatre, London, 1960; ensemble, *The Lord Chamberlain Regrets* (revue), Saville Theatre, 1961; Judy, *State of Emergency*, Pembroke Theatre, Croydon, U.K., 1962; Tweenie, *Our Man Crichton*, Shaftesbury Theatre, London, 1964; title role, *Peter Pan*, Scala Theatre, London, 1967; Sabina, *The Skin of Our Teeth*, Chichester Festival Theatre, Chichester, U.K., 1968; various roles, *Tonight at Eight*, Hampstead Theatre Club, London, 1970, then Fortune Theatre, London, 1971; Polly Peachum, *The Beggar's Opera*, Chichester Festival Theatre, 1972; Ruth Earp, *The Card*, Queen's Theatre, London, 1973; Marion, *Absurd Person Singular*, Vaudeville Theatre, London, 1975; ensemble, *Side by Side by Sondheim*, Mermaid Theatre, London, 1976, then Wyndham's Theatre, London, later Music Box Theatre, New York City, then Huntington Hartford Theatre, Los Angeles, CA, all 1977; Madeleine, *King of Hearts*, Minskoff Theatre, New York City, 1978; Dorothy Brock, *Forty-Second Street*, Winter Garden Theatre, then Majestic Theatre, both New York City, 1985; Dottie Otley, *Noises Off*, Brooks Atkinson Theatre, New York City, 1987; Phyllis Stone, *Follies*, Shaftesbury Theatre, 1988. Also appeared in *Two into One*, 1988; and productions of *Puss 'n' Boots*, *Aladdin*, *Move Over Mrs. Markham*, and *Meet Mr. Stewart*.

MAJOR TOURS—Polly Brown, *The Boy Friend*, U.S. cities, 1954-57; Dorothy Brock, *Forty-Second Street*, U.S. cities, 1983-84.

PRINCIPAL FILM APPEARANCES—Maisie, *Libel*, Metro-Goldwyn-Mayer (MGM), 1959; Sister Kay Manning, *Invasion Quartet*, MGM, 1961; Billie Bennett, *The Girl on the Boat*, Knightsbridge, 1962; Ann Horton, *Nothing but the Best*, Royal, 1964; airline hostess, *Those Magnificent Men in Their Flying Machines*, Twentieth Century-Fox, 1965; Siddie, *Alfie*, Paramount, 1966; Evie, Anya, Ara, and Ginnie, *Stop the World—I Want to Get Off*, Warner Brothers, 1966. Also appeared in *The Horsemaster*.

PRINCIPAL TELEVISION APPEARANCES—Series: Co-host, *The Piccadilly Palace*, ABC, 1967; Millie Grover, *From a Bird's Eye View*, NBC, 1971; Harriet Conover, *Downtown*, CBS, 1986; also *Millicent TV*, 1966; *International Detective*; and *Millie*. Episodic: Arlene Sabrett, *L.A. Law*, NBC, 1986; Sylvia, *Newhart*, CBS, 1986; also *Espionage*, NBC; *That Was the Week That Was, Harry Moorings, London Palladium Color Show, The Danny Kaye Show*, and *Englebert Humperdinck Show*. Specials: *The Tom Jones Christmas Special*, syndicated, 1971; *Song by Song by Ira Gershwin*, PBS, 1978; *The Stars Salute Israel at Thirty*, ABC, 1978; *Song by Song* (seven episodes), PBS, 1980. Also appeared in *Mainly Millicent*.

AWARDS: Ondus Television Award (Spain), 1963; Light Entertainment Award, 1964; also TV Society Award.

SIDELIGHTS: FAVORITE ROLES—Polly Peachum in *The Beggar's Opera* and parts in *Side by Side by Sondheim*. RECREATIONS—Swimming, diving, music, and cooking.

ADDRESSES: AGENT—London Management, 235-241 Regent Street, London W1, England.

*   *   *

MASON, Marsha   1942-

PERSONAL: Born April 3, 1942, in St. Louis, MO; daughter of James Joseph and Jacqueline Helena (Rachowsky) Mason; married Gary Campbell (divorced, 1964); married Neil Simon (a playwright), October 25, 1973 (divorced). EDUCATION: Received B.A. in speech and drama from Webster College.

VOCATION: Actress and director.

CAREER: BROADWAY DEBUT—Botticelli's Springtime, *Cactus Flower*, Royale Theatre, 1965. PRINCIPAL STAGE APPEARANCES—Bobby, *The Deer Park*, Theatre De Lys, New York City, 1967; Joanna Dibble, *It's Called the Sugar Plum*, Astor Place Theatre, New York City, 1968; Penelope Ryan, *Happy Birthday, Wanda June*, Theatre De Lys, 1970; Lady Anne, *Richard III*, New York Shakespeare Festival, Mitzi E. Newhouse Theatre, New York City, 1972; various roles, *The Good Doctor*, Eugene O'Neill Theatre, New York City, 1973; title role, *Mary Stuart*, Ahmanson Theatre, Los Angeles, CA, 1981; Viola, *Twelfth Night*, Old Globe Theatre, San Diego, CA, 1983; Kate, *Old Times*, Roundabout Theatre, New York City, 1983; Melissa Gardner, *Love Letters*, Promenade Theatre, New York City, 1989. Also appeared in *Private Lives*, American Conservatory Theatre, San Francisco, CA, 1971; *You Can't Take It with You* and *The Merchant of Venice*, both American Conservatory Theatre, 1972; in productions of *Cyrano de Bergerac, A*

Doll's House, and *The Crucible,* all 1972; and in *The Heiress,* 1975.

PRINCIPAL STAGE WORK—Director, *Juno's Swans*, Second Stage, New York City, 1985.

MAJOR TOURS—*Cactus Flower*, U.S. cities, 1968.

FILM DEBUT—*Hot Rod Hullabaloo*, Allied Artists, 1966. PRINCIPAL FILM APPEARANCES—Arlene, *Blume in Love*, Samuel Bronston, 1973; Maggie Paul, *Cinderella Liberty*, Twentieth Century-Fox, 1973; Janice Templeton, *Audrey Rose*, United Artists, 1977; Paula McFadden, *The Goodbye Girl*, Warner Brothers, 1977; Georgia Merkle, *The Cheap Detective*, Columbia, 1978; Jennie MacLaine, *Chapter Two*, Columbia, 1979; Dr. Alexandra Kenda, *Promises in the Dark*, Warner Brothers, 1979; Georgia Hines, *Only When I Laugh* (also known as *It Hurts Only When I Laugh*), Columbia, 1981; Nora McPhee, *Max Dugan Returns*, Twentieth Century-Fox, 1983; Aggie, *Heartbreak Ridge*, Warner Brothers, 1986.

PRINCIPAL TELEVISION APPEARANCES—Series: Nurse Marsha Lord, *Young Dr. Kildare*, syndicated, 1972; also Judith Cole, *Love of Life*, CBS. Episodic: Courtney Woods, *Hothouse*, ABC, 1988; host, *Shortstories*, Arts and Entertainment, 1988. Movies: Title role, *Lois Gibbs and the Love Canal*, CBS, 1982; Lois, *Surviving*, ABC, 1985; Jennifer Hubbell, *Trapped in Silence*, CBS, 1986. Specials: Roxanne, *Cyrano de Bergerac*, PBS, 1974; *The American Film Institute Salute to Henry Fonda*, CBS, 1978; co-host, *Oscar's Best Actors*, ABC, 1978; *Variety '77—The Year in Entertainment*, CBS, 1978. Also appeared in *The Clinic*, 1987; and in *Brewsie and Willie*.

PRINCIPAL TELEVISION WORK—Director, *Little Miss Perfect*, 1987.

AWARDS: Academy Award nomination, Best Supporting Actress, Golden Globe Award, Best Motion Picture Actress, both 1974, for *Cinderella Liberty;* Academy Award nomination, Best Actress, British Academy Award, Best Actress, Golden Globe Award, Best Motion Picture Actress, all 1978, for *The Goodbye Girl;* Academy Award nomination, Best Actress, 1980, for *Chapter Two;* Academy Award nomination, Best Actress, 1982, for *Only When I Laugh.*

MEMBER: Actors' Equity Association, Screen Actors Guild, American Federation of Television and Radio Artists.

ADDRESSES: AGENT—Ron Meyer, Creative Artists Agency, 1888 Century Park E., Suite 1400, Los Angeles, CA 90067.*

*   *   *

MASTERSON, Mary Stuart   1967-

PERSONAL: Born in 1967 in New York, NY; daughter of Peter Masterson (an actor and writer) and Carlin Glynn (an actress). EDUCATION: Attended New York University; trained for the stage with Estelle Parsons.

VOCATION: Actress.

CAREER: PRINCIPAL STAGE APPEARANCES—Small White Rabbit and Four of Hearts, *Alice in Wonderland*, Virginia Theatre, New

York City, 1982; Margaret, *Been Taken*, Ensemble Studio Theatre, New York City, 1985; Cassidy Smith, *The Lucky Spot*, Manhattan Theatre Club, New York City, 1987; also appeared in *Lily Dale*, Samuel Beckett Theatre, 1987.

FILM DEBUT—Kim, *The Stepford Wives*, Columbia, 1975. PRINCIPAL FILM APPEARANCES—Danni, *Heaven Help Us* (also known as *Catholic Boys*), Tri-Star, 1984; Terry, *At Close Range*, Orion, 1985; Franny Bettinger, *My Little Girl*, Hemdale, 1986; Rachel Feld, *Gardens of Stone*, Tri-Star, 1987; Watts "Drummer Girl," *Some Kind of Wonderful*, Paramount, 1987; Elspeth Skeel, *Mr. North*, Samuel Goldwyn, 1988; Miranda Jeffries, *Chances Are*, Tri-Star, 1989.

PRINCIPAL TELEVISION APPEARANCES—Episodic: Cynthia, *Amazing Stories*, NBC, 1986. Movies: Susan Wallace, *Love Lives On*, ABC, 1985; also *City in Fear*, ABC, 1980.

RELATED CAREER—Attended the Sundance Institute for two summers and the Stage Door Manor, NY, for one summer.

ADDRESSES: AGENTS—David Lewis and Paul Matins, International Creative Management, 8899 Beverly Boulevard, Los Angeles, CA 90048.*

*   *   *

MATTHAU, Walter   1920-

PERSONAL: Born Walter Matthow, October 1, 1920, in New York, NY; son of Milton (an electrician) and Rose (Berolsky) Matthow; married Grace Geraldine Johnson, 1948 (divorced, 1958); married Carol Grace Marcus Saroyan, August 21, 1959; children: David, Jenny (first marriage); Charles (second marriage). EDUCATION: Attended Columbia University and Oxford University; studied acting with Erwin Piscator at the Dramatic Workshop of the New School for Social Research, 1946-47, and with Raiken Ben-Ari. MILITARY: U.S. Army Air Force, staff sergeant, 1942-45.

VOCATION: Actor.

CAREER: STAGE DEBUT—*Ten Nights in a Bar Room*, Erie County Playhouse, Erie, PA, 1946. OFF-BROADWAY DEBUT—Sadovsky, *The Aristocrats*, President Theatre, 1946. BROADWAY DEBUT—Bishop Fisher, *Anne of the 1000 Days*, Shubert Theatre, 1948. PRINCIPAL STAGE APPEARANCES—All in New York City, unless indicated: First soldier, *The Flies*, President Theatre, 1947; Venetian guard, *The Liar*, Broadhurst Theatre, 1950; John Colgate, *Season in the Sun*, Cort Theatre, 1951; Sam Dundee, *Twilight Walk*, Fulton Theatre, 1951; Sinclair Heybore, *Fancy Meeting You Again*, and George Lawrence, *One Bright Day*, both Royale Theatre, 1952; Charlie Hill, *In Any Language*, Cort Theatre, 1952; John Hart, *The Grey-Eyed People*, Martin Beck Theatre, 1952; Paul Osgood, *The Ladies of the Corridor*, Longacre Theatre, 1953; Tony Lack, *The Burning Glass*, Longacre Theatre, 1954; Yancy Loper, *The Wisteria Trees*, and Nathan Detroit, *Guys and Dolls*, both City Center Theatre, 1955; Michael Freeman, *Will Success Spoil Rock Hunter?*, Belasco Theatre, 1955; Odysseus, *Maiden Voyage*, Forrest Theatre, Philadelphia, PA, 1957; Maxwell Archer, *Once More with Feeling*, National Theatre, 1958; Potemkin, *Once There Was a Russian*, Music Box Theatre, 1961; Benjamin Beaurevers, *A Shot in the Dark*, Booth Theatre, 1961; Herman Halpern, *My Mother, My Father, and Me*, Plymouth Theatre, 1963;

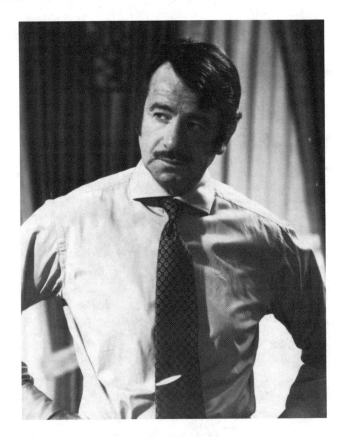

WALTER MATTHAU

Oscar Madison, *The Odd Couple*, Plymouth Theatre, 1965; Captain Jack Boyle, *Juno and the Paycock*, Mark Taper Forum, Los Angeles, CA, 1974.

MAJOR TOURS—Andrew Lamb, *A Certain Joy*, U.S. cities, 1953; also *The Glass Menagerie*, U.S. cities, 1952.

FILM DEBUT—Bodine, *The Kentuckian*, United Artists, 1955. PRINCIPAL FILM APPEARANCES—Wes Todd, *The Indian Fighter*, United Artists, 1955; Wally, *Bigger Than Life*, Twentieth Century-Fox, 1956; Mel Miller, *A Face in the Crowd*, Warner Brothers, 1957; Al Dahlke, *Slaughter on Tenth Avenue*, Universal, 1957; Maxie Fields, *King Creole*, Warner Brothers, 1958; Red Wildoe, *Onionhead*, Warner Brothers, 1958; Judge Kyle, *Ride a Crooked Trail*, Universal, 1958; Doctor Leon Karnes, *Voice in the Mirror*, Universal, 1958; Jack Martin, *Gangster Story*, Releasing Corporation of Independent Producers, 1959; Felix Anders, *Strangers When We Meet*, Columbia, 1960; Sheriff Johnson, *Lonely Are the Brave*, Universal, 1962; Tony Gagoots, *Who's Got the Action?*, Paramount, 1962; Hamilton Bartholomew, *Charade*, Universal, 1963; Tony Dallas, *Island of Love* (also known as *Not on Your Life*), Warner Brothers, 1963; Groeteschele, *Fail Safe*, Columbia, 1964; Doc, *Ensign Pulver*, Warner Brothers, 1964; Sir Leopold Sartori, *Goodbye Charlie*, Twentieth Century-Fox, 1964; Ted Caselle, *Mirage*, Universal, 1965; Willie Gingrich, *The Fortune Cookie* (also known as *Meet Whiplash Willie*), United Artists, 1966; Paul Manning, *A Guide for the Married Man*, Twentieth Century-Fox, 1967; General Smight, *Candy*, Cinerama, 1968; Oscar Madison, *The Odd Couple*, Paramount, 1968; Charlie, *The Secret Life of an American Wife*, Twentieth Century-Fox, 1968; Julian Winston,

Cactus Flower, Columbia, 1969; Horace Vandergelder, *Hello, Dolly!*, Twentieth Century-Fox, 1969.

Henry Graham, *A New Leaf*, Paramount, 1971; Sam Nash, Jesse Kiplinger, and Roy Hubley, *Plaza Suite*, Paramount, 1971; Joseph P. Kotcher, *Kotch*, Cinerama, 1971; Pete Seltzer, *Pete 'n' Tillie*, Universal, 1972; title role, *Charley Varrick*, Universal, 1973; Jake Martin, *The Laughing Policeman* (also known as *An Investigation of Murder*), Twentieth Century-Fox, 1973; Walter Burns, *The Front Page*, Universal, 1974; Lieutenant Garber, *The Taking of Pelham One-Two-Three*, United Artists, 1974; Willie Clark, *The Sunshine Boys*, United Artists, 1975; Buttermaker, *The Bad News Bears*, Paramount, 1976; Marvin Michaels, *California Suite*, Columbia, 1978; Lloyd Bourdelle, *Casey's Shadow*, Columbia, 1978; Dr. Charley Nichols, *House Calls*, Universal, 1978; Miles Kendig, *Hopscotch*, AVCO-Embassy, 1980; Sorrowful Jones, *Little Miss Marker*, Universal, 1980; Trabucco, *Buddy Buddy*, Metro-Goldwyn-Mayer/United Artists (MGM/UA), 1981; Dan Snow, *First Monday in October*, Paramount, 1981; Herbert Tucker, *I Ought to Be in Pictures*, Twentieth Century-Fox, 1982; Sonny Paulso, *The Survivors*, Columbia, 1983; Joe Mulholland, *Movers and Shakers*, MGM/UA, 1985; Captain Thomas Bartholomew Red, *Pirates*, Cannon, 1986; Donald Becker, *The Couch Trip*, Orion, 1988.

PRINCIPAL FILM WORK—Director, *Gangster Story*, Releasing Corporation of Independent Producers, 1959.

PRINCIPAL TELEVISION APPEARANCES—Series: Lex Rogers, *Tallahassee 7000*, syndicated, 1961. Episodic: *Danger*, CBS; *Motorola TV Theatre*, ABC; *Plymouth Playhouse*, ABC; *Philco TV Playhouse*, NBC; *Campbell Soundstage*, NBC; *Alfred Hitchcock Presents*, CBS; *Center Stage*, NBC; *Goodyear TV Playhouse*, NBC; *The Alcoa Hour*, NBC; *DuPont Show of the Week*, NBC. Specials: *We the People 200: The Constitutional Gala*, CBS, 1987.

NON-RELATED CAREER—File clerk, boxing instructor, basketball coach, radio operator.

AWARDS: New York Drama Critics Award and Antoinette Perry Award nomination, Best Supporting or Featured Actor in a Play, 1959, both for *Once More with Feeling*; Antoinette Perry Award, Best Supporting or Featured Actor in a Play, 1962, for *A Shot in the Dark*; Film Daily Award, 1962, for *Lonely Are the Brave*; Antoinette Perry Award, Best Actor in a Play, and New York Drama Critics Award, both 1965, for *The Odd Couple*; Academy Award, Best Supporting Actor, 1967, for *The Fortune Cookie*; Academy Award nomination, Best Actor, 1972, for *Kotch*; British Academy Award, Best Actor, 1973, for *Pete 'n' Tillie* and *Charley Varrick*; Academy Award nomination, Best Actor, 1976, for *The Sunshine Boys*. Military honors include six battle stars.

MEMBER: Actors' Equity Association, Screen Actors Guild, American Federation of Television and Radio Artists.

ADDRESSES: OFFICE—10100 Santa Monica Boulevard, Suite 2200, Los Angeles, CA 90067. AGENT—Leonard Hirshan, William Morris Agency, 151 El Camino Drive, Beverly Hills, CA 90212.

McANALLY, Ray   1926-

PERSONAL: Full name, Raymond McAnally; born March 30, 1926, in Buncrana, Ireland; son of James William Anthony and Winifred (Ward) McAnally; married Ronnie Masterton. EDUCATION: Attended St. Eunan's College and St. Patrick's College; received M.A. in literature and philosophy; trained for the stage at the Abbey Theatre, Dublin.

VOCATION: Actor.

CAREER: STAGE DEBUT—*Strange House*, Town Hall Theatre, Malin Town, Ireland, 1942. LONDON DEBUT—Bud Connor, *A Cheap Bunch of Nice Flowers*, New Arts Theatre, 1962. PRINCIPAL STAGE APPEARANCES—Becket, *Murder in the Cathedral*, Dublin Theatre Festival, St. Patrick's Cathedral, Dublin, Ireland, 1962; first merchant, *The Countess Cathleen*, Paris International Festival, Paris, France, 1962; Pastor John Earls, *The Evangelist*, Belfast Opera House, Belfast, Ireland, 1963; Phil Kerrigan, *Carrie*, Dublin Theatre Festival, Olympia Theatre, Dublin, 1963; George, *Who's Afraid of Virginia Woolf?*, Piccadilly Theatre, London, 1964; "The Bull" McCabe, *The Field*, Olympia Theatre, 1965; Lopakhin, *The Cherry Orchard*, and Macduff, *Macbeth*, both Chichester Festival Theatre, Chichester, U.K., 1966; John Kerr, *Cemented with Love*, Gaiety Theatre, Dublin, 1966; Dron, *The Mighty Reservoy*, Jeanetta Cochrane Theatre, London, 1967; Quentin, *After the Fall*, Dublin Festival, Dublin, 1968; lawyer, *Tiny Alice*, Royal Shakespeare Company, Aldwych Theatre, London, 1970; Ted, *Lorna and Ted*, Greenwich Theatre, London, 1970; Reverend Anthony Anderson, *The Devil's Disciple*, Dolphin Theatre Festival, Shaw Theatre, London, 1971; title role, *Da*, Dublin Festival, Olympia Theatre, 1971; Bernard Shaw, *Best of Friends*, Apollo Theatre, London, 1988. Also appeared in *The Devil's Own People*, Dublin Festival, Gaiety Theatre, 1976.

With the Abbey Theatre Company, all at the Abbey Theatre, Dublin, Ireland, unless indicated: Michael Gillane, *Cathleen Ni Houlihan*, 1948; Leonardo, *Blood Wedding*, and O'Flingsley, *Shadow and Substance*, both 1949; Denis, *The Whiteheaded Boy*, and Hugh O'Cahan, *Professor Tim*, both 1950; Blanco, *The Shewing Up of Blanco Posnet*, and Davoran, *The Shadow of a Gunman*, both 1951; Fred Byrne, *Grogan and the Ferret*, 1952; Darrell Blake, *The Moon in the Yellow River*, 1953; Colm, *Knockavain*, 1954; Dacey Adam, *Twilight of a Warrior*, 1955; Superintendent Brownrigg, *Strange Occurrence on Ireland's Eye*, and MacDara, *Winter Wedding*, both 1956; Christy Mahon, *The Playboy of the Western World*, and Bartholomew Mulchrone, *The Wanton Tide*, both 1957; Sergeant Tinley, *The Plough and the Stars*, Sarah Bernhardt Theatre, Paris Festival, Paris, France, 1957; Sergeant Garside, *A Right Rose Tree*, 1958; Eddie, *The Country Boy*, 1959; George John Lee, *The Shaws of Synge Street*, 1960; Justin McHenry, *The Evidence I Shall Give*, and Gaffur, *The Post Office*, both 1961; title role, *Macbeth*, 1971; also appeared as Willy Loman, *Death of a Salesman*, and in *The Quare Fellow*.

MAJOR TOURS—Grantley Lewis, *A Little Winter Love*, U.S. cities, 1964.

PRINCIPAL STAGE WORK—Director: *The Gingerbread Lady*, Eblana Theatre, Dublin, Ireland, 1974; *Of Mice and Men*, Peacock Theatre, Dublin, 1980; also *Out of Town*, Cork, Ireland, 1974; and *Kennedy's Children*, Dublin, 1975.

PRINCIPAL FILM APPEARANCES—Hugh O'Cahan, *Professor Tim*, RKO, 1957; Paddy Nolan, *Shake Hands with the Devil*, United

Artists, 1959; Donald Heath, *The Naked Edge*, United Artists, 1961; O'Daniel, *Billy Budd*, United Artists, 1962; Sergeant Hardy, *Desert Patrol* (also known as *Sea of Sand*), Universal, 1962; Inspector Sharkey, *Murder in Eden*, Colorama/Schoenfeld, 1962; Jim Power, *She Didn't Say No!*, Warner Brothers, 1962; orphanage superintendent, *He Who Rides a Tiger*, Sigma III, 1966; Starr, *The Looking Glass War*, Columbia, 1970; Ruthven, *Fear Is the Key*, Paramount, 1973; MacWhirter, *The Outsider*, Paramount, 1980; Bloom, *Angel*, British Film Institute, 1982; Cyril Dunlop, *Cal*, Warner Brothers, 1984; Cardinal Altamirano, *The Mission*, Warner Brothers, 1986; Billy McRacken, *No Surrender*, Norstar, 1986; Frank, *Empire State*, Virgin-Miracle, 1987; General Karpov, *The Fourth Protocol*, Lorimar, 1987; Minister Trezza, *The Sicilian*, Twentieth Century-Fox, 1987; Morris, *White Mischief*, Columbia, 1987; O'Rourke, *Taffin*, Metro-Goldwyn-Mayer/United Artists, 1988; Plunkett Senior (ghost), *High Spirits* (also known as *Ghost Tours*), Tri-Star, 1988; grandfather, *Venus Peter*, Atlantic, 1989. Also appeared in *My Left Foot*, Ferndale/Miramax, 1989.

TELEVISION DEBUT—*A Leap in the Dark*, 1959. PRINCIPAL TELEVISION APPEARANCES—Series: *The Little Father* and *Court Martial*. Mini-Series: Rick Pym, *The Perfect Spy*, BBC, then *Masterpiece Theatre*, PBS, 1988; Prime Minister Harry Perkins, *A Very British Coup*, Channel Four, then *Masterpiece Theatre*, PBS, 1989. Movies: Sir William Gull, *Jack the Ripper*, CBS, 1988.

RELATED CAREER—Member, Abbey Theatre Company, Dublin, Ireland, 1947—; drama teacher.

AWARDS: *Evening Herald* Actor of the Year Award, 1959, for *The Country Boy;* British Television Society Award, 1988, for *A Perfect Spy.*

SIDELIGHTS: FAVORITE ROLES—George in *Who's Afraid of Virginia Woolf?* and Dacey Adam in *Twilight of a Warrior*. RECREATIONS—Reading and golf.*

*   *   *

McCALLUM, David   1933-

PERSONAL: Born September 19, 1933, in Glasgow, Scotland; married Jill Ireland (an actress), 1957 (divorced, 1967); married Katherine Carpenter; children: Paul, Jason, Valentine (first marriage); Peter, Sophie (second marriage). EDUCATION: Attended Chapman College; studied acting at the Royal Academy of Dramatic Art, 1949-51.

VOCATION: Actor and director.

CAREER: BROADWAY DEBUT—Julian, *The Flip Side*, Booth Theatre, 1968. PRINCIPAL STAGE APPEARANCES—William Warren, "Visitor from New York," Sidney Nichols, "Visitors from London," and Stu Franklyn, "Visitors from Chicago," *California Suite*, Eugene O'Neill Theatre, New York City, 1976; Inspector, *The Mousetrap*, Arlington Park Theatre, Arlington Heights, IL, 1976; Brian, *After the Prize*, Phoenix Theatre, Marymount Manhattan Theatre, New York City, 1981; Philip, *The Philanthropist*, Manhattan Theatre Club, New York City, 1983; Martin Dysart, *Equus*, Missouri Repertory Theatre, Kansas City, MO, 1986. Also appeared in *Run for Your Wife*, Paper Mill Playhouse, Millburn, NJ, 1986; in productions of *Camelot, Crown Matrimonial, Deathtrap, Donkey's Years, Night Must Fall, Outward Bound, Romantic*

Comedy, Salome, Sleuth, Signpost to Murder, Stage Struck, and *Alfie;* and with the Glyndebourne Opera Company, U.K.

MAJOR TOURS—*Run for Your Wife*, U.S. and Australian cities, 1988.

FILM DEBUT—Jimmy Yately, *Hell Drivers*, Rank, 1958. PRINCIPAL FILM APPEARANCES—Bride, *A Night to Remember*, Rank, 1958; Jim Marston, *Robbery under Arms*, Rank, 1958; Mike Wilson, *The Secret Place*, Rank of America, 1958; Johnny Murphy, *Violent Playground*, Rank, 1958; Private Whitaker, *The Long and the Short and the Tall* (also known as *Jungle Fighters*), Warner/Pathe, 1961; Carl von Schlosser, *Freud* (also known as *The Secret Passion*), Universal, 1962; Ashley-Pitt, *The Great Escape*, United Artists, 1963; Terry Collins, *Jungle Street Girls*, Ajay, 1963; Judas Iscariot, *The Greatest Story Ever Told*, United Artists, 1965; Dr. Phil Volker, *Around the World under the Sea*, Metro-Goldwyn-Mayer (MGM), 1966; Illya Kuryakin, *One of Our Spies Is Missing*, MGM, 1966; Illya Kuryakin, *One Spy Too Many*, MGM, 1966; Illya Kuryakin, *The Spy in the Green Hat*, MGM, 1966; Illya Kuryakin, *The Spy with My Face*, MGM, 1966; Illya Kuryakin, *To Trap a Spy*, MGM, 1966; Illya Kuryakin, *The Karate Killers*, MGM, 1967; Stanley Thrumm, *Three Bites of the Apple*, MGM, 1967; Illya Kuryakin, *The Helicopter Spies*, MGM, 1968; title role, *Sol Madrid* (also known as *The Heroin Gang*), MGM, 1968; Quint Munroe, *Mosquito Squadron*, United Artists, 1970; Harlan Thompson, *Dogs*, La Quinta Film Partners, 1976; Benedict, *The Kingfish Caper* (also known as *The Kingfisher Caper*), Cinema Shares International, 1976; Sir Henry Curtis, *King Solomon's Treasure*, Canafox Towers, 1978; Paul Curtis, *The Watcher in the Woods*, Buena Vista, 1980; Dr. Dodson, *Terminal Choice*, Almi, 1985; John, *The Wind*, Omega, 1987. Also appeared in *Night Ambush* (also known as *Ill Met by Moonlight*), Rank, 1958; *Billy Budd*, United Artists, 1962; and in *The Diamond Hunters, Critical List,* and *La Cattura.*

PRINCIPAL TELEVISION APPEARANCES—Series: Illya Kuryakin, *The Man from U.N.C.L.E.*, NBC, 1964-68; Dr. Daniel Westin, *The Invisible Man*, NBC, 1975-76; also *The Colditz Story*, BBC, 1973-74; *Sapphire and Steel* ATV, 1987. Pilots: Tone Hobart, *The Form of Things Unknown* (broadcast as an episode of *The Outer Limits*), ABC, 1964; Alexi Kaslov, *The Six Million Dollar Man*, ABC, 1973; Dr. Daniel Westin, *The Invisible Man*, NBC, 1975; Illya Kuryakin, *Return of the Man from U.N.C.L.E.: The Fifteen Years Later Affair*, CBS, 1983; Lieutenant Colonel Shelley Flynn, *Behind Enemy Lines*, NBC, 1985. Episodic: Gwyllm Griffiths, "The Sixth Finger," *The Outer Limits*, ABC, 1963; Ivan Tregorin, *The A-Team*, NBC, 1986; Phillip Dudley, *Matlock*, NBC, 1987; Fever Man, *Monsters*, syndicated, 1988; Cyril Grantham, *Murder, She Wrote*, CBS, 1989; also "The Phantom Farmhouse," *Rod Serling's Night Gallery* (also known as *Night Gallery*), NBC, 1971; *Profiles in Courage*, NBC; *Perry Mason*, CBS; *The Travels of Jamie McPheeters*, ABC. Movies: Hillel Mondoro, *Hauser's Memory*, NBC, 1970; Mark Wilson, *She Waits*, CBS, 1972; Henri Clerval, *Frankenstein: The True Story*, NBC, 1973; Sergeant Hans Kemper, *Freedom Fighter* (also known as *The Wall of Tyranny*), NBC, 1987; Charley Ritz, *The Man Who Lived at the Ritz*, syndicated, 1988. Specials: *An Evening with Carol Channing*, CBS, 1966; Kenneth Canfield, "The File on Devlin," *Hallmark Hall of Fame*, NBC, 1969; Hamilton Cade, "Teacher, Teacher," *Hallmark Hall of Fame*, NBC, 1969. Also appeared in *Kidnapped.*

PRINCIPAL TELEVISION WORK—Episodic: Director, *Ten Who Dared*, BBC, 1974.

RELATED CAREER—Director of productions for British Army Entertainment; child actor with the BBC; stage manager, Glyndebourne Opera Company.

SIDELIGHTS: RECREATIONS—Computers and golf.

ADDRESSES: AGENT—Don Buchwald and Associates, Inc., 10 E. 44th Street, New York, NY 10017.*

*   *   *

McCANN, Donal

VOCATION: Actor.

CAREER: PRINCIPAL STAGE APPEARANCES—Vladimir, *Waiting for Godot,* Abbey Theatre, Dublin, Ireland, 1969; Jean, *Miss Julie,* Royal Shakespeare Company, Place Theatre, London, 1971; Seumus Shields, *Shadow of a Gunman,* Abbey Theatre Company, Summerfare '81, State University of New York at Purchase, NY, 1981; Captain Boyle, *Juno and the Paycock,* Gate Theatre, Dublin, Ireland, then John Golden Theatre, New York City, both 1988; also appeared in *Shadow of a Gunman,* Abbey Theatre, Dublin, then International Theatre Festival, Baltimore, MD, both 1981; and as Captain Boyle, *Juno and the Paycock,* Edinburgh, Scotland, then Jerusalem, Israel.

PRINCIPAL FILM APPEARANCES—Sean O'Toole, *The Fighting Prince of Donegal,* Buena Vista, 1966; Sir James Graham, *Sinful Davey,* United Artists, 1969; second agent, *Poitin,* Cinegael, 1979; Bonner, *Angel,* British Film Institute, 1982; Edward Lawless, *Reflections,* Artificial Eye, 1984; Shamie, *Cal,* Warner Brothers, 1984; doctor, *Out of Africa,* Universal, 1985; Leo, *Mr. Love,* Warner Brothers/Goldcrest, 1986; priest, *Budawanny,* Channel Four, 1987; Gabriel Conroy, *The Dead,* Vestron/Zenith, 1987; as himself, *John Huston and the Dubliners* (documentary), Gray City, 1987; Tom Garron, *Rawhead Rex,* Empire, 1987; Eamon, *High Spirits* (also known as *Ghost Tours*), Tri-Star, 1988.

PRINCIPAL TELEVISION APPEARANCES—Mini-Series: Phineas Finn, *The Pallisers,* PBS, 1977. Specials: Jeff, "Screamer," *Thriller,* ABC, 1974.

PRINCIPAL RADIO APPEARANCES—Plays: Captain Boyle, *Juno and the Paycock,* BBC.*

*   *   *

McCUTCHEON, Bill

PERSONAL: Full name, James William McCutcheon; born May 23, in Russell, KY; son of Robert Kenna (a railroad conductor) and Florence Louise (Elam) McCutcheon; married wife, Anne, March 27, 1952; children: Carol, Jay, Kenna. EDUCATION: Ohio University, B.F.A., 1948.

VOCATION: Actor.

CAREER: PRINCIPAL STAGE APPEARANCES—Skeeter Roach, *Out West of Eighth,* Ethel Barrymore Theatre, New York City, 1952; ensemble, *New Faces of 1956* (revue), Ethel Barrymore

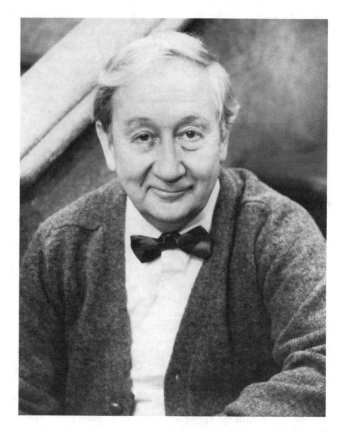

BILL McCUTCHEON

Theatre, 1956; ensemble, *Wet Paint* (revue), Renata Theatre, New York City, 1965; Gladhand, *West Side Story,* Music Theatre of Lincoln Center, State Theatre, New York City, 1968; Daddy Ellis, *My Daughter, Your Son,* Booth Theatre, New York City, 1969; ensemble, *Ben Bagley's Shoestring Revue,* Casa Manana Theatre, Fort Worth, TX, 1970; Pulcinella, *Comedy,* Colonial Theatre, Boston, MA, 1972; Colonel Freeleigh and Jonas the junkman, *Dandelion Wine,* Phoenix Sideshows, Playhouse II Theatre, New York City, 1975; Androcles, *Androcles and the Lion,* Denver Center Theatre Company, Denver, CO, 1981; John, *The Man Who Came to Dinner,* Circle in the Square, New York City, 1980; Mr. DePinna, *You Can't Take It with You,* Plymouth Theatre, New York City, 1983; Paul Brennan, *The Marriage of Bette and Boo,* New York Shakespeare Festival, Public Theatre, New York City, 1985; Mr. Pincus, *The Front Page,* Vivian Beaumont Theatre, New York City, 1986; William H. Gallagher, *Light Up the Sky,* Center Theatre Group, Ahmanson Theatre, Los Angeles, CA, 1987; Moonface, *Anything Goes,* Vivian Beaumont Theatre, 1987. Also appeared in *How to Steal an Election,* Pocket Theatre, New York City, 1968; *Over Here!,* Shubert Theatre, New York City, 1974; *The Miser,* Center Stage, Baltimore, MD, 1982; *Where's Charley* and *Girl Crazy,* both Goodspeed Opera House, East Haddam, CT; *The Taming of the Shrew,* Philadelphia Drama Guild, Philadelphia, PA; *One's a Crowd* and *The Little Revue,* both in New York City; and in productions at Upstairs at the Downstairs, New York City.

PRINCIPAL FILM APPEARANCES—Dropo, *Santa Claus Conquers the Martians,* Embassy, 1964; Desmond Miller, *Viva Max!,* Commonwealth United, 1969; (as William McCutcheon) gas station proprietor, *The Stoolie,* Continental, 1972; gas station attendant, *W.W. and the Dixie Dancekings,* Twentieth Century-Fox, 1975;

Paully, *Hot Stuff*, Columbia, 1979; used car dealer, *Deadhead Miles*, filmed in 1970, released by Paramount, 1982; Mr. Van Der Meer, *Vibes*, Columbia, 1988; Owen, *Steel Magnolias*, Tri-Star, 1989; Doheny, *Family Business*, Tri-Star, 1989.

PRINCIPAL TELEVISION APPEARANCES—Series: Dudley B. Dudley, *Mr. Mayor*, CBS, 1964-65; regular, *The Dom DeLuise Show*, CBS, 1968; Coach Pinky Pinkney, *Ball Four*, CBS, 1976; also Uncle Wally, *Sesame Street*, PBS. Episodic: Bailiff, *Spenser: For Hire*, ABC, 1985; also *Kojak*, CBS; *Forever Fernwood*, syndicated; *All My Children*, ABC; *Search for Tomorrow*, NBC; *Nurse*, CBS; *Person to Person*, CBS. Specials: Uncle Wally, *Sesame Street Special*, PBS, 1988.

AWARDS: Obie Award from the *Village Voice*, 1985, for *The Marriage of Bette and Boo;* Antoinette Perry Award, Best Featured Actor in a Musical, 1988, for *Anything Goes;* also received three Emmy Awards for *Sesame Street*.

ADDRESSES: AGENT—J. Michael Bloom, 233 Park Avenue S., New York, NY 10003.

*   *   *

McDORMAND, Frances   1958-

PERSONAL: Born in 1958. EDUCATION: Graduated from the Yale University School of Drama.

VOCATION: Actress.

CAREER: PRINCIPAL STAGE APPEARANCES—Hennie Berger, *Awake and Sing!*, Circle in the Square, New York City, 1984; Ann Deever, *All My Sons*, Long Wharf Theatre, New Haven, CT, 1986; Stella Kowalski, *A Streetcar Named Desire*, Circle in the Square, 1988. Also appeared in "Rococo" in *Winterset: Four New American Plays*, Yale Repertory Theatre, New Haven, CT, 1980; *Mrs. Warren's Profession*, Yale Repertory Theatre, 1981; *Twelfth Night*, Alliance Theatre Company, Atlanta, GA, 1982; *Painting Churches*, Lambs Theatre, New York City, 1984; and *The Three Sisters*, Tyrone Guthrie Theatre, Minneapolis, MN, 1985.

FILM DEBUT—Abby, *Blood Simple*, Circle, 1984. PRINCIPAL FILM APPEARANCES—Dot, *Raising Arizona*, Twentieth Century-Fox, 1987; Mrs. Pell, *Mississippi Burning*, Orion, 1988; also *Crimewave*, Columbia, 1986.

PRINCIPAL TELEVISION APPEARANCES—Series: Willie Pipal, *Legwork*, CBS, 1986-87. Episodic: Amanda Strickland, "The Need to Know," *The Twilight Zone*, CBS, 1986; Jessie Moore, *The Equalizer*, CBS, 1986. Movies: Brigette, *Vengeance: The Story of Tony Cimo*, CBS, 1986; also *Scandal Sheet*, ABC, 1985.

AWARDS: Antoinette Perry Award nomination, Best Actress in a Play, 1988, for *A Streetcar Named Desire*.

ADDRESSES: AGENT—Smith-Freedman and Associates, 850 Seventh Avenue, New York, NY 10019.*

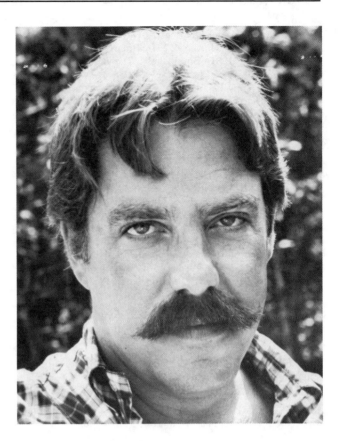

BRUCE McGILL

McGILL, Bruce   1950-

PERSONAL: Full name, Bruce Travis McGill; born July 11, 1950, in San Antonio, TX; son of Woodrow Wilson (an insurance and real estate agent) and Adriel Rose (an artist; maiden name, Jacobs) McGill. EDUCATION: University of Texas, Austin, B.F.A., acting, 1973.

VOCATION: Actor.

CAREER: OFF-BROADWAY DEBUT—Francisco, Bernardo, and Osric, *Hamlet*, New York Shakespeare Festival, Delacorte Theatre, for twenty-eight performances. PRINCIPAL STAGE APPEARANCES—Reynaldo, *Hamlet*, New York Shakespeare Festival (NYSF), Delacorte Theatre, New York City, 1975; Osric, *Hamlet*, Vivian Beaumont Theatre, New York City, 1975; French Ambassador and Orleans, *Henry V*, NYSF, Delacorte Theatre, 1976; Michael Wall, *Museum*, NYSF, Public Theatre, New York City, 1978; Alton, *End of the War*, Ensemble Studio Theatre, New York City, 1978; Lodovico, *Othello*, NYSF, Delacorte Theatre, 1979; Prince Nicolai Erraclyovitch Tchatchavadze and Achmed, *My One and Only*, St. James Theatre, New York City, 1983; Hotspur, *Henry IV, Part I*, Kennedy Center for the Performing Arts, Washington, DC, 1985. Also appeared in *Tom Jones, Peer Gynt, Lady Audley's Secret, Sherlock Holmes*, and *Tooth of Crime*, all Trinity Square Repertory Company, Providence, RI, 1973-75; *As You Like It, St. John*, and *Kiss Me Kate*, all National Shakespeare Company, Washington, DC, 1973; and with the Manhattan Theatre Club.

FILM DEBUT—Dean Lovejoy/"Blood," *Citizens Band* (also known as *Handle with Care*), Paramount, 1977. PRINCIPAL FILM

APPEARANCES—Daniel Simpson "D-Day" Day, *National Lampoon's Animal House,* Universal, 1978; Brian Ferguson, *The Hand,* Warner Brothers, 1981; Bill Blakely, *The Ballad of Gregorio Cortez,* Embassy, 1983; Mace Hurley, *Silkwood,* Twentieth Century-Fox, 1983; Tony Fallon, *Tough Enough,* Twentieth Century-Fox, 1983; Charlie, *Into the Night,* Universal, 1985; Lieutenant Hall, *No Mercy,* Tri-Star, 1986; Dan Darwell, *Wildcats,* Warner Brothers, 1986; Ernest Hemingway, *Waiting for the Moon,* Skouras, 1987; Ernie Cannald, *Out Cold,* Hemdale, 1989.

TELEVISION DEBUT—Daniel Simpson "D-Day" Day, *Delta House,* ABC, 1979. PRINCIPAL TELEVISION APPEARANCES—Series: Billy Clyde Pucket, *Semi-Tough,* ABC, 1980; Jack Dalton, *McGyver,* ABC, 1986—. Episodic: Hank Weldon, "Out Where the Buses Don't Run," *Miami Vice,* NBC, 1984. Movies: Glenn, *A Whale for the Killing,* ABC, 1981; V.D. Skinner, *As Summers Die,* HBO, 1986; Matson, *The Last Innocent Man,* HBO, 1987; Harold Cassady, *Baby M,* ABC, 1988; Charlie, *Fugitives,* Disney Channel, 1988; also *The Man Who Fell to Earth,* ABC, 1987.

MEMBER: Actors' Equity Association, Screen Actors Guild, American Federation of Television and Radio Artists.

SIDELIGHTS: RECREATIONS—Guitar, piano, golf, and ocean sailing.

ADDRESSES: AGENT—Ken Kaplan, Agency for the Performing Arts, 888 Seventh Avenue, New York, NY 10106.

*   *   *

McGINNIS, Scott   1958-

PERSONAL: Born November 19, 1958, in Glendale, CA.

VOCATION: Actor.

CAREER: PRINCIPAL FILM APPEARANCES—Jefferson Bailey, *Joysticks* (also known as *Video Madness*), Jensen Farley, 1983; Norman, *Wacko,* Jensen Farley, 1983; Bif, *Making the Grade* (also known as *Preppies*), Metro-Goldwyn-Mayer/Cannon/United Artists, 1984; Michael, *Racing with the Moon,* Paramount, 1984; "Mr. Adventure," *Star Trek III: The Search for Spock,* Paramount, 1984; Steve Powers, *Secret Admirer,* Orion, 1985; Donnie, *Thunder Alley,* Cannon, 1985; Chris, *3:15, The Moment of Truth* (also known as *3:15*), Dakota Entertainment, 1986; Woody, *Odd Jobs,* Tri-Star, 1986; Barney, *Sky Bandits,* Galaxy International, 1986; Skip, *You Can't Hurry Love,* Lightning, 1988.

PRINCIPAL TELEVISION APPEARANCES—Series: Seaman Dixon, *Operation Petticoat,* ABC, 1978-79. Pilots: Ronny, *All Night Radio,* HBO, 1982; Craig, *The Staff of "Life",* ABC, 1985. Movies: Paul, *Survival of Dana,* CBS, 1979.

ADDRESSES: AGENT—Scott Zimmerman, William Morris Agency, 151 El Camino Drive, Beverly Hills, CA 90212.*

McKECHNIE, Donna   1940-

PERSONAL: Born November, 1940 (some sources say 1944), in Detroit, MI; married Michael Bennett (a dancer, choreographer, and director), December, 1976 (divorced, 1977).

VOCATION: Actress, dancer, choreographer, and singer.

CAREER: BROADWAY DEBUT—Dancer, *How to Succeed in Business without Really Trying,* 46th Street Theatre, 1961. LONDON DEBUT—Kathy, *Company,* Her Majesty's Theatre, 1972. PRINCIPAL STAGE APPEARANCES—Kathy McKenna, *The Education of H*Y*M*A*N K*A*P*L*A*N,* Alvin Theatre, New York City, 1968; Vivien Della Hoya, *Promises, Promises,* Shubert Theatre, New York City, 1968; Kathy, *Company,* Alvin Theatre, 1970, then Ahmanson Theatre, Los Angeles, CA, 1971; Ivy Smith, *On the Town,* Imperial Theatre, New York City, 1971; ensemble, *Sondheim: A Musical Tribute* (revue), Shubert Theatre, 1973; ensemble, *Music! Music!* (revue), City Center Theatre, New York City, 1974; Cassie, *A Chorus Line,* New York Shakespeare Festival, Public Theatre, New York City, then Shubert Theatre, both 1975; Lillian, *Wine Untouched,* Harold Clurman Theatre, New York City, 1979; Cassie, *A Chorus Line,* Shubert Theatre, 1986.

PRINCIPAL STAGE WORK—Choreographer, *Sondheim: A Musical Tribute* (revue), Shubert Theatre, New York City, 1973.

MAJOR TOURS—Philia, *A Funny Thing Happened on the Way to the Forum,* U.S. cities, 1963-64; Cassie, *A Chorus Line,* U.S. cities, 1975.

PRINCIPAL FILM APPEARANCES—The Rose, *The Little Prince,* Paramount, 1974.

PRINCIPAL TELEVISION APPEARANCES—Series: Amanda Harris and Olivia Corey, *Dark Shadows,* ABC. Episodic: Sandra Wall, *Scarecrow and Mrs. King,* CBS, 1986; Anemone, "The Little Mermaid," *Faerie Tale Theatre,* Showtime, 1987; also *Cheers,* NBC, 1982. Movies: Louise Jordan, *Twirl,* NBC, 1981. Specials: *I'm a Fan,* CBS, 1972; *Hotel 90,* CBS, 1973; *The Kraft Seventy-Fifth Anniversary Special,* CBS, 1978; *Sylvia Fine Kaye's Musical Comedy Tonight III,* PBS, 1985; *Broadway Sings: The Music of Jule Styne,* PBS, 1987.

AWARDS: Antoinette Perry Award, Best Actress in a Musical, 1976, for *A Chorus Line.*

MEMBER: Actors' Equity Association.

ADDRESSES: AGENT—William Morris Agency, 151 El Camino Drive, Beverly Hills, CA 90210.*

*   *   *

McMURRAY, Sam   1952-

PERSONAL: Born April 15, 1952, in New York, NY; son of Richard (an actor) and Jane (an actress; maiden name, Hoffman) McMurray; married Elizabeth Collins (an actress); children: Hannah Jane, Rachel Elizabeth. EDUCATION: Studied English literature and acting at Washington University.

VOCATION: Actor.

CAREER: OFF-BROADWAY DEBUT—Lonnie, *The Taking of Miss Janie*, New York Shakespeare Festival, Mitzi E. Newhouse Theatre, 1975. PRINCIPAL STAGE APPEARANCES—Otis Fitzhugh, *Ballymurphy*, Manhattan Theatre Club, New York City, 1976; Bobby Wheeler, *Clarence*, Roundabout Theatre, New York City, 1976; Doalty, *Translations*, Manhattan Theatre Club, 1981; Mick Connor, *Comedians*, Manhattan Punch Line, New York City, 1983; Benjamin "Kid Purple" Schwartz, *Kid Purple*, Manhattan Punch Line, 1984; Phil, "Desperadoes" in *Marathon '85*, Ensemble Studio Theatre, New York City, 1985; Mike Connor, *The Philadelphia Story*, Hartman Theatre, Stamford, CT, 1985. Also appeared in *The Great Magoo*, Hartford Stage Company, Hartford, CT, 1982; *Man Overboard*, Sargent Theatre, New York City, 1983; *Homesteaders*, Long Wharf Theatre, New Haven, CT, 1984; *Union Boys*, Yale Repertory Theatre, New Haven, CT, 1985; *L.A. Freewheeling*, Hartley House Theatre, New York City, 1986; *Savage in Limbo*, O'Neill Theatre Center, New London, CT, 1987, then CAST Theatre, Los Angeles, CA; as Phil, *The Dumping Ground*, and in *Welfare, The Store*, and *Lucky Star*, all Ensemble Studio Theatre; in productions of *A Soldier's Play, The Merry Wives of Windsor*, and *The Connection*, all in New York City; and with the O'Neill Playwrights Conference, New London, CT, for five years.

FILM DEBUT—Young man at party, *The Front*, Columbia, 1976. PRINCIPAL FILM APPEARANCES—Young vagrant, *Union City*, Kinesis, 1980; Mr. McManus, *Baby, It's You*, Paramount, 1983; Crespi, *C.H.U.D.*, New World, 1984; Clem Friedkin, *Fast Forward*, Columbia, 1985; Glen, *Raising Arizona*, Twentieth Century-Fox, 1987; Peter Harriman, *Ray's Male Heterosexual Dance Hall* (short film), Discovery Program/Chanticleer, 1988.

PRINCIPAL TELEVISION APPEARANCES—Series: Wes Leonard, *Ryan's Hope*, ABC, 1975; Officer Harvey Schoendorf, *Baker's Dozen*, CBS, 1982; regular, *The Tracey Ullman Show*, Fox, 1987—. Mini-Series: *Hands of a Stranger*, CBS, 1987. Pilots: Regular, *Not Necessarily the News*, HBO, 1982; Frank McGee, *Hope Division*, ABC, 1987; also *Dads*, ABC. Episodic: Ned, "The Devil's Work," *Ourstory*, PBS, 1976; Gann, *Hill Street Blues*, NBC, 1986; Stu Angry, *You Again?*, NBC, 1986; Michael Saxon, *Ohara*, ABC, 1987; Mike, *Dear John*, NBC, 1988; Lieutenant Tony Brandt, *21 Jump Street*, Fox, 1988; Coach Finelli, *Head of the Class*, ABC, 1988; Brent, *Empty Nest*, NBC, 1988; Mark Harper, *Who's the Boss?*, NBC, 1989; Bart Hess, *Matlock*, NBC, 1989; also *Moonlighting*, ABC; *Miami Vice*, NBC; *Easy Street*, CBS; *Kojak*, CBS. Movies: Morrison, *Out of the Darkness*, CBS, 1985; police lieutenant, *Adam: His Song Continues*, NBC, 1986; David Thomas, *Take My Daughters, Please* (also known as *All My Darling Daughters*), NBC, 1988; also *Tracey Ullman Backstage*, 1988.

ADDRESSES: AGENT—Harris/Goldberg, 2121 Avenue of the Stars, Suite 950, Los Angeles, CA 90067. PUBLICIST—Max Green, Sumski/Green, 8380 Melrose Avenue, Suite 200, Los Angeles, CA 90069.

*   *   *

MEEKER, Ralph   1920-1988

PERSONAL: Born Ralph Rathgeber, November 21, 1920, in Minneapolis, MN; died of a heart attack, August 5, 1988, in Woodland Hills, CA; son of Ralph and Magnhild Senovia Haavig Meeker Rathgeber; married Salome Jens (an actress), July 20, 1964 (divorced, 1966); married Colleen Rose Neary (marriage ended); third wife's name, Millicent. EDUCATION: Attended Northwestern University, 1938-42; studied acting with Alvina Krauss, 1941-42. MILITARY: U.S. Navy.

VOCATION: Actor.

CAREER: STAGE DEBUT—Bellboy, *Doughgirls*, Selwyn Theatre, Chicago, IL, 1943. BROADWAY DEBUT—Chuck, *Strange Fruit*, Royale Theatre, 1945. PRINCIPAL STAGE APPEARANCES—All in New York City, unless indicated: Mannion, *Mister Roberts*, Alvin Theatre, 1947; Stanley Kowalski, *A Streetcar Named Desire*, Ethel Barrymore Theatre, 1949; Hal Carter, *Picnic*, Music Box Theatre, 1953; Frank Copley, *Top Man*, Shubert Theatre, New Haven, CT, 1955; Newton Reece, *Cloud 7*, John Golden Theatre, 1958; Berenger, *Rhinocerous*, Longacre Theatre, 1961; Sergeant Toat, *Something about a Soldier*, Ambassador Theatre, 1962; Bernie Slovenk, *Natural Affection*, Sombrero Playhouse, Phoenix, AZ, 1962; Mickey, *After the Fall*, and Charles Taney, *But for Whom Charlie*, both Lincoln Center Repertory Theatre Company, American National Theatre Academy Washington Square Theatre, 1964; Sam, *Mrs. Dally*, John Golden Theatre, 1965; Artie Shaughnessy, *The House of Blue Leaves*, Truck and Warehouse Theatre, 1971. Also appeared in *Cyrano de Bergerac*, Alvin Theatre, 1946; and in *Streamers*, Westwood Playhouse, Los Angeles, CA, then Cannery Theatre, San Francisco, CA, both 1977.

PRINCIPAL STAGE WORK—Assistant stage manager, *Strange Fruit*, Royale Theatre, New York City, 1945; assistant stage manager, *Cyrano de Bergerac*, Alvin Theatre, New York City, 1946.

PRINCIPAL TOURS—Bellboy, *The Doughgirls*, U.S. cities, 1943; Anthony Marston, *Ten Little Indians*, U.S.O. tour, Mediterranean area, 1944; Stanley Kowalski, *A Streetcar Named Desire*, U.S. cities, 1950; Hal Carter, *Picnic*, U.S. cities, 1954; also appeared in *Mrs. Dally Has a Lover*, U.S. cities, 1965.

FILM DEBUT—Sergeant Dobbs, *Teresa*, Metro-Goldwyn-Mayer, 1951. PRINCIPAL FILM APPEARANCES—Sergeant William Long, *Four in a Jeep*, Praesens Film Zurich, 1951; Burt, *Shadow in the Sky*, Metro-Goldwyn-Mayer (MGM), 1951; Socks Barbarrosa, *Glory Alley*, MGM, 1952; Benny Fields, *Somebody Loves Me*, Paramount, 1952; Chuck O'Flair, *Code Two*, MGM, 1953; Lawson, *Jeopardy*, MGM, 1953; Roy Anderson, *The Naked Spur*, MGM, 1953; Jerry Barker, *Big House, U.S.A.*, United Artists, 1955; David Malcolm, *Desert Sands*, United Artists, 1955; Mike Hammer, *Kiss Me Deadly*, United Artists, 1955; Trevor Stevenson, *A Woman's Devotion* (also known as *War Shock* and *Battleshock*), Republic, 1956; Mike Valla, *The Fuzzy Pink Nightgown*, United Artists, 1957; Corporal Paris, *Paths of Glory*, United Artists, 1957; Lieutenant Driscoll, *Run of the Arrow*, Universal, 1957.

Colonel Yancy, *Ada*, MGM, 1961; Mike, *Something Wild*, United Artists, 1961; Matt Rubio, *Wall of Noise*, Warner Brothers, 1963; Captain Stuart Kinder, *The Dirty Dozen*, MGM, 1967; Fog Hanson, *Gentle Giant*, Paramount, 1967; George "Bugs" Moran, *The St. Valentine's Day Massacre*, Twentieth Century-Fox, 1967; Lieutenant Curran, *The Detective*, Twentieth Century-Fox, 1968; Burl, *The Devil's 8*, American International, 1969; Carl McCain, *I Walk the Line*, Columbia, 1970; Delaney, *The Anderson Tapes*, Columbia, 1971; the Major, *The Happiness Cage* (also known as *The Mind Snatchers*), Cinerama, 1972; Captain Moretti, *Brannigan*, United Artists, 1975; Bensington, *The Food of the Gods*, American International, 1976; Gameboy Baker, *Winter Kills,* AVCO-Embassy, 1979; Dave, *Without Warning* (also known as *It Came . . . Without Warning*), Filmways, 1980. Also appeared in *Love Comes Quietly,* 1974; *Johnny Firecloud,* 1975; *The Alpha Incident,* 1976; *The Hi-Riders,* Dimension, 1978; and *My Boys Are Good Boys,* Peter Perry, 1978.

PRINCIPAL FILM WORK—Executive producer, *My Boys Are Good Boys,* Peter Perry, 1978.

PRINCIPAL TELEVISION APPEARANCES—Episodic: "Fifty Grand," *Kraft Television Theatre,* NBC, 1958; *The Loretta Young Show,* NBC, 1964; *Route 66,* CBS, 1966; *The Doctors and the Nurses,* CBS, 1964; *Kraft Suspense Theatre,* NBC, 1964; *Moment of Fear,* NBC, 1965; *The Long, Hot Summer,* ABC, 1966; *The F.B.I.,* ABC, 1966, then 1967; *The Green Hornet,* ABC, 1967; *Custer,* ABC, 1967; *Tarzan,* NBC, 1967; *The High Chaparral,* NBC, 1967; *The Name of the Game,* NBC, 1968; *Ironside,* NBC, 1968; *The Men from Shiloh,* NBC, 1970; *Police Surgeon,* syndicated, 1971; "Hard Traveling," *NET Playhouse,* NET, 1971; *The Rookies,* ABC, 1975. Movies: Captain Luke Danvers, *The Reluctant Heroes,* ABC, 1971; Bernie Jenks, *The Night Stalker,* ABC, 1972; Will Alden, *You'll Never See Me Again,* ABC, 1973; Chief Harry Stahlgaher, *Police Story,* NBC, 1973; Jim McAndrew, *Birds of Prey,* CBS, 1973; Chuck Braswell, *Cry Panic,* ABC, 1974; Inspector DeBiesse, *The Girl on the Late, Late Show,* NBC, 1974; Dutch Armbreck, *Night Games,* NBC, 1974; Lieutenant Reardon, *The Dead Don't Die,* NBC, 1975. Specials: Sergeant Dekker, *Not for Hire,* NBC, 1960; also *The Lost Flight.*

NON-RELATED CAREER—Soda jerk.

MEMBER: Actors' Equity Association, Screen Actors Guild, American Federation of Television and Radio Artists, Ancient Mystical Order Rosae Crucis (Rosicrucian Order).

OBITUARIES AND OTHER SOURCES: New York Times, August 6, 1988; *Variety,* August 10, 1988.*

*   *   *

MENGES, Chris   1941-

PERSONAL: Born in 1941 in Herefordshire, England; son of Herbert Menges (a composer and conductor); married second wife, Judy Freeman (a sound recordist); children: five (first marriage).

VOCATION: Cinematographer and director.

CAREER: FIRST FILM WORK—Cinematographer, *If . . . ,* Paramount, 1968. PRINCIPAL FILM WORK—All as cinematographer, unless indicated. *Kes,* United Artists, 1970; *Black Beauty,* Paramount, 1971; *Gumshoe,* Columbia, 1972; *Black Jack,* National Film Finance, 1979; *Before the Monsoon,* BFV, 1979; *Babylon,* Diversity Music Production, 1980; *The Gamekeeper,* ATV Network, 1980; camera operator (second unit), *The Empire Strikes Back,* Twentieth Century-Fox, 1980; *Couples and Robbers,* Warner Brothers, 1981; *Angel,* Motion Picture Company, 1982; *Battletruck* (also known as *Warlords of the Twenty-First Century*), New World, 1982; *Looks and Smiles,* Artificial Eye, 1982; *Bloody Kids,* Palace/British Film Institute, 1983; *Local Hero,* Warner Brothers, 1983; *Comfort and Joy,* Universal, 1984; *The Killing Fields,* Warner Brothers, 1984; *Winter Flight,* Enigma/Goldcrest, 1984;

Marie, Metro-Goldwyn-Mayer/United Artists, 1985; *A Sense of Freedom,* Handmade/Island, 1985; *Fatherland,* Film Four International, 1986; *The Mission,* Warner Brothers, 1986; *High Season,* Hemdale, 1987; *Shy People,* Cannon, 1987; *Singing the Blues in Red,* Angelika, 1988; director, *A World Apart,* Atlantic, 1988. Also cinematographer, *The Tribe That Hides from Man* (documentary).

PRINCIPAL TELEVISION WORK—All as cinematographer, unless indicated. Series: *World in Action,* BBC. Mini-Series: *Loving Walter,* Central Television, 1983. Specials: *The Opium Warlords* (documentary), BBC, 1973; (also producer and director) *East 103rd Street* (documentary), Central Television, 1983; and *Opium Trail,* BBC.

RELATED CAREER—Cutting-room trainee to director Alan Forbes, Jr.; documentary filmmaker for Granada Television in South Africa, 1963; also made documentaries in Southeast Asia, 1968-69, and in Brazil, Tibet, Burma, Rhodesia, Angola, Congo, Cyprus, and Algeria.

AWARDS: Academy Award and British Academy Award, both Best Cinematography, and New York Film Critics Circle Award, all 1984, for *The Killing Fields;* Academy Award and British Academy Award, both Best Cinematography, and Los Angeles Film Critics Association Award, all 1987, for *The Mission.*

ADDRESSES: AGENT—Leading Artists, 445 N. Bedford Drive, Penthouse, Beverly Hills, CA 90210.*

*   *   *

MERCER, Marian   1935-

PERSONAL: Born November 26, 1935, in Akron, OH; daughter of Samuel Lewis and Nelle (Leggatt) Mercer; married Martin Joseph Cassidy (an actor), November 9, 1964. EDUCATION: University of Michigan, B.Mus., 1957; studied singing with Frances Greer.

VOCATION: Actress and singer.

CAREER: STAGE DEBUT—*The Happiest Millionaire,* Palmtree Playhouse, Sarasota, FL, 1957. OFF-BROADWAY DEBUT—Marcelle, *Hotel Paradiso,* Equity Library Theatre, Lenox Hill Playhouse, 1959. PRINCIPAL STAGE APPEARANCES—Title role, *Little Mary Sunshine,* Orpheum Theatre, New York City, 1959; chorus, *Greenwillow,* Alvin Theatre, New York City, 1960; Mrs. Peterson, *Bye Bye Birdie,* Musicarnival, Palm Beach, FL, 1962; title role, *Little Mary Sunshine,* Ann Arbor Dramatic Festival, Ann Arbor, MI, 1962; ensemble, *New Faces of '62,* Alvin Theatre, New York City, 1962; Tessie Tura, *Gypsy,* Kenley Players, Warren, OH, 1962; Beatrice, *Much Ado about Nothing,* Shakespeare Summer Festival, Washington, DC, 1963; title role, *Little Mary Sunshine,* Nutmeg Playhouse, Storrs, CT, 1963; Helena, *A Midsummer Night's Dream,* and Beatrice, *Much Ado about Nothing,* both Shakespeare Summer Festival, Washington, DC, 1964; Marcelle Paillardin, *Hotel Passionato,* East 74th Street Theatre, New York City, 1965; Helena, *A Midsummer Night's Dream,* and Blanche Du Bois, *A Streetcar Named Desire,* both Repertory Theatre of St. Louis, Loretto-Hilton Center, St. Louis, MO, 1966; Olivia, *Your Own Thing,* Orpheum Theatre, 1968; Marge MacDougall, *Promises, Promises,* Shubert Theatre, New York City, 1968.

Desdemona, *Othello,* Loretto-Hilton Center, 1970; Polly, *A Place for Polly,* Ethel Barrymore Theatre, New York City, 1970; Myra Arundel, *Hay Fever,* Helen Hayes Theatre, New York City, 1970; Katherina, *The Taming of the Shrew,* Trinity Square Repertory Company, Providence, RI, 1970; woman and Dinah Darling, *The Good and Bad Times of Cady Francis McCullum and Friends,* Trinity Square Repertory Company, 1971; Colomba, *Volpone,* Center Theatre Group, Mark Taper Forum, Los Angeles, CA, 1972; Colleen, *Tadpole,* New Theatre for Now, Stage B, Twentieth Century-Fox, Los Angeles, 1973; Lillian, *Travellers,* Playhouse in the Park, Cincinnati, OH, 1974; Gwendolen Fairfax, *Nobody's Earnest,* Williamstown Festival Theatre, Williamstown, MA, 1973; Masha, *The Seagull,* Williamstown Festival Theatre, 1974; Lorene, Ilse, and Evie, *Stop the World—I Want to Get Off,* State Theatre, New York City, 1978; Deidre, *Bosoms and Neglect,* Goodman Theatre, Chicago, 1978, then Longacre Theatre, New York City, 1979; Masha Chekhov, *Chekhov in Yalta,* and Olivia, *Twelfth Night,* both Center Theatre Group, Mark Taper Forum, 1981; *Female Parts* (one-woman play), Los Angeles Actors Theatre, Los Angeles, 1982.

Also appeared in *Holiday for Lovers* and *A Hole in the Head,* both Palmtree Playhouse, Sarasota, FL, 1958; *The Ballad of Baby Doe, Show Boat,* and *The Most Happy Fella,* all Musicarnival, Cleveland, OH, 1958; *The Waltz of the Toreadors,* Rickaway Theatre, Newark, NJ, 1958; *Guys and Dolls, The Pajama Game,* and *The Student Prince,* all Musicarnival, Palm Beach, FL, 1958; *Fiorello!,* Broadhurst Theatre, New York City, 1960; *The Tunnel of Love, Odd Man In,* and *Lady Be Good,* all Totem Pole Playhouse, Fayetteville, PA, 1960; *Come to the Palace of Sin,* American National Theatre and Academy Matinee Theatre Series, Theatre De Lys, New York City, 1963; *And in This Corner* and *The Game Is Up,* both Upstairs at the Downstairs, New York City, 1964; *Twelfth Night* and *Oh, What a Lovely War!,* Repertory Theatre of St. Louis, Loretto-Hilton Center, 1966; *The Hostage,* Loretto-Hilton Center, 1967; *The Wanderers* (series of short plays), Orpheum Theatre, 1971; *And Miss Reardon Drinks a Little,* Seattle Repertory Theatre, Seattle, WA, 1972; *Three Men on a Horse,* Seattle Repertory Theatre, 1973; *Petrified Man,* Theatre Vanguard, Los Angeles, 1974; *The Waltz of the Toreadors,* Seattle Repertory Theatre, 1975.

MAJOR TOURS—Mrs. Peterson, *Bye Bye Birdie,* U.S. cities, 1962-63; Ilse, Lorene, and Evie, *Stop the World—I Want to Get Off,* U.S. cities, 1978; also in *Bells Are Ringing,* U.S. cities, 1959; *Gypsy* and *Little Mary Sunshine,* U.S. cities, both 1962-63; *Lovers and Other Strangers,* U.S. cities, 1973.

PRINCIPAL FILM APPEARANCES—Mags Elliot, *John and Mary,* Twentieth Century-Fox, 1969; Evie, *Sammy Stops the World* (also known as *Stop the World—I Want to Get Off*), Special Entertainment, 1978; Missy Hart, *Nine to Five,* Twentieth Century-Fox, 1980. Also appeared in *Oh God! Book II,* Warner Brothers, 1980.

TELEVISION DEBUT—*The Dave Garroway Show,* NBC, 1961. PRINCIPAL TELEVISION APPEARANCES—Series: Regular, *The Andy Williams Show,* NBC, 1962-63; regular, *The Dom DeLuise Show,* CBS, 1968; regular, *The Dean Martin Show,* NBC, 1971-72; Kay Fox, *The Sandy Duncan Show,* CBS, 1972; regular, *The Wacky World of Jonathan Winters,* syndicated, 1972-74; Myra Bradley, *A Touch of Grace,* ABC, 1973; Wanda Jeeter, *Mary Hartman, Mary Hartman,* syndicated, 1976-77, retitled *Forever Fernwood,* syndicated, 1977-78; Nancy Beebe, *It's a Living,* ABC, 1980-82, then syndicated, 1985—; Mrs. Griffin, *Foot in the Door,* CBS, 1983. Pilots: Reporter, *Comedy News,* ABC, 1972; reporter, *Comedy News II,* ABC, 1973; Maggie Barbour, *Calling Dr. Storm, M.D.,* NBC, 1977; Mildred Braffman, *King of the*

Road, CBS, 1978; Nancy Beebe, *Making a Living,* ABC, 1982; also *What's Up?,* NBC, 1971. Episodic: Masha, "The Seagull," *Great Performances,* PBS, 1975; Dr. Woods, *You Again?,* NBC, 1986; Nurse Eve Leighton, *St. Elsewhere,* NBC, 1986 and 1987; also *The Mike Wallace Show,* 1961. Movies: Eleanor, *The Cracker Factory,* ABC, 1979; Rita, *Life of the Party: The Story of Beatrice,* CBS, 1982; Daisy Eastman, *Agatha Christie's "Murder in Three Acts,"* CBS, 1986; also *Zero Hour,* ABC, 1967. Specials: *Johnny Carson's Repertory Company in an Evening of Comedy,* NBC, 1969; *What's Up, America?,* NBC, 1971; *Ladies and Gentlemen /. . . Bob Newhart,* CBS, 1980; *Ladies and Gentlemen . . . Bob Newhart, Part II,* CBS, 1981; *Dom DeLuise and Friends, Part II,* ABC, 1984; *Dom DeLuise and Friends, Part III,* ABC, 1985; Sister Regina, "Are You My Mother?," *ABC Afterschool Special,* ABC, 1986.

RELATED CAREER—Nightclub performer, *Prickly Pair,* the Showplace, New York City, 1961.

AWARDS: Variety New York Drama Critics Poll, Best Supporting Actress, and Antoinette Perry Award, Best Supporting Actress in a Musical, both 1969, for *Promises, Promises;* Theatre World Award, 1969; Drama Desk Award.

SIDELIGHTS: RECREATIONS—Music, reading, antiques, and art collecting.

ADDRESSES: AGENT—Cunningham, Escott, Dipere, and Associates, 261 S. Robertson Boulevard, Beverly Hills, CA 90211. HOME—1 W. 72nd Street, New York, NY 10023.*

*   *   *

METCALF, Laurie   1955-

PERSONAL: Born June 16, 1955, in Edwardsville, IL; children: Zoe. EDUCATION: Attended Illinois State University.

VOCATION: Actress.

CAREER: OFF-BROADWAY DEBUT—Darlene, *Balm in Gilead,* Steppenwolf Theatre Company, Circle Repertory Theatre, then Minetta Lane Theatre, 1984. PRINCIPAL STAGE APPEARANCES—Honey, *Who's Afraid of Virginia Woolf?,* North Light Repertory Theatre, Evanston, IL, 1982; Scarlet, *Coyote Ugly,* Steppenwolf Theatre Company, Terrace Theatre, Kennedy Center for the Performing Arts, Washington, DC, 1985; Beth, *Bodies, Rest, and Motion,* Steppenwolf Theatre Company, Mitzi E. Newhouse Theatre, New York City, 1986; Rita, *Educating Rita,* Steppenwolf Theatre Company, Westside Arts Theatre, New York City, 1987; Faye, *Little Egypt,* Steppenwolf Theatre Company, Steppenwolf Theatre, Chicago, IL, 1987; Faye, *Killers,* Steppenwolf Theatre Company, Steppenwolf Theatre, 1988. Also appeared as the mother in *True West* and in *The Fifth of July,* both with the Steppenwolf Theatre Company, Chicago.

FILM DEBUT—Leslie Glass, *Desperately Seeking Susan,* Orion, 1984. PRINCIPAL FILM APPEARANCES—Sandy, *Making Mr. Right,* Orion, 1987; Melissa, *Stars and Bars,* Columbia, 1988; Alice, *Candy Mountain,* Xanadu, 1988; exotic dancer, *Miles from Home,* Cinecom International, 1988.

PRINCIPAL TELEVISION APPEARANCES—Series: Regular, *Satur-*

day Night Live, NBC, 1981; Jackie Harris, *Roseanne,* ABC, 1988—. Episodic: Theresa, *The Equalizer,* CBS, 1986. Movies: Carol Graham, *The Execution of Raymond Graham,* ABC, 1985.

RELATED CAREER—Founding member, Steppenwolf Theatre Company, Chicago, IL.

AWARDS: Theatre World Award, 1984, for *Balm in Gilead;* Joseph Jefferson Award, Best Performance by a Principal Actress in a Play, 1987, for *Educating Rita.*

OTHER SOURCES: Premiere, February, 1988.

ADDRESSES: OFFICE—Steppenwolf Theatre, 2851 N. Halsted Street, Chicago, IL 60657. AGENT—Elaine Goldsmith, William Morris Agency, 151 El Camino Drive, Beverly Hills, CA 90212.*

*   *   *

METCALFE, Stephen   1953-

PERSONAL: Born July 4, 1953, in New Haven, CT; son of Stephen B., Jr. and Marylouise (Brigham) Metcalfe. EDUCATION: Attended Westminster College; graduate work, Boston University, 1976.

VOCATION: Writer.

CAREER: See *WRITINGS* below. RELATED CAREER—Associate editor, *Racquet* magazine, New York City, 1976-79; member of the Playwright's Unit, Manhattan Theatre Club, New York City, 1980; also associate artist, Old Globe Theatre, San Diego, CA; and actor in regional productions and in New York City.

WRITINGS: STAGE—*Baseball Play* and *Jacknife,* both Quaigh Theatre, New York City, 1980; *Vikings,* Manhattan Theatre Club, New York City, 1980; *Strange Snow,* Manhattan Theatre Club, 1982, published by Theatre Communications Group, 1982; *White Linen,* Boarshead Theatre, Lansing, MI, 1982; *Half a Lifetime,* Manhattan Theatre Club, 1983; *Loves and Hours,* Playhouse in the Park, Cincinnati, OH, 1984; *The Incredibly Famous Willy Rivers,* WPA Theatre, New York City, 1984; "Sorrows and Sons," "Spittin' Image," and "Pilgrims," all in *Sorrows and Sons,* Vineyard Theatre, New York City, 1986; *Emily,* Old Globe Theatre, San Diego, CA, 1987, then Manhattan Theatre Club, 1988.

FILM—*Cousins,* Paramount, 1989; *Jacknife,* Cineplex Odeon, 1989.

TELEVISION—Episodic: *The Comedy Zone,* CBS, 1984. Plays: *Half a Lifetime,* HBO, 1987.

AWARDS: Award from the Double Image Theatre, 1978, for *Spittin' Image;* playwrighting commissions from the Manhattan Theatre Club, 1980-82; grant in playwriting from the Creative Artists Public Service Program, 1982; National Endowment for the Arts grant, 1983; San Diego Drama Critics Award for *Emily.*

MEMBER: Dramatists Guild.

ADDRESSES: AGENT—Jeremy Zimmer, International Creative Management, 8899 Beverly Boulevard, Los Angeles, CA 90048.

MILES, Sylvia   1932-

PERSONAL: Born September 9, 1932, in New York, NY; married Gerald Price (an actor), 1952 (divorced, 1958); married Ted Brown (a radio and television performer), 1963 (divorced). EDUCATION: Graduated from Pratt Institute, 1947; studied acting with Erwin Piscator, Ben Ari, and Stella Adler at the Dramatic Workshop of the New School for Social Research; with Harold Clurman and the Group Theatre; with N. Richard Nash; and with Lee Strasberg and Frank Corsaro at the Actors Studio.

VOCATION: Actress.

CAREER: STAGE DEBUT—Lampito, *Lysistrata,* Dramatic Workshop, President Theatre, New York City. BROADWAY DEBUT—Rosie, *The Riot Act,* Cort Theatre, 1963. PRINCIPAL STAGE APPEARANCES—Arlene, *A Stone for Danny Fisher,* Downtown National Theatre, New York City, 1954; Ruthie, *Wedding Breakfast,* Capri Theatre, Long Island, NY, 1955; shoplifter, *Detective Story,* Great Neck Summer Theatre, Long Island, NY, 1955; Margie, *The Iceman Cometh,* Circle in the Square, New York City, 1956; Lizzie Curry, *The Rainmaker,* Drury Lane Theatre, Chicago, IL, 1959; Ninotchka, *Silk Stockings,* Casa Manana Theatre, Fort Worth, TX, 1959; Rita Marlowe, *Will Success Spoil Rock Hunter?,* Candlelight Theatre, Washington, DC, 1959; thief, *The Balcony,* Circle in the Square, 1960; Bessie, *Man Around the House,* Bucks County Playhouse, New Hope, PA, 1961; Katrin, *The Marriage-Go-Round,* British Colonial Theatre, Nassau, Bahamas, then Coconut Grove Playhouse, Miami, FL, both 1961; Raisa, "The Witch" in *A Chekhov Sketchbook,* Gramercy Arts Theatre, New York City, 1962; Mrs. Boker, "Infancy," and the Nurse, "Pullman Car Hiawatha," in *Plays for Bleecker Street,* Olney Playhouse, Olney, MD, 1963; Mildred Turner, *Oh Men! Oh, Women!,* North Shore Playhouse, Beverly, MA, 1963; Stella Rizzo, *Matty and the Moron and Madonna,* Orpheum Theatre, New York City, 1965; Monique, *The Kitchen,* 81st Street Theatre, New York City, 1966; title role, *The Killing of Sister George,* Santa Fe Theatre, Santa Fe, NM, 1969.

Sylvie, *Rosebloom,* East Side Playhouse, New York City, 1972; Martha, *Who's Afraid of Virginia Woolf?,* Pittsburgh Playhouse, Pittsburgh, PA, 1972; title role, *Nellie Toole and Co.,* Theatre Four, New York City, 1973; Maxine Faulk, *The Night of the Iguana,* Circle in the Square, New York City, 1976; Mrs. Wire, *Vieux Carre,* Nottingham Playhouse, Piccadilly Theatre, London, 1978; *It's Me, Sylvia!* (one-woman show), Playhouse Theatre II, New York City, 1981; Lucille, "The Cemetery Club" in *Winterfest Seven,* Yale Repertory Theatre, New Haven, CT, 1986. Also appeared at the Taminent Playhouse, Taminent, PA, 1949; in *Play That on Your Old Piano,* Renata Theatre, New York City, 1965; in *Luv* and *The Owl and the Pussycat,* both Hampton Playhouse, Hampton, NY, 1967; in "This Bird of Longing Singeth All Night Long," *American Night Cry,* Actors Studio, New York City, 1974; and in *Employment Agency* and *Before Breakfast,* both Chichester Festival Theatre, Chichester, U.K., 1978.

MAJOR TOURS—June, *Made in Heaven,* U.S. cities, 1949; Windy Hill, *The Glass Rooster,* U.S. cities, 1964; also *Show Boat,* U.S. cities, 1950.

FILM DEBUT—Sadie, *Murder, Inc.,* Twentieth Century-Fox, 1960. PRINCIPAL FILM APPEARANCES—Eileen, *Parrish,* Warner Brothers, 1961; Rose, *Pie in the Sky* (also known as *Terror in the City* and *The Truant*), Allied Artists, 1964; Silvia, *Psychomania* (also known as *Violent Midnight*), Victoria/Emerson, 1964; Cass,

Midnight Cowboy, United Artists, 1969; script girl, *The Last Movie* (also known as *Chinchero*), Universal, 1971; Christine, *Who Killed Mary What's 'er Name?* (also known as *Death of a Hooker*), Cannon, 1971; Sally, *Heat,* Levitt-Pickman, 1972; Mrs. Jessie Florian, *Farewell, My Lovely,* AVCO-Embassy, 1975; Bella Knowles, *92 in the Shade,* United Artists, 1975; Mike, *The Great Scout and Cathouse Thursday,* American International, 1976; Gerde, *The Sentinel,* Universal, 1977; Flo, *Zero to Sixty* (also known as *Repo*), First Artists, 1978; Madame Zena, *The Funhouse,* Universal, 1981; Myra Gardener, *Evil under the Sun,* Universal, 1982; Maggie, *Critical Condition,* Paramount, 1987; Sylvie Drimmer, *Wall Street,* Twentieth Century-Fox, 1987; Red Fairy, *Sleeping Beauty,* Cannon, 1987; Hannah Mandelbaum, *Crossing Delancey,* Warner Brothers, 1988; congresswoman, *Spike of Bensonhurst,* FilmDallas, 1988. Also appeared in *Shalimar,* 1978; and *Hammett,* Warner Brothers, 1982.

TELEVISION DEBUT—*The Bob Hope Show,* NBC, 1950. PRINCI-PAL TELEVISION APPEARANCES—Pilots: Sally Rogers, "Head of the Family," *Comedy Spot,* CBS, 1960. Episodic: As herself, "I Was Always Sylvia," *51st State,* PBS, 1974; mother, *The Equaliz-er,* CBS, 1986; Allison Kennedy, *Tattinger's,* NBC, 1988; also *Car 54, Where Are You?,* NBC; "Uncle Harry," *Play of the Week,* WNTA; *Route 66,* CBS; *The Defenders,* CBS; *The Mask,* ABC; *Naked City,* ABC; *CBS Workshop,* CBS; *Love of Life,* CBS; *The Edge of Night,* NBC; *U.S. Steel Hour,* CBS; *Sergeant Bilko,* CBS; *Search for Tomorrow,* CBS; *The Tonight Show,* NBC; *All My Children,* ABC; *The Sid Caesar Show,* ABC; *The Mike Douglas Show,* syndicated; *The Merv Griffin Show,* CBS; *The David Frost Show,* syndicated; *The Bob Hope Show,* NBC; *The Steve Allen Show,* NBC; *Girl Talk; The Doctors.* Specials: Sweet Susie, "Cindy Eller: A Modern Fairy Tale," *ABC Afterschool Special,* ABC, 1985.

RELATED CAREER—Member, Actors Studio, 1968—.

WRITINGS: STAGE—Book and lyrics, *It's Me, Sylvia!* (one-woman show), Playhouse Theatre II, New York City, 1981.

AWARDS: Academy Award nomination, Best Supporting Actress, 1970, for *Midnight Cowboy;* Academy Award nonimation, Best Supporting Actress, 1976, for *Farewell, My Lovely;* Society of West End Theatres Award nomination, Actress of the Year in a New Play, 1978, for *Vieux Carre.*

MEMBER: Screen Actors Guild, Actors' Equity Association, Ameri-can Federation of Radio and Television Artists, Manhattan Chess Club.

SIDELIGHTS: RECREATIONS—Chess (U.S. female champion-ship contender), antiquing and finishing furniture, carpentry, and construction of apartments.

ADDRESSES: AGENT—Milton Goldman, International Creative Management, 40 W. 57th Street, New York, NY 10019.*

                              *   *   *

MILLER, George

PERSONAL: Born in Australia.

VOCATION: Director, producer, and screenwriter.

CAREER: PRINCIPAL FILM WORK—All as director, unless indi-cated: First assistant director, *In Search of Anna,* Storm/Australian Film Commission/Victorian Film Corporation, 1978; associate producer and second unit director, *The Chain Reaction,* Columbia/EMI/Warner/Hoyts, 1980; *The Man from Snowy River,* Twentieth Century-Fox, 1981; *The Aviator,* Metro-Goldwyn-Mayer/United Artists, 1985; *Cool Change,* Hoyts, 1986; *Les Patterson Saves the World,* Hoyts, 1987. Also *The Year My Voice Broke,* 1987.

PRINCIPAL TELEVISION WORK—All as director, unless indicated. Mini-Series: (With Pino Amenta) *All the Rivers Run,* HBO, 1984; co-producer, *Vietnam,* Network Ten (Australia), 1987. Movies: *The Far Country,* Seven Network (Australia), 1987; *The Christmas Visitor,* Disney Channel, 1987; *Anzacs: The War Down Under,* syndicated, 1987; *Bushfire Moon,* Disney Channel, 1987. Also *Cash and Company, Against the Wind, The Last Outlaw,* and *Bodyline.*

WRITINGS: TELEVISION—*Bodyline.**

                              *   *   *

MILLER, George   1945-

PERSONAL: Born in Brisbane, Australia, March 3, 1945. EDUCA-TION: Received M.D. from the University of New South Wales.

VOCATION: Director, producer, and screenwriter.

CAREER: Also see *WRITINGS* below. FIRST FILM WORK—Direc-tor, *Violence in the Cinema: Part I* (short film), 1971. PRINCIPAL FILM WORK—All as director, unless indicated: *Mad Max,* Ameri-can International, 1979; associate producer, *Chain Reaction,* Hoyt Distribution, 1980; *The Road Warrior* (also known as *Mad Max II*), Warner Brothers, 1982; "Nightmare at 20,000 Feet," *Twilight Zone—The Movie,* Warner Brothers, 1983; (with George Ogilvie; also producer with Doug Mitchell and Terry Hayes) *Mad Max Beyond Thunderdome,* Warner Brothers, 1985; *The Witches of Eastwick,* Warner Brothers, 1987. Also director, *The Devil in Evening Dress* (documentary), 1973; and editor, *Frieze, an Under-ground Film* (short film), 1973.

PRINCIPAL TELEVISION WORK—Series: Executive producer, *The Dismissal,* 1982. Episodic: Director, *The Dismissal,* 1982.

RELATED CAREER—Jury president, Avoriaz Festival du film fantastique, 1983.

NON-RELATED CAREER—Physician, St. Vincent's Hospital, Sydney, Australia.

WRITINGS: See production credits above. (With Byron Kennedy) *Violence in the Cinema* (short film), 1971; *Devil in Evening Dress* (documentary), 1973; (with James McCausland) *Mad Max,* 1979; (with Terry Hayes and Brian Hannat) *The Road Warrior,* 1982; (with Hayes) *Mad Max Beyond Thunderdome,* 1985.

ADDRESSES: AGENT—Dale Olson, Dale Olson and Associates, 292 S. La Cienga Boulevard, Suite 315, Beverly Hills, CA 90211.*

MILLER, J.P. 1919-

PERSONAL: Full name, James P. Miller; born December 18, 1919, in San Antonio, TX; son of Rolland James (a builder) and Rose Jetta (Smith) Miller; married Ayers Elizabeth Fite (marriage ended); married Juanita Marie Currie (marriage ended); married Liane Nicolaus, October 18, 1964; children: James P., Jr. (first marriage); John R., Montgomery A. (second marriage); Lisa Marie, Anthony Milo, Sophie Jetta (third marriage). EDUCATION: Rice Institute (now Rice University), B.A., 1941; studied drama at Yale University, 1946-47, and with the American Theatre Wing. POLITICS: ''Non-aligned Centrist Humanist.'' MILITARY: U.S. Navy, lieutenant, 1941-46.

VOCATION: Writer.

CAREER: See *WRITINGS* below. RELATED CAREER—Creative writing teacher. NON-RELATED CAREER—Professional boxer under the name ''Ted Frontier.''

WRITINGS: FILM—*The Rabbit Trap*, United Artists, 1959; (with Edward Anhalt) *The Young Savages*, United Artists, 1961; *Days of Wine and Roses*, Warner Brothers, 1962; *Behold a Pale Horse*, Columbia, 1964; *The People Next Door*, AVCO-Embassy, 1970, published by Dell, 1970.

TELEVISION—Episodic: ''The Rabbit Test,'' *Philco TV Playhouse*, CBS, 1954; ''Days of Wine and Roses,'' *Playhouse 90*, CBS, 1958; ''The People Next Door,'' *CBS Television Playhouse*, CBS, 1968; also ''Hide and Seek,'' ''Old Tasslefoot,'' and ''The Pardon-Me Boy,'' all *Philco TV Playhouse*, CBS. Movies: *Your Money or Your Wife*, CBS, 1972; *The Lindbergh Kidnapping Case*, NBC, 1976; *Helter Skelter*, CBS, 1976; *Gauguin the Savage*, CBS, 1980. Also *The Preppie Killing* and *The Unwanted*.

OTHER—*The Race for Home* (novel), Dial, 1968; *Liv* (novel), Dial, 1973; *The Skook* (novel), Warner Books, 1984. Has also written short stories and poetry for periodicals.

AWARDS: Emmy Award, Outstanding Writing Achievement in Drama, 1969, for ''The People Next Door,'' *CBS Television Playhouse;* special award from the Mystery Writers of America, 1974, for *Your Money or Your Wife;* Emmy Award nomination, Outstanding Writing in a Special Program—Comedy or Drama (Original Teleplay), 1976, for *The Lindbergh Kidnapping Case.* Military honors: Presidential Unit Citation and Purple Heart.

MEMBER: Writers Guild, Dramatists Guild, P.E.N., Academy of Motion Picture Arts and Sciences.

ADDRESSES: HOME—Stockton, NJ.*

*   *   *

MILLER, Joan 1910-1988

PERSONAL: Born in 1910 in Nelson, BC, Canada; moved to England, 1935; died August 31, 1988, in London, England; daughter of Richard Wallace and Rhoda (Tingle) Miller; married John Godfrey (died); married Peter Cotes (a theatrical director), 1948.

VOCATION: Actress.

CAREER: STAGE DEBUT—*When Knights Were Bold*, Empress Theatre, Vancouver, BC, Canada, 1930. LONDON DEBUT—*Josephine*, His Majesty's Theatre, 1934. BROADWAY DEBUT—Julia Almond, *A Pin to See the Peepshow*, Playhouse Theatre, 1953. PRINCIPAL STAGE APPEARANCES—Mistress Quickly and Lady Tree (understudy), *Henry IV, Part I*, His Majesty's Theatre, London, 1935; May Stokes, *Golden Arrow*, Whitehall Theatre, London, 1935; the Maid, *The Soldier's Fortune*, Ambassadors' Theatre, London, 1935; Louise Michel, *The Tiger*, Embassy Theatre, London, 1936; Hennie Berger, *Awake and Sing*, Vaudeville Theatre, London, 1938; Eliza Doolittle, *Pygmalion*, Vaudeville Theatre, then Alexandra Theatre, Birmingham, U.K., both 1942; Rebecca West, *Rosmersholm*, Torch Theatre, London, 1945; Branwen Elder, *The Long Mirror*, and Eva, *For Services Rendered*, New Lindsey Theatre, London, 1946; Mrs. Collins, *Pick-Up Girl*, New Lindsey Theatre, then Prince of Wales' Theatre, London, both 1946, later Casino Theatre, London, 1947; Gisela Waldstein, *Dark Summer*, Lyric Hammersmith Theatre, London, 1947, then St. Martin's Theatre, London, 1948; Frances Shelley, *The Rising Wind*, Embassy Theatre, 1949; title role, *Miss Julie*, Lyric Hammersmith Theatre, 1949.

Helen Winthrop, *Birdcage*, People's Palace, London, 1950; Karen Wright, *The Children's Hour*, New Boltons Theatre, London, 1950; Mrs. Fitzgerald, *Loaves and Fishes*, Julia Almond, *A Pin to See the Peepshow*, Helen, *Mrs. Basil Farrington*, and Godiva, *The Importance of Wearing Clothes*, all New Boltons Theatre, 1951; Mrs. Gillis, *The Man*, Her Majesty's Theatre, London, 1952, then St. Martin's Theatre, 1953; Clara Dennison, *The Wooden Dish*, Phoenix Theatre, London, 1954; title role, *Medea*, Oxford Playhouse, Oxford, U.K., 1957; Constane, *King John*, Portia, *Julius Caesar*, the Queen, *Cymbeline*, and Juno, *The Tempest*, all Shakespeare Memorial Theatre Company, Shakespeare Memorial Theatre, Stratford-on-Avon, U.K., 1957; Nell Palmer, *Hot Summer Night*, New Theatre, London, 1958; Margaret Hyland, *The Rope Dancers*, Arts Theatre, London, 1959; Hannah Kingsley, QC, *Girl on the Highway*, Princes' Theatre, London, 1960; Helen Baird, *A Loss of Roses*, Pembroke Theatre, Croydon, U.K., 1962; Contessa Catherine Minadoli, *Hidden Stranger*, Longacre Theatre, New York City, 1963; *A Woman Alone* (one-woman show), Theatre Royal, Bristol, U.K., 1963; Nora Melody, *A Touch of the Poet*, Ashcroft Theatre, Croydon, U.K., 1963; Marya, *Uncle's Dream*, Phoenix Theatre, Leicester, U.K., 1965; Sally, *Staring at the Sun*, Vaudeville Theatre, 1968; Lucy Amorest, *The Old Ladies*, Yvonne Arnaud Theatre, Guildford, U.K., then Westminster Theatre, London, both 1969, later Duchess Theatre, London, 1970.

Mrs. Morland, *Mary Rose*, Yvonne Arnaud Theatre, 1971; Mrs. Warren, *Mrs. Warren's Profession*, Theatre Royal, York, U.K., 1972; Mrs. George, *Getting Married*, Theatre Royal, York, U.K., 1974; Madame Raquin, *Therese*, Yvonne Arnaud Theatre, 1974; title role, *The Dame of Sark*, Theatre Royal, York, U.K., 1976; Madame d'Alvarez, *Gigi*, Swan Theatre, Worcester, U.K., 1977; Judith Bliss, *Hay Fever*, Watermill Theatre, Newbury, U.K., 1977; Amanda Wingfield, *The Glass Menagerie*, Liverpool Playhouse, Liverpool, U.K., 1978. Also appeared in repertory at the Open Air Theatre, London, 1935; as Ella Rentheim, *John Gabriel Borkman*, and in *Candida*, both in Manchester, U.K., 1948; in *Candida*, New Boltons Theatre, 1951.

MAJOR TOURS—Lola, *Come Back, Little Sheba*, U.K. cities, 1952; Margaret Pardee, *The Odd Ones*, U.K. cities, 1963; Mrs. Laurentz, *So Wise, So Young*, U.K. cities, 1964; Lavinia Penniman, *The Heiress*, U.K. cities, 1975.

PRINCIPAL FILM APPEARANCES—Secretary, *Take It from Me* (also known as *Transatlantic Trouble*), Warner Brothers/First National, 1937; Vera, *Cry of the City*, Twentieth Century-Fox, 1948; reporter, *One Touch of Venus*, Universal, 1948; lush, *Criss Cross*, Universal, 1949; woman, *The Great Sinner*, Metro-Goldwyn-Mayer (MGM), 1949; Susan, *The Woman in the Hall*, General Films Distributors/Eagle-Lion, 1949; Claire, *Caged*, Warner Brothers, 1950; Mabel Spooner, *The Jackpot*, Twentieth Century-Fox, 1950; Mac, *Something for the Birds*, Twentieth Century-Fox, 1952; woman on the bridge, *The Story of Three Loves*, MGM, 1953; Barker, *Blonde Sinner* (also known as *Yield to the Night*), Allied Artists, 1956; Frank, *Over-Exposed*, Columbia, 1956; Mrs. Canaday, *Fire Down Below*, Columbia, 1957; Victor's wife, *Menace in the Night*, United Artists, 1958; Mrs. Collins, *Too Young to Love*, Rank, 1960; Mrs. Smith-Gould, *Heavens Above!*, British Lion/Romulus/Janus, 1963; Jess, *No Tree in the Street*, Seven Arts, 1964.

PRINCIPAL TELEVISION APPEARANCES—Series: *Picture Page Girl*, BBC, 1936. Specials: *Candida*, Australian television. Also title role, *Jane Clegg;* and in *Woman in a Dressing Gown.*

RELATED CAREER—Actress and writer for various radio productions.

WRITINGS: Television in the Making, 1956; *The Woman Poet,* 1977.

AWARDS: Bessborough Trophy from the Dominion Drama Festival, Best Actress, 1934.

MEMBER: Lansdowne Club.

SIDELIGHTS: FAVORITE ROLES—Rebecca West in *Rosmersholm.*

OBITUARIES AND OTHER SOURCES: Variety, September 7, 1988.*

*   *   *

MILNER, Martin   1931-

PERSONAL: Born December 28, 1931 (some sources say 1927 or 1932), in Detroit, MI. EDUCATION: Attended the University of Southern California. MILITARY: U.S. Army, 1952-54.

VOCATION: Actor.

CAREER: PRINCIPAL STAGE APPEARANCES—George, *Doubles,* tour of U.S. cities, 1986-87.

FILM DEBUT—John, *Life with Father,* Warner Brothers, 1947. PRINCIPAL FILM APPEARANCES—Private Mike McHugh, *The Sands of Iwo Jima,* Republic, 1949; Bob Stewart, *Louisa,* Universal, 1950; Bert, *Our Very Own,* RKO, 1950; Al Prescott, *Fighting Coast Guard,* Republic, 1951; Private Whitney, *The Halls of Montezuma,* Twentieth Century-Fox, 1951; George Kress, Jr., *I Want You,* RKO, 1951; Caldwell, *Operation Pacific,* Warner Brothers, 1951; Andy, *Battle Zone,* Allied Artists, 1952; Al Lynch, *Belles on Their Toes,* Twentieth Century-Fox, 1952; Phil Harding, *The Captive City,* United Artists, 1952; Billy Creel, *Last of the Comanches* (also known as *The Sabre and the Arrow*), Columbia, 1952; Buddy Chamberlain, *My Wife's Best Friend,* Twentieth Century-Fox, 1952; Olie Larsen, *Springfield Rifle,* Warner Broth-

ers, 1952; Elwood Halsey, *Destination Gobi,* Twentieth Century-Fox, 1953; Rick, *Francis in the Navy,* Universal, 1955; Jim O'Carberry, *The Long Gray Line,* Columbia, 1955; shore patrol officer, *Mister Roberts,* Warner Brothers, 1955; Joey Firestone, *Pete Kelly's Blues,* Warner Brothers, 1955; Lieutenant Morton Glenn, *On the Threshold of Space,* Twentieth Century-Fox, 1956; Corliss, *Screaming Eagles,* Allied Artists, 1956; Waco, *Pillars of the Sky* (also known as *The Tomahawk and the Cross*), Universal, 1956; James Earp, *Gunfight at the O.K. Corral,* Paramount, 1957; Ship Hamilton, *Man Afraid,* Universal, 1957; Steve Dallas, *Sweet Smell of Success,* United Artists, 1957; Wally, *Marjorie Morningstar,* Warner Brothers, 1958; Lincoln Forrester, *Too Much, Too Soon,* Warner Brothers, 1958; Sid, *Compulsion,* Twentieth Century-Fox, 1959.

George Barton, *Sex Kittens Go to College* (also known as *Beauty and the Robot* and *Beauty and the Brain*) Allied Artists, 1960; Ben Rush, *Thirteen Ghosts,* Columbia, 1960; (as Marty Milner) Ad Simms and Adam, *The Private Lives of Adam and Eve,* Universal, 1961; Dr. Del Hartwood, *Zebra in the Kitchen,* Metro-Goldwyn-Mayer, 1965; John Sullivan, Jr., *Sullivan's Empire,* Universal, 1967; Mel Anderson, *Valley of the Dolls,* Twentieth Century-Fox, 1967; MacMillan, *Three Guns for Texas,* Universal, 1968; Brian Davis, *Ski Fever* (also known as *Liebe Spiele im Schnee*), Allied Artists, 1979.

PRINCIPAL TELEVISION APPEARANCES—Series: Jimmy Clark, *The Stu Erwin Show,* ABC, 1954-55; Don Marshall, *The Life of Riley,* NBC, 1957-58; Tod Stiles, *Route 66,* CBS, 1960-64; Officer Pete Malloy, *Adam-12,* NBC, 1968-75; Karl Robinson, *Swiss Family Robinson,* ABC, 1975-76. Pilots: Joe Starr, *Starr, First Baseman,* CBS, 1965; Officer Pete Malloy, *Emergency!,* NBC, 1972; Karl Robinson, *Swiss Family Robinson,* ABC, 1975. Mini-Series: Tom Gray, *Black Beauty,* NBC, 1978; Sergeant Drabic, *The Last Convertible,* NBC, 1979. Episodic: Paul Grinstead, "Mirror Image," *The Twilight Zone,* CBS, 1960; guest host, *The Golddiggers,* syndicated, 1971; Sheriff Bodine, *Murder, She Wrote,* CBS, 1985; Turk Donner, *MacGyver,* NBC, 1988; Clint Phelps, *Murder, She Wrote,* CBS, 1988; also *Kraft Television Theatre,* NBC, 1949; as Kahuna, *Gidget,* ABC; Jimmy Clark, *The Trouble with Father,* ABC; *The Lone Ranger,* ABC; *The Dupont Show of the Week,* NBC; *TV Readers Digest,* ABC; *The Sheriff of Cochise,* syndicated; *Navy Log.* Movies: John Shedd, *Runaway!* (also known as *The Runaway Train*), ABC, 1973; Major Stoddard, *Hurricane,* ABC, 1974; Lyle Kingman, *SST: Death Flight* (also known as *SST: Disaster in the Sky*), ABC, 1977; Paul Blake, *Flood!,* NBC, 1978; Folsom, *Little Mo,* NBC, 1978; Dr. Denvers, *Crisis in Mid-Air,* CBS, 1979; Philip Kent, *The Seekers,* syndicated, 1979; Peter Belton, *The Ordeal of Bill Carney,* CBS, 1981. Specials: *The Rowan and Martin Special,* NBC, 1973. Also appeared in *True Confessions,* ABC, 1986.

RELATED CAREER—Director of training films for the U.S. Army, 1952-54.

ADDRESSES: AGENT—Agency for the Performing Arts, 9000 Sunset Boulevard, Suite 1200, Los Angeles, CA 90069.*

*   *   *

MILSTEAD, Harris Glenn   1945-1988
See DIVINE

MOKAE, Zakes   1935-

PERSONAL: Born August 5, 1935, in Johannesburg, South Africa. EDUCATION: Attended St. Peter's College; studied acting at the Royal Academy of Dramatic Art.

VOCATION: Actor and director.

CAREER: OFF-BROADWAY DEBUT—Old African, *Boesman and Lena,* Circle in the Square, 1969. PRINCIPAL STAGE APPEAR-ANCES—Waiter, *Fingernails as Blue as Flowers,* American Place Theatre, New York City, 1971; Firs, *The Cherry Orchard,* New York Shakespeare Festival, Public Theatre, New York City, 1973; Steve Daniels, *A Lesson from Aloes,* Playhouse Theatre, New York City, 1980; Sam, *Master Harold . . . and the boys,* Yale Repertory Theatre, New Haven, CT, 1981, then Lyceum Theatre, New York City, 1982, later Plaza Theatre, Dallas, TX, 1983; Zachariah, *The Blood Knot,* Yale Repertory Theatre, 1985, then John Golden Theatre, New York City, 1986; M. Gerard de Villefort, *The Count of Monte Cristo,* John F. Kennedy Center for the Performing Arts, Washington, DC, 1986. Also appeared as Zachariah, *Blood Knot,* West End production, London, 1961; at the Long Wharf Theatre, New Haven, CT, 1970-71; in *Boesman and Lena,* Trinity Square Repertory Company, Providence, RI, 1978; in *Boesman and Lena* and *An Attempt at Flying,* both Yale Repertory Theatre, 1980; in *Last Days of British Honduras,* American Place Theatre; in *Trial of Vessay,* New Dramatists, New York City; in *Lion and Jewel* and *Brother Jero,* both Inglewood Playhouse, Inglewood, CA; and in productions of *Othello, Macbeth, Waiting for Godot, Krapp's Last Tape, Tall Maidens, No Good Friday,* and *The Tempest,* all in Europe.

PRINCIPAL STAGE WORK—Director, *Boesman and Lena,* in Canada; director, *Angel Feathers on the Roof,* in Johannesburg, South Africa; director, *I'm a Come Home Chile,* in London.

PRINCIPAL FILM APPEARANCES—Michel, *The Comedians,* Metro-Goldwyn-Mayer, 1967; Father Kani, *Cry Freedom,* Universal, 1987; Dargent Peytraud, *The Serpent and the Rainbow,* Universal, 1988. Also appeared in *Darling,* Embassy, 1965; *The River Niger,* Cine Artists, 1976; *The Island,* Universal, 1980; *Roar,* 1981; and in *Tremor, Dilemma, Legends of Fear,* and *Darkest Africa.*

PRINCIPAL TELEVISION APPEARANCES—Movies: Pee Wee Parker, *One in a Million: The Ron LeFlore Story,* CBS, 1978; Captain Daventry, *Agatha Christie's "A Caribbean Mystery,"* CBS, 1983. Specials: *Master Harold . . . and the boys,* Showtime, 1984; also Zachariah, *The Blood Knot,* BBC.

RELATED CAREER—Teacher, American Conservatory Theatre, San Francisco, CA; directing fellow, American Film Institute.

AWARDS: Antoinette Perry Award, Best Actor in a Play, 1982, for *Master Harold . . . and the boys.*

MEMBER: British Drama League.*

MONTAGUE, Lee   1927-

PERSONAL: Born October 16, 1927, in London, England; married Ruth Goring. EDUCATION: Trained for the stage at the Old Vic Theatre School, London, 1948-50.

VOCATION: Actor.

CAREER: STAGE DEBUT—*Twelfth Night,* Old Vic Theatre, London, 1950. BROADWAY DEBUT—Gregory Hawke, *The Climate of Eden,* Martin Beck Theatre, 1952. PRINCIPAL STAGE APPEAR-ANCES—Usumcasane, *Tamburlaine the Great,* Edmund, *King Lear,* and Flaminius, *Timon of Athens,* all Old Vic Theatre, London, 1951-52; Ben, *Love for Love,* Bristol Old Vic Company, Bristol Old Vic Theatre, Bristol, U.K., 1953; the Dauphin, *Henry V,* Bristol Old Vic Company, Bristol Old Vic Theatre, then Old Vic Theatre, London, both 1953; Francis X. Gibbons, *Mrs. Gibbons' Boys,* Westminster Theatre, London, 1956; Demetrius, *Titus Andronicus,* Stoll Theatre, London, 1957; Rocky Pioggi, *The Iceman Cometh,* Arts Theatre, then Winter Garden Theatre, both London, 1958; Shylock, *The Merchant of Venice,* and Face, *The Alchemist,* both Old Vic Theatre, London, 1962; Angelo, *Measure for Measure,* Old Vic Theatre, London, 1963; Charles Smith, *Meals on Wheels,* Royal Court Theatre, London, 1965; Ed, *Entertaining Mr. Sloan,* Lyceum Theatre, New York City, 1965; Irving Spaatz, *The Latent Heterosexual,* Aldwych Theatre, London, 1968; Iago, *Othello,* Oxford Playhouse, Oxford, U.K., 1970; Lopakhin, *The Cherry Orchard,* Oxford Playhouse, 1971; title role, *Volpone,* and Grigory Charnota, *Flight,* both Bristol Old Vic Company, Bristol Old Vic Theatre, 1972; Jack Rawlings, *Who Saw Him Die?,* Royal Haymarket Theatre, London, 1974; title role, *The Father,* Stratford East Theatre, London, 1976; Dr. Prentice, *What the Butler Saw,* and Mr. Antrobus, *The Skin of Our Teeth,* both Royal Exchange Theatre, Manchester, U.K., 1977; O'Connor, *Cause Celebre,* Her Majesty's Theatre, London, 1977; Barney Cashman, *Last of the Red Hot Lovers,* Royal Exchange Company, Criterion Theatre, London, 1979.

MAJOR TOURS—The Dauphin, *Henry V,* Bristol Old Vic Company, Swiss cities, 1953; Iago, *Othello,* U.K. cities, 1970; Lopakhin, *The Cherry Orchard,* U.K. cities, 1971; Jack Rawlings, *Who Killed Jack Robin?,* U.K. cities, 1972.

FILM DEBUT—Maurice Joyant, *Moulin Rouge,* United Artists, 1952. PRINCIPAL FILM APPEARANCES—Miguel's mate, *The Silent Enemy,* Universal, 1959; Michael, *Another Sky,* Harrison, 1960; Sergeant Farrow, *Chance Meeting* (also known as *Blind Date*), Paramount, 1960; Aberle, *Foxhole in Cairo,* British Lion, 1960; Itti, *The Savage Innocents,* Paramount, 1960; Tim Jordan, *The Man at the Carlton Tower,* Anglo Amalgamated, 1961; Detective Inspector Henderson, *The Secret Partner* (also known as *The Street Partner*), Metro-Goldwyn-Mayer, 1961; Pepe, *The Singer, Not the Song,* Warner Brothers, 1961; Squeak, *Billy Budd,* United Artists, 1962; Miklos Tabori, *Operation Snatch,* Continental Distributing, 1962; Larry Hart, *Five to One,* Allied Artists, 1963; Levy, *The Secret of Blood Island,* Universal, 1965; Staff Sergeant Mansfield, *You Must Be Joking!,* Columbia, 1965; Box, *Deadlier Than the Male,* Universal, 1967; Sergeant Transom, *How I Won the War,* United Artists, 1967; Denzil, *The High Commissioner* (also known as *Nobody Runs Forever*), Cinerama, 1968; Cipriani, *Eagle in a Cage,* National General, 1971; Father, *Brother Sun, Sister Moon,* Paramount, 1973; Bernhard Mahler, *Mahler,* Visual Programme Systems, 1974; Lucky Luciano, *Brass Target,* United Artists, 1978; Jacques, *The Legacy* (also known as *The Legacy of Maggie Walsh*), Universal, 1979; Jack Freeman, *Silver Dream Racer,* Almi

Films, 1982; Lee, *Red Monarch,* Goldcrest, 1983; Renard, *Lady Jane,* Paramount, 1986; also appeared in *A London Affair.*

PRINCIPAL TELEVISION APPEARANCES—Series: *Feet First.* Mini-Series: Uncle Sasha, *Holocaust,* NBC, 1978. Episodic: *Space: 1999,* syndicated, 1977. Movies: Igor, *The Spy Killer,* ABC, 1969; Habbukuk, *Jesus of Nazareth,* NBC, 1977; Kozelski, *Kim,* CBS, 1984; Marshal Konev, *Pope John Paul II,* CBS, 1984; Slavsky, *Sakharov,* HBO, 1984. Also appeared in *Eleanor Marx, Darwin's Dream,* and *Comrades.*

SIDELIGHTS: FAVORITE ROLES—Iago in *Othello,* Face in *The Alchemist,* Irving Spaatz in *The Latent Heterosexual,* and Barney Cashman in *Last of the Red Hot Lovers.* RECREATIONS—Squash, bridge, music, tennis, and travel.*

*   *   *

MORANIS, Rick

PERSONAL: Born April 18, in Toronto, ON, Canada.

VOCATION: Actor, director, writer, and comedian.

CAREER: Also see *WRITINGS* below. FILM DEBUT—Bob McKenzie, *Strange Brew,* Metro-Goldwyn-Mayer/United Artists, 1983. PRINCIPAL FILM APPEARANCES—Louis Tully, *Ghostbusters,* Columbia, 1984; Billy Fish, *Streets of Fire,* Universal/RKO, 1984; Harry, *The Wild Life,* Universal, 1984; Morty King, *Brewster's Millions,* Universal, 1985; Gross, *Head Office,* Tri-Star, 1985; Barry Nye, *Club Paradise,* Warner Brothers, 1986; Seymour Krelborn, *Little Shop of Horrors,* Warner Brothers, 1986; Lord Dark Helmet, *Spaceballs,* Metro-Goldwyn-Mayer/United Artists, 1987.

PRINCIPAL FILM WORK—Director (with Dave Thomas), *Strange Brew,* Metro-Goldwyn-Mayer/United Artists, 1983.

PRINCIPAL TELEVISION APPEARANCES—Series: Regular, *Second City TV,* syndicated, 1980-81; regular, *SCTV Network 90,* NBC, 1981-82. Pilots: Regular, *Twilight Theatre II,* NBC, 1982. Episodic: Coach Willi Liepert, "Hockey Night," *Wonderworks,* PBS, 1987. Specials: Doug McKenzie, *A Funny Thing Happened on the Way to the Olympics,* City-TV (Canada), 1988; also *The Last Polka,* HBO, 1985.

RELATED CAREER—Radio engineer, writer, then performer on his own radio show, Toronto, ON, Canada; performed comedy routines in nightclubs and cabarets in Canada.

WRITINGS: FILM—(With Dave Thomas and Steven DeJarnatt) *Strange Brew,* Metro-Goldwyn-Mayer/United Artists, 1983. TELEVISION—Series: *Second City TV,* syndicated, 1980-81; *SCTV Network 90,* NBC, 1981-82. Specials: (With Thomas) *A Funny Thing Happened on the Way to the Olympics,* City-TV (Canada), 1988.

RECORDINGS: ALBUMS—(With Dave Thomas, as Bob and Doug McKenzie) *Great White North,* Mercury, 1981; (with Thomas, as Bob and Doug McKenzie) *Strange Brew* (original soundtrack), Mercury, 1983. SINGLES—(With Thomas, as Bob and Doug McKenzie) "Take Off," Mercury, 1981.

AWARDS: Emmy Award, Best Writing for a Comedy Program, 1982, for *SCTV Network 90;* Grammy Award nomination (with Dave Thomas), Best Comedy Album of the Year, for *Great White North.*

ADDRESSES: AGENT—John Gaines, Agency for the Performing Arts, 9000 Sunset Boulevard, Los Angeles, CA 90069.*

*   *   *

MORGENSTERN, S.
See GOLDMAN, William

*   *   *

MORLEY, Robert 1908-

PERSONAL: Full name, Robert Adolph Wilton Morley; born May 26, 1908, in Semley, England; son of Robert Wilton (an officer in the British Army) and Gertrude Emily (Fass) Morley; married Joan Buckmaster, 1940; children: Sheridan, Annbel, Wilton. EDUCATION: Attended Wellington College; trained for the stage at the Royal Academy of Dramatic Art.

VOCATION: Actor, director, producer, and writer.

CAREER: Also see *WRITINGS* below. STAGE DEBUT—*Dr. Syn,* Hippodrome Theatre, Margate, U.K., 1928. LONDON DEBUT—Pirate, *Treasure Island,* Strand Theatre, 1929. BROADWAY DEBUT—Title role, *Oscar Wilde,* Fulton Theatre, 1938. PRINCIPAL STAGE APPEARANCES—Oakes, *Up in the Air,* Royalty Theatre, London, 1933; title role, *Oscar Wilde,* Gate Theatre, London, 1936; Alexandre Dumas, *The Great Romancer,* Strand Theatre, then New Theatre, both London, 1937; Henry Higgins, *Pygmalion,* Old Vic Theatre, London, 1937; Decius Hess, *Play with Fire* (also known as *The Shop at Sly Corner*), Theatre Royal, Brighton, U.K., 1941; Sheridan Whiteside, *The Man Who Came to Dinner,* Savoy Theatre, London, 1941; Prince Regent of England, *The First Gentleman,* New Theatre, 1945, then Savoy Theatre, 1946; Arnold Holt, *Edward, My Son,* His Majesty's Theatre, London, 1947, then Martin Beck Theatre, New York City, 1948; Philip, *The Little Hut,* Lyric Theatre, London, 1950; title role, *Hippo Dancing,* Lyric Theatre, 1954; Oswald Petersham, *A Likely Tale,* Globe Theatre, London, 1956; Panisse, *Fanny,* Drury Lane Theatre, London, 1956; Sebastian Le Boeuf, *Hook, Line, and Sinker,* Piccadilly Theatre, London, 1958; Mr. Asano, *A Majority of One,* Phoenix Theatre, London, 1960; title role, *Mr. Rhodes,* Theatre Royal, Windsor, U.K., 1961; the Bishop, *A Time to Laugh,* Piccadilly Theatre, 1962; *An Evening with Robert Morley* (one-man show), 92nd Street YM-YWHA, New York City, 1964; Prince Regent, *Son et lumiere* (pageant), Royal Pavilion Grounds, Brighton, U.K., 1965; Sir Mallalieu Fitzbuttress, *Halfway up the Tree,* Queen's Theatre, London, 1967; Frank Foster, *How the Other Half Loves,* Lyric Theatre, 1970; Barnstable, *A Ghost on Tiptoe,* Savoy Theatre, 1974; Pound, *Banana Ridge,* Savoy Theatre, 1976; Hilary, *The Old Country,* Theatre Royal, Sydney, Australia, 1980. Also appeared as Henry Dewlip, *Springtime for Henry,* Perranporth, U.K., 1939; in repertory at the Oxford Playhouse, Oxford, U.K., 1931; at the Cambridge Arts Festival, Cambridge, U.K., 1933; and in Perranporth, U.K., 1935.

PRINCIPAL STAGE WORK—Producer (with H.M. Tennent, Ltd.), *A Likely Tale,* Globe Theatre, London, 1956; director, *The Full Treatment,* Q Theatre, London, 1957; director, *The Tunnel of Love,* Her Majesty's Theatre, London, 1957; director, *Once More, with Feeling,* New Theatre, London, 1959. Also director at the Cambridge Arts Festival, Cambridge, U.K., 1933.

MAJOR TOURS—Assistant stage manager, *And So to Bed,* U.K. cities, 1930; Reverend Vernon Isopod, *Late Night Final,* U.K. cities, renamed *Five Star Final,* U.S. cities, both 1934; Gloucester, *Richard of Bordeaux,* U.K. cities, 1935; Sheridan Whiteside, *The Man Who Came to Dinner,* U.K. cities, 1943; Charles, *Staff Dance,* U.K. cities, 1944; Arnold Holt, *Edward, My Son,* Australian and New Zealand cities, 1949-50; *The Sound of Morley* (one-man show), Australian cities, 1966-67; Frank Foster, *How the Other Half Loves,* U.S. and Canadian cities, 1972, then Australian cities, 1973; *Robert Morley Talks to Everyone* (one-man show), U.K. cities, 1978; also with H.V. Nielson's Shakespearean company, U.K. cities, 1934; and in *Picture of Innocence,* Canadian cities, 1978.

FILM DEBUT—Louis XVI, *Marie Antoinette,* Metro-Goldwyn-Mayer, 1938. PRINCIPAL FILM APPEARANCES—Tom Barrett/ Leslie Stuart, *You Will Remember,* British Lion, 1941; Andrew Undershaft, *Major Barbara,* United Artists, 1941; Von Geiselbrecht, *The Big Blockade,* Ealing, 1942; Van Der Stuyl, *This Was Paris* (also known as *So This Was Paris*), Warner Brothers, 1942; Charles James Fox, *The Young Mr. Pitt,* Twentieth Century-Fox, 1942; French mayor, *Somewhere in France* (also known as *The Foreman Went to France*), United Artists, 1943; Duke of Exmoor, *A Yank in London* (also known as *I Live in Grosvenor Square*), Twentieth Century-Fox, 1946; General Burlap, *Ghosts in Berkeley Square,* British National, 1947; Arnold Holt, *Edward, My Son,* Metro-Goldwyn-Mayer (MGM), 1949; minister, *Hour of Glory* (also known as *The Small Back Room*), British Lion, 1949.

Reverend Samuel Sayer, *The African Queen,* United Artists, 1951; Harry, *Curtain Up,* Rank/General Films Distributors, 1952; Mr. Almayer, *Outcasts of the Islands,* British Lion, 1952; Peterson, *Beat the Devil,* United Artists, 1953; Alexander Whitehead, *The Final Test,* General Films Distributors, 1953; W.S. Gilbert, *Gilbert and Sullivan* (also known as *The Great Gilbert and Sullivan*), United Artists, 1953; Oscar Hammerstein, *Melba,* United Artists, 1953; King George III, *Beau Brummell,* MGM, 1954; Sir Francis Ravenscourt, *The Good Die Young,* United Artists/International Films, 1954; Lord Logan, *The Rainbow Jacket,* General Films Distributors, 1954; King Louis XI, *Quentin Durward* (also known as *The Adventures of Quentin Durward*), MGM, 1955; Ralph, *Around the World in Eighty Days,* United Artists, 1956; Druether, *Loser Takes All,* British Lion, 1956; Sir Ralph Bloomfield-Bonington, *The Doctor's Dilemma,* MGM, 1958; Sir Edward Crichton, *Law and Disorder,* Continental, 1958; Uncle Lucius, *The Sheriff of Fractured Jaw,* Twentieth Century-Fox, 1958; Hugh Deverill, *The Journey,* MGM, 1959; Sir Wilfred, *Libel,* MGM, 1959.

Robert MacPherson, *The Battle of the Sexes,* Continental, 1960; title role, *Oscar Wilde,* Four City, 1960; Montgomery, *The Boys,* Gala, 1962; Arson Eddie, *Go to Blazes,* Warner Brothers/Pathe, 1962; the Leader, *The Road to Hong Kong,* United Artists, 1962; Potiphar, *The Story of Joseph and His Brethren* (also known as *Joseph and His Brethren* and *Joseph Sold by His Brothers*), Colorama/CAP, 1962; Hamilton Black, *Wonderful to Be Young!* (also known as *The Young Ones*), Paramount, 1962; Colonel Conliffe, *Agent 8 3/4* (also known as *Hot Enough for June*),

Continental, 1963; Hector Enderby, *Murder at the Gallop,* MGM, 1963; P.K. Mussadi, *Nine Hours to Rama* (also known as *Nine Hours to Live*), Twentieth Century-Fox, 1963; Roderick Femm, *The Old Dark House,* Columbia, 1963; Pope-Jones, *Take Her, She's Mine,* Twentieth Century-Fox, 1963; Colonel Whitforth, *Ladies Who Do,* Continental, 1964; Dr. Jacobs, *Of Human Bondage,* MGM, 1964; Cedric Page, *Topkapi,* United Artists, 1964; Tiffield, *Life at the Top,* Columbia, 1965; Sir Ambrose Abercrombie, *The Loved One,* MGM, 1965; Emperor of China, *Genghis Khan,* Columbia, 1965; Lord Rawnsley, *Those Magnificent Men in Their Flying Machines, or How I Flew from London to Paris in 25 Hours and 11 Minutes* (also known as *Those Magnificent Men in Their Flying Machines*), Twentieth Century-Fox, 1965; Hastings, *The Alphabet Murders* (also know as *The ABC Murders*), MGM, 1966; Colonel Roberts, *Finders Keepers,* United Artists, 1966; Henri Cot, *Hotel Paradiso,* MGM, 1966; Mycroft Holmes, *A Study in Terror* (also known as *Sherlock Holmes Grosster Falls* and *Fog*), Columbia, 1966; Harold Quonset, *Way . . . Way Out,* Twentieth Century-Fox, 1966; Lord Swift, *Tender Scoundrel* (also known as *Tender voyou* and *Un avventuriero a Tahiti*), Embassy, 1967; Dr. Xavier, *Woman Times Seven,* Embassy, 1967; Caesar Smith, *Hot Millions,* MGM, 1968; Duke of Argyll, *Sinful Davey,* United Artists, 1969; Miss Mary, *Some Girls Do,* United Artists, 1969; Hubert Hamlyn, *The Trygon Factor,* Warner Brothers, 1969.

Earl of Manchester, *Cromwell,* Columbia, 1970; Captain George Spratt, *Doctor in Trouble,* Rank, 1970; Berg, *Song of Norway,* Cinerama, 1970; Judge Roxburgh, *Lola* (also known as *Twinky*), American International, 1971; Sir Arthur Arnold-Jones, *When Eight Bells Toll,* Cinerama, 1971; Meredith Merridew, *Theatre of Blood,* United Artists, 1973; Pumblechook, *Great Expectations,* Transcontinental, 1975; Father Time, *The Blue Bird,* Twentieth Century-Fox, 1976; voice characterization, *Hugo the Hippo* (animated), Twentieth Century-Fox, 1976; Max, *Who Is Killing the Great Chefs of Europe?* (also known as *Someone Is Killing the Great Chefs of Europe* and *Too Many Chefs*), Warner Brothers, 1978; Percival, *The Human Factor,* Metro-Goldwyn-Mayer/ United Artists, 1979; Bernstein, *Scavenger Hunt,* Twentieth Century-Fox, 1979; Bernie, *Oh, Heavenly Dog!,* Twentieth Century-Fox, 1980; Godfrey, *Loophole,* Brent Walker, 1981; Bentik, *High Road to China,* Warner Brothers, 1983; God, *Second Time Lucky,* United International, 1984; Lord Decimus Barnacle, *Little Dorrit,* Sands Film/Cannon Screen Entertainment, 1987; Angus Watking, *The Trouble with Spies,* De Laurentiis Entertainment Group/Home Box Office, 1987; Elias Appleby, *The Wind,* Omega, 1987. Also appeared in *The Great Muppet Caper,* Universal, 1981.

PRINCIPAL TELEVISION APPEARANCES—Series: *Charge,* BBC, 1952; *Bringing Up Parents,* BBC, 1952. Mini-Series: Alistair Tudsbury, *War and Remembrance,* ABC, 1988-89. Episodic: Arnold Holt, "Edward, My Son," *U.S. Steel Hour,* CBS, 1955; "An Evening with Robert Morley," *The Creative Urge,* BBC-2, 1965; also "Misalliance," *Playhouse 90,* CBS, 1959; "Oliver Twist," *Dupont Show of the Month,* CBS, 1959; "Heaven Can Wait," *Dupont Show of the Month,* CBS, 1960; *The Bluffers,* NBC, 1971; *Alfred Hitchcock Presents,* CBS; *Dick Powell Theatre,* NBC; *Espionage,* NBC; *The Jack Paar Show,* NBC; *The Danny Kaye Show,* CBS; *The Today Show,* NBC; *The Mike Douglas Show,* syndicated; *The David Susskind Show,* syndicated; *Book Beat,* PBS; *The Festival of Performing Arts,* WNEW (New York). Movies: Pumblechook, *Great Expectations,* NBC, 1974; King of Hearts, *Alice in Wonderland,* CBS, 1985. Specials: *The Jo Stafford Show,* syndicated, 1964; host, *Golden Drama Special,* ATV, 1965; Bernard Laroque, *Deadly Game,* HBO, 1982.

PRINCIPAL TELEVISION WORK—Series: Producer, *Captain Gallant;* producer, *Scene of the Crime;* producer and director, *Closeup.* Also executive producer (with Leon Fromkess), *The Long Corridor.*

RELATED CAREER—Founder (with Peter Bull) of a repertory company, Perranporth, U.K., 1935; appeared in cabaret at Cafe de Paris, London, 1957, and the Mandarin, Hong Kong, 1976; also advisor, Telepictures of Morocco; advisor, Telerama, Ltd.; producer, Telerama, Inc.; producer, Georgetown Films, Inc.; founder, Alliance of Television Film Producers; president, Creative Association, Inc.; commercial spokesperson for British Airways.

WRITINGS: STAGE—*Short Story,* Queen's Theatre, London, 1935, then Heckscher Theatre, New York City, 1940, published by H.F.W. Deane, 1936; *Goodness, How Sad!,* Vaudeville Theatre, London, 1938, published by English Theatre Guild, 1939; *Staff Dance,* first produced on a tour of U.K. cities, 1944; (with Noel Langley) *Edward, My Son,* His Majesty's Theatre, 1947, then Martin Beck Theatre, 1948, published by Samuel French, Inc., 1948; (adaptor) *Hippo Dancing,* Lyric Theatre, London, 1954; (with Ronald Gow) *The Full Treatment,* Q Theatre, London, 1957; (with Dundas Hamilton) *Six Months' Grace,* Phoenix Theatre, London, 1957; (adaptor) *Hook, Line, and Sinker,* Piccadilly Theatre, London, 1958; (with Rosemary Ann Sisson) *A Ghost on Tiptoe,* Savoy Theatre, London, 1974; (co-writer) *Picture of Innocence,* first produced on a tour of Canadian cities, 1978.

OTHER—*A Musing Morely,* Robson Books, 1974, published in the United States as *The Robert Morley Bedside Reader,* Regnery, 1976; *Morley Marvels,* Robson Books, 1976, published in the United States by Barnes, 1979; *Robert Morley's Book of Bricks,* Weidenfeld and Nicolson, 1978; *Robert Morley's Book of Worries,* Weidenfeld and Nicolson, 1979; *Pardon Me, But You're Eating My Doily and Other Embarrassing Moments of Famous People,* St. Martin's Press, 1983; also (with Sewell Stokes) *Robert Morley: A Responsible Gentleman* (autobiography), 1966, published in the United States as *Robert Morley: A Reluctant Autobiography,* 1967; *More Morely,* 1978; *Morley Matters,* 1980; *Robert Morley's Second Book of Bricks,* 1981; *The Best of Robert Morley,* 1981. Also writer of poetry, articles, and short stories.

AWARDS: Academy Award nomination, Best Supporting Actor, 1938, for *Marie Antoinette;* Delia Austrian Medal from the Drama League of New York, 1949, for *Edward, My Son;* Commander of the Order of the British Empire, 1957. Honorary degrees: D.Litt., Reading University, 1979.

MEMBER: British Actors' Equity Association, Garrick Club, Buck's Club.

SIDELIGHTS: RECREATIONS—Conversation and horse racing.

ADDRESSES: HOME—Fairmans Cottage, Wargrave, Berkshire, England. OFFICE—London Management, 235 Regent Street, London W1, England.*

*   *   *

MORRICONE, Ennio   1928-
(Leo Nichols)

PERSONAL: Born November 10, 1928, in Rome, Italy. EDUCATION: Studied with Goffredo Petrassi at the Academy of Santa Cecilia.

VOCATION: Composer, music director, orchestrator, and conductor.

CAREER: Also see WRITINGS below. PRINCIPAL FILM WORK—All as music director, unless indicated: *Le Monachine* (also known as *The Little Nuns*), 1963, released in the United States by Embassy, 1965; *Once Upon a Time in the West* (also known as *C'era una volta il west*), 1968, released in the United States by Paramount, 1969; *Hornets' Nest,* United Artists, 1970; *My Name Is Nobody* (also known as *Il mio nome e nessuno*), 1973, released in the United States by Universal, 1974; music conductor, *The End of the Game* (also known as *Murder on the Bridge* and *Der Richter und Sein Henker*), 1975, released in the United States by Twentieth Century-Fox, 1975; *Exorcist II: The Heretic,* Warner Brothers, 1977; *Orca* (also known as *La Orca* and *Orca—Killer Whale*), Paramount, 1977; *Days of Heaven,* Paramount, 1978; (also music conductor) *Bloodline* (also known as *Sidney Sheldon's "Bloodline"*), Paramount, 1979; *The Island,* Universal, 1980; *La Cage aux folles II,* United Artists, 1981; *Il miestero della quattro corona* (also known as *Treasure of the Four Crowns* and *El tesora de las cuatro coronas*), Cannon, 1983; *La Chiave* (also known as *The Key*), 1983, released in the United States by Enterprise, 1985; *Sahara,* Metro-Goldwyn-Mayer/United Artists, 1984; *La Cage aux folles III: The Wedding,* Warner Brothers/Columbia/Tri-Star, 1985; (also orchestrator) *The Mission,* Warner Brothers, 1986; (also orchestrator) *The Untouchables,* Warner Brothers, 1987; (also music conductor and orchestrator) *Frantic,* Warner Brothers, 1988; *A Time of Destiny,* Columbia, 1988. Also music director for *Centomila dollari per Ringo,* 1965; *Quien sabe?* (also known as *A Bullet for the General*), 1966; and *Gentleman Jo . . . uccidi,* 1967.

WRITINGS: FILM—All as composer. Scores: *Il federale* (also known as *The Fascist*), 1961, released in the United States by Embassy, 1965; *Diciotteni al sole* (also known as *Eighteen in the Sun* and *Beach Party Italian Style*), 1962, released in the United States by Goldstone, 1964; *La Voglia matta* (also known as *Crazy Desire*), 1962, released in the United States by Embassy, 1964; *Le monachine* (also known as *The Little Nuns*), 1963, released in the United States by Embassy, 1965; *I malamondo* (also known as *Malamondo*), Titanis, 1964; (as Leo Nichols) *A Fistful of Dollars* (also known as *Per un pugno di dollari*), 1964, released in the United States by United Artists, 1964; (with Gino Paoli) *Before the Revolution* (also known as *Prima della revoluzione*), 1964, released in the United States by New Yorker, 1964; *I marziani hanno dodici mani* (also known as *Siammo quattro marziani, Llegaron los marcianos,* and *The Twelve-Handed Men of Mars*), 1964, released in the United States by Epoca, 1964; *I pugni in tasca* (also known as *Fist in the Pocket* and *Fists in the Pocket*), 1964, released in the United States by Peppercorn-Wormser, 1968.

El Greco, Twentieth Century-Fox, 1965; *Amanti d'oltretomba* (also known as *Nightmare Castle, Night of the Doomed, The Faceless Monsters,* and *Lovers from Beyond the Tomb*), 1965, released in the United States by Allied Artists, 1966; *For a Few Dollars More* (also known as *Per qualche dollaro in piu*), 1965, released in the United States by United Artists, 1967; *The Good, the Bad, and the Ugly* (also known as *Il buono, il brutto, il cattivo*), 1966, released in the United States by United Artists, 1966; (with Gino Pontecorvo) *La battaglia di Algeri* (also known as *The Battle of Algiers*), 1966, released in the United States by Rizzoli, 1967; *Uccelacci e uccellini* (also known as *The Hawks and the Sparrows*), 1966, released in the United States by Brandon, 1967; (with Piero Piccioni and Gino Marinuzzi, Jr.) *Matchless,* 1966, released in the United States by United Artists, 1967; (as Leo Nichols) *Navajo Joe* (also known as *Un dollaro a testa* and *Joe, El implacable*), 1966, released in the United States by United Artists, 1967; *Up the

MacGregors (also known as *Sette donne per i MacGregor* and *Siete mujeres para los MacGregor*), 1966, released in the United States by Columbia, 1967; *Lutring . . . reveille-toi et meurs* (also known as *Svegliati e uccidi [Lutring]* and *Wake Up and Die*), 1966, released in the United States by Rizzoli, 1967; *Seven Guns for the MacGregors* (also known as *Sette pistole per i MacGregor* and *Siete pistolas para los MacGregor*), 1966, released in the United States by Columbia, 1968.

Operation Kid Brother (also known as *O.K. Connery*), United Artists, 1967; *The Rover* (also known as *The L' aventuriero* and *The Adventurer*), Cinerama, 1967; *La ragazza e il generale* (also known as *The Girl and the General*), 1967, released in the United States by Metro-Goldwyn-Mayer (MGM), 1967; (with Piccioni) *Le streghe* (also known as *The Witches*), 1967, released in the United States by Lopert, 1967; *Da uomo a uomo* (also known as *Death Rides a Horse*), 1967, released in the United States by United Artists, 1967; (as Leo Nichols) *I crudeli* (also known as *The Hellbenders*), 1967, released in the United States by Embassy, 1967; *La resa dei conti* (also known as *The Big Gundown*), 1967, released in the United States by Columbia, 1968; *La Cina e vicina* (also known as *China Is Near*), 1967, released in the United States by Royal Films International, 1968; *Ad ogni costo* (also known as *Grand Slam, Top Job,* and *Diamantes a go-go*) 1967, released in the United States by Paramount, 1968; *La Bataille de San Sebastian* (also known as *Guns for San Sebastian, Los canones de San Sebastian,* and *I cannoni di San Sebastian*), 1967, released in the United States by MGM, 1968; *Arabella,* 1967, released in the United States by Universal, 1969.

Danger: Diabolik (also known as *Diabolik*), Paramount, 1968; *Galileo,* Fenice Cinematografica/Rizzoli/Kinozenter, 1968; *Ruba al prossimo tuo* (also known as *Una coppia tranquilla* and *A Fine Pair*), 1968, released in the United States by National General, 1969; *Gospodjica Doktor—Spijunka bez imena* (also known as *Fraulein Doktor*), 1968, released in the United States by Paramount, 1969; *Scusi, facciamo l'amore?* (also known as *Et Si on faisait l'amour?* and *Listen, Let's Make Love*), 1968, released in the United States by Lopert, 1969; *Once Upon a Time in the West* (also known as *C'era una volta il west*), 1968, released in the United States by Paramount, 1969; *Teorema* (also known as *Theorem*), 1968, released in the United States by Continental Distributing, 1969; *Grazia, zia* (also known as *Thank You, Aunt* and *Come Play with Me*), 1968, released in the United States by AVCO-Embassy, 1969; *La monaca di Monza* (also known as *Una storia Lombarda, The Lady of Monza,* and *The Nun of Monza*), 1968, released in the United States by Tower, 1970; (with Bruno Nicolai) *Il mercenario* (also known as *Salario para matar* and *The Mercenary*), 1968, released in the United States by United Artists, 1970; *Un tranquillo posto di campagna* (also known as *Un Tranquille a la campagne* and *A Quiet Place in the Country*), 1968, released in the United States by Lopert, 1970; (with Bruno Nicolai) *La dalle ardenne all' inferno* (also known as *Dirty Heroes*), 1968, released in the United States by Golden Eagle, 1971; *Un Bellissima novembre* (also known as *That Splendid November*), 1968, released in the United States by United Artists, 1971; *Gli intoccabili* (also known as *Machine Gun McCain*), 1969, released in the United States by Columbia, 1969; *The Bird with the Crystal Plumage* (also known as *L'ucello dalle plume di cristallo* and *The Phantom of Terror*), 1969, released in the United States by UM, 1970; *Quemimada!* (also known as *Burn*), 1969, released in the United States by United Artists, 1970; *The Sicilian Clan* (also known as *Le Clan des Siciliens*), 1969, released in the United States by Twentieth Century-Fox, 1970; *Un esercito di cinque uomini* (also known as *The Five Man Army*), 1969, released in the United States by MGM, 1970.

I cannibali (also known as *The Cannibals*), Dori-San Marco, 1970; *La califfa* (also known as *Lady Califfa*), Titanus, 1970; *Hornets' Nest,* United Artists, 1970; *Indagine su un cittadino al di sopra di ogni sospetto* (also known as *Investigation of a Citizen above Suspicion*), 1970, released in the United States by Columbia, 1970; *Two Mules for Sister Sara,* Universal, 1970; *Quando le donne avevano la coda* (also known as *When Women Had Tails*), 1970, released in the United States by Film Ventures, 1970; *Maddalena,* International Co-Production, 1970; *Vamos a matar, companeros* (also known as *Companeros*), 1970, released in the United States by GSF, 1970; *Citta violenta* (also known as *The Family* and *Violent City*), 1970, released in the United States by International Co-Production/EDP Films, 1974; *Chi l'ha vista morire?* (also known as *Who Saw Her Die?*), Assonitis-Romeo, 1971; *La classe operaia in paradiso* (also known as *The Working Class Goes to Heaven* and *Lulu the Tool*), Euro International, 1971; *Cat O'Nine Tails* (also known as *Il gatto a nove code*), 1971, released in the United States by National General, 1971; *The Decameron* (also known as *Il decamerone*), Roma Film, 1971; *Una lucertola con la pelle di donna* (also known as *A Lizard in a Woman's Skin*), Fida Cinematografica, 1971; *Krasnaya palatka* (also known as *La tenda rossa* and *The Red Tent*), 1971, released in the United States by Paramount, 1971; *Oceano* (also known as *The Wind Blows Free*), PEA, 1971; *Sacco and Vanzetti,* UMC, 1971; *Le Tueur* (also known as *The Killer*), Societe nouvelle prodis, 1971; *Le Casse* (also known as *The Burglars*), 1971, released in the United States by Columbia, 1972; *Quatro mosche di velluto grigio* (also known as *Four Flies on Grey Velvet*), 1971, released in the United States by Paramount, 1972.

Anche se volessi lavorare, che faccio? (also known as *Even If I Wanted to Work What Could I Do?*), Titanus, 1972; *Bluebeard* (also known as *Barbe-bleue*), 1972, released in the United States by Cinerama, 1972; *D'amore si muore* (also known as *For Love One Dies*), Euro International, 1972; *Duck, You Sucker* (also known as *Giu la testa* and *A Fistful of Dynamite*), 1972, released in the United States by United Artists, 1972; *Quando le donne persero la coda* (also known as *When Women Lost Their Tails*), 1972, released in the United States by Film Ventures, 1972; *Without Apparent Motive* (also known as *Sans mobile apparent*), 1972, released in the United States by Twentieth Century-Fox, 1972; *Il Maestro e Margherita* (also known as *The Master and Margherite*), Euro International, 1972; *Les Deux saisons de la vie* (also known as *Two Seasons of Life*), De L'aube, 1972; *Questa specie d'amore* (also known as *This Kind of Love*), Titanus, 1972; *L'ultimo uomo di Sara* (also known as *Sarah's Last Man*), Italnoleggio Cinematografica, 1972; *Sbatti il mostro in prima pagina* (also known as *Slap the Monster on Page One*), Euro International, 1972; *La tarantola dal ventro nero* (also known as *The Black Belly of the Tarantula*), 1972, released in the United States by MGM, 1972; *Das Geheimnis der Gruenen Stecknadel,* (also known as *The Secret of the Green Pins*), 1972, released in the United States by Constantin Films, 1972; *L'attentat* (also known as *The French Conspiracy* and *The Assassination*), 1972, released in the United States by Cine Globe, 1973; *The Serpent* (also known as *Night Flight from Moscow*), 1972, released in the United States by AVCO-Embassy, 1973; *Ci risiamo, vero Provvidenza?* (also known as *La vita, a volte e molto dura, vero provvidenza?* and *Life Is Tough, Eh Providence?*), 1972, released in the United States by Euro International, 1973; *La banda J. & S. (cronaca criminale del far west)* (also known as *Sonny and Jed* and *Far West Story*), 1972, released in the United States by Loyola Cinematography/Terra K-Tel, 1974.

La cosa buffa (also known as *La Drole de chose* and *The Funny Thing*), Euro International, 1973; *Giordano Bruno,* Euro International, 1973; *Le Moine* (also known as *The Monk*), Maya Films, 1973; *Rappresaglia* (also known as *Massacre in Rome*) National General, 1973; *Addio fratello crudele* (also known as *'Tis a Pity She's a Whore*), Euro International, 1973; *La proprieta non e piu un furto* (also known as *Property Is No Longer a Theft*), Quasars Film/ Labrador, 1973; *Libera, amore mio* (also known as *Libera, My Love*), Italnoleggio Cinematografica, 1973; *Un uomo da rispettare* (also known as *Hearts and Minds* and *The Master Touch*), 1973, released in the United States by Warner Brothers, 1974; *Il mio nome e nessuno* (also known as *My Name Is Nobody*), 1973, released in the United States by Universal, 1974; *Il fiore delle mille e una notte* (also known as *A Thousand and One Nights* and *Arabian Nights*), United Artists, 1974; *Il giro del mondo degli "innamorati" di Peynet* (also known as *A World Tour Made by Peynet's "Lovers"*), NOC, 1974; *Mussolini: Ultimo atto* (also known as *Last Days of Mussolini* and *The Last Four Days*), Paramount, 1974; *Milano odia: la polizia no puo sparare* (also known as *Almost Human*), Joseph Brenner, 1974; *Le Secret,* Valoria Films, 1974; *The Tempter,* Euro International/Lifeguard, 1974; *Le Trio infernal,* Levitt-Pickman, 1974; *Peur sur la ville* (also known as *Fear on the City* and *Night Caller*), AMLF, 1974; *Il sorriso del grande tentatore* (also known as *The Devil Is a Woman*), 1974, released in the United States by Twentieth Century-Fox, 1975; *Fatti di gente per bene* (also known as *La Grande bourgeoise* and *Drama of the Rich*), 1974, released in the United States by Production Artistique Cinematographique, 1975; *Anticristo* (also known as *L'anticristo* and *The Tempter*), 1974, released in the United States by AVCO-Embassy, 1978; *Allonsanfan,* 1974, released in the United States by Italoons-Wonder Movies, 1985.

Blood in the Streets (also known as *The Revolver*), Independent International, 1975; *La Faille* (also known as *La smagliature* and *The Weak Stop*), Gaumont, 1975; *The Human Factor,* Bryanston, 1975; *The End of the Game* (also known as *Murder on the Bridge* and *Der Richter und Sein Henker*), Twentieth Century-Fox, 1975; *Salo, o le 120 giornate di Sodoma* (also known as *Pasolini's 120 Days of Sodom* and *Salo—The 120 Days of Sodom*), United Artists, 1975; *La donna della domenica* (also known as *The Sunday Woman*), Fox Europa, 1975; *Attenti al buffone* (also known as *Eye of the Cat*), Medusa Distributors, 1975; *Leonor,* 1975, released in the United States by New Line, 1977; *Divina creatura* (also known as *The Divine Nymph*), 1975, released in the United States by Film Releasing Corporation, 1979; *Il deserto dei Tartari* (also known as *Le Desert des Tartares* and *The Desert of the Tartars*), Gaumont, 1976; *Un genio, due compari, un pollo* (also known as *The Genius*), Titanus, 1976; *1900* (also known as *Novecento*), Paramount/United Artists/Twentieth Century-Fox, 1976; *Rene la Canne* (also known as *Rene the Cane*), AMLF, 1976; *Per le antiche scale* (also known as *Down the Ancient Staircase*), Twentieth Century-Fox, 1976; *Todo modo,* Nu-Image, 1976; *Eredita Ferramonti* (also known as *The Inheritance*), 1976, released in the United States by S.J. International, 1978.

L'Arriviste (also known as *The Thruster*), Elan Films, 1977; *Exorcist II: The Heretic,* Warner Brothers, 1977; *Orca* (also known as *Orca—Killer Whale* and *La Orca*), Paramount, 1977; *Il gatto* (also known as *The Cat*), United Artists, 1977; *Il prefetto di ferro* (also known as *The Iron Perfect*), Cineriz, 1977; *Autostop rosso sangue* (also known as *Death Drive*), Watchgrove, 1977; *The Chosen* (also known as *Holocaust 2000*), 1977, released in the United States by American International, 1978; *Days of Heaven,* Paramount, 1978; *Deutschland im Herbst* (also known as *Germany in Autumn*), Osiris, 1978; *Corleone* (also known as *Father of the Godfathers*), Cineriz, 1978; *Cosi comme sei* (also known as *Stay as You Are* and *Bleib wie du Bist*), Columbia-Warner Distribution, 1978; *122 rue de Provence,* Columbia-Warner Distribution, 1978; *La Cage aux folles* (also known as *Birds of a Feather* and *The Mad Cage*), 1978, released in the United States by United Artists, 1979; *Viaggio con Anita* (also known as *Lovers and Liars, A Trip with Anita,* and *Travels with Anita*), 1978, released in the United States by Levitt-Pickman, 1981; *Bloodline* (also known as *Sidney Sheldon's Bloodline*), Paramount, 1979; *L'umanoide* (also known as *The Humanoid*), Columbia, 1979; *Il prato* (also known as *The Meadow*), Sacis, 1979; *I . . . comme Icare* (also known as *I as in Icarus*), AMLF, 1979; *Le buone notizie* (also known as *Good News*), Medusa Distribution, 1979; *Ogro* (also known as *Operation Ogre*), Vides Cinematografica, 1979; *Un sacco bello* (also known as *Fun Is Beautiful*), Medusa Distribution, 1979; *Il ladrone* (also known as *The Thief*), Italian International Films, 1979; *La Luna* (also known as *Luna*), 1979, released in the United States by Twentieth Century-Fox, 1979; *Windows,* 1979, released in the United States by United Artists, 1980.

Arabian Nights, United Artists, 1980; *La banquiere* (also known as *The Woman Banker*), Gaumont, 1980; *The Island,* Universal, 1980; *Uomini e no* (also known as *Men or Not Men*), Italnoleggio Cinematografica, 1980; *La Cage aux folles II,* 1980, released in the United States by United Artists, 1981; *Bianco, rosso, e verdone* (also known as *White, Red, and Verdon Green*), Medusa Distributors, 1981; *So Fine,* Warner Brothers, 1981; *La tragedia di un uomo ridicolo* (also known as *The Tragedy of a Ridiculous Man*), 1981, released in the United States by Warner Brothers, 1982; *Butterfly,* Analysis, 1982; *The Thing,* Universal, 1982; *White Dog* (also known as *Trained to Kill*), Paramount, 1982; *Le Ruffian,* Roissy Films/AMLF, 1982; *Nana,* 1982, released in the United States by Cannon, 1983; *Porca vacca!* (also known as *Dammit!*), Filmexport Group, 1982; *Le Marginal* (also known as *The Outsider*), Roissy Films/Gaumont, 1983; (with Robert O. Ragland) *A Time to Die* (also known as *Seven Graves for Rogan*), Almi, 1983; *Il miestero della quattro corona* (also known as *Treasure of the Four Crowns* and *El tesora de las cuatro coronas*), Cannon, 1983; *Corrupt* (also known as *Order of Death* and *Cop Killer*), 1983, released in the United States by New Line, 1984; *Hundra,* 1983, released in the United States by GTO, 1984; *La Chiave* (also known as *The Key*), 1983, released in the United States by Enterprise, 1985.

Don't Kill God, Armand Rubin/Europex, 1984; *Once Upon a Time in America,* Warner Brothers, 1984; *Sahara,* Metro-Goldwyn-Mayer/United Artists (MGM/UA), 1984; *Les Voleurs de la nuit* (also known as *Thieves After Dark*), Parafrance, 1984; *Il pentito* (also known as *The Repenter*), Columbia, 1985; *La Cage aux folles III: The Wedding,* Warner Brothers/Columbia/Tri-Star, 1985; *The Forester's Sons* (also known as *Die Forstenbuben*), MR-Films, 1985; *La Gabbia* (also known as *The Cage*), A.C.T.A.-Filman, 1985; *Die Einsteiger,* Tivoli, 1985; *Kommando Leopard,* Ascot, 1985; *The Link,* Zadar, 1985; *Red Sonja,* MGM/UA, 1985; *La Venexiana* (also known as *The Venetian Woman*), Titanus, 1986; *The Mission,* Warner Brothers, 1986; *Gli occhiali d'oro* (also known as *The Gold Spectacles*), D.M.V., 1987; *Il giorno prima* (also known as *The Day Before*), Columbia, 1987; *Masca addio* (also known as *Moscow Farewell*), Istituto Luce-Italnoleggio, 1987; *Quartiere* (also known as *Another Day*), Istituto Luce-Italnoleggio, 1987; *Rampage,* De Laurentiis Entertainment Group, 1987; *The Untouchables,* Warner Brothers, 1987; *Frantic,* Warner Brothers, 1988; *Nuovo cinema paradiso* (also known as *New Paradise Cinema*), Titanus, 1988; *A Time of Destiny,* Columbia, 1988.

Also as composer: *La cuccagna*, 1962; *I basilischi* (also known as *The Lizards*), 1963; *Il successo* (also known as *The Success*), 1963; *Le ore dell'amore*, 1963; *Una pistola per Ringo* (also known as *A Pistol for Ringo*), 1965; *Centomila dollari per Ringo*, 1965; *Il trionfo di Ringo*, 1965; *Quin sabe* (also known as *A Bullet for the General*), 1966; *Un fiume di dollari* (also known as *The Hills Run Red*), 1966; *Il giardino delle delizie*, 1967; *L'harem*, 1967; *Faccia a faccia*, 1967; *Gentleman Jo . . . uccidi*, 1967; *Escalation*, 1968; *Comandamenti per un gangster*, 1968; *Partner*, 1968; *Vergogna Schifosi* (also known as *The Dirty Angels*), 1968; *Il grande silenzio*, 1968; *Roma come Chicago*, 1968; *L'alibi*, 1968; *Corri uomo corri*, 1968; *H. 2S.*, 1968; *Et per tetto un cielo di stelle*, 1968; *Metti, une sera a cena*, 1969; *Una breve stagione* (also known as *Brief Season*), 1969; *Metello*, 1969; *Tepepa*, 1969; *La stagione dei sensi*, 1969; *Cuore di mamma*, 1969; *L'assoluto naturale*, 1969; *Mangiala*, 1969; *Ecce homo—I soparavvisuti*, 1969; *Sai cosa faceva Stalin alle donne*, 1969; *La donna invisibile*, 1969; *Senza sapere niente di lei*, 1969.

Gott mit uns, 1970; *La moglie piu bella*, 1970; *Uccidete il vitello grasso ed arrostitelo*, 1970; *Giocchi particolari*, 1970; *Forza G*, 1971; *Veruschka—Poesia di una donna*, 1971; *Incontro*, 1971; *Tre nel mille*, 1971; *Gli occhi freddi della paura*, 1971; *Le foto proibite di una signora per bene*, 1971; *La corta notte delle bambole di vetro*, 1971; *Lui per lei*, 1971; *L'istruttoria e chiusa, dimentichi!*, 1971; *Il diavolo nel cervello* (also known as *Devil in the Brain*), 1972; *Correva l'anno di grazia 1870 . . .*, 1972; *Violenza: quinto potere*, 1972; *Cosa avete fatto a solange*, 1972; *Giornata nera per l'ariete*, 1972; *Mio caro assassino*, 1972; *I bambini chiedono perche*, 1972; *Il retorno di Clint il solitario*, 1972; *I racconti di Canterbury*, 1972; *Chi l'ha vista morire?*, 1972; *Sepolta viva*, 1973; *Crescete e moltiplicatevi*, 1973; *Spogliati, protesta, uccidi!*, 1973; *Che c'entriamo noi con la rivoluzione?*, 1973; *Fiorina la vacca*, 1973; *La cugina*, 1974; *Sesso in confessionale*, 1974; *Spasmo*, 1974; *Macchie solari*, 1974.

Storie di vita e malavita, 1975; *L'ultimo treno della notte*, 1975; *Gente di rispetto*, 1975; *Labbra di lurido blu*, 1976; *San Babila ore 20: un delitto inutile*, 1976; *Per amore*, 1976; *L'agnese va a morire*, 1977; *Pedro Peramo*, 1977; *Una vita venduta*, 1977; *Stato interessante*, 1977; *Il mostro*, 1977; *Forza Italia!*, 1978; *L'immoralita*, 1978; "*Saro tuto per te*" in *Dove vai in vacanza?*, 1978; *Dedicato al mare Eglo*, 1979; *Il giocattalo*, 1979; *La vera storia della signora delle Camelie* (also known as *The True Story of Camille*), 1980; *Stark System*, 1980; *Si salvi chi vuole*, 1980; *Professione Figlio*, 1980; *Le Professionel*, 1981; *Espion, Leve-toi*, 1981; *Occhio alla penna*, 1981; *La disubbidienza*, 1981; *The Seven Magnificent Gladiators*, 1984.

TELEVISION—All as composer. Mini-Series: *Moses: The Lawgiver*, CBS, 1975; *Marco Polo*, NBC, 1982. Movies: *The Scarlet and the Black*, CBS, 1983; *C.A.T. Squad: Python Wolf*, NBC, 1988. Episodic: *Space 1999*, syndicated, 1974; "*Control*," *HBO Showcase*, HBO, 1987. Specials: *Le mani sporche*, 1978.

RECORDINGS: ALBUMS—All original soundtrack recordings: *A Fistful of Dollars*, RCA, 1967; *The Good, the Bad, and the Ugly*, Liberty, 1967; *Guns for San Sebastian*, MCA, 1968; *Once Upon a Time in the West*, Mercury, 1969; *Bloodline*, Varese/Sarabande, 1979; *Sahara*, Varese/Sarabande, 1984; *Once Upon a Time in America*, RCA, 1984; *Red Sonja*, Varese/Sarabande, 1985; *The Mission*, Virgin, 1986; *The Untouchables*, A&M, 1987.

AWARDS: Academy Award nomination, Best Original Score, 1978, and British Academy Award, Anthony Asquith Award for

Best Original Film Music, 1979, both for *Days of Heaven;* Golden Globe Award, Best Original Score for a Motion Picture, Academy Award nomination, Best Original Score, and Los Angeles Film Critics Association Award nomination, Best Original Score, all 1987, for *The Mission;* Academy Award nomination, Best Original Score, and Golden Globe Award nomination, Best Original Score for a Motion Picture, both 1988, for *The Untouchables;* London Film Critics Award, Best Music, 1988, for *The Mission* and *The Untouchables;* London Film Critics Award, 1988, for his career work; Annual Cable Excellence (ACE) Award, Best Original Score, 1988, for "*Control*," *HBO Showcase.**

*   *   *

MORSE, David   1953-

PERSONAL: Born October 11, 1953, in Beverly, MA; son of Charles (a sales manager) and Gacquelin (a teacher) Morse; married Susan Wheeler Duff (an actress), June 19, 1982. EDUCATION: Trained for the stage with William Esper.

VOCATION: Actor.

CAREER: PRINCIPAL STAGE APPEARANCES—Jim, *The Trading Post*, WPA Theatre, New York City, 1981; Nub and Clyde, *Threads*, Circle Repertory Company, New York City, 1981. Also appeared as the reporter, *How I Got That Story*, Los Angeles Public Theatre, Los Angeles, CA; in *A Death in the Family*, Off-Broadway production; in *Of Mice and Men*, Los Angeles; and as the junkie, *A Hatful of Rain*, in the title role, *The Night Thoreau Spent in Jail*, in *The Point*, and in more than thirty other productions, all with the Boston Repertory Company, Boston, MA, 1971-77.

PRINCIPAL FILM APPEARANCES—Jerry Maxwell, *Inside Moves*, Associated, 1980; shoe store cop, *Max Dugan Returns*, Twentieth Century-Fox, 1983; Ben, *Personal Foul*, Personal Foul, Ltd., 1987.

PRINCIPAL TELEVISION APPEARANCES—Series: Dr. Jack Morrison, *St. Elsewhere*, NBC, 1982-88; host and narrator, *Knowzone*, PBS, 1987. Pilots: Phil, *Our Family Business*, ABC, 1981. Movies: Michael, *Prototype*, CBS, 1983; Father Tim, *Shattered Vows*, NBC, 1984; Robert Wynton, *When Dreams Come True*, ABC, 1985; Marvin Hubbard, *Six Against the Rock*, NBC, 1987; Detective Jackson, *Downpayment on Murder*, NBC, 1987; Tom Williams, *A Place at the Table*, NBC, 1988; Thomas, *Winnie* (also known as *Winnie: My Life in the Institution*), NBC, 1988; Chris Kilmoonie, *Brotherhood of the Rose*, NBC, 1989.

PRINCIPAL TELEVISION WORK—Episodic: Director, *St. Elsewhere* (two episodes), NBC, 1987.

NON-RELATED CAREER—Waiter.

AWARDS: *Drama-Logue* Award for *Of Mice and Men*.

ADDRESSES: AGENT—Yvette Bikoff Agency, 9255 Sunset Boulevard, Suite 510, Los Angeles, CA 90069.*

MORSE, Robert 1931-

PERSONAL: Full name, Robert Alan Morse; born May 18, 1931, in Newton, MA; son of Charles (an assistant manager of a record store) and May (Silver) Morse; married Carole Ann D'Andrea, April 8, 1961; children: three daughters. EDUCATION: Trained for the stage with the American Theatre Wing, New York City. MILITARY: U.S. Navy, 1951.

VOCATION: Actor.

CAREER: STAGE DEBUT—*Our Town,* Peterborough Players, Peterborough, NH, 1949. BROADWAY DEBUT—Barnaby Tucker, *The Matchmaker,* Royale Theatre, 1955. PRINCIPAL STAGE APPEARANCES—Ted Snow, *Say, Darling,* American National Theatre Academy Theatre, New York City, 1958; Richard Miller, *Take Me Along,* Shubert Theatre, New York City, 1959; J. Pierpont Finch, *How to Succeed in Business without Really Trying,* 46th Street Theatre, New York City, 1961; Jerry, *Sugar,* Majestic Theatre, New York City, 1972; ensemble, *Milliken Breakfast Show* (revue), Waldorf-Astoria, New York City, 1973; Mr. Applegate, *Damn Yankees,* Meadowbrook Dinner Theatre, Cedar Grove, NJ, 1973; Jerry, *Sugar,* Dorothy Chandler Pavilion, Los Angeles, CA, 1974; J. Pierpont Finch, *How to Succeed in Business without Really Trying,* Dorothy Chandler Pavilion, 1975; David, *So Long, 174th Street,* Harkness Theatre, New York City, 1976; Sidney Black, *Light Up the Sky,* Ahmanson Theatre, Los Angeles, 1986; Scooter Malloy, *Mike,* Walnut Street Theatre, Philadelphia, PA, 1988. Also appeared with the Folger Theatre, Washington, DC, 1985; and in the Off-Broadway productions *More of Loesser* and *Eileen in Concert.*

PRINCIPAL STAGE WORK—Director, *How to Succeed in Business without Really Trying,* Dorothy Chandler Pavilion, Los Angeles, CA, 1975.

MAJOR TOURS—Barnaby Tucker, *The Matchmaker,* U.S. cities, 1957; Bobby, *Sugar Babies,* U.S. cities, 1980.

FILM DEBUT—Casualty, *The Proud and the Profane,* Paramount, 1956. PRINCIPAL FILM APPEARANCES—Barnaby Tucker, *The Matchmaker,* Paramount, 1958; Bobby, *The Cardinal,* Columbia, 1963; Jay Menlow, *Honeymoon Hotel,* Metro-Goldwyn-Mayer (MGM), 1964; Oliver Cromwell Cannon, *Quick, Before It Melts,* MGM, 1964; Dennis Barlow, *The Loved One,* MGM, 1965; Jonathan, *Oh Dad, Poor Dad, Mama's Hung You in the Closet and I'm Feeling So Sad,* Paramount, 1967; J. Pierpont Finch, *How to Succeed in Business without Really Trying,* United Artists, 1967; Ed Stander, *A Guide for the Married Man,* Twentieth Century-Fox, 1967; Waldo Zane, *Where Were You When the Lights Went Out?,* MGM, 1968; Ensign Garland, *The Boatniks,* Buena Vista, 1970; Henry, *The Emperor's New Clothes,* Cannon, 1987; Garrison Gaylord, *Hunk,* Crown International, 1987.

PRINCIPAL TELEVISION APPEARANCES—Series: Robert Dickson, *That's Life,* ABC, 1968-69. Episodic: Larry, "Midnight Mystery," *Matinee Theater,* NBC, 1957; Cupid, "Ye Gods," *Twilight Zone,* CBS, 1985; also Wayne McIntyre, *Trapper John, M.D.,* CBS; *Naked City,* ABC; *The Perry Como Show,* NBC; *The Jack Paar Show,* NBC; *People and Other Animals,* syndicated; *To Tell the Truth,* CBS; *The Mike Douglas Show,* syndicated; *The Red Skelton Show,* CBS; *The Clay Cole Show,* syndicated; *I've Got a Secret,* CBS; *The Hollywood Squares,* NBC; *The Smothers Brothers Comedy Hour,* CBS; *Alias Smith and Jones,* ABC; *Alfred Hitchcock Presents; The Shirley Temple Show.* Movies: Nat Couray,

The Calendar Girl Murders, ABC, 1984. Specials: *Leslie,* ABC, 1968; *Marlo Thomas and Friends in Free to Be . . . You and Me,* ABC, 1974; voice of Stuffy, *The First Easter Rabbit* (animated), CBS, 1978; title role, *Jack Frost,* NBC, 1980.

AWARDS: Theatre World Award, 1958, and Antoinette Perry Award nomination, Best Supporting or Featured Actor, 1959, both for *Say, Darling;* Antoinette Perry Award nomination, Best Actor in a Musical, 1960, for *Take Me Along;* Antoinette Perry Award, Best Actor in a Musical, 1962, for *How to Succeed in Business without Really Trying;* Antoinette Perry Award nomination, Best Actor in a Musical, 1973, for *Sugar.*

MEMBER: Actors' Equity Association, Screen Actors Guild, American Federation of Television and Radio Artists.

SIDELIGHTS: RECREATIONS—Sports, cooking, and photography.*

*   *   *

MORTON, Joe 1947-

PERSONAL: Born October 18, 1947, in New York, NY; father, in the U.S. Army. EDUCATION: Studied drama at Hofstra University.

VOCATION: Actor.

CAREER: OFF-BROADWAY DEBUT—Jesse, *A Month of Sundays,* Theatre De Lys, 1968. BROADWAY DEBUT—*Hair,* New York Shakespeare Festival, Biltmore Theatre. PRINCIPAL STAGE APPEARANCES—Mark, *Salvation,* Village Gate Theatre, then Jan Hus Playhouse, both New York City, 1969; Willy Thomas, *Prettybelle,* Shubert Theatre, Boston, MA, 1971; title role, *Charlie Was Here and Now He's Gone,* Eastside Playhouse, New York City, 1971; Sam (Samuel Adams), *Two If by Sea,* Circle in the Square, New York City, 1972; Walter Lee Younger, *Raisin,* Arena Stage, Washington, DC, 1972, then 46th Street Theatre, New York City, 1973; Arlecchino, *Tricks,* Alvin Theatre, New York City, 1973; Shoulders, *G.R. Point,* Marymount Manhattan Theatre, New York City, 1977; Lucius, *Johnny on a Spot,* and Autolycus, *The Winter's Tale,* both Brooklyn Academy of Music, Brooklyn, NY, 1980; Eastern Habim, *Oh, Brother!,* American National Theatre Academy Theatre, New York City, 1981; Lysander, *A Midsummer Night's Dream,* Kite, *The Recruiting Officer,* naval officer, *The Wild Duck,* and title role, *Oedipus the King,* all Brooklyn Academy of Music, 1981; Sam Dodd, *Rhinestone,* Richard Allen Center, New York City, 1982; Peter, *Souvenirs,* Cubiculo Theatre, New York City, 1984; Ty Fletcher, *Tamer of Horses,* Crossroads Theatre Company, New Brunswick, NJ, 1985, then Los Angeles Theatre Center, Los Angeles, CA, 1986; Cutting Ball, *Cheapside,* Roundabout Theatre, New York City, 1986; Mama Zaza, *Almost by Chance a Woman: Elizabeth,* Yale Repertory Theatre, New Haven, CT, 1986; Barney Walker, *Honky Tonk Nights,* Biltmore Theatre, New York City, 1986. Also appeared in *I Paid My Dues,* Astor Place Theatre, New York City, 1976; *Two Gentlemen of Verona,* Pennsylvania Stage Company, Allentown, PA, 1982; *How I Got That Story,* GeVa Theatre, Rochester, NY, 1982; and with the Actors Theatre of Louisville, Louisville, KY, 1984-85.

PRINCIPAL FILM APPEARANCES—Ahmad, *Between the Lines,* Midwest Films, 1977; doctor, *. . . And Justice for All,* Columbia, 1970; title role, *The Brother from Another Planet,* Cinecom, 1984; Scratch's assistant, *Crossroads,* Columbia, 1985; Solo, *Trouble in*

Mind, Alive, 1985; Earl, *Zelly and Me,* Columbia, 1988; Frank Williams, *The Good Mother,* Buena Vista, 1988; Nicky, *Tap,* Tri-Star, 1989. Also appeared in *The Killing Hour,* Lansbury-Berun, 1979.

PRINCIPAL TELEVISION APPEARANCES—Series: Dr. Jason, *Feeling Good,* PBS, 1974-75; Hal Marshall, *Grady,* NBC, 1975-76; also in *Raymond Geeter, Watch Your Mouth,* PBS, 1978; as Dr. Joe Foster, *Search for Tomorrow,* CBS; and as Dr. Abel Marsh, *Another World,* NBC. Pilots: Elgin Jones, *We're Fighting Back,* CBS, 1981. Episodic: "Der Tag," *M*A*S*H,* CBS, 1976. Movies: William Terry, *Death Penalty,* NBC, 1980; Lionel Zachary, *A Good Sport,* CBS, 1984; also *This Man Stands Alone,* NBC, 1979; and *Alone in the Neon Jungle,* CBS, 1988.

AWARDS: Theatre World Award and Antoinette Perry Award nomination, Best Actor in a Musical, both 1974, for *Raisin.*

ADDRESSES: AGENT—Artists Agency, 10000 Santa Monica Boulevard, Suite 305, Los Angeles, CA 90067.*

*   *   *

MOST, Donald   1953-

PERSONAL: Born August 8, 1953, in Brooklyn, NY; father, an accountant. EDUCATION: Attended Lehigh University; trained for the stage with Elinor Raab; studied voice with Warren Barigian.

VOCATION: Actor and singer.

CAREER: PRINCIPAL STAGE APPEARANCES—Shoeless Joe, *Damn Yankees,* Theatre of the Stars, Civic Center, Atlanta, GA, 1982; Chris, *Hello Dali,* Actors Outlet, New York City, 1985; also appeared as Bo, *Bus Stop,* Austin, TX; in *Wait Until Dark,* Omaha, NE; and in *Barefoot in the Park,* Skowhega, ME.

MAJOR TOURS—Shoeless Joe, *Damn Yankees,* U.S. cities, 1982.

PRINCIPAL FILM APPEARANCES—Shawn, *Crazy Mama,* New World, 1975; Leo Green, *Leo and Loree,* United Artists, 1980; George Bunkle, *Stewardess School,* Columbia, 1986.

PRINCIPAL TELEVISION APPEARANCES—Series: Ralph Malph, *Happy Days,* ABC, 1974-80; voice of Ralph Malph, *Fonz and the Happy Days Gang* (animated), ABC, 1980-82; voice of Eric, *Dungeons and Dragons* (animated), CBS, 1983. Episodic: T.J. Holt, *Murder, She Wrote,* CBS, 1986; also *Emergency,* NBC; *Room 222,* ABC. Movies: Tom Sawyer, *Huckleberry Finn,* ABC, 1975; James, *With This Ring,* ABC, 1978. Specials: Henry Cooper, "$1,000 Bill," *ABC Weekend Special,* ABC, 1978.

RELATED CAREER—Singer and dancer in a specialty review on the Catskill circuit, New York; actor in television commercials.

RECORDINGS: ALBUMS—*Donny Most,* United Artists, 1986. SINGLES—"All Roads (Lead Back to You)," "Better to Forget Him," and "Here's Some Love," all United Artists.

ADDRESSES: AGENT—Mark Levin and Associates, 1341 Ocean Avenue, Suite 206, Santa Monica, CA 90401.*

MOYERS, Bill   1934-

PERSONAL: Born Billy Don Moyers (name legally changed), June 5, 1934, in Hugo, OK; son of John Henry (a laborer) and Ruby (Johnson) Moyers; married Judith Suzanne Davidson, December 18, 1954; children: William Cope, Alice Suzanne, John Davidson. EDUCATION: Attended North Texas State University, 1952-54; University of Texas, B.J. (honors), journalism, 1956; graduate work at University of Edinburgh, 1956-57; Southwest Baptist Theological Seminary, B.D., 1959.

VOCATION: Journalist, commentator, and producer.

CAREER: Also see WRITINGS below. PRINCIPAL TELEVISION APPEARANCES—All as correspondent and commentator, unless indicated. Series: *This Week,* PBS, 1971; *Bill Moyers' Journal,* PBS, 1972-74 and 1978-81; *Bill Moyers' International Report,* PBS, 1975; *CBS Evening News,* CBS, 1981-86; *Creativity with Bill Moyers,* PBS, 1982; *Our Times with Bill Moyers,* CBS, 1983; *The American Parade* (also known as *Crossroads*), CBS, 1984; *A Walk through the Twentieth Century,* CBS Cable, then PBS, 1984; *Bill Moyers: In Search of the Constitution,* PBS, 1987; *Moyers: God and Politics,* PBS, 1987; *Philadelphia Journal,* PBS, 1987; *Moyers: The Wisdom of Joseph Campbell,* PBS, 1987; *The World of Ideas,* PBS, 1988; *Moyers: A Second Look,* PBS, 1989. Specials: *World Hunger! Who Will Survive?,* PBS, 1975; "The Last Ballot," "The World Turned Upside Down," and "The Peach Gang," all *Ourstory,* PBS, 1975; *Eliza,* PBS, 1975; *The Erie War,* PBS, 1976; *Jade Snow,* PBS, 1976; *The Devil's Work,* PBS, 1976; "The Queen's Destiny," *Ourstory,* PBS, 1976; "The Aliens," *CBS Reports,* CBS, 1977; "The Fire Next Door," *CBS Reports,* CBS, 1977, updated and rebroadcast, 1978; "The Battle for South Africa," *CBS Reports,* CBS, 1978; *The Edelin Conviction,* PBS, 1978; "Goodbye, Congress," *CBS Reports,* CBS, 1978; "Into the Mouths of Babes," *CBS Reports,* 1978; "New Orleans," *CBS Reports,* CBS, 1978; "The Politics of Abortion," *CBS Reports,* CBS, 1978; "The Soul of Freedom," *CBS Reports,* CBS, 1978; "Who's Minding the Bank," *CBS Reports,* CBS, 1978; *The Vanishing Family: Crisis in Black America,* CBS, 1986; *Moyers: In Search of the Constitution Special,* PBS, 1987; *Promises! Promises!,* PBS, 1988; *The Secret Government,* PBS, 1988.

PRINCIPAL TELEVISION WORK—Editor, *CBS Reports,* CBS, 1976-78.

RELATED CAREER—Reporter and sports editor, *News Messenger,* Marshall, TX, 1949-54; assistant news editor, KTBS Radio and Television, Austin, TX, 1954-56; White House press secretary, Washington, DC, 1965-67; publisher, *Newsday* (daily newspaper), Garden City, NY, 1967-70; contributing editor, *Newsweek,* 1974-75; executive editor, Public Affairs Television, Inc. (a production company), 1987—.

NON-RELATED CAREER—Student minister in churches in Texas and Oklahoma, 1954-57; special assistant to Senator Lyndon B. Johnson, 1959-60; executive assistant to Johnson during vice-presidential campaign, 1960, and after election, 1961; associate director for public affairs, Peace Corps, Washington, DC, 1961, then deputy director, 1962-63; special assistant to President Johnson, 1963-65.

WRITINGS: TELEVISION—(With Tom Spain) "The Aliens," *CBS Reports,* CBS, 1977; (with Spain) "The Fire Next Door," *CBS Reports,* CBS, 1977, updated and rebroadcast, 1978; (with Janet Roach) "Into the Mouths of Babes," *CBS Reports,* CBS, 1978.

OTHER—*Listening to America: A Traveler Rediscovers His Country,* Harpers Magazine Press, 1971; *The Secret Government,* Seven Locks Press, 1988; (with Joseph Campbell) *The Power of Myth,* Doubleday, 1988; *The World of Ideas,* Doubleday, 1989.

AWARDS: Emmy Awards, Best News Segments, 1974, 1980, 1982, 1983, 1984, 1985, 1986, and 1987, Achievement in Broadcast Journalism, 1978; Peabody Awards, 1976, 1980, 1985, and 1986; DuPont Columbia Awards, 1979 and 1986; George Polk Awards, 1981 and 1986; Ralph Lowell Medal for contributions to public television; Silver Gavel Award from American Bar Association; fellow, Aspen Institute for Humanistic Studies.

SIDELIGHTS: With two decades of award-winning television journalism, Bill Moyers has established himself as the acknowledged "conscience of American television," in the words of the *Christian Science Monitor.* Alternating between the Public Broadcasting Service (PBS), where he at times has felt limited resources and small audiences diminished the impact of his work, and the CBS network news division, where irregular scheduling and a sensitivity to commercial interests frustrated him, he has continually sought the best forum for his efforts.

Although Moyers was trained as a journalist, his television career began almost accidentally. He had already served in Washington, first as a special assistant to Senator and then Vice-President Lyndon B. Johnson, and later, after a stint in the public affairs office of the Peace Corps, as Johnson's press secretary when he became president. Next Moyers took the reins as publisher of the Long Island, New York, daily, *Newsday,* which garnered two Pulitzer Prizes during his tenure. When his bid to buy the paper failed, it was a phone call inviting him to host a new PBS series, *This Week,* that brought the commentator to television.

After dealing with television reporters in the White House, as Moyers recalled in *Broadcasting,* the opportunity to sit on the other side of the camera "intrigued me." So much so that he accepted the job without even asking what it paid. After one season, he assumed the title of editor-in-chief on the weekly half-hour series, now known as *Bill Moyers' Journal.* Richard Schickel in *Time* described the three types of programs that comprised most of the series: profiles of citizens' groups trying to better their communities; *cinema verite* examinations of such subjects as an encounter group for clergymen; and conversations on public life with a broad spectrum of people, including not only an economist and labor leader, but a poet and historian.

This last category, according to Schickel, comprised about half the *Journal* shows; it has remained a favorite Moyers genre. The series exhibited other hallmarks of its creator's method as well. "Moyers does not hide his own biases while drawing out those of his guests," the critic observed. "[The *Journal*] is distinguished by the host's dogged pursuit of matters that are not only of wide general interest but that he seems to care more deeply about than does the typical TV talking head." Moyers himself has criticized the medium as in his remark to *People,* "TV makes stars out of people who stand for nothing by standing in front of a camera acting agreeable." In contrast, he has relished television's power to set the national agenda, while characterizing his own role with the *Journal* as "helping to keep the conversation of America going," Schickel reported.

By 1974, however, Moyers came to a conclusion. "Quite frankly I have said all I have to say for now in current affairs and do not wish to be merely carried along by the relentless momentum of the media

when I no longer have anything really compelling to say," Kay Gardella quoted from his retirement statement in the *Daily News.* Nevertheless, by the end of the year he announced a new series on international affairs, again for PBS; and when public television was suffering a financial squeeze, an offer from CBS to lead its prestigious *CBS Reports* documentary unit lured Moyers to the network. There he turned out an award-winning list of programs, including *The Fire Next Door* on arson in the South Bronx, *The Politics of Abortion,* and *Into the Mouths of Babes,* an examination of western countries' sales of infant formula in third world nations ill equipt to handle them appropriately. He yielded to network pressure to soften his attack in the latter program, but it prompted him to remark, "You've just turned *Jaws* into *Gums,*" *People* reported.

Not long after, Moyers returned to PBS and *Bill Moyers' Journal,* which received partial sponsorship from the Weyerhaeuser Company at a time when federal support for public broadcasting was shrinking. After the *Journal* ran three shows on critics of big business, its corporate sponsor backed out. With all three networks making him offers, in 1981 Moyers announced, "I can no longer do my best work at PBS. You have to keep moving where you can do your best work," and rejoined CBS (*Daily News,* June 26, 1981). He felt that the increasing costs of entertainment programming would make the kind of reality shows he produced more attractive to the network, although he recognized that the return to commercial television was a risk. As the *Daily News* recorded, he told Dick Cavett, ". . . My beat always has been ideas, and commercial television deals with events. It does not allow for any attention span."

Moyers was to act as commentator on the regular evening newscast as well as to turn out documentary specials. With the support of anchorman Dan Rather, he was able to take relatively long stretches of the half-hour show to cover topics in depth and with feeling. For example, he closed a scathing expose of the Congressional influence peddling behind an Alaska pipeline appropriation with the declaration, "The two-party system is not only up for grabs—it's up for sale," as the *Village Voice* noted. Consumer activist Ralph Nader credited Moyers' coverage with turning fifty votes in the Congress against the bill, although it still passed. The broadcaster answered politicians' protests over his story, "It's one thing to be impartial and another to be indifferent."

His CBS contract this time allowed him to take on projects outside the network, so he also initiated his *Creativity* series on PBS and *A Walk through the Twentieth Century* for CBS Cable, which later aired on PBS after the cable network was dropped. Moyers told *People,* "I want to produce television that engages the viewer instead of passively feeding him." Television critic John Corry analyzed the purpose of *A Walk through the Twentieth Century* in the *New York Times:* "We are meant to look at the connective tissue of our time. . . . Much of the tissue has been shaped by film, as seen in newsreels, movies and television, and sometimes the film does not so much shape the tissue as become the tissue itself." Among the subjects of various segments were Teddy Roosevelt's use of the media and the birth of the public relations industry.

The latitude to work outside the network did not outweigh the frustrations Moyers reportedly felt within it. He found spending months putting together a special that would be poorly scheduled or promoted self-defeating, even when it might earn a prestigious award, as *The Vanishing Family* did the DuPont Columbia Award. The October 14, 1985 *New York Times* had carried his statement, "I have concluded that serious public affairs reporting isn't going to make it in the entertainment milieu of prime time." A year later he resigned from the network, saying, "Broadcasting is going through an incredible transformation and I am out of synch" (*New York Times,* September 9, 1986).

By January, 1987, he formed his own production company, Public Affairs Television, and announced several projects, including three related to the United States Constitution, which was approaching its two-hundredth anniversary. In addition to a ninety-minute special, he planned a series of hour-long shows, and *Philadelphia Journal,* daily three-minute spots that presented the events in the development of the Constitution from a contemporary viewpoint. Moyers told *Variety,* "It's a wonderful way to focus your journalism in a particular period of time on something that has to be rescued from the glitz and superficiality in which these occasions are often treated."

Other projects made public at the same time reveal the consistency of Moyers' interests and technique. One was the series *The World of Ideas,* which he described as "a forum for news of the mind" (*Variety*). Once again he saw an opportunity to "broaden and enhance the conversation of democracy," as the September 12, 1988 *New York Times* quoted him. The commentator again assembled a wide variety of people—a filmmaker, a pediatrician, an ethicist, a historian, a surgeon, an environmental scientist—and in one-on-one conversations explored with them the issues of the day. Another series, *Joseph Campbell and the Power of Myth* gave six hours to one man's lifelong study of the human effort to understand the cosmos. Though even public television stations at first hesitated to book the Campbell series, it went on to become such a hit that it was issued on video cassette and a book was spun off from it.

Both these series also exemplify the part of Moyers' technique most often criticized by media professionals—his simple, focus-on-the-speaker direction that eschews graphics, music, and elaborate camera work or artistic editing. Moyers defends what critics dismiss as "talking heads," saying, "The only thing more beautiful than the spoken word is the human face—the talking head combines both" (*New York Times,* May 14, 1989). Others fault his approach as sanctimonious, and he himself has acknowledged, "I prefer the role of teacher and illuminator" and in *Broadcasting* cited with pleasure a professor's letter counseling, "You have the best classroom in America. Don't ever give it up." Moreover, the commentator sees a program as a reflection of its producer's view of the audience. "If he sees them as consumers, then the truth becomes that which sells, nothing more. If he sees them as citizens, he sees them as yearning to know, to matter, to signify," he was quoted in the May 5, 1989 *New York Times.*

Jack Newfield in the *Village Voice* credited Moyers' success to these particular talents: "The ability to translate abstract concepts into emotions and images. The sixth sense that anticipates the timely subject. And the intellect that thinks systematically." In 1989 PBS reprised fourteen of his past programs on topics ranging from his own hometown of Marshall, Texas, to Aristotle, Southern Baptists and the religious right, and the plight of the poor, in a series called *Moyers: A Second Look.* In the *Times,* Ken Burns assessed: ". . . If anything, his work improves with age; we become aware of what national treasures he and [his programs] are."

OTHER SOURCES: *Broadcasting,* November 19, 1984; *Christian Science Monitor,* February 20, 1981; [New York] *Daily News,* May 13, 1974, June 26, 1981; *New York Times,* June 25, 1983, January 8, 1984, August 14, 1985, September 9, 1986, January 14, 1987, May 5, 1987, September 12, 1988, October 31, 1988, May 14,

1989; *People,* January 26, 1976, February 22, 1982; *Time,* January 14, 1974; *Village Voice,* January 20, 1982; *Variety,* January 21, 1987.

ADDRESSES: OFFICE—Public Affairs Television, Inc., 524 W. 57th Street, New York, NY 10019.

*   *   *

MUELLERLEILE, Marianne   1948-

PERSONAL: Surname is pronounced "Mull-ler-lie-lee"; born November 26, 1948, in St. Louis, MO; daughter of Cecil E. (an oil company executive) and Margaret (Keany) Muellerleile; married Joseph T. Norris, Jr. (an officer in the U.S. Air Force), May 7, 1988. EDUCATION: St. Louis University, B.A., 1971; University of Minnesota, M.F.A., 1974; studied tap and jazz dancing with Bob Audy; studied acting with Barbara Byrne and Joan Darling; studied voice with J. Peck, H. Mombo, and E. Thorendahl. RELIGION: Roman Catholic.

VOCATION: Actress.

CAREER: STAGE DEBUT—*Member of the Wedding,* Meadow Brook Theatre, Rochester, MI, 1973, for twenty-seven performances. OFF-BROADWAY DEBUT—Susan Brady, *The Playboy of the Western World,* Playwrights Horizons, Queens Festival Theatre, 1977, for twelve performances. PRINCIPAL STAGE APPEARANCES—Mary, *How the Other Half Loves,* and Eunice, *A Streetcar Named Desire,* both Meadow Brook Theatre, Rochester, MI, 1973-74; Sabetella, *April Fish,* Joseph Jefferson Theatre Company, Little Church around the Corner, New York City, 1975; Trudy, *The Last Christians,* New Dramatists, New York City, 1975; Mrs. Hedges, *Born Yesterday,* Meadow Brook Theatre, 1976; Mrs. Watty, *The Corn Is Green,* Mrs. Shandig, *The Runner Stumbles,* and Myrtle Keller, *The Male Animal,* all Meadow Brook Theatre, 1977-78; Mrs. Candour, *School for Scandal,* Meadow Brook Theatre, 1979; Mrs. Soames, *Our Town,* Beline, *The Imaginary Invalid,* and Grace, *Bus Stop,* all Meadow Brook Theatre, 1980-81; Audry, *As You Like It,* Miss Felloes, *Night of the Iguana,* and Eugenie, *A Flea in Her Ear,* all Coconut Grove Playhouse, Coconut Grove, FL; Countess, *Humulus the Mute,* Direct Theatre, New York City; Kakonyi/Palivec, *Good Soldier Schweik,* and Madame, *The Threepenny Opera,* both Minnesota Opera Company, MN; Ceres, *The Tempest,* Maria, *Twelfth Night,* Sylvia, *Two Gentlemen of Verona,* and Beatrice, *Much Ado about Nothing,* all Shakespeare-in-the-Streets; in *Spoon River Anthology* and *Tonight at 8:30,* both Meadow Brook Theatre, 1974; *The Tempest* Meadow Brook Theatre, 1977; *A Summer Remembered* and *Night Must Fall,* both Meadow Brook Theatre, 1979; and in a musical version of *The Drunkard,* Coconut Grove Playhouse.

PRINCIPAL FILM APPEARANCES—Waitress, *Going Berserk,* Universal, 1983; nurse, *Stitches,* International Film Marketing, 1985; Betty, *The Trouble with Dick,* Frolix, 1987; Wrong Sarah, *The Terminator,* Orion, 1984; woman, *Revenge of the Nerds,* Twentieth Century-Fox, 1984; also appeared in *The Heartbreak Kid,* Twentieth Century-Fox, 1972; *An Unmarried Woman,* Twentieth Century-Fox, 1978; *Manhattan,* United Artists, 1979; *Stardust Memories,* United Artists, 1980; *Endless Love,* Universal, 1981; *Independence Day,* Warner Brothers, 1982; *Whatever It Takes,* Aquarius, 1986; and in *The Bite, Dirty Business,* and *Captain Avenger.*

PRINCIPAL TELEVISION APPEARANCES—Mini-Series: Gloria, *Fresno*, CBS, 1986; also *Seventh Avenue*, NBC, 1977. Pilots: Nurse, *I'd Rather Be Calm*, CBS, 1982; Betty Jo, *P.O.P.*, NBC, 1984; nurse, "Puppetman," *CBS Summer Playhouse*, CBS, 1987; also *House Detective*. Episodic: Olga, *Magnum, P.I.*, CBS, 1981; first woman, "A Matter of Minutes," *The Twilight Zone*, CBS, 1986; Harriet, *You Again?*, NBC, 1986; Rosie Feeney, *Hooperman*, ABC, 1987; Big Mabel, *Sledge Hammer!*, ABC, 1988; Margo, *The Bronx Zoo*, NBC, 1988; eighth secretary, *Murphy Brown*, CBS, 1988; matron, *thirtysomething*, ABC, 1988; Nurse Hawkins, *Mr. Belvedere*, ABC, 1988; Gretchen, *Day by Day*, NBC, 1989; Miss Bauer, *Growing Pains*, ABC, 1989; Cecelia, *Family Ties*, NBC, 1989; also *Amanda's*, ABC, 1983; *Blacke's Magic*, NBC, 1986; *Roxie*, CBS, 1987; *The A-Team*, NBC; *The Jeffersons*, CBS; *Highway to Heaven*, NBC; *Amen*, NBC; *Falcon Crest*, CBS; *Perfect Strangers*, ABC; *Hotel*, ABC; *Night Court*, NBC; *Moonlighting*, ABC; *Santa Barbara*, NBC; *Knot's Landing*, CBS; *Remington Steele*, NBC; *The Greatest American Hero*, ABC; *Gimme a Break*, NBC; *The Doctors*, NBC; *Double Trouble*, NBC; *One Day at a Time*, CBS; *One Big Family*, syndicated. Movies: Eric's teacher, *Child's Cry*, CBS, 1986; also *To Kill a Cop*, NBC, 1978; *Disaster at Silo 7* (also known as *Silo*), ABC, 1988; *Going to the Chapel* (also known as *Wedding Bells*), NBC, 1988; *She Knows Too Much* (also known as *Lady Be Good*), NBC, 1989; and *Promised a Miracle*. Specials: *American Night*, PBS; *Martin Mull: A History of White America*.

RELATED CAREER—Appeared in television commercials and industrial films.

MEMBER: Screen Actors Guild, American Federation of Television and Radio Artists, Actors' Equity Association.

SIDELIGHTS: Marianne Muellerleile told *CTFT:* "Although encouraged by my mentor, Charles Nolte, to become a professional actor, I was getting an M.F.A. at the University of Minnesota to become a better teacher. Not until meeting Tennessee Williams at a cast party where he had seen me do Eunice in *Streetcar* and having him tell me, 'My dear, you will always work,' did I decide I'd go for it. Shortly thereafter, Terence Kilburn of the Meadow Brook Theatre saw the same university production and offered me a seven-play contract and my equity card."

ADDRESSES: AGENT—Gage Group, Inc., 1650 Broadway, New York, NY 10019 and 9255 Sunset Boulevard, Suite 515, Los Angeles, CA 90069.

*   *   *

MULLAVEY, Greg   1939-

PERSONAL: Born September 10, 1939, in Buffalo, NY; son of Greg Mullavey, Sr. (a baseball scout and coach); married Meredith MacRae (an actress and singer). EDUCATION: Attended Hobart College; trained for the stage with Sanford Meisner and Herbert Berghof in New York City.

VOCATION: Actor.

CAREER: STAGE DEBUT—Ricky, *Ah, Wilderness!*, New York City. PRINCIPAL STAGE APPEARANCES—Leo Janowitz, *Romantic Comedy*, Ethel Barrymore Theatre, New York City, 1979; also appeared in *City Lights*, Burbank Theatre, Los Angeles, CA; *I*

Won't Dance, Gene Dynarski Theatre; and in production of *Special Occasions*, *Barefoot in the Park*, and *The Owl and the Pussycat*.

PRINCIPAL FILM APPEARANCES—Phelps, *The Shakiest Gun in the West*, Universal, 1968; group leader, *Bob and Carol and Ted and Alice*, Columbia, 1969; Harry, *Marigold Man*, Emerson, 1970; Robin Schwartz, *The Christian Licorice Store*, National General, 1971; Bob Summers, *The Love Machine*, Columbia, 1971; Private Peter Brown, *Raid on Rommel*, Universal, 1971; Harley Burton, *Stand Up and Be Counted*, Columbia, 1972; detective, *I Dismember Mama* (also known as *Poor Albert and Little Annie*), Europix, 1974; Morrison, *The Hindenberg*, Universal, 1975; Harold Green, *I'm Going to Be Famous*, International Film Sales, 1982; George, *The Census Taker*, Seymour Borde, 1984; Gene Kline, *My Friends Need Killing*, Nick Felix, 1984; Harry Danvers, *The Check Is in the Mail*, Ascot Entertainment, 1986; Ralph Duris, *Body Count*, Manson International, 1988. Also appeared in *C.C. and Company*, Embassy, 1970; *Single Girls*, Dimension, 1973; and in *Vultures in Paradise*.

PRINCIPAL TELEVISION APPEARANCES—Series: David Goldberg, *Wednesday Night Out*, NBC, 1972; Tom Hartman, *Mary Hartman, Mary Hartman*, syndicated, 1976-77, then retitled *Forever Fernwood*, syndicated, 1977-78; Sam Wilder, *Wilder and Wilder*, CBS, 1978; Max Quintzel, *Number 96*, NBC, 1980-81; Eddie Gallagher, *Rituals*, NBC, 1984-85. Mini-Series: Mule Canby, *Centennial*, NBC, 1978-79. Pilots: Mike, *Quarantined*, ABC, 1970; Chuck Powell, *Switch* (also known as *Las Vegas Roundabout*), CBS, 1975; Ritter, *Big Eddie*, CBS, 1975; Mickey Paterno, *Having Babies*, NBC, 1976; Happy Burleso, *Crash Island*, NBC, 1981; Ed Fiore, *This Is Kate Bennett*, ABC, 1982; Mr. Rogers, *She's with Me*, CBS, 1982.

Episodic: "Bob and Rhoda and Teddy and Mary," *The Mary Tyler Moore Show*, CBS, 1970; "Mike's Friend," *All in the Family*, CBS, 1974; "Major Ego," *M*A*S*H*, CBS, 1978; Allen Powell, *The Fall Guy*, ABC, 1985; Russell, "A Little Peace and Quiet," *The Twilight Zone*, CBS, 1985; Walter Nash, *Spenser: For Hire*, ABC, 1986; Biff, *Tales from the Darkside*, syndicated, 1986; Jerry McDonague, *Hill Street Blues*, NBC, 1986; Randy, *Life with Lucy*, ABC, 1986; Sam Quigley, *Highway to Heaven*, NBC, 1986; editor, *Dynasty*, ABC, 1986; sheriff, *Dynasty*, ABC, 1987; Clay Graham, *Matlock*, NBC, 1987; Fisher, *Houston Knights*, CBS, 1988; Edward Travers, *The Highwayman*, NBC, 1988. Movies: Man in funeral parlor, *Companions in Nightmare*, NBC, 1968; Sparrow, *The Birdmen* (also known as *Escape of the Birdmen*), ABC, 1971; Liam Price, *Cry Rape!*, CBS, 1973; Lieutenant Tony Podryski, *The Disappearance of Flight 412*, NBC, 1974; Tom Malik, *Children of Divorce*, NBC, 1980; Charlie Greene, *Who Gets the Friends?*, CBS, 1988. Specials: *The National Love, Sex, and Marriage Test*, NBC, 1978.

NON-RELATED CAREER—In insurance and advertising.*

*   *   *

MURPHY, Michael   1938-

PERSONAL: Full name, Michael George Murphy; born May 5, 1938, in Los Angeles, CA; son of Bearl Branton (a salesman) and Georgia Arlyn (a teacher; maiden name, Money) Murphy. EDUCATION: University of Arizona, B.A., 1961. MILITARY: U. S. Marine Corps, 1956-57.

VOCATION: Actor.

CAREER: STAGE DEBUT—*Take Her, She's Mine,* Valley Music Theatre, Los Angeles, CA, 1966. PRINCIPAL STAGE APPEARANCES—Hank, *Goodbye, Freddy,* Manhattan Punch Line, Intar Theatre, New York City, 1985; also *Our Town,* Huntington Hartford Theatre, Los Angeles, CA, 1970; *The Hotel Play,* La Mama Experimental Theatre Club, New York City, 1981; *Playing in Local Bands,* Yale Repertory Theatre, New Haven, CT, 1983; and *Curse of the Starving Class,* Portland Stage Company, Portland, ME, 1985.

PRINCIPAL STAGE WORK—Director, *Rat's Nest,* Vandam Theatre, then Grove Street Theatre, both New York City, 1978.

PRINCIPAL FILM APPEARANCES—Morley, *Double Trouble,* Metro-Goldwyn-Mayer (MGM), 1967; Rick, *Countdown,* Warner Brothers, 1968; Mark Peter Sheehan, *The Legend of Lylah Clare,* MGM, 1968; Father Draddy, *The Arrangement,* Warner Brothers, 1969; Frank Shaft, *Brewster McCloud,* MGM, 1970; Paul, *Count Yorga, Vampire,* American International, 1970; Me Lay, *M*A*S*H,* Twentieth Century-Fox, 1970; Sears, *McCabe and Mrs. Miller,* Warner Brothers, 1971; Mr. Smith, *What's Up, Doc?,* Warner Brothers, 1972; Ted, *The Thief Who Came to Dinner,* Warner Brothers, 1973; James Lasko, *Phase IV,* Paramount, 1974; John Triplette, *Nashville,* Paramount, 1975; Alfred Miller, *The Front,* Columbia, 1976; Manigma, *The Great Bank Hoax* (also known as *The Great Georgia Bank Hoax* and *Shenanigans*), Jacoby, 1977; Martin, *The Class of Miss MacMichael,* Brut, 1978; Martin, *An Unmarried Woman,* Twentieth Century-Fox, 1978; Yale, *Manhattan,* United Artists, 1979; Brody, *Dead Kids* (also known as *Strange Behavior*), South Street, 1981; Pete Curtis, *The Year of Living Dangerously,* MGM, 1982; Rice, *Cloak and Dagger,* Universal, 1984; Ambassador Thomas Kelly, *Salvador,* Hemdale, 1986. Also appeared in *That Cold Day in the Park,* Commonwealth United Entertainment, 1969.

TELEVISION DEBUT—*Saints and Sinners,* 1962. PRINCIPAL TELEVISION APPEARANCES—Series: Dr. Art Armstrong, *Two Marriages,* ABC, 1983-1984; Jack Tanner, *Tanner '88: The Dark Horse,* HBO, 1988. Episodic: *Ben Casey,* ABC; *Dr. Kildare,* NBC; *Bonanza,* NBC; *Combat!,* ABC. Movies: Frank Adamic, *The Crooked Hearts,* ABC, 1972; Alec Shield, *I Love You . . . Goodbye,* CBS, 1974; Quentin Lerner, *The Autobiography of Miss Jane Pittman,* CBS, 1974; attendant, *Born to Be Sold,* NBC, 1981; Alan Murray, *The Rules of Marriage,* CBS, 1982; process server, *Right of Way,* HBO, 1983; chief judge, *The Caine Mutiny Court-Martial,* CBS, 1988. Also *John Cheever's "Oh Youth and Beauty,"* 1979.

NON-RELATED CAREER—English and drama teacher, Los Angeles, CA, 1962-64.

ADDRESSES: AGENT—Joe Funicello, International Creative Management, 8899 Beverly Boulevard, Los Angeles, CA 90048.*

*   *   *

MURPHY, Rosemary   1927-

PERSONAL: Born January 13, 1927, in Munich, Germany; daughter of Robert D. (a diplomat) and Mildred (Taylor) Murphy. EDUCATION: Received B.A. from Manhattanville College; trained for the stage at the Neighborhood Playhouse School of the Theatre

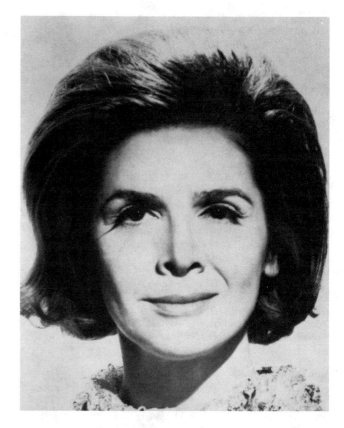

ROSEMARY MURPHY

with Sanford Meisner and at the Actors Studio. RELIGION: Roman Catholic.

VOCATION: Actress.

CAREER: STAGE DEBUT—*Claudia,* Olney Theatre, Olney, MD, 1946. BROADWAY DEBUT—Townsperson, *The Tower beyond Tragedy,* American National Theatre and Academy Theatre, 1950. LONDON DEBUT—Harriet, Edith, and Muriel, *You Know I Can't Hear You When the Water's Running,* New Theatre, 1968. PRINCIPAL STAGE APPEARANCES—Woman in Green, *Peer Gynt,* Schlosspark Theatre, Berlin, West Germany, 1949; Mary Boleyn, *Anne of the Thousand Days,* Flatbush Theatre, Brooklyn, NY, 1950; Jane Pugh, *Clutterbuck,* and Liserle, *Candle-Light,* both Arena Theatre, Memphis, TN, 1952; Lizzie Curry, *The Rainmaker,* and Rosemary Sydney, *Picnic,* both Myrtle Beach Playhouse, Myrtle Beach, SC, 1955; Lady Isabel Welwyn, *The Ascent of F6,* Davenport Theatre, New York City, 1955; Lady Macduff, *Macbeth,* Rooftop Theatre, New York City, 1955; Helen Gant Barton, *Look Homeward, Angel,* Ethel Barrymore Theatre, New York City, 1957; Hannah Jelkes, *The Night of the Iguana,* Festival of the Two Worlds, Spoleto, Italy, 1959.

Dorothea Bates, *Period of Adjustment,* Helen Hayes Theatre, New York City, 1960; ensemble, *Brecht on Brecht* (revue), Theatre De Lys, New York City, 1962; Goneril, *King Lear,* and a courtesan, *The Comedy of Errors,* both American Shakespeare Festival, Stratford, CT, 1963; Dorothy Cleves, *Any Wednesday,* Music Box Theatre, New York City, 1964; Claire, *A Delicate Balance,* Martin Beck Theatre, New York City, 1966; Estelle MacGruder, *Weekend,* Broadhurst Theatre, New York City, 1968; the Nurse, *The*

Death of Bessie Smith, Billy Rose Theatre, New York City, 1968; Mrs. Bakcr, *Butterflies Are Free,* Booth Theatre, New York City, 1969; Lady Macbeth, *Macbeth,* American Shakespeare Festival, 1973; Joanne Remington, *Ladies at the Alamo,* Martin Beck Theatre, 1977; Monica, *Cheaters,* Biltmore Theatre, New York City, 1978; Lillian Hellman, *Are You Now or Have You Ever Been?,* Promenade Theatre, New York City, 1978; Mrs. Gunhild Borkman, *John Gabriel Borkman,* Circle in the Square, New York City, 1980; Philaminte, *The Learned Ladies,* Raft Theatre, New York City, 1982; M.J. Adams, *Coastal Disturbances,* Second Stage Theatre, New York City, 1986, then Circle in the Square, 1987; Mrs. Dudgeon, *The Devil's Disciple,* Circle in the Square, 1988. Also appeared in *Red Sky at Morning,* Olney Theatre, Olney, MD, 1953; *The Women,* Norwich Playhouse, Norwich, CT, 1954; *Ring 'round the Moon,* Ahmanson Theatre, Los Angeles, CA, 1975; *Mourning Becomes Electra,* Goodman Theatre, Chicago, IL, 1976; *Medea,* Clarence Brown Company, Knoxville, TN, 1982; and in *The Importance of Being Earnest,* Alliance Theatre Company, Atlanta, GA, 1985.

MAJOR TOURS—Mary Boleyn, *Anne of the Thousand Days,* U.S. cities, 1950; Olivia, *The Chalk Garden,* U.S. cities, 1956; Claire, *A Delicate Balance,* U.S. cities, 1966-67.

FILM DEBUT—*Berlin Express,* RKO, 1948. PRINCIPAL FILM APPEARANCES—Nurse Chornis, *That Night,* Universal, 1957; Miss Graves, *The Young Doctors,* United Artists, 1961; Miss Maudie Atkinson, *To Kill a Mockingbird,* Universal, 1962; Dorothy Cleves, *Any Wednesday* (also known as *Bachelor Girl Apartment*), Warner Brothers, 1966; Beth Garrison, *Ben,* Cinerama, 1972; Moms, *A Fan's Notes,* Warner Brothers, 1972; Mrs. Kinsolving, *You'll Like My Mother,* Universal, 1972; Hannah, *Ace Eli and Rodger of the Skies,* Twentieth Century-Fox, 1973; Mrs. Latham, *Forty Carats,* Columbia, 1973; Callie Hacker, *Walking Tall,* Cinerama, 1973; Dorothy Parker, *Julia,* Twentieth Century-Fox, 1977; Mrs. Perkins, *The Attic,* Atlantic, 1979; Karen Wagner, *The Hand,* Warner Brothers, 1981; Mrs. Mason, *September,* Orion, 1987; also appeared in the German film *Der Ruf,* 1949.

PRINCIPAL TELEVISION APPEARANCES—Series: Nola Hollister, *The Secret Storm,* CBS, 1969; Margaret Blumenthal, *Lucas Tanner,* NBC, 1974-75; Maureen Teller, *All My Children,* ABC, 1977-78; also Loretta Fowler, *Another World,* NBC. Mini-Series: Mary Ball Washington, *George Washington,* CBS, 1984. Pilots: Margaret Blumenthal, *Lucas Tanner,* NBC, 1974. Episodic: "The Long Way Home," *Robert Montgomery Presents,* NBC, 1956; "Way Out," *Studio One,* CBS, 1962; *Cannon,* CBS, 1972; *Banyon,* NBC, 1973; *Medical Center,* CBS, 1973; *The Streets of San Francisco,* ABC, 1973; *Columbo,* NBC, 1974; also *Thriller,* NBC; *The Virginian,* NBC; *The Wide Country,* NBC; *Murder, She Wrote,* CBS; *Magnum, P.I.,* CBS; *Kate and Allie,* CBS. Movies: Muriel Dyer, *A Case of Rape,* NBC, 1974; Sara Delano Roosevelt, *Eleanor and Franklin,* ABC, 1976; Sara Delano Roosevelt, *Eleanor and Franklin: The White House Years,* ABC, 1977; Helen, *Before and After,* ABC, 1979. Plays: *The Lady's Not for Burning,* PBS, 1974.

RELATED CAREER—Member, Actors Studio, New York City, 1954—.

AWARDS: Clarence Derwent Award, Outer Circle Critics Award, *Variety* New York Critics Poll Award, and Antoinette Perry Award nomination, Best Supporting or Featured Actress in a Drama, all 1961, for *Period of Adjustment;* Antoinette Perry Award nomination, Best Supporting or Featured Actress in a Drama, 1964, for *Any Wednesday;* Motion Picture Arts Club Award, 1966; *Variety* New

York Critics Poll Award and Antoinette Perry Award nomination, Best Actress in a Drama, both 1967, for *A Delicate Balance;* Emmy Award, Best Supporting Actress in a Drama Special, 1976, for *Eleanor and Franklin.*

MEMBER: Actors' Equity Association, Screen Actors Guild, American Federation of Television and Radio Artists.

ADDRESSES: HOME—220 E. 73rd Street, New York, NY 10021.

*   *   *

MUSANTE, Tony   1936-

PERSONAL: Full name, Anthony Peter Musante, Jr.; born June 30, 1936, in Bridgeport, CT; son of Anthony Peter (an accountant) and Natalie Anne (a school teacher; maiden name, Salerno) Musante; married Jane Ashley Sparkes (a writer), June 2, 1962. EDUCATION: Attended Northwestern University, 1957; Oberlin College, B.A., psychology, 1958; trained for the stage at the HB Studios with Walt Witcover and with Will Geer and Tucker Ashworth.

VOCATION: Actor, director, and screenwriter.

CAREER: OFF-BROADWAY DEBUT—(As Anthony Musante) Soldier and villager, *Borak,* Martinique Theatre, 1960. BROADWAY DEBUT—Vito, *P.S. Your Cat Is Dead,* John Golden Theatre, 1975. PRINCIPAL STAGE APPEARANCES—George, *Kiss Mama,* Actors Playhouse, New York City, 1964; Marty, "Match Play," in

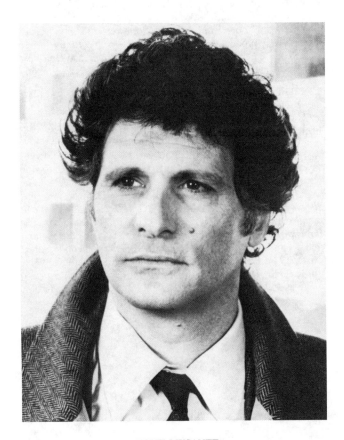

TONY MUSANTE

A Party for Divorce [and] Match-Play (double-bill), Province-town Playhouse, New York City, 1966; David Byron, *Night of the Dunce*, Cherry Lane Theatre, New York City, 1966; Wallace, *A Gun Play*, Cherry Lane Theatre, 1971; Stanley Kowalski, *A Streetcar Named Desire*, Hartford Stage Company, Hartford, CT, 1972; Vito, *P.S. Your Cat Is Dead*, Studio Arena Theatre, Buffalo, NY, 1974; Silva Vicarro, "27 Wagons Full of Cotton," and Larry, "A Memory of Two Mondays," in *27 Wagons Full of Cotton [and] A Memory of Two Mondays* (double-bill), Phoenix Theatre Company, Playhouse Theatre, New York City, 1976; Mark Sanders, *Souvenir*, Shubert Theatre, Century City, CA, 1975; Calogero Di Spelta, *Grand Magic*, Manhattan Theatre Club, New York City, 1979.

Sam, *The Lady from Dubuque*, Morosco Theatre, New York City, 1980; Edgar Degas, *Cassatt*, Playhouse 46, New York City, 1980; Petruchio, *The Taming of the Shrew*, Old Globe Theatre, San Diego, CA, 1982; Charlie, *The Big Knife*, Berkshire Theatre Festival, MA, 1983; Coach Dean, *Dancing in the End Zone*, Coconut Grove Playhouse, Coconut Grove, FL, 1983; Charlie, *The Big Knife*, Walnut Street Theatre Company, Philadelphia, PA, 1986. Also appeared in *L'Histoire du soldat*, 1967; *The Archbishop's Ceiling*, Kennedy Center, Washington, DC, 1977; *Two Brothers*, Long Wharf Theatre, Hartford, CT, 1978; *Double Play*, Westwood Playhouse, Los Angeles, CA, 1984; *Widows*, Williamstown Theatre Festival, NY, 1988; *Frankie & Johnnie in the Clair de Lune*, Westside Arts Theatre, New York City, 1988; in *Madame Mousse*, Westport Country Playhouse, Westport, CT; *The Tender Heel*, Curran Theatre, San Francisco, CA; *Miss Julie* and *APA Shakespeare Repertory*, both McCarter Theatre, Princeton, NJ; *Falling Man*, Florida State University; *The Glass Menagerie* and *Traveller without Luggage*, both Branford Theatre; *Desire under the Elms*, *Ring around the Moon*, and *Death of a Salesman*, all Clinton Theatre; *Love's Labour Lost*, Northwestern University; in Off-Broadway productions including *The Zoo Story*, *Pinter Plays*, *The Balcony*, *Theatre of the Absurd*, *Benito Cereno*, and *Half Past Wednesday*; and at the McCarter Theatre, Princeton, NJ, 1965-66.

PRINCIPAL STAGE WORK—Assistant stage manager, *Borak*, Martinique Theatre, New York City, 1960; stage manager, *Whisper into My Good Ear* and *Mrs. Dally Has a Lover*, both Cherry Lane Theatre, New York City, 1962.

FILM DEBUT—Cleve Schoenstein, *Once a Thief*, Metro-Goldwyn-Mayer (MGM), 1965. PRINCIPAL FILM APPEARANCES—Joe Ferrone, *The Incident*, Twentieth Century-Fox, 1967; Felix, *The Detective*, Twentieth Century-Fox, 1968; Sam Dalmas, *The Bird with the Crystal Plumage* (also known as *L'Ucello dalle plume di cristallo* and *The Phantom of Terror*), UM, 1970; Eufemio, *The Mercenary* (also known as *Il mercenario* and *Salario para matar*), United Artists, 1970; Enrico, *The Anonymous Venetian*, Allied Artists, 1971; Eddie Hagen, *The Grissom Gang*, Cinerama, 1971; Paul Richard, *The Last Run*, MGM, 1971; Paolo, *Break Up* (also known as *Eutanasia de amore*), Rizzoli Films, 1978; Pete Grillo,

The Pope of Greenwich Village, Metro-Goldwyn-Mayer/United Artists, 1984; Tommaso Buscetta, *The Repenter*, Columbia, 1985; also appeared in *One Night at Dinner*, 1970; *Nocturne*, RTA/RAI, 1981; *The Trap*, 1984; *The Cage*, 1985; *The Pisciotta Case*, Columbia; and *Goodbye and Amen*, Rizzoli Films.

TELEVISION DEBUT—Joe Ferrone, "Ride with Terror," *DuPont Show of the Month*, NBC, 1963. PRINCIPAL TELEVISION APPEARANCES—Series: Detective David Toma, *Toma*, ABC, 1973-74. Mini-Series: *Nutcracker: Money, Madness, and Murder*, NBC, 1986; *Devil's Hill*, RAI-TV (Italy), 1987; *Appointment in Trieste*, RAI-TV, 1987; *The Legend of the Black Hand*, ABC. Pilots: Dave Toma, *Toma*, ABC, 1973; Joey Faber, *Nowhere to Hide*, NBC, 1977; King, *The 13th Day: The Story of Esther*, ABC, 1979. Episodic: George, "Weekend," *American Playhouse*, PBS, 1982; John Parker, *The Equalizer*, CBS, 1986; Roy, *Night Heat*, CBS, 1987; also *Police Story*, NBC, 1974-76; *Bob Hope Presents the Chrysler Theatre*, NBC; *The Fugitive*, ABC; *N.Y.P.D.*, ABC; *The Trials of O'Brien*, CBS; *Medical Story*, NBC; *The Alfred Hitchcock Hour*. Movies: Joe Larkin, *The Desperate Miles*, ABC, 1975; Derek MacKenzie, *My Husband Is Missing*, NBC, 1978; Sal Falcone, *Breaking Up Is Hard to Do*, ABC, 1979; Lieutenant Colonel Harris Thatcher, *High Ice*, NBC, 1980; Vince Martino, *Rearview Mirror*, NBC, 1984; Brad Baxter, *Last Waltz on a Tightrope*, PBS, 1986; also *The Quality of Mercy*, ABC, 1975; title role, *Judgement: The Court-Martial of Lt. William Calley*, ABC.

RELATED CAREER—Director of community theatres in Connecticut, Ohio, and Illinois; president of jury, International Film Festival, Coruna, Spain, 1983.

WRITINGS: TELEVISION—Episodic: (With Jane Sparkes) *Toma*, ABC, 1973-74.

AWARDS: Hollywood Women's Press Club Award, 1973, Golden Apple Award, 1973, and *Photoplay* (magazine) Gold Medal Award, 1974, all for *Toma*; New York Drama Desk Award nomination, Best Actor, 1975, for *P.S. Your Cat Is Dead*; Emmy Award nomination, Outstanding Performance, 1976, for *The Quality of Mercy*; Silver Screen Award (Italy), 1977; Rudolfo Valentino Award (Italy), 1980; Il carro d'oro award (Italy), 1988; also South American International Film Festival Award, Best Actor, for *The Incident*.

MEMBER: Academy of Motion Picture Arts and Sciences, Actors' Equity Association, Screen Actors Guild, American Federation of Television and Radio Artists, Writers Guild of America-West, Academy of Television Arts and Sciences.

ADDRESSES: HOMES—New York, NY; Los Angeles, CA. AGENT—Don Wolff, The Artists Agency, 10000 Santa Monica Boulevard, Los Angeles, CA 90067.

N

NAPIER, Alan   1903-1988

PERSONAL: Born Alan Napier-Clavering, January 7, 1903, in Birmingham, England; died of pneumonia, August 8, 1988, in Santa Monica, CA; son of Claude Gerald and Millicent Mary (Kendrick) Napier-Clavering; married Emily Nancy Bevill Pethybridge; children: one daughter, one stepdaughter. EDUCATION: Trained for the stage at the Royal Academy of Dramatic Art.

VOCATION: Actor.

CAREER: STAGE DEBUT—Policeman, *Dandy Dick,* Oxford Playhouse, Oxford, U.K., 1924. LONDON DEBUT—Professor Boland, *Storm,* Ambassadors' Theatre, 1924. PRINCIPAL STAGE APPEARANCES—All in London, unless indicated: Reverend John Williams, *A Comedy of Good and Evil,* Ambassadors' Theatre, 1925; Leonid Gayef, *The Cherry Orchard,* Lyric Hammersmith Theatre, 1925; Pick-purse, *And So to Bed,* Queen's Theatre, 1926; colonel, *The Spook Sonata,* Globe Theatre, 1927; Boris Waberski, *The House of the Arrow,* Vaudeville Theatre, 1928; Colonel Tripp, *Down Wind,* Arts Theatre, 1928; Episcopal vicar, *Ginevra,* Everyman Theatre, 1928; Ernie Dunstan, *Out of the Sea,* and title role, *Doctor Knock,* both Strand Theatre, 1928; Marquis of Shayne, *Bitter Sweet,* His Majesty's Theatre, 1929; Everard Webley, *This Way to Paradise,* Daly's Theatre, 1930; professor, *Brain,* Savoy Theatre, 1930; Pharmaceutis, *The Devil and the Lady,* Arts Theatre, 1930; Edward IV, *Richard III,* New Theatre, 1930; Earl of Dorincourt, *Little Lord Fauntleroy,* Gate Theatre, 1931; Claude Spencer, *Marry at Leisure,* Haymarket Theatre, 1931; Venetian ambassador, *The Immortal Lady,* Royalty Theatre, 1931; Sir Henry Cosham, *A-Hunting We Will Go,* Savoy Theatre, 1931; Nasmyth Sheldon, *The Home Front,* Grafton Theatre, 1931; Mark Elliott, *The Green Pack,* Wyndham's Theatre, 1932; Lovasdy, *Firebird,* Playhouse Theatre, 1932; Absalon, *The Witch,* Little Theatre, 1933; John Clayne, *The Lake,* Arts Theatre, then Westminster Theatre, both 1933; Richard Greatham, *Hay Fever,* Shaftesbury Theatre, 1933; Mr. Wise, *Private Room,* Westminster Theatre, 1934; Sir John Craig, *Forsaking All Others,* Fulham Theatre, 1934; Mr. Lennox, *The Roof,* Embassy Theatre, 1934; Lord Farrington, *Sweet Aloes,* Wyndham's Theatre, 1934.

Prince of Verona, *Romeo and Juliet,* New Theatre, 1935; Gray Blackett, *Gentle Rain,* Vaudeville Theatre, 1936; Hyalmar Ekdal, *The Wild Duck,* Westminster Theatre, 1936; Sir Basil Graham, *Because We Must,* Wyndham's Theatre, 1937; Hector Hushabye, *Heartbreak House,* Westminster Theatre, 1937; General Rakovski, *Judgment Day,* Strand Theatre, 1937; Hugh Gifford, *Land's End,* and Michael, *The Zeal of Thy House,* both Westminster Theatre, 1938; Boris Rachinoff, *No Sky So Blue,* Savoy Theatre, 1938; king, *The Shoemaker's Holiday,* Playhouse Theatre, 1938; Sir Francis Chesney, *Charley's Aunt,* Haymarket Theatre, 1938; Sir William

Warring, *Lady in Waiting,* Martin Beck Theatre, New York City, 1940; Charles II, *And So to Bed,* Las Palmas Theatre, Los Angeles, CA, 1948; Mr. Ritchie, *Gertie,* Plymouth Theatre, New York City, 1952; Menenius Agrippa, *Coriolanus,* Phoenix Theatre, New York City, 1954; Captain Massingham, *Too Late the Phalarope,* Belasco Theatre, New York City, 1956. Also appeared in repertory at the Theatre Royal, Huddersfield, U.K., 1926; and in Glasgow, Scotland, 1927.

MAJOR TOURS—Inspector Hubbard, *Dial "M" for Murder,* U.S. cities, 1952; also *Loyalties* and *Justice,* U.K. cities, both 1929.

PRINICPAL FILM APPEARANCES—Captain Hawtree, *Caste,* United Artists, 1930; Bouchier, *Stamboul,* Paramount, 1931; General Canynge, *Loyalties,* Harold Auten, 1934; Count Romano, *In a Monastery Garden,* Associated Producers and Distributors, 1935; general, *For Valor,* General Films Distributors, 1937; governor, *The Wife of General Ling* (also known as *The Revenge of General Ling*), Gaumont, 1938; archdeacon, *We Are Not Alone,* Warner Brothers, 1939; Redfern, *Wings over Africa,* Merit, 1939; Fuller, *The House of the Seven Gables,* Universal, 1940; Willie Spears, *The Invisible Man Returns,* Universal, 1940; Sir Haymar Ryman, M.P., *The Secret Four* (also known as *The Four Just Men*), Monogram, 1940; Updyke, *Confirm or Deny,* Twentieth Century-Fox, 1941; Carver, *Cat People,* RKO, 1942; Black Watch officer, *Eagle Squadron,* Universal, 1942; Julian, *Random Harvest,* Metro-Goldwyn-Mayer (MGM), 1942; Captain Blackstone, *We Were Dancing,* MGM, 1942; restaurateur, *A Yank at Eton,* MGM, 1942; Colonel Patterson, *Appointment in Berlin,* Columbia, 1943; Andrew, *Lassie, Come Home,* MGM, 1943; Doctor Bladh, *Madame Curie,* MGM, 1943; psychiatrist, *The Song of Bernadette,* Twentieth Century-Fox, 1943; Latimer, *Action in Arabia,* RKO, 1944; doctor, *Dark Waters,* United Artists, 1944; MacDougald, *The Hairy Ape,* United Artists, 1944; Doctor Woodring, *Lost Angel,* MGM, 1944; Count de Breville, *Mademoiselle Fifi,* RKO, 1944; Mr. Parker, *Thirty Seconds Over Tokyo,* MGM, 1944; Doctor Scott, *The Uninvited,* Paramount, 1944.

Sir Henry Chapman, *Hangover Square,* Twentieth Century-Fox, 1945; Mr. St. Aubyn, *Isle of the Dead,* RKO, 1945; Doctor Forrester, *Ministry of Fear,* Paramount, 1945; F. Holmes Harmon, *House of Horrors* (also known as *Joan Medford Is Missing*), Universal, 1946; Houdon, *A Scandal in Paris* (also known as *Thieves' Holiday*), United Artists, 1946; Judge Saladine, *The Strange Woman,* United Artists, 1946; Shackleford, *Three Strangers,* Warner Brothers, 1946; Mr. Atwater, *Adventure Island,* Paramount, 1947; Doctor Adams, *Driftwood,* Republic, 1947; tourist, *Fiesta,* MGM, 1947; Landale, *Forever Amber,* Twentieth Century-Fox, 1947; Thomas, *High Conquest,* Monogram, 1947; Sir Jonathan Wright, *Ivy,* Universal, 1947; Monty Beresford, *Lone Wolf in London,* Columbia, 1947; Inspector Gordon, *Lured* (also known as

Personal Column), United Artists, 1947; Aga, *Sinbad the Sailor*, RKO, 1947; Sir William Johnson, *Unconquered*, Paramount, 1947; Sir George, *Hills of Home* (also known as *Master of Lassie*), MGM, 1948; Earl of Warwick, *Joan of Arc*, RKO, 1948; defense attorney, *Johnny Belinda*, Warner Brothers, 1948; Holy Father, *Macbeth*, Republic, 1948; Kittredge, *My Own True Love*, Paramount, 1948; Lord Provost, *Challenge to Lassie*, MGM, 1949; high executioner, *A Connecticut Yankee in King Arthur's Court*, Paramount, 1949; Finchley, *Criss Cross*, Universal, 1949; Alton Bennett, *Manhandled*, Paramount, 1949; Doctor Druzik, *Master Minds*, Monogram, 1949; general, *The Red Danube*, MGM, 1949; Jessup, *Tarzan's Magic Fountain*, RKO, 1949.

Captain Kidd, *Double Crossbones*, Universal, 1950; Khalil, *Tripoli* (also known as *The First Marines*), Paramount, 1950; Captain Humberstone Lyon, *Across the Wide Missouri*, MGM, 1951; Professor Carter, *The Blue Veil*, RKO, 1951; Jean de Reszke, *The Great Caruso*, MGM, 1951; Barton, *The Highwayman*, Monogram, 1951; Count Grassin, *The Strange Door*, Universal, 1951; Peters, *Tarzan's Peril* (also known as *Tarzan and the Jungle Queen*), RKO, 1951; Sturak, *Big Jim McLain*, Warner Brothers, 1952; Cicero, *Julius Caesar*, MGM, 1953; Robert Tyrwhitt, *Young Bess*, MGM, 1953; Despereaux, *Desiree*, Twentieth Century-Fox, 1954; Parson Glennie, *Moonfleet*, MGM, 1955; Sir Brockhurst, *The Court Jester*, Paramount, 1956; Raymond Sheridan, *Miami Expose*, Columbia, 1956; Elinu high priest, *The Mole People*, Universal, 1956; prosecuting attorney, *Until They Sail*, MGM, 1957; Doctor Lujan, *Island of Lost Women*, Warner Brothers, 1959; Dean, *Journey to the Center of the Earth*, Twentieth Century-Fox, 1959; Pardo, *Tender Is the Night*, Twentieth Century-Fox, 1961; Professor Larson, *Wild in the Country*, Twentieth Century-Fox, 1961; Doctor Gideon Gault, *The Premature Burial*, American International, 1962; voice of Sir Pelinore, *The Sword in the Stone* (animated), Buena Vista, 1963; Mr. Rutland, *Marnie*, Universal, 1964; ambassador, *My Fair Lady*, Warner Brothers, 1964; vicar, *Signpost to Murder*, MGM, 1964; club official, *The Loved One*, MGM, 1965; Colonel Peter MacLean, *36 Hours*, MGM, 1965; Alfred Pennyworth, *Batman*, Twentieth Century-Fox, 1966. Also appeared in *The Paper Chase*, Twentieth Century-Fox, 1973.

PRINCIPAL TELEVISION APPEARANCES—Series: General Steele, *Don't Call Me Charlie*, NBC, 1962-63; Alfred Pennyworth, *Batman*, ABC, 1966-68. Mini-Series: Lord Venneford, *Centennial*, NBC, 1979. Episodic: *The Late Show*, Fox, 1988. Movies: John, *Crime Club*, CBS, 1973; Semple, *QB VII*, ABC, 1974; Briarton, *The Monkey Mission*, NBC, 1981; also *The Bastard*, syndicated, 1978. Also appeared in *The Contest Kid Strikes Again*.

OBITUARIES AND OTHER SOURCES: New York Times, August 9, 1988; *Variety*, August 17, 1988.*

*   *   *

NATWICK, Mildred   1908-

PERSONAL: Born June 19, 1908, in Baltimore, MD; daughter of Joseph and Mildred Marion (Dawes) Natwick.

VOCATION: Actress.

CAREER: STAGE DEBUT—Widow Quin, *The Playboy of the Western World*, Vagabond Theatre, Baltimore, MD, 1929. BROADWAY DEBUT—Mrs. Noble, *Carry Nation*, Biltmore Theatre,

1932. LONDON DEBUT—Aunt Mabel, *The Day I Forgot*, Globe Theatre, 1933. PRINCIPAL STAGE APPEARANCES—Drusilla Thorpe, *Amourette*, and Pura, *Spring in Autumn*, both Henry Miller's Theatre, New York City, 1933; Mrs. McFie, *The Wind and the Rain*, Ritz Theatre, New York City, 1934; Mrs. Venables, *The Distaff Side*, Booth Theatre, New York City, 1934; May Beringer, *Night in the House*, Booth Theatre, 1935; Mrs. Wyler, *End of Summer*, Guild Theatre, New York City, 1936; Ethel, *Love from a Stranger*, Fulton Theatre, New York City, 1936; Proserpine Garnett, *Candida*, and Mrs. Rutledge, *The Star Wagon*, both Empire Theatre, New York City, 1937; Widow Weeks, *Missouri Legend*, Empire Theatre, 1938; Bess, *Stars in Your Eyes*, Majestic Theatre, New York City, 1939; Mother McGlory, *Christmas Eve*, Henry Miller's Theatre, 1939.

Milly, *The Lady Who Came to Stay*, Maxine Elliott's Theatre, New York City, 1941; Madame Arcati, *Blithe Spirit*, Morosco Theatre, New York City, 1941; Proserpine Garnett, *Candida*, Shubert Theatre, New York City, 1942; Widow Quin, *The Playboy of the Western World*, Booth Theatre, 1946; Proserpine Garnett, *Candida*, Cort Theatre, New York City, 1946; Dolly Talbo, *The Grass Harp*, Martin Beck Theatre, New York City, 1952; Volumnia, *Coriolanus*, Phoenix Theatre, New York City, 1954; Madame St. Pe, *The Waltz of the Toreadors*, Coronet Theatre, New York City, 1957; Kathie Morrow, *The Day the Money Stopped*, Belasco Theatre, New York City, 1958; Miriam, *The Firstborn*, Coronet Theatre, 1958; Marie-Paule's mother, Angele, and Armand's mother, *The Good Soup*, Plymouth Theatre, New York City, 1960; Charlotte Orr, *Critic's Choice*, Ethel Barrymore Theatre, New York City, 1960; Mrs. Banks, *Barefoot in the Park*, Biltmore Theatre, New York City, 1963-65, then Piccadilly Theatre, London, 1965; Mrs. Gibbs, *Our Town*, American National Theatre and Academy Theatre, New York City, 1969; Beth, *Landscape*, Forum Theatre, New York City, 1970; Ida, *70 Girls 70*, Broadhurst Theatre, New York City, 1971; Delia, *Bedroom Farce*, Brooks Atkinson Theatre, New York City, 1979. Also appeared with the National Junior Theatre Company, Washington, DC.

PRINCIPAL FILM APPEARANCES—Freda, *The Long Voyage Home*, United Artists, 1940; Abigail Minnett, *The Enchanted Cottage*, RKO, 1945; Aunt Amarilla, *Yolanda and the Thief*, Metro-Goldwyn-Mayer (MGM), 1945; Amelia Newcombe, *The Late George Apley*, Twentieth Century-Fox, 1947; Nurse Braddock, *A Woman's Vengeance*, Universal, 1947; Isabella, *The Kissing Bandit*, MGM, 1948; the mother, *The Three Godfathers*, MGM, 1948; Mrs. Abby Allshard, *She Wore a Yellow Ribbon*, RKO, 1949; Mrs. McBane, *Cheaper by the Dozen*, Twentieth Century-Fox, 1950; Molvina MacGregor, *Against All Flags*, Universal, 1952; Mrs. Sarah Tillane, *The Quiet Man*, Republic, 1952; Miss Graveley, *The Trouble with Harry*, Paramount, 1956; Griselda, *The Court Jester*, Paramount, 1956; Grace Hewitt, *Teenage Rebel*, Twentieth Century-Fox, 1956; Aunt Renie, *Tammy and the Bachelor* (also known as *Tammy*), Universal, 1957; Mrs. Ethel Banks, *Barefoot in the Park*, Paramount, 1967; Jenny Grant, *If It's Tuesday, This Must Be Belgium*, United Artists, 1969; Molly Fletcher, *The Maltese Bippy*, MGM, 1969; Miss Miller, "Miriam" in *Truman Capote's Trilogy*, Allied Artists, 1969; Mrs. Costello, *Daisy Miller*, Paramount, 1974; Mabel Pritchard, *At Long Last Love*, Twentieth Century-Fox, 1975; Mrs. Reilly, *Kiss Me Goodbye*, Twentieth Century-Fox, 1982; Madame DeRosemonde, *Dangerous Liaisons*, Warner Brothers, 1988; also appeared as herself, *The Thrill of Genius* (also known as *Hitchcock, Il brivido del genio*; documentary), 1985.

PRINCIPAL TELEVISION APPEARANCES—Series: Gwendolyn Snoop, *The Snoop Sisters*, NBC, 1973-74; Aunt Kathryn March,

Little Women, NBC, 1979. Pilots: Grandmother Mills, *The House without a Christmas Tree,* CBS, 1972; Gwendolyn Snoop, *Female Instinct,* NBC, 1972; Grandmother Mills, *The Thanksgiving Treasure,* CBS, 1973; Grandmother Mills, *The Easter Promise,* CBS, 1975; Grandmother Mills, *Addie and the King of Hearts,* CBS, 1976. Episodic: Beatrice McMillan, *McMillan and Wife,* NBC, 1971; Aunt Agatha, *Alice,* CBS, 1976; May Hardcastle, *Hardcastle and McCormick,* ABC, 1983; Carrie McKittrick, *Murder, She Wrote,* CBS, 1986; also *Magnavox Theatre,* CBS, 1950; *Love Story,* Dumont, 1954; *The Bob Newhart Show,* CBS, 1977; *Cameo Theater,* NBC; *The Loretta Young Theatre,* NBC; *Starlight Theatre,* CBS; *Pulitzer Prize Playhouse,* ABC; *The Doctor* (also known as *The Visitor*), NBC; *Suspense,* CBS; *The Love Boat,* ABC; *The Web,* CBS; *The Clock,* CBS; *Hawaii Five-O,* CBS. Movies: Shelby Saunders, *Do Not Fold, Spindle, or Mutilate,* ABC, 1971; Emily Finnegan, *Money to Burn,* ABC, 1973; Mrs. Angstrom, *Maid in America,* CBS, 1982; Sarah Cleason, *Deadly Deception* (also known as *Shattered Dreams*), CBS, 1987. Specials: Madame Arcati, *Blithe Spirit,* CBS, 1956; Martha Brewster, "Arsenic and Old Lace," *Hallmark Hall of Fame,* NBC, 1962; Olga, *You Can't Take It with You,* CBS, 1979; also in "The 75th," *The Booth,* PBS, 1985.

PRINCIPAL RADIO APPEARANCES—Episodic: "Diary of a Saboteur," *Cavalcade of America,* NBC, 1943.

AWARDS: Emmy Award nomination, 1956, for *Blithe Spirit;* Antoinette Perry Award nomination, Best Supporting or Featured Actress in a Play, 1957, for *The Waltz of the Toreadors;* Academy Award nomination, Best Supporting Actress, 1967, for *Barefoot in the Park;* Antoinette Perry Award nomination, Best Actress in a Musical, 1972, for *70 Girls 70;* Emmy Award, Best Lead Actress in a Limited Series, 1974, for *The Snoop Sisters;* also Barter Theatre Award for *Blithe Spirit.*

ADDRESSES: OFFICE—1001 Park Avenue, New York, NY 10028. AGENT—Fred Westheimer, William Morris Agency, 151 El Camino Drive, Beverly Hills, CA 90212.*

*   *   *

NEAME, Christopher   1942-

PERSONAL: Born in 1942 in Windsor, England.

VOCATION: Actor, director, producer, and screenwriter.

CAREER: Also see *WRITINGS* below. PRINCIPAL STAGE APPEARANCES—Phebe, *As You Like It,* National Theatre Company, Mark Hellinger Theatre, New York City, 1974; Edmund, *King Lear,* and Captain Absolute, *The Rivals,* both Prospect Theatre Company, Old Vic Theatre, London, 1978; Dr. Prentice, *What the Butler Saw,* Los Angeles Theatre Center, Los Angeles, CA, 1988.

PRINCIPAL FILM APPEARANCES—Locke, *No Blade of Grass,* Metro-Goldwyn-Mayer, 1970; Hans, *Lust for a Vampire* (also known as *To Kill a Vampire*), Levitt-Pickman, 1971; Johnny Alucard, *Dracula A.D. 1972* (also known as *Dracula Today*), Warner Brothers, 1972; Sho, *Steel Dawn,* Vestron, 1987; Bernard, *D.O.A.,* Touchstone, 1988; Van Hoeven, *Bloodstone,* Omega, 1989.

PRINCIPAL FILM WORK—Production manager, *Monique,* Tigon,

1970; production supervisor, *Blue Blood,* Impact Quadrant, 1973; production supervisor, *Malachi Cove* (also known as *The Seaweed Children*), Impact Quadrant, 1973; producer, *Emily,* Emily Productions, 1976; European consultant, *Power Play,* Rank Film Distributors, 1978; executive producer, *Foreign Body,* Orion/Rank Film Distributors, 1986; producer, *Bellman and True,* Island/Handmade, 1987.

PRINCIPAL TELEVISION APPEARANCES—Mini-Series: John Curtis, *Secret Army,* Entertainment Channel, 1982. Pilots: *Lily,* CBS, 1986. Episodic: Max, *Benson,* ABC, 1985; Jack Scarlett, *The A-Team,* NBC, 1985; Jason Gottlieb, *Lime Street,* ABC, 1985; Barrett Terrell, *The Fall Guy,* ABC, 1986; Quayle, *MacGyver,* ABC, 1986; Gunter, *Riptide,* NBC, 1986; Hans Von Sykes, *Spies,* CBS, 1987; Shakespeare, *Second Chance,* Fox, 1987; Hamilton Stone, *Dynasty,* ABC, 1988 and 1989; Collin, *Beauty and the Beast,* CBS, 1989; Gustav Helstrom, *Dallas,* CBS, 1989; Krupp, *Dallas,* CBS, 1989. Movies: Ian, *Love among Thieves,* ABC, 1987; Kiowski, *The Great Escape: The Untold Story* (also known as *The Great Escape: The Final Chapter*), NBC, 1988; Max Dolpho, *Case Closed,* CBS, 1988.

PRINCIPAL TELEVISION WORK—Series: Producer, *Q.E.D.,* CBS, 1982. Mini-Series: Producer, *The Flame Trees of Thika,* 1979, then *Masterpiece Theatre,* PBS, 1982; producer, "The Irish R.M.," *Masterpiece Theatre,* PBS, 1983-84; producer, "The Irish R.M., Part II," *Masterpiece Theatre,* PBS, 1986; also associate producer, "Danger UXB," *Masterpiece Theatre,* PBS. Specials: Producer, "Monsignor Quixote," *Great Performances,* PBS, 1987. Also producer, *The Knowledge,* 1979.

RELATED CAREER—Production manager, Hammer Films; production supervisor, Quadrant Films.

WRITINGS: TELEVISION—Specials: "Monsignor Quixote," *Great Performances,* PBS, 1987.

ADDRESSES: OFFICE—9 Kensington Court Mews, London W8 5DR, England. AGENT—Scott Manners, Stone/Manners Agency, 9113 Sunset Boulevard, Los Angeles, CA 90069.*

*   *   *

NEESON, Liam

PERSONAL: Born in Ballymena, Northern Ireland.

VOCATION: Actor.

CAREER: STAGE DEBUT—*The Risen,* Lyric Players Theatre, Belfast, Northern Ireland, 1976. PRINCIPAL STAGE APPEARANCES—*The Informer,* Dublin Theatre Festival, Dublin Ireland; *Translations,* National Theatre, London, England; also appeared with the Lyric Players Theatre, Belfast, Northern Ireland, 1976-78; and with the Abbey Theatre, Dublin.

FILM DEBUT—Gawain, *Excalibur,* Warner Brothers, 1981. PRINCIPAL FILM APPEARANCES—Kegan, *Krull,* Columbia, 1983; Churchill, *The Bounty,* Orion, 1984; Carns, *The Innocent,* TVS-Curzon, 1984; Michael Lamb/Brother Sebastian, *Lamb,* Flickers-Limehouse, 1985; Harry Totter, *Duet for One,* Cannon, 1986; Fielding, *The Mission,* Warner Brothers, 1986; Liam Dougherty, *A Prayer for the Dying,* Goldwyn, 1987; Carl Wayne Anderson,

Suspect, Tri-Star, 1987; Martin Falcon, *Satisfaction,* Twentieth Century-Fox, 1988; Peter Swan, *The Dead Pool,* Warner Brothers, 1988; Martin Brogan (ghost), *High Spirits,* Tri-Star, 1988; Leo Cutter, *The Good Mother,* Buena Vista, 1988.

PRINCIPAL TELEVISION APPEARANCES—Mini-Series: Kevin Murray, *Ellis Island,* CBS, 1984; Blackie O'Neill, *A Woman of Substance,* syndicated, 1984; Inspector Trignant, *If Tomorrow Comes,* CBS, 1986. Episodic: Sean Carroon, *Miami Vice,* NBC, 1986. Movies: Grak, *Arthur the King,* CBS, 1985; Blackie O'Neill, *Hold That Dream,* syndicated, 1986; Vincent Cauley, *Sworn to Silence,* ABC, 1987. Also appeared in *Across the War,* BBC; and *Sweet As You Are.*

NON-RELATED CAREER—Forklift truck driver for a brewery.

ADDRESSES: PUBLICIST—Susan Patricola, 518 N. La Cienega Boulevard, Los Angeles, CA 90048.*

*   *   *

NELLIGAN, Kate   1951-

PERSONAL: Born Patricia Colleen Nelligan, March 16, 1951, in London, ON, Canada; daughter of Patrick Joseph (a municipal employee) and Josephine Alice (a school teacher; maiden name, Dier) Nelligan; married Robert Reale (a pianist and arranger), February 19, 1989. EDUCATION: Attended York University (Cana-

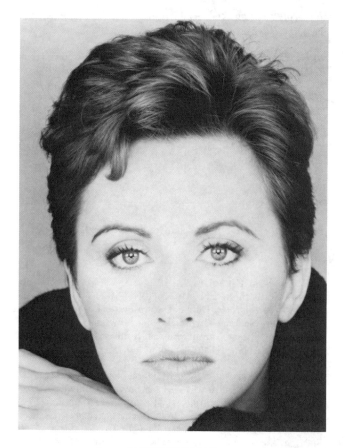

KATE NELLIGAN

da); trained for the stage at the Central School of Speech and Drama.

VOCATION: Actress.

CAREER: STAGE DEBUT—Corrie Bratter, *Barefoot in the Park,* Little Theatre, Bristol, U.K., 1972. LONDON DEBUT—Jenny, *Knuckle,* Comedy Theatre, 1974. BROADWAY DEBUT—Susan Traherne, *Plenty,* New York Shakespeare Festival, Plymouth Theatre, 1983. PRINCIPAL STAGE APPEARANCES—Hypatia, *Misalliance,* Stella Kowalski, *A Streetcar Named Desire,* Pegeen Mike, *The Playboy of the Western World,* Grace Harkaway, *London Assurance,* title role, *Lulu,* and Sybil Chase, *Private Lives,* all Bristol Old Vic Company, Bristol, U.K., 1972-73; Ellie Dunn, *Heartbreak House,* National Theatre Company, Old Vic Theatre, London, 1975; Marianne, *Tales from the Vienna Woods,* National Theatre Company, Olivier Theatre, London, 1977; Rosalind, *As You Like It,* Royal Shakespeare Company, Royal Shakespeare Theatre, Stratford-on-Avon, U.K., 1977; Susan Traherne, *Plenty,* National Theatre Company, Lyttelton Theatre, London, 1978, then New York Shakespeare Festival (NYSF), Public Theatre, New York City, 1982; Josie Hogan, *A Moon for the Misbegotten,* American Repertory Theatre, Cambridge, MA, then Cort Theatre, New York City, both 1984; title role, *Virginia,* NYSF, Public Theatre, 1985; Marylou Baines, *Serious Money,* Royale Theatre, New York City, 1988; Elise, *Spoils of War,* Second Stage Theatre, then Music Box Theatre, both New York City, 1988.

PRINCIPAL FILM APPEARANCES—Isabel, *The Romantic Englishwoman,* New World, 1975; Mercedes, *The Count of Monte Crisco,* ITC, 1976; Anna Seaton, *Licking Hitler,* British Film Institute, 1977; Lucy Seward, *Dracula,* Universal, 1979; Peabody, *Mr. Patman,* Film Consortium of Canada, 1980; Lucy, *Eye of the Needle,* United Artists, 1981; Susan Selky, *Without a Trace,* Twentieth Century-Fox, 1983; title role, *Eleni,* Warner Brothers, 1985. Also appeared in *Bethune,* 1977; *Agent,* 1980; *Forgive Our Foolish Ways,* 1980; *The Mystery of Henry Moore* (documentary), TV Arts, 1985; and in *Il giorno prima* (also known as *The Day Before*), Columbia, 1987.

PRINCIPAL TELEVISION APPEARANCES—Series: Leonora Biddulph, *The Onedin Line,* syndicated, 1976. Mini-Series: Title role, "Therese Raquin," *Masterpiece Theatre,* PBS, 1981. Movies: Mercedes, *The Count of Monte Cristo,* NBC, 1975; Ruth Hession, *Victims,* NBC, 1982; Kitty Keeler, *Kojak: The Price of Justice,* CBS, 1987; Sarah Howell, *Control,* HBO, 1987. Specials: Laura, "The Arcata Promise," *Great Performances,* PBS, 1977; Isabella, "Measure for Measure," *The Shakespeare Plays,* PBS, 1979. Also appeared in *The Lady of the Camellias* and *Dreams of Leaving.*

AWARDS: London Critics' Most Promising Actress Award for *Knuckle; Evening Standard* Award, Best Actress, 1978, for *Plenty;* Antoinette Perry Award nomination, Best Actress in a Play, 1983, for *Plenty;* Antoinette Perry Award nomination, Best Actress in a Play, 1984, for *A Moon for the Misbegotten;* Antoinette Perry Award nomination, Best Actress in a Play, 1988, for *Serious Money.*

SIDELIGHTS: FAVORITE ROLES—Josie in *A Moon for the Misbegotten.* RECREATIONS—Reading, cooking, and gardening.

ADDRESSES: AGENTS—Sam Cohn, International Creative Management, 40 W. 57th Street, New York, NY 10019; Larry Dalzell Associates, 3 Goodwin's Court, London WC2, England.*

NELSON, Gene   1920-

PERSONAL: Born Eugene Leander Berg, March 24, 1920, in Seattle, WA.

VOCATION: Actor, dancer, singer, and director.

CAREER: PRINCIPAL STAGE APPEARANCES—(As Gene Berg) *It Happens on Ice*, Center Theatre, New York City, 1940, then 1941; (as Gene Berg) ensemble, *This Is the Army* (revue), Broadway Theatre, New York City, 1942; ensemble, *Lend an Ear* (revue), National Theatre, New York City, 1948; Will Parker, *Oklahoma!*, City Center Theatre, New York City, 1958; Buddy Plummer, *Follies*, Winter Garden Theatre, New York City, 1971, then Shubert Theatre, Century City, CA, 1972, later City Center Theatre, 1974; Master of Ceremonies, *Music! Music!*, City Center Theatre, 1974; Bill Johnson, *Good News*, St. James Theatre, New York City, 1974.

PRINCIPAL STAGE WORK—Director, *Period of Adjustment*, American Theatre Arts, Hollywood, CA, 1983.

MAJOR TOURS—*Hit the Deck*, U.S. cities, 1960.

PRINCIPAL FILM APPEARANCES—Tommy Yale, *I Wonder Who's Kissing Her Now*, Twentieth Century-Fox, 1947; Jerry, *Apartment for Peggy*, Twentieth Century-Fox, 1948; assistant prosecutor, *Walls of Jericho*, Twentieth Century-Fox, 1948; Doug Martin, *The Daughter of Rosie O'Grady*, Warner Brothers, 1950; Tommy Trainor, *Tea for Two*, Warner Brothers, 1950; Hal Courtland, *The West Point Story* (also known as *Fine and Dandy*), Warner Brothers, 1950; Tom Farnham, *The Lullaby of Broadway*, Warner Brothers, 1951; as himself, *Starlift*, Warner Brothers, 1951; Ted Lansing, *Painting the Clouds with Sunshine*, Warner Brothers, 1951; Don Weston, *She's Working Her Way through College*, Warner Brothers, 1952; Gordon Evans, *She's Back on Broadway*, Warner Brothers, 1953; Twitch, *Three Sailors and a Girl*, Warner Brothers, 1953; Steve Lacey, *Crime Wave* (also known as *The City Is Dark*), Warner Brothers, 1954; Al Howard, *So This Is Paris*, Universal, 1954; Mike Delaney, *The Atomic Man* (also known as *Timeslip*), Allied Artists, 1955; Will Parker, *Oklahoma*, Magna Theatres, 1955; Greg Carradine, *The Way Out* (also known as *Dial 999*), RKO, 1956; Gil Shepard, *The Purple Hills*, Twentieth Century-Fox, 1961; Dan Warren, *20,000 Eyes*, Twentieth Century-Fox, 1961; Billy Poole, *Thunder Island*, Twentieth Century-Fox, 1963; Clive Lytell, *S.O.B.*, Paramount, 1981.

PRINCIPAL FILM WORK—Choreographer (with LeRoy Prinz), *Three Sailors and a Girl*, Warner Brothers, 1953; choreographer (with Lee Scott), *So This Is Paris*, Universal, 1954; director, *Hand of Death* (also known as *Five Fingers of Death*), Twentieth Century-Fox, 1962; director, *Hootenanny Hoot*, Metro-Goldwyn-Mayer (MGM), 1963; director, *Kissin' Cousins*, MGM, 1964; director, *Your Cheatin' Heart*, MGM, 1964; director, *Harum Scarum* (also known as *Harem Holiday*), MGM, 1965; director, *The Cool Ones*, Warner Brothers, 1967.

PRINCIPAL TELEVISION APPEARANCES—Pilots: Tom Fellows, *Tom, Dick, and Harry*, CBS, 1960. Episodic: Mr. Metcalf, *Murder, She Wrote*, CBS, 1987; also *The Kaiser Aluminum Hour*, NBC. Movies: Aircraft carrier captain, *Family Flight*, ABC, 1972;

Harry, *A Brand New Life*, ABC, 1973. Specials: Roy Lane, "Broadway," *The Best of Broadway*, CBS, 1955; Robert, "Shangri-La," *The Hallmark Hall of Fame*, NBC, 1960; Burbage, *Married Alive*, NBC, 1970.

PRINCIPAL TELEVISION WORK—All as director. Pilots: *I and Claudie*, CBS, 1964; *Where's Everett?*, CBS, 1966; (with Paul Krasny) *The Letters*, ABC, 1973. Episodic: *Dan August*, ABC, 1970; *Get Christie Love!*, ABC, 1974; *McNaughton's Daughter*, NBC, 1976; *The San Pedro Beach Bums*, ABC, 1977; *The New Operation Petticoat*, ABC, 1978; *Shirley*, NBC, 1979; *Salvage I*, ABC, 1979; *The Bad News Bears*, CBS, 1979; also *Burke's Law*, ABC; *The Cara Williams Show*, CBS; *The Donna Reed Show*, ABC; *The Farmer's Daughter*, ABC; *The Rifleman*, ABC; *The Felony Squad*, ABC; *Lancer*, CBS; *The F.B.I.*, ABC; *The Mod Squad*, ABC; *I Dream of Jeannie*, NBC; *Hawaii Five-O*, CBS; *Fantasy Island*, ABC. Movies: *Wake Me When the War Is Over*, ABC, 1969.

RELATED CAREER—Toured with Sonja Henie ice shows, 1940-41.

WRITINGS: FILM—(With Gerald Drayson Adams) *Kissin' Cousins*, Metro-Goldwyn-Mayer, 1964; (with Robert Kaufman) *The Cool Ones*, Warner Brothers, 1967. OTHER—"Is There Room in Your World for Me?" (song), *Son Rise: A Miracle of Love*, NBC, 1979.

ADDRESSES: OFFICE—Actors Equity Association, 165 W. 46th Street, New York, NY 10036.*

*   *   *

NELSON, Richard

VOCATION: Lighting designer.

CAREER: PRINCIPAL STAGE WORK—All as lighting designer, unless indicated: *Hamlet of Stepney Green*, Cricket Theatre, New York City, 1958; *Vincent*, Cricket Theatre, 1959; *Curtains Up!*, East 74th Street Theatre, New York City, 1959; *Guitar*, Jan Hus Auditorium, New York City, 1959; *Time of Vengeance*, York Playhouse, New York City, 1959; *Marching Song*, Gate Theatre, New York City, 1959; *Oh, Kay!*, East 74th Street Theatre, 1960; *The Idiot*, *Man and Superman*, and *Emmanuel*, all Gate Theatre, 1960; *Nat Turner*, Casa Galicia, New York City, 1960; *Montserrat*, *Five Posts in the Market Place*, and *Hobo*, all Gate Theatre, 1961; *The Caucasian Chalk Circle*, Vivian Beaumont Theatre, New York City, 1966; *Crimes of Passion*, Astor Place Theatre, New York City, 1969; *Uncle Vanya*, Center Theatre Group, Mark Taper Forum, Los Angeles, CA, 1969.

Water Color and *Criss-Crossing*, both American National Theatre and Academy (ANTA) Theatre, New York City, 1970; lighting supervisor, *Gloria and Esperanza*, ANTA Theatre, 1970; *All Over*, Martin Beck Theatre, New York City, 1971; *Macbeth*, Mercer-O'Casey Theatre, then Soho Theatre, both New York City, 1971; *Six*, Cricket Playhouse, 1971; *Any Resemblance to Persons Living or Dead*, Gate Theatre, 1971; *Drat!*, McAlpin Rooftop Theatre, New York City, 1971; *The Sign in Sidney Brustein's Window*, Longacre Theatre, New York City, 1972; *The Real Inspector Hound* and *After Magritte*, both Theatre Four, New York City,

1972; *Anna K.*, Actors Playhouse, New York City, 1972; *The Mother of Us All*, Guggenheim Museum, New York City, 1972; *The Magic Show*, Cort Theatre, New York City, 1974.

The Taking of Miss Janie, New York Shakespeare Festival (NYSF), Mitzi E. Newhouse Theatre, 1975; *Finn Mackool, The Grand Distraction*, Theatre De Lys, New York City, 1975; *Zalmen, or the Madness of God*, Lyceum Theatre, New York City, 1976; *So Long, 174th Street*, Harkness Theatre, New York City, 1976; *Showboat*, Jones Beach Theatre, Long Island, NY, 1976; *Every Night When the Sun Goes Down*, American Place Theatre, New York City, 1976; *Finian's Rainbow*, Jones Beach Theatre, 1977; *The Trip Back Down*, Longacre Theatre, 1977; *Annie Get Your Gun*, Jones Beach Theatre, 1978; *The End of the War*, Ensemble Studio Theatre, New York City, 1978; *Murder at the Howard Johnson's*, John Golden Theatre, New York City, 1979; *Bruce Forsyth on Broadway*, Winter Garden Theatre, New York City, 1979; *Englebert on Broadway*, Minskoff Theatre, New York City, 1979; *The Price*, Playhouse Theatre, New York City, 1979; *King of Schnorrers*, Harold Clurman Theatre, New York City, 1979; *Holeville*, Brooklyn Academy of Music, Attic Theatre, Brooklyn, NY, 1979.

Onward Victoria, Martin Beck Theatre, 1980; *Mornings at Seven*, Lyceum Theatre, 1980, then Center Theatre Group, Ahmanson Theatre, Los Angeles, 1981; *The Lady from Dubuque*, Morosco Theatre, New York City, 1980; *Censored Scenes from King Kong*, Princess Theatre, New York City, 1980; *Changes*, Theatre De Lys, 1980; *Beyond Therapy*, Marymount Manhattan Theatre, New York City, 1981; *The Supporting Cast*, Biltmore Theatre, New York City, 1981; *Oh, Brother!*, ANTA Theatre, 1981; *Henry IV, Part I*, NYSF, Delacorte Theatre, New York City, 1981; *Solomon's Child*, Little Theatre, New York City, 1982; *Present Laughter*, Circle in the Square, New York City, 1982; *The Misunderstanding*, Open Space Theatre Experiment, Main Stage Theatre, New York City, 1982; *A Little Family Business*, Martin Beck Theatre, 1982, then Center Theatre Group, Ahmanson Theatre, 1983; *Pump Boys and Dinettes*, Fisher Theatre, Detroit, MI, 1982; *The Price of Genius*, Lambs Theatre, New York City, 1982; *The Death of Von Richthofen as Witnessed from Earth*, NYSF, Public Theatre, New York City, 1982; *5-6-7-8 . . . Dance!*, Radio City Music Hall, New York City, 1983; *The Corn Is Green*, Lunt-Fontanne Theatre, New York City, 1983; *The Tap Dance Kid*, Broadhurst Theatre, New York City, then Minskoff Theatre, both 1983; *The Misanthrope* and *The Caine Mutiny Court-Martial*, both Circle in the Square, 1983; *Sunday in the Park with George*, Playwrights Horizons, New York City, 1983, then Booth Theatre, New York City, 1984; *Awake and Sing!*, Circle in the Square, 1984; *Serenading Louie*, NYSF, Public Theatre, 1984; *Danny and the Deep Blue Sea*, Circle in the Square Downtown, New York City, 1984; *Total Eclipse*, Westside Arts Theatre, New York City, 1984.

Harrigan 'n Hart, Longacre Theatre, 1985; *Arms and the Man*, Circle in the Square, 1985; *Personals*, Minetta Lane Theatre, New York City, 1985; *Oliver Oliver*, Manhattan Theatre Club, City Center Theatre Space, New York City, 1985; *Measure for Measure*, NYSF, Delacorte Theatre, 1985; *Miami*, Playwrights Horizons, 1986; *You Never Can Tell*, Circle in the Square, 1986; *Brownstone*, Roundabout Theatre, New York City, 1986; *Precious Sons*, Longacre Theatre, 1986; *Loot*, Manhattan Theatre Club, then Music Box Theatre, New York City, both 1986; *Long Day's Journey into Night*, Broadhurst Theatre, 1986; *The Boys in Autumn*, Circle in the Square, 1986; *Into the Woods*, Old Globe Theatre, San Diego, CA, then Martin Beck Theatre, both 1987; *Blithe Spirit*, Neil Simon Theatre, New York City, 1987; *Sleight of Hand*, Cort Theatre, 1987; *Hunting Cockroaches*, Manhattan Theatre Club,

1987; *The Night of the Iguana*, Circle in the Square, 1988. Also lighting designer, Seattle Repertory Theatre, Seattle, WA, 1965-66, 1972-75, and 1980-82; lighting designer, McCarter Theatre Company, Princeton, NJ, 1977-79.

MAJOR TOURS—Lighting designer: *The Magic Show*, U.S. cities, 1974-75; *Sarah in America*, U.S. cities, 1981.

AWARDS: Antoinette Perry Award and Drama Desk Award, both Best Lighting Design, 1984, for *Sunday in the Park with George;* Antoinette Perry Award nomination, Best Lighting Design, 1988, for *Into the Woods.*

ADDRESSES: AGENT—Kip Gould, Broadway Play Publishing Company, 357 W. 20th Street, New York, NY 10011.*

*   *   *

NICHOLS, Leo
See MORRICONE, Ennio

*   *   *

NIMOY, Leonard   1931-

PERSONAL: Born March 26, 1931, in Boston, MA; son of Max and Dora (Spinner) Nimoy; married Sandra Zober (an actress), February 21, 1954 (divorced); children: Julie, Adam. EDUCATION: Received B.A. in drama from Boston College; received M.A. from Antioch University; studied acting with Jeff Corey at the Pasadena Playhouse, 1960-63. POLITICS: Democrat. RELIGION: Jewish. MILITARY: U.S. Army, 1954-56.

VOCATION: Actor, director, producer, and writer.

CAREER: Also see *WRITINGS* below. BROADWAY DEBUT—Rohde, *Full Circle*, American National Theatre and Academy Theatre, 1973. PRINCIPAL STAGE APPEARANCES—Stanley Kowalski, *A Streetcar Named Desire*, Atlanta Theatre Guild, Atlanta, GA, 1955; Brick, *Cat on a Hot Tin Roof*, Town and Gown Repertory Theatre, Birmingham, AL, 1959; Arthur, *Camelot*, North Shore Music Theatre, Beverly, MA, 1973; Rohde, *Full Circle*, Kennedy Center for the Performing Arts, Washington, DC, then American National Theatre and Academy Theatre, New York City, both 1973; King Monghut, *The King and I*, Melody Top Theatre, Milwaukee, WI, 1974; Tevye, *Fiddler on the Roof*, Opera House, Atlanta, GA, 1974; He, *The Fourposter*, Drury Lane North Theatre, Chicago, IL, 1975; Henry Higgins, *My Fair Lady*, Melody Top Theatre, 1976; Dysart, *Equus*, Helen Hayes Theatre, New York City, 1977. Also appeared in *Awake and Sing!*, Elizabeth Peabody Playhouse, Boston, MA, 1948; *Dr. Faustus*, Orchard Gables Repertory Theatre, Los Angeles, CA, 1950; *Stalag 17*, Pasadena Playhouse, Pasadena, CA, 1951; *Deathwatch*, Cosmo Alley Gallery, Los Angeles, 1960; *Monserrat*, Los Angeles, 1963; *Irma La Douce*, Valley Music Theatre, Woodland Hills, CA, 1965; *The Man in the Glass Booth*, Old Globe Theatre, San Diego, CA, 1971; *One Flew over the Cuckoo's Nest*, Little Theatre on the Square, Sullivan, IL, 1974; *Caligula*, St. Edward's University Theatre, Austin, TX, 1975; *Twelfth Night*, Pittsburgh Public Theatre, Pittsburgh, PA, 1975.

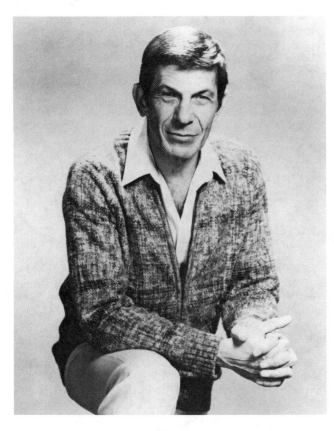

LEONARD NIMOY

PRINCIPAL STAGE WORK—Director, *A Streetcar Named Desire,* Atlanta Theatre Guild, Atlanta, GA, 1955.

MAJOR TOURS—Tevye, *Fiddler on the Roof,* U.S. cities, 1971; Paul Friedman, *6 Rms Riv Vu,* U.S. cities, 1973; title role, *Sherlock Holmes,* U.S. cities, 1976; Vincent van Gogh (also producer and director), *Vincent: The Story of a Hero,* U.S. cities, 1978-80; also in *Oliver!,* U.S. cities, 1972-73.

FILM DEBUT—Chief, "High Diver" in *Queen for a Day* (also known as *Horsie*), United Artists, 1951. PRINCIPAL FILM APPEARANCES—Ball player, *Rhubarb,* Paramount, 1951; football player, *Francis Goes to West Point,* Universal, 1952; Paul "Monk" Baroni, *Kid Monk Baroni,* Real Art, 1952; Black Hawk, *Old Overland Trail,* Republic, 1953; sergeant, *Them!,* Warner Brothers, 1954; Protector, *The Brain Eaters,* American International, 1958; Narab, *Satan's Satellites* (also known as *Zombies of the Stratosphere*), Republic, 1958; Roger, *The Balcony,* Continental, 1963; Jules LaFranc, *Deathwatch,* Beverly, 1966; Spence Atherton, *Valley of Mystery,* Universal, 1967; Miller, *Catlow,* Metro-Goldwyn-Mayer, 1971; Dr. David Kibner, *Invasion of the Body Snatchers,* United Artists, 1978; Spock, *Star Trek: The Motion Picture,* Paramount, 1979; Spock, *Star Trek II: The Wrath of Khan,* Paramount, 1982; Spock, *Star Trek III: The Search for Spock,* Paramount, 1984; Spock, *Star Trek IV: The Voyage Home,* Paramount, 1986; voice of Galvatron, *Transformers: The Movie* (animated), De Laurentiis Entertainment Group, 1986; Spock, *Star Trek V: The Final Frontier,* Paramount, 1989. Also appeared in *Just One Step: The Great Peace March,* Peace Films, Inc., 1988.

PRINCIPAL FILM WORK—Producer (with Vic Morrow), *Death-*

watch, Beverly, 1966; co-producer, *Valley of Mystery,* Universal, 1967; director, *Star Trek III: The Search for Spock,* Paramount, 1984; director, *Star Trek IV: The Voyage Home,* Paramount, 1986; director, *Three Men and a Baby,* Buena Vista, 1987; director, *The Good Mother,* Buena Vista, 1988.

PRINCIPAL TELEVISION APPEARANCES—Series: Mr. Spock, *Star Trek,* NBC, 1966-69; Paris, *Mission: Impossible,* CBS, 1969-71; voice of Mr. Spock, *Star Trek* (animated), NBC, 1973-75; host and narrator, *The Coral Jungle* (documentary), syndicated, 1976; host and narrator, *In Search of . . .,* syndicated, 1976-82. Mini-Series: Achmet, *Marco Polo,* NBC, 1982. Pilots: Tom Kovack, *Baffled,* NBC, 1973; Mick, *Kiss Me Again, Stranger* (broadcast as an episode of *Rex Harrison Presents Short Stories of Love*), NBC, 1974. Episodic: Hansen, "A Quality of Mercy," *The Twilight Zone,* CBS, 1961; Judson Ellis, "I, Robot," *The Outer Limits,* ABC, 1964; Konig, "The Production and Decay of Strange Particles," *The Outer Limits,* ABC, 1964; evil genie, "Aladdin and His Wonderful Lamp," *Faerie Tale Theatre,* Showtime, 1986; also *The Lieutenant,* NBC, 1964; "She'll Be Company for You," *Rod Serling's Night Gallery* (also known as *Night Gallery*), NBC, 1972; Mr. Burr Jones, "Richard T. Ely," *Profiles in Courage,* NBC; *Cain's Hundred,* NBC; *Sea Hunt,* syndicated; *Rawhide,* CBS; *Eleventh Hour,* NBC; *Kraft Suspense Theatre,* NBC; *Perry Mason,* CBS; *Dragnet,* NBC; *Gunsmoke,* CBS; *The Man from U.N.C.L.E.,* NBC; *Dr. Kildare,* NBC; *Bonanza,* NBC; *The Virginian,* NBC; *Columbo,* NBC; *Navy Log; Matinee Theatre; Wagon Train; Get Smart.*

Movies: Commander Phil Kettenring, *Assault on the Wayne,* ABC, 1971; Mitch, *The Alpha Caper* (also known as *Inside Job*), ABC, 1973; Dr. Durov, *The Missing Are Deadly,* ABC, 1975; Dr. Richard Connought, *Seizure: The Story of Kathy Morris,* CBS, 1980; Morris Meyerson, *A Woman Called Golda,* syndicated, 1982; the Count, *Ernest Hemingway's "The Sun Also Rises,"* NBC, 1984. Specials: *Mitzi and a Hundred Guys,* CBS, 1975; "You're a Poet and Don't Know It! . . . The Poetry Power Hour," *CBS Festival of Lively Arts for Young People,* CBS, 1976; host and narrator, *Snakes: Eden's Deadly Charmers,* CBS, 1988.

PRINCIPAL TELEVISION WORK—All as director, unless indicated. Episodic: "Death on a Barge," *Rod Serling's Night Gallery* (also known as *Night Gallery*), NBC, 1972; *T.J. Hooker,* ABC, 1983; also *The Powers of Matthew Star,* NBC. Specials: Producer, *If the Mind Is Free* (documentary), 1971.

RELATED CAREER—Director and teacher at a drama studio, North Hollywood, CA, 1962-65; teacher, Synanon, Santa Monica, CA, 1964-65; owner, Adajul Music Publishing Company.

NON-RELATED CAREER—Delegate, Democratic Central Committee, 1971 and 1972; also cab driver, pet shop clerk, soda jerk, and movie usher.

WRITINGS: STAGE—*Vincent: The Story of a Hero,* first produced on a tour of U.S. cities, 1978. FILM—(Story only) *Star Trek IV: The Voyage Home,* Paramount, 1986. OTHER—*You and I* (poetry), Celestial Arts, 1973; *Will I Not Think of You* (poetry), Celestial Arts, 1974; *I Am Not Spock* (autobiography), Celestial Arts, 1975; *Warmed by Love* (poetry), Blue Mountain Press, 1983; also (contributor) *Bio-Cosmos,* by James Christian, 1975; *We Are All Children Searching for Love* (poetry), 1977; *Come Be with Me* (poetry), 1978; *These Words Are for You* (poetry), 1981.

RECORDINGS: ALBUMS—*Leonard Nimoy Presents Mr. Spock's*

Music from Outer Space, Dot, 1967; also *Two Sides of Leonard Nimoy,* Dot; *The Way I Feel,* Dot; *The Touch of Leonard Nimoy,* Dot; *The New World of Leonard Nimoy,* Dot; *The Martian Chronicles,* Caedmon; *The Illustrated Man,* Caedmon; *The Green Hills of Earth,* Caedmon; *Gentlemen, Be Seated.*

MEMBER: American Federation of Television and Radio Artists, Screen Actors Guild, Actors' Equity Association, American Civil Liberties Union.

SIDELIGHTS: RECREATIONS—Photography and writing poetry.

ADDRESSES: PUBLICIST—Francis and Freedman, 328 S. Beverly Drive, Beverly Hills, CA 90212.

*   *   *

NIXON, Cynthia   1966-

PERSONAL: Born April 9, 1966, in New York, NY.

VOCATION: Actress.

CAREER: STAGE DEBUT—Dinah Lord, *The Philadelphia Story,* Vivian Beaumont Theatre, New York City, 1980. BROADWAY DEBUT—Debbie, *The Real Thing,* Plymouth Theatre, 1984. PRINCIPAL STAGE APPEARANCES—Lydie Hickman, *Lydie Breeze,* American Place Theatre, New York City, 1982; Donna, *Hurlyburly,* Goodman Theatre, Chicago, IL, then Promenade Theatre, New

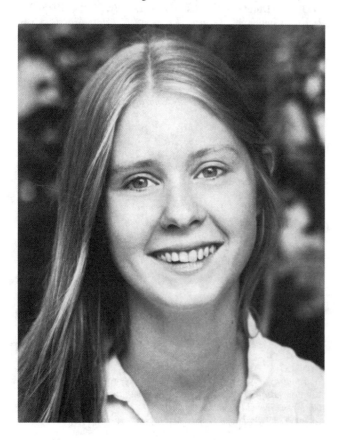

CYNTHIA NIXON

York City, later Ethel Barrymore Theatre, New York City, all 1984; Sally Decker, *Sally's Gone, She Left Her Name,* Perry Street Theatre, New York City, 1985; Carol, *Lemon Sky,* Second Stage Theatre, New York City, 1986; Phoebe, *Alterations,* WPA Theatre, Chelsea Playhouse, New York City, 1986; Piper, *Cleveland and Half-Way Back,* Ensemble Studio Theatre, New York City, 1987; Juliet, *Romeo and Juliet,* New York Shakespeare Festival, Public Theatre, New York City, 1988. Also appeared in *The Heidi Chronicles,* Playwrights Horizons, then Plymouth Theatre, both New York City, 1989.

PRINCIPAL FILM APPEARANCES—Sunshine Walker, *Little Darlings,* Paramount, 1980; Cindy, *Tattoo,* Twentieth Century-Fox, 1981; Jeannie, *Prince of the City,* Warner Brothers, 1981; Amy, *I Am the Cheese,* Almi, 1983; Lorl, *Amadeus,* Orion, 1984; Jenny, *The Manhattan Project* (also known as *Manhattan Project: The Deadly Game*), Twentieth Century-Fox, 1986; Michelle, *O.C. and Stiggs,* Metro-Goldwyn-Mayer/United Artists, 1987; Evangeline, *Let It Ride,* Alleged Productions, 1989.

PRINCIPAL TELEVISION APPEARANCES—Series: Alex Tanner, *Tanner '88,* HBO, 1988. Episodic: Jackie, "Silent Fury," *The Equalizer,* CBS, 1989; Alison Slocum, *Gideon Oliver,* ABC, 1989. Movies: Nancy, *My Body, My Child,* ABC, 1982; Alice, *Rascals and Robbers—The Secret Adventures of Tom Sawyer and Huck Finn,* CBS, 1982; Doreen Camp, *The Murder of Mary Phagan,* NBC, 1988. Specials: Melanie Gamble, "Three Wishes of a Rich Kid," *ABC Afterschool Special,* ABC, 1979; Shirley, *Fifth of July,* Showtime, 1982, then PBS, 1983; Ann Cassidy, "It's No Crush, I'm in Love," *ABC Afterschool Special,* ABC, 1983.

AWARDS: Theatre World Award, 1980, for *The Philadelphia Story.*

ADDRESSES: AGENT—International Creative Management, 40 W. 57th Street, New York, NY 10019.

*   *   *

NOBLE, James   1922-

PERSONAL: Full name, James Wilkes Noble; born March 5, 1922, in Dallas, TX; son of Ralph Byrne and Lois Frances (Wilkes) Noble; married Carolyn Owen Coates, May 19, 1956; children: Jessica Katherine. EDUCATION: Attended North Texas College, 1939-41, and Southern Methodist University, 1941-43 and 1946-47. MILITARY: U.S. Naval Reserve, 1943-46.

VOCATION: Actor and mime.

CAREER: BROADWAY DEBUT—Professor Pearson, *The Velvet Glove,* Booth Theatre, 1949. PRINCIPAL STAGE APPEARANCES—Professor Pearson, *The Velvet Glove,* John Golden Theatre, New York City, 1950; friend of the woman, *Come of Age,* City Center Theatre, New York City, 1952; Aegisthus, *Electra,* Henry Street Playhouse, New York City, 1954; Gordon Douglas, *A Far Country,* Music Box Theatre, New York City, 1961; soldier, *Dynamite Tonight,* Actors Studio, York Playhouse, New York City, 1964; Malcolm Supley, *Night of the Dunce,* Cherry Lane Theatre, New York City, 1966; judge and preacher, *Rimers of Eldritch,* Cherry Lane Theatre, 1967; Stephen Chenier, *The Death of the Well-Loved Boy,* St. Mark's Playhouse, New York City, 1967; Sam, "The Acquisition" in *Trainer, Dean, Liepolt, and Company,* American

Place Theatre, Theatre at St. Clement's Church, New York City, 1968; David, *A Scent of Flowers,* Martinique Theatre, New York City, 1969; Frank Kroner, Sr., *Siamese Connections,* Actors Studio Theatre, New York City, 1972; Toby Felker, *The Runner Stumbles,* Hartman Theatre, Stamford, CT, 1975, then Little Theatre, New York City, 1976; Stubbs, *The Vienna Notes,* Second Stage, New York City, 1985. Also appeared in *Helen's Room,* in New York City, 1947; *The Big Knife,* National Theatre, New York City, 1949; *Medea,* in New York City, 1951; *Strange Interlude,* Hudson Theatre, New York City, 1963; *1776,* 46th Street Theatre, New York City, 1969; *Harvey,* Playhouse in the Park, Cincinnati, OH, 1973; *A Touch of the Poet,* Manhattan Theatre Club, New York City, 1974; *The Show-Off,* Long Wharf Theatre, New Haven, CT, 1975; *Tom Jones,* Hartman Theatre Company, 1975; *Born Yesterday,* Pasadena Playhouse, Pasadena, CA, 1988; and in more than two hundred other plays.

PRINCIPAL FILM APPEARANCES—Canon Pritchard, *The Sporting Club,* AVCO-Embassy, 1971; priest, *Been Down So Long It Looks Like Up to Me,* Paramount, 1971; John Witherspoon, *1776,* Columbia, 1972; General Deptford, *Who?* (also known as *Man Without a Face, Prisoner of the Skull,* and *The Man in the Steel Mask*), Lorimar, 1975; Norman, *Death Play,* New Line Cinema, 1976; Dr. Leo Cooper, *One Summer Love* (also known as *Dragonfly*), American International, 1976; Presidential Advisor Kaufman, *Being There,* United Artists, 1979; Dr. Blankenship, *Promises in the Dark,* Warner Brothers, 1979; Fred Miles, *10,* Warner Brothers, 1979; secretary of defense, *The Nude Bomb* (also known as *The Return of Maxwell Smart*), Universal, 1980; Father of Flanagan, *Airplane II: The Sequel,* Paramount, 1982; Peter Archer, *You Talkin' to Me?,* Metro-Goldwyn-Mayer/United Artists, 1987; Sinclair, *A Tiger's Tale,* Atlantic Entertainment, 1987; Chief Wilkins, *Paramedics,* Vestron, 1988.

TELEVISION DEBUT—Title role, *The Egoist,* DuMont, 1943. PRINCIPAL TELEVISION APPEARANCES—Series: Edward Simms, *A World Apart,* ABC, 1970-71; Governor James Gatling, *Benson,* ABC, 1979-86; Raymond Voss, *First Impressions,* CBS, 1988; also Dr. Bill Winters, *The Doctors,* NBC. Pilots: Dr. Metz, *Hart to Hart,* ABC, 1979; Tom Fairmont, *This Is Kate Bennett,* ABC, 1982; Dr. Gilmore Blount, "The Absent-Minded Professor," *Magical World of Disney,* NBC, 1988. Episodic: Allen Carlisle, *Murder, She Wrote,* CBS, 1987; Harry Beaumont, *Scarecrow and Mrs. King,* CBS, 1987. Movies: Haberle, *Breaking Up,* ABC, 1978; Ed, *Lovey: A Circle of Children, Part II,* CBS, 1978; Pierce, *Summer of My German Soldier,* NBC, 1978; Dr. Elliot Losen, *Baby Comes Home,* CBS, 1980; Gavin McNab, *Dempsey,* CBS, 1983; Dr. Warren Towle, *When the Bough Breaks,* NBC, 1986; Ed Shoat, *Deadly Deception,* CBS, 1987; Leonard Weeks, *Perry Mason: The Case of the Murdered Madam,* NBC, 1987. Specials: Dr. Edwards, "The Woman Who Willed a Miracle," *ABC Afterschool Special,* ABC, 1983; *Life's Most Embarrassing Moments,* ABC, 1986; Max Smiley, "The Day My Kid Went Punk," *ABC Afterschool Special,* ABC, 1987.

RELATED CAREER—Member, Lydia Tarnower Modern Dance Company, 1937-39; member, American Mime Theatre, 1952-59; lecturer on acting and mime, American Academy of Dramatic Art, 1956-59; life member, Actors Studio; writer of journal articles on American mime.

AWARDS: Named Honorary Governor of New Jersey and New York, 1982; American Heart Association Appreciation Award, 1983.

MEMBER: Actors' Equity Association, Screen Actors Guild, American Federation of Television and Radio Artists.

SIDELIGHTS: RECREATIONS—Photography.*

*   *   *

NOURI, Michael   1945-

PERSONAL: Born December 9, 1945, in Washington, DC; son of Edward and Gloria (Montgomery) Nouri. EDUCATION: Attended Rollins College and Emerson College; studied acting with Larry Moss, Lee Strasberg, Bill Alderson, and Bob Modica.

VOCATION: Actor.

CAREER: OFF-BROADWAY DEBUT—*The Crucible,* 1964. BROADWAY DEBUT—Peter Latham, *Forty Carats,* Morosco Theatre, 1968. PRINCIPAL STAGE APPEARANCES—Hap, *Nefertiti,* Blackstone Theatre, Chicago, IL, 1977; Edwin Booth, *Booth,* South Street Theatre, New York City, 1982.

MAJOR TOURS—*Forty Carats,* U.S. cities, 1970.

FILM DEBUT—Don Farber, *Goodbye, Columbus,* Paramount, 1969. PRINCIPAL FILM APPEARANCES—Nick Hurley, *Flashdance,* Paramount, 1982; Roger Blackwell, *The Imagemaker,* Castle Hill/Manson, 1986; voice of Boulder, *Gobots: Battle of the Rock Lords* (animated), Clubhouse/Atlantic, 1986; Tom Beck, *The Hidden,* New Line Cinema/Heron Communications, 1987.

TELEVISION DEBUT—Giorgio Bellonci, *Beacon Hill,* CBS, 1975. PRINCIPAL TELEVISION APPEARANCES—Series: Count Dracula, *The Curse of Dracula* (also known as *Dracula '79*), NBC, 1979; Charles "Lucky" Luciano, *The Gangster Chronicles,* NBC, 1981; Joe Rohner, *Bay City Blues,* NBC, 1983; Detective John Forney, *Downtown,* CBS, 1986-87; also Steve Kaslo, *Search for Tomorrow,* CBS; *Somerset,* NBC. Mini-Series: Jean R.G.R. des Barres, *The Last Convertible,* NBC, 1979. Pilots: Nick Macazie, *Nick and the Dobermans,* NBC, 1980; Michael Spraggue, *Spraggue,* ABC, 1984. Movies: Lou Savage, *Contract on Cherry Street,* NBC, 1977; Greg, *Fun and Games,* ABC, 1980; Alex Shepherd, *Secrets of a Mother and Daughter,* CBS, 1983; James Moretti, *Rage of Angels: The Story Continues,* NBC, 1986; Harry Petherton, *Between Two Women,* ABC, 1986. Specials: *After Hours: From Janice, John, Mary, and Michael, with Love,* CBS, 1976.

AWARDS: Emmy Award nomination, 1976.

ADDRESSES: AGENT—The Light Company, 901 Bringham Avenue, Brentwood, CA 90049. MANAGER—Bernie Brillstein, The Brillstein Company, 9200 Sunset Boulevard, Suite 428, Los Angeles, CA 90069. PUBLICIST—Freeman and Sutton Public Relations, 8961 Sunset Boulevard, Suite 2-A, Los Angeles, CA 90069.

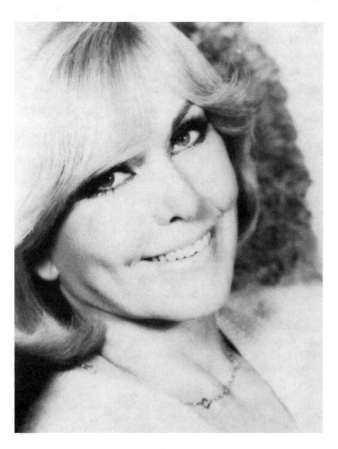

KIM NOVAK

NOVAK, Kim   1933-

PERSONAL: Born Marilyn Pauline Novak, February 13, 1933, in Chicago, IL; daughter of Joseph A. and Blanche (Kral) Novak; married Richard Johnson (an actor), April, 1965 (divorced, 1966); married Robert Malloy (a doctor), January, 1978. EDUCATION: Los Angeles City College, A.A., 1958; also attended Wright Junior College.

VOCATION: Actress.

CAREER: FILM DEBUT—(As Marilyn Novak) Model, *The French*

Line, RKO, 1954. PRINCIPAL FILM APPEARANCES—Janis, *Phfft!,* Columbia, 1954; Lona McLane, *Pushover,* Columbia, 1954; Molly, *The Man with the Golden Arm,* United Artists, 1955; raider, *Son of Sinbad* (also known as *Nights in a Harem*), RKO, 1955; Kay Greylek, *Five Against the House,* Columbia, 1955; Madge Owens, *Picnic,* Columbia, 1956; Marjorie Oelrichs, *The Eddie Duchin Story,* Columbia, 1956; title role, *Jeanne Eagels,* Columbia, 1957; Linda English, *Pal Joey,* Columbia, 1957; Gillian Holroyd, *Bell, Book, and Candle,* Columbia, 1958; Madeleine Elster and Judy Barton, *Vertigo,* Paramount, 1958; Betty Preisser, *Middle of the Night,* Columbia, 1959; as herself, *Pepe,* Columbia, 1960; Maggie Gault, *Strangers When We Meet,* Columbia, 1960; Cathy, *Boys' Night Out,* Metro-Goldwyn-Mayer (MGM), 1962; Carlye Hardwicke, *The Notorious Landlady,* Columbia, 1962; Polly the Pistol, *Kiss Me, Stupid,* Lopert, 1964; Mildred Rogers, *Of Human Bondage,* MGM, 1964; title role, *The Amorous Adventures of Moll Flanders,* Paramount, 1965; Lylah Clare and Elsa Brinkmann, *The Legend of Lylah Clare,* MGM, 1968; Lyda Kabanov, *The Great Bank Robbery,* Warner Brothers, 1969; Auriol Pageant, ''Luau'' in *Tales That Witness Madness,* Paramount, 1973; Poker Jenny Shermerhorn, *The White Buffalo* (also known as *Hunt to Kill*), United Artists, 1977; Helga, *Just a Gigolo,* United Artists, 1979; Lola Brewster, *The Mirror Crack'd,* Associated Film Distribution, 1980. Also appeared in *The Celebrity Art Portfolio* (short film), 1974.

PRINCIPAL FILM WORK—Costume designer (with Elizabeth Courtney), *The Notorious Landlady,* Columbia, 1962.

PRINCIPAL TELEVISION APPEARANCES—Series: Kit Marlowe, *Falcon Crest,* CBS, 1986-87. Pilots: Billie Farnsworth, *Malibu,* ABC, 1983. Episodic: Rosa, ''Man from the South,'' *Alfred Hitchcock Presents,* NBC, 1985. Movies: Gloria Joyce, *The Third Girl from the Left,* ABC, 1973; Eva, *Satan's Triangle,* ABC, 1975. Specials: *Light's Diamond Jubilee,* ABC, CBS, DuMont, and NBC, 1954; *The Bob Hope Show,* NBC, 1956; also *This Land Is Mine* (documentary), 1970.

RELATED CAREER—Professional model; founder, Kimco (a production company), 1961.

MEMBER: Screen Actors Guild.

ADDRESSES: MANAGER—Susan Cameron Enterprises, 29 1/2 Mast Street, Marina Del Rey, CA 90292.

O

O'CONNOR, Pat

PERSONAL: Born in Ardmore, Ireland. EDUCATION: Received B.A. from the University of California, Los Angeles; studied film and television at Ryerson Institute, Toronto.

VOCATION: Director.

CAREER: PRINCIPAL FILM WORK—Director: Cal, Warner Brothers, 1984; A Month in the Country, Orion Classics, 1987; Stars and Bars, Columbia, 1988; The January Man, Metro-Goldwyn-Mayer/United Artists, 1989.

PRINCIPAL TELEVISION WORK—Producer and director with Radio Telefis Eirann (RTE): The Four Roads, The Shankhill, Kiltycogher, One of Ourselves, A Ballroom of Romance, Night in Ginitia, and more than forty other productions, 1970-78.

NON-RELATED CAREER—Road paver and wine corker.

AWARDS: British Academy of Film and Television Arts Award, 1981, for A Ballroom of Romance.*

*   *   *

O'HARA, Catherine

PERSONAL: Born March 4, in Toronto, ON, Canada.

VOCATION: Actress and writer.

CAREER: Also see WRITINGS below. PRINCIPAL FILM APPEARANCES—Gail, After Hours, Warner Brothers, 1985; Betty, Heartburn, Paramount, 1986; Delia Deetz, Beetlejuice, Warner Brothers, 1988; also appeared in Rock 'n' Rule (also known as Rock and Rule), Metro-Goldwyn-Mayer/United Artists, 1983.

PRINCIPAL TELEVISION APPEARANCES—Series: Regular, Second City TV, syndicated, 1977-80; regular, The Steve Allen Comedy Hour, NBC, 1980-81; regular, SCTV Network 90, NBC, 1981-82; regular, SCTV, Cinemax, 1984; voice of Miss Malone, The Completely Mental Misadventures of Ed Grimley, NBC, 1988-89. Mini-Series: Really Weird Tales, HBO, 1986. Pilots: Regular, From Cleveland, CBS, 1980. Episodic: Sally Hayes, George Burns Comedy Week, CBS, 1985; Rebecca, "Get a Job," Trying Times, PBS, 1987. Specials: Late Night Film Festival, NBC, 1985; The Last Polka, HBO, 1985; Comic Relief, HBO, 1986; Marie Antoinette, Dave Thomas: The Incredible Time Travels of Henry Osgood, Showtime, 1986; Comic Relief '87 (also known as Comic Relief II),

HBO, 1987; Second City [Toronto] Fifteenth Anniversary Special (also known as The Second City Anniversary Reunion), Showtime, 1988; Andrea Martin: Together Again, Showtime, 1989; Comic Relief III, HBO, 1989; Martin Short's Hollywood, HBO, 1989.

WRITINGS: TELEVISION—All as co-writer. Series: Second City TV, syndicated, 1977-80; The Steve Allen Comedy Hour, NBC, 1980-81; SCTV Network 90, NBC, 1981-82; SCTV, Cinemax, 1984. Mini-Series: Really Weird Tales, HBO, 1986. Pilots: From Cleveland, CBS, 1980.

AWARDS: Emmy Award, Best Writing for a Comedy Program, 1983, for SCTV Network 90.

ADDRESSES: AGENT—Nancy Geller, International Creative Management, 8899 Beverly Boulevard, Los Angeles, CA 90048.

*   *   *

O'KEEFE, Miles

VOCATION: Actor.

CAREER: PRINCIPAL FILM APPEARANCES—Title role, Tarzan, The Ape Man, Metro-Goldwyn-Mayer/United Artists (MGM/UA), 1981; title role, Ator: The Blade Master, Comworld/Continental/Eureka/New Line Cinema, 1982; SAS Malko Linge, SAS a San Salvador (also known as SAS— Terminate with Extreme Prejudice), Union Generale Cinematographique, 1982; title role, Ator: The Fighting Eagle, Trans World Entertainment, 1983; title role, Ator: The Invincible, Trans World Entertainment, 1984; Sir Gawain, Sword of the Valiant—The Legend of Gawain and the Green Knight, Cannon, 1984; title role, Ator: Iron Warrior, Trans World Entertainment, 1987; Garrett, The Lone Runner (also known as Fistful of Diamonds), Trans World Entertainment, 1987; Cactus Jack, Campus Man, Paramount, 1987; Trey, The Drifter, MGM/UA, 1988; Count Dracula, Waxwork, Vestron, 1988. Also appeared in Fuga dall'inferno (also known as Fuite de l'enfer and Double Target), Variety, 1987.

ADDRESSES: MANAGER—Chris Trainor, Chris Trainor and Associates, Los Angeles, CA.*

O'LOUGHLIN, Gerald S. 1921-

PERSONAL: Full name, Gerald Stuart O'Loughlin; born December 23, 1921, in New York, NY; son of Gerald S., Sr., and Laura (Ward) O'Loughlin; married Meryl Abeles (a television casting director), 1967; children: one son, one daughter. EDUCATION: Attended the University of Rochester, 1943-44; Lafayette College, B.S., 1948; trained for the stage with Sanford Meisner, David Pressman, and Martha Graham at the Neighborhood Playhouse, 1948-50, with Lee Strasberg and Alice Hermes at the Actors Studio, 1951, and with Nick Colasanto; studied voice with Albert Malver and singing with David Craig. MILITARY: U.S. Marine Corps, first lieutenant, 1942-46.

VOCATION: Actor.

CAREER: STAGE DEBUT—Harry Brock, *Born Yesterday,* Crystal Lake Lodge, Crystal Lake, NY, 1949. BROADWAY DEBUT—Sam, *Golden Boy,* American National Theatre and Academy Theatre, 1952. PRINCIPAL STAGE APPEARANCES—Joe Keller, *All My Sons,* Crystal Lake Lodge, Crystal Lake, NY, 1949; Stanley Kowalski, *A Streetcar Named Desire,* City Center Theatre, New York City, 1956; Morris Lacey, *The Dark at the Top of the Stairs,* Music Box Theatre, New York City, 1958; Seamus Shields, *Shadow of a Gunman,* Bijou Theatre, New York City, 1958; Mickey Maloy, *A Touch of the Poet,* Helen Hayes Theatre, New York City, 1959; Rubin Flood, *The Dark at the Top of the Stairs,* Playhouse-in-the-Park, Philadelphia, PA, 1960; Richard Roe, *Machinal,* Gate Theatre, New York City, 1960; Goober, *A Cook for Mister General,* Playhouse Theatre, New York City, 1961; William Medlow, *Calculated Risk,* Ambassador Theatre, New York City, 1962; Albert Cobb, *Who'll Save the Plowboy?,* Phoenix Theatre, New York City, 1962; Charles Cheswick, *One Flew over the Cuckoo's Nest,* Cort Theatre, New York City, 1963; Archer, *Harry, Noon, and Night,* Pocket Theatre, New York City, 1965; Harry Mills, *Happily Never After,* Eugene O'Neill Theatre, New York City, 1966; Johnny, *Lovers and Other Strangers,* Brooks Atkinson Theatre, New York City, 1968. Also appeared in *Flowering Peach,* Belasco Theatre, New York City, 1954.

MAJOR TOURS—Gooper, *Cat on a Hot Tin Roof,* U.S. cities, 1956.

FILM DEBUT—Larry, *Lovers and Lollipops,* Trans-Lux, 1956. PRINCIPAL FILM APPEARANCES—Chuck, *A Hatful of Rain,* Twentieth Century-Fox, 1957; Mike Maguire, *Cop Hater,* United Artists, 1958; LaSueur, *Ensign Pulver,* Warner Brothers, 1964; Chester Quirk, *A Fine Madness,* Warner Brothers, 1966; Harold Nye, *In Cold Blood,* Columbia, 1967; Lieutenant Commander Bob Raeburn, *Ice Station Zebra,* Filmways/Metro-Goldwyn-Mayer, 1968; Grossman, *Riot,* Paramount, 1969; Charlie, *Desperate Characters,* Paramount, 1971; Lieutenant Jack Pecora, *The Organization,* United Artists, 1971; F.B.I. Agent Ryan, *The Valachi Papers* (also known as *Joe Valachi: I segretti di cosa nostra*), Columbia, 1972; Brigadier General Michael O'Rourke, *Twilight's Last Gleaming,* Allied Artists, 1977; lobotomy doctor, *Frances,* Universal, 1982; counterman Louie, *City Heat,* Warner Brothers, 1984; Ben, *Crimes of Passion,* New World, 1984; Mr. Casey, *Quicksilver,* Columbia, 1986. Also appeared in *A Man Called Adam,* Embassy, 1966.

TELEVISION DEBUT—*Cameo Theatre,* NBC, 1950. PRINCIPAL TELEVISION APPEARANCES—Series: Peter Bonds, *The Doctors,* NBC, 1963; Devlin McNeil, *Storefront Lawyer,* CBS, 1970, renamed *Men at Law,* CBS, 1971; Lieutenant Eddie Ryker, *The Rookies,* ABC, 1972-76; Captain Boyd, *Automan,* ABC, 1983-84; Joe Kaplan, *Our House,* NBC, 1986-88. Mini-Series: Rusty Horton, *Arthur Hailey's "Wheels"* (also known as *Wheels*), NBC, 1978; Richard Payson, *Women in White,* NBC, 1979; Sergeant O'Toole, *The Blue and the Gray,* CBS, 1982; John J. Caulfield, *Blind Ambition,* CBS, 1979; Captain Bowker, *Roots: The Next Generations,* ABC, 1979. Pilots: Russ Faine, "Lassiter," *Premiere,* CBS, 1968; Andrushian, *The D.A.: Murder One,* NBC, 1969; Mr. Medwick, *Sparrow,* CBS, 1978; Tim Halloran, *Dusty,* NBC, 1983; Sam Gains, *London and Davis in New York,* CBS, 1984; Bud Oliver, *Brothers-in-Law,* ABC, 1985.

Episodic: Dave Brandon, *Lassiter,* NBC, 1980; Sid Lammon, *McClain's Law,* NBC, 1981; Jack Allword, *Bridges to Cross,* CBS, 1986; Mr. Callahan, *Dirty Dancing,* CBS, 1988; also "A Piece of Blue Sky," *Play of the Week,* WNTA, 1960; "A Clearing in the Woods," *Play of the Week,* WNTA, 1961; *Ben Casey,* NBC, 1962; *The Defenders,* CBS, 1963; *Naked City,* ABC, 1963; *Alcoa Premiere,* ABC, 1963; *The Guiding Light,* CBS, 1963; *Dr. Kildare,* NBC, 1964; *For the People,* CBS, 1965; *Run for Your Life,* NBC, 1966; *The Green Hornet,* ABC, 1966; *The F.B.I.,* ABC, 1966, 1969, and 1971; *Judd, for the Defense,* ABC, 1968; *Felony Squad,* ABC, 1967; *Cimarron Strip,* CBS, 1967; *Mission: Impossible,* CBS, 1968 and 1971; *Mannix,* CBS, 1968; *Hawaii Five-O,* CBS, 1968 and 1970; *The Virginian,* NBC, 1969; *Medical Center,* CBS, 1969; *Then Came Bronson,* NBC, 1969; *Ironside,* NBC, 1969 and 1970; *The Young Lawyers,* ABC, 1970; *Dan August,* ABC, 1970; *The Senator,* NBC, 1970; *Sarge,* NBC, 1971; *Owen Marshall, Counselor at Law,* ABC, 1971; *Cade's County,* CBS, 1971; *Nichols,* NBC, 1971; *Room 222,* ABC, 1972, 1973, and 1974; *Cannon,* CBS, 1972, 1973, and 1974; as Max, *The Powers of Matthew Star,* NBC; Jack Schwartz, *Fame;* in *The Mod Squad,* ABC; *Highway to Heaven,* NBC; *Murder, She Wrote,* CBS; *Riptide,* NBC; *Quincy, M.E.,* NBC; *Going My Way,* ABC; *Twelve O'Clock High,* ABC; *Too Close for Comfort.*

Movies: John Cappelletti, Sr., *Something for Joey,* CBS, 1977; Moe Gold, *Murder at the World Series,* ABC, 1977; Larry Cross, *Crash,* ABC, 1978; Joe McCarthy, *A Love Affair: The Eleanor and Lou Gehrig Story,* NBC, 1978; Martin Brain, *Detour to Terror,* NBC, 1980; Benny Moffo, *Pleasure Palace,* CBS, 1980; Duffy, *A Matter of Life and Death,* CBS, 1981; Sam, *Child's Cry,* CBS, 1986; General Lord, *Under Siege,* NBC, 1986; Monsignor Kyser, *Perry Mason: The Case of the Notorious Nun,* NBC, 1986. Specials: Ginger Ted Wilson, *Wilson's Reward,* syndicated, 1984; voice of Ben McMasters, *Alvin Goes Back to School* (animated), NBC, 1986.

PRINCIPAL TELEVISION WORK—Episodic: Director, *The Rookies,* ABC, 1972.

RELATED CAREER—Faculty member, Lee Strasberg Theatre Institute, Hollywood, CA.

NON-RELATED CAREER—Cabinet maker, mechanical engineer, photographer, and auto mechanic.

AWARDS: Obie Award from the *Village Voice,* Distinguished Performance, 1962, for *Who'll Save the Plowboy?.*

MEMBER: Actors' Equity Association, Screen Actors Guild, American Federation of Television and Radio Artists, Theta Delta Chi.*

OLSON, Nancy   1928-

PERSONAL: Full name, Nancy Ann Olson; born July 14, 1928, in Milwaukee, WI; daughter of Henry J. (a physician) and Evelyn (Bergstrom) Olson; married Alan Jay Lerner (a playwright and lyricist), March 19, 1950 (divorced, 1957); married Alan W. Livingston (a record company executive), September 1, 1962; children: two daughters (first marriage); one son (second marriage). EDUCATION: Attended the University of Wisconsin, 1946-47, and the University of California, Los Angeles, 1947-49.

VOCATION: Actress.

CAREER: BROADWAY DEBUT—Isolde Poole, *The Tunnel of Love*, Royale Theatre, 1957. PRINCIPAL STAGE APPEARANCES—Judy Kimball, *Send Me No Flowers*, Brooks Atkinson Theatre, New York City, 1960; Mary McKellaway, *Mary, Mary*, Helen Hayes Theatre, New York City, 1962.

FILM DEBUT—Cecille Gautier, *Canadian Pacific*, Twentieth Century-Fox, 1949. PRINCIPAL FILM APPEARANCES—Katherine Holbrook, *Mr. Music*, Paramount, 1950; Betty Schaefer, *Sunset Boulevard*, Paramount, 1950; Joyce Willecombe, *Union Station*, Paramount, 1950; Eleanor, *Force of Arms* (also known as *A Girl for Joe*), Warner Brothers, 1951; Carol, *Submarine Command*, Paramount, 1951; Nancy Vallon, *Big Jim McLain*, Warner Brothers, 1952; Dallas O'Mara, *So Big*, Warner Brothers, 1953; Katie Brannigan, *The Boy from Oklahoma*, Warner Brothers, 1954; Pat, *Battle Cry*, Warner Brothers, 1955; Nancy Furman, *Pollyanna*, Buena Vista, 1960; Betsy Carlisle, *The Absent-Minded Professor*, Buena Vista, 1961; Betsy Brainard, *Son of Flubber*, Buena Vista, 1963; Norah Smith, *Smith*, Buena Vista, 1969; Sue Baxter, *Snowball Express*, Buena Vista, 1972; Mrs. Abbott, *Airport 1975*, Universal, 1974; Christine, *Making Love*, Twentieth Century-Fox, 1982.

PRINCIPAL TELEVISION APPEARANCES—Series: Jessica Frazier, *Kingston: Confidential*, NBC, 1977; Marjorie Harper, *Paper Dolls*, ABC, 1984. Episodic: Jessica Landon, *Channing*, ABC. Specials: Gwen Cavendish, "The Royal Family," *The Best of Broadway*, CBS, 1954; Peggy Day, *The Women*, NBC, 1955; Judith, *High Tor*, CBS, 1956.

AWARDS: Academy Award nomination, Best Supporting Actress, 1950, for *Sunset Boulevard*.

MEMBER: Actors' Equity Association, Screen Actors Guild, American Federation of Television and Radio Artists.

SIDELIGHTS: RECREATIONS—Music and playing the piano.*

*   *   *

OPATOSHU, David   1918-

PERSONAL: Born David Opatovsky, January 30, 1918; son of Joseph (a novelist; known as Joseph Opatoshu) and Adele (a teacher) Opatovsky; married Lillian Weinberg (a psychiatric social worker; divorced); married Peggy O'Shea (an author), May 25, 1979; children: one son (first marriage). EDUCATION: Trained for the stage at the Benno Schneider Studio. MILITARY: U.S. Army Air Forces, 1942-45.

VOCATION: Actor and writer.

CAREER: Also see *WRITINGS* below. STAGE DEBUT—Mr. Carp, *Golden Boy*, Shubert Theatre, Newark, NJ, 1938. BROADWAY DEBUT—Sleeping man and blind man, *Night Music*, Broadhurst Theatre, 1940. PRINCIPAL STAGE APPEARANCES—Dan, *Clinton Street*, Mercury Theatre, New York City, 1940; Ralph, *Man of Tomorrow*, National Theatre, New York City, 1941; Mr. Mendel, *Me and Molly*, Belasco Theatre, New York City, 1948; Tewfik Bey, *Flight into Egypt*, Music Box Theatre, New York City, 1952; Denesco, *Reclining Figure*, Lyceum Theatre, New York City, 1954; Bibinski, *Silk Stockings*, Imperial Theatre, New York City, 1955; Luca, *At the Grand*, Philharmonic Auditorium, Los Angeles, CA, 1958; Maxwell Archer, *Once More, with Feeling*, National Theatre, 1958; Pan Apt, *The Wall*, Billy Rose Theatre, New York City, 1960; Amedeo, *Bravo Giovanni*, Broadhurst Theatre, 1962; Filippo, *Lorenzo*, Plymouth Theatre, New York City, 1963; Dr. Werner, *Does a Tiger Wear a Necktie?*, Belasco Theatre, 1969; Rabbi Reb Melech, *Yoshe Kalb*, Eden Theatre, New York City, 1972; Shimele Soroker, *The Big Winner*, Eden Theatre, 1974. Also appeared in *Mexican Mural: Moonlight Scene*, 1942; *The Devils*, Mark Taper Forum, Los Angeles, 1967; and in *Scream*, Alley Theatre, Houston, TX, 1978.

PRINCIPAL STAGE WORK—Director, *The Big Winner*, Eden Theatre, New York City, 1974.

MAJOR TOURS—Bibinski, *Silk Stockings*, U.S. cities, 1956; Luca, *At the Grand*, U.S. cities, 1958.

FILM DEBUT—*The Light Ahead*, Ultra, 1939. PRINCIPAL FILM APPEARANCES—Ben Miller, *The Naked City*, Universal, 1948; Frenchy, *Thieves' Highway*, Twentieth Century-Fox, 1949; Mr. Dutton, *The Goldbergs* (also known as *Molly*), Paramount, 1950; Captain Snegiryov, *The Brothers Karamazov*, Metro-Goldwyn-Mayer (MGM), 1958; Lou Forbes, *Party Girl*, MGM, 1958; Sol Levy, *Cimarron*, MGM, 1960; Akiva, *Exodus*, United Artists, 1960; Captain Bernasconi, *The Best of Enemies*, Columbia, 1962; President Rivera, *Guns of Darkness*, Warner Brothers, 1962; Slim, *The Most Wanted Man* (also known as *L'Ennemi public no. 1, Il nemico pubblico n. 1*, and *The Most Wanted Man in the World*), Astor, 1962; Daoud, *Rebels against the Light* (also known as *Sands of Beersheba*), David, 1964; Orlovsky, *The Defector* (also known as *Lautlose Waffen* and *L'Espion*), Warner Brothers/Seven Arts, 1966; Kavon, *One Spy Too Many*, MGM, 1966; Vinaro, *Tarzan and the Valley of Gold*, American International, 1966; Mr. Jacobi, *Torn Curtain*, Universal, 1966; Mr. Kolowitz, *Enter Laughing*, Columbia, 1967; Latke, *The Fixer*, MGM, 1968; Edward Rosenbloom, *Death of a Gunfighter*, Universal, 1969; Schloime Kradnik, *Romance of a Horse Thief*, Allied Artists, 1971; Bender, *Who'll Stop the Rain?* (also known as *Dog Soldiers*), United Artists, 1978; first Hebrab, *Americathon*, United Artists, 1979; Dr. Solomon, *Beyond Evil*, Scope III, 1980; Herod, *In Search of Historic Jesus*, Sunn Classic, 1980; Sam Paschal, *Forced Vengeance*, Metro-Goldwyn-Mayer/United Artists, 1982; Henry Morgenthau, Sr., *Forty Days of Musa Dagh*, High Investments, 1987. Also appeared in *Crowded Paradise*, Tudor, 1956; and *Almonds and Raisins* (documentary), Contemporary Films, Ltd./Teleculture, 1983.

TELEVISION DEBUT—Mr. Dutton, *The Goldbergs*, CBS, 1949. PRINCIPAL TELEVISION APPEARANCES—Series: Walter Rogers, *Bonino*, NBC, 1953; Hator, *The Secret Empire*, NBC, 1979. Mini-Series: Shimon, *Masada*, ABC, 1981. Pilots: Sam Mitschner, *Man against Crime* (broadcast as an episode of *Decision*), NBC, 1958; Dr. Grainger, *The D.A.: Murder One*, NBC, 1969; Herschel

Rosen, *Incident in San Francisco*, ABC, 1971; Arthur Horowitz, *Conspiracy of Terror*, NBC, 1975; Ed Miles, *Woman on the Run*, CBS, 1977; voice of Dr. Hans Zarkov, *Flash Gordon--The Greatest Adventure of All*, NBC, 1983. Episodic: Father, "Big Deal," *Goodyear Playhouse*, NBC, 1953; Finkle, "Finkle's Comet," *Alcoa Hour*, NBC, 1956; brother-in-law, "The Mother," *Philco Television Playhouse*, NBC, 1956; father, "Bricoe: Mayor Dublin," *Playhouse 90*, CBS, 1957; bookie, "On the Nose," *Alfred Hitchcock Presents*, CBS, 1958; mayor, "Hidden Valley," *Alfred Hitchcock Presents*, CBS, 1962; diplomat, "The Traitor," *Alcoa Premiere*, ABC, 1962; Dulong, "The Magic Show," *Alfred Hitchcock Presents*, CBS, 1963; Dorn, "Valley of the Shadow," *The Twilight Zone*, CBS, 1963; Ralph Cashman, "A Feasibility Study," *The Outer Limits*, ABC, 1964; Anan 7, "A Taste of Armageddon," *Star Trek*, NBC, 1967; also "Rivierra," *Studio One*, CBS, 1949; *Ellery Queen*, NBC, 1958; "Earthquake," *One Step Beyond*, ABC, 1959; "The Price of Doom," *Voyage to the Bottom of the Sea*, ABC, 1964; "Reign of Terror," *The Time Tunnel*, ABC, 1966; *Perry Mason*, CBS; *Mission: Impossible*, CBS; *Kojak*, CBS. Movies: Alfredo Faggio, *The Smugglers*, NBC, 1968; Grinev, *Francis Gary Powers: The True Story of the U-2 Spy Incident*, NBC, 1976; Menachem Begin, *Raid on Entebbe*, NBC, 1977; Dr. Ziegfeld, *Ziegfeld: The Man and His Women*, NBC, 1978; Ambassador Sajid Moktasanni, *Under Siege*, NBC, 1986; Judge Julius Hoffman, *Conspiracy: The Trial of the Chicago Eight*, HBO, 1987. Also appeared as the friend, *Six O'Clock Call*, ABC, 1954.

RELATED CAREER—Newscaster, WEVD, New York City, 1941, then 1946-55.

NON-RELATED CAREER—Silk screen printer.

WRITINGS: STAGE—*The Big Winner*, Eden Theatre, New York City, 1974. FILM—*Romance of a Horse Thief*, Allied Artists, 1971. OTHER—*Mid Sea and Sand*, 1947.

AWARDS: Limelight Award, Best Supporting Actor, 1961, for *Exodus;* Distinguished Artist Award from the State of Israel Bonds, Los Angeles, CA, 1961.

MEMBER: Actors' Equity Association, American Federation of Television and Radio Artists, Screen Actors Guild.

ADDRESSES: AGENT—Harry Abrams, Abrams Artists and Associates, 9200 Sunset Boulevard, Suite 625, Los Angeles, CA 90069.*

*   *   *

OPPENHEIMER, Alan   1930-

PERSONAL: Born April 23, 1930, in New York, NY; son of Louis E. (a stockbroker) and Irene (Rothschild) Oppenheimer; married Marianna Elliott (a costume designer), September 12, 1958 (divorced); married Marilyn Greenwood (a professional tennis player), March 22, 1984; children: Michael, Jane, Jennifer. EDUCATION: Carnegie-Mellon University, B.F.A., 1951.

VOCATION: Actor.

CAREER: PRINCIPAL STAGE APPEARANCES—Grandpa and Kapush, *The American Clock: A Mural for the Theatre*, Center Theatre Group, Mark Taper Forum, Los Angeles, CA, 1983; also

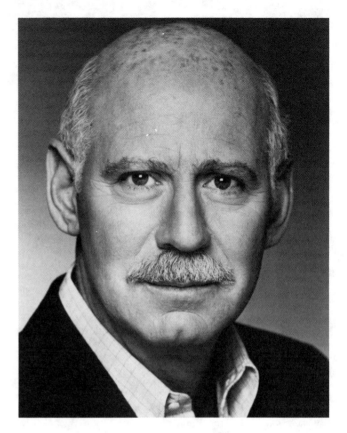

ALAN OPPENHEIMER

appeared in *The Devils*, Center Theatre Group, Mark Taper Forum, 1967; *The Hot l Baltimore*, Center Theatre Group, Mark Taper Forum, 1971; *The Taking Away of Little Willie*, Center Theatre Group, Mark Taper Forum, 1979; "Spared" in *The Quannapowitt Quartet*, Los Angeles Actors Theatre, Los Angeles, 1983; and with Arena Stage, Washington, DC, 1954-65.

PRINCIPAL FILM APPEARANCES—Ted Appleton, *In the Heat of the Night*, United Artists, 1967; Everett Bauer, *How to Save a Marriage—And Ruin Your Life* (also known as *Band of Gold*), Columbia, 1968; Andre Charlot, *Star!* (also known as *Those Were the Happy Times*), Twentieth Century-Fox, 1968; Adolph Springer, *The Maltese Bippy*, Metro-Goldwyn-Mayer, 1969; major, *Little Big Man*, National General, 1970; Hackett, *The Groundstar Conspiracy*, Universal, 1972; chief supervisor, *Westworld*, Metro-Goldwyn-Mayer, 1973; insurance agent, *The Thief Who Came to Dinner*, Warner Brothers, 1973; narrator, *Gentleman Tramp* (documentary), Fox/Rank, 1974; Albert Breslau, *The Hindenberg*, Universal, 1975; Lieutenant Mannite, *Win, Place, or Steal* (also known as *Three for the Money* and *Just Another Day at the Races*), Cinema National, 1975; Mr. Joffert, *Freaky Friday*, Buena Vista, 1976; blind man, *Record City*, American International, 1978; rabbi, *Private Benjamin*, Warner Brothers, 1980; voice of Folker, *The Never Ending Story*, Warner Brothers, 1984; voice of Bo, *The Secret of the Sword*, Atlantic, 1985. Also appeared in *A Pleasure Doing Business*, 1979; and *Moving*, Warner Brothers, 1987.

PRINCIPAL TELEVISION APPEARANCES—Series: Murray Mouse, *He and She*, CBS, 1967-68; voice characterization, *Inch High, Private Eye* (animated), NBC, 1973-74; voice characterization, *Butch Cassidy and the Sundance Kids* (animated), NBC, 1973-74;

voice characterization, *Speed Buggy* (animated), CBS, 1973-74, then ABC, 1975-76; voice characterization, *Partridge Family: 2200 A.D.* (animated), CBS, 1974-75; Dr. Rudy Wells, *The Six Million Dollar Man*, ABC, 1974-75; voice of Gorak, *Valley of the Dinosaurs* (animated), CBS, 1974-76; Jessie Smith, *Big Eddie*, CBS, 1975; voice characterization, *Tarzan: Lord of the Jungle* (animated), CBS, 1976; voice of Sidney Merciless, *The C.B. Bears* (animated), CBS, 1977-78; Captain Finnerty, *Eischied*, NBC, 1979-80; voice of Mighty Mouse and Oilcan Harry, *The New Adventures of Mighty Mouse and Heckle and Jeckle* (animated), CBS, 1979-82; voice of Dr. Hans Zarkov and Ming the Merciless, *The New Animated Adventures of Flash Gordon* (animated), NBC, 1979, then 1982-83; voice characterization, *The Heathcliff and Dingbat Show* (animated), ABC, 1980-81; voice characterization, *Thundarr the Barbarian* (animated), ABC, 1980-82; voice of Big D (Dracula), *The Drak Pack* (animated), CBS, 1980-82; voice of Sheriff Pudge Trollsom, *Trollkins* (animated), CBS, 1981-82; voice of Mr. Sampson, *The Kid Super Power Hour with Shazam* (animated), NBC, 1981-82; voice characterization, *Blackstar* (animated), CBS, 1981-84; voice of Vanity Smurf, *The Smurfs* (animated), NBC, 1981-89; voice of Skeletor and Man-at-Arms, *He-Man and the Masters of the Universe* (animated), syndicated, 1982-84; voice characterization, *She-Ra: Princess of Power* (animated), 1985; voice characterization, *The Thirteen Ghosts of Scooby-Doo*, ABC, 1985-86; voice characterization, *The Wuzzles* (animated), CBS, 1985-86, then ABC, 1986-87; voice characterization, *Chuck Norris Karate Kommandos* (animated), syndicated, 1986; voice characterization, *Rambo* (animated), syndicated, 1986; voice characterization, *The Centurions—PowerXtreme!* (animated), syndicated, 1986; voice characterization, *Ghostbusters* (animated), syndicated, 1986; voice characterization, *BraveStarr* (animated), syndicated, 1987; voice characterization, *The New Adventures of the Snorks* (animated), syndicated, 1987.

Mini-Series: Simon Cappell, *Washington: Behind Closed Doors*, ABC, 1977; George Simonson, *Blind Ambition*, CBS, 1979. Pilots: Cecil Barrett, *Three for Tahiti*, ABC, 1970; Dr. Bryan Dorman, *The Shameful Secrets of Hastings Corners*, NBC, 1970; Edgar Winston, *Inside O.U.T.*, CBS, 1971; Mr. Hansen, *Margie Passes* (broadcast as episode of *Of Men Of Women*), ABC, 1973; Bennett, *Daddy's Girl*, CBS, 1973; Dr. Rudy Wells, *The Six Million Dollar Man*, ABC, 1973; Springfield, *The Lives of Jenny Dolan*, NBC, 1975; Mr. Frederick, *Maureen*, CBS, 1976; Hilly, *Susan and Sam*, NBC, 1977; Captain Finnerty, *To Kill a Cop*, NBC, 1978; Mel Adamson, *Living in Paradise*, NBC, 1981; Chris Mantock, *Stopwatch: Thirty Minutes of Investigative Ticking*, HBO, 1983; Reuben Ziskind, "Sirens," *CBS Summer Playhouse*, CBS, 1987. Episodic: Mr. Ruskin, "Barney Hosts a Summit Meeting," *The Andy Griffith Show*, CBS, 1968; Judge Crockett, *Night Court*, NBC, 1987; Dr. Linder, *Matlock*, NBC, 1988; Dean Brown, *Who's the Boss?*, ABC, 1988 and 1989; Eugene Kinsella, *Murphy Brown*, CBS, 1989; also Mickey Malph, *Happy Days*, ABC; mayor, *Mama's Family*, syndicated; *Barney Miller*, ABC, 1982; *L.A. Law*, NBC, 1988.

Movies: Dr. Otto Ludwig, *What Are Best Friends For?*, ABC, 1973; Lubell, *Death Sentence*, ABC, 1974; Aaron Stovitz, *Helter Skelter*, CBS, 1976; Barton, *The Ghost of Flight 401*, NBC, 1978; Arthur Lazar, *Divorce Wars*, ABC, 1982; Conroy, *Memorial Day*, CBS, 1983; Jerry Gersler, *My Wicked, Wicked Ways . . . The Legend of Errol Flynn*, CBS, 1985; Max Langbein, *The Execution*, NBC, 1985; Dr. Noah Townsend, *Arthur Hailey's "Strong Medicine,"* syndicated, 1986; Sam Rosenthal, *The Two Mrs. Grenvilles*, NBC, 1987; also *Tail Gunner Joe*, NBC, 1977; *Raid on Entebbe*,

NBC, 1987. Specials: Voice characterization, *Cyrano* (animated), ABC, 1974; *How to Survive the Seventies and Maybe Even Bump into Happiness*, CBS, 1978; voice, *The Fabulous Funnies*, NBC, 1978; John Hocker, "Dinky Hocker," *ABC Afterschool Special*, ABC, 1979; Miles Rathbourne, *Peeping Times*, NBC, 1978; Watson, *Close Ties*, Entertainment Channel, 1983; voice of Vanity Smurf, *My Smurfy Valentine* (animated), NBC, 1983; voice of Skeletor, *He-Man and She-Ra: A Christmas Special* (animated), syndicated, 1985; voice of Mr. Dithers, *Blondie and Dagwood* (animated), CBS, 1987; Monty Gladstone, "Tales from the Hollywood Hills: The Old Reliable," *Great Performances*, PBS, 1988. Also appeared as General Reynolds, *Court-Martial of General Yamisita*, 1974.

ADDRESSES: AGENT—The Gage Group, 9229 Sunset Boulevard, Suite 306, Los Angeles, CA 90069.

*   *   *

ORBACH, Jerry   1935-

PERSONAL: Full name, Jerome Orbach; born October 20, 1935, in Bronx, NY; son of Leon (a restaurant manager) and Emily (a greeting card manufacturer; maiden name, Olexy) Orbach; married Marta Curro (an actress and writer), June 21, 1958 (divorced); married Elaine Cancilla, 1979; children: Anthony Nicholas, Christopher Ben (first marriage). EDUCATION: Attended the University of Illinois, 1952-53, and Northwestern University, 1953-55; trained for the stage with Herbert Berghof, Mira Rostova, and Lee Strasberg; studied singing with Hazel Schweppe.

VOCATION: Actor.

CAREER: STAGE DEBUT—Typewriter man, *Room Service*, Chevy Chase Tent Theatre, Wheeling, IL, 1952. OFF-BROADWAY DEBUT—Streetsinger and various roles, *The Threepenny Opera*, Theatre De Lys, 1955. PRINCIPAL STAGE APPEARANCES—Mannion, *Mister Roberts*, Kralhome, *The King and I*, Dr. Sanderson, *Harvey*, and Benny, *Guys and Dolls*, all Dayton Municipal Auditorium, Dayton, OH, then Shubert Theatre, Cincinnati, OH, both 1959; El Gallo (the narrator), *The Fantasticks*, Sullivan Street Playhouse, New York City, 1960; Paul Berthalet, *Carnival!*, Imperial Theatre, New York City, 1961, then Shubert Theatre, Chicago, IL, 1963; Larry Foreman, *The Cradle Will Rock*, Theatre Four, New York City, 1964; Sky Masterson, *Guys and Dolls*, City Center Theatre, New York City, 1965; Jigger Craigin, *Carousel*, State Theatre, New York City, 1965; Charlie Davenport, *Annie Get Your Gun*, State Theatre, 1966; Malcolm, *The Natural Look*, Longacre Theatre, New York City, 1967; Harold Wonder, *Scuba Duba*, New Theatre, New York City, 1967; Chuck Baxter, *Promises, Promises*, Shubert Theatre, New York City, 1968; Paul Friedman, *6 Rms Riv Vu*, Helen Hayes Theatre, New York City, 1972; Billy Flynn, *Chicago*, 46th Street Theatre, New York City, 1975; Julian Marsh, *42nd Second Street*, Winter Garden Theatre, New York City, 1980, then Majestic Theatre, New York City, 1981. Also appeared in *Picnic* and *The Caine Mutiny Court-Martial*, both Gristmill Playhouse, Andover, NJ, 1955; *The Student Prince*, Dayton Municipal Auditorium, then Shubert Theatre, Cincinnati, both 1959; *The Rose Tattoo*, Philadelphia Drama Guild, Walnut Street Theatre, Philadelphia, PA, 1973; *The Trouble with People . . . and Other Things*, Coconut Grove Theatre, Miami, FL, 1974; and in more than forty productions with the Show Case Theatre, Evanston, IL, 1953-54.

MAJOR TOURS—Paul Friedman, *6 Rms Riv Vu*, U.S. cities, 1973; Billy Flynn, *Chicago*, U.S. cities, 1977-78; George Schneider, *Chapter Two*, U.S. cities, 1978-79.

PRINCIPAL FILM APPEARANCES—Joe, *Mad Dog Coll*, Columbia, 1961; Pinkerton, *John Goldfarb, Please Come Home*, Twentieth Century-Fox, 1964; Kid Sally Palumbo, *The Gang That Couldn't Shoot Straight*, Metro-Goldwyn-Mayer, 1971; Fred, *A Fan's Notes*, Warner Brothers, 1972; Lorsey, *Foreplay*, Cinema National, 1975; film director, *The Sentinel*, Universal, 1977; Gus Levy, *Prince of the City*, Warner Brothers, 1981; Charley Pegler, *Brewster's Millions*, Universal, 1985; Nicholas DeFranco, *F/X*, Orion, 1986; Byron Caine, *The Imagemaker*, Castle Hill/Manson, 1986; Dr. Jake Houseman, *Dirty Dancing*, Vestron, 1987; Leo, *I Love N.Y.*, Manley, 1987; Lieutenant Garber, *Someone to Watch Over Me*, Columbia, 1987. Also appeared in *Cop Hater*, United Artists, 1958.

PRINCIPAL TELEVISION APPEARANCES—Series: Voice characterization, *Adventures of the Galaxy Rangers* (animated), syndicated, 1986; Harry McGraw, *Murder, She Wrote* (recurring role), CBS, 1986—; Harry McGraw, *The Law and Harry McGraw*, CBS, 1987-88. Mini-Series: John Sutter, *Dream West*, CBS, 1986; Mort Viner, *Out on a Limb*, ABC, 1987. Pilots: Sergeant Max Grozzo, *The Streets*, NBC, 1984. Episodic: Brian Merrick, *Our Family Honor*, ABC, 1985; Malcolm Shanley III, *Simon and Simon*, CBS, 1988; also *The Nurses*, CBS, 1963; *Bob Hope Presents the Chrysler Theatre*, NBC, 1964; *Diana*, NBC, 1973; as Brubaker, *Kojak*, CBS; in *Love, American Style*, ABC; *The Shari Lewis Show*, NBC; *The Jack Paar Show*, NBC. Movies: Sam Bianchi, *An Invasion of Privacy*, CBS, 1983; Spicer, *Love among Thieves*, ABC, 1987. Specials: Cristol, *Twenty-Four Hours in a Woman's Life*, CBS, 1961; Charles Davenport, *Annie Get Your Gun*, NBC, 1967; *Mitzi: A Tribute to the American Housewife*, CBS, 1974; *The Way They Were*, syndicated, 1981; Sam Nash, "Visitor from Mamaroneck," Jesse Kiplinger, "Visitor from Hollywood," and Rob Hubley, "Visitor from Forest Hills," *Plaza Suite*, HBO, 1982; *Irving Berlin's One Hundredth Birthday Celebration*, CBS, 1988; "A Salute to Broadway: The Shows," *In Performance at the White House*, PBS, 1988.

RECORDINGS: SINGLES—"Love Stolen," Take Home Tunes, 1976. ALBUMS—*The Fantasticks* (original cast recording), MGM, 1960, reissued by Polydor; *Carnival!* (original cast recording), MGM, 1961; *Jerry Orbach Off-Broadway*, MGM, 1961; *The Cradle Will Rock* (cast recording), MGM, 1965; *Carousel* (cast recording), RCA Victor, 1965; *Annie Get Your Gun* (cast recording), RCA Victor, 1966; *Promises, Promises* (original cast recording), United Artists Records, 1969, reissued by Liberty; *Alan Jay Lerner Revisited*, Crewe, 1966, reissued by Painted Smiles; *Chicago* (original cast recording), Arista, 1975; *42nd Street* (original cast recording), RCA Red Seal, 1980.

AWARDS: New March of Dimes Horizon Award and Actor's Fund Award of Merit, both 1961; Antoinette Perry Award nomination, Best Supporting or Featured Actor in a Musical, 1965, for *Guys and Dolls*; Antoinette Perry Award, Best Actor in a Musical, 1969, for *Promises, Promises*; Antoinette Perry Award nomination, Best Actor in a Musical, 1976, for *Chicago*.

MEMBER: Actors' Equity Association, Screen Actors Guild, American Federation of Television and Radio Artists, Lone Star Boat Club.

SIDELIGHTS: RECREATIONS—Pocket billiards, fishing, poker, golf, and tennis.

ADDRESSES: AGENT—Contemporary Artists, 132 Lasky Drive, Beverly Hills, CA 90212.*

* * *

OSBORN, Paul 1901-1988

PERSONAL: Born September 4, 1901, in Evansville, IN; died May 12, 1988, in New York, NY; son of Edwin Faxon (a minister) and Bertha (Judson) Osborn; married Millicent Green (an actress and writer), May 10, 1939; children: Judith. EDUCATION: University of Michigan, B.A., 1923, M.A., 1924; graduate work, Yale University, 1927.

VOCATION: Playwright, screenwriter, and teacher.

CAREER: See *WRITINGS* below. RELATED CAREER—English instructor, University of Michigan, Ann Arbor, MI, 1925-27; English instructor, Yale University, New Haven, CT, 1928.

NON-RELATED CAREER—Worked with the Long Island Railroad during the 1920s.

WRITINGS: STAGE—*Hotbed*, Klaw Theatre, New York City, 1928; *A Ledge*, Assembly Theatre, New York City, 1929; *The Vinegar Tree*, Playhouse Theatre, New York City, 1930, published by Farrar and Rinehart, 1931, then Samuel French, Inc., 1932 and 1959; *Oliver, Oliver*, Playhouse Theatre, 1934, published by Samuel French, Inc., 1934; *On Borrowed Time*, Longacre Theatre, New York City, 1938, published by Knopf, 1938, then Dramatists Play Service, 1942; *Morning's at Seven*, Longacre Theatre, 1939, then Lyceum Theatre, New York City, 1980, and in London, 1984, published by Samuel French, Inc., 1940; *The Innocent Voyage*, Belasco Theatre, New York City, 1943, published by Brandt and Brandt, 1946; *A Bell for Adano*, Cort Theatre, New York City, 1944, published by Knopf, 1945; *Point of No Return*, Alvin Theatre, New York City, 1951, published by Random House, 1952, then Samuel French, Inc., 1954; *The World of Suzie Wong*, Broadhurst Theatre, New York City, 1958; (co-writer) *Hot September*, Shubert Theatre, Boston, MA, 1965. Also *Tomorrow's Monday*, New York City, 1936; *Maiden Voyage*, Philadelphia, PA, 1957; and *Film of Memory*, London, 1965.

FILM—*The Young in Heart*, United Artists, 1938; *Madame Curie*, Metro-Goldwyn-Mayer (MGM), 1943; *Cry Havoc*, MGM, 1943; *The Yearling*, MGM, 1946; *Homecoming*, MGM, 1948; (with Peter Berneis and Leonardo Bercovici) *Portrait of Jennie* (also known as *Jennie* and *Tidal Wave*), Selznick International, 1949; *Invitation*, MGM, 1952; *East of Eden*, Warner Brothers, 1955; *Sayonara*, Warner Brothers, 1957; *South Pacific*, Twentieth Century-Fox, 1958; *Wild River*, Twentieth Century-Fox, 1960; *Dunbar's Cove*, Twentieth Century-Fox, 1960. Also wrote the unproduced screenplays *Forever*, MGM, 1948; and *John Brown's Body*, Twentieth Century-Fox, 1967.

AWARDS: Academy Award nomination, Best Screenplay, 1955, for *East of Eden*; Academy Award nomination, Best Screenplay, 1957, for *Sayonara*; Antoinette Perry Award, Best Reproduction, 1980, for *Morning's at Seven*; Laurel Award for Screen from the Writers Guild of America, 1982, in recognition of outstanding contributions to the profession of the screenwriter and of notable work which has advanced the literature of the motion picture.

OBITUARIES AND OTHER SOURCES: New York Times, May 13, 1988; *Variety,* May 18, 1988.*

*   *   *

OXENBERG, Catherine   1961-

PERSONAL: Born September 22, 1961, in New York, NY; daughter of Princess Elizabeth of Yugoslavia; father, in business. EDUCATION: Studied acting with Stanley Zaraff in New York City.

VOCATION: Actress.

CAREER: PRINCIPAL FILM APPEARANCES—Eve Trent, *The Lair of the White Worm,* Vestron, 1988; also appeared in *Walking after Midnight,* Kay Film, 1988.

TELEVISION DEBUT—Lady Diana Spencer, *The Royal Romance of Charles and Diana,* CBS, 1982. PRINCIPAL TELEVISION APPEARANCES—Series: Amanda Carrington, *Dynasty,* ABC, 1984-86. Episodic: Host, *Saturday Night Live,* NBC, 1986; also *The Love Boat,* ABC; *Cover Up,* CBS. Movies: Nancy Church, *Still Crazy Like a Fox,* CBS, 1987; Princess Alisa, *Roman Holiday,* CBS, 1987; also *Swimsuit,* NBC, 1989. Specials: *That's What Friends Are For: AIDS Concert '88,* Showtime, 1988.

RELATED CAREER—Professional model.

ADDRESSES: AGENT—John Gaines, Agency for the Performing Arts, 9000 Sunset Boulevard, Suite 1200, Los Angeles, CA 90069.*

*   *   *

OZ, Frank   1944-

PERSONAL: Born Frank Richard Oznowicz, May 24, 1944, in Hereford, England; son of Isidore and Frances Oznowicz. EDUCATION: Attended Oakland City College, 1962.

VOCATION: Puppeteer, actor, producer, director, and screenwriter.

CAREER: Also see *WRITINGS* below. PRINCIPAL FILM APPEARANCES—Puppeteer and voice of Miss Piggy, Fozzie Bear, Animal, and Sam the Eagle, *The Muppet Movie,* Associated Film Distributors, 1979; corrections officer, *The Blues Brothers,* Universal, 1980; voice of Yoda, *The Empire Strikes Back,* Twentieth Century-Fox, 1980; Mr. Collins and voice of Miss Piggy, *An American Werewolf in London,* Universal, 1981; puppeteer and voice of Miss Piggy, Fozzie Bear, Animal, and Sam the Eagle, *The Great Muppet Caper,* Universal, 1981; puppet operator for Aughra and Skeksis Chamberlain, *The Dark Crystal,* Universal/Associated Film Distributors/ITC Entertainment, 1982; voice of Yoda, *Return of the Jedi,* Twentieth Century-Fox, 1983; corrupt cop, *Trading Places,* Paramount, 1983; puppeteer and voice of Miss Piggy, Fozzie Bear, and Animal, *The Muppets Take Manhattan,* Tri-Star, 1984; puppeteer and voice of Cookie Monster, Bert, and Grover, *Sesame Street Presents: Follow That Bird!,* Warner Brothers, 1985; test monitor, *Spies Like Us,* Warner Brothers, 1985; Wiseman, *Labyrinth,* Tri-Star, 1986.

PRINCIPAL FILM WORK—Producer and creative consultant (with David Lazer), *The Great Muppet Caper,* Universal, 1981; director (with Jim Henson), *The Dark Crystal,* Universal/Associated Film Distributors/ITC Entertainment, 1982; director, *The Muppets Take Manhattan,* Tri-Star, 1984; director, *Little Shop of Horrors,* Warner Brothers, 1986; director, *Dirty Rotten Scoundrels,* Orion, 1988.

PRINCIPAL TELEVISION APPEARANCES—All as puppeteer and voice characterizations with the Muppets. Series: *Sesame Street,* PBS, 1969—; Fozzie Bear, Animal, Miss Piggy, Sam the Eagle, Swedish Chef, and others, *The Muppet Show,* syndicated, 1976-81. Episodic: The Mighty Favag, *Saturday Night Live,* NBC, 1975-76. Specials: Miss Piggy, *The Fantastic Miss Piggy Show,* ABC, 1982; Miss Piggy, *San Francisco Ballet in Cinderella,* PBS, 1985; also *Julie Andrews: One Step into Spring,* CBS, 1978; *The Muppets—A Celebration of Thirty Years,* CBS, 1986; *A Muppet Family Christmas* (also known as *Christmas at Home with the Muppets*), ABC, 1987; *Sesame Street Special,* PBS, 1988; *Sesame Street . . . Twenty and Still Counting,* PBS, 1989.

RELATED CAREER—Puppeteer with the Muppets, 1963—; vice-president and producer, Henson Associates, New York City.

WRITINGS: FILM—(With Tom Patchett) *The Muppets Take Manhattan,* Tri-Star, 1984.

AWARDS: Emmy Award, Best Performer in a Comedy-Variety or Music Series, 1978, for *The Muppet Show.*

MEMBER: American Federation of Television and Radio Artists, Screen Actors Guild, Academy of Television Arts and Sciences.

ADDRESSES: OFFICE—Henson Associates, 117 E. 69th Street, New York, NY 10024.*

P

PACKER, David

VOCATION: Actor.

CAREER: PRINCIPAL FILM APPEARANCES—Emergency doctor, Robocop, 1987; Eddie, You Can't Hurry Love, Lightning, 1988.

PRINCIPAL TELEVISION APPEARANCES—Series: Neil "Trout" Troutman, The Best Times, 1985. Mini-Series: Daniel Bernstein, V: The Final Battle, NBC, 1984. Pilots: Danny, High School U.S.A., NBC, 1983; Jeff, What's Alan Watching?, CBS, 1989. Episodic: Derry, Thirtysomething, ABC, 1985; also "U.N. the Night and the Music," M*A*S*H, CBS, 1983. Movies: Daniel Bernstein, V, NBC, 1983; CBS, 1985; Brian, First Steps, CBS, 1985.

ADDRESSES: AGENT—Triad Artists, 10100 Santa Monica Boulevard, 16th Floor, Los Angeles, CA 90067.*

*   *   *

PAGE, Harrison

PERSONAL: Born August 27, in Atlanta, GA.

VOCATION: Actor.

CAREER: PRINCIPAL FILM APPEARANCES—Beyond the Valley of the Dolls, Twentieth Century-Fox, 1970.

PRINCIPAL TELEVISION APPEARANCES—Series: Ferguson Bruce, Love Thy Neighbor, ABC, 1973; Chief Robinson, C.P.O. Sharkey, NBC, 1976-78; George Boone, Supertrain, NBC, 1979; Captain Trunk, Sledge Hammer!, ABC, 1986-88. Mini-Series: Wheatley Parks, Backstairs at the White House, NBC, 1979. Pilots: Arnold Jackson, Adventuring with the Chopper, NBC, 1976; Al Cook, High Five, NBC, 1982; George Link, Generation, ABC, 1985. Episodic: Louis Hurley, 227, NBC, 1985; Lieutenant Gowans, Murder, She Wrote, CBS, 1988; also Monday, Benson, ABC. Movies: Josh, Sergeant Matlovich versus the U.S. Air Force, NBC, 1978; Walter Newell, The Kid with the 200 I.Q., NBC, 1983.

ADDRESSES: AGENT—Twentieth Century Artists, 3800 Barham Boulevard, Suite 303, Los Angeles, CA 90068.*

PALMER, Gregg   1927-
(Palmer Lee)

PERSONAL: Born Palmer Lee, January 25, 1927, in San Francisco, CA. EDUCATION: Attended the University of Utah. MILITARY: U.S. Air Force, 1945-46.

VOCATION: Actor.

CAREER: PRINCIPAL FILM APPEARANCES—Attendant, My Friend Irma Goes West, Paramount, 1950; (as Palmer Lee) Grat Dalton, The Cimarron Kid, Universal, 1951; (as Palmer Lee) William Norton, Francis Goes to West Point, Universal, 1952; (as Palmer Lee) tank lieutenant, Red Ball Express, Universal, 1952; (as Palmer Lee) Marty Smith, The Raiders (also known as Riders of Vengeance), Universal, 1952; (as Palmer Lee) Farouk, Son of Ali Baba, Universal, 1952; (as Palmer Lee) Johnny Evans, Sally and Saint Anne, Universal, 1952; (as Palmer Lee) Joe Bent, The Battle at Apache Pass, Universal, 1952; (as Palmer Lee) Captain White, Back at the Front (also known as Willie and Joe Back at the Front), Universal, 1952; (as Palmer Lee) Chet Dunne, It Happens Every Thursday, Universal, 1953; (as Palmer Lee) Chalmers, Column South, Universal, 1953; (as Palmer Lee) Oaman, The Veils of Bagdad, Universal, 1953; (as Palmer Lee) Hal Jessup, The Redhead from Wyoming, Universal, 1953; Cameron, The All-American (also known as The Winning Way), Universal, 1953; Tom Masterson, Magnificent Obsession, Universal, 1954; Tom Bradley, Playgirl, Universal, 1954; Captain Burnett, Taza, Son of Cochise, Universal, 1954; Lieutenant Manning, To Hell and Back, Universal, 1955; Jed Grant, The Creature Walks among Us, Universal, 1956; Dink, Hilda Crane, Twentieth Century-Fox, 1956; Pat Orvello, Footsteps in the Night, Allied Artists, 1957; Kimo, From Hell It Came, Allied Artists, 1957; Captain James Tenslip, Revolt at Fort Laramie, United Artists, 1957; Jeff Clark, Zombies of Mora Tau, Columbia, 1957; Piggy, The Female Animal, Universal, 1958; Captain Dexter, Thundering Jets, Twentieth Century-Fox, 1958; John Mapes, The Rebel Set (also known as Beatsville), Allied Artists, 1959; Bart Connors, The Sad Horse, Twentieth Century-Fox, 1959.

Reed Taylor, The Cat Burglar, United Artists, 1961; Brad Santley, Gun Fight, United Artists, 1961; Lieutenant Fisher, The Most Dangerous Man Alive, Columbia, 1961; Piper, Forty Pounds of Trouble, Universal, 1962; Swedish commentator, The Prize, Metro-Goldwyn-Mayer (MGM), 1963; gambler, Advance to the Rear (also known as Company of Cowards?), MGM, 1964; Donovan, The Quick Gun, Columbia, 1964; Union guard, Shenandoah, Universal, 1965; Rodenbush, The Rare Breed, Universal, 1966; special officer, If He Hollers, Let Him Go, Cinerama, 1968; Parker, The Undefeated, Twentieth Century-Fox, 1969; Riker, Chisum, Warner Brothers, 1970; Berger, The McKenzie Break, United

Artists, 1970; John Goodfellow, *Big Jake*, National General, 1971; Hurricane Kid, *La vita, a volte e molto dura, vera provvidenza?* (also known as *Life Is Tough Enough, Eh Providence?*), Euro International, 1972; burly man, *The Shootist,* Paramount, 1976; Jeff, *Hot Lead and Cold Feet,* Buena Vista, 1978; Sergeant Hacksaw, *The Man with Bogart's Face* (also known as *Sam Marlow, Private Eye*), Twentieth Century-Fox, 1980; Ross, *Scream* (also known as *The Outing*), Cal-Com Releasing, 1981. Also appeared in *The Golden Blade,* Universal, 1953; *Five Guns to Tombstone,* United Artists, 1961.

PRINCIPAL TELEVISION APPEARANCES—Series: Harry, *Run Buddy Run*, CBS, 1966-67. Mini-Series: Bull Run colonel, *The Blue and the Gray,* CBS, 1982. Pilots: Payne, *Go West, Young Girl!*, ABC, 1978. Movies: Szabo, *Mongo's Back in Town*, CBS, 1971; Slatter, *True Grit (A Further Adventure)*, ABC, 1978; also *The Daughters of Joshua Cabe,* ABC, 1976; *Beggarman, Thief,* NBC, 1979.

RELATED CAREER—Radio announcer and disc jockey.*

*　　*　　*

PANKIN, Stuart　1946-

PERSONAL: Born April 8, 1946, in Philadelphia, PA; children: one son. EDUCATION: Dickinson College, B.A., 1968; Columbia University, M.F.A., 1971.

VOCATION: Actor.

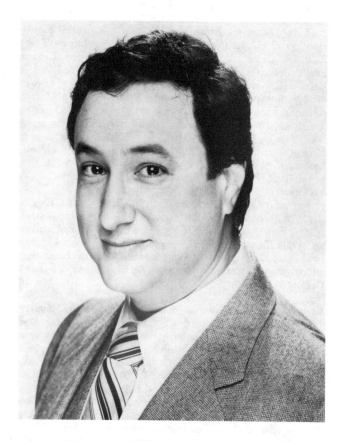

STUART PANKIN

CAREER: OFF-BROADWAY DEBUT—*The Wars of the Roses,* 1968. PRINCIPAL STAGE APPEARANCES—Jeweler, *Timon of Athens,* and beast, *The Tale of Cymbeline,* both New York Shakespeare Festival, Delacorte Theatre, New York City, 1971; Sheriff of Northampton, *Mary Stuart,* Vivian Beaumont Theatre, New York City, 1971; Hopkins, *The Crucible,* peasant, soldier, and tribesman, *Narrow Road to the Deep North,* and Orsino's attendant, *Twelfth Night,* all Vivian Beaumont Theatre, 1972; Blacksmith and Bear, *The Glorious Age,* Theatre Four, New York City, 1975; Zeus, *Wings,* Eastside Playhouse, New York City, 1975; Gavrillo and offstage speaking patient, *Gorky,* American Place Theatre, New York City, 1975; Reuben, *Joseph and the Amazing Technicolor Dreamcoat,* Brooklyn Academy of Music, Opera House, Brooklyn, NY, 1976; Second Lieutenant Fedotik, *The Three Sisters,* Brooklyn Academy of Music, Helen Carey Playhouse, Brooklyn, NY, 1977. Also appeared in productions of *Richard III, The Inspector General,* and *The Winter's Tale,* all in New York City.

PRINCIPAL FILM APPEARANCES—Duane, *Scavenger Hunt,* Twentieth Century-Fox, 1979; Sam, *Hangar 18* (also known as *Invasion Force*), Sunn Classic, 1980; Dudley Laywicker, *The Hollywood Knights,* Columbia, 1980; Nicky LaBelle, *An Eye for an Eye,* AVCO-Embassy, 1981; Sweeny, *Earthbound,* Taft International, 1981; Ronnie, *Irreconcilable Differences,* Warner Brothers, 1984; Mr. Hodgkins, *The Dirt Bike Kid,* Concorde/Cinema Group, 1986; Jimmy, *Fatal Attraction,* Paramount, 1987; Judge Samuel John, *Love at Stake* (also known as *Burnin' Love*), Tri-Star, 1987; Preston Picket, Ph.D., *Second Sight,* Lorimar, 1989.

PRINCIPAL TELEVISION APPEARANCES—Series: Stuf, *The San Pedro Beach Bums,* ABC, 1977; Al Tuttle, *No Soap, Radio,* ABC, 1982; Bob Charles and various other roles, *Not Necessarily the News,* HBO, 1983-88; Mike Dooley, *Nearly Departed,* NBC, 1989—. Pilots: Stuf, *The San Pedro Beach Bums,* ABC, 1977; Last Chance, *Car Wash,* NBC, 1979; Harvey Kreppler, *The Eyes of Texas II,* NBC, 1979; Harvey, *Valentine Magic on Love Island* (also known as *Magic on Love Island*), NBC, 1980; Lyle Floon, *The Wonderful World of Philip Malley,* CBS, 1981. Episodic: Dr. Melnick, *Night Court,* NBC, 1985; Plato, *Scarecrow and Mrs. King,* CBS, 1985; as himself, *Comedy Break with Mack and Jamie,* syndicated, 1985; Gary Weed, *Crazy Like a Fox,* CBS, 1986; Jacques, *Golden Girls,* NBC, 1986; Morgan, *Stingray,* NBC, 1986; Adelman, *Night Court,* NBC, 1987; Claude Jenkins, *The New Mike Hammer,* CBS, 1987; Marv, *Family Ties,* NBC, 1987; the Devil, *Hooperman,* ABC, 1989; Gary's brain, *It's Gary Shandling's Show,* Showtime, then Fox, both 1989; also *Barney Miller,* ABC, 1978 and 1980; *Trapper John, M.D.,* CBS; *Three's a Crowd,* ABC. Movies: Robert, *A Different Affair,* CBS, 1987. Specials: Host, *Stuart Pankin,* Cinemax, 1987; *Comic Relief II,* HBO, 1987; also *American Comedy Awards,* 1988; *9th Annual ACE Awards,* 1988.

PRINCIPAL TELEVISION WORK—Co-executive producer, *Stuart Pankin,* Cinemax, 1987.

WRITINGS: TELEVISION—Co-writer and writer of songs, *Stuart Pankin,* Cinemax, 1987.

AWARDS: ACE (Awards for Cablecasting Excellence) Award, Best Actor, for *Not Necessarily the News.*

SIDELIGHTS: RECREATIONS—Fencing, joggling, scuba diving, performing magic tricks, and playing piano.

ADDRESSES: AGENT—Dade/Rosen/Schultz, 15010 Ventura Boulevard, Suite 219, Sherman Oaks, CA 91403.

PARKER, Sarah Jessica 1965-

PERSONAL: Born March 25, 1965, in Nelsonville, OH.

VOCATION: Actress.

CAREER: PRINCIPAL STAGE APPEARANCES—Flora, The Innocents, Morosco Theatre, New York City, 1976; July, then title role, Annie, Alvin Theatre, New York City, 1978; Rachel, To Gillian on Her 37th Birthday, Ensemble Studio Theatre, New York City, 1983, then Circle in the Square Downtown, New York City, 1984; Darlene Magnum, "Terry Neal's Future" in Marathon '86, Ensemble Studio Theatre, 1986. Also appeared in The War Brides, New Dramatists, New York City, 1981; The Death of a Miner, Portland Stage Company, Portland, ME, 1982; The Heidi Chronicles, Playwrights Horizons, then Plymouth Theatre, both New York City, 1989; and in By Strouse, Off-Broadway production.

PRINCIPAL FILM APPEARANCES—Lisa, Firstborn, Paramount, 1984; Rusty, Footloose, Paramount, 1984; Janey Glenn, Girls Just Want to Have Fun, New World, 1985; Carolyn McAdams, Flight of the Navigator, Buena Vista, 1986. Also appeared in Rich Kids, United Artists, 1979.

PRINCIPAL TELEVISION APPEARANCES—Series: Patty Greene, Square Pegs, CBS, 1982-83; Kay Erickson Gardner, A Year in the Life, NBC, 1987-88. Pilots: Samantha Cooper, The Alan King Show, CBS, 1986; Kay Erickson, A Year in the Life, NBC, 1986. Episodic: Rachel Sutton, Hotel, ABC, 1986; Amy-Beth, "Life under Water," American Playhouse, PBS, 1989; also 3-2-1 Contact, PBS; Another World, NBC. Movies: Katy, My Body, My Child, ABC, 1982; Maggie, Going for the Gold: The Bill Johnson Story, CBS, 1985; Rachel Goldman, Dadah Is Death (also known as A Long Way Home, A Long Way from Home, and Deadly Decision), CBS, 1988; Laura, The Ryan White Story, ABC, 1989; Miriam Kleiman, Twist of Fate, NBC, 1989; also Pursuit, NBC. Specials: Suzanne Henderson, "The Almost Royal Family," ABC Afterschool Special, ABC, 1984; Mandy, "The Room Upstairs," Hallmark Hall of Fame, CBS, 1987. Also appeared in Do Me a Favor . . . Don't Vote for My Mom, Kennedy Center Tonight, The Little Match Girl, and Meanwhile, Back at the Castle.

RELATED CAREER—Ballet dancer.

ADDRESSES: AGENT—Creative Artists Agency, 1888 Century Park E., Suite 1400, Los Angeles, CA 90067. PUBLICIST—Jimmy Dobson and Associates, 1917 1/2 Westwood Boulevard, Suite 2, Los Angeles, CA 90025.*

*   *   *

PARKS, Michael 1938-

PERSONAL: Born April 4, 1938, in Corona, CA; father, a truck driver.

VOCATION: Actor and director.

CAREER: FILM DEBUT—Fargo, Wild Seed, Universal, 1965. PRINCIPAL FILM APPEARANCES—Title role, Bus Riley's Back in Town, Universal, 1965; Adam, The Bible . . . In the Beginning, Twentieth Century-Fox, 1966; Marco, The Idol, Embassy, 1966; Sureshot, The Happening, Columbia, 1967; Toby, Get Back, Clearwater, 1973; Sheriff Noel Nye, The Last Hard Men, Twentieth Century-Fox, 1976; J.W. Wyatt, Sidewinder One, AVCO-Embassy, 1977; Sergeant Anderson, Breakthrough (also known as Sergeant Steiner), Maverick, 1978; Duke, Love and the Midnight Auto Supply, Producers Capital, 1978; Robert F. Kennedy, The Private Files of J. Edgar Hoover, American International, 1978; Ben Watkins, The Evictors, American International, 1979; Shulman, Ffolkes (also known as North Sea Hijack and Assault Force), Universal, 1980; Royce Richardson, Hard Country, Universal, 1981; Lieutenant Savage, Savannah Smiles, Gold Coast, 1983; Tank, Club Life, Troma Team, 1987; title role, The Return of Josey Wales, Reel Movies International, 1987; Larry Kapinski, Arizona Heat, Spectrum Entertainment, 1988. Also appeared in French Quarter Undercover, Shapiro Entertainment, 1985; King of the City, 1985; and Spiker, Seymour Borde, 1987.

PRINCIPAL FILM WORK—Director, The Return of Josey Wales, Reel Movies International, 1987.

PRINCIPAL TELEVISION APPEARANCES—Series: Jim Bronson, Then Came Bronson, NBC, 1969-70; Hoyt Parker/Phillip Colby, The Colbys, ABC, 1987. Pilots: Tack Reynolds, The Mob Riders (shown as an episode of Stoney Burke), ABC, 1962; Dr. Daniel Dana, Diagnosis: Danger (shown as an episode of The Alfred Hitchcock Hour), CBS, 1963; Jim Bronson, Then Came Bronson, NBC, 1969; Ron Baron, The Young Lawyers, ABC, 1969; Blair Mabry, Royce, CBS, 1976; Jim Spanner, Hunters of the Reef, NBC, 1978; Michael Dolan, Reward, ABC, 1980; Lieutenant Brophy, Turnover Smith, ABC, 1980. Episodic: Candel Logen, The Equalizer, CBS, 1986; Jonathan Grey, The Equalizer, CBS, 1988; Ben Aaron, Murder, She Wrote, CBS, 1989; also The Detectives, NBC; The Asphalt Jungle, ABC; Bus Stop, ABC; Wagon Train, ABC. Movies: Vince McKay, Stranger on the Run, NBC, 1967; Bradley Floyd, The Story of Pretty Boy Floyd, ABC, 1974; Joseph, Can Ellen Be Saved?, ABC, 1974; Dr. Jeff DuRand, The Savage Bees, NBC, 1976; Antonio DeLeon, Perilous Voyage, NBC, 1976; Jack Kern, Escape from Bogen County, CBS, 1977; Larry Marshall, Murder at the World Series, ABC, 1977; Mitch Haskins, Night Cries, ABC, 1978; Roger Edens, Rainbow, NBC, 1978; David York, Fast Friends, NBC, 1979; Max Halliday, Dial M for Murder, NBC, 1981; Larry Butler, Chase, CBS, 1985; Wicks, Dangerous Affection, NBC, 1987. Specials: Johnny Pope, A Hatful of Rain, ABC, 1968.*

*   *   *

PATTON, Will 1954-

PERSONAL: Born June 14, 1954, in Charleston, SC.

VOCATION: Actor.

CAREER: PRINCIPAL STAGE APPEARANCES—Chicken, Kingdom of Earth, Staircase Theatre Company, Impossible Ragtime Theatre (IRT), New York City, 1976; Goldie, Heaven and Earth, Off-Center Theatre, New York City, 1977; Billy Cavanaugh, Scenes from Country Life, Perry Street Theatre, New York City, 1978; Officer Gruber, Salt Lake City Skyline, New York Shakespeare Festival (NYSF), Public Theatre, New York City, 1980; thief, Dark Ride, Soho Repertory Theatre, New York City, 1981; Bingo, Goose and Tomtom, NYSF, Public Theatre, 1982; Ward and Dauphin, Joan of Lorraine, Mirror Theatre, New York City, 1983; Eddie, Fool for Love, Circle Repertory Theatre, then Douglas Fairbanks Theatre, both New York City, 1983; Mike, *A Lie of the Mind,* Promenade Theatre, New York City, 1985. Also appeared in *Rearrangements* (mime/puppet show), Winter Project, Other Theatre Company, La Mama Experimental Theatre Club (E.T.C.), New York City, 1979; *After the Revolution,* American Place Theatre, New York City, 1980; *Tourists and Refugees, 1 [and] 2,* both Winter Project, La Mama E.T.C.; and in productions of *Cops, Pedro Paramo, Limbo Tales,* and *The Red Snake,* all in New York City.

PRINCIPAL FILM APPEARANCES—Bar customer, priest in diner, man in dream, and radio preacher, *King Blank,* Metafilms, 1983; Joe, *Silkwood,* Twentieth Century-Fox, 1983; Lang Marsh, *Chinese Boxes,* Palace, 1984; Mark, *Variety,* Horizon, 1984; Horst, *After Hours,* Warner Brothers, 1985; Wayne Nolan, *Desperately Seeking Susan,* Orion, 1986; Matthew Perry, *Belizaire the Cajun,* Skouras/Norstar, 1986; Scott Pritchard, *No Way Out,* Orion, 1987; Duane, *Stars and Bars,* Columbia, 1988; Mike, *Wildfire,* Zupnik Enterprises/Roadshow, 1988; Mr. Coughlin, Sr., *Signs of Life,* Avenue, 1989.

PRINCIPAL TELEVISION APPEARANCES—Series: Ox Knowles, *Ryan's Hope,* ABC. Episodic: Braxton, *The Equalizer,* CBS, 1985. Movies: Lou Dimes, *A Gathering of Old Men,* CBS, 1987; also *Kent State,* NBC, 1981. Specials: Ben Moody, "Robbers, Rooftops, and Witches," *CBS Library,* CBS, 1982.

RELATED CAREER—Member, Winter Project (an experimental theatre group), New York City.

WRITINGS: STAGE—(With Winter Project) *Rearrangements,* La Mama Experimental Theatre Club (E.T.C.), New York City, 1979; also *Tourists and Refugees 1 [and] 2,* both La Mama E.T.C.

AWARDS: Obie Award from the *Village Voice,* Best Actor, 1983, for *Fool for Love;* Obie Award, Best Actor, for *Tourists and Refugees 2;* Villager Awards for *Dark Ride* and *Goose and Tomtom.*

ADDRESSES: AGENT—Smith-Freedman and Associates, 121 N. San Vicente Boulevard, Beverly Hills, CA 90211.*

*　　　*　　　*

PAYS, Amanda   1959-

PERSONAL: Born in 1959 in Berkshire, England; father, a talent agent; mother, an actress; married Peter Kohn (a production manager; divorced); married Corbin Bernsen (an actor), 1988; children: Oliver (second marriage). EDUCATION: Attended Hammersmith Polytechnic; studied acting at the Academy of Live and Recorded Arts.

VOCATION: Actress.

CAREER: PRINCIPAL FILM APPEARANCES—Lady Victoria, *Oxford Blues,* Metro-Goldwyn-Mayer/United Artists, 1984; Melissa Leftridge, *The Kindred,* F-M Entertainment, 1987; Nicole, *Off Limits,* Twentieth Century-Fox, 1988; also appeared in *Leviathan,* 1989.

PRINCIPAL TELEVISION APPEARANCES—Series: Theora Jones, *Max Headroom,* ABC, 1987. Mini-Series: Sarah, *A.D.,* NBC, 1985. Pilots: Alex, "The Pretenders," *CBS Summer Playhouse,*

CBS, 1988. Movies: Carla Martin and Christa Bruchner, *The Cold Room,* HBO, 1984; Geraldine Marsh, *Agatha Christie's "Thirteen at Dinner,"* CBS, 1985.

RELATED CAREER—Fashion model.

SIDELIGHTS: RECREATIONS—Bicycling, working out with a trainer.*

*　　　*　　　*

PEARLMAN, Stephen   1935-

PERSONAL: Born February 26, 1935, in New York, NY. EDUCATION: Dartmouth College, B.A., philosophy, 1956; studied acting with Stella Adler, 1957-59.

VOCATION: Actor.

CAREER: OFF-BROADWAY DEBUT—Walt Dreary, *The Threepenny Opera,* Theatre De Lys, 1959. BROADWAY DEBUT—Telephone repairman, *Barefoot in the Park,* Biltmore Theatre, 1964. PRINCIPAL STAGE APPEARANCES—Earl of Northumberland and Ralph Mouldy, *Falstaff (Henry IV, Part II),* Antonio, *Twelfth Night,* and Popilius Lena and Messala, *Julius Caesar,* all American Shakespeare Festival, Stratford, CT, 1966; the Innkeeper, *Man of La Mancha,* Martin Beck Theatre, New York City, 1968; Zampano, *La Strada,* Lunt-Fontanne Theatre, New York City, 1969; Ike,

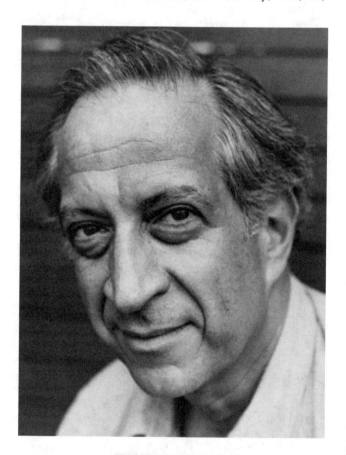

STEPHEN PEARLMAN

Richie, Orpheum Theatre, New York City, 1980; Simon Blumberg, *Isn't It Romantic?,* Playwrights Horizons, then Lucille Lortel Theatre, both New York City, 1984; Jake Abrams, *The Bloodletters,* Ensemble Studio Theatre, New York City, 1984; Sidney Black, *Light Up the Sky,* Jewish Repertory Theatre, New York City, 1986; Sam Maidman, *Miami,* Playwrights Horizons, 1986; Wes Wellman, *The Perfect Party,* Playwrights Horizons, then Astor Place Theatre, New York City, later Eisenhower Theatre, John F. Kennedy Center for the Performing Arts, Washington, DC, all 1986; Mordecai Weiss, *A Shayna Maidel,* Westside Arts Theatre, New York City, 1988. Also appeared in *A Time of the Key,* Sheridan Square Playhouse, New York City, 1963; *Pimpernel!,* Gramercy Arts Theatre, New York City, 1964; *In White America,* Players Theatre, New York City, 1965; *Viet Rock,* Martinique Theatre, New York City, 1966; *Chocolates,* Gramercy Arts Theatre, 1967; *Bloomers,* Master Theatre, New York City, 1974; and in *The Front Page,* Long Wharf Theatre, New Haven, CT, 1982.

MAJOR TOURS—Sergei Alexandrovitch, *On Your Toes,* U.S. cities, 1984.

FILM DEBUT—Chuck Morello, *The Iceman Cometh,* American Film Theatre, 1973. PRINCIPAL FILM APPEARANCES—Russ Rothman, *Audrey Rose,* United Artists, 1977; Lyons, *Rollercoaster,* Universal, 1977; also appeared in *Serpico,* Paramount, 1973; *American Hot Wax,* Paramount, 1978; *Xanadu,* Universal, 1980.

PRINCIPAL TELEVISION APPEARANCES—Series: Murray Zuckerman, *Husbands, Wives, and Lovers,* CBS, 1978. Mini-Series: Arnold, *Celebrity,* NBC, 1984. Pilots: Dorfman, *Future Cop,* ABC, 1976; Nick Wolf, *Corey: For the People,* NBC, 1977; prosecutor, *Ethel Is an Elephant,* CBS, 1980. Episodic: *Barney Miller,* ABC, 1977. Movies: Dr. Hotfield, *Return to Earth,* ABC, 1975; Murray Rosenman, *Perfect Gentlemen,* CBS, 1978; Dr. Rosenthal, *Trapped in Silence,* CBS, 1986; Martin Prager, *A Deadly Business,* CBS, 1986; also *A Question of Guilt,* CBS, 1978.

ADDRESSES: AGENT—Don Buchwald & Associates, 10 E. 44th Street, New York, NY 10017.

*   *   *

PENN, Christopher

PERSONAL: Son of Leo Penn (an actor and director) and Eileen Ryan (an actress).

VOCATION: Actor.

CAREER: FILM DEBUT—B.J., *Rumble Fish,* Universal, 1983. PRINCIPAL FILM APPEARANCES—Brian, *All the Right Moves,* Twentieth Century-Fox, 1983; Willard, *Footloose,* Paramount, 1984; Tom Drake, *The Wild Life,* Universal, 1984; Josh LaHood, *Pale Rider,* Warner Brothers, 1985; Tommy Whitewood, *At Close Range,* Orion, 1986; Tuck, *Made in U.S.A.,* De Laurentiis Entertainment Group, 1987.

PRINCIPAL TELEVISION APPEARANCES—Episodic: Mark Edwards, *Riptide,* NBC, 1986; Kirby, *Houston Knights,* CBS, 1987; Sean Bracken, *Simon and Simon,* CBS, 1988; Larry Rassy, *High Mountain Rangers,* CBS, 1988; also in "Rip Van Winkle," *Faerie Tale Theatre,* Showtime, 1987. Movies: Dan Donnelly, *North Beach and Rawhide,* CBS, 1985.

ADDRESSES: AGENT—Eileen Feldman, Herb Tobias and Associates, 1901 Avenue of the Stars, Suite 840, Los Angeles, CA 90067.*

*   *   *

PENNY, Joe   1956-

PERSONAL: Born September 14, 1956, in London, England; father, a pilot.

VOCATION: Actor.

CAREER: PRINCIPAL FILM APPEARANCES—Dean Berger, *Our Winning Season,* American International, 1978; Phil, *S.O.B.,* Paramount, 1981; Mr. Harding, *Bloody Birthday* (also known as *Creeps*), Judica, 1986. Also appeared in *Life Pod,* 1980.

PRINCIPAL TELEVISION APPEARANCES—Series: Sal DiVito, *Forever Fernwood,* syndicated, 1977; Benny Siegel, *The Gangster Chronicles,* NBC, 1981; Nick Ryder, *Riptide,* NBC, 1984-86; Jake Stiles, *Jake and the Fat Man,* CBS, 1987—. Pilots: Joe Ed, *Delta County, U.S.A.,* ABC, 1977; Speed, *Mother, Juggs, and Speed,* ABC, 1978; Lee Cantrell, *Samurai,* ABC, 1979; Rocco Spinelli, *The Home Front,* CBS, 1980; Peter Savage, *Savage: In the Orient,* CBS, 1983. Episodic: Rick Walsh, *The Twilight Zone,* CBS, 1986; Paul Baron, *Matlock,* NBC, 1987; also *The Nancy Drew Mysteries,* ABC, 1977; *Vega$,* ABC. Movies: Rick Bladen, *Death Moon,* CBS, 1978; Beau Galloway, *The Girls in the Office,* syndicated, 1980; Paul Cameron, *The Gossip Columnist,* syndicated, 1980; Robert McKay, *Perry Mason: The Case of the Shooting Star,* NBC, 1986; Lloyd Murphy, *Roses Are for the Rich,* CBS, 1987; Edward Moran, *Blood Vows: The Story of a Mafia Wife* (also known as *The Story of a Mafia Wife* and *The Godfather's Wife*), NBC, 1987; Dan Walker, *A Whisper Kills,* ABC, 1988. Specials: *Richard Lewis' "I'm in Pain" Concert,* Showtime, 1985; *The NBC All-Star Hour,* NBC, 1985; Detroit host, *CBS All-American Thanksgiving Day Parade,* CBS, 1987; Hawaii host, *CBS All-American Thanksgiving Day Parade,* CBS, 1988.

ADDRESSES: AGENTS—Pam Prince and Joan Hyler, William Morris Agency, 151 El Camino Drive, Beverly Hills, CA 90212. PUBLICISTS—Connie Morris, Freeman and Sutton Public Relations, 8961 Sunset Boulevard, Suite 2-A, Los Angeles, CA 90069; Scotti Brothers, Moress, and Nanas, 2128 Pico Boulevard, Santa Monica, CA 90405.*

*   *   *

PERKINS, Elizabeth   1960-

PERSONAL: Born November 18, 1960, in Queens, NY; daughter of Jo Williams (a drug treatment counselor); father, a farmer, writer, and in business; married Terry Kinney (an actor and director). EDUCATION: Trained for the stage at the Goodman Theatre School for three years.

VOCATION: Actress.

CAREER: BROADWAY DEBUT—Nora, *Brighton Beach Memoirs,* Alvin Theatre, 1984. PRINCIPAL STAGE APPEARANCES—Ann

Green, neighbor, nurse, and Maureen, *The Arbor,* La Mama Experimental Theatre Club, New York City, 1983; Juliet, *Measure for Measure,* New York Shakespeare Festival, Delacorte Theatre, New York City, 1985; Robin, "Between Cars" in *Marathon '85,* Ensemble Studio Theatre, New York City, 1985; Effie, *Life and Limb,* Playwrights Horizons, New York City, 1985. Also appeared in *A Christmas Carol,* Goodman Theatre, Chicago, IL, 1981; *Gardenia* and *A Christmas Carol,* both Goodman Theatre, 1982; and *Les Belles Soeurs,* North Light Repertory Theatre, Evanston, IL, 1982.

MAJOR TOURS—Nora, *Brighton Beach Memoirs,* U.S. cities, 1983.

PRINCIPAL FILM APPEARANCES—Joan, *About Last Night,* Tri-Star, 1986; JoAnn, *From the Hip,* De Laurentiis Entertainment Group, 1987; Susan Lawrence, *Big,* Twentieth Century-Fox, 1988; Adie Nims, *Sweetheart's Dance,* Tri-Star, 1988.

SIDELIGHTS: RECREATIONS—Writing poetry and reading.

ADDRESSES: AGENT—Kevin Huvane, Creative Artists Agency, 1888 Century Park E., Suite 1400, Los Angeles, CA 90067.*

*   *   *

PERLOFF, Carey

PERSONAL: Full name, Carey Elizabeth Perloff. EDUCATION: Stanford University, B.A., classics and comparative literature, 1980; Oxford University, M.A., 1981.

VOCATION: Director and playwright.

CAREER: Also see *WRITINGS* below. PRINCIPAL STAGE WORK— All as director, unless indicated: *The Boor* and *Sexual Perversity in Chicago,* both Nitery Theatre, Stanford University, Stanford, CA, 1980; *Out at Sea,* Oxford Playhouse, Oxford, U.K., 1980; *Satyricon: A Grotesque Farce in Seven Courses,* Lindsay Theatre, Oxford, 1981; (also set designer) *The Bed Bug,* Edinburgh Festival Fringe, Edinburgh, U.K., 1981; associate director, *Greek,* Los Angeles Theatre Works, Los Angeles, CA, 1982; *The Silver Tassie,* Soho Repertory Theatre, New York City, 1982; *Gunplay,* White Barn Theatre, Westport, CT, 1983; *Second Lady,* Production Company, Theatre Guinevere, New York City, then Edinburgh Festival Fringe, both 1983; *The Man Who Could See through Time,* Ark Theatre, New York City, 1984; *Candy and Shelley Go to the Desert,* Women's Project, American Place Theatre, New York City, 1984; *Charlotte's Web,* Lincoln Center Institute, Juilliard Opera Theatre, New York City, 1984; *Hearts on Fire,* New York Shakespeare Festival, Public Theatre, New York City, 1984; "Leverage" in *Leverage/Babysteps* (double-bill), Production Company, Theatre Guinevere, 1985; *Cheapside,* White Barn Theatre, 1985, then Roundabout Theatre, New York City, 1986; *St. Joan of the Stockyards,* Minor Latham Playhouse, Columbia University, New York City, 1986; *The Skin of Our Teeth,* Classic Stage Company (CSC) Repertory Ltd., New York City, 1986; *Uncle Maroje,* New Dramatists, New York City, 1987; *Sand and Thunder,* Bond Street Theatre Coalition, New York City, 1987; *E & O Line,* workshop production at the Musical Theatre Works, New York City, 1987; *Elektra,* CSC Repertory Ltd., 1987; *The Birthday Party,* CSC Repertory Ltd., 1988; *Phaedra Britannica,* Chautauqua Institute, Chautauqua, NY, then CSC Repertory Ltd., both 1988; *The Scoun-*

drel of Seville, CSC Repertory Ltd., 1989. Also director of three plays in workshop productions for the Young Playwrights Festival, Playwrights Horizons, New York City, 1985.

RELATED CAREER—Auditor, New York State Council of the Arts, Theatre Program and Presenting Program, 1981—; program manager, International Theatre Institute, New York City, 1981-82; casting assistant, New York Shakespeare Festival, New York City, 1982-83; managing director, New York Tent, Edinburgh Festival Fringe, Edinburgh, Scotland, 1983; teaching artist, Lincoln Center Institute, New York City, 1983—; artistic director, Classic Stage Company (CSC) Repertory Ltd., New York City, 1986—; International Theatre Institute representative from the United States to the Theater de Welt, Stuttgart, West Germany, 1987; dramatic writing instructor, Tisch School of the Arts, New York University, New York City; member, Women's Project, American Place Theatre, New York City.

WRITINGS: STAGE—(Adaptor) *Satyricon: A Grotesque Farce in Seven Courses* and *Vladimir Mayakovsky: A Collage,* both Lindsay Theatre, Oxford, U.K., 1981; (adaptor) *The Bed Bug,* Edinburgh Festival Fringe, Edinburgh, Scotland, 1981; *Interviewing Djuna,* Women's Project, American Place Theatre, New York City, 1985; *The Colossus of Rhodes,* workshop production at the New York Theatre Workshop and reading at the Double Image Theatre, both New York City, 1986; (adaptor) *Helen,* workshop production at the Classic Stage Company (CSC) Repertory Ltd., New York City, 1987. Also *El Grosso's Daughter.*

AWARDS: Fulbright Fellowship, 1981; Los Angeles Drama Critics Circle Award, Best Production, 1983, for *Greek;* Observership Grant from the Theatre Communications Group, 1986; National Theatre Conference Award as Theatrician with Outstanding Career Promise, 1987; Obie Award from the *Village Voice,* Artistic Excellence, 1988, for Classic Stage Company (CSC) Repertory Ltd.

MEMBER: Dramatists Guild.

ADDRESSES: OFFICE—CSC Repertory Theatre, 136 E. 13th Street, New York, NY 10003.

*   *   *

PERRY, Felton

PERSONAL: Born October 11, in Evanston, IL. EDUCATION: Attended Wilson Junior College; received B.A. in Spanish and French from Roosevelt University; graduate work, University of Chicago. MILITARY: U.S. Marine Corps.

VOCATION: Actor and playwright.

CAREER: Also see *WRITINGS* below. PRINCIPAL STAGE APPEARANCES—Dr. Martin Luther King, Jr., *The Meeting,* New Federal Theatre, Harry DeJur Henry Street Settlement Playhouse, New York City, 1987; also appeared in *MacBird,* Candlelight Dinner Theatre, Chicago, IL, 1968; *Chemin de Fer,* Center Theatre Group, Mark Taper Forum, Los Angeles, CA, 1969; and in *Tiger, Tiger Burning Bright,* Chicago, IL.

MAJOR TOURS—*No Place to Be Somebody,* U.S. cities; also with the Second City touring company, U.S. cities.

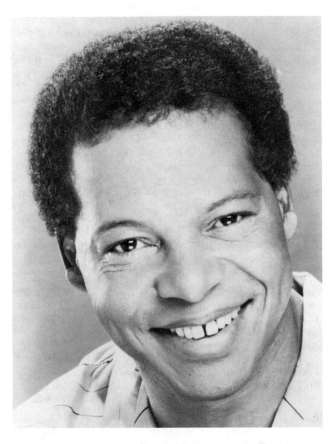

FELTON PERRY

FILM DEBUT—Black militant, *Medium Cool*, Paramount, 1969. PRINCIPAL FILM APPEARANCES—Bobby, *Trouble Man*, Twentieth Century-Fox, 1972; Early Smith, *Magnum Force*, Warner Brothers, 1973; Deputy Obra Eaker, *Walking Tall*, Cinerama, 1973; Jude, *Night Call Nurses*, New World, 1974; Scott, *The Towering Inferno*, Twentieth Century-Fox/Warner Brothers, 1974; Jake Turner, *Mean Dog Blues*, American International, 1978; Al, *Down and Out in Beverly Hills*, Buena Vista, 1986; Johnson, *Robocop*, Orion, 1987; associate warden, *Weeds*, De Laurentiis Entertainment Group, 1987; Dr. Duffin, *Checking Out*, Warner Brothers, 1989. Also appeared in *Sudden Death*, 1977.

PRINCIPAL TELEVISION APPEARANCES—Series: Jimmy, *Matt Lincoln*, ABC, 1970-71; Inspector Clarence McNeil, *Hooperman*, ABC, 1987—. Pilots: Jimmy, *Dial Hot Line*, ABC, 1970; cab driver, *Jigsaw* (also known as *Man on the Move*), ABC, 1972; Detective Luther Prince, *The Fuzz Brothers*, ABC, 1973; Winston L.T. St. Andrew, *Hunters of the Reef*, NBC, 1978; Dr. Hill, *The Critical List*, NBC, 1978. Episodic: Bobby Castro, *Hill Street Blues*, NBC, 1985; Lieutenant Lester Tuttle, *L.A. Law*, NBC, 1986-87; Al, *Down and Out in Beverly Hills*, Fox, 1987; Lieutenant McKenzie, *Harry*, ABC, 1987; Floyd Jackson, *Stingray*, ABC, 1987; also *Cagney and Lacey*, CBS. Movies: Dr. Hank Cullen, *The City*, NBC, 1977; Cinque, *The Ordeal of Patty Hearst*, ABC, 1979; Randall Perkins, *Seduced*, CBS, 1985; Reverend Avery, *The Atlanta Child Murders*, CBS, 1985.

RELATED CAREER—Founder, YAY (a production company); actor in television commercials.

WRITINGS: STAGE—*by the bi and bye*, Theatre at Holy Name House, New York City, 1979, and in Los Angeles, CA; also *Or* and *Sleep No More*, both produced in Los Angeles.

MEMBER: Actors' Equity Association, American Federation of Television and Radio Artists, Screen Actors Guild.

ADDRESSES: PUBLICIST—The Garrett Company, 6922 Hollywood Boulevard, Los Angeles, CA 90028.

*　　　*　　　*

PERSKY, Lester　1927-

PERSONAL: Born July 6, 1927, in New York, NY; son of Louis (in business) and Dora (Linden) Persky. EDUCATION: Received B.A. from Brooklyn College. POLITICS: Democrat. MILITARY: U.S. Coast Guard, 1945-48.

VOCATION: Producer.

CAREER: PRINCIPAL FILM WORK—Producer: (With Donald Ginsberg and Lewis M. Allen) *Fortune and Men's Eyes*, Metro-Goldwyn-Mayer, 1971; (with Elliott Kastner) *Equus*, United Artists, 1977; (with Joseph Janni) *Yanks*, Universal, 1979; (with Michael Butler) *Hair*, United Artists, 1979. Also producer, *Lone Star*, 1983; *Eye of the Tiger*, Scotti Brothers, 1986; and *Handcarved Coffins* (unreleased).

As principal in Persky-Bright Organization, has provided financing for numerous films including: *The Last Detail*, Columbia, 1974; *For Pete's Sake*, Columbia, 1974; *The Golden Voyage of Sinbad*, Columbia, 1974; *California Split*, Columbia, 1974; *Bite the Bullet*, Columbia, 1975; *The Killer Elite*, Columbia, 1975; *Funny Lady*, Columbia, 1975; *The Wind and the Lion*, Metro-Goldwyn-Mayer/United Artists, 1975; *The Front*, Columbia, 1976; *The Missouri Breaks*, United Artists, 1976; *Bound for Glory*, United Artists, 1977; *Shampoo*, Columbia, 1975; *The Man Who Would Be King*, Allied Artists, 1976; and *Taxi Driver*, Columbia, 1976.

PRINCIPAL TELEVISION WORK—Movies: Executive producer, *Poor Little Rich Girl*, NBC, 1987.

RELATED CAREER—President, Product Service, Inc. (an advertising agency), New York City, 1953-63; Curtice-York Advertising, New York City, 1964-71; theatrical producer, 1966-69; president, Persky-Bright Organization (a film financing company), 1973—; member, Mayor's Council on Motion Pictures, Radio, and Television, New York City, 1978-83; president, Lester Persky Productions, 1980—.

NON-RELATED CAREER—Member, National Finance Council of the Democratic National Committee, 1977-80; pentathlon delegate, U.S. Olympic House of Delegates, Los Angeles, CA, 1984.

MEMBER: Academy of Motion Picture Arts and Sciences.

ADDRESSES: OFFICE—c/o Lester Persky Productions, 485 Madison Avenue, New York, NY 10022.*

PERSOFF, Nehemiah 1920-

PERSONAL: Born August 14, 1920, in Jerusalem, Palestine; son of Samuel (a jeweler) and Puah (Holman) Persoff; married Thia Persov, August 22, 1951; children: three sons, one daughter. EDUCATION: Graduated from the Hebrew Technical Institute, New York City, 1937; studied acting at the Actors Studio with Stella Adler, Lee Strasberg, and Elia Kazan. MILITARY: U.S. Army, Airborne Infantry, 1942-45.

VOCATION: Actor.

CAREER: OFF-BROADWAY DEBUT—Minister of State, *The Emperor's New Clothes*, Heckscher Foundation, 1940. PRINCIPAL STAGE APPEARANCES—Candy, *Of Mice and Men*, Dean Frederick Damon, *The Male Animal*, and Dick Dudgeon, *The Devil's Disciple*, all Haverhill Playhouse, Haverhill, MA, 1947; Tutor, *The Flies*, President Theatre, New York City, 1947; Andrea, *Galileo*, Maxine Elliott's Theatre, New York City, 1947; Cecil, *Sundown Beach*, Belasco Theatre, New York City, 1948; Tyrell, *Richard III*, Booth Theatre, New York City, 1949; Antonanzas, *Montserrat*, Fulton Theatre, New York City, 1949; Cecco, *Peter Pan*, Imperial Theatre, New York City, 1950; Duke of Cornwall, *King Lear*, National Theatre, New York City, 1950; Ingrid's father and the Troll King, *Peer Gynt*, American National Theatre Academy Theatre, New York City, 1951; Fowzi, *Flahooley*, Broadhurst Theatre, New York City, 1951; Tom, *The Glass Menagerie*, and Mosca, *Volpone*, both Chamber Theatre, Tel Aviv, Israel, 1951; Street Cleaner, *Camino Real*, National Theatre, 1953; Charlie, *Detective Story*, Playhouse in the Park, Philadelphia, PA, 1953; the Hairdresser, *Mademoiselle Colombe*, Longacre Theatre, New York City, 1954; Eddie Fuseli, *Golden Boy*, Playhouse in the Park, 1954; Dr. Hickey, *Reclining Figure*, Lyceum Theatre, New York City, 1954; Topman, *Tiger at the Gates*, Plymouth Theatre, New York City, 1955; Harry Golden, *Only in America*, Cort Theatre, New York City, 1959; Harry, *Rosebloom*, Mark Taper Forum, Los Angeles, CA, 1970; *Aleichem Sholem—Sholem Aleichem* (one-man show), Oxford Theatre, Los Angeles, CA, 1971; Rabbi Azrielke, *The Dybbuk*, Mark Taper Forum, 1975. Also appeared in *Hay Fever*, Haverhill Playhouse, 1947; *The Road to Rome*, Playhouse in the Park, 1953; and as Fagin, *Oliver!*, summer theatre production.

MAJOR TOURS—John, "Snowangel," and Man, "Epiphany," on a bill as *Cages* (renamed *Last of the Great Jelly Bellies*), U.S. cities, 1974.

FILM DEBUT—*Naked City*, Universal, 1948. PRINCIPAL FILM APPEARANCES—Taxi driver, *On the Waterfront*, Columbia, 1954; Leo, *The Harder They Fall*, Columbia, 1956; Kicks Johnson, *The Wild Party*, United Artists, 1956; Gene Conforti, *The Wrong Man*, Warner Brothers, 1956; Sergeant Lewis, *Men in War*, United Artists, 1957; Leon, *Street of Sinners*, United Artists, 1957; Vincente, *Badlanders*, Metro-Goldwyn-Mayer (MGM), 1958; Albert, *This Angry Age* (also known as *The Sea Wall* and *La Diga sul Pacifico*), Columbia, 1958; Pinneli, *Never Steal Anything Small*, Universal, 1959; Don Panta, *Green Mansions*, MGM, 1959; Johnny Torrio, *Al Capone*, Allied Artists, 1959; Little Bonaparte, *Some Like It Hot*, United Artists, 1959; Dan, *Day of the Outlaw*, United Artists, 1959; Graile, *The Comanchero*, Twentieth Century-Fox, 1961; Bruno Everard, *The Big Show*, Twentieth Century-Fox, 1961; Captain Van Ryn, *The Hook*, MGM, 1962; Segura, *A Global Affair*, MGM, 1964; Ben Sawyer, *Fate Is the Hunter*, Twentieth Century-Fox, 1964.

Shemiah, *The Greatest Story Ever Told*, United Artists, 1965; Pizzuco, *The Day of the Owl* (also known as *Mafia* and *Il Giorno della civetta*), Euro-International, 1968; Lieutenant Dow Reeves, *The Money Jungle* (also known as *The Silken Trap* and *The Billion Dollar Caper*), Commonwealth United, 1968; August Best, *Panic in the City*, Commonwealth United, 1968; Carl Melniker, *The Power*, MGM, 1968; Lieutenant Crawford, *The Girl Who Knew Too Much*, Commonwealth United, 1969; Dr. Salazar, *The People Next Door*, AVCO-Embassy, 1970; General Berisha, *Mrs. Pollifax, Spy*, Warner Brothers, 1970; Amadeo Montoya, *Red Sky at Dawn*, Universal, 1970; Dr. Gubner, *Psychic Killer*, AVCO-Embassy, 1975; Mr. Hausner, *Voyage of the Damned*, AVCO-Embassy, 1976; Herod Antipas, *In Search of Historic Jesus*, Sunn Classics, 1980; Dr. Fischer, *O'Hara's Wife*, Davis-Panzer, 1983; Papa, *Yentl*, Metro-Goldwyn-Mayer/United Artists, 1983; voice of Papa Mousekewitz, *An American Tail*, Universal, 1986; Also appeared in *A Double Life*, Universal, 1948; *Too Many Thieves*, MGM, 1968; *Deadly Harvest*, 1972; *The Kirlian Effect*, Mars, 1974; and *St. Helens*, Parnell, 1981.

PRINCIPAL TELEVISION APPEARANCES—Series: Victor Tauss, *High Hopes*, syndicated, 1978. Mini-Series: Colonel Schreiner, *The French Atlantic Affair*, ABC, 1979. Pilots: Skoda, *The Dangerous Days of Kiowa Jones*, ABC, 1966; El Primero, *The Hellcats*, ABC, 1967; Earl Stone, *Killing Stone*, NBC, 1978; Mordecai, *The 13th Day: The Story of Esther*, ABC, 1979; Ashmed Amad, *Turnover Smith*, ABC, 1980; also *Manley and the Mob; The Barbara Eden Show*.

Episodic: Marty's friend, "Marty," *The Goodyear TV Playhouse*, NBC, 1953; Pablo, "For Whom the Bell Tolls," *Playhouse 90*, CBS, 1958; Langer, "Judgment Night," *The Twilight Zone*, CBS, 1959; Jake "Greasy Thumb" Guzik, *The Untouchables*, ABC, 1961-63; Ernest Dettmer, *Rich Man, Poor Man—Book II*, ABC, 1976-77; also "The Fingers of Fear," *Thriller*, NBC, 1961; *Route 66*, CBS, 1961; *Naked City*, ABC, 1961-63; *Rawhide*, CBS, 1963-64; *Bob Hope Presents*, NBC, 1964; *Convoy*, NBC, 1965; "Deadly Creature Below," *Voyage to the Bottom of the Sea*, ABC, 1966; "Secret Weapon," *Time Tunnel*, ABC, 1966; "Land of the Lost," *Land of the Giants*, ABC, 1969; "The Ghost," *Barney Miller*, ABC, 1978; "Middle Age," *Barney Miller*, ABC, 1979; "Riot," *Barney Miller*, ABC, 1981; "The Last Days of Benito Mussolini," *Playhouse 90*, CBS; *Captain Video*, Dumont; *The Red Buttons Show*, CBS; *Producers' Showcase*, NBC; *Playwrights '56*, NBC; *Philco-Goodyear Playhouse*, NBC; *Kraft Television Theatre*, NBC; *Dick Powell Theatre*, NBC; *You Are There*, CBS; *Danger*, CBS; *Appointment with Adventure*, CBS; *Five Fingers*, NBC; *Shirley Temple's Storybook*, NBC; *Mr. Lucky*, CBS; *Disney's Wonderful World of Color*, NBC; *The Danny Thomas Show*, CBS; *Alfred Hitchcock Presents*, NBC; *Burke's Law*, ABC; *The Trials of O'Brien*, CBS; *Ben Casey*, ABC; *Wagon Train*, NBC; *The Big Valley*, ABC; *Mr. Novak*, NBC; *Bus Stop*, ABC; *Gilligan's Island*, CBS; *The Man from U.N.C.L.E.*, NBC; *Honey West*, ABC; *Dan August*, ABC; *It Takes a Thief*, ABC; *I Spy*, NBC; *Wild, Wild West*, CBS; *Gunsmoke*, CBS; *The Flying Nun*, ABC; *Tarzan*, NBC; *The Joey Bishop Show*, ABC; *The Merv Griffin Show*, CBS; *The Virginia Graham Show*, syndicated; *Love, American Style*, ABC; *The Bill Cosby Show*, NBC; *The New Breed*, ABC; *The Mod Squad*, ABC; *The Chicago Teddy Bears*, CBS; *Search*, NBC; *Mission: Impossible*, CBS; *Hawaii Five-O*, CBS; *Marcus Welby, M.D.*, ABC; *Adam-12*, NBC; *Mannix*, CBS; *Name of the Game*, NBC; *Cool Million*, NBC; *McCloud*, NBC; *McMillan and Wife*, NBC; *Police Surgeon*, ABC; *Police Story*, NBC; *The Streets of San Francisco*, ABC.

Movies: Captain Kramer, *Escape to Mindanao*, NBC, 1968; Santillo, *Cutter's Trail*, CBS, 1970; Champagne Joe Carroll, *Lieutenant Schuster's Wife*, ABC, 1972; Nikos Fortis, *The Sex Symbol*, ABC, 1974; Dr. Edward Klein, *The Stranger Within*, ABC, 1974; Dr. Duchesnes, *Eric*, NBC, 1975; Rudenko, *Francis Gary Powers: The True Story of the U-2 Spy Incident*, NBC, 1976; Abbot Petropolus, *The Word*, CBS, 1978; Charles Frohman, *Ziegfeld: The Man and His Women*, NBC, 1978; Baron Von Steuben, *The Rebels*, syndicated, 1979; Professor Leo Tedeschi, *The Henderson Monster*, CBS, 1980; Josef Stalin, *F.D.R.—The Last Year*, NBC, 1980; Conlaw, *Condominium*, syndicated, 1980; Leonid Brezhnev, *Sadat*, syndicated, 1983. Specials: Strup, *Reunion in Vienna*, NBC, 1955; Dr. Salazar, *The People Next Door*, CBS, 1968; also *Tiger at the Gates*, CBC, 1958; *Dracula*, CBC. Also appeared as Jerry, *Clash by Night*, BBC, 1958.

NON-RELATED CAREER—Electrician and signal maintenance worker, New York City subway system, 1939-41.

AWARDS: Sylvania Award, 1958, for "For Whom the Bell Tolls," *Playhouse 90;* Los Angeles Critics Circle awards, 1971, for *Aleichem Sholem—Sholem Aleichem* and 1975, for *The Dybbuk.*

MEMBER: Screen Actors Guild, Actors' Equity Association, American Federation of Television and Radio Artists.

SIDELIGHTS: FAVORITE ROLES—Tom in *The Glass Menagerie* and Jerry in *Clash by Night*. RECREATIONS—Tennis, chess, gardening, and swimming.

ADDRESSES: AGENT—Contemporary Artists, 132 Lasky Drive, Beverly Hills, CA 90212.*

*   *   *

PETHERBRIDGE, Edward   1936-

PERSONAL: Born August 3, 1936, in Bradford, England; son of William and Hannah (Harrison) Petherbridge; married Louise Durant Harris (divorced). EDUCATION: Studied acting at the Northern Theatre School, Bradford, England; studied mime with Claude Chagrin.

VOCATION: Actor, director, and playwright.

CAREER: Also see *WRITINGS* below. STAGE DEBUT—Gaveston, *Edward II*, Ludlow Festival, Ludlow, U.K., 1956. LONDON DEBUT—Demetrius, *A Midsummer Night's Dream*, Open Air Theatre, 1962. PRINCIPAL STAGE APPEARANCES—Geoffrey Fitton, *All in Good Time*, Mermaid Theatre, then Phoenix Theatre, both London, 1963; the Soldier, *The Soldier's Tale*, Bath Festival, Bath, U.K., 1968; Alceste, *The Misanthrope*, Nottingham Playhouse, Nottingham, U.K., 1970; Alwa, *Lulu*, Royal Court Theatre, London, 1970, then Apollo Theatre, London, 1971; Laurence Caldecott, *Morality*, Royal Court Theatre Upstairs, London, 1971; Laurence Doyle, *John Bull's Other Island*, Mermaid Theatre, 1971; Nikita, *Swan Song*, Crucible Theatre, Sheffield, U.K., 1971; *Who Thought It?* (one-man show), Arts Theatre, London, 1972; Soranzo, *'Tis Pity She's a Whore*, Actors' Company, Edinburgh Festival, Edinburgh, Scotland, 1972; Prospero, *The Tempest*, Northcott Theatre, Exeter, U.K., 1973; Fool, *King Lear*, Simon, *The Wood Demon*, and Mirabell, *The Way of the World*, all Actors' Company, Brooklyn Academy of Music, Brooklyn, NY, 1974; Soranzo, *'Tis Pity*

She's a Whore, Fool, *King Lear*, Simon, *The Wood Demon*, and Hotel Manager, *Ruling the Roost*, all Actors' Company, Wimbledon Theatre, London, 1974; Valere, *Tartuffe*, and Teiresias, *The Bacchae*, both Edinburgh Festival, 1974.

Erik, *The Phantom of the Opera*, title role, *Tartuffe*, and Ring Master, *The Beanstalk*, all Actors' Company, Wimbledon Theatre, 1975; the Compere and Museum Attendant, *Do You Love Me?*, and Dr. Chasuble, *The Importance of Being Earnest*, both Actors' Company, Round House Theatre, London, 1977; Captain St. Clare, *The Crucifer of Blood*, Royal Haymarket Theatre, London, 1979; Vershinin, *The Three Sisters*, Royal Shakespeare Company, Other Place Theatre, Stratford-on-Avon, U.K., 1979; Newman Noggs, *The Life and Adventures of Nicholas Nickleby*, Aldwych Theatre, London, 1980, then Plymouth Theatre, New York City, 1981; Charles Marsden, *Strange Interlude*, Nederlander Theatre, New York City, 1985. Also appeared in *Knots*, Actors' Company, Edinburgh Festival, 1973, then Brooklyn Academy of Music, Brooklyn, NY, 1974.

With the National Theatre Company, London: Ferdinand Gadd, *Trelawny of the Wells*, 1965; Guildenstern, *Rosencrantz and Guildenstern Are Dead*, 1967; Voltore, *Volpone*, Spencer, *Edward II*, and Lorenzo, *The Advertisement*, all 1968; Harlequin and Pierrot, *Scrabble*, Waitwell, *The Way of the World*, and Lodovico, *The White Devil*, all 1969.

PRINCIPAL STAGE WORK—Director: *Flow* and *Knots*, both Actors' Company, Edinburgh Festival, Edinburgh, Scotland, 1973; *The Bacchae*, Edinburgh Festival, 1974; *Do You Love Me?*, Actors' Company, Round House Theatre, London, 1977.

MAJOR TOURS—Fool, *King Lear*, Actors' Company, U.K. cities, 1973; Dobson, *Dog's Dinner*, Cambridge Theatre Company, U.K. cities, 1977; the Compere and Museum Attendant, *Do You Love Me?*, and Dr. Chasuble, *The Importance of Being Earnest*, both Actors' Company, U.K. cities, 1977; the Brigadier, *Game of Kings*, U.K. cities, 1978; Orsino, *Twelfth Night*, Vershinin, *The Three Sisters*, both Royal Shakespeare Company (RSC), U.K. cities, 1978. Also appeared in *Flow* and *Knots*, both Actors' Company, U.K. cities, 1973; *The Hollow Crown* and *Pleasure and Repentance*, both RSC, Australian and New Zealand cities, 1976; and in *Is There Honey Still for Tea?*, RSC, U.K. cities, 1978.

Director: *Knots*, Actors' Company, U.K. cities, 1973; *Uncle Vanya*, Cambridge Theatre Company, U.K. cities, 1977; *Do You Love Me?*, Actors' Company, U.K. cities, 1977.

PRINCIPAL FILM APPEARANCES—*Knots*, 1975.

PRINCIPAL TELEVISION APPEARANCES—Episodic: Charles Marsden, "Strange Interlude," *American Playhouse*, PBS, 1988. Movies: *No Strings*, Yorkshire Television. Also appeared in *The Soldier's Tale*, *After Magritte*, *A True Patriot*, *Schubert*, and *Pyramid of Fire*.

RELATED CAREER—Member, National Theatre Company, London, 1964-70; founding member, Actors' Company, 1972; teacher in acting workshops and mime demonstrations.

WRITINGS: STAGE—(Adaptor) *Knots*, Actors' Company, Edinburgh Festival, Edinburgh, Scotland, 1973; (adaptor) *Do You Love Me?*, Actors' Company, U.K. tour, then Round House Theatre, London, both 1977.

SIDELIGHTS: RECREATIONS—Listening to music; the country-side; photography.

ADDRESSES: AGENT—French's, 26 Binney Street, London W1, England.*

*　　*　　*

PETTET, Joanna　1944-

PERSONAL: Born November 16, 1944, in London, England. EDUCATION: Trained for the stage at the Neighborhood Playhouse.

VOCATION: Actress.

CAREER: PRINCIPAL STAGE APPEARANCES—Catherine Shaw, *Poor Richard,* Helen Hayes Theatre, New York City, 1964; Roxane, *The Chinese Prime Minister,* Royale Theatre, New York City, 1964.

MAJOR TOURS—Mollie Michaelson, *Take Her, She's Mine,* U.S. cities, 1962.

PRINCIPAL FILM APPEARANCES—Kay Strong, *The Group,* United Artists, 1966; Mata Bond, *Casino Royale,* Columbia, 1967; Ulrike von Seidlitz-Garbler, *The Night of the Generals* (also known as *La Nuit de generaux*), Columbia, 1967; Kate Clifton, *Robbery,* Embassy, 1967; Joanne Morton, *Blue,* Paramount, 1968; Josephine Pacefoot, *The Best House in London,* Metro-Goldwyn-Mayer, 1969; Grace Henry, *Tender Flesh* (also known as *Welcome to Arrow Beach*), Warner Brothers, 1976; Caroline, *The Evil,* New World, 1978; Desdemona, *Othello* (also known as *Black Commando*), MB Diffusion/Eurocine, 1982; Monica Araya, *Sweet Country,* Cinema Group, 1987. Also appeared in *Double Exposure,* Crown, 1982.

PRINCIPAL TELEVISION APPEARANCES—Series: Janet Baines, *Knots Landing,* CBS, 1983. Mini-Series: Katherine Hennessey, *Captains and the Kings,* NBC, 1976. Pilots: Serena, *Three for Danger,* NBC, 1967; Kate Stewart, *Miss Stewart, Sir,* CBS, 1972; Jesse Breton, *The Dark Side of Innocence* (also known as *The Hancocks*), NBC, 1976; Allison Nash, *Winner Take All,* CBS, 1977; Joanna St. John, *All That Glitters* (broadcast as an episode of *Knight Rider*), NBC, 1984. Episodic: Sylvia, "A Killer in Every Corner," *Thriller,* ABC, 1974; Jody Baxter, "Appointment with a Killer" (also know as "Midsummer Nightmare"), *Thriller,* ABC, 1975; Virginia McCormack, *Murder, She Wrote,* CBS, 1987; also "The House" and "Keep in Touch—We'll Think of Something," *Night Gallery,* NBC, 1970; "The Caterpiller," *Night Gallery,* NBC, 1971; "The Girl with the Hungry Eyes," *Night Gallery,* NBC, 1972; Judy Stratton, *The Doctors,* NBC; Chris Verdon, *Banacek,* NBC; Tina Andresen, *The Fugitive,* ABC; Glenna, *Harry O,* ABC; *Police Woman,* NBC. Movies: Sister Mary Damian/ Marjorie Walker, *The Weekend Warrior,* ABC, 1972; Sarah Allison, *Footsteps,* CBS, 1972; Maggie Sergeant, *Pioneer Woman,* ABC, 1973; Delda Hadley, *A Cry in the Wilderness,* ABC, 1974; Ruth Merrick, *The Desperate Miles,* ABC, 1975; Leslie Fitch, *Sex and the Married Woman,* NBC, 1977; Cynthia Donigan/Candia Leighton, *Cry of the Innocent,* NBC, 1980; Alana Richardson, *The Return of Frank Cannon,* CBS, 1980. Specials: *Battle of the Network Stars,* ABC, 1976.

AWARDS: Theatre World Award, 1965, for *Poor Richard.*

ADDRESSES: AGENT—Gores/Fields Agency, 10100 Santa Monica Boulevard, Suite 700, Los Angeles, CA 90067.*

*　　*　　*

PEYSER, Penny

PERSONAL: Full name, Penelope Allison Peyser; born February 9, in Irvington, NY; daughter of Peter Peyser (a former congressman).

VOCATION: Actress.

CAREER: PRINCIPAL STAGE APPEARANCES—Girl, *Hot l Baltimore,* Circle in the Square, New York City, 1973; Carol, *Lemon Sky,* Chelsea Theatre Center, New York City, 1976; also appeared in *Diamond Studs,* Chelsea Theatre Center; and with the Proposition Group, Cambridge, MA.

PRINCIPAL FILM APPEARANCES—Sharon Lyons, *All the President's Men,* Warner Brothers, 1976; Rosalie, *The Frisco Kid* (also known as *No Knife*), Warner Brothers, 1979; Barbara Kornpett, *The In-Laws,* Warner Brothers, 1979; jewelry salesgirl, *Unfaithfully Yours,* Twentieth Century-Fox, 1984; Trudy Pike, *Messenger of Death,* Cannon, 1988.

PRINCIPAL TELEVISION APPEARANCES—Series: Ramona Scott, *Rich Man, Poor Man, Book II,* ABC, 1976-77; Roberta "Bobby" Franklin, *The Tony Randall Show,* CBS, 1977-78; Cindy Fox, *Crazy Like a Fox,* CBS, 1984-86; also *Knots Landing,* CBS, 1989-

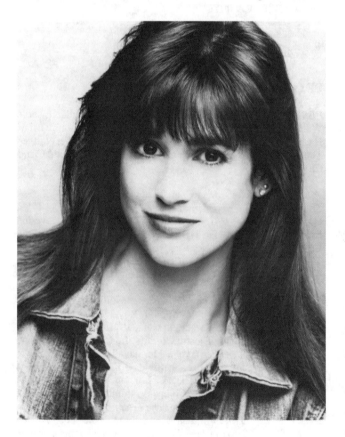

PENNY PEYSER

90. Mini-Series: Emma Geyser, *The Blue and the Grey,* CBS, 1982. Pilots: Stilts, *B.J. and the Bear,* NBC, 1978; waitress, *National Lampoon's Two Reelers,* NBC, 1981. Movies: Janice Zimmer, *Off Sides,* NBC, 1974; Laurie O'Neill, *The Quinns,* ABC, 1977; Tracy Beaumont, *The Girls in the Office,* ABC, 1979; Libby Tyree, *Wild Times,* syndicated, 1980; Nicky Tice, *Emergency Room,* syndicated, 1983; Cindy Fox, *Still Crazy Like a Fox,* CBS, 1987. Specials: *Battle of the Network Stars,* ABC, 1982.

RELATED CAREER—Actress in television commercials.

ADDRESSES: AGENTS—J. Michael Bloom Agency, 9200 Sunset Boulevard, Beverly Hills, CA 90069; (commercials) Talent Group, Inc., 9250 Wilshire Boulevard, Beverly Hills, CA 90212.

*   *   *

PHILLIPS, Lou Diamond

PERSONAL: Born Lou Upchurch, c. 1962 in the Philippines; son of Gerald and Lucy Upchurch; took his stepfather's name when his mother married George Phillips (a U.S. Naval officer); married Julie Cypher (an assistant director), June 27, 1987. EDUCATION: University of Texas, Arlington, B.A., theatre, 1984; studied acting at Adam Rourke's Film Actors Lab.

VOCATION: Actor.

CAREER: PRINCIPAL FILM APPEARANCES—Ritchie Valens, *La Bamba,* Columbia, 1987; drifter, *Trespasses,* Shapiro, 1987; Angel, *Stand and Deliver,* Warner Brothers, 1988; Jose Chavez y Chavez, *Young Guns,* Twentieth Century-Fox, 1988; title role, *Dakota,* Miramax, 1988; Ray Forgy, *Disorganized Crime,* Touchstone, 1989; also appeared in *Renegades,* 1989. PRINCIPAL FILM WORK—Associate producer, *Dakota,* Miramax, 1988.

PRINCIPAL TELEVISION APPEARANCES—Episodic: Detective Diaz, *Miami Vice,* NBC, 1987; also *Dallas,* CBS. Movies: Tag, *The Three Kings,* ABC, 1987. Specials: Host, *Teen Times,* syndicated, 1988; also *An All-Star Celebration: The '88 Vote,* ABC, 1988.

WRITINGS: FILM—(With Loren Bivens and Jo Carol Pierce) *Trespasses,* Shapiro, 1987.

ADDRESSES: AGENT—Harris and Goldberg, 2121 Avenue of the Stars, Suite 950, Los Angeles, CA 90067. PUBLICIST—Joe Sutton, Freeman and Sutton Public Relations, 8961 Sunset Boulevard, Suite 2-A, Los Angeles, CA 90069.*

*   *   *

PHILLIPS, Mackenzie   1959-

PERSONAL: Full name, Laura Mackenzie Phillips; born November 10, 1959, in Alexandria, VA; daughter of John Phillips (a singer).

VOCATION: Actress and singer.

CAREER: PRINCIPAL FILM APPEARANCES—Carol, *American Graffiti,* Universal, 1973; Frisbee, *Rafferty and the Gold Dust Twins* (also known as *Rafferty and the Highway Hustlers*), Warner

Brothers, 1975; Carol Rainbow, *More American Graffiti,* Universal, 1979; J.J., *Love Child,* Warner Brothers, 1982.

PRINCIPAL TELEVISION APPEARANCES—Series: Julie Cooper Horvath, *One Day at a Time,* CBS, 1975-80, then 1981-83. Pilots: *That's TV,* NBC, 1982. Episodic: Carol, *Murder, She Wrote,* CBS, 1985; also "Mary's Delinquent," *The Mary Tyler Moore Show,* CBS, 1975; *Movin' On,* NBC; *Baretta,* ABC. Movies: Doris, *Go Ask Alice,* ABC, 1973; Robin Williams, *Miles to Go before I Sleep,* CBS, 1975; Eleanor Roosevelt at age fourteen, *Eleanor and Franklin,* ABC, 1976; Susan, *Fast Friends,* NBC, 1979; Lillian Gish, *Moviola: The Silent Lovers,* NBC, 1980; Deyna, *Kate's Secret,* NBC, 1986. Specials: *Battle of the Network Stars,* ABC, 1977 and 1978; *Things We Did Last Summer,* NBC, 1978; *Circus of the Stars,* CBS, 1979.

RELATED CAREER—Singer with the New Mammas and Papas.

NON-RELATED CAREER—Lecturer on drug abuse.

ADDRESSES: AGENT—Helen Barkan, Aimee Entertainment, 13743 Victor Boulevard, Van Nuys, CA 91401.*

*   *   *

PHILLIPS, Michael   1943-

PERSONAL: Full name, Michael Steven Phillips; born June 29, 1943, in Brooklyn, NY; son of Lawrence Ronald and Shirley Lee (Fischer) Phillips; wife's name, Julia (a producer; divorced); children: Kate Elizabeth. EDUCATION: Dartmouth College, A.B., 1965; New York University Law School, J.D., 1968.

VOCATION: Producer.

CAREER: PRINCIPAL FILM APPEARANCES—Commune member, *Electra Glide in Blue,* United Artists, 1973. PRINCIPAL FILM WORK—Producer: (With Tony Bill and Julia Phillips) *Steelyard Blues* (also known as *The Final Crash*), Warner Brothers, 1973; (with Bill and Phillips) *The Sting,* Universal, 1973; *The Big Bus,* Paramount, 1976; (with Phillips) *Taxi Driver,* Columbia, 1976; (with Phillips) *Close Encounters of the Third Kind,* Columbia, 1977; *Heartbeeps,* Universal, 1981; *Cannery Row,* Metro-Goldwyn-Mayer/United Artists, 1982; *The Flamingo Kid,* Twentieth Century-Fox, 1984.

RELATED CAREER—Founder (with Tony Bill and Julia Phillips), Bill/Phillips Productions, 1971-73.

NON-RELATED CAREER—Securities analyst, 1968-70.

AWARDS: Academy Award, Best Picture, 1973, for *The Sting;* Academy Award nomination, Best Picture, British Academy Award nomination, Best Picture, and Golden Palm from the Cannes Film Festival, all 1976, for *Taxi Driver;* British Academy Award nomination, Best Picture, 1978, for *Close Encounters of the Third Kind.*

MEMBER: Academy of Motion Picture Arts and Sciences, New York Bar Association.

ADDRESSES: OFFICE—Mercury Entertainment Corporation, 1901 Avenue of the Stars, 20th floor, Los Angeles, CA 90067.*

PICKETT, Cindy   1947-

PERSONAL: Born April 18, 1947, in Norman, OK; daughter of Cecil Pickett (a director and drama teacher); married Lyman Ward (an actor), 1986; children: Clay.

VOCATION: Actress.

CAREER: PRINCIPAL FILM APPEARANCES—Valerie St. John, *Night Games,* AVCO-Embassy, 1980; Kate, *Hysterical,* Embassy, 1983; Lyn Nilsson, *Mystique,* Televicin International/Qui Production, 1983; Katie Bueller, *Ferris Bueller's Day Off,* Paramount, 1986; Hannah, *The Men's Club,* Atlantic Releasing, 1986; Victoria Peyton, *Hot to Trot,* Warner Brothers, 1988. Also appeared in *Brainwash,* 1982; and *Circle of Power,* 1984.

PRINCIPAL TELEVISION APPEARANCES—Series: Vanessa Sarnac, *Call to Glory,* ABC, 1984-85; Dr. Carol Novino, *St. Elsewhere,* NBC, 1986-88; also Jackie Spaulding, *The Guiding Light,* CBS. Mini-Series: Amanda Bradford, *Amerika,* ABC, 1987. Pilots: Mary Breydon, *The Cherokee Trail,* CBS, 1981; Tina Royce, *Family in Blue,* CBS, 1982; Catherine, *Cocaine and Blue Eyes,* NBC, 1983. Episodic: Marcia Loomis, *Alfred Hitchcock Presents,* NBC, 1986; also *Magnum, P.I.,* CBS. Movies: Lil Taylor, *The Ivory Ape,* ABC, 1980; Velda, *Mickey Spillane's Margin for Murder,* CBS, 1981; Elaine Russell, *Cry for the Strangers,* CBS, 1982; Sue Meyers, *Echoes in the Darkness,* CBS, 1987; Rye Swallow, *Into the Heartland,* HBO, 1987; Kay Stayner, *I Know My First Name Is Steven,* NBC, 1989.

ADDRESSES: MANAGER—Mike Gursey, Larry Thompson Organization, 1440 S. Sepulveda Boulevard, Suite 118, Los Angeles, CA 90025.*

*   *   *

PLEASENCE, Donald   1919-

PERSONAL: Born October 5, 1919, in Worksop, England; son of Thomas Stanley (a railway station master) and Alice (Armitage) Pleasence; married Miriam Raymond (an actress), August 8, 1941 (divorced, 1957); married Josephine Martin Crombie, May 15, 1958 (divorced, 1971); married Meira Shore, 1971; children: Angela, Jean (first marriage); Lucy Maria, Polly Jo (second marriage); Alexis Helena (third marriage). MILITARY: Royal Air Force, flight lieutenant, 1942-46.

VOCATION: Actor.

CAREER: STAGE DEBUT—Hareton, *Wuthering Heights,* Playhouse Theatre, Jersey, U.K., 1939. LONDON DEBUT—Curio, *Twelfth Night,* Arts Theatre, 1942. BROADWAY DEBUT—Majordomo, *Caesar and Cleopatra,* Ziegfeld Theatre, 1951. PRINCIPAL STAGE APPEARANCES—Mavriky, *The Brothers Karamazov,* Lyric Hammersmith Theatre, London, 1946; bellboy, *Vicious Circle* (also known as *No Exit*), Arts Theatre, London, 1946; Steen, *Tangent,* Mercury Theatre, London, 1946; Starkey, *Peter Pan,* Scala Theatre, London, 1946; Sherman, *Right Side Up,* and Reverend Giles Aldus, *Saint's Day,* both Arts Theatre, 1951; Lemprius Euphronius, *Antony and Cleopatra,* Ziegfeld Theatre, New York City, 1951; William Mossop, *Hobson's Choice,* Arts Theatre, 1952; Huish, *Ebb Tide,* Edinburgh Festival, Edinburgh, Scotland, then Royal Court Theatre, London, both 1952; Horst Bratsch, *High*

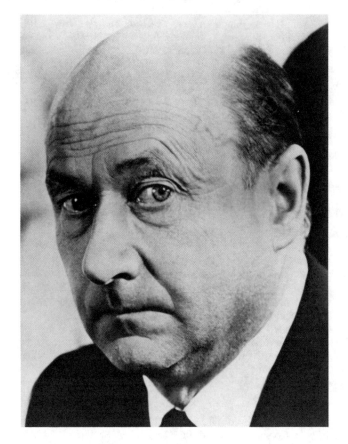

DONALD PLEASENCE

Balcony, Embassy Theatre, London, 1952; Launcelot Gobbo, *The Merchant of Venice,* and Grumio, *The Taming of the Shrew,* both Memorial Theatre Company, Shakespeare Memorial Theatre, Stratford-on-Avon, U.K., 1953; Diomedes and Lepidus, *Antony and Cleopatra,* Memorial Theatre Company, Shakespeare Memorial Theatre, then Prince's Theatre, London, both 1953; Maccario, *The Impressario from Smyrna,* Arts Theatre, 1954; Leone Gola, *The Rules of the Game,* Arts Theatre, 1955; Dauphin, *The Lark,* Lyric Hammersmith Theatre, 1955; Gunner, *Misalliance,* Lyric Hammersmith Theatre, 1956; Monsieur Tarde, *Restless Heart,* St. James's Theatre, London, 1957.

Davies, *The Caretaker,* Arts Theatre, then Duchess Theatre, London, both 1960, later Lyceum Theatre, New York City, 1961; title role, *Poor Bitos,* New Arts Theatre, London, 1963, then Duke of York's Theatre, London, 1964, later Cort Theatre, New York City, 1964; Arthur Goldman, *The Man in the Glass Booth,* St. Martin's Theatre, London, 1967, then Royale Theatre, New York City, 1968; Disson, *Tea Party,* and Law, *The Basement* (double-bill), Eastside Playhouse, New York City, 1968, then Duchess Theatre, London, 1970; Artminster, *Wise Child,* Helen Hayes Theatre, New York City, 1972; George Greive, *Reflections,* Royal Haymarket Theatre, London, 1980. Also appeared as with the Perth Repertory Theatre, 1947; Birmingham Repertory Theatre, Birmingham, U.K., 1948-50; and the Bristol Old Vic Company, Royal Theatre, Bristol, U.K., 1950-51.

PRINCIPAL STAGE WORK—Co-producer, *Poor Bitos,* Arts Theatre, London, 1963, then Duke of York's Theatre, London, 1964, later Cort Theatre, New York City, 1964.

FILM DEBUT—Tromp, *The Beachcomber*, 1953, released in the United States by United Artists, 1955. PRINCIPAL FILM APPEARANCES—Ali, *The Black Tent*, Rank, 1956; Parsons, *1984*, Columbia, 1956; Crabtree, *Decision against Time* (also known as *The Man in the Sky*), Metro-Goldwyn-Mayer (MGM), 1957; Evans, *Stowaway Girl* (also known as *Manuela*), Paramount, 1957; Limpy, *Value for Money*, Rank, 1957; bank teller, *All at Sea* (also known as *Barnacle Bill*), MGM, 1958; Speil, *Heart of a Child*, Rank, 1958; organ grinder, *The Man Inside*, Columbia, 1958; Barsad, *A Tale of Two Cities*, Rank, 1958; doctor, *The Wind Cannot Read*, Twentieth Century-Fox, 1958; Hurst, *Look Back in Anger*, Warner Brothers, 1959; Lance-Corporal Martin, *Orders Are Orders*, British Lion, 1959; General Hardt, *The Two-Headed Spy*, Columbia, 1959.

Major Pinksy, *The Horsemasters*, Buena Vista, 1960; Irwin Hoffman, *The Battle of the Sexes*, Continental, 1960; Victor Partridge, *The Big Day*, Bryanston, 1960; Vanet, *Circus of Horrors*, American International, 1960; Gus Hawkins, *Hell Is a City*, Columbia, 1960; captain, *Killers of Kilimanjaro*, Columbia, 1960; Jessel, *The Shakedown*, Universal, 1960; Pappleworth, *Sons and Lovers*, Twentieth Century-Fox, 1960; Nabal, *The Story of David*, British Lion, 1960; William Hare, *Mania* (also known as *The Flesh and the Fiends*, *Psycho Killers*, and *The Fiendish Ghouls*), Valiant/Pacemaker, 1961; Roger Renfrew, *No Love for Johnnie*, Embassy, 1961; Brown, *The Risk* (also known as *Suspect*), Kingsley International, 1961; Mr. Jenkins, *Spare the Rod*, British Lion, 1961; Pop, *The Wind of Change*, Brynaston, 1961; Sergeant Wolters, *Lisa* (also known as *The Inspector*), Twentieth Century-Fox, 1962; Everett Sloane, *Solicitor, What a Carve Up!* (also known as *No Place Like Homicide*), Embassy, 1962; Dr. Hawley Harvey Crippen, *Dr. Crippen*, Warner Brothers, 1963; Blythe ("The Forger"), *The Great Escape*, United Artists, 1963; Davies, *The Caretaker* (also known as *The Guest*), Janus, 1963; Coates, *The Hands of Orlac*, Continental Distributing, 1964; Dark Hermit, *The Greatest Story Ever Told*, United Artists, 1965; Oracle Jones, *The Hallelujah Trial*, United Artists, 1965; George, *Cul-de-Sac*, Filmways, 1966; Dr. Michaels, *Fantastic Voyage* (also known as *Microscopia* and *Strange Journey*), Twentieth Century-Fox, 1966; Pere Dominic, *Eye of the Devil* (also known as *13*), MGM, 1967; Andreanu, *Matchless*, United Artists, 1967; General Kahlenberge, *The Night of the Generals* (also known as *La Nuit de gereraux*), Columbia, 1967; Ernst Stavro Blofeld, *You Only Live Twice*, United Artists, 1967; Preacher Quint, *Will Penny*, Paramount, 1968; the Prospector, *The Madwoman of Chaillot*, Warner Brothers, 1969.

Dr. Freedom, *Mister Freedom*, Grove, 1970; Isaac Q. Cumber, *Soldier Blue*, AVCO-Embassy, 1970; Ebenezer Balfour, *Kidnapped*, American International, 1971; Doc Tydon, *Outback*, United Artists, 1971; SEN 5241, *THX 1138*, Warner Brothers, 1971; Thomas Cromwell, *Henry VIII and His Six Wives* (also known as *The Six Wives of Henry VIII*), MIGM/EMI, 1972; Major Samuels, *The Jerusalem File*, MGM, 1972; Baron, *The Pied Piper*, Paramount, 1972; Jim, *Wedding in White*, AVCO-Embassy, 1972; Inspector Calhoun, *Death Line* (also known as *Raw Meat*), American International, 1973; Loomis, *Innocent Bystanders*, Paramount, 1973; Logan, *The Rainbow Boys*, Mutual, 1973; Dr. Tremayne, *Tales That Witness Madness*, Paramount, 1973; Cedric Harper, *The Black Windmill*, Universal, 1974; Dr. Nolter, *The Mutations* (also known as *The Mutation*), Columbia, 1974.

Erich, Count Plasma, *Barry McKenzie Holds His Own*, Roadshow, 1975; Deranian, *Escape to Witch Mountain*, Buena Vista, 1975; A.J. Nietz, *Hearts of the West* (also known as *Hollywood Cowboy*), Metro-Goldwyn-Mayer/United Artists (MGM/UA), 1975; Dr. Finch, *The Devil within Her* (also known as *I Don't Want to Be Born*), American International, 1976; Sir Giles Marley, *Dirty Knight's Work* (also known as *Trial by Combat* and *A Choice of Arms*), Gamma III, 1976; Heinrich Himmler, *The Eagle Has Landed*, Columbia, 1976; Kuvetli, *Journey into Fear* (also known as *Burn Out*), Sterling Gold, 1976; Father Roche, *Land of the Minotaur* (also known as *The Devil's Men*, *The Devil's People*, and *Minotaur*), Crown International, 1976; Boxley, *The Last Tycoon*, Paramount, 1976; Pontius Pilate, *The Passover Plot*, Atlas, 1976; Dr. Harmon, *Oh, God!*, Warner Brothers, 1977; Nicolai Dalchimsky, *Telefon*, MGM/UA, 1977; Valentine De'Ath, "Hollywood, 1936" in *The Uncanny*, Rank, 1977; Doniac, *Blood Relatives* (also known as *Les Liens de sang*), SNS, 1978; Sam Loomis, *Halloween*, Compass, 1978; Blair, *Power Play*, Robert Cooper, 1978; B.D. Brockhurst, *Sergeant Pepper's Lonely Hearts Club Band*, Universal, 1978; Dr. Todd, *Tomorrow Never Comes*, Rank, 1978; Pumpelmayer, *The Angry Man* (also known as *L'Homme en colere* and *Jigsaw*), United Artists, 1979; Jack Seward, *Dracula*, Universal, 1979; Dr. Steiner, *Good Luck Miss Wyckoff*, Bel Air/Gradison, 1979; General Villanova, *Jaguar Lives!*, American International, 1979; Axel MacGregor, *Night Creature* (also known as *Out of the Darkness* and *Fear*), Dimension, 1979.

President of the United States, *Escape from New York*, AVCO-Embassy, 1981; Sam Loomis, *Halloween II*, Universal, 1981; Pickering, "The Vampire Story" in *The Monster Club*, ITC, 1981; Dr. Leo Bain, *Alone in the Dark*, New Line Cinema, 1982; Dr. Warley, *The Devonsville Terror*, New West, 1983; Defense Minister Eretz, *The Ambassador* (also known as *Peacemaker*), Cannon, 1984; J.P. Whittier, *A Breed Apart*, Orion, 1984; Gilbert "Gibbie" Gibson, *Treasure of the Yankee Zephyr* (also known as *Race for the Yankee Zephyr*), Film Ventures, 1984; Mackintosh, *Where Is Parsifal?* Terence Young, 1984; John McGregor, *Creepers* (also known as *Phenomena*), New Line, 1985; Inspector, *Sotto il vestito niente* (also known as *Under the Dress, Nothing*), Titanus/Filmexport, 1985; Colonel Kostik, *To Kill a Stranger* (also known as *To Murder a Stranger*), VCL/Media Home Entertainment, 1985; Klaus, *The Treasure of the Amazons* (also known as *El tesoro del Amazones*), Videocine/S.A., 1985; Prosper Gaffney, *Ground Zero*, Hoyts, 1987; Professor Lasky, *Specters* (also known as *Spettri*), Intra, 1987; Claudius, *Warrior Queen*, Seymour Borde, 1987; Rosza, *Hanna's War*, Cannon, 1988. Also appeared in *Arthur! Arthur?*, 1969; *Malachi's Cove* (also known as *The Seaweed Children*), Impact Quadrant, 1973; as a peddler, *Tales from beyond the Grave*, 1973; Rothko, *The Order and Security of the World* (also known as *L'Ordre et la securite du monde*), 1978; in *Puma Man*, 1980; as Prosser, *Warrior of the Lost World*, 1985; Victor Frankenstein/Old Baron Frankenstein, *Frankenstein's Great Aunt Tilly*, 1985; narrator, *Terror in the Aisles*, 1985; in *Cobra Mission* (also known as *The Rainbow Professional* and *Mission Cobra*), Vip/Delta, 1986; *Fuga dall'inferno*, 1987; as Don Alvise, *Nosferatu a Venezia*, 1987; priest, *Prince of Darkness*, 1987; Inspector Downey, *Phantom of Death*, 1988; and in *La loba y la paloma*, *Wake in Fright*, *Animale Metropolitani*, *Black Rock*, *Altrimenti ci Arabiano*, *Dick Turpin*, *Honour Thy Father*, *Catacomb*, *Pompeii*, *Devil Cat*, *Gula and Rick*, *Imbalances*, *Search and Destroy*, *Night Trap*, *River of Death*, and *Buried Alive*.

PRINCIPAL FILM WORK—Co-producer, *The Caretaker* (also known as *The Guest*), Janus, 1963.

TELEVISION DEBUT—*I Want to Be a Doctor*, 1946. PRINCIPAL TELEVISION APPEARANCES—Series: Prince John, *The Adventures of Robin Hood* (also known as *Adventures in Sherwood Forest*), CBS, 1955-56; also host, *Armchair Mystery Theatre*, 1960; *Fate and Mr. Browne*. Mini-Series: Melchior, *Jesus of*

Nazareth, NBC, 1977; Samuel Purchase, *Centennial,* NBC, 1978-79; Max Dechambre, *The French Atlantic Affair,* ABC, 1979; Salomon Van der Merwe, *Master of the Game,* CBS, 1984; also Reverend Septimus Harding, *Barchester Chronicles,* BBC, then *Masterpiece Theatre,* PBS. Pilots: George Dettler, *Computercide,* NBC, 1982. Episodic: Professor Ellis Fowler, "The Changing of the Guard," *The Twilight Zone,* CBS, 1962; Harold J. Finley, "The Man with the Power," *The Outer Limits,* ABC, 1963; also "The Confession," *One Step Beyond,* ABC, 1961; *Mrs. Columbo,* NBC, 1979; *Columbo,* NBC; *Omnibus.* Movies: Danglars, *The Count of Monte Cristo,* NBC, 1975; John Tyler Jones, *Goldenrod,* CBS, 1977; Captain Vladimir Popov, *The Defection of Simas Kudirka,* CBS, 1978; Solomon Sholto, *The Bastard* (also known as *The Kent Family Chronicles*), syndicated, 1978; narrator, *The Dark Secret of Harvest Home,* NBC, 1978; Kantorek, *All Quiet on the Western Front,* CBS, 1979; Colonel Riddle, *Better Late Than Never,* NBC, 1979; Clarence Blasko, *Gold of the Amazon Women,* NBC, 1979; Haake, *Arch of Triumph,* CBS, 1985; Chancellor, *The Corsican Brothers,* CBS, 1985; Oates, *Black Arrow,* Disney Channel, 1985; Dr. Absalon, *The Great Escape II: The Untold Story,* NBC, 1988; also *Witness for the Prosecution.*

Specials: Mr. Dusseli, *The Diary of Anne Frank,* ABC, 1967; Smudge, *Dr. Jekyll and Mr. Hyde,* NBC, 1973; Mr. Kidd, *The Room,* ABC, 1987. Also appeared in *Blade on the Feather,* London Weekend Television (LWT); *The Cafeteria,* BBC; *The Captain of Kopenick,* Canadian television; *Death,* Canadian television; *Falklands Factor,* BBC; *Future of All Evil,* Thames; *The Joke,* BBC; *The Man Outside,* BBC; *Orson Welles's Great Mysteries,* Anglia; *Punishment without Crime,* Granada; *Rivals of Sherlock Holmes,* Thames; *Scoop,* LWT; *Valuation for the Purposes of . . . ,* BBC; and in *Ambrose, The Bandstand, Bi Centennial, Call Me Daddy, Captain Rogers, The Cupboard, Double Indemnity, The Fox Trot, The Hatchet Man, Hindle Lakes, A House of His Own, It's Never Too Late, Julius Caesar, Machinal, Man in a Moon, The Millionairess, Misalliance, Moment of Truth, Montserrat, 1984, No Flags for Geebang, Occupations, One, The Scarf, The Silk Purse, Skin Deep, Small Fish Are Sweet, Taste, Thou Good and Faithful Servant,* and *The Traitor.*

PRINCIPAL TELEVISION WORK—Series: Producer, *Armchair Mystery Theatre,* 1960.

RELATED CAREER—Assistant stage manager and stage manager, Jersey, U.K.; founder (with Harold Pinter and Robert Shaw), Glasshouse Productions.

NON-RELATED CAREER—Railway station master, Swinton, U.K.

WRITINGS: STAGE—*Ebb Tide,* Edinburgh Festival, Edinburgh, Scotland, then Royal Court Theatre, London, both 1952. OTHER—*Scouse the Mouse,* 1977; *Scouse in New York,* 1978.

AWARDS: Actor of the Year Award from the London Guild of Film and Television Producers, 1958; London Critics Award, Best Stage Performance, 1961, and Antoinette Perry Award nomination, Best Actor in a Play, 1962, both for *The Caretaker;* Antoinette Perry Award nomination, Best Actor in a Play, 1965, for *Poor Bitos;* Variety Club Award, Best Stage Actor, 1967; Antoinette Perry Award nomination, Best Actor in a Play, 1969, for *The Man in the Glass Booth; Time* (magazine) Award, Best Stage Performance, 1969, for *The Caretaker;* Antoinette Perry Award nomination, Best Actor in a Play, 1972, for *Wise Child;* also received an Emmy Award for *Call Me Daddy* and an Emmy Award nomination for *The Defection of Simas Kudirka.*

MEMBER: Actors' Equity Association, British Actors' Equity Association, Screen Actors Guild, Arts Club (London), Royal Automobile Club (London), White Elephant Club.

SIDELIGHTS: FAVORITE ROLES—Gunner in *Misalliance* and Davies in *The Caretaker.*

CTFT learned that Donald Pleasence spent a year in a German prisoner of war camp during World War II.

ADDRESSES: AGENT—Joy Jameson Ltd., 7 W. Eaton Place Mews, London SW1X 8LY, England.

*   *   *

PLESHETTE, Suzanne

PERSONAL: Born January 31, in New York, NY; daughter of Eugene (a theatre manager and network executive) and Geraldine (an artist and dancer; maiden name, Rivers) Pleshette; married Troy Donahue (an actor; divorced); married Thomas Joseph Gallagher III (in business), March 16, 1968. EDUCATION: Attended the High School of Performing Arts, Syracuse University, and Finch College; studied acting at the Neighborhood Playhouse School of Theatre.

VOCATION: Actress.

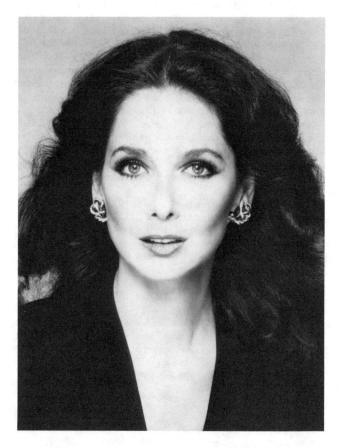

SUZANNE PLESHETTE

CAREER: STAGE DEBUT—*Truckline Cafe.* BROADWAY DEBUT—*Compulsion,* Ambassador Theatre, 1957. PRINCIPAL STAGE APPEARANCES—Leah, *The Cold Wind and the Warm,* Morosco Theatre, New York City, 1958; Julie, *The Golden Fleecing,* Henry Miller's Theatre, New York City, 1959; Annie Sullivan, *The Miracle Worker,* Playhouse Theatre, New York City, 1961; Amy Ruskin, *Special Occasions,* Music Box Theatre, New York City, 1982; also appeared as Gittel Mosca, *Two for the Seesaw,* Booth Theatre, New York City; and in a production of *A Streetcar Named Desire.*

FILM DEBUT—Private Betty Pearson, *The Geisha Boy,* Paramount, 1958. PRINCIPAL FILM APPEARANCES—Chris Lockwood, *Forty Pounds of Trouble,* Universal, 1962; Prudence Bell, *Rome Adventure* (also known as *Lovers Must Learn*), Warner Brothers, 1962; Annie Hayworth, *The Birds,* Universal, 1963; Laura Rubio, *Wall of Noise,* Warner Brothers, 1963; Kitty, *A Distant Trumpet,* Warner Brothers, 1964; Martha Webster, *Fate Is the Hunter,* Twentieth Century-Fox, 1964; Jeanne Green, *Youngblood Hawke,* Warner Brothers, 1964; Grace Caldwell, *A Rage to Live,* United Artists, 1965; Fiddle, *Mister Buddwing* (also known as *Woman without a Face*), Metro-Goldwyn-Mayer (MGM), 1966; Pilar, *Nevada Smith,* Paramount, 1966; Fran Garrison, *The Ugly Dachshund,* Buena Vista, 1966; Arabella Flagg, *The Adventures of Bullwhip Griffin,* Buena Vista, 1967; Jo Anne Baker, *Blackbeard's Ghost,* Buena Vista, 1968; Margery Lansing, *The Power,* MGM, 1968; Samantha, *If It's Tuesday, This Must Be Belgium,* United Artists, 1969; Ramona, *Suppose They Gave a War and Nobody Came?* (also known as *War Games*), Cinerama, 1970; Patience Barton, *Support Your Local Gunfighter,* United Artists, 1971; Betty Daniels, *The Shaggy D.A.,* Buena Vista, 1976; Louise Webster, *Hot Stuff,* Columbia, 1979; Paula, *Oh, God! Book II,* Warner Brothers, 1980; Diane Reed, *Target: Harry* (also known as *How to Make It* and *What's in It for Harry?*), filmed in 1969, released by Roger Corman, 1980; as herself, *Sanford Meisner—The Theatre's Best Kept Secret* (documentary), Columbia, 1984.

PRINCIPAL TELEVISION APPEARANCES—Series: Emily Hartley, *The Bob Newhart Show,* CBS, 1972-78; title role, *Suzanne Pleshette Is Maggie Briggs,* CBS, 1984; Tracy Bridges, *Bridges to Cross,* CBS, 1986; Chris Broderick, *Nightingales,* 1989—. Pilots: Renee Fontaine, *Band of Gold* (broadcast as an episode of *The General Electric Theatre*), CBS, 1961; Anita King, *Corridor 400* (broadcast as an episode of *The Bob Hope Chrysler Theatre*), NBC, 1963; Elizabeth Morton, *Richie Brockelman: Missing 24 Hours,* NBC, 1976; Kate Bliss, *Kate Bliss and the Ticker Tape Kid,* ABC, 1978. Episodic: "Delusion," *One Step Beyond,* ABC, 1959; "The Mutation," *The Invaders,* ABC, 1967; "The Pursued," *The Invaders,* ABC, 1968; *Relatively Speaking,* syndicated, 1988; also as Lori Moore, *Channing,* ABC; in *The Dick Powell Show,* NBC; *Dr. Kildare,* NBC; *Route 66,* CBS; *The Fugitive,* ABC; *The Name of the Game,* NBC; *Ironside,* NBC; *Bonanza,* NBC. Movies: Kitty Sanborn, *Wings of Fire,* NBC, 1967; Barbara Soline, *Hunters Are for Killing,* 1970; Anne Banning/Janet Furie, *Along Came a Spider,* ABC, 1970; Anna, *River of Gold,* ABC, 1971; Kate Todd, *In Broad Daylight,* ABC, 1971; June Mathis, *The Legend of Valentino,* ABC, 1975; Karen Day, *Law and Order,* NBC, 1976; Kate Fallon, *Flesh and Blood,* CBS, 1979; Janet Langford, *If Things Were Different,* CBS, 1980; Margot Murray, *The Star Maker,* NBC, 1981; Laura Bingham, *Help Wanted: Male,* CBS, 1982; Carla Webber, *Fantasies,* ABC, 1982; Joanne Boone, *One Cooks the Other Doesn't,* CBS, 1983; Dixie Cabot, *Dixie: Changing Habits,* CBS, 1983; Joanna Piper, *For Love or Money,* CBS, 1984; Dana Sutton, *Kojak: The Belarus File,* CBS, 1985; Kate Bennington, *A Stranger Waits,* CBS, 1987; Captain Janet Hamil-

ton, *Alone in the Neon Jungle,* CBS, 1988. Specials: Nona, *Flesh and Blood,* NBC, 1968; *Mitzie: A Tribute to the American Housewife,* CBS, 1974; *Memories Then and Now,* CBS, 1988.

PRINCIPAL TELEVISION WORK—Series: Co-creator, *Suzanne Pleshette Is Maggie Briggs,* CBS, 1984; co-creator, *Bridges to Cross,* CBS, 1986.

NON-RELATED CAREER—Designer of home furnishings and linens.

AWARDS: Emmy Award nomination for *Dr. Kildare;* also received three additional Emmy Award nominations.

ADDRESSES: AGENT—William Morris Agency, 151 El Camino Drive, Beverly Hills, CA 90212.

*   *   *

POITIER, Sidney   1927-

PERSONAL: Born February 20, 1927, in Miami, FL; son of Reginald James (a tomato farmer) and Evelyn (a tomato farmer; maiden name, Outten) Poitier; married Juanita Hardy (a dancer), April 29, 1950 (divorced, 1965); married Joanna Shimkus (an actress), January 23, 1976; children: Beverly, Pamela, Sherri, Gina (first marriage); Anika, Sydney (second marriage). EDUCATION: Trained for the stage with Paul Mann and Lloyd Richards. MILITARY: U.S. Army, physiotherapist, 1941-45.

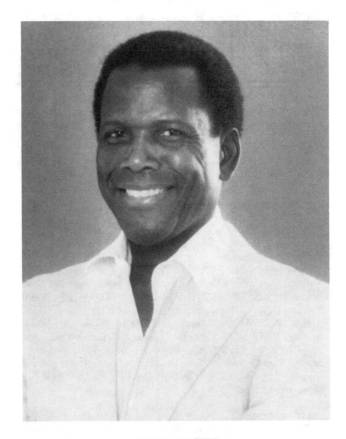

SIDNEY POITIER

VOCATION: Actor and director.

CAREER: STAGE DEBUT—*Days of Our Youth,* American Negro Theatre Playhouse, New York City, 1945. BROADWAY DEBUT—Polydorus, *Lysistrata,* Belasco Theatre, 1946. PRINCIPAL STAGE APPEARANCES—Lester, *Anna Lucasta,* National Theatre, New York City, 1947; Walter Lee Younger, *A Raisin in the Sun,* Ethel Barrymore Theatre, New York City, 1959; also appeared in *On Striver's Row,* American National Theatre Playhouse, New York City, 1946; and in productions of *You Can't Take It with You, Rain, Freight, The Fisherman, Hidden Horizon, Sepia Cinderella,* and *Riders to the Sea,* all with the American Negro Theatre.

PRINCIPAL STAGE WORK—Director, *Carry Me Back to Morningside Heights,* John Golden Theatre, New York City, 1968.

MAJOR TOURS—Lester, *Anna Lucasta,* U.S. cities, 1948.

FILM DEBUT—Dr. Luther Brooks, *No Way Out,* Twentieth Century-Fox, 1950. PRINCIPAL FILM APPEARANCES—Reverend Maimangu, *Cry, the Beloved Country* (also known as *African Fury*), Lopert, 1952; Corporal Andrew Robertson, *Red Ball Express,* Universal, 1952; Inman Jackson, *Go, Man, Go!,* United Artists, 1954; Gregory W. Miller, *The Blackboard Jungle,* Metro-Goldwyn-Mayer (MGM), 1955; Gates, *Goodbye, My Lady,* Warner Brothers, 1956; Tommy Tyler, *Edge of the City* (also known as *A Man Is Ten Feet Tall*), MGM, 1957; Kimani, *Something of Value,* MGM, 1957; Rau-Ru, *Band of Angels,* Warner Brothers, 1957; Noah Cullen, *The Defiant Ones,* United Artists, 1958; Oban, *The Mark of the Hawk* (also known as *Accused*), Universal, 1958; Porgy, *Porgy and Bess,* Columbia, 1959.

Towler, *All the Young Men,* Columbia, 1960; Marcus, *Virgin Island* (also known as *Our Virgin Island*), Films-Around-the-World, 1960; Eddie Cook, *Paris Blues,* United Artists, 1961; Walter Lee Younger, *A Raisin in the Sun,* Columbia, 1961; doctor, *Pressure Point,* United Artists, 1962; Homer Smith, *Lilies of the Field,* United Artists, 1963; El Mansuh, *The Long Ships* (also known as *Dugi Brodovi*), Columbia, 1964; Ben Munceford, *The Bedford Incident,* Columbia, 1965; Simon of Cyrene, *The Greatest Story Ever Told,* United Artists, 1965; Gordon Ralfe, *A Patch of Blue,* MGM, 1965; Alan Newell, *The Slender Thread,* Paramount, 1965; Toller, *Duel at Diablo,* United Artists, 1966; John Prentice, *Guess Who's Coming to Dinner,* Columbia, 1967; Virgil Tibbs, *In the Heat of the Night,* United Artists, 1967; Mark Thackeray, *To Sir, with Love,* Columbia, 1967; Jack Parks, *For Love of Ivy,* Cinerama, 1968; Jason Higgs, *The Lost Man,* Universal, 1969.

Virgil Tibbs, *They Call Me Mister Tibbs,* United Artists, 1970; John Kane, *Brother John,* Columbia, 1971; Lieutenant Virgil Tibbs, *The Organization,* United Artists, 1971; Buck, *Buck and the Preacher,* Columbia, 1972; Dr. Matt Younger, *A Warm December,* National General, 1973; Steve Jackson, *Uptown Saturday Night,* Warner Brothers, 1974; Clyde Williams, *Let's Do It Again,* Warner Brothers, 1975; Shack Twala, *The Wilby Conspiracy,* United Artists, 1975; Manny Durrell, *A Piece of the Action,* Warner Brothers, 1977; Warren Stantin, *Shoot to Kill,* Buena Vista, 1988; Roy Parmenter, *Little Nikita,* Columbia, 1988. Also appeared in *From Whom Cometh My Help* (documentary), U.S. Army Signal Corps, 1949; and *King: A Filmed Record . . . Montgomery to Memphis,* Marion, 1970.

FIRST FILM WORK—Director, *Buck and the Preacher,* Columbia, 1972. PRINCIPAL FILM WORK—Director: *A Warm December,* National General, 1973; *Uptown Saturday Night,* Warner Brothers,

1974; *Let's Do It Again,* Warner Brothers, 1975; *A Piece of the Action,* Warner Brothers, 1977; *Stir Crazy,* Columbia, 1980; *Hanky Panky,* Columbia, 1982; *Fast Forward,* Columbia, 1985.

PRINCIPAL TELEVISION APPEARANCES—Episodic: "Parole Chief," *Philco Television Playhouse,* NBC, 1952; "A Man Is Ten Feet Tall," *Philco Television Playhouse,* NBC, 1955; "Fascinating Stranger," *Ponds Theatre,* ABC, 1955; "A Tribute to Eleanor Roosevelt on Her Diamond Jubilee," *Sunday Showcase,* NBC, 1959; "A Time for Laughter," *ABC Stage '67,* ABC, 1967; *The Strolling '20s,* CBS, 1966; *The New Bill Cosby Show,* CBS, 1972. Specials: *The American Film Institute Tenth Anniversary Special,* CBS, 1977; *The Spencer Tracy Legacy: A Tribute by Katharine Hepburn,* PBS, 1986; narrator, *Bopha!,* PBS, 1987.

RELATED CAREER—Founder (with Paul Newman, Barbra Streisand, Steve McQueen, and Dustin Hoffman), First Artists Film Production Company, 1969.

NON-RELATED CAREER—Janitor, dishwasher, construction worker, messenger, and longshoreman.

WRITINGS: This Life (autobiography), Knopf, 1980.

AWARDS: Georgio Cini Award from the Venice Film Festival, 1958, for *Something of Value;* Academy Award nomination, Silver Bear Award from the Berlin Film Festival, New York Film Critics Award, all Best Actor, and British Academy Award, Best Foreign Actor, all 1958, for *The Defiant Ones;* Academy Award, Best Actor, 1963, for *Lilies of the Field;* William J. German Human Relations Award from the American Jewish Congress, 1966; San Sebastian Film Festival Award, Best Actor, 1968, for *For Love of Ivy;* Knight Commander of the British Empire, 1974; Cecil B. De Mille Award from the Hollywood Foreign Press Association, 1982.

MEMBER: American Federation of Television and Radio Artists, Actors' Equity Association, Screen Actors Guild, Directors Guild of America, Writers Guild of America, Center Theatre Group, American Film Institute, Martin Luther King, Jr. Center for Non-violent Social Change, NAACP (life member), Charles Drew Medical Group, Los Angeles Olympic Committee.

SIDELIGHTS: Actor/director Sidney Poitier was the first black man to be given a succession of serious, dignified roles in Hollywood films; he was also the first black to win an Academy Award for a leading role in a movie. An *American Film* commentator observes that Poitier's career "conveniently marks a turning point in the fortune of blacks on the screen and in Hollywood. . . . The movies were at last responding to the changing social winds, and Poitier . . . was there to sail with them." The son of poor West Indian farmers, Poitier has chosen for the most part to play the sort of respectable roles that once were denied minorities—doctor, teacher, businessman, psychiatrist, and detective, to name a few. According to Patricia Bosworth in the *Washington Post Book World,* Poitier is a pioneer who is "celebrated as the first black actor to break through the sterotyping and racism of Hollywood" who also "has individualized and humanized the black experience with [his] powerful performances."

Poitier, the youngest child in a large family, grew up in the Bahamas, helping his parents to subsist on their small tomato farm. As a teenager, he moved to Miami to find work, but instead he found racial prejudice and communications difficulties arising from his West Indian accent. He hopped freight trains to New York City, and there, in the early 1940s, he found odd jobs as a dishwasher and busboy in restaurants. After seeing an advertisement for black actors in the newspaper, he auditioned for the American Negro Theatre. He was turned down, again because of his accent and his near illiteracy (he spent only four years in school). Seized with determination, Poitier bought a radio and practiced reading and speaking more like a North American. On his second application to the American Negro Theatre, he was given a three-month trial position. Even then his success was not assured. Hearing that the director planned to oust him after his three months were up, he struck a bargain—if he could stay and study, he said, he would perform the theatre's janitorial duties for free. The offer was accepted and Poitier was allowed to continue with the theatre group.

Eventually Poitier began to land small speaking roles in all-black cast plays. Some of these included *Lysistrata, You Can't Take It with You, Hidden Horizon,* and *Sepia Cinderella.* His first major film credit came in 1950, when he appeared in *No Way Out* as a black doctor encountering hostility in an all-white hospital staff. Once established, Poitier politely demanded serious roles that flew in the face of the racist sterotype of a shuffling, silly black man. According to David Zinman in *Fifty from the Fifties,* it was Poitier's "searing, sensative performance in *The Blackboard Jungle* (1955)" that "established his credentials as a dramatic actor." In that film, Poitier plays a bitter youth in a tough city school who gradually learns to respect authority. After *The Blackboard Jungle,* Zinman concludes, "when a part called for a tense, brooding young black, first call went to Poitier."

Poitier received his first Academy Award nomination in 1958 for his work in *The Defiant Ones.* In that film Poitier and Tony Curtis appear as convicts, chained together at the ankles, who must learn to cooperate in order to make good a desperate escape attempt. Although Poitier did not win the Oscar for that role, he did make history by winning one for *Lilies of the Field,* in which he plays a stubborn handyman who builds a chapel for a persistent group of nuns. By the mid-1960s, notes *New York Times Book Review* contributor Mel Watkins, Poitier was "an accepted and bankable star." Unlike many Hollywood performers, however, Poitier used his bankability in an adventurous manner. If offered a good script, he would agree to wave his six-figure fee in lieu of a percentage of the film's profits. By that means Poitier earned a sizable sum for *Lilies of the Field* and for the low budget movie *To Sir, with Love,* released in 1967. He also received wide notice for his work in *Guess Who's Coming to Dinner?,* a comedy about interracial marriage, and the adventure-drama *In the Heat of the Night.*

Even at the height of his career, however, Poitier had to endure the scorn of some critics. *American Film* correspondent Thomas Cripps writes that the actor's "high visibility made him an easy target for critics in search of a heavy on whom to lay blame for the long history of Hollywood's contempt for blacks." James Powers addresses this issue, also in *American Film*: "The times have put the burden on Poitier's films; and his blacks are often derided for being overly high-minded. . . . It has fallen to other black actors—for whom his presence in Hollywood paved the way—to explore more complex aspects of black life." Whether stung by the critics or not, Poitier turned more and more toward directing as the 1970s progressed. At first he directed movies in which he appeared, including *Buck and the Preacher, A Warm December,* and *Uptown Saturday Night.* Then he began simply to direct others, scoring his biggest success with the 1980 Richard Pryor-Gene Wilder comedy *Stir Crazy.* Poitier returned to acting in 1988 with two films, *Shoot to Kill* and *Little Nikita,* both action-adventure dramas.

To hear Poitier tell it, the years have not changed his desire to

innovate—and to be taken seriously. "I want to take risks, and I want to be my own man—as I have been—to the extent of saying, 'I'll work at what I want to work at,'" Poitier told *American Way.* "I don't have to direct or act in films, I don't have to write films. I can do all three. . . . I think that after all these years and after this life, I'm entitled to make choices on a purer basis than people are generally afforded. It's not for financial reasons. It's for reasons that have to do with an honest look at my life." Powers concludes that a "smoldering energy, coupled with an alert intelligence, marks Poitier's major roles. . . . The alertness, the presence have such a force that the debate that flies around the hero seems intolerably petty."

OTHER SOURCES: American Film, September, 1976, September, 1980; *American Way,* July, 1980; *Contemporary Literary Criticism,* Volume 26, Gale, 1983; [New York] *Daily News,* March 6, 1989; *Fifty from the Fifties,* by David Zinman, Arlington, 1979; *The Films of Sidney Poitier,* by Alvin H. Marill, Citadel, 1978; *Los Angeles Times Book Review,* June 1, 1980; *New Republic,* May, 1980; *New York Times,* August 17, 1950, March 21, 1955, May 11, 1957, September 25, 1958, March 12, 1959, March 29, 1959, June 25, 1959, August 27, 1960, March 30, 1961, October 2, 1963, June 15, 1967, August 3, 1967, December 12, 1967, February 29, 1968, July 18, 1968, April 29, 1972, June 17, 1974, June 2, 1980, December 12, 1980, June 4, 1982, February 15, 1985; *New York Times Book Review,* August 17, 1980, March 29, 1981; *New Yorker,* June 17, 1974, September 15, 1975, November 3, 1975; *Newsweek,* June 24, 1974, December 15, 1980; *People,* August 4, 1980, July 5, 1982; *This Life,* by Sidney Poitier, 1980; *Time,* October 6, 1975, October 27, 1975, June 7, 1982; *Washington Post Book World,* May 25, 1980.

ADDRESSES: OFFICE—Verdon Productions, 9350 Wilshire Boulevard, Suite 310, Beverly Hills, CA 90212.*

*   *   *

POLIC, Henry II

PERSONAL: Born February 20, in Pittsburgh, PA. EDUCATION: Received M.A. in speech and drama.

VOCATION: Actor.

CAREER: PRINCIPAL STAGE APPEARANCES—*Room Service,* Pasadena Playhouse, Pasadena, CA, 1987; also appeared in stage productions in Sarasota, FL, Miami, FL, and Phoenix, AZ.

PRINCIPAL FILM APPEARANCES—Captain Merdmanger, *The Last Remake of Beau Geste,* Universal, 1977; also appeared in *Scavenger Hunt,* Twentieth Century-Fox, 1979.

TELEVISION DEBUT—Sheriff of Nottingham, *When Things Were Rotten,* ABC, 1975. PRINCIPAL TELEVISION APPEARANCES—Series: Regular, *The Late Summer Early Fall Bert Convy Show,* CBS, 1976; Count Dracula, *The Monster Squad,* NBC, 1976-77; Jerry Silver, *Webster,* ABC, 1983-87; host, *Double Talk,* ABC, 1986. Mini-Series: Mark Steiner, *Scruples,* ABC, 1981. Pilots: Pierre Ritz, *Heck's Angels,* CBS, 1976; Schnell, *McNamara's Band,* ABC, 1977. Episodic: Alan Dupree, *Murder, She Wrote,* CBS, 1986; also "Something Old, Something New," *Brothers,* syndicated, 1989. Specials: *How to Survive the 70s and Maybe Even Bump into Happiness,* CBS, 1978.

ADDRESSES: AGENT—Bauman, Hiller, and Strain, 9220 Sunset Boulevard, Suite 202, Los Angeles, CA 90069. PUBLICIST—Brad Lemack, Lemack and Company, 7060 Hollywood Boulevard, Suite 320, Los Angeles, CA 90028.*

*   *   *

POLLACK, Sydney   1934-

PERSONAL: Born July 1, 1934, in Lafayette, IN; son of David and Rebecca (Miller) Pollack; married Claire Griswold, September 22, 1958; children: Steven, Rebecca, Rachel. EDUCATION: Trained for the stage at the Neighborhood Playhouse. MILITARY: U.S. Army, 1957-59.

VOCATION: Director, producer, and actor.

CAREER: PRINCIPAL STAGE APPEARANCES—Rusti, *The Dark Is Light Enough,* American National Theatre and Academy Theatre, New York City, 1955; also appeared in *A Stone for Danny Fisher,* Downtown National Theatre, New York City, 1954.

MAJOR TOURS—*Stalag 17,* U.S. cities.

PRINCIPAL FILM APPEARANCES—Sergeant Van Horn, *War Hunt,* United Artists, 1962; George Fields, *Tootsie,* Columbia, 1982.

PRINCIPAL FILM WORK—All as director, unless indicated: *The*

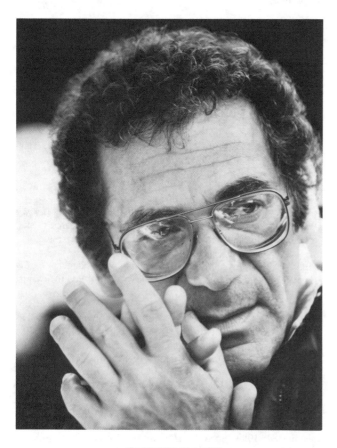

SYDNEY POLLACK

Slender Thread, Paramount, 1965; *This Property Is Condemned,* Paramount, 1966; *The Scalphunters,* United Artists, 1968; *The Swimmer,* Columbia, 1968; *Castle Keep,* Columbia, 1969; (also producer with Irwin Wrinkler and Robert Chartoff) *They Shoot Horses Don't They,* ABC-Cinerama, 1969; *Jeremiah Johnson,* Warner Brothers, 1972; *The Way We Were,* Columbia, 1973; *Three Days of the Condor,* Paramount, 1975; (also producer) *The Yakuza* (also known as *Brotherhood of the Yakuza*), Warner Brothers/Toei, 1975; (also producer) *Bobby Deerfield,* Columbia, 1976; *The Electric Horseman,* Columbia, 1979; executive producer, *Honeysuckle Rose,* Warner Brothers, 1980; (also producer) *Absence of Malice,* Columbia, 1981; (also producer with Dick Richards) *Tootsie,* Columbia, 1982; producer, *Songwriter,* Tri-Star, 1984; executive producer, *Sanford Meisner—The Theatre's Best Kept Secret,* Columbia, 1984; (also producer) *Out of Africa,* Universal, 1985; producer (with Mark Rosenberg), *Bright Lights, Big City,* United Artists, 1988.

PRINCIPAL TELEVISION APPEARANCES—Episodic: *Alcoa Presents* (also known as *One Step Beyond*), ABC; *Playhouse 90,* CBS; *Shotgun Slade,* syndicated; *Ben Casey,* ABC. Also appeared in *A Cardinal Act of Mercy.*

PRINCIPAL TELEVISION WORK—All as director. Pilots: *Diagnosis: Danger,* CBS, 1963; *The Watchman* (broadcast as an episode of *Kraft Suspense Theatre*), NBC, 1964; *The Fliers,* NBC, 1965. Episodic: *Ben Casey,* ABC, 1962-63; "The Game," *Bob Hope Presents the Chrysler Theatre,* NBC, 1965; also *Something about Lee Wiley,* 1963-64; *Target: The Corrupters,* ABC.

RELATED CAREER—Assistant to Sanford Meisner, Neighborhood Playhouse Theatre, New York City, 1954; acting instructor, 1954-60; supervisor of dubbed American version of *The Leopard,* Twentieth Century-Fox, 1963; executive director, Actors Studio (West coast branch); dialogue coach.

AWARDS: Emmy Award, Outstanding Directorial Achievement in Drama, 1966, for "The Game," *Bob Hope Presents the Chrysler Theatre;* Academy Award nomination, Best Director, 1969, for *They Shoot Horses, Don't They?;* New York Film Critics Circle Award and Academy Award nomination, both Best Director, 1982, for *Tootsie;* Academy Award, Best Director, 1986, for *Out of Africa.*

ADDRESSES: OFFICE—Mirage Enterprises, 100 Universal Plaza, Building 414, Universal City, CA 91608.

*   *   *

POLLAN, Tracy

PERSONAL: Full name, Tracy Jo Pollan; daughter of Steven (a financial consultant and writer) and Corky (a magazine editor) Pollan; married Michael J. Fox (an actor), July 17, 1988. EDUCATION: Trained for the stage with Lee Strasberg and at the Herbert Berghof Studios; studied dance at the Alvin Ailey School and the Martha Meredith School.

VOCATION: Actress.

CAREER: PRINCIPAL STAGE APPEARANCES—Peggy, *Album,* Cherry Lane Theatre, New York City, 1980; Julie Jackson, *Pack of Lies,* Royale Theatre, New York City, 1985; also appeared in

Women in Mind, Manhattan Theatre Club, City Center Theatre, New York City, 1988.

FILM DEBUT—Leslie, *Baby, It's You,* Paramount, 1983. PRINCIPAL FILM APPEARANCES—Mary, *Promised Land,* Vestron, 1988; Vicky, *Bright Lights, Big City,* United Artists, 1988.

PRINCIPAL TELEVISION APPEARANCES—Series: Ellen Reed, *Family Ties,* NBC, 1985-86. Pilots: *For Lovers Only,* ABC, 1982. Episodic: Nicki Davis, "The Little Sister," *American Playhouse,* PBS, 1985. Movies: Leslie Churchill, *Sessions,* ABC, 1983; Eileen Grafton, *Trackdown: Finding the Goodbar Killer,* CBS, 1983; Mary Beth Phillips, *The Baron and the Kid,* CBS, 1984; Suzanne Tenney, *A Good Sport,* CBS, 1984; title role, *The Abduction of Kari Swenson,* NBC, 1987; Elizabeth Van Lew, *A Special Friendship,* CBS, 1987. Specials: Jen Robbins, "The Great Love Experiment," *ABC Afterschool Special,* ABC, 1984.

ADDRESSES: AGENT—Triad Artists, 10100 Santa Monica Boulevard, Los Angeles, CA 90067.*

*   *   *

POLLARD, Michael J.   1939-

PERSONAL: Born May 30, 1939, in Passaic, NJ; son of Michael John and Sonia (Dubanowich) Pollard; married Beth Howland (an actress), November, 1961 (divorced); children: Holly.

VOCATION: Actor.

CAREER: STAGE DEBUT—*Anniversary Waltz,* Nutley, NJ, 1955. BROADWAY DEBUT—Joe Glover, *Comes a Day,* Ambassador Theatre, 1958. PRINCIPAL STAGE APPEARANCES—Wally Webb, *Our Town,* Circle in the Square, New York City, 1959; Geoffrey Beamis, *A Loss of Roses,* Eugene O'Neill Theatre, New York City, 1959; Hugo Peabody, *Bye Bye Birdie,* Martin Beck Theatre, New York City, 1960; Marvin, *Enter Laughing,* Henry Miller's Theatre, New York City, 1963; Headmaster, *Leda Had a Little Swan,* Cort Theatre, New York City, 1968; Emerson, *Curse of the Starving Class,* Public Theatre, New York City, 1978.

PRINCIPAL FILM APPEARANCES—George, *Adventures of a Young Man* (also known as *Hemingway's Adventures of a Young Man*), Twentieth Century-Fox, 1962; Jelly, *The Stripper* (also known as *Woman of Summer*), Twentieth Century-Fox, 1963; Digby Popham, *Summer Magic,* Buena Vista, 1963; Stanley, *The Russians Are Coming, The Russians Are Coming,* United Artists, 1966; Pigmy, *The Wild Angels,* American International, 1966; C.W. Moss, *Bonnie and Clyde,* Warner Brothers, 1967; Barney, *Caprice,* Twentieth Century-Fox, 1967; Marvin, *Enter Laughing,* Columbia, 1967; Dill, *Jigsaw,* Universal, 1968; Packy, *Hannibal Brooks,* United Artists, 1969; Little Fauss, *Little Fauss and Big Halsey,* Paramount, 1970; Marshal, *The Legend of Frenchie King* (also known as *Les Petroleuses, The Petroleum Girls,* and *The Oil Girls*), Hemdale, 1971; Billy Bonnery, *Dirty Little Billy,* Columbia, 1972; Leroy, *Sunday in the Country,* American International, 1975; hawker, *Between the Lines,* Midwest Films, 1977; Little Red, *Melvin and Howard,* Universal, 1980; Bob Jolly, *America,* ASA, 1986; Howard, *The Patriot,* Crown International, 1986; Andy, *Roxanne,* Columbia, 1987; Bob, *Season of Fear,* Metro-Goldwyn-Mayer/United Artists (MGM/UA), 1989; Stanley Willard, *Night*

Visitor, MGM/UA, 1989. Also appeared in *Heated Vengeance,* 1984; and *Scrooged,* Paramount, 1988.

PRINCIPAL TELEVISION APPEARANCES—Series: Leonard, *Leo and Liz in Beverly Hills,* CBS, 1986. Pilots: Spider, *The Miss and the Missiles,* CBS, 1964. Episodic: Cousin Virgil, *The Andy Griffith Show,* CBS, 1962; alien boy, *Lost in Space,* CBS, 1966; Jahn, "Miri," *Star Trek,* NBC, 1967; Mr. Mxyzptlk, *Superboy,* syndicated, 1989; also Jerome Krebs, *Dobie Gillis,* CBS; Ted Mooney, Jr., *The Lucy Show,* CBS; *Gunsmoke,* CBS; *The Nurses,* CBS; *Alfred Hitchcock Presents.* Movies: Piero, *The Smugglers,* NBC, 1968. Specials: *Henry Fonda and the Family,* CBS, 1962. Also appeared in *Five Fingers.*

AWARDS: Academy Award nomination, Best Supporting Actor, 1967, for *Bonnie and Clyde.*

MEMBER: American Federation of Television and Radio Artists, Actors' Equity Association, Screen Actors Guild.

ADDRESSES: AGENT—International Creative Management, 40 W. 57th Street, New York, NY 10019.*

*   *   *

POSTER, Steven

PERSONAL: Born in Chicago, IL; married Lynne Griffin (an actress). EDUCATION: Graduated from the Illinois Institute of Technology; also attended Southern Illinois University and the Los Angeles Art College of Design.

VOCATION: Cinematographer.

CAREER: PRINCIPAL FILM WORK—All as cinematographer, unless indicated: Second unit photographer, *Close Encounters of the Third Kind,* Columbia, 1977; *Blood Beach,* AVCO-Embassy, 1981; *Dead and Buried,* AVCO-Embassy, 1981; second unit photographer, *Blade Runner,* Warner Brothers, 1982; second unit photographer, *Best Little Whorehouse in Texas,* Universal, 1982; *Strange Brew,* Metro-Goldwyn-Mayer/United Artists, 1983; *Spring Break,* Columbia, 1983; *Testament,* Paramount, 1983; *The New Kids,* Columbia, 1985; *The Heavenly Kid,* Orion, 1985; *Blue City,* Paramount, 1986; (with Adam Holender) *The Boy Who Could Fly,* Twentieth Century-Fox, 1986; *Someone to Watch Over Me,* Columbia, 1987; *Big Top Pee Wee,* Paramount, 1988; also *Aloha Summer.*

PRINCIPAL TELEVISION WORK—All as cinematographer. Series: *The Duke,* NBC, 1979. Pilots: *The Night Rider,* NBC, 1979. Movies: *The Grass Is Always Greener,* CBS, 1978; *Coward of the County,* CBS, 1981; *The Cradle Will Fall,* CBS, 1983; *Courage,* CBS, 1986; *I'll Take Manhattan,* CBS, 1987.

RELATED CAREER—Cinematographer for television commercials, industrial films, and documentaries in Chicago, IL, and for worldwide television commercials for Pepsi Cola, Ford, Bank Indo-Suez, and Snickers candy bars.

MEMBER: International Alliance of Theatrical Stage Employees, American Society of Cinematographers.

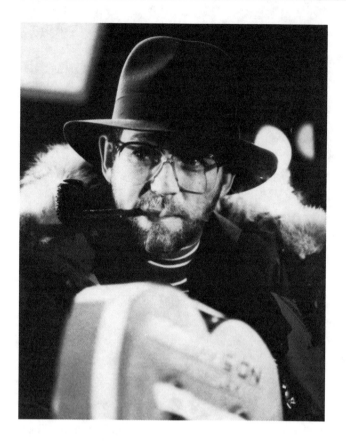

STEVEN POSTER

ADDRESSES: PUBLICIST—The Garrett Company, 6922 Hollywood Boulevard, Los Angeles, CA 90028.

*　　*　　*

POTTS, Annie

PERSONAL: Born October 28, in Nashville, TN; children: Clay. EDUCATION: Attended Stephens College.

VOCATION: Actress.

CAREER: FILM DEBUT—Vanessa, *Corvette Summer* (also known as *The Hot One*), United Artists, 1978. PRINCIPAL FILM APPEARANCES—Persa, *King of the Gypsies*, Dino De Laurentiis/Paramount, 1978; Bonnie Howard, *Heartaches*, Rising Star, 1981; Amy Grady, *Crimes of Passion*, New World, 1984; Janine Melnitz, *Ghostbusters*, Columbia, 1984; Liz Carlson, *Jumpin' Jack Flash*, Twentieth Century-Fox, 1985; Iona, *Pretty in Pink*, Paramount, 1986; Darla, *Pass the Ammo*, New Century, 1988; Helen Downing, *Who's Harry Crumb?*, Tri-Star, 1989. Also appeared in *Stick*, Universal, 1985.

PRINCIPAL TELEVISION APPEARANCES—Series: Edith Bedelmeyer, *Goodtime Girls*, ABC, 1980; Mary Jo Shively, *Designing Women*, CBS, 1986—. Pilots: Phoebe, *Hollywood High*, NBC, 1977; Paula

Lundell, *Hollywood High*, NBC, 1977; Flatbed Annie, *Flatbed Annie and Sweetiepie: Lady Truckers*, CBS, 1979; Annie Leighton, *In Security*, CBS, 1982; Annie, *Hearts of Steel*, ABC, 1986. Episodic: Kathy Lawry, "Wordplay," *The Twilight Zone*, CBS, 1985; Tracy Spencer, *Magnum P.I.*, CBS, 1986; also *Lime Street*, ABC, 1985. Movies: Linda Cleary, *Black Market Baby*, ABC, 1977; Sunday, *Something So Right*, CBS, 1982; D.G., *Cowboy*, CBS, 1983; Cindy Mills, *It Came Upon the Midnight Clear*, syndicated, 1984; Daria, *Why Me?*, ABC, 1984; Louise, *The Man Who Fell to Earth*, ABC, 1987. Specials: Host, *CBS Tournament of Roses Parade*, CBS, 1987; Kathy Sanders, *My Dissident Mom*, CBS, 1987; also *Miss Ruby's Southern Holiday Dinner*, PBS, 1988.

RELATED CAREER—Actress in summer theatre productions; also set and costume designer for stage productions.

NON-RELATED CAREER—Spokesperson for the Arthritis Foundation; auxiliary board member, Mothers Against Drunk Drivers (M.A.D.D.).

SIDELIGHTS: RECREATIONS—Swimming and yoga.

ADDRESSES: AGENT—Triad Artists, 10100 Santa Monica Boulevard, 16th Floor, Los Angeles, CA 90067. PUBLICIST—Karen Samfilippo, P/M/K Public Relations, 8436 W. Third Street, Suite 650, Los Angeles, CA 90048.

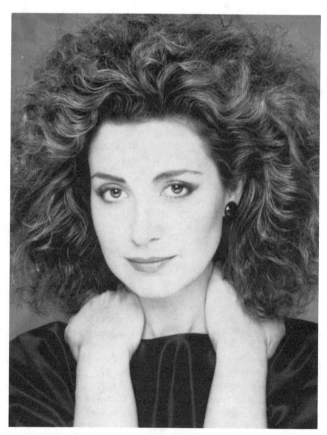

ANNIE POTTS

POWELL, Jane   1929-

PERSONAL: Born Suzanne Burce, April 1, 1929 (some sources say 1928), in Portland, OR; daughter of Paul and Eileen Burce; married Geary Steffen, 1953 (divorced); married Pat Nerney (divorced, 1963); married James Fitzgerald, June 27, 1965 (marriage ended); married David Parlour, 1978 (marriage ended); married Dick Moore (a public relations executive and former child actor), 1988; children: Geary, Suzanne (first marriage); Lindsay (second marriage).

VOCATION: Actress and singer.

CAREER: PRINCIPAL STAGE APPEARANCES—Irene O'Dare, *Irene,* Minskoff Theatre, New York City, 1973.

MAJOR TOURS—In productions of *South Pacific, Oklahoma!, My Fair Lady,* and *The Sound of Music.*

FILM DEBUT—As herself, *Song of the Open Road,* United Artists, 1944. PRINCIPAL FILM APPEARANCES—Cheryl Williams, *Delightfully Dangerous,* United Artists, 1945; Christine Evans, *Holiday in Mexico,* Metro-Goldwyn-Mayer (MGM), 1946; Judy Foster, *A Date with Judy,* MGM, 1948; Polly Bradford, *Luxury Liner,* MGM, 1948; Tess Morgan, *Three Daring Daughters* (also known as *The Birds and the Bees*), MGM, 1948; Nancy Barklay, *Nancy Goes to Rio,* MGM, 1950; Patti Robinson, *Two Weeks with Love,* MGM, 1950; Elizabeth Rogers, *Rich, Young, and Pretty,* MGM, 1951; Ellen Bowen, *Royal Wedding* (also known as *Wedding Bells*), MGM, 1951; Cindy Kimbell, *Small Town Girl,* MGM, 1953; Penny Weston, *Three Sailors and a Girl,* Warner Brothers, 1953; title role, *Athena,* MGM, 1954; as herself, *Deep in My Heart,* MGM, 1954; Milly, *Seven Brides for Seven Brothers,* MGM, 1954; Susan Smith, *Hit the Deck,* MGM, 1955; Dodie, *The Girl Most Likely,* Universal, 1957; Fayaway, *The Enchanted Island,* Warner Brothers, 1958; Penny Windsor, *The Female Animal,* Universal, 1958; singer at rally, *Marie,* Metro-Goldwyn-Mayer/United Artists, 1985.

PRINCIPAL TELEVISION APPEARANCES—Series: Regular, *Turn of Fate,* NBC, 1957-58; also *Alcoa/Goodyear Theatre,* NBC, 1957-58; *Loving,* ABC. Pilots: Elaine Anderson, *The Letters,* ABC, 1973. Episodic: *Fantasy Island,* ABC, 1978; *The Love Boat,* ABC, 1981; also *The Dick Powell Show,* NBC; *The June Allyson Show,* CBS. Movies: Kitty Douglass, *Mayday at 40,000 Feet!,* CBS, 1976. Specials: Clementine, *Ruggles of Red Gap,* NBC, 1957; *Standard Oil Anniversary Show,* NBC, 1957; *Give My Regards to Broadway,* NBC, 1959; Esther, *Meet Me in St. Louis,* CBS, 1959; *The Victor Borge Show,* NBC, 1960; *The Victor Borge Special,* NBC, 1960; *Hooray for Love,* CBS, 1960; Julie Balfour, *Feathertop,* ABC, 1961; host, *The Jane Powell Show,* NBC, 1961; *The Danny Thomas Special,* NBC, 1967.

RELATED CAREER—Hostess of her own program on KOIN-Radio, Portland, OR; singer on various network radio programs; singer in nightclubs and touring stage shows; has produced and appears in an exercise video for arthritis patients.

WRITINGS: The Girl Next Door . . . and How She Grew (autobiography), Morrow, 1988.

ADDRESSES: AGENT—Hal Stalmaster, The Artists Group, 1930 Century Park W., Suite 303, Los Angeles, CA 90067.*

PRENTISS, Paula   1939-

PERSONAL: Born Paula Ragusa, March 4, 1939, in San Antonio, TX; married Richard Benjamin (an actor and director); children: Ross Thomas. EDUCATION: Northwestern University, B.A., drama, 1959.

VOCATION: Actress.

CAREER: PRINCIPAL STAGE APPEARANCES—Stewardess, *The Great Airplane Snatch,* and Fido, *Arf,* both Stage 73, New York City, 1969; also appeared in a production of *As You Like It.*

PRINCIPAL FILM APPEARANCES—Tuggle Carpenter, *Where the Boys Are,* Metro-Goldwyn-Mayer (MGM), 1960; Linda Delavane, *Bachelor in Paradise,* MGM, 1961; Pam Dunstan, *The Honeymoon Machine,* MGM, 1961; Lieutenant Molly Blue, *The Horizontal Lieutenant,* MGM, 1962; Toni Denham, *Follow the Boys,* MGM, 1963; as herself, *Looking for Love,* MGM, 1964; Abigail Page, *Man's Favorite Sport(?),* Universal, 1964; Stella, *The World of Henry Orient,* United Artists, 1964; Bev McConnel, *In Harm's Way,* Paramount, 1965; Liz, *What's New Pussycat?,* United Artists, 1965; Nurse Duckett, *Catch-22,* Filmways, 1970; Dolly Jaffe, *Move,* Twentieth Century-Fox, 1970; Veronica, *Born to Win,* United Artists, 1971; Bobbi Michele, *Last of the Red Hot Lovers,* Paramount, 1972; Anne, *Crazy Joe,* Columbia, 1974; Lee Carter, *The Parallax View,* Paramount, 1974; Bobby, *The Stepford Wives,* Columbia, 1975; Sergeant Natalie Zimmerman, *The Black Marble,* AVCO-Embassy, 1980; Celia Clooney, *Buddy Buddy,* Metro-Goldwyn-Mayer/United Artists, 1981; Mary, *Saturday the 14th,* New World, 1981. Also appeared in *Scraping Bottom.*

PRINCIPAL TELEVISION APPEARANCES—Series: Paula Hollister, *He and She,* CBS, 1967-68. Pilots: Trish Canfield, *Having Babies II,* ABC, 1977. Movies: Barbara Hamilton, *The Couple Takes a Wife,* ABC, 1972; Sandy MacIntosh, *Friendships, Secrets, and Lies,* NBC, 1979; Norma Cully, *Top of the Hill,* syndicated, 1980; Lynne Wiley, *M.A.D.D.: Mothers against Drunk Drivers,* NBC, 1983; Diana Webber, *Packin' It In,* CBS, 1983.

ADDRESSES: AGENT—Phil Gersh, The Gersh Agency, Inc., 222 N. Canon Drive, Beverly Hills, CA 90210.*

*   *   *

PRESSBURGER, Emeric   1902-1988
(Richard Imrie)

PERSONAL: Born Imre Pressburger, December 5, 1902, in Miskolc, Hungary (now Romania); died of bronchial pneumonia, February 5, 1988, in Saxstead, England; married; children: Angela. EDUCATION: Attended the University of Prague and the University of Stuttgart.

VOCATION: Writer, producer, and director.

CAREER: Also see *WRITINGS* below. PRINCIPAL FILM WORK—Director, *One of Our Aircraft Is Missing,* United Artists, 1942; producer, *Colonel Blimp* (also known as *The Life and Death of Colonel Blimp*), Archers/General, 1943; producer and director, *A Canterbury Tale,* Eagle/Lion, 1944; producer (with Michael Powell and Ralph Richardson), *The Silver Fleet,* Producers Releasing Corporation, 1945; producer (with Powell) and director, *I Know*

Where I'm Going, Universal, 1945; producer (with Powell) and director, *Stairway to Heaven* (also known as *A Matter of Life and Death*), Universal, 1946; producer (with Powell) and director, *Black Narcissus,* Universal, 1947; producer (with Powell), *The End of the River,* General Films Distributors, 1947; producer (with Powell) and director, *The Red Shoes,* Eagle/Lion, 1948; producer (with Powell) and director, *Hour of Glory* (also known as *The Small Back Room*), British Lion, 1949; director, *The Fighting Pimpernel* (also known as *The Elusive Pimpernel*), British/Lion, 1950; director, *The Wild Heart* (also known as *Gone to Earth*), RKO, 1950; producer (with Powell) and director, *The Tales of Hoffman,* Lopert, 1951; producer (with Powell) and director, *Pursuit of the Graf Spee* (also known as *Battle of the River Plate*), Rank, 1956; (with Powell) *Night Ambush,* Rank, 1957. Also producer and director, *Twice upon a Time,* 1953; producer and director, *Oh Rosalinda!,* 1955; producer, *Miracle in Soho,* 1957.

RELATED CAREER—Founder (with Michael Powell), Archers Film Producing Company, 1942-57; founder (with Powell), Vega Productions, Ltd.; writer, Universum-Film Aktien-Gesellschaft, Berlin, Germany; journalist in Hungary and Germany.

WRITINGS: FILM—(With Reinhold Schuenzel) *Beautiful Adventure,* Deutsche Universum-Film, 1932; (co-writer) *Spy for a Day,* Paramount, 1939; *The Spy in Black* (also known as *U-Boat Twenty-Nine*), Columbia, 1939; *Contraband* (also known as *Blackout*), Anglo-American, 1940; (with Gordon Welesley and Edward Dryhurst) *Sons of the Sea* (also known as *Atlantic Ferry*), Warner Brothers, 1941; *The Invaders* (also known as *The Forty-Ninth Parallel*), Columbia, 1942; (with Michael Powell) *One of Our Aircraft Is Missing,* United Artists, 1942; *Colonel Blimp* (also known as *The Life and Death of Colonel Blimp*), Archers/General, 1943; (with Powell) *A Canterbury Tale,* Eagle/Lion, 1944; (with Powell) *I Know Where I'm Going,* Universal, 1945; (with Powell) *Stairway to Heaven* (also known as *A Matter of Life and Death*), Universal, 1946; (with Rodney Ackland and Maurice Cowan) *Wanted for Murder* (also known as *A Voice in the Night*), Twentieth Century-Fox, 1946; (with Powell) *Black Narcissus,* Universal, 1947; (with Powell) *The Red Shoes,* Eagle/Lion, 1948, published by Avon, 1978; (with Powell) *The Wild Heart* (also known as *Gone to Earth*), RKO, 1950; (with Powell) *The Fighting Pimpernel* (also known as *The Elusive Pimpernel*), British/Lion, 1950; (with Powell) *The Tales of Hoffman,* Lopert, 1951; (with Powell) *Pursuit of the Graf Spee* (also known as *Battle of the River Plate*), Rank, 1956; (with Powell) *Night Ambush,* Rank, 1957; (as Richard Imrie; with Derry Quinn and Ray Rigby) *Operation Crossbow* (also known as *The Great Spy Mission*), Metro-Goldwyn-Mayer, 1965; *They're a Weird Mob,* British Empire, 1966; also (co-writer) *Abschied* (also known as *Farewell*), 1930; (co-writer) *Emil and the Detectives,* 1932; (co-writer) *La Vie Parisienne,* 1935; *Twice upon a Time,* 1952; *Oh Rosalinda!,* 1955; *Miracle in Soho,* 1957; *The Boy Who Turned Yellow,* 1972.

OTHER—(With Michael Powell) *Story of the Film: One of Our Aircraft Is Missing* (nonfiction), H.M.S.O., 1942; *Killing a Mouse on Sunday* (fiction), Harcourt, 1961, published in England as *Behold a Pale Horse,* Collins, 1964; *The Glass Pearls* (fiction), Heinemann, 1966.

AWARDS: Academy Award, Best Original Story, 1942, for *The Invaders* (also known as *The Forty-Ninth Parallel*); British Film Institute Special Award, 1978.

MEMBER: British Academy of Film and Television Arts, British Film Insititute.

OBITUARIES AND OTHER SOURCES: New York Times, February 6, 1988.*

*   *   *

PRINCE, William 1913-

PERSONAL: Full name, William LeRoy Prince; born January 26, 1913, in Nichols, NY; son of Gorman (in sales) and Myrtle (a nurse; maiden name, Osborne) Prince; married Dorothy Huass, October 27, 1934 (divorced, 1964); married Augusta Dapney; children: two sons, two daughters (first marriage). EDUCATION: Attended Cornell University, 1930-34; studied acting with Tamara Daykarhanova, 1936-37.

VOCATION: Actor.

CAREER: PRINCIPAL STAGE APPEARANCES—Servant to York, *Richard II,* St. James Theatre, New York City, 1937; page, *Hamlet,* St. James Theatre, 1938; John of Lancaster, *Henry IV, Part I,* St. James Theatre, 1939; Richard, *Ah! Wilderness,* Guild Theatre, New York City, 1941; Dan Proctor, *Guest in the House,* Plymouth Theatre, New York City, 1942; Callaghan Mallory, *Across the Board on Tomorrow Morning,* Belasco Theatre, New York City, 1942; Private Quizz West, *The Eve of St. Mark,* Cort Theatre, New York City, 1942; David Rice, *Judy O'Connor,* Shubert Theatre, New Haven, CT, then Copely Theatre, Boston, MA, 1946; John Lawrence, *John Loves Mary,* Booth Theatre, New York City, 1947; David Gibbs, *Forward the Heart,* 48th Street Theatre, New York City, 1949; Orlando, *As You Like It,* Cort Theatre, New York City, 1950; Christopher Isherwood, *I Am a Camera,* Empire Theatre, New York City, 1951; Captain Tom Cochran, *Affair of Honor,* Ethel Barrymore Theatre, New York City, 1956; Dr. Jonas Lockwood, *Third Best Sport,* Ambassador Theatre, New York City, 1958; Dr. Robert Leigh, *The Highest Tree,* Longacre Theatre, New York City, 1959.

Alec Grimes, *Venus at Large,* Morosco Theatrae, New York City, 1962; Charles Marsden, *Strange Interlude,* Hudson Theatre, New York City, 1963; Henry Macy, *The Ballad of the Sad Cafe,* Martin Beck Theatre, New York City, 1963; Bob McKellaway, *Mary, Mary,* Helen Hayes Theatre, New York City, 1964; Father Arnall and Preacher, *Stephen D.,* East 74th Street Theatre, New York City, 1967; William Marshall, *The Little Foxes,* Vivian Beaumont Theatre, New York City, 1967; Arthur, *Mercy Street,* American Place Theatre, St. Clement's Church Theatre, New York City, 1969; James Tyrone, *Long Day's Journey into Night,* Center Stage, Baltimore, MD, 1970; Gracie, *The Silent Partner,* Actors Studio, New York City, 1972; Davies, *The Caretaker,* Roundabout Theatre, New York City, 1973; Charlie, *Seascape,* Ahmanson Theatre, Los Angeles, CA, 1975; He, *Counting the Ways,* and Man, *Listening,* both Hartford Stage Company, Hartford, CT, 1976; Weller Martin, *The Gin Game,* Studio Arena Theatre, Buffalo, NY, 1979; title role, *The Man Who Had Three Arms,* Lyceum Theatre, New York City, 1983; Mazzini Dunn, *Heartbreak House,* Circle in the Square, New York City, 1983. Also appeared in *The Eternal Road,* Manhattan Opera House, New York City, 1937; *In the Matter of J. Robert Oppenheimer,* Goodman Theatre, Chicago, IL, 1973; and in summer theatre productions at the Barter Theatre, Abingdon, VA, 1937, and the Playhouse Theatre, Eagles Mere, PA, 1940.

MAJOR TOURS—Servant to York, *Richard II*, U.S. cities, 1937-38; Bob McKellaway, *Mary, Mary*, U.S. cities, 1964.

FILM DEBUT—Pills, *Destination Tokyo*, Warner Brothers, 1943. PRINCIPAL FILM APPEARANCES—As himself, *Hollywood Canteen*, Warner Brothers, 1944; Fred, *The Very Thought of You*, Warner Brothers, 1944; Lieutenant Jacobs, *Objective Burma!*, Warner Brothers, 1945; Lieutenant Don Mallory, *Pillow to Post*, Warner Brothers, 1945; Bart Williams, *Cinderella Jones*, Warner Brothers, 1946; David MacKellar, *Shadow of a Woman*, Warner Brothers, 1946; Tony Salerno, Jr., *Carnegie Hall*, United Artists, 1947; Johnny Drake, *Dead Reckoning*, Columbia, 1947; Barry Storm, *Lust for Gold*, Columbia, 1949; Christian, *Cyrano de Bergerac*, United Artists, 1950; Robert Kendall, *Secret of Treasure Mountain*, Columbia, 1956; Rene, *The Vagabond King*, Paramount, 1956; Dr. Rodney Barrett, *Macabre*, Allied Artists, 1958.

William Thompson, *Sacco and Vanzetti* (also known as *Sacco e Vanzetti*), UMC, 1971; Colorado man, *The Heartbreak Kid*, Twentieth Century-Fox, 1972; Powers, *Blade*, Pintoff, 1973; artist, *The Stepford Wives*, Columbia, 1975; Bishop, *Family Plot*, Universal, 1976; Edward George Ruddy, *Network*, Metro-Goldwyn-Mayer/United Artists (MGM/UA), 1976; Mr. Cooper, *Fire Sale*, Twentieth Century-Fox, 1977; Blakelock, *The Gauntlet*, Warner Brothers, 1977; Quinlan, *Rollercoaster*, Universal, 1977; Olympus, *The Cat from Outer Space*, Buena Vista, 1978; George Calloway, *The Promise* (also known as *Face of a Stranger*), Universal, 1979; Edgar, *Bronco Billy*, Warner Brothers, 1980; Reverend Hollis, *Kiss Me Goodbye*, Twentieth Century-Fox, 1982; Ambassador Paultz, *Love and Money*, Paramount, 1982; President of the United States, *The Soldier* (also known as *Codename: The Soldier*), Embassy, 1982; Mitchell, *Fever Pitch*, MGM/UA, 1985; Louis Martin, *Movers and Shakers*, MGM/UA, 1985; Mr. Keyes, *Spies Like Us*, Warner Brothers, 1985; H.H. Royce, *Assassination*, Cannon, 1987; Clarence Middleton, *Nuts*, Warner Brothers, 1987. Also appeared in *Roughly Speaking*, Warner Brothers, 1945; and in *Vice Versa*, Columbia, 1988.

PRINCIPAL TELEVISION APPEARANCES—Series: Peter Guilfoyle, *The Mask*, ABC, 1954; Richard Adams, *Justice*, NBC, 1955-56; Dr. Jerry Malone, *Young Dr. Malone*, NBC, 1958-63; Jason Cook, *The American Girls*, CBS, 1978; also Ken Baxter, *Another World*, NBC; judge, *Where the Heart Is*, CBS; Russell Barry, *A World Apart*, ABC. Mini-Series: Jay Regan, *Captains and the Kings*, NBC, 1976; Robert Wheeler, *The Best of Families*, PBS, 1977; Judge Kendrick, *Aspen* (also known as *The Innocent and the Damned*), NBC, 1977; Alex Spaulding, *The Rhinemann Exchange*, NBC, 1977; William Fairfax, *George Washington*, CBS, 1984. Pilots: Senator, *Key West*, NBC, 1973; Clayton Nichols, *Night Games*, NBC, 1974; Thomas Marshall Bibb/Mr. White, *Moonlight*, CBS, 1982; Asa Lamar, *Joe Dancer: Murder One, Dancer 0*, NBC, 1983. Episodic: "The Second Oldest Profession," *Philco Playhouse*, NBC, 1950; "Pretend I Am a Stranger," *Philco Playhouse*, NBC, 1951; "Night of the Vulcan," *Philco Playhouse*, NBC, 1951; "A Man and His Conscience," *Armstrong Circle Theatre*, NBC, 1952; "A Volcano Is Dancing Here," *Armstrong Circle Theatre*, NBC, 1952; "Two Prisoners," *Armstrong Circle Theatre*, NBC, 1953; "Babylon Revisited," *Theatre for You*, 1953; *Modern Romances*, NBC, 1956, 1957, and 1958; *True Story*, NBC, 1957; "John Doe 154," *Armstrong Circle Theatre*, NBC, 1957; "The Meanest Crime in the World," *Armstrong Circle Theatre*, CBS, 1958; "All the King's Men," *Kraft Television Theatre*, NBC, 1958; *The Nurses*, CBS, 1964; also *The Chevrolet Tele-Theatre*, NBC; *Starlight Theatre*, CBS; "The Waxworks," *Suspense*, CBS.

Movies: Willard Dorsett, *Sybil*, NBC, 1976; Ambassador Joseph P. Kennedy, *Johnny, We Hardly Knew Ye*, NBC, 1977; O.A.U. chairman, *The Jericho Mile*, ABC, 1979; Harrison Crawford II, *City in Fear*, ABC, 1980; Supreme Court justice, *Gideon's Trumpet*, CBS, 1980; Milo Spears, *Make Me an Offer*, ABC, 1980; prefect, *A Time for Miracles*, ABC, 1980; Dr. Burgess, *A Matter of Life and Death*, CBS, 1981; George Peterson, *Found Money* (also known as *My Secret Angel*), NBC, 1983; Archbishop Stefan Corro, *Perry Mason: The Case of the Notorious Nun*, NBC, 1986. Specials: Mortimer Brewster, *Arsenic and Old Lace*, CBS, 1949; Bert Jefferson, "The Man Who Came to Dinner," *The Best of Broadway*, NBC, 1954; "An Enemy of the People," *NET Playhouse*, PBS, 1966; "Father Uxbridge Wants to Marry," *New York Television Theatre*, PBS, 1970; "All Over," *Great Performances*, PBS, 1978.

RELATED CAREER—Radio announcer, National Broadcasting Company.

MEMBER: Actors' Equity Association (council member, 1949-52), Screen Actors Guild, American Federation of Television and Radio Artists (board member, 1954-56).

ADDRESSES: OFFICE—Fred Amsel and Associates, 6310 San Vicente Boulevard, Suite 407, Los Angeles, CA 90048.*

*   *   *

PROCHNOW, Jurgen   1941-

PERSONAL: Born Juergen Prochnow, June 10, 1941, in Berlin, Germany; father, an engineer; married; children: one son. EDUCATION: Trained for the stage at the Folkswangschule, Essen, 1963-66.

VOCATION: Actor.

CAREER: FILM DEBUT—*Zoff* (also known as *The Hitch of It*), Gloria, 1971. PRINCIPAL FILM APPEARANCES—Franz Blum, *Die Verrohung des Franz Blum* (also known as *The Brutalization of Franz Blum*), Bioskop, 1975; Ludwig Gotten, *Die Verlorene Ehre der Katharina Blum* (also known as *The Lost Honor of Katharina Blum*), Cinema International/Nelson Entertainment, 1975; Martin Kurath, *Die Konsequenz* (also known as *The Consequence*), Almi Cinema 5/Prestige, 1977; Dr. Volker Schwartz, *Unter Verschluss* (also known as *Under Lock and Key*), Artus, 1979; Alex, *So Weit das Auge Reicht* (also known as *As Far as the Eye Sees*), Cactus, 1980; captain, *Das Boot* (also known as *The Boat*), Columbia, 1982; General Siegfried Kapler, *Comeback*, Twentieth Century-Fox, 1982; Woermann, *The Keep*, Paramount, 1983; Kevin, *Krieg und Frieden* (also known as *War and Peace*), Teleculture, 1983; Duke Leto Atreides, *Dune*, Dino De Laurentiis/Universal, 1984; cop, *Der Bulle und das Madchen* (also known as *The Cop and the Girl*), Atlas, 1985; Ralph Korda, *Killing Cars*, Sentana, 1986; Maxwell Dent, *Beverly Hills Cop II*, Paramount, 1987; Escher, *Devil's Paradise*, Overview, 1987; doctor, monsieur, and driver of "Little Brother," *Terminus*, Hemdale, 1987; boarder, *The Seventh Sign*, Tri-Star, 1988. Also appeared in *Zaertlichkeit der Woelfe* (also known as *The Tenderness of Wolves*), Filmverlag der Autoren, 1973; *Einer von uns Beiden* (also known as *One or the Other*), Transocean International, 1978.

PRINCIPAL TELEVISION APPEARANCES—Series: *Harbour at the*

River Rhine, 1970. Movies: General Serge Kapler, *Love Is Forever,* NBC, 1983; Fritz Friedlander, *Forbidden,* HBO, 1985; Adam Berwid, *Murder: By Reason of Insanity,* CBS, 1985.

RELATED CAREER—Stage actor in West Germany for seven years.

NON-RELATED CAREER—Bank clerk.

ADDRESSES: AGENT—Paul Schwartzman, International Creative Management, 8899 Beverly Boulevard, Los Angeles, CA 90048.*

*   *   *

PRYCE, Jonathan   1947-

PERSONAL: Born June 1, 1947, in Wales. EDUCATION: Trained for the stage at the Royal Academy of Dramatic Art.

VOCATION: Actor.

CAREER: BROADWAY DEBUT—Gethin Price, *Comedians,* Music Box Theater, 1976. PRINCIPAL STAGE APPEARANCES—Rainer, *Heroes,* Royal Court Theatre Upstairs, London, 1975; Gethin Price, *Comedians,* and Belvawny, *Engaged,* both National Theatre Company, Old Vic Theatre, London, 1975; Count Ludovico, *The White Devil,* Old Vic Theatre, 1976; Rainer, *Heroes,* Theatre Upstairs, London, 1975; Jakob Lenz, *Lenz,* Hampstead Theatre Club, London, 1976; Angelo, *Measure for Measure,* Royal Shakespeare Company (RSC), Royal Shakespeare Theatre, Stratford-on-Avon, U.K., 1978; Petruchio, *The Taming of the Shrew,* and Octavius Caesar, *Antony and Cleopatra,* both RSC, Royal Shakespeare Theatre, 1978, then Aldwych Theatre, London, 1979; the Fool, *Accidental Death of an Anarchist,* Belasco Theatre, New York City, 1984; Astrov, *Uncle Vanya,* Vaudeville Theatre, London, 1988. Also appeared in the title role, *Macbeth,* with the Royal Shakespeare Company.

PRINCIPAL FILM APPEARANCES—Joseph Manasse, *Voyage of the Damned,* AVCO-Embassy, 1977; Ken, *Breaking Glass,* Paramount, 1980; Taylor, *Loophole,* Brent Walker, 1981; Christian Magny, *Praying Mantis,* Channel Four, 1982; Mr. Dark, *Something Wicked This Way Comes,* Buena Vista, 1983; James Penfield, *The Ploughman's Lunch,* Samuel Goldwyn, 1984; Sam Lowry, *Brazil,* Universal, 1985; Robert Fallon, *The Doctor and the Devils,* Twentieth Century-Fox, 1985; Charles, *Haunted Honeymoon,* Orion, 1986; Jack, *Jumpin' Jack Flash,* Twentieth Century-Fox, 1986; Michael, *Man on Fire,* Tri-Star, 1987; Sean, *Hotel London,* Retake Film and Video Collective, 1987; Farris, *Consuming Passions,* Samuel Goldwyn, 1988; Horatio Jackson, *The Adventures of Baron Munchausen,* Columbia, 1989.

PRINCIPAL TELEVISION APPEARANCES—Series: Roger Flower, *Roger Doesn't Live Here Anymore,* Entertainment Channel, 1982-83. Movies: King Herod, *The Day Christ Died,* CBS, 1980; Mr. Ellsworthy, *Agatha Christie's "Murder Is Easy,"* CBS, 1982. Also appeared in *Comedians, Playthings, Partisans, For Tea on Sunday,* and *Timon of Athens.*

AWARDS: Theatre World Award, 1977, for *Comedians.*

ADDRESSES: AGENT—Tom Korman, Agency for the Performing Arts, 9000 Sunset Boulevard, Suite 1200, Los Angeles, CA 90069.*

*   *   *

PULLMAN, Bill

PERSONAL: Born in Delhi, NY; father, a physician; mother, a nurse. EDUCATION: Attended State University of New York, Oneonta; received M.F.A. in directing from the University of Massachusetts, Amherst.

VOCATION: Actor.

CAREER: PRINCIPAL STAGE APPEARANCES—Robinson, *The Old Flag,* George Street Playhouse, New Brunswick, NJ, 1983; Reuben, "Simon of Cyrene" in *Dramathon '84,* Quaigh Theatre, New York City, 1984; Wesley, *Curse of the Starving Class,* INTAR Theatre, New York City, 1985; Chris Keller, *All My Sons,* and title role, *Barabbas,* both Los Angeles Theatre Center, Los Angeles, CA, 1986. Also appeared under the name William Pullman in *The Rover,* Folger Theatre Group, Washington, DC, 1981; and as Bill Pullman in *Ah, Wilderness!,* GeVa Theatre, Rochester, NY, 1983; with Playwrights Horizons, New York City; and with the Ensemble Studio Theatre, New York City.

PRINCIPAL FILM APPEARANCES—Earl, *Ruthless People,* Touchstone, 1986; Lone Starr, *Spaceballs,* Metro-Goldwyn-Mayer/United Artists, 1987; Dennis Alan, *The Serpent and the Rainbow,* Universal, 1988; Julian Hedge, *The Accidental Tourist,* Warner Brothers, 1989.

RELATED CAREER—Co-founder, Jam Center (theatre company), Los Angeles, CA; theatre instructor, Montana State University, Bozeman, MT.

NON-RELATED CAREER—Worked in a liquor store.

ADDRESSES: AGENT—J.J. Morris and Elaine Goldsmith, William Morris Agency, 151 El Camino Drive, Beverly Hills, CA 90212.*

Q

QUARRY, Robert 1924-

PERSONAL: Born November 3, 1924, in Santa Rosa, CA. EDUCATION: Trained for the stage at the Actors' Lab.

VOCATION: Actor.

CAREER: BROADWAY DEBUT—Silvius, As You Like It, Cort Theatre, 1950. PRINCIPAL STAGE APPEARANCES—Lucentio, The Taming of the Shrew, City Center Theatre, New York City, 1951.

PRINCIPAL FILM APPEARANCES—Phil, House of Bamboo, Twentieth Century-Fox, 1955; Frank Stewart, Soldier of Fortune, Twentieth Century-Fox, 1955; Dwight Powell, A Kiss Before Dying, United Artists, 1956; reporter, Crime of Passion, United Artists, 1957; Borg, Agent for H.A.R.M., Universal, 1966; Sam Jagin, Winning, Universal, 1969; title role, Count Yorga, Vampire, American International, 1970; title role, The Return of Count Yorga, American International, 1971; Khorda, The Deathmaster, American International, 1972; Biederbeck, Doctor Phibes Rises Again, American International, 1972; Oliver Quayle, Madhouse, American International, 1974; Dr. Pritchet, The Midnight Man, Universal, 1974; Morgan, Sugar Hill (also known as The Voodoo Girl and The Zombies of Sugar Hill), American International, 1974; mayor, Rollercoaster, Universal, 1977; Milo, Commando Squad, Trans World, 1987; Knowles, Cyclone, Cinetel, 1987; Dr. Khorda, Moon in Scorpio, Trans World, 1987. Also appeared in WUSA, Paramount, 1970.

PRINCIPAL TELEVISION APPEARANCES—Series: Assistant, Hollywood Screen Test, ABC, 1949. Pilots: Michael Anthony, The Millionaire, CBS, 1978. Episodic: Mumphrey, Fortune Dane, ABC, 1986.*

* * *

QUINN, Anthony 1915-

PERSONAL: Full name, Anthony Rudolph Oaxaca Quinn; born April 21, 1915, in Chihuahua, Mexico; naturalized U.S. citizen, 1947; son of Frank and Manuela (Oaxaca) Quinn; married Katherine de Mille, October 2, 1937 (divorced, 1965); married Iolanda Addolori, January, 1966; children: Christina, Kathleen, Duncan, Valentina (first marriage); Francesco, Daniele, Lorenzo (second marriage).

VOCATION: Actor.

CAREER: STAGE DEBUT—Clean Beds, 1936. BROADWAY DE-

BUT—Stephen S. Christopher, The Gentleman from Athens, Mansfield Theatre, 1947. PRINCIPAL STAGE APPEARANCES—Stanley Kowalski, A Streetcar Named Desire, City Center Theatre, New York City, 1950; Texas, Borned in Texas, Fulton Theatre, New York City, 1950; Alvin Connors, Let Me Hear the Melody, Playhouse Theatre, Wilmington, DE, 1951; Henry II, Becket, St. James Theatre, New York City, 1960; Caesario Grimaldi, Tchin-Tchin, Plymouth Theatre, New York City, 1962; King del Rey, The Red Devil Battery Sign, Shubert Theatre, Boston, MA, 1975; title role, Zorba!, Broadway Theatre, New York City, 1983.

MAJOR TOURS—Stanley Kowalski, A Streetcar Named Desire, U.S. cities, 1948-49; title role, Zorba!, U.S. cities, 1983-86.

FILM DEBUT—Zingo Browning, Parole, Universal, 1936. PRINCIPAL FILM APPEARANCES—A hood, Night Waitress, RKO, 1936; a gangster, Sworn Enemy, Metro-Goldwyn-Mayer (MGM), 1936; Harry Morgan, Daughter of Shanghai, Paramount, 1937; Captain Ricardo Alvarez, The Last Train from Madrid, Paramount, 1937; Nicholas Mazaney, Partners in Crime, Paramount, 1937; Cheyenne warrior, The Plainsman, Paramount, 1937; the Don, Swing High, Swing Low, Paramount, 1937; Kimo, Waikiki Wedding, Paramount, 1937; Beluche, The Buccaneer, Paramount, 1938; Deane Fordline, Bulldog Drummond in Africa, Paramount, 1938; Nicholas Kusnoff, Dangerous to Know, Paramount, 1938; Legs, Hunted Men (also known as Crime Gives Orders), Paramount, 1938; Lou Gedney, King of Alcatraz, Paramount, 1938; Marty, Tip-Off Girls, Paramount, 1938; Chang Tai, Island of Lost Men, Paramount, 1939; Mike Gordon, King of Chinatown, Paramount, 1939; Forbes, Television Spy, Paramount, 1939; Jack Cordray, Union Pacific, Paramount, 1939.

Nick Buller, Emergency Squad, Paramount, 1940; Ramon and Francisco Maderos, The Ghost Breakers, Paramount, 1940; Francis "Big Boy" Bradmore, Parole Fixer, Paramount, 1940; Caesar, Road to Singapore, Paramount, 1940; Joe Yuma, Texas Rangers Ride Again, Paramount, 1940; Manolo de Palma, Blood and Sand, Twentieth Century-Fox, 1941; Tony Van Dyne, Bullets for O'Hara, Warner Brothers, 1941; Murray Burns, City for Conquest, Warner Brothers, 1941; Trego, Knockout, Warner Brothers, 1941; Alex Moreno, The Perfect Snob, Twentieth Century-Fox, 1941; Chic Collins, Thieves Fall Out, Warner Brothers, 1941; Wogan, The Black Swan, Twentieth Century-Fox, 1942; Leo Dexter, Larceny, Inc., Warner Brothers, 1942; Mullay Kasim, Road to Morocco, Paramount, 1942; Crazy Horse, They Died with Their Boots On, Warner Brothers, 1942; Jesus "Soose" Alvarez, Guadalcanal Diary, Twentieth Century-Fox, 1943; Juan Martines, The Ox-Bow Incident (also known as Strange Incident), Twentieth Century-Fox, 1943; Yellow Hand, Buffalo Bill, Twentieth Century-Fox, 1944; Al Jackson, Irish Eyes Are Smiling, Twentieth Century-Fox, 1944; Michael Romanescue, Ladies of Washington, Twentieth Century-

Fox, 1944; George Carroll, *Roger Touhy, Gangster!* (also known as *The Last Gangster*), Twentieth Century-Fox, 1944; Captain Andres Bonifacio, *Back to Bataan*, RKO, 1945; Chen Ta, *China Sky*, RKO, 1945; Indian chief, *Where Do We Go from Here?*, Twentieth Century-Fox, 1945; Don Luis Rivera y Hernandez, *California*, Paramount, 1946; Charley Eagle, *Black Gold*, Monogram, 1947; Jose Martinez, *The Imperfect Lady*, Paramount, 1947; Emir, *Sinbad the Sailor*, RKO, 1947; Enrique "Ricky" Vargas, *Tycoon*, RKO, 1947.

Raul Fuentes, *The Brave Bulls*, Columbia, 1951; Giovanni LaRocca, *Mask of the Avenger*, Columbia, 1951; Roc Brasiliano, *Against All Flags*, Universal, 1952; Prince Ramon, *The Brigand*, Columbia, 1952; Eufemio Zapata, *Viva Zapata!*, Twentieth Century-Fox, 1952; Portugee, *The World in His Arms*, Universal, 1952; Paco, *Blowing Wild*, Warner Brothers, 1953; Tony Bartlett, *City beneath the Sea* (also known as *One Hour to Doomsday*), Universal, 1953; Kiang, *East of Sumatra*, Universal, 1953; Alfio, *Fatal Desire* (also known as *Cavalleria rusticana*), Ultra, 1953; Jose Esqueda, *Ride, Vaquero!*, MGM, 1953; Osceola/John Powell, *Seminole*, Universal, 1953; Johnny McBride, *The Long Wait*, United Artists, 1954; Luis Santos, *The Magnificent Matador* (also known as *The Brave and the Beautiful*), Twentieth Century-Fox, 1955; Phil Regal, *The Naked Street*, United Artists, 1955; Captain Gaspar de Portola, *Seven Cities of Gold*, Twentieth Century-Fox, 1955; Antinous, *Ulysses*, Paramount, 1955; Francesco Caserto, *Angels of Darkness* (also known as *Forbidden Women* and *Donne proibite*), Supra, 1956; Zampano, *La Strada* (also known as *The Road*), Trans-Lux, 1956; Paul Gauguin, *Lust for Life*, MGM, 1956; Dave Robles, *The Man from Del Rio*, United Artists, 1956; Big Tom Kupfen, *The Wild Party*, United Artists, 1956; Quasimodo, *The Hunchback of Notre Dame*, Allied Artists, 1957; Bob Kallen, *The Ride Back*, United Artists, 1957; Ben Cameron, *The River's Edge*, Twentieth Century-Fox, 1957; Gino, *Wild Is the Wind*, Paramount, 1957; title role, *Attila*, Universal, 1958; Dominique, *The Buccaneer*, Paramount, 1958; Jack Duval, *Hot Spell*, Paramount, 1958; Frank Valentine, *The Black Orchid*, Paramount, 1959; Craig Belden, *The Last Train from Gun Hill*, Paramount, 1959; Tom Morgan, *Warlock*, Twentieth Century-Fox, 1959.

Tom Healy, *Heller in Pink Tights*, Paramount, 1960; Dr. David Rivera, *Portrait in Black*, Universal, 1960; Inuk, *The Savage Innocents*, Paramount, 1960; Colonel Andrea Stavros, *The Guns of Navarone*, Columbia, 1961; title role, *Barabbas*, Columbia, 1962; Auda Abu Tayi, *Lawrence of Arabia*, Columbia, 1962; Mountain Rivera, *Requiem for a Heavyweight*, Columbia, 1962; Captain Vinolas, *Behold a Pale Horse*, Columbia, 1964; Serge Miller, *The Visit* (also known as *Der Besuch*, *La Rancune*, and *La vendetta della signora*), Twentieth Century-Fox, 1964; Alexis Zorba, *Zorba the Greek*, International Classics, 1964; Juan Chavez, *A High Wind in Jamaica*, Twentieth Century-Fox, 1965; Lieutenant Colonel Pierre Raspeguy, *The Lost Command*, Columbia, 1966; Kublai Khan, *Marco the Magnificent* (also known as *Le meravigliose avventure di Marco Polo*, *La Fabuleuse aventure de Marco Polo*, and *Marco Polo*), MGM, 1966; Roc Delmonico, *The Happening*, Columbia, 1967; Peyrol, *The Rover* (also known as *L'avventuriero* and *The Adventurer*), Cinerama, 1967; Johann Moritz, *The 25th Hour* (also known as *La 25e Heure* and *La venticinquesima ora*), MGM, 1967; Leon Alastray, *Guns for San Sebastian* (also known as *La Bataille de San Sebastian*, *Los canones de San Sebastian*, and *I cannoni di San Sebastian*), MGM, 1968; Maurice Conchis, *The Magus*, Twentieth Century-Fox, 1968; Kiril Lakota, *The Shoes of the Fisherman*, MGM, 1968; Matsoukas, *A Dream of Kings*, National General, 1969; Italo Bombolini, *The Secret of Santa Vittoria*, United Artists, 1969.

Flapping Eagle, *Flap* (also known as *The Last Warrior*, *Nobody Loves a Drunken Indian*, and *Nobody Loves a Flapping Eagle*), Warner Brothers, 1970; Will Cade, *A Walk in the Spring Rain*, Columbia, 1970; Professor F.W.J. "Paco" Perez, *R.P.M.* (also known as *Revolutions per Minute*), Columbia, 1970; Captain Frank Matteli, *Across 110th Street*, United Artists, 1972; Erastus "Deaf" Smith, *Deaf Smith and Johnny Ears* (also known as *Los amigos*), MGM, 1973; Don Angelo, *The Don Is Dead* (also known as *Beautiful but Deadly*), Universal, 1973; Steve Ventura, *The Destructors* (also known as *The Marseilles Contract*), American International, 1974; Hamza, *Mohammad: Messenger of God* (also known as *Al-Risalah* and *The Message*), Tarik-Irwin Yablans, 1976; Zulfigar, *Caravans*, Ibex, 1978; Theo Tomasis, *The Greek Tycoon*, Universal, 1978; Gregorio Ferramonti, *The Inheritance* (also known as *L'Eredita Ferramonti*), S.J. International, 1978; the Basque, *The Passage*, United Artists, 1979; Bang, *The Con Artists* (also known as *The Con Man*), S.J. International, 1981; Mariano, *High Risk*, American Cinema, 1981; Omar Mukhtar, *Lion of the Desert*, United Film Distribution, 1981; Bruno Manzini, *The Salamander*, ITC, 1983. Also appeared in *The Milky Way*, Paramount, 1936; *High Treason*, General Film Distributors/Pacemaker-Mayer-Kingsley, 1951; narrator, *Arruza*, 1971; narrator, *The Voice of La Raza*, 1972; in *High Rollers* (also known as *Bluff*), 1976; *Tigers Don't Cry*, 1976; *Target of an Assassin*, 1978; as Sanchez, *The Children of Sanchez*, 1978; as Mosen Joaquin, *Valentina*, 1983; and as himself, *Ingrid* (documentary), 1985.

PRINCIPAL FILM WORK—Director, *The Buccaneer*, Paramount, 1958; executive producer, *Across 110th Street*, United Artists, 1972; also executive producer, *Mystique*, 1981.

PRINCIPAL TELEVISION APPEARANCES—Series: Mayor Thomas Jefferson Alacala, *The Man and the City*, ABC, 1971-72. Mini-Series: Narrator, *Ten Who Dared*, syndicated, 1977; Caiaphas, *Jesus of Nazareth*, NBC, 1977; Long John Silver, *Treasure Island* (also known as *L'isola del tesoro*), RAI-2 (Italian television), 1987; title role, *Onassis: The Richest Man in the World*, ABC, 1988. Pilots: Thomas Alacala, *The City*, ABC, 1971. Episodic: *Danger*, CBS; *Schlitz Playhouse*, CBS; *Lights Out*, NBC; *Ford Theater Hour*, NBC; *Philco Television Playhouse*, NBC; *The Dick Cavett Show*, ABC. Movies: *King: A Filmed Record . . . Montgomery to Memphis* (documentary), ABC, 1970. Specials: *Salute to Lady Liberty*, CBS, 1984; *Gregory Peck—His Own Man*, Cinemax, 1988; *The American Film Institute Salute to Gregory Peck*, NBC, 1989; also *Remembering Bing*, 1987.

NON-RELATED CAREER—As an artist, has had eight major exhibitions of his oil paintings, sculptures, and serigraphs throughout the United States.

WRITINGS: The Original Sin: A Self-Portrait (autobiography), Little Brown, 1972.

AWARDS: Academy Award, Best Supporting Actor, 1953, for *Viva Zapata!*; Academy Award, Best Supporting Actor, 1957, for *Lust for Life;* Academy Award nomination, Best Actor, 1958, for *Wild Is the Wind;* Antoinette Perry Award nomination, Best Actor in a Drama, 1961, for *Becket;* Academy Award nomination, Best Actor, 1965, for *Zorba the Greek;* Cecil B. DeMille Award from the Hollywood Foreign Press Association, 1987, for Outstanding Contribution to the World of Entertainment.

ADDRESSES: AGENT—Johnnie Planco, William Morris Agency, 1350 Avenue of the Americas, New York, NY 10019.*

R

RACHINS, Alan

PERSONAL: Born October 10, in Cambridge, MA; married Joanna Frank (an actress); children: Robby. EDUCATION: Attended the Wharton School of Finance; trained for the stage with William Ball, Warren Robertson, Kim Stanley, and Harvey Lembeck in New York City; studied film directing and writing with the American Film Institute, 1972.

VOCATION: Actor, director, and screenwriter.

CAREER: Also see WRITINGS below. PRINCIPAL STAGE AP-PEARANCES—*After the Rain*, John Golden Theatre, New York City, 1967; *Hadrian the Seventh*, Helen Hayes Theatre, New York City, 1969; *Oh, Calcutta!*, Eden Theatre, New York City, 1969; also appeared in *The Trojan Women*, New York City.

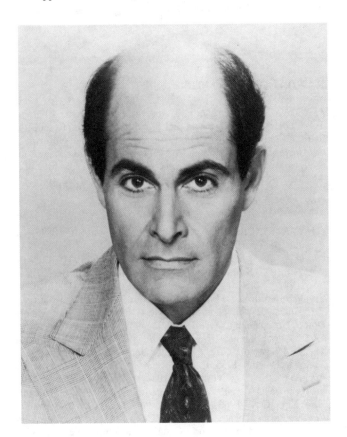

ALAN RACHINS

PRINCIPAL FILM APPEARANCES—Eddie, *Always*, Samuel Gold-wyn, 1985; Carlos, *Thunder Run*, Cannon, 1986.

PRINCIPAL TELEVISION APPEARANCES—Series: Douglas Brackman, Jr., *L.A. Law*, NBC, 1986—; also *Paris*, CBS, 1979. Episodic: Pasban Bapu, "Enlightened," *J.J. Starbuck*, NBC, 1988; also *D.C. Follies*, syndicated, 1988. Movies: Ben Washburn, *Mistress*, CBS, 1987; also *Fear on Trial*, CBS, 1975. PRINCIPAL TELEVI-SION WORK—Episodic: Director, *Paris*, CBS, 1979.

RELATED CAREER—Studio script reader for two years.

NON-RELATED CAREER—Operator of an ice cream topping and cake decorating business, Boston, MA.

WRITINGS: TELEVISION—Episodic: *Hill Street Blues*, NBC; *The Fall Guy*, ABC; *Hart to Hart*, ABC; *Knight Rider*, NBC; *Quincy, M.E.*, NBC.

ADDRESSES: AGENT—The Artists Agency, 10000 Santa Monica Boulevard, Suite 305, Los Angeles, CA 90067. PUBLICIST—Baker/Winokur/Ryder Public Relations, 9348 Civic Center Drive, Suite 407, Beverly Hills, CA 90210.

*   *   *

RAMSAY, Remak   1937-

PERSONAL: Born February 2, 1937, in Baltimore, MD; son of John Breckinridge, Jr. and Caroline Voorhees (Remak) Ramsay. EDUCATION: Princeton University, B.A., architecture, 1958; trained for the stage at the Neighborhood Playhouse and with David Craig.

VOCATION: Actor.

CAREER: OFF-BROADWAY DEBUT—Ensemble, *Hang Down Your Head and Die* (revue), Mayfair Theatre, 1964. PRINCIPAL STAGE APPEARANCES—Young Walsingham, *Half a Sixpence*, Broadhurst Theatre, New York City, 1965; Jack, *Everything in the Garden*, Charles Playhouse, Boston, MA, 1968; Edward Snelling, *Sheep on the Runway*, Helen Hayes Theatre, New York City, 1970; Captain McLean, *Lovely Ladies, Kind Gentlemen*, Majestic Thea-tre, New York City, 1970; Ozzie, *On the Town*, Imperial Theatre, New York City, 1971; Foot, *After Magritte*, and Magnus, *The Real Inspector Hound*, both Theatre Four, New York City, 1972; Archie, *Jumpers*, Billy Rose Theatre, New York City, 1974; Victor Prynne, *Private Lives*, 46th Street Theatre, New York City, 1975; Hector Hushabye, *Heartbreak House*, Williamstown Festival Theatre, Williamstown, MA, 1976; Cocklebury-Smythe, *Dirty Linen*, John

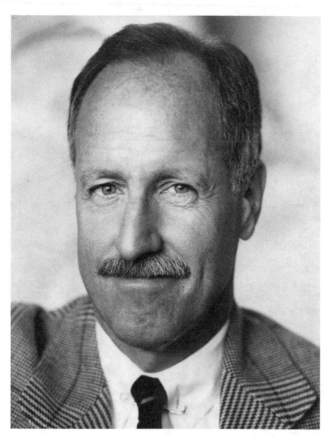

REMAK RAMSAY

Golden Theatre, New York City, 1977; Durwood Peach, *Landscape of the Body,* New York Shakespeare Festival (NYSF), Public Theatre, New York City, 1977; King of France, *All's Well That Ends Well,* NYSF, Delacorte Theatre, New York City, 1978; Major E.M. Barttelot, *The Rear Column,* Manhattan Theatre Club, New York City, 1978; Major Frederick Lowndes, *Home and Beauty,* Eisenhower Theatre, Kennedy Center for the Performing Arts, Washington, DC, 1978; doctor, *Every Good Boy Deserves Favour,* Metropolitan Opera House, New York City, then Kennedy Center for the Performing Arts, both 1979; Sir Robert Morton, *The Winslow Boy,* Roundabout Theatre, New York City, 1981; St. John Quartermaine, *Quartermaine's Terms,* Long Wharf Theatre, New Haven, CT, 1982, then Playhouse 91, New York City, 1983; Anthony Anderson, *The Devil's Disciple,* Circle in the Square, New York City, 1988. Also appeared in *Save Grand Central,* New York City, 1980; *The Dining Room,* Playwrights Horizons Theatre, then Astor Place Theatre, both New York City, 1982; *A Little Bit More of Pygmalion* (concert performance), Parsons/May Auditorium, New York City, 1984; *Woman in Mind,* Manhattan Theatre Club, City Center Theatre, 1988; *The Rehearsal* and *Tonight at 8:30,* both Phoenix Theatre, New York City; in summer theatre productions, 1963-64; and with the Phoenix Theatre, John Drew Theatre, Easthampton, NY, 1975.

MAJOR TOURS—Ken Powell, *Generation,* U.S. cities, 1967; Norman Cornell, *The Star-Spangled Girl,* U.S. cities, 1967-68; Gordon Lowther, *The Prime of Miss Jean Brodie,* U.S. cities, 1969; Chrysalde, *School for Wives,* U.S. cities, 1973; Hysterium, *A Funny Thing Happened on the Way to the Forum,* U.S. cities, 1973; doctor, *Every Good Boy Deserves Favour,* U.S. cities, 1978; Sir

Robert Morton, *The Winslow Boy,* U.S. cities, 1981. Also in *The Matchmaker,* U.S. cities, 1964.

PRINCIPAL FILM APPEARANCES—Housing guard, *The Tiger Makes Out,* Columbia, 1967; Mr. Atkinson, *The Stepford Wives,* Columbia, 1975; Hennessey, *The Front,* Columbia, 1976; television newscaster, *Simon,* Warner Brothers, 1980; Kennedy, *Class,* Orion, 1983; Senator Byington, *The House on Carroll Street,* Orion, 1988; Hilary Knowles, *The Money Juggler,* Archer, 1989. Also appeared in *The Great Gatsby,* Paramount, 1974; and as Andrew Mellon, *Mellon,* 1981.

PRINCIPAL TELEVISION APPEARANCES—Series: *As the World Turns,* CBS; *All My Children,* ABC; *One Life to Live,* ABC; *Another World,* NBC; *The Guiding Light,* CBS. Mini-Series: Richard Bissell, *Kennedy,* NBC, 1983; Carl Binger, "Concealed Enemies," *American Playhouse,* PBS, 1984. Pilots: "Baby on Board," *CBS Summer Playhouse,* CBS, 1988. Episodic: *On Our Own,* CBS. Movies: Henry Gebhardt, *Dream House,* CBS, 1981; John LaFarge, *Liberty,* NBC, 1986. Plays: Hector Hushabye, *Heartbreak House,* PBS, 1986; also "The Dining Room," *Great Performances,* PBS, 1983. Specials: *Funny Papers,* CBS, 1972.

AWARDS: Obie Award from the *Village Voice* and Drama Desk Award nomination, both for *Quartermaine's Terms;* Drama Desk Award nomination for *The Winslow Boy.*

SIDELIGHTS: FAVORITE ROLES—Barttelot in *The Rear Column,* Quartermaine in *Quartermaine's Terms,* and Sir Robert Morton in *The Winslow Boy.*

ADDRESSES: HOME—New York, NY.

*   *   *

RANDALL, Tony   1920-

PERSONAL: Born Leonard Rosenberg, February 26, 1920, in Tulsa, OK; son of Philip (an art dealer) and Julia (Finston) Rosenberg; married Florence Gibbs, 1939. EDUCATION: Attended Northwestern University and Columbia University; trained for the stage with Sanford Meisner at the Neighborhood Playhouse, 1938-40. MILITARY: U.S. Army, Signal Corps, first lieutenant, 1942-46.

VOCATION: Actor.

CAREER: STAGE DEBUT—Upper Ferndale Country Club, Upper Ferndale, NY, 1939. OFF-BROADWAY DEBUT—Brother, *The Circle of Chalk,* New School for Social Research, 1941. BROADWAY DEBUT—Scarus, *Antony and Cleopatra,* Martin Beck Theatre, 1947. PRINCIPAL STAGE APPEARANCES—Marchbanks, *Candida,* North Shore Players, Marblehead, MA, 1941; Adam, *To Tell You the Truth,* New Stages, New York City, 1948; Major-Domo, *Caesar and Cleopatra,* National Theatre, New York City, 1949; Arthur Turner, *Oh, Men! Oh, Women!,* Henry Miller's Theatre, New York City, 1954; E.K. Hornbeck, *Inherit the Wind,* National Theatre, 1955; Captain Henry St. James, *Oh, Captain!,* Alvin Theatre, New York City, 1958; J. Francis Amber, *UTBU* (also known as *Unhealthy to Be Unpleasant*), Helen Hayes Theatre, New York City, 1966; Frank Fay, *Parade of Stars Playing the Palace,* Palace Theatre, New York City, 1983. Also appeared in *Arms and the Man,* Westport Country Playhouse, Westport, CT, 1960; in *Goodbye Again,* summer theatre productions in Detroit,

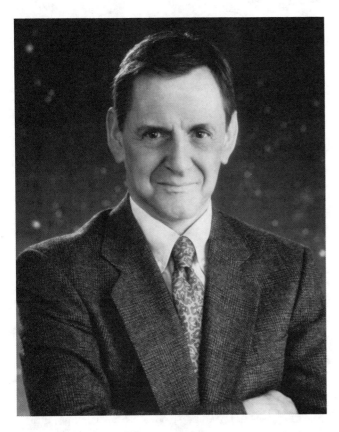

TONY RANDALL

MI, then Chicago, IL, both 1961; and in productions of *The Sea Gull* and *The Master Builder*.

MAJOR TOURS—Miner, *The Corn Is Green*, New York and New Jersey cities, 1942; Octavius Moulton-Barrett, *The Barretts of Wimpole Street*, U.S. cities, 1947; Felix Unger, *The Odd Couple*, various tours of U.S. cities, 1970-76; Professor Harold Hill, *The Music Man*, U.S. cities, 1978.

FILM DEBUT—Grant Cobbler, *Oh, Men! Oh, Women!*, Twentieth Century-Fox, 1957. PRINCIPAL FILM APPEARANCES—Title role, *Will Success Spoil Rock Hunter?* (also known as *Oh! For a Man*), Twentieth Century-Fox, 1957; Jerry Flagg, *No Down Payment*, Twentieth Century-Fox, 1957; Jonathan Forbes, *Pillow Talk*, Universal, 1959; Lorenzo Charlton, *The Mating Game*, Metro-Goldwyn-Mayer (MGM), 1959; the King, *The Adventures of Huckleberry Finn*, MGM, 1960; Howard Coffman, *Let's Make Love*, Twentieth Century-Fox, 1960; Peter Ramsey, *Lover Come Back*, Universal, 1961; George Drayton, *Boys' Night Out*, MGM, 1962; Paul Ferris, *Island of Love* (also known as *Not on Your Life*), Warner Brothers, 1963; hood, *Robin and the Seven Hoods*, Warner Brothers, 1964; Arnold Nash, *Send Me No Flowers*, Universal, 1964; Harold Ventimore, *The Brass Bottle*, Universal, 1964; Dr. Lao, Merlin the Magician, Pan, the Abominable Snowman, Medusa, the Giant Serpent, and Apollonius of Tyana, *The Seven Faces of Dr. Lao*, MGM, 1964; Daniel Potter, *Fluffy*, Universal, 1965; Hercule Poirot, *The Alphabet Murders* (also known as *The ABC Murders*), MGM, 1966; Andrew Jessel, *Bang, Bang, You're Dead* (also known as *Our Man in Marrakesh* and *Marrakesh*), American International, 1966; Fred Miller, *Hello Down There* (also known as *Sub-a-Dub-Dub*), Paramount, 1969; operator, *Everything You Always Wanted to Know about Sex* (*but were afraid to ask)*, United Artists, 1972; Henry Motley, *Scavenger Hunt*, Twentieth Century-Fox, 1979; Peddicord, *Foolin' Around*, Columbia, 1980; as himself, *The King of Comedy*, Twentieth Century-Fox, 1983; as himself, *Sanford Meisner—The Theatre's Best Kept Secret* (documentary), Columbia, 1984; voice of Moonchick, *My Little Pony* (animated), DeLaurentiis Entertainment Group, 1986. Also appeared in *Two Weeks in Another Town*, MGM, 1962; as the director, *Save the Dog*, 1988; in *That's Adequate*, 1988; *Going Hollywood: The War Years*, 1988; and *It Had to Be You*, 1988.

PRINCIPAL TELEVISION APPEARANCES—Series: Mac, *One Man's Family*, NBC, 1950-52; Harvey Weskit, *Mr. Peepers*, NBC, 1952-55; Felix Unger, *The Odd Couple*, ABC, 1970-75; host, *Top of the Month*, syndicated, 1972; Judge Walter O. Franklin, *The Tony Randall Show*, ABC, 1976-77, then CBS, 1977-78; Sidney Shorr, *Love, Sidney*, NBC, 1981-83; also host, *Live from the Met*, PBS. Pilots: Willie Coogan, *Coogan's Reward*, CBS, 1965; title role, *Sidney Shorr: A Girl's Best Friend*, NBC, 1981. Episodic: Inspector Berry and Geoffrey Judge, "The Wide Open Door," *Stage '67*, ABC, 1967; Rodney Wonderful, *That's Life*, ABC, 1969; also *Hippodrome*, CBS, 1966; *The Flip Wilson Show*, NBC, 1970; *The Sonny and Cher Comedy Hour*, CBS, 1972; *The Hanna-Barbera Happy Hour*, NBC, 1978; *The Big Show*, NBC, 1980; *General Electric Theatre*, CBS; *Captain Video and His Video Rangers*, Dumont; *Short, Short Drama*, NBC; *Sunday Showcase*, NBC; *Philco Playhouse*, NBC; *Pepsi-Cola Playhouse*, ABC; *The Web*, CBS; *Kraft Television Theatre*, NBC; *Goodyear Television Playhouse*, NBC; *Motorola Television Hour*, ABC; *Armstrong Circle Theatre*, NBC; *Appointment with Adventure*, CBS; *Alcoa Hour*, NBC; *Studio One*, CBS; *Playhouse 90*, CBS; *Checkmate*, CBS; *Here's Lucy*, CBS; *Love, American Style*, ABC; *The Carol Burnette Show*, CBS. Movies: Rambaba Organimus, *Off Sides*, NBC, 1974; Lord Seymour Devery, *Kate Bliss and the Ticker-Tape Kid*, ABC, 1978; Putzi, *Hitler's SS: Portrait in Evil*, NBC, 1985; Uncle Bill, *Sunday Drive*, ABC, 1986; Minks, *Agatha Christie's "The Man in the Brown Suit*," CBS, 1989.

Specials: *Panorama*, NBC, 1956; *Heaven Will Protect the Working Girl*, NBC, 1956; *Holiday in Las Vegas*, NBC, 1957; *The Sid Caesar Special*, CBS, 1959; Ernest, *So Help Me Aphrodite*, NBC, 1960; *Hooray for Love*, CBS, 1960; *The Man in the Moon*, NBC, 1960; *Sound of the 60s*, NBC, 1961; *The Chevrolet Golden Anniversary Show*, CBS, 1961; Jonathan Brewster, "Arsenic and Old Lace," *Hallmark Hall of Fame*, NBC, 1962; *The Bob Hope Show*, NBC, 1964; *The Bob Hope Show*, NBC, 1965; *The Alan King Show*, ABC, 1969; Democritus, "The Littlest Angel," *Hallmark Hall of Fame*, NBC, 1969; *The Wonderful World of Aggravation*, ABC, 1972; *The Bob Hope Show*, NBC, 1973; *Cos: The Bill Cosby Comedy Special*, CBS, 1975; *Celebrity Challenge of the Sexes*, CBS, 1977; *The Paul Lynde Comedy Hour*, ABC, 1977; *Battle of the Network Stars*, ABC, 1978; *Bob Hope on Campus*, NBC, 1979; *Bob Hope for President*, NBC, 1980; *Doug Henning: Magic on Broadway*, NBC, 1982; *Parade of Stars*, ABC, 1983; *Circus of the Stars*, CBS, 1984; *Bob Hope Lampoons the New TV Scene*, NBC, 1986; Mr. LaTort, *NBC Investigates Bob Hope*, NBC, 1987; *Bob Hope's Christmas Special*, NBC, 1987; *Happy Birthday Bob—50 Stars Salute Your 50 Years with NBC*, NBC, 1988; *Hope News Network*, NBC, 1988; also *Curtain's Up*, 1985; *Walt Disney World Celebrity Circus*, 1987; voice characterization, *Lyle, Lyle, Crocodile—The Musical: "The House on 88th Street"* (animated), 1988.

PRINCIPAL RADIO APPEARANCES—Series: Reggie, *I Love a Mystery;* also *Portia Faces Life, When a Girl Marries,* and *Life's True Story*. Also announcer, WTAG, Worcester, MA, 1941-42.

RELATED CAREER—Director and actor in various productions at the Olney Theatre, Olney, MD, 1946, and at the Sussex County Playhouse, Culvers Lake, NJ.

RECORDINGS: ALBUMS—(With Jack Klugman) *The Odd Couple Sings,* London, 1973; also *Vo, Vo, De, Oh, Do,* 1967.

AWARDS: Emmy Award, Best Actor in a Comedy Series, 1975, for *The Odd Couple.*

MEMBER: Actors' Equity Association, Screen Actors Guild, American Federation of Television and Radio Artists, Association of the Metropolitan Opera Company.

SIDELIGHTS: RECREATIONS—Studying opera and collecting antiques, paintings, and classical records.

ADDRESSES: OFFICE—145 Central Park W., New York, NY 10023. PUBLICIST—John Springer Associates, 130 E. 67th Street, New York, NY 10021.

*   *   *

RAPPAPORT, David

PERSONAL: Born November 23, in London, England; married; children: one son. EDUCATION: Received degree in psychology from Bristol University.

VOCATION: Actor.

CAREER: PRINCIPAL STAGE APPEARANCES—Nano, *Volpone,* National Theatre Company, Olivier Theatre, London, 1977; also appeared as Markov Chaney, *Illuminatus,* National Theatre Company, Science Fiction Theatre, Liverpool, U.K., then National Theatre, London; in *The Warp,* Regent Theatre, Edinburgh Festival, Edinburgh, Scotland, 1979; *Little Brother Is Watching You* (one-man show), 1979; *Dr. Faustus* and *Exit the King,* both Lyric Hammersmith Theatre, London.

MAJOR TOURS—*Bristol Revue,* U.K. cities.

PRINCIPAL FILM APPEARANCES—Jesus, *Cuba,* United Artists, 1979; Tom Thumb's Army member, *Black Jack,* Kestral/National Film Finance, 1979; Minuut, *Mysteries,* Cine-Vog, 1979; Randall, *Time Bandits,* AVCO-Embassy, 1981; Sage, *Sword of the Valiant,* Cannon, 1984; Rinaldo, *The Bride,* Columbia, 1985. Also appeared in *The Secret Policeman's Ball,* Tigon/Amnesty International, 1979; and *The Secret Policeman's Other Ball,* Almi Cinema 5, 1981.

PRINCIPAL TELEVISION APPEARANCES—Series: Simon McKay, *The Wizard,* CBS, 1986-87. Episodic: Augie Briscoe, *Fortune Dane,* ABC, 1986; Cluracan, *Hardcastle and McCormick,* ABC, 1986; troll, *Amazing Stories,* NBC, 1986; Schuyler, *L.A. Law,* NBC, 1987; Galen Belvedere, *Mr. Belvedere,* ABC, 1988; Nick Derringer, *Hooperman* (two episodes), ABC, 1988. Movies: Arthur, *Unfair Exchanges,* BBC, 1984. Specials: Toronto host, *CBS All-American Thanksgiving Day Parade,* CBS, 1986. Also appeared in *File on Harry Jordan,* Yorkshire Television; *The Young Ones,* BBC; *Beauty and the Beast,* Thames; *Mr. Stabs,* Thames; *The Illustrated Wednesday Revue,* Central Television; *The Satur-*

day Show, 09 and 10, Not the Nine O'Clock News, History of Pantomime, Tales from 1,001 Nights, Jigsaw, and *Grapevine.*

RELATED CAREER—Comedian.

NON-RELATED CAREER—Teacher and cemetery gardener.

ADDRESSES: MANAGER—Frankie Leigh, 1515 N. Hayworth, Los Angeles, CA 90046.*

*   *   *

RAWLINS, Lester   1924-1988

PERSONAL: Born September 24, 1924, in Sharon, PA; died of a heart attack, March 22, 1988, in New York, NY. son of Leona Verier. EDUCATION: Carnegie Institute of Technology (now Carnegie-Mellon University), B.F.A., drama, 1950; trained for the stage at the American Shakespeare Festival and Academy School and with Mary Morris, Henry Boettcher, Lawrence Carra, and Edith Skinner. MILITARY: U.S. Army Air Forces, first sergeant, 1943-46.

VOCATION: Actor.

CAREER: STAGE DEBUT—Hunchback dwarf, *Birthday of the Infanta,* Farrell Auditorium, Farrell, PA, 1930. OFF-BROADWAY DEBUT—Lodovico, *Othello,* City Center Theatre, 1955. PRINCIPAL STAGE APPEARANCES—Scrooge, *A Christmas Carol,* Farrell Auditorium, Farrell, PA, 1935; Maxie, *June Moon,* Chapel Playhouse, Guildford, CT, 1948; the Nephew, *The Golden State,* Pasadena Playhouse, Pasadena, CA, 1953; Lodovico, *Othello,* Conrade, *Much Ado about Nothing,* and Worcester, *Henry IV, Part One,* all Brattle Theatre, Cambridge, MA, 1955; Worcester, *Henry IV, Part One,* City Center Theatre, New York City, 1955; Lennox, *Macbeth,* Jan Hus Playhouse, New York City, 1955; Gloucester, *King Lear,* City Center Theatre, 1956; Friar Lawrence, *Romeo and Juliet,* Jan Hus Playhouse, 1956; Escavalon, *The Lovers,* Martin Beck Theatre, New York City, 1956; Dogberry, *Much Ado about Nothing,* Angelo, *Measure for Measure,* and Gloucester, *King Lear,* all Antioch Shakespeare Festival, Antioch, OH, 1956; Polonius, *Hamlet,* Shakespearewrights Theatre, New York City, 1956; the Cardinal, *The Prisoner,* Arena Stage, Washington, DC, 1957; Pop, *The Pajama Game,* the Artist, *Can-Can,* Mr. Moon, *Anything Goes,* Jeff, *Brigadoon,* Mr. Applegate, *Damn Yankees,* and Luther Billis, *South Pacific,* all Flint Musical Tent, Flint, MI, then Detroit Musical Tent, Detroit, MI, 1957; David Slater, *The Moon Is Blue,* North Jersey Playhouse, Fort Lee, NJ, 1957; Clarence, *Richard III,* New York Shakespeare Festival, Heckscher Theatre, New York City, 1957; Hamm, *Endgame,* Cherry Lane Theatre, New York City, 1958; Shunderson, *Dr. Praetorius,* North Jersey Playhouse, 1958; Ensign Pulver, *Mister Roberts,* Flint Musical Tent, 1958; Regan, *The Quare Fellow,* Circle in the Square, New York City, 1958; Sir Nathaniel, *Love's Labour's Lost,* Library of Congress, Washington, DC, 1959.

Papa, *The Happy Time,* Coconut Grove Playhouse, Coconut Grove, FL, 1960; Lord Byron, *Camino Real,* St. Mark's Playhouse, New York City, 1960; Poppet, *Redhead,* and Bennie, *The Desert Song,* both Rochester Musical Theatre, Rochester, NY, then Syracuse Musical Theatre, Syracuse, NY, 1960; Fender, *The Bespoke Overcoat,* Grigson, *Shadow of a Gunman,* and Beggar, *Elektra,* all Olney Theatre, MD, 1960; Tesman, *Hedda Gabler,* Fourth Street

Theatre, New York City, 1960; Cranmer, *A Man for All Seasons,* American National Theatre and Academy Theatre, New York City, 1961; Don Felipe, *We Take the Town,* Shubert Theatre, New Haven, CT, then Shubert Theatre, Philadelphia, PA, 1962; the Fool, *King Lear,* Angelo, *Comedy of Errors,* and Fluellen, *Henry V,* all American Shakespeare Festival, Stratford, CT, 1963, then Festival of the Two Worlds, Spoleto, Italy, 1964; title role, *Hamlet,* American Shakespeare Festival, 1964; Captain Amasa Delano, *Benito Cereno,* American Place Theatre, New York City, 1964; Wissey Jones, *The Child Buyer,* Garrick Theatre, New York City, 1964; Trock, *Winterset,* Jan Hus Playhouse, 1966; Leonard, *In the Bar of a Tokyo Hotel,* Eastside Playhouse, New York City, 1969; Governor, *The Reckoning,* St. Mark's Playhouse, 1969.

He, *He Who Gets Slapped,* Playhouse in the Park, Cincinnati, OH, 1970; Jon Bristow, *Nightride,* Van Dam Theatre, New York City, 1971; Count Paul Nevlinski, *Herzl,* Palace Theatre, New York City, 1976; Capulet, *Romeo and Juliet,* Circle in the Square, 1977; Drumm, *Da,* Hudson Guild Theatre, then Morosco Theatre, both New York City, 1978. Also appeared in *The Glass Menagerie,* City Center Theatre, 1956; as the title role, *Richard III,* summer theatre production, 1960; in *The Golden Age* (concert reading), Lyceum Theatre, New York City, 1963; in summer theatre productions at the Chapel Playhouse, Guildford, CT, 1949; and in thirty productions at Arena Stage, Washington, DC, 1950-52 and 1954-55.

MAJOR TOURS—Mr. Applegate, *Damn Yankees,* U.S. cities, 1958; Jack Jordan, *Say, Darling,* and Papa, *Happy Time,* U.S. cities, both 1959.

FILM DEBUT—Reporter, *Mr. Congressman,* Metro-Goldwyn-Mayer, 1951. PRINCIPAL FILM APPEARANCES—Editor, *Within Man's Power,* National Tuberculosis Association, 1954; Dr. Linstrom, *Diary of a Mad Housewife,* Universal, 1970; Blevins Playfair, *They Might Be Giants,* Universal, 1971; board chairman, *God Told Me To* (also known as *Demon*), New World, 1976; silent patient, *Lovesick,* Warner Brothers, 1983.

TELEVISION DEBUT—Dancer, *The Dinah Shore Show,* CBS, 1953. PRINCIPAL TELEVISION APPEARANCES—Series: Rysdale, *Secret Storm,* CBS, 1962-63; also Spencer Smith, *Ryan's Hope,* ABC; Orin Hellyer, *The Edge of Night,* CBS. Pilots: Brown, *Nick and Nora,* ABC, 1975. Episodic: Dr. Timms, *The Equalizer,* CBS, 1985; also "The Life of Samuel Johnson," *Omnibus,* CBS, 1956; *Studio One,* CBS, 1956; *Look Up and Live,* CBS, 1961; "Salome," *Omnibus,* CBS; *The Defenders,* CBS; *The Nurses,* CBS; *Camera Three,* CBS; *Eye on New York,* CBS; *Portraits in Verse,* CBS; *John Brown's Body,* CBS; *Russian Special,* CBS; *Banacek,* NBC; *Apple's Way,* CBS; *The Snoop Sisters,* NBC; *Police Woman,* NBC; *Starsky and Hutch,* ABC. Specials: *The Waste Land* (dramatic reading), NTA, 1965.

RELATED CAREER—Stage manager, Chapel Playhouse, Guildford, CT, 1949; founding member, Arena Stage, Washington, DC, 1950-55.

NON-RELATED CAREER—Waiter, salesman, and file clerk.

AWARDS: Norman Apell Award and Goldbloom Memorial Award from the Carnegie Institute of Technology, both 1950; Obie Award from the *Village Voice,* 1958, for *The Quare Fellow;* Obie Award, 1960, for *Hedda Gabler;* Obie Award, 1965, for *Benito Cereno;*

Drama Desk Award, 1972, for *Nightride;* Antoinette Perry Award, Best Featured Actor in a Play, 1978, for *Da.*

OBITUARIES AND OTHER SOURCES: Variety, March 30, 1988.*

*   *   *

RAYMOND, Gene   1908-
(Raymond Guion)

PERSONAL: Born Raymond Guion, August 13, 1908, in New York, NY; son of LeRoy D. and Mary (Smith) Guion; married Jeanette MacDonald (a singer and actress), June 16, 1937 (died, January 14, 1965); married Nel Bentley Hees, September 8, 1974. MILITARY: U.S. Army Air Forces, 1942-45, then U.S. Air Force Reserve, colonel, 1945-68.

VOCATION: Actor.

CAREER: BROADWAY DEBUT—(As Raymond Guion) *The Piper,* Fulton Theatre, 1920. PRINCIPAL STAGE APPEARANCES—As Raymond Guion: Shepherd boy, *Eyvind of the Hills,* Greenwich Village Theatre, New York City, 1921; Billy Thompson, *Why Not?,* 48th Street Theatre, New York City, 1922; Bill Potter, *The Potters,* Plymouth Theatre, New York City, 1923; Oscar Nordholm, *Cradle Snatchers,* Music Box Theatre, New York City, 1925; Bud Weaver, *Take My Advice,* Belmont Theatre, New York City, 1927; Calvin Trask, *Mirrors,* Forrest Theatre, New York City, 1928; Billy, *Sherlock Holmes,* Cosmopolitan Theatre, New York City, 1928; Michael Graham, *Say When,* Morosco Theatre, New York City, 1928; Sid Swanson, *The War Song,* National Theatre, New York City, 1928; Wilbur Jones, *Jonesy,* Bijou Theatre, New York City, 1929; Gene Gibson, *Young Sinners,* Morosco Theatre, 1929.

As Gene Raymond: Mercutio, *Romeo and Juliet,* Community Playhouse, Pasadena, CA, 1957; Horace Smith, *A Shadow of My Enemy,* American National Theatre and Academy Theatre, New York City, 1957; Edward Burgeon, *Madly in Love,* Playhouse in the Park, Philadelphia, PA, 1963. Also appeared in *The Man in Possession,* Dennis, MA, 1946; *The Greatest of These,* Chicago, IL, 1947; *Call Me Madam,* Dallas, TX, 1952; *The Detective Story,* 1954; *The Devil's Disciple,* 1954; *Holiday for Lovers,* Drury Lane Theatre, Chicago, 1959; *Diplomatic Relations,* Ogunquit Playhouse, Ogunquit, ME, 1965; and in summer theatre productions of *Candida, Mr. Roberts, Kiss Me Kate, Write Me a Murder,* and *A Majority of One.*

MAJOR TOURS—The Actor, *The Guardsman,* U.S. cities, 1950-51; Joseph Cantwell, *The Best Man,* U.S. cities, 1960; *The Voice of the Turtle,* U.S. cities, 1952; *Angel Street,* U.S. cities, 1952; *The Petrified Forest,* U.S. cities, 1952; *Private Lives,* U.S. cities, 1953; *The Moon Is Blue,* U.S. cities, 1953; *Be Quiet, My Love,* U.S. cities, 1953; *The Fifth Season,* California cities, 1955; *Will Success Spoil Rock Hunter?,* California cities, 1956.

FILM DEBUT—Dick Gary, *Personal Maid,* Paramount, 1931. PRINCIPAL FILM APPEARANCES—Paul Ossip, *Forgotten Commandments,* Paramount, 1932; John Wallace, *If I Had a Million,* Paramount, 1932; Standish McNeil, *Ladies of the Big House,* Paramount, 1932; Herbert Morrow, *The Night of June 13,* Paramount, 1932; Gary Willis, *Red Dust,* Metro-Goldwyn-Mayer (MGM), 1932; Bill Graham, *Ann Carver's Profession,* Columbia, 1933; Rodney Deane, *Brief Moment,* Columbia, 1933; Don Peterson,

Ex-Lady, Warner Brothers, 1933; Roger Bond, *Flying down to Rio,* RKO, 1933; Monte Van Tyle, *The House on 56th Street,* Warner Brothers, 1933; Zani, *Zoo in Budapest,* Twentieth Century-Fox, 1933; Chris Hansen, *Coming Out Party,* Twentieth Century-Fox, 1934; Tony, *I Am Suzanne,* Twentieth Century-Fox, 1934; Tommy Wallace, *Sadie McKee,* MGM, 1934; Jimmy Brett, *Transatlantic Merry-Go-Round,* United Artists, 1934; Michael Carter, *Behold My Wife,* Paramount, 1935; Doug, *Hooray for Love,* RKO, 1935; Magee, *Seven Keys to Baldpate,* RKO, 1935; Carey Marshall, *Transient Lady,* Universal, 1935; Johnnie Wyatt, *The Woman in Red,* Warner Brothers/First National, 1935; Michael Martin, *The Bride Walks Out,* RKO, 1936; Michael, *Love on a Bet,* RKO, 1936; Dick Smith, *The Smartest Girl in Town,* RKO, 1936; Pete Quinlan, *Walking on Air,* RKO, 1936; Barry Saunders, *The Life of the Party,* RKO, 1937; Windy McLean, *That Girl from Paris,* RKO, 1937; Jerry Martin, *There Goes My Girl,* RKO, 1937; Fuller Partridge, *She's Got Everything,* RKO, 1938; Carl, *Stolen Heaven,* Paramount, 1938.

Larry, *Cross Country Romance,* RKO, 1940; Jeff Custer, *Mr. and Mrs. Smith,* RKO, 1941; Kenneth Wayne/Jeremy Wayne, *Smilin' Through,* MGM, 1941; John Willis, *The Locket,* RKO, 1946; Dan Sullivan, *Assigned to Danger,* Eagle-Lion, 1948; Nicholas Lawrence, *Million Dollar Weekend,* Eagle-Lion, 1948; Steve Roark, *Sofia,* Film Classics, 1948; Wendell Craig, *Hit the Deck,* MGM, 1955; Eddie, *Plunder Road,* Twentieth Century-Fox, 1957; Dan Cantwell, *The Best Man,* United Artists, 1964; Martin Wood, *I'd Rather Be Rich,* Universal, 1964; voice of death, *The Gun Riders* (also known as *Five Bloody Graves,* *Lonely Man,* and *Five Bloody Days to Tombstone*), Independent International, 1969. Also appeared in *The Way of the West,* Superior, 1934.

PRINCIPAL FILM WORK—Director, *Million Dollar Weekend,* Eagle-Lion, 1948.

PRINCIPAL TELEVISION APPEARANCES—Series: Host, *Fireside Theatre,* NBC, 1953-55; panelist, *What's Going On?,* CBS, 1954; host, *Hollywood Summer Theatre,* CBS, 1956; host, *TV Reader's Digest,* ABC, 1956; Robert Stevens, *Paris 7000,* ABC, 1970. Pilots: Ben Solomon, *The Old Man and the City* (broadcast as an episode of *The Dick Powell Show*), NBC, 1963. Episodic: Benson Sawyer, "The Borderland," *The Outer Limits,* ABC, 1963; also *G.E. Summer Originals,* ABC, 1956; *Matinee Theatre,* NBC; *Robert Montgomery Presents,* NBC; *Climax,* CBS; *Playhouse 90,* CBS; *The Red Skelton Show,* CBS; *The Man from U.N.C.L.E.,* NBC; *The Girl from U.N.C.L.E.,* NBC; *Laredo,* NBC; *Ironside,* NBC; *Julia,* NBC; *Judd for the Defense,* ABC; *The Defenders,* CBS; *Mannix,* CBS; *The Name of the Game,* NBC; *The Bold Ones,* NBC; also *Lux Video Theatre,* *Kraft Television Theatre,* *U.S. Steel Hour.* Movies: Whitey Devlin, *The Hanged Man,* NBC, 1964.

PRINCIPAL TELEVISION WORK—Episodic: Director, *Matinee Theatre,* ABC.

RELATED CAREER—Founder, Masque Productions, 1949; president, Motion Picture and Television Fund, 1980.

NON-RELATED CAREER—Past vice-president, Arthritis Foundation of Southern California; president, Los Angeles chapter of the Air Force Association; trustee, Falcon Foundation of the United States Air Force Academy.

WRITINGS: FILM—*Million Dollar Weekend,* Eagle-Lion, 1949. TELEVISION—Plays: *Prima Donna.* OTHER—Songs: "Will You?" and "Let Me Always Sing."

AWARDS: Bronze Halo Award from the Southern California Motion Picture Council, Distinguished Service Award from the Arthritis Foundation, Humanitarian Award from the Air Force Association, Better World Award from the Veterans of Foreign Wars, Legion of Merit from the United States Air Force Reserve.

MEMBER: Screen Actors Guild (board member), Academy of Television Arts and Sciences (board member), Players Club, New York Athletic Club, Bel Air Country Club, Los Angeles Tennis Club, Army and Navy Club, Order of Daedalians.

ADDRESSES: OFFICE—9570 Wilshire Boulevard, Beverly Hills, CA 90212.*

*   *   *

REDGRAVE, Lynn   1943-

PERSONAL: Full name, Lynn Rachel Redgrave; born March 8, 1943, in London, England; daughter of Sir Michael (an actor) and Rachel (an actress; professional name, Rachel Kempson) Redgrave; married John Clark (a producer and director), April 2, 1967; children: Benjamin, Kelly, Annabel. EDUCATION: Trained for the stage at the Central School of Speech and Drama, London.

VOCATION: Actress.

CAREER: STAGE DEBUT—Helena, *A Midsummer Night's Dream,* Royal Court Theatre, London, 1962. BROADWAY DEBUT—Carol Melkett, *Black Comedy,* Ethel Barrymore Theatre, 1967. PRINCIPAL STAGE APPEARANCES—Portia, *The Merchant of Venice,* Dundee Repertory Theatre, Dundee, Scotland, 1962; Sarah Elliott, *The Tulip Tree,* Haymarket Theatre, London, 1962; court lady, *Hamlet,* National Theatre, London, 1963; court lady, *Saint Joan,* and Rose, *The Recruiting Officer,* both National Theatre, 1963; Barblin, *Andorra,* and Jackie Coryton, *Hay Fever,* both National Theatre, 1964; Margaret, *Much Ado about Nothing,* Kattrin, *Mother Courage,* and Miss Prue, *Love for Love,* all National Theatre, 1965; Maeve, *Zoo, Zoo, Widdershins Zoo,* Edinburgh Festival, Lyceum Theatre, Edinburgh, Scotland, 1969; Joanne, *Slag,* Royal Court Theatre, London, 1971; Stella, *A Better Place,* Gate Theatre, Dublin, Ireland, 1972; Billie Dawn, *Born Yesterday,* Greenwich Theatre, London, 1973; Vicky, *My Fat Friend,* Brooks Atkinson Theatre, New York City, 1974; Vivie, *Mrs. Warren's Profession,* Vivian Beaumont Theatre, New York City, 1976; Joan, *Knock Knock,* Biltmore Theatre, New York City, 1976; title role, *Saint Joan,* Goodman Theatre, Chicago, IL, then Circle in the Square, New York City, both 1977; Viola, *Twelfth Night,* American Shakespeare Festival, Stratford, CT, 1978; Sarah Siddons, *The Actor's Nightmare,* and title role, *Sister Mary Ignatius Explains It All for You,* both Westside Arts Theatre, New York City, 1982; the Honorable Mrs. William Tatham, *Aren't We All?,* Brooks Atkinson Theatre, 1985; Susan Too, *Sweet Sue,* Music Box Theatre, then Royale Theatre, both New York City, 1987; and as La Marquise de Merteuil, *Les Liaisons Dangereuses,* Ahmanson Theatre, Los Angeles, CA, 1988. Also appeared in *The Two of Us,* Garrick Theatre, London, 1970; *Misalliance,* Lake Forest, IL, 1976; and as Anna Leonowens, *The King and I,* St. Louis, MO, 1983.

MAJOR TOURS—Barbara, *Billy Liar,* U.K. cities, 1962; Miss Prue, *Love for Love,* National Theatre Company, Moscow and Berlin, 1965; Vicky, *My Fat Friend,* U.S. cities, 1974; also *The Two of Us,* U.S. cities, 1975; *Hellzapoppin',* U.S. cities, 1976-77.

FILM DEBUT—Susan, *Tom Jones*, United Artists, 1963. PRINCIPAL FILM APPEARANCES—Baba Brenan, *The Girl with the Green Eyes*, Lopert, 1964; title role, *Georgy Girl*, Columbia, 1966; Virgin, *The Deadly Affair*, Columbia, 1967; Yvonne, *Smashing Time*, Paramount, 1967; Phillipa Raskin, *The Virgin Soldiers*, Columbia, 1970; Myrtle, *The Last of the Mobile Hot-Shots*, Warner Brothers, 1970; Miss Poole, *Every Little Crook and Nanny*, Metro-Goldwyn-Mayer, 1972; the Queen, *Everything You Always Wanted to Know about Sex* (*but were afraid to ask)*, United Artists, 1972; Nurse Sweet and Betty Martin, *The National Health, or Nurse Norton's Affair*, Columbia, 1973; Mary, *Don't Turn the Other Cheek* (also known as *Viva la muerta . . . tua*), International Amusement Corporation, 1974; Xaviera Hollander, *The Happy Hooker*, Cannon, 1975; Camille Levy, *The Big Bus*, Paramount, 1976; Lady Davina, ''An Englishman's Home'' in *Sunday Lovers*, United Artists, 1980; Nancy Stewart, *Morgan Stewart's Coming Home* (also known as *Home Front*), New Century/Vista, 1987; Joan, *Getting It Right*, MCEG, 1989. Also appeared as Pauline Williams, *Death of a Son*, 1988; and in *Midnight*, 1988.

TELEVISION DEBUT—*The Power and the Glory*, ABC (British television), 1963. PRINCIPAL TELEVISION APPEARANCES—Series: Host, *Not for Women Only*, syndicated, 1972; Ann Anderson, *House Calls*, CBS, 1979-81; Diana Swanson, *Teachers Only*, NBC, 1982-83; also host, *Weight Watchers Magazine*, 1984. Mini-Series: Charlotte Buckland Lloyd Seccombe, *Centennial*, NBC, 1978-79. Pilots: *Hellzapoppin'*, ABC, 1972. Episodic: Eliza, ''Pygmalion,'' *Play of the Month*, BBC, 1973; Audrey Beck, *Hotel*, ABC, 1986; also *The Shape of Things*, NBC, 1982; Tango, *The Edge of Night*, ABC; *The Muppet Show*, syndicated. Movies: Jane Cubberly, *Turn of the Screw*, ABC, 1974; teacher, *Sooner or Later*, NBC, 1979; Kate Jordache, *Beggarman, Thief*, NBC, 1979; Leona De Vos, *The Seduction of Miss Leona*, CBS, 1980; Mette Gad, *Gauguin the Savage*, CBS, 1980; Monica Welles, *Rehearsal for Murder*, CBS, 1982; Monica Breedlove, *The Bad Seed*, ABC, 1985; Marjorie Lloyd, *My Two Loves*, ABC, 1986; also *The Fainthearted Feminist*, BBC, 1984. Specials: *The National Love, Sex, and Marriage Test*, NBC, 1978; *Linda in Wonderland*, CBS, 1980; *Steve Martin's Best Show Ever*, NBC, 1981; *Musical Comedy Tonight*, PBS, 1981; *Battle of the Network Stars*, ABC, 1982; *Circus of the Stars*, CBS, 1983; *All Star Party for Clint Eastwood*, CBS, 1986; *All Star Party for Joan Collins*, CBS, 1987; *Candid Camera Christmas*, CBS, 1987; also in *Battle of the Video Games*, 1983; *The Screen Actors Guild 50th Anniversary Celebration*, 1984; *Silent Mouse*, 1988. Also appeared as Queen Victoria, *Hall of Kings*, ABC (British television), 1973; Berta, *Vienna 1900: Games with Love and Death*, BBC-2, 1974; Sarah Cotter, *The Shooting*, 1982; Mrs. Hepp, *Walking on Air*, 1987; and in *Pretty Polly, Ain't Afraid to Dance, The End of the Tunnel, I Am Osango, What's Wrong with Humpty Dumpty?, Egg on the Face of the Tiger, Blank Pages, A Midsummer Night's Dream, William, Antony and Cleopatra, Daft As a Brush*, and *The Old Reliable*.

RELATED CAREER—Commercial spokesperson for Weight Watchers (food products).

RECORDINGS: ALBUMS—*Make Mine Manhattan*, 1978; *Cole Porter Revisited*, 1979.

AWARDS: Golden Globe Award, New York Film Critics Award, Independent Film Importers and Distributors of America Award, and Academy Award nomination, all Best Actress, 1967, for *Georgy Girl*; Antoinette Perry Award nomination, Best Actress in a Play, 1976, for *Mrs. Warren's Profession*; Sarah Siddons Awards,

Best Stage Actress in Chicago, 1977 and 1978; also Emmy Award nomination for *House Calls*.

ADDRESSES: OFFICE—Box 1207, Topanga, CA 90290.*

*　　*　　*

REDGRAVE, Vanessa　1937-

PERSONAL: Born January 30, 1937, in London, England; daughter of Sir Michael (an actor) and Rachel (an actress; professional name, Rachel Kempson); married Tony Richardson (a director), April 29, 1962 (divorced, 1967); children: Natasha Jane, Joely Kim (with Richardson); Carlo Gabriel (with Franco Nero). EDUCATION: Trained for the stage at the Central School of Speech and Drama, 1955-57.

VOCATION: Actress.

CAREER: STAGE DEBUT—Clarissa, *The Reluctant Debutante*, Frinton Summer Theatre, Frinton, U.K., 1957. LONDON DEBUT—Caroline Lester, *A Touch of the Sun*, Saville Theatre, 1958. PRINCIPAL STAGE APPEARANCES—Mrs. Spottsworth, *Come On, Jeeves*, Arts Theatre, Cambridge, U.K., 1957; Sarah Undershaft, *Major Barbara*, Royal Court Theatre, London, 1958; principal boy, *Mother Goose*, Leatherhead Theatre, Surrey, U.K., 1958; Helena, *A Midsummer Night's Dream*, and Valeria, *Coriolanus*, both Shakespearean Memorial Theatre Company, Shakespeare Memorial Theatre, Stratford-on-Avon, U.K., 1959.

Rose Sinclair, *Look on Tempests*, Comedy Theatre, London, 1960; Stella Dean, *The Tiger and the Horse*, Queen's Theatre, London, 1960; Boletta, *The Lady from the Sea*, Queen's Theatre, 1961; Rosalind, *As You Like It*, Royal Shakespeare Company (RSC), Royal Shakespeare Theatre, Stratford-on-Avon, U.K., 1961, then Aldwych Theatre, London, 1962; Katharina, *The Taming of the Shrew*, RSC, Aldwych Theatre, 1961, then Royal Shakespeare Theatre, 1962; Imogen, *Cymbeline*, RSC, Royal Shakespeare Theatre, 1962; Nina, *The Seagull*, Queen's Theatre, 1964; title role, *The Prime of Miss Jean Brodie*, Wyndham's Theatre, London, 1966; Gwendolen Harleth, *Daniel Deronda*, University Theatre, Manchester, U.K., 1969; Susan Thistlewood, *Cato Street*, Young Vic Theatre, London, 1971; Polly Peachum, *The Threepenny Opera*, Prince of Wales Theatre, London, 1972; Viola, *Twelfth Night*, Shaw Theatre, London, 1972; Cleopatra, *Antony and Cleopatra*, Bankside Globe Theatre, London, 1973; Gilda, *Design for Living*, Phoenix Theatre, London, 1973; Ellida, *The Lady from the Sea*, Circle in the Square, New York City, 1976, then Royal Exchange Theatre, Manchester, U.K., 1978, later Round House Theatre, London, 1979; Nora, *A Touch of the Poet*, Young Vic Theatre, then Royal Haymarket Theatre, London, 1988. Also appeared in *Macbeth*, 1975; *The Aspern Papers*, 1984; *The Seagull*, London, 1985; and in *Antony and Cleopatra* and *The Taming of the Shrew*, both 1986.

FILM DEBUT—Pamela Gray, *Behind the Mask*, GW, 1958. PRINCIPAL FILM APPEARANCES—Jane, *Blow-Up*, Premier, 1966; Anne Boleyn, *A Man for All Seasons*, Columbia, 1966; Leonie Delt, *Morgan!* (also known as *Morgan: A Suitable Case for Treatment* and *A Suitable Case for Treatment*), Cinema V, 1966; Guinevere, *Camelot*, Warner Brothers/Seven Arts, 1967; Sheila, *The Sailor from Gibraltar*, Lopert, 1967; Clarissa, *The Charge of the Light Brigade*, United Artists, 1968; Isadora Duncan, *Isadora* (also known as *The Loves of Isadora*), Universal, 1968; Nina, *The Sea Gull,* Warner Brothers, 1968; Sylvia Pankhurst, *Oh! What a Lovely War,* Paramount, 1969; Flavia, *A Quiet Place in the Country* (also known as *Un tranquillo posto di campagna* and *Un coin tranquille a la campagne*), Lopert, 1970; narrator, *The Body,* Metro-Goldwyn-Mayer, 1970; title role, *Mary, Queen of Scots,* Universal, 1971; Andromache, *The Trojan Women,* Cinerama, 1971; Immacolata, *La Vacanza* (also known as *The Vacation* and *Vacation Dropout*), Lion, 1971; Sister Jeanne, *The Devils,* Warner Brothers, 1971; Mary Debenham, *Murder on the Orient Express,* Paramount, 1974.

Ann, *Out of Season* (also known as *Winter Rates*), Athenaeum/EMI, 1975; title role, *Julia,* Twentieth Century-Fox, 1977; Lola Deveraux, *The Seven Percent Solution,* Universal, 1977; narrator, *The Palestinians,* 1977; Agatha Christie, *Agatha,* Warner Brothers, 1979; Helen, *Yanks,* Universal, 1979; Hedi Lindquist, *Bear Island,* Columbia, 1980; Cosima Wagner, *Wagner,* Alan Landsburg, 1983; Olive Chancellor, *The Bostonians,* Almi, 1984; Nancy, *Steaming,* Columbia, 1985; Jean Travers, *Wetherby,* Metro-Goldwyn-Mayer/United Artists Classics, 1985; Mrs. Carlyle, *Comrades,* Curzon, 1987; Peggy Ramsay, *Prick Up Your Ears,* Samuel Goldwyn, 1987; Mrs. Garza, *Consuming Passions,* Samuel Goldwyn, 1988. Also appeared as Anne-Marie, *La Musica,* 1965; Jacky, *Red and Blue,* 1967; guest, *Let's All Make Love in London,* 1968; and in *Dropout,* 1969.

PRINCIPAL FILM WORK—Producer, *The Palestinians,* Battersby, 1977.

PRINCIPAL TELEVISION APPEARANCES—Mini-Series: Sarah Cloyce, "Three Sovereigns for Sarah," *American Playhouse,* PBS, 1985; Sophia, *Peter the Great,* NBC, 1986. Episodic: Wicked queen, "Snow White and the Seven Dwarfs," *Faerie Tale Theatre,* Showtime, 1985. Movies: Fania Fenelon, *Playing for Time,* CBS, 1980; Leenie Cabrezi, *My Body, My Child,* ABC, 1982; Richard Radley/Renee Richards, *Second Serve,* CBS, 1986. Plays: Title role, *Katherine Mansfield,* BBC, 1973; Lady Alice More, *A Man for All Seasons,* TNT, 1988; also Helena, *A Midsummer Night's Dream,* 1962; Rosalind, *As You Like It,* 1962; Maggie, *Sally,* 1964. Also appeared in *A Farewell to Arms.*

RELATED CAREER—Member of the board of governors, Central School of Speech and Drama, London, 1963—.

WRITINGS: Editor, *Pussies and Tigers* (writings by children), 1964.

AWARDS: *Evening Standard* Drama Award, Actress of the Year, 1961; Variety Club of Great Britain Award, Best Actress, 1961; Cannes Film Festival Award and Academy Award nomination, both Best Actress, 1966, for *Morgan!;* Variety Club of Great Britain Award, Best Actress, 1966; British Guild of Television Producers and Directors Award, 1966; Commander, Order of the British Empire (CBE), 1967; *Evening Standard* Drama Award, Actress of the Year, 1967; Academy Award nomination and Cannes Film Festival Award, both Best Actress, 1968, National Society of Film Critics Award, Leading Actress, 1969, and Film Critics' Guild (U.K.) Award, Best Actress, 1969, all for *Isadora;* Academy Award nomination, Best Actress, 1971, for *Mary, Queen of Scots;* Academy Award, Best Supporting Actress, 1977, for *Julia;* Golden Globe Award, 1978; Emmy Award, Best Actress in a Limited Series or Special, 1981, for *Playing for Time;* Laurence Olivier Award, 1984; Academy Award nomination, Best Actress, 1984, for *The Bostonians;* Emmy Award nomination, 1986, for *Peter the*

Great; Emmy Award nomination, Outstanding Actress in a Drama, 1986, for *Second Serve;* New York Film Critics Circle Award, Best Supporting Actress, 1987, and Golden Globe Award nomination, Best Actress in a Supporting Role, 1988, both for *Prick Up Your Ears.*

MEMBER: Workers' Revolutionary Party.

SIDELIGHTS: FAVORITE ROLES—Rosalind, in *As You Like It.*

ADDRESSES: MANAGER—Marina Martin Management, Ltd., 7 Windmill Street, London W1P 1HF, England. AGENT—Agency for the Performing Arts, 9000 Sunset Boulevard, Suite 1200, Los Angeles, CA 90069.*

*   *   *

REDINGTON, Michael   1927-

PERSONAL: Born May 18, 1927, in Leicester, England; son of Clarence John (a surveyor) and Kathleen (Mawby) Redington; married Ann Connell (a horticulturist), July 28, 1950; children: Mandy Jane, Simon John.

VOCATION: Producer and actor.

CAREER: STAGE DEBUT—Ghost of Christmas Past, *A Christmas Carol,* Leicester Repertory Company, Theatre Royal, Leicester, U.K., 1943. PRINCIPAL STAGE APPEARANCES—Snug the Joiner, *A Midsummer Night's Dream,* Old Vic Theatre Company, Metropolitan Opera House, New York City, 1954. Also appeared in productions of *Richard III, Antigone,* and *The School for Scandal,* all Old Vic Theatre Company, New Theatre, London, 1949.

PRINCIPAL STAGE WORK—Producer: *Heartaches of an English Pussycat,* Old Vic Theatre, London, 1980; *The Flying Karamazov Brothers,* May Fair Theatre, London, 1981; *84 Charing Cross Road,* Ambassadors' Theatre, London, 1981, then (with Alexander Cohen) Nederlander Theatre, New York City, 1982; *This Thing Called Love,* Ambassadors' Theatre, 1983; *Pack of Lies,* Lyric Theatre, London, 1983, then (with Arthur Cantor) Royale Theatre, New York City, 1985; *Breaking the Code,* Royal Haymarket Theatre, London, then (with James Nederlander) Neil Simon Theatre, New York City, both 1987; *Mr. and Mrs. Nobody,* Garrick Theatre, London, 1987; *The Best of Friends,* Apollo Theatre, London, 1987; *Mrs. Klein,* Apollo Theatre, 1988. Also produced *The Flying Karamazov Brothers,* Edinburgh Festival, Edinburgh, Scotland; productions of the Arena Stage Company, Washington, DC, at the Hong Kong Arts Festival; and productions of the Abbey Theatre Company, Dublin, Ireland, at the Baltimore International Theatre Festival, Baltimore, MD.

MAJOR TOURS—Snug the Joiner, *A Midsummer Night's Dream,* U.S. cities, 1954.

ADDRESSES: OFFICE—Michael Redington Ltd., 10 Maunsel Street, Westminster, London SW1P 2QL, England.

REED, Pamela   1949-

PERSONAL: Born April 2, 1949, in Tacoma, WA. EDUCATION: Graduated from the University of Washington.

VOCATION: Actress.

CAREER: BROADWAY DEBUT—Kathleen, *The November People*, Billy Rose Theatre, 1978. PRINCIPAL STAGE APPEARANCES—Merry Sue Tinglehoff, *Getting Through the Night*, Ensemble Studio Theatre, New York City, 1976; Emma, *Curse of the Starving Class*, New York Shakespeare Festival (NYSF), Public Theatre, New York City, 1978; Helena, *All's Well That Ends Well*, NYSF, Delacorte Theatre, New York City, 1978; Arlie, *Getting Out*, Phoenix Theatre, Marymount Manhattan Theatre, New York City, 1978; Luna, *Seduced*, American Place Theatre, New York City, 1979; Christine, *Sorrows of Stephen*, NYSF, Public Theatre, 1979; Sophia Zubritsky, *Fools*, Eugene O'Neill Theatre, New York City, 1981; Billy Marie, *Criminal Minds*, The Production Company, Theatre Guinevere, New York City, 1984; boy, Angela, Deb, and Mrs. Finch, *Fen*, NYSF, Public Theatre, 1984; Aunt Dan, *Aunt Dan and Lemon*, NYSF, Public Theatre, 1985; Vivie Warren, *Mrs. Warren's Profession*, Roundabout Theatre, New York City, 1985, then Haft Theatre, New York City, 1986. Also appeared in *Standing on My Knees.*

PRINCIPAL FILM APPEARANCES—Belle Starr, *The Long Riders*, United Artists, 1980; Bonnie Dummar, *Melvin and Howard*, Universal, 1980; Linda Mercer, *Eyewitness* (also known as *The Janitor*), Twentieth Century-Fox, 1981; Norine Sprockett, *Young Doctors in Love*, Twentieth Century-Fox, 1982; Trudy Cooper, *The Right Stuff*, Warner Brothers, 1983; Nancie "Shirley" Scot, *The Goodbye People*, Embassy, 1984; Gigi Hightower, *The Best of Times*, Universal, 1986; Iza, *The Clan of the Cave Bear*, Warner Brothers, 1986; Mary Graving, *Rachel River*, Taurus Entertainment, 1989.

PRINCIPAL TELEVISION APPEARANCES—Series: Sandi Farrell, *The Andros Targets*, CBS, 1977; T.J. Cavanaugh, *Tanner '88: The Dark Horse*, HBO, 1988. Episodic: Norma Heisler, *L.A. Law*, NBC, 1988. Movies: Sunny, *Inmates: A Love Story*, ABC, 1981; Edie Bannister, *I Want to Live*, ABC, 1983; Valerie Driscoll, *Heart of Steel*, ABC, 1983; Helen Grant, *Scandal Sheet*, ABC, 1985; Mary Welsh, *Hemingway*, syndicated, 1988; Grace, "Caroline?," *Hallmark Hall of Fame*, CBS, 1989. Specials: *Until She Talks*, PBS, 1983.

AWARDS: Drama Desk Award, Outstanding Featured Actress in a Play, 1979, for *Getting Out;* ACE Award, Best Actress in a Dramatic Role, 1989, for *Tanner '88: The Dark Horse.*

ADDRESSES: AGENT—Triad Artists, 888 Seventh Avenue, Suite 1602, New York, NY 10019.*

*   *   *

REID, Sheila

PERSONAL: EDUCATION: Trained for the stage at the Rose Bruford School.

VOCATION: Actress.

CAREER: PRINCIPAL STAGE APPEARANCES—Mavis Price, *The Gentle Avalanche*, Royal Court Theatre, London, 1963; Lucienne, *Ruling the Roost*, Philotis, *'Tis Pity She's a Whore*, Sonya, *The Wood Demon*, and Regan, *King Lear*, all Actors' Company, Wimbledon Theatre, London, 1974; chorus leader, "The Bacchae," and cow and shadow play puppeteer, "The Bean Stalk," in *The Bacchae and the Bean Stalk* (double-bill), Emily, *The Last Romantic*, La Carlotta, *The Phantom of the Opera*, and Elmire, *Tartuffe*, all Actors' Company, Wimbledon Theatre, 1975; Widow Leocadia Begbick, *A Man's a Man*, Hampstead Theatre Club, London, 1975; Gladys, *If You're Glad, I'll Be Frank*, and Mrs. Drudge, *The Real Inspector Hound*, both Young Vic Theatre, London, 1977; Smidge, Cousin Vladimir, and Olivia Alston, *Saratoga*, both Royal Shakespeare Company, Aldwych Theatre, London, 1978. Also appeared as Natasha, *The Three Sisters*, Mrs. Elvsted, *Hedda Gabler*, Dorinda, *The Beaux' Stratagem*, Bianca, *Othello*, and Mrs. Fainall, *The Way of the World*, all National Theatre Company, London; in *Wakefield Mystery Plays*, *Eastward Ho!*, and *The Bed Bug*, all Mermaid Theatre, London; Sonya, *Uncle Vanya*, Welsh National Theatre Company, Wales; as Flo Bates, *Half a Sixpence;* with the Bristol Old Vic Company, Bristol, U.K.; and in repertory in Colchester, U.K., Perth, U.K., and Farnham, U.K.

MAJOR TOURS—Nurse, *Romeo and Juliet*, British Council, Far Eastern cities, 1963; also as Pamela, *Five Finger Exercise*, U.K. cities.

PRINCIPAL FILM APPEARANCES—Bianca, *Othello*, Warner Brothers, 1965; Sara Kovac, *The Touch* (also known as *Be Roringen*), Cinerama, 1971; June, *I Want What I Want*, Cinerama, 1972; Dr. Mary Herrick, *Z.P.G.* (also known as *Zero Population Growth*), Paramount, 1972; Natasha, *The Three Sisters*, American Film Theatre, 1974; "Mother," *Big Wheels and Sailor*, Associates/Children's Film Foundation, 1979; Florrie, *Sir Henry at Rawlinson End*, Charisma, 1980; Gillian Pierce, *Five Days One Summer*, Warner Brothers, 1982; Lydia Gibson, *The Dresser*, Columbia, 1983; Mrs. Buttle, *Brazil*, Universal, 1985; Miss Friel, *The Lonely Passion of Judith Hearne*, Island, 1987; Doris, *The Raggedy Rawney* (also known as *The Rawney*), Island/Handmade, 1988. Also appeared in *Vroom*, Film Four International, 1988.

PRINCIPAL TELEVISION APPEARANCES—Mini-Series: Jenny, *Moll Flanders*, BBC, 1975, then PBS, 1980.

AWARDS: Most Promising Actress of the Year, 1963, for *The Gentle Avalanche.**

*   *   *

REID, Tim   1944-

PERSONAL: Born December 19, 1944, in Norfolk, VA; second wife's name, Daphne Maxwell (an actress); children: Tim, Jr., Tori (first marriage); Christopher (stepson). EDUCATION: Received B.S. in business and marketing from Norfolk State College.

VOCATION: Actor.

CAREER: PRINCIPAL FILM APPEARANCES—*Mother, Jugs, and Speed*, Twentieth Century-Fox, 1976; *Uptown Saturday Night*, Warner Brothers, 1974; also appeared in *The Union*.

PRINCIPAL TELEVISION APPEARANCES—Series: Regular, *Easy*

Does It . . . Starring Frankie Avalon, CBS, 1976; regular, *The Marilyn McCoo and Billy Davis, Jr. Show,* CBS, 1977; regular, *The Richard Pryor Show,* NBC, 1977; Gordon "Venus Flytrap" Sims, *WKRP in Cincinnati,* CBS, 1978-82; Michael Horne, *Teachers Only,* NBC, 1983; Detective Marcel "Downtown" Brown, *Simon and Simon,* CBS, 1983-84; host, *CBS Summer Playhouse,* CBS, 1987; Frank Parrish, *Frank's Place,* CBS, 1987-88; also *The Snoops,* CBS, 1989—. Pilots: Jay, *Bumpers,* NBC, 1977. Episodic: *Matlock,* NBC, 1987; also *Rhoda,* CBS; *Maude,* CBS; *Lou Grant,* CBS; *What's Happening?,* ABC; *Solid Gold,* syndicated; *Fernwood 2-Night,* syndicated. Specials: Counselor Tilson, "Little Lulu," *ABC Weekend Special,* ABC, 1978; Donald, *You Can't Take It with You,* CBS, 1979; *Battle of the Network Stars,* ABC, 1978, 1981, and 1984; Philadelphia host, *CBS All-American Thanksgiving Day Parade,* CBS, 1984; host, *CBS Cotton Bowl Parade,* CBS, 1987; host, *CBS All-American Thanksgiving Day Parade,* CBS, 1987; *Fourth Annual CBS Easter Parade,* CBS, 1988; *The Hollywood Christmas Parade,* syndicated, 1988.

PRINCIPAL TELEVISION WORK—Executive producer, *Frank's Place,* CBS, 1987-88; executive producer, *The Snoops,* CBS, 1989—.

RELATED CAREER—Comedian (with Tom Dreeson) appearing as "Tim and Tom," Chicago, IL, then U.S. cities, 1971-75; active in entertainment industry anti-drug programs.

NON-RELATED CAREER—Sales representative, DuPont Corporation.

WRITINGS: TELEVISION—Episodic: *WKRP in Cincinnati,* CBS, 1978-82. OTHER—*As I Feel It* (poetry and photography), 1982.

ADDRESSES: AGENT—The Garrett Company, 6922 Hollywood Boulevard, Los Angeles, CA 90028.*

*　　　*　　　*

REITMAN, Ivan   1946-

PERSONAL: Born October 27, 1946, in Komarmo, Czechoslovakia; immigrated to Canada in 1951; son of Leslie and Klara Reitman; married Genevieve Robert, September 12, 1976; children: Jason, Catherine, Carolyn. EDUCATION: McMaster University, Mus.B., 1969.

VOCATION: Producer, director, and composer.

CAREER: PRINCIPAL STAGE WORK—Producer: (With Edgar Lansbury and Joseph Beruh) *The Magic Show,* Cort Theatre, New York City, 1974; *The National Lampoon Show,* New Palladium Theatre, New York City, 1975; (also director) *Merlin,* Mark Hellinger Theatre, New York City, 1983.

PRINCIPAL FILM APPEARANCES—*The Canadian Conspiracy,* Schtick/HBO Pictures/Canadian Broadcasting Company, 1986. PRINCIPAL FILM WORK—Producer, director, and editor, *Foxy Lady,* Cinepix, 1971; executive producer and director, *Cannibal Girls,* American International, 1973; producer, *They Came from Within* (also known as *Shivers, Frissons,* and *The Parasite Murders*), American International, 1975; executive producer, *Rabid* (also known as *Rage*), Alpha/New World, 1976; producer and music supervisor, *House by the Lake* (also known as *Death Weekend*), American International, 1977; executive producer, *Blackout*

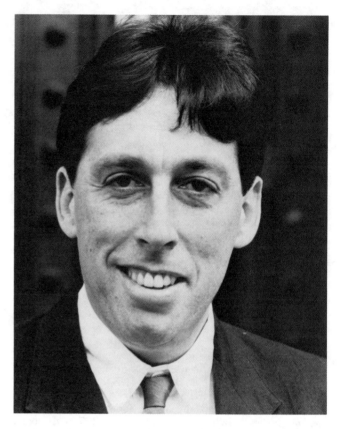

IVAN REITMAN

(also known as *Et la terreur commence*), Cinepix/New World, 1978; producer (with Matty Simmons), *National Lampoon's Animal House,* Universal, 1978; director, *Meatballs,* Paramount, 1979; producer (with Dan Goldberg) and director, *Stripes,* Columbia, 1981; producer, *Heavy Metal,* Columbia, 1981; executive producer, *Spacehunter: Adventures in the Forbidden Zone* (also known as *Road Gangs* and *Adventures in the Creep Zone*), Columbia, 1983; producer and director, *Ghostbusters,* Columbia, 1984; producer and director, *Legal Eagles,* Universal, 1986; executive producer, *Big Shots,* Twentieth Century-Fox, 1987; executive producer, *Feds,* Warner Brothers, 1988; executive producer, *Casual Sex?,* Universal, 1988; producer and director, *Twins,* Universal, 1988; producer and director, *Ghostbusters II,* Columbia, 1989.

PRINCIPAL TELEVISION WORK—Series: Executive producer (with Matty Simmons), *Delta House,* ABC, 1979; executive consultant, *The Real Ghostbusters* (animated; also known as *Slimer and the Real Ghostbusters*), ABC, 1986—. Episodic: Director, *Delta House,* ABC, 1979.

WRITINGS: FILM—Composer (with Doug Riley), *Foxy Lady,* Cinepix, 1971; composer, *They Came from Within* (also known as *Shivers, Frissons,* and *The Parasite Murders*), American International, 1975; composer, *Rabid* (also known as *Rage*), Alpha/New World, 1976.

AWARDS: Golden Reel Award, 1979, for *Meatballs;* Golden Reel Award, 1981, for *Heavy Metal;* Antoinette Perry Award nominations, Best Musical and Best Director, both 1983, for *Merlin;* Academy Award nomination, Best Director, 1984, for *Ghostbusters.*

MEMBER: Directors Guild of America, Academy of Motion Picture Arts and Sciences.

ADDRESSES: OFFICE—Ivan Reitman Productions, Columbia Plaza, Producers' Building 7, Room 8, Burbank, CA 91505.

*   *   *

REMICK, Lee   1935-

PERSONAL: Full name, Lee Ann Remick; born December 14, 1935, in Boston, MA; daughter of Frank E. (owner of a retail store) and Margaret Patricia (an actress; maiden name, Waldo) Remick; married William A. Colleran (a television director and producer), August 3, 1957 (divorced, November 23, 1969); married William Rory "Kip" Gowans (a producer), December 18, 1970; children: Kate, Matthew (first marriage). EDUCATION: Attended Barnard College, 1953; studied dancing at the Swoboda Ballet School, New York City, and with Charles Weidman.

VOCATION: Actress.

CAREER: BROADWAY DEBUT—Lois Holly, *Be Your Age,* 48th Street Theatre, 1953. LONDON DEBUT—Grace, *Bus Stop,* Phoenix Theatre, 1976. PRINCIPAL STAGE APPEARANCES—Dancer, *Paint Your Wagon,* State Fair Music Hall, Dallas, TX, 1953; Ado Annie, *Oklahoma!,* Fox River Valley Theatre, St. Charles, IL, 1954; Fay Apple, *Anyone Can Whistle,* Majestic Theatre, New York City, 1964; Susy Hendrix, *Wait until Dark,* Ethel Barrymore Theatre,

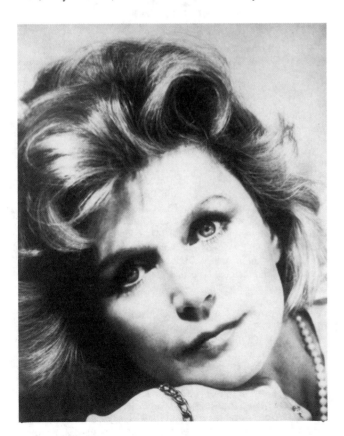

LEE REMICK

New York City, 1966. Also appeared in *Brigadoon,* Cape Cod Melody Tent, Cape Cod, MA, then South Shore Music Circus, Cohasset, MA, both 1953; *Show Boat* and *Annie Get Your Gun,* both Fox River Valley Theatre, 1954; in *I Do, I Do,* 1983; and in *Follies in Concert,* 1985.

MAJOR TOURS—Title role, *Jenny Kissed Me,* U.S. cities, 1955; the Girl, *The Seven Year Itch,* U.S. cities, 1956; also in *Brigadoon,* U.S. cities, 1953.

FILM DEBUT—Betty Lou Fleckum, *A Face in the Crowd,* Warner Brothers, 1957. PRINCIPAL FILM APPEARANCES—Eula Varner, *The Long Hot Summer,* Twentieth Century-Fox, 1958; Laura Manion, *Anatomy of a Murder,* Columbia, 1959; Callie, *These Thousand Hills,* Twentieth Century-Fox, 1959; Carol Baldwin, *Wild River,* Twentieth Century-Fox, 1960; Temple Drake, *Sanctuary,* Twentieth Century-Fox, 1961; Kirsten, *Days of Wine and Roses,* Warner Brothers, 1962; Kelly Sherwood, *Experiment in Terror* (also known as *Grip of Fear*), Columbia, 1962; Stella Black, *The Running Man,* Columbia, 1963; Molly Thatcher, *The Wheeler Dealers* (also known as *Separate Beds*), Metro-Goldwyn-Mayer, 1963; Georgette Thomas, *Baby, the Rain Must Fall* (also known as *Traveling Lady*), Columbia, 1965; Cora Templeton Massingale, *The Hallelujah Trail,* United Artists, 1965; Karen Leland, *The Detective,* Twentieth Century-Fox, 1968; Kate Palmer, *No Way to Treat a Lady,* Paramount, 1968; Sheila, *Hard Contract,* Twentieth Century-Fox, 1969.

Fay, *Loot,* Cinevision, 1971; Antonia Lynch-Gibbon, *A Severed Head,* Columbia, 1971; Viv Stamper, *Sometimes a Great Notion* (also known as *Never Give an Inch*), Universal, 1971; Julia, *A Delicate Balance,* American Film Theatre, 1973; Kate Brook, *Hennessy,* American International, 1975; Katherine Thorn, *The Omen* (also known as *Birthmark*), Twentieth Century-Fox, 1976; Barbara, *Telefon,* Metro-Goldwyn-Mayer/United Artists, 1977; Dr. Zonfeld, *The Medusa Touch,* Warner Brothers, 1978; Eugenia, *The Europeans,* Levitt-Pickman, 1979; Greta Vandemann, *The Competition,* Columbia, 1980; Maggie Stratton, *Tribute,* Twentieth Century-Fox, 1980; Anne Grange, *Emma's War,* Curzon, 1985. Also appeared as herself, *Montgomery Clift* (documentary), 1982.

PRINCIPAL TELEVISION APPEARANCES—Mini-Series: Lady Margaret Alexander Weidman, *QB VII,* ABC, 1974; Jennie Jerome, *Jennie: Lady Randolph Churchill,* Thames, then PBS, both 1975; Erica Trenton, *Wheels* (also known as *Arthur Hailey's "Wheels"*), NBC, 1978; Kay Summersby, *Ike: The War Years,* ABC, 1979; Kate Browning, *Mistral's Daughter,* CBS, 1984; Sandra Bernhardt, *Around the World in 80 Days,* NBC, 1989. Pilots: Host and wife in "All Her Own" segment, *Of Men, Of Women,* ABC, 1972. Episodic: Katrin Holstrom, "The Farmer's Daughter," *Theater '62,* NBC, 1962; also *Kraft Television Theater,* NBC; *Robert Montgomery Presents,* NBC; *Studio One,* CBS; *Armstrong Circle Theatre,* NBC; *Playhouse 90,* CBS.

Movies: Cassie Walters, *The Blue Knight,* NBC, 1973; Fern O'Neil, *And No One Could Save Her,* ABC, 1973; Elizabeth McHenry, *A Girl Named Sooner,* NBC, 1975; Fran Morrison, *Hustling,* ABC, 1975; JoAnn Hammil, *Breaking Up,* ABC, 1978; Diane Conti, *Torn between Two Lovers,* CBS, 1979; Mira Adams, *The Women's Room,* ABC, 1980; Margaret Sullavan, *Haywire,* CBS, 1980; Leslie Crosbie, *The Letter,* ABC, 1982; Janet Broderick, *The Gift of Love: A Christmas Story,* CBS, 1983; Terry Seton, *Rearview Mirror,* NBC, 1984; Michelle Tenney, *A Good Sport,* CBS, 1984; Jan Charters, *Toughlove,* ABC, 1985; Alicia Browning, *Of Pure Blood,* CBS, 1986; Frances Bradshaw Schreuder, *Nutcracker: Money, Madness, and Murder,* NBC, 1987; Grace Gardner, *The Vision,* BBC, 1987; Jesse Maloney, *Jesse,* CBS, 1988; Marge Duffield, *A Bridge to Silence,* CBS, 1989; also *The Snow Queen,* 1985; as Gene LePere, *Dark Holiday,* 1989. Specials: Miranda, "The Tempest," *Hallmark Hall of Fame,* NBC, 1960; *The Andy Williams Special,* NBC, 1963; Lola, *Damn Yankees,* NBC, 1967; Maggie, "The Man Who Came to Dinner," *Hallmark Hall of Fame,* NBC, 1972; *James Stewart: A Wonderful Life,* PBS, 1987; host, *Remembering Marilyn,* ABC, 1988; *The Kennedy Center Honors: A Celebration of the Performing Arts,* CBS, 1988; *Gregory Peck—His Own Man,* Cinemax, 1988; also *An American Portrait,* 1984; *Follies in Concert,* 1986; *A Star Spangled Celebration,* 1987; and as Eleanor Roosevelt, *Eleanor: In Her Own Words,* 1987.

AWARDS: Academy Award nomination, Best Actress, 1963, for *Days of Wine and Roses;* Hasty Pudding Woman of the Year Award from the Harvard Hasty Pudding Theatricals, 1965; Antoinette Perry Award nomination, Best Actress in a Drama, 1966, for *Wait until Dark;* Golden Globe Award, Best Television Actress—Drama, and Emmy Award nomination, both 1974, for *The Blue Knight;* Emmy Award nomination, 1975, for *QB VII;* British Academy of Film and Television Arts Award, Best Actress—Television, 1975, and Golden Globe Award, Best Television Actress—Drama, 1976, both for *Jennie: Lady Randolph Churchill.* Honorary degrees: Doctor of Humane Letters, Emerson College, 1975.

MEMBER: Actors' Equity Association, Screen Actors Guild, American Federation of Television and Radio Artists.

ADDRESSES: AGENT—Ben Benjamin, International Creative Management, 8899 Beverly Boulevard, Los Angeles, CA 90048.*

*   *   *

RHYS-DAVIES, John   1944-

PERSONAL: Born May 5, 1944, in Salisbury, England; son of Rhys Davies (a mechanical engineer) and Mary Margretta Phyllis Jones (a nurse); married Suzanne A.D. Wilkinson (a translator), 1966; children: Ben, Tom. EDUCATION: University of East Anglia, B.A., English and history, 1966; graduated from the Royal Academy of Dramatic Art, 1968.

VOCATION: Actor.

CAREER: PRINCIPAL STAGE APPEARANCES—Sebastian, *The Tempest,* Mermaid Theatre, London, 1970; Captain Vitelli, *The Lorenzaccio Story,* Royal Shakespeare Company (RSC), Other Place Theatre, Stratford-on-Avon, U.K., 1977, then Warehouse Theatre, London, 1978; Duke Frederick, *As You Like It,* RSC, Royal Shakespeare Theatre, Stratford-on-Avon, 1977; Monatond, *The Sons of Light,* RSC, Other Place Theatre, 1977; Henry Beaufort, *Henry IV, Part One,* RSC, Royal Shakespeare Theatre, 1977, then Aldwych Theatre, London, 1978; Cardinal Beaufort, *Henry IV, Part Two,* RSC, Aldwych Theatre, 1978. Also appeared in *Under Milk Wood,* Dolphin Theatre Company, Shaw Theatre, London, 1974; as Falstaff, *The Merry Wives of Windsor;* in *The Misanthrope, A Servant of Two Masters, It Happened in Venice, Hedda Gabler, Desire Caught by the Tail, Love on the Dole, How the Other Half Loves, Royal Hunt of the Sun, Macbeth, Hamlet, The Shop at Sly Corner, A Month in the Country, The Revenger's*

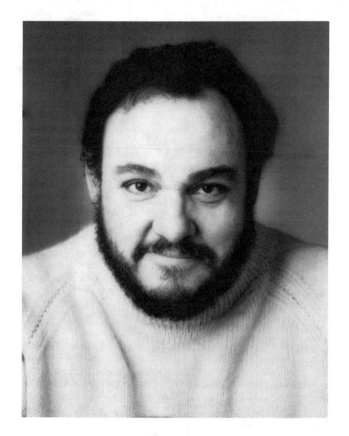

JOHN RHYS-DAVIES

Tragedy, Women Beware Women, Murder at the Vicarage, The Cherry Orchard, Troilus and Cressida, Volpone, and *Othello,* all in the U.K.

PRINCIPAL FILM APPEARANCES—Special policeman, *The Black Windmill,* Universal, 1974; Sallah, *Raiders of the Lost Ark,* Paramount, 1981; Stephanos Markoulis, *Sphinx,* Warner Brothers, 1981; Andre Cassell, *Victor/Victoria,* Metro-Goldwyn-Mayer/United Artists (MGM/UA), 1982; Rasoul, *Sahara,* MGM/UA, 1984; Baron Fortinbras, *Sword of the Valiant,* Cannon, 1984; Mustapha, *Best Revenge,* Black Cat/RKR Releasing, 1984; Dogati, *King Solomon's Mines,* Cannon Group, 1985; Corky Taylor, *Firewalker,* Cannon, 1986; Chris Tucker, *In the Shadow of Kilimanjaro,* Scotti Brothers, 1986; General Leonid Pushkin, *The Living Daylights,* MGM/UA, 1987; Claudio Rossi, *Il Giovane Toscanini* (also known as *The Young Toscanini*), Carthogo/Canal Plus, 1988; Anton Weber, *Waxwork,* Vestron, 1988; Sallah, *Indiana Jones and the Last Crusade,* Paramount, 1989. Also appeared in *Predator* and *Fire in Eden.*

PRINCIPAL TELEVISION APPEARANCES—Series: Sir Edward, *The Quest,* ABC, 1982. Mini-Series: Vasco Rodriguez, *Shogun,* NBC, 1980; Quillant Gornt, *Noble House,* NBC, 1988; Sammy Mutterperl, *War and Remembrance,* ABC, 1988; also *I, Claudius,* BBC, 1976, then *Masterpiece Theatre,* PBS, 1977; "Reilly, Ace of Spies," *Mystery,* PBS; *Great Expectations,* Disney Channel, 1989. Pilots: John Grimshaw, *No Man's Land,* NBC, 1984; Dr. Paul Boardman, *Blessed,* NBC, 1989. Episodic: Lancaster, *Murder, She Wrote,* CBS, 1988; also "School for Scandal," *Play of the Week,* BBC. Movies: Nestor, *The Nativity,* ABC, 1978; Silas, *Peter and Paul,* CBS, 1981; Reginald Front de Boeuf, *Ivanhoe,* CBS, 1982;

Gamal Abdel Nasser, *Sadat,* syndicated, 1983; Babu, *Kim,* CBS, 1984; Simon, *Nairobi Affair,* CBS, 1984; Police Chief Murphy, *The Little Match Girl,* NBC, 1987; Edward Tremayne, *Perry Mason: The Case of the Murdered Madam,* NBC, 1987; Zeus, *The Goddess of Love,* NBC, 1988; Lieutenant Smight, *Higher Ground,* CBS, 1988; also *The Naked Civil Servant,* BBC. Plays: *The Merchant of Venice,* BBC; *Henry VII,* BBC. Also appeared in *Robin Hood.*

RELATED CAREER—President, Talisman Productions, 1988.

NON-RELATED CAREER—Teacher, Walton County Secondary School, Norfolk, U.K., 1967; director, Hardy Research Laboratories, Whitefish, MT, 1988.

SIDELIGHTS: RECREATIONS—Collecting classic cars, contemporary art, and books; chess.

ADDRESSES: AGENT—Russ Lyster, The Agency, 10351 Santa Monica Boulevard, Suite 211, Los Angeles, CA 90025. PUBLICIST—Sharry Manning, Baker/Winokur/Ryder Public Relations, 9348 Civic Center Drive, Suite 407, Beverly Hills, CA 90210.

*   *   *

RICHARDS, Beah

PERSONAL: Born in Vicksburg, MS; married Hugh Harrell. EDUCATION: Attended Dillard University; trained for the stage at San Diego Community Theatre.

VOCATION: Actress.

CAREER: OFF-BROADWAY DEBUT—Grandmother, *Take a Giant Step,* Jan Hus House, 1956. PRINCIPAL STAGE APPEARANCES— Understudy for Lena Younger, *A Raisin in the Sun,* Ethel Barrymore Theatre, New York City, 1959; Viney, *The Miracle Worker,* Playhouse Theatre, New York City, 1959; Idella Landy, *Purlie Victorious,* Cort Theatre, New York City, 1961; Sister Margaret, *The Amen Corner,* Robertson Playhouse, Los Angeles, CA, 1963; the Woman, *Arturo Ui,* Lunt-Fontanne Theatre, New York City, 1963; Sister Margaret, *The Amen Corner,* Ethel Barrymore Theatre, 1965, then Theatre of Being, Los Angeles, 1966; Addie, *The Little Foxes,* Vivian Beaumont Theatre, New York City, 1967; Lena Younger, *A Raisin in the Sun,* Inner City Repertory Theatre, Los Angeles, 1968; Lena Younger, *A Raisin in the Sun,* Yale Repertory Theatre, New Haven, CT, 1983; also appeared in *The Crucible,* Center Theatre Group, Ahmanson Theatre, Los Angeles, 1972; *One Is a Crowd,* Inner City Repertory Theatre, 1970, then 1973; *A Black Woman Speaks,* Inner City Repertory Theatre, 1975, then 1976; *Iago,* Inner City Cultural Center, 1979; and in *An Evening with Beah Richards* (one-woman show).

PRINCIPAL FILM APPEARANCES—May Scott, *Take a Giant Step,* United Artists, 1959; Viney, *The Miracle Worker,* United Artists, 1962; Idella, *Gone Are the Days* (also known as *The Man from C.O.T.T.O.N.* and *Purlie Victorious*), Hammer, 1963; Mrs. Prentice, *Guess Who's Coming to Dinner,* Columbia, 1967; Rose Scott, *Hurry Sundown,* Paramount, 1967; Mrs. Bellamy (Mama Caleba), *In the Heat of the Night,* United Artists, 1967; Mama Tiny, *The Great White Hope,* Twentieth Century-Fox, 1970; Charity Tomlin, *The Biscuit Eater,* Buena Vista, 1972; Florence, *Mahogany,* Para-

mount, 1975; Verna, *Inside Out,* Hemdale, 1986; Miss Hanks, *Big Shots,* Twentieth Century-Fox, 1987.

PRINCIPAL TELEVISION APPEARANCES—Series: Rose Kincaid, *The Bill Cosby Show,* NBC, 1970-71; Aunt Ethel, *Sanford and Son,* NBC, 1972. Mini-Series: Cynthia Harvey Palmer, *Roots: The Next Generations,* ABC, 1979. Pilots: Grandma Bessie, *A Dream for Christmas,* ABC, 1973; Grandma, *Just an Old Sweet Song,* CBS, 1976; Aunt Velvet, *Down Home,* CBS, 1978; Mona Rainey, *Too Good to Be True,* ABC, 1983; Edna, *Generation,* ABC, 1985; Miss Aldrich, *Time Out for Dad* (also known as *Kowalski Loves Ya* and *Kowalski's Way*), NBC, 1987; Katherine, "Barrington," *CBS Summer Playhouse,* CBS, 1987. Episodic: Jamaican woman, "The Curse," *The Hitchhiker,* HBO, 1986; Carolyn Hurley, *227,* NBC, 1986 and 1987; Pockets, *Hunter,* NBC, 1986 and 1988; Olive Varden, *Frank's Place,* CBS, 1987; Narcissa, *Beauty and the Beast,* CBS, 1987, 1988, and 1989; Grandmother Rogers, *The Facts of Life,* NBC, 1988; Ola Mae, *Murder, She Wrote,* CBS, 1988; also Lois, *Benson,* ABC; *Dr. Kildare,* NBC; *The Big Valley,* ABC; *I Spy,* NBC; *Hawaii Five-O,* CBS; *Ironside,* NBC; *Room 222,* ABC; *It Takes a Thief,* ABC; *On Stage,* ABC. Movies: Jessie Blake, *Footsteps* (also known as *Footsteps: Nice Guys Finish Last*), CBS, 1972; Thelma, *Outrage!,* ABC, 1973; Lilly Brooks, *Ring of Passion,* NBC, 1978; Wendell's Grandma, *A Christmas without Snow,* CBS, 1980; Miz Porter, *The Sophisticated Gents,* NBC, 1981; Sally Framm, *Acceptable Risks,* ABC, 1986; Elvira Backus, *As Summers Die,* HBO, 1986; also *The Autobiography of Miss Jane Pittman,* CBS, 1974. Specials: *Inner Visions—Beah Richards,* PBS, 1978; voice of Zazu, *Banjo, the Woodpile Cat* (animated), ABC, 1982.

WRITINGS: STAGE—*One Is a Crowd,* Inner City Repertory Theatre, Los Angeles, CA, 1970; *A Black Woman Speaks,* Inner City Repertory Theatre, 1975. OTHER—*A Black Woman Speaks and Other Poems.*

AWARDS: Best Plays' citation and Theatre World Award, both 1964, for *The Amen Corner;* Academy Award nomination, Best Supporting Actress, 1967, for *Guess Who's Coming to Dinner;* All-American Press Association Award, 1968; inducted into Black Filmmakers Hall of Fame, 1974.

MEMBER: Actors' Equity Association, Screen Actors Guild, Congress of Racial Equality, National Association for the Advancement of Colored People.

ADDRESSES: AGENT—Jack Fields and Associates, 9255 Sunset Boulevard, Suite 1105, Los Angeles, CA 90069.*

*   *   *

RICHARDSON, Lee   1926-

PERSONAL: Born September 11, 1926, in Chicago, IL. EDUCATION: Trained for the stage at the Goodman Theatre.

VOCATION: Actor.

CAREER: BROADWAY DEBUT—Reverend Phipps, *The Legend of Lizzie,* 54th Street Theatre, New York City, 1959. PRINCIPAL STAGE APPEARANCES—Percival, *Misalliance,* Theatre Guild-American Theatre Society, Locust Theatre, Philadelphia, PA, then Erlanger Theatre, Buffalo, NY, both 1954; Bertrand De Poulengey,

Saint Joan, Phoenix Theatre, New York City, 1956; Leone, *Volpone,* Rooftop Theatre, New York City, 1957; Ben Gant, *Look Homeward Angel,* The Playhouse, Wilmington, DE, 1960; intern, *The Death of Bessie Smith,* York Playhouse, then Cherry Lane Theatre, both New York City, 1961; Father Francis, "Someone from Assisi" in *Plays for Bleecker Street,* Circle in the Square, New York City, 1962; Wilfred Oliver, *Lord Pingo,* Royale Theatre, New York City, 1962; Edgar, *King Lear,* and Bassanio, *The Merchant of Venice,* both New York Shakespeare Festival, Delacorte Theatre, New York City, 1962; Claudius, *Hamlet,* and Lieutenant Fedotik, *The Three Sisters,* both Minnesota Theatre Company, Tyrone Guthrie Theatre, Minneapolis, MN, 1963; Sir Politic Wouldbe, *Volpone,* Peter Cauchon, *Saint Joan,* and the Son, *The Glass Menagerie,* all Minnesota Theatre Company, Tyrone Guthrie Theatre, 1964.

Iago, *Othello,* American National Theatre Academy Theatre, New York City, 1970; Lord Bothwell, *Vivat! Vivat Regina!,* Broadhurst Theatre, New York City, 1972; the Elephant, "Louis and the Elephant," and title role, "The Adventures of Eddie Greshaw" both in *Louis and the Elephant,* Sheridan Square Playhouse, New York City, 1971; Lord Green, *The Jockey Club Stakes,* Cort Theatre, New York City, then Kennedy Center for the Performing Arts, Washington, DC, both 1973; Alan Harrison, *Find Your Way Home,* Brooks Atkinson Theatre, New York City, 1974; Floyd Kinkaid, "The Oldest Living Graduate" in *A Texas Trilogy,* Broadhurst Theatre, 1976; Andrew Creed, *Trick,* Playhouse Theatre, New York City, 1979; Richard, *Father's Day,* American Place Theatre, New York City, 1979; Alvaro, *Goodbye Fidel,* Ambassador Theatre, New York City, 1980; Howard, *Tricks of the Trade,* Brooks Atkinson Theatre, 1980; Becket, *Murder in the Cathedral,* St. Malachy's Theatrespace, New York City, 1981; Sir Harry Sims, *The Twelve-Pound Look,* and Andrew Crocker-Harris, *The Browning Version,* both Roundabout Theatre, New York City, 1982; St. John Quartermaine, *Quartermaine's Terms,* Playhouse 91, New York City, 1983; Ephraim Cabot, *Desire Under the Elms,* Roundabout Theatre, 1984; General St. Pe, *The Waltz of the Toreadors,* Roundabout Theatre, 1985.

Also appeared in *Beckett,* St. James Theatre, New York City, 1960; *Bartleby* and *The American Dream,* both York Playhouse, 1961; *House of Atreus,* Minnesota Theatre Company, Billy Rose Theatre, 1968; *The Devil's Disciple,* American Shakespeare Festival, Stratford, CT, 1970; *The Merry Wives of Windsor* and *Mourning Becomes Electra,* both American Shakespeare Festival, 1971; *Major Barbara,* American Shakespeare Festival, 1972; *Semmelweiss, Hedda Gabler,* and *The Millionairess,* all Hartman Theatre, Stamford, CT, 1981; *Meetings with Mustapha Mutura,* Crossroads Theatre Company, New Brunswick, NJ, 1982; *Uncommon Women and Others,* Huntington Theatre Company, Boston, MA, 1983; *Slow Dance on the Killing Ground,* Crossroads Theatre Company, 1984; *The Devil's Disciple,* Circle in the Square, New York City, 1989; and in *Thieves Carnival;* also appeared with the Minnesota Theatre Company, Tyrone Guthrie Theatre, 1965; and with the Yale Repertory Theatre, New Haven, CT, 1970-71.

PRINCIPAL STAGE WORK—Director, *The Colored Museum,* Crossroads Theatre Company, 1985; also stage director, Crossroads Theatre Company, 1982.

PRINCIPAL FILM APPEARANCES—Narrator, *Network,* Metro-Goldwyn-Mayer/United Artists, 1976; Warden Renfrew, *Brubaker,* Twentieth Century-Fox, 1980; Sam Heinsdorff, *Prince of the City,* Warner Brothers, 1981; Jack Fein, *Daniel,* Paramount, 1983; Mr. Grey, *I Am the Cheese,* Almi, 1983; Dominic Prizzi, *Prizzi's*

Honor, Twentieth Century-Fox, 1985; Jeffries, *Amazing Grace and Chuck,* Tri-Star, 1987; Sam, *Sweet Lorraine,* Angelika, 1987; Dennis Maslow, *The Believers,* Orion, 1987; Mitchell Warsaw, *Tiger Warsaw,* Sony, 1988; Anton Bartok, *The Fly II,* Twentieth Century-Fox, 1989.

PRINCIPAL TELEVISION APPEARANCES—Series: Jim Swanson, *The Guiding Light,* CBS. Episodic: Bayard, "The Last Ballot," *Ourstory,* PBS, 1975; Everett Norman, *The Insiders,* ABC, 1985; Dr. Ernst Decker, *Stingray,* NBC, 1986; also "The Joy That Kills," *American Playhouse,* PBS, 1985; *Kate and Allie,* CBS. Movies: Sam Vogul, *Country Gold,* CBS, 1982; Chief Jim Hart, *Doubletake,* CBS, 1985; Larry Baumgarten, *Laura Lansing Slept Here,* NBC, 1988; Chief of Detectives Hart, *Internal Affairs,* CBS, 1988. Specials: Narrator, *Francis of Assisi: A Search for the Man and His Meaning,* NBC, 1977; Lou, *After the Fall,* NBC, 1974.

RELATED CAREER—Founder and artistic director, Crossroads Theatre Company.

ADDRESSES: OFFICE—Crossroads Theatre Company, 320 Memorial Parkway, New Brunswick, NJ 08901.*

*   *   *

RICHARDSON, Miranda

PERSONAL: Born in Lancashire, England; father, a marketing executive. EDUCATION: Trained for the stage at the Bristol Old Vic Theatre School, 1977-79.

VOCATION: Actress.

CAREER: PRINCIPAL STAGE APPEARANCES—*The Changeling* and *Mountain Language,* both National Theatre, London, 1988; also appeared in *Moving,* Queen's Theatre, London; and in productions of *All My Sons, Who's Afraid of Virginia Woolf?, The Life of Einstein,* and *Educating Rita.*

FILM DEBUT—Ruth Ellis, *Dance with a Stranger,* Twentieth Century-Fox, 1985. PRINCIPAL FILM APPEARANCES—Oriel, *Underworld,* Limehouse/Green Man, 1985; Mary Turner, *The Innocent,* TVS/Curzon, 1985; DHSS blond, *Eat the Rich,* New Line Cinema, 1987; Mrs. Victor, *Empire of the Sun,* Warner Brothers, 1987.

PRINCIPAL TELEVISION APPEARANCES—Series: Queen Elizabeth I, *The Black Adder II,* BBC, then Arts and Entertainment, 1986. Mini-Series: Paula Amory, *A Woman of Substance,* syndicated, 1984; also "Sorrel and Son," *Masterpiece Theatre,* PBS. Movies: Daphne Heccomb, *The Death of the Heart,* Granada, 1986, then *Masterpiece Theatre,* PBS, 1987; Penny Newhouse, *After Pilkington,* BBC, 1986, then Arts and Entertainment, 1988. Also appeared in *The Hard Word.*

ADDRESSES: AGENT—Kerry Gardner, 15 Kensington High Street, London W8 5NP, England.*

RICHMOND, John Peter
See CARRADINE, John

*   *   *

RICHMOND, Peter
See CARRADINE, John

*   *   *

RICHTER, Deborah

PERSONAL: Married Charles Haid (an actor), February 17, 1985.

VOCATION: Actress.

CAREER: PRINCIPAL FILM APPEARANCES—Dolly, *Hometown, U.S.A.,* Film Ventures International, 1979; Susan, *Swap Meet,* Dimension, 1979; Barbara, *Gorp,* American International/Filmways, 1980; Pammie, *Promised Land,* Vestron, 1987; Gwen, *Square Dance,* Island, 1987; Cindy Wickes, *Winners Take All,* Manson/Apollo, 1987; Nady Simmons, *Cyborg* (also known as *Cyborg Attack from the Future*), Cannon Releasing, 1989. Also appeared in *Hot Moves,* Cardinal Film Releasing, 1984; *The Banker,* 1989.

PRINCIPAL TELEVISION APPEARANCES—Series: Sherry Levy, *All Is Forgiven,* NBC, 1986. Mini-Series: Lizabeth, *Testimony of Two Men,* syndicated, 1977; Angela Morelli, *Aspen* (also known as *The Innocent and the Damned,* NBC, 1977; Val, *Arthur Hailey's "Wheels,"* NBC, 1978; Rebecca Stolfitz, *Centennial,* NBC, 1978. Pilots: Meredith Gilhooley, *Last Chance,* NBC, 1978; Holly Brannigan, "Roughhouse" (also known as "House and Home"), *CBS Summer Playhouse,* CBS, 1988. Episodic: Kathy, *Alfred Hitchcock Presents,* NBC, 1985; Daryl Ann, *Hill Street Blues,* NBC, 1986-88; also *Cheers,* NBC, 1985. Movies: Bonnie, *Portrait of a Stripper,* CBS, 1979; Molly, *The Rebels,* syndicated, 1979; Brigit Kummel, *Twirl,* NBC, 1981; Lucille Hartley, *My Wicked, Wicked Ways . . . The Legend of Errol Flynn,* CBS, 1985; Patti, *Christmas Eve,* NBC, 1986.

RELATED CAREER—Professional model.

ADDRESSES: AGENT—The Light Company, 901 Bringham Avenue, Brentwood, CA 90049.

*   *   *

ROBARDS, Jason   1922-

PERSONAL: Full name, Jason Nelson Robards, Jr.; early in his career known as Jason Robards, Jr.; born July 26, 1922, in Chicago, IL; son of Jason, Sr. (an actor) and Hope Maxine (Glanville) Robards; married Eleanor Pitman, 1948 (divorced, 1958); married Rachel Taylor (divorced); married Lauren Bacall (an actress), July 4, 1961 (divorced, 1969); married Lois O'Connor (a producer), 1970; children: Jason III, Sarah Louise, David (first marriage); Sam (third marriage); Shannon, Jake (fourth marriage). EDUCATION: Trained for the stage at the American Academy of

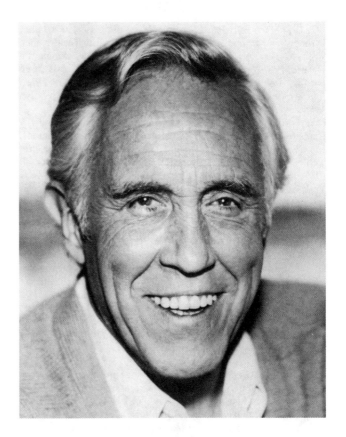

JASON ROBARDS

Dramatic Arts, 1946-47; also studied acting with Uta Hagen. MILITARY: U.S. Navy, radioman, 1939-46.

VOCATION: Actor.

CAREER: STAGE DEBUT—*Out of the Frying Pan,* Delyork Theatre, Rehoboth Beach, DE, 1947. BROADWAY DEBUT—*The Mikado,* D'Oyly Carte Opera Company, Century Theatre, 1947. PRINCIPAL STAGE APPEARANCES—Rear end of the cow, *Jack and the Beanstalk,* Children's World Theatre, New York City, 1947; Buoyant, *Buoyant Billions,* 23rd Street YMCA, New York City, 1947; Ed Moody, *American Gothic,* Circle in the Square, New York City, 1953; Hickey, *The Iceman Cometh,* Circle in the Square, 1956; Jamie, *Long Day's Journey into Night,* Helen Hayes Theatre, New York City, 1956; Hotspur, *Henry IV, Part I,* and Polixenes, *The Winter's Tale,* both Stratford Shakespearean Festival, Stratford, ON, Canada, 1958; Manley Halliday, *The Disenchanted,* Coronet Theatre, New York City, 1958; title role, *Macbeth,* Metropolitan Boston Arts Center, Cambridge, MA, 1959; Julian Berniers, *Toys in the Attic,* Hudson Theatre, New York City, 1960; William Baker, *Big Fish, Little Fish,* American National Theatre and Academy Theatre, New York City, 1961; Murray Burns, *A Thousand Clowns,* Eugene O'Neill Theatre, New York City, 1962; Quentin, *After the Fall,* and Seymour Rosenthal, *But for Whom Charlie,* both Washington Square Theatre, New York City, 1964; Erie Smith, *Hughie,* Royale Theatre, New York City, 1964; Vicar of St. Peter's, *The Devils,* Broadway Theatre, New York City, 1965; Captain Starkey, *We Bombed in New Haven,* Ambassador Theatre, New York City, 1968.

Frank Elgin, *The Country Girl,* Eisenhower Theatre, Washington,

DC, 1971, then Billy Rose Theatre, New York City, 1972; James Tyrone, Jr., *A Moon for the Misbegotten,* Eisenhower Theatre, then Morosco Theatre, New York City, both 1973, later Ahmanson Theatre, Los Angeles, CA, 1974; Erie Smith, *Hughie,* Zellerbach Theatre, Los Angeles, 1975; James Tyrone, Sr., *Long Day's Journey into Night,* Eisenhower Theatre, 1975, then Brooklyn Academy of Music, Brooklyn, NY, 1976; Erie Smith, *Hughie,* Lake Forest Theatre, Lake Forest, IL, 1976; Cornelius Melody, *A Touch of the Poet,* Helen Hayes Theatre, 1977; Martin Vanderhof, *You Can't Take It with You,* Booth Theatre, then Plymouth Theatre, both New York City, later Kennedy Center, Washington, DC, all 1983; Hickey, *The Iceman Cometh,* Lunt-Fontanne Theatre, New York City, 1985, then James A. Doolittle Theatre, UCLA Center for the Arts/The Theatre Group, Los Angeles, 1986; Cooper, *A Month of Sundays,* Ritz Theatre, New York City, 1987; James Tyrone, Sr., *Long Day's Journey into Night,* and Nat Miller, *Ah, Wilderness,* both Neil Simon Theatre, New York City, 1988. Also appeared in *Iolanthe* and *The Yeoman of the Guard,* both with the D'Oyly Carte Opera Company, Century Theatre, 1948; in *Stalag 17,* 48th Street Theatre, New York City, 1951; in summer theatre productions of *Stalag 17, The Philadelphia Story,* and *Oh, Men! Oh, Women!,* in Pennsylvania, New Jersey, and Connecticut, all 1955; in *O'Neill and Carlotta,* Public Theatre, New York City, 1979; and in *You Can't Take It with You,* Paper Mill Playhouse, Millburn, NJ.

PRINCIPAL STAGE WORK—Assistant stage manager, *Stalag 17,* 48th Street Theatre, New York City, 1951; assistant stage manager, *The Chase,* Playhouse Theatre, New York City, 1952; director, *Long Day's Journey into Night,* Eisenhower Theatre, Washington, DC, 1975, then Brooklyn Academy of Music, Brooklyn, NY, 1976.

MAJOR TOURS—Witherspoon (also stage manager), *Stalag 17,* U.S. cities, 1952-53; Erie Smith, *Hughie,* U.S. cities, 1965.

FILM DEBUT—Paul Kedes and Fleming, *The Journey,* Metro-Goldwyn-Mayer, 1959. PRINCIPAL FILM APPEARANCES—Julius Penrose, *By Love Possessed,* United Artists, 1961; Dick Diver, *Tender Is the Night,* Twentieth Century-Fox, 1961; James Tyrone, Jr., *Long Day's Journey into Night,* Embassy, 1962; George S. Kaufman, *Act One,* Warner Brothers, 1964; Murray Burns, *A Thousand Clowns,* United Artists, 1965; John Cleves, *Any Wednesday* (also known as *Bachelor Girl Apartment*), Warner Brothers, 1966; Henry Drummond, *A Big Hand for the Little Lady* (also known as *Big Deal at Dodge City*), Warner Brothers, 1966; Nelson Downes, *Divorce American Style,* Columbia, 1967; Doc Holliday, *Hour of the Gun,* United Artists, 1967; Al "Scarface" Capone, *The St. Valentine's Day Massacre,* Twentieth Century-Fox, 1967; Paris Singer, *Isadora* (also known as *The Loves of Isadora*), Universal, 1968; Raymond Paine, *The Night They Raided Minsky's* (also known as *The Night They Invented Striptease*), United Artists, 1968; Cheyenne, *Once Upon a Time in the West,* Paramount, 1969.

Title role, *The Ballad of Cable Hogue,* Warner Brothers, 1970; Matthew South, *Fools,* Cinerama, 1970; Brutus, *Julius Caesar,* American International, 1970; General Walter C. Short, *Tora! Tora! Tora!,* Twentieth Century-Fox, 1970; Joe's father, *Johnny Got His Gun,* Cinemation, 1971; Cesar Charron, *Murders in the Rue Morgue,* American International, 1971; Stephen Kozlenko, *The War between Men and Women,* National General, 1972; Governor Lew Wallace, *Pat Garrett and Billy the Kid,* Metro-Goldwyn-Mayer, 1973; Mr. Craddock, *A Boy and His Dog,* LQJAF, 1975; John Gwilt, *Mr. Sycamore,* Film Venture, 1975; Ben Bradlee, *All the President's Men,* Warner Brothers, 1976;

Dashiell Hammett, *Julia,* Twentieth Century-Fox, 1977; Jacob Ewing, *Comes a Horseman,* United Artists, 1978; Captain Bruckner, *Hurricane* (also known as *Forbidden Paradise*), Paramount, 1979; Howard Hughes, *Melvin and Howard,* Universal, 1980; Admiral James Sandecker, *Raise the Titanic,* Associated Film Distribution, 1980; Gunther Beckdorff, *Caboblanco,* AVCO-Embassy, 1981; President Grant, *The Legend of the Lone Ranger,* Associated Film Distribution, 1981; as himself, *Burden of Dreams* (also known as *Die Last der Traume;* documentary about the making of the film *Fitzcarraldo*), Contemporary Films, Ltd., 1982; title role, *Max Dugan Returns,* Twentieth Century-Fox, 1983; Charles Halloway, *Something Wicked This Way Comes,* Buena Vista, 1983; Dillard, *Square Dance,* Island, 1987; Alex Hardy, *Bright Lights, Big City,* United Artists, 1988; Muth, *The Good Mother,* Buena Vista, 1988; Coleman Ettinger, *Dream a Little Dream,* Vestron, 1989. Also appeared in *Jud,* Maron, 1971; and voice characterization, *America and Lewis Hine* (documentary), 1984.

PRINCIPAL TELEVISION APPEARANCES—Mini-Series: President Richard Monckton, *Washington: Behind Closed Doors,* ABC, 1977. Pilots: James Mills, *The House without a Christmas Tree,* CBS, 1972; James Mills, *The Thanksgiving Treasure,* CBS, 1973; James Mills, *The Easter Promise,* CBS, 1975; James Mills, *Addie and the King of Hearts,* CBS, 1976. Episodic: Roberto, "For Whom the Bell Tolls," *Playhouse 90,* CBS, 1959; Hickey, "The Iceman Cometh," *Play of the Week,* WNTA, 1960; title role, "One Day in the Life of Ivan Denisovitch," *Bob Hope Chrysler Theatre,* NBC, 1963; also "People Kill People Sometimes," *Sunday Showcase,* NBC, 1959; *Ghost Story,* NBC, 1970; *The Alcoa Hour,* NBC; *Studio One,* CBS; *The Web,* CBS; *Philco Television Playhouse,* NBC; *Suspense,* CBS; *Treasury Men in Action,* NBC; *Armstrong Circle Theatre,* NBC; *Justice,* NBC; *Appointment with Adventure,* CBS; *The Deputy,* ABC; *Goodyear Playhouse,* NBC; *Westinghouse Presents,* CBS; *Omnibus,* ABC.

Movies: Daniel Larson, *A Christmas to Remember,* CBS, 1978; Franklin Delano Roosevelt, *F.D.R.—The Last Year,* NBC, 1980; Leland Hayward, *Haywire,* CBS, 1980; Dr. Russell Oakes, *The Day After,* ABC, 1983; Andrei Sakharov, *Sakharov,* HBO, 1984; Will Varner, *The Long Hot Summer,* NBC, 1985; Alvin Binder, *The Atlanta Child Murders,* CBS, 1985; Stephan Kovacs, *Johnny Bull,* ABC, 1986; Ed Stenning, *The Last Frontier,* CBS, 1986; Lloyd Welles, *Norman Rockwell's "Breaking Home Ties,"* ABC, 1987; Wade Shepherd, *Laguna Heat,* HBO, 1987; Henry Drummond, *Inherit the Wind,* NBC, 1988; John Tanner, *The Christmas Wife,* HBO, 1988. Specials: Dr. Rank, "A Doll's House," *Hallmark Hall of Fame,* NBC, 1959; title role, "Abe Lincoln in Illinois," *Hallmark Hall of Fame,* NBC, 1964; Frank Elgin, "The Country Girl," *Hallmark Hall of Fame,* NBC, 1974; narrator, "Polar Bear Alert," *National Geographic Special,* PBS, 1982; also *Barbra Streisand: The Belle of 14th Street,* CBS, 1967; *The Magic of David Copperfield,* CBS, 1981; host, *The Unknown Soldier,* 1985; *Happy Birthday Hollywood,* ABC, 1987; "Robert Frost," *Voices and Visions,* PBS, 1988; and narrator, *The Making of "Gorillas in the Mist,"* 1988.

RELATED CAREER—Actor on radio serials, 1948-50; member of board of directors, American Academy of Dramatic Arts, 1957—.

RECORDINGS: VIDEO—Narrator, *The World of Tomorrow,* Tom Johnson and Lance Bird, 1984.

AWARDS: Obie Award from the *Village Voice,* 1956, for *The Iceman Cometh;* Theatre World Award, 1957, for *Long Day's Journey into Night;* Antoinette Perry Award, Best Actor in a

Drama, 1959, for *The Disenchanted;* American National Theatre and Academy Award, 1959, for outstanding contribution to living theatre; New York Drama Critics Award, Most Promising Actor, 1960, for *Toys in the Attic;* award for ensemble performance from the Cannes Film Festival, 1962, for *Long Day's Journey into Night;* Antoinette Perry Award nomination, Best Actor in a Drama, 1964, for *After the Fall;* Antoinette Perry Award nomination, Best Actor in a Drama, 1972, for *The Country Girl;* Antoinette Perry Award nomination, Best Actor in a Play, 1978, for *A Touch of the Poet;* Academy Award and New York Film Critics Award, both Best Supporting Actor, 1976, for *All the President's Men;* Academy Award, Best Supporting Actor, 1977, for *Julia;* Emmy Award nomination, Best Actor, 1980, for *F.D.R.—The Last Year;* Academy Award nomination, Best Supporting Actor, 1980, for *Melvin and Howard;* Los Angeles Drama Critics Award nomination, Best Lead Performance, 1987, for *The Iceman Cometh;* presidential citation. Honorary degrees: D.H.L., Fairfield University, 1982; D.F.A., Williams College, 1983.

MEMBER: American Federation of Television and Radio Artists, Actors' Equity Association, Screen Actors Guild, Players Club (New York City).

SIDELIGHTS: FAVORITE ROLES—Hickey in *The Iceman Cometh,* Hotspur in *Henry IV, Part I,* Manley Halliday in *The Disenchanted,* and Macbeth. RECREATIONS—Guitar, banjo, photography.

ADDRESSES: AGENT—Fred Specktor, Creative Artists Agency, 1888 Century Park E., Suite 1400, Los Angeles, CA 90067.*

*   *   *

ROBB, David   1947-

PERSONAL: Born August 23, 1947, in London, England; married Briony McRoberts. EDUCATION: Trained for the stage at the Central School of Speech and Drama.

VOCATION: Actor.

CAREER: PRINCIPAL STAGE APPEARANCES—Nimming Ned and servant, *The Beggar's Opera,* and Nicholas, *The Taming of the Shrew,* both Chichester Festival Theatre, Chichester, U.K., 1972; Honorable George Carstairs, *Betzi,* Royal Haymarket Theatre, London, 1975; Ferdinand, *An Audience Called Edouard,* Greenwich Theatre, London, 1978; Hastings, *She Stoops to Conquer,* Greenwich Theatre, 1979. Also appeared in *Cowardly Custard.*

PRINCIPAL FILM APPEARANCES—Alex Zendor, *The Swordsman,* Twentieth Century-Fox/Rank, 1974; Second Lieutenant Winters, *Conduct Unbecoming,* Allied Artists, 1975; George Anglesmith, *The Deceivers,* Cinecom International, 1988. Also appeared in *The Wars,* Spectrafilm, 1983.

PRINCIPAL TELEVISION APPEARANCES—Series: Sir Lancelot, *King Arthur,* syndicated, 1987. Mini-Series: Germanicus, "I, Claudius," *Masterpiece Theatre,* BBC, then PBS, 1977; Captain Charles Tennant, *Fanny by Gaslight,* Entertainment Channel, 1982; Robin Grant, "The Flame Trees of Thika," *Masterpiece Theatre,* PBS, 1982; Sallust, *The Last Days of Pompeii,* ABC, 1984; Lancelot, "The Legend of King Arthur," *Once Upon a Classic,* PBS, 1985; Andrew Fraser, *First Among Equals,* Granada, then PBS, 1987. Movies: Thomas Willoughby, *The Four Feathers,*

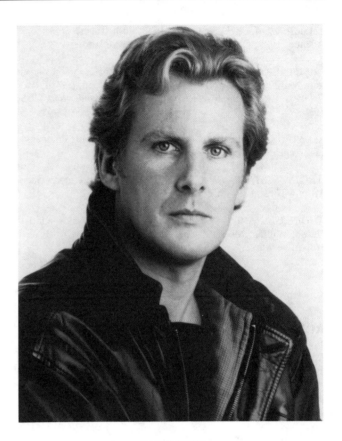

DAVID ROBB

NBC, 1978; Prince Charles, *Charles and Diana: A Royal Love Story,* ABC, 1982; Robin Hood, *Ivanhoe,* CBS, 1982; Per Anger, *Wallenberg: A Hero's Story,* NBC, 1985; Lieutenant Karl Pressler, *Freedom Fighter,* NBC, 1987; Ross Fleming, *Dreams Lost, Dreams Found,* Showtime, 1987; De Forrestiere, *The Man Who Lived at the Ritz,* syndicated, 1988. Also appeared in *Off-Peak* and *Dangerous Corner.*

ADDRESSES: AGENT—William Morris Agency, 31-32 Soho Square, London W1, England.*

*   *   *

ROBBINS, Tim

PERSONAL: EDUCATION: Attended the University of California, Los Angeles.

VOCATION: Actor.

CAREER: PRINCIPAL STAGE WORK—Director, *Carnage,* Actor's Gang, Tiffany Theatre, in California, 1988.

PRINCIPAL FILM APPEARANCES—Nelson, *No Small Affair,* Columbia, 1984; Boe, *Toy Soldiers,* New World, 1984; Larry "Mother" Tucker, *Fraternity Vacation,* New World, 1985; Gary Cooper, *The Sure Thing,* Embassy, 1985; Phil Blumburtt, *Howard the Duck,* Universal, 1986; Sam Wills, *Top Gun,* Paramount, 1986; Harry, *Five Corners,* Cineplex Odeon, 1987; Ebby Calvin "Nuke"

LaLoosh, *Bull Durham*, Orion, 1988; Josh Tager, *Tapeheads*, Avenue, 1989; Delmount, *Miss Firecracker*, Corsair, 1989.

PRINCIPAL TELEVISION APPEARANCES—Episodic: Jordon's phantom, *Amazing Stories*, NBC, 1986. Movies: Marvin, *Quarterback Princess*, CBS, 1983; Joseph Cotten, *Malice in Wonderland*, CBS, 1985.

RELATED CAREER—Founder, Actor's Gang (a theatre company), Los Angeles, CA, 1981.

WRITINGS: STAGE—(With Adam Simon) *Carnage*, Actor's Gang, Tiffany Theatre, in California, 1988.

ADDRESSES: AGENTS—Elaine Goldsmith, Cary Woods, and J.J. Harris, William Morris Agency, 151 El Camino Drive, Beverly Hills, CA 90212.*

*　　*　　*

ROBERTS, Eric   1956-

PERSONAL: Full name, Eric Anthony Roberts; born April 18, 1956, in Biloxi, MS; father, founder of the Actor's and Writer's Workshop. EDUCATION: Trained for the stage at the Royal Academy of Dramatic Art, 1973-74, and the American Academy of Dramatic Arts, 1974-75.

VOCATION: Actor.

CAREER: PRINCIPAL STAGE APPEARANCES—First soldier, *Rebel Women*, New York Shakespeare Festival, Public Theatre, New York City, 1976; Mark Dolson, *Mass Appeal*, Manhattan Theatre Club, New York City, 1980; Pale, *Burn This*, Plymouth Theatre, New York City, 1988; also appeared in *A Streetcar Named Desire*, McCarter Theatre Company, Princeton, NJ, 1976; *The Glass Menagerie*, Hartford Stage Company, Hartford, CT, 1983; *Alms for the Middle Class*, Long Wharf Theatre, New Haven, CT; and as a child in *The Member of the Wedding, Charley's Aunt,* and *The Taming of the Shrew,* all Actor's and Writer's Workshop, Atlanta, GA.

FILM DEBUT—Dave Stepanowitz, *King of the Gypsies*, Paramount, 1978. PRINCIPAL FILM APPEARANCES—Judge, *The Alternative Miss World* (documentary), Tigon, 1980; Teddy, *Raggedy Man*, Universal, 1981; Paul Snider, *Star 80*, Warner Brothers, 1983; Paulie, *The Pope of Greenwich Village*, Metro-Goldwyn-Mayer, 1984; Buck, *Runaway Train*, Cannon, 1985; Becker, *The Coca-Cola Kid*, Cinecom/Film Gallery, 1985; Riley, *Nobody's Fool*, Island, 1986; narrator, *Dear America: Letters Home from Vietnam*, HBO Productions, 1988.

PRINCIPAL TELEVISION APPEARANCES—Series: *Another World,* NBC, 1976-77. Episodic: Title role, "Miss Lonelyhearts," *American Playhouse*, PBS, 1983; also "Paul's Case," *American Short Story*, PBS. Movies: Jacob Asch, *Slow Burn*, Showtime, 1986; Jan Scruggs, *To Heal a Nation*, NBC, 1988.

ADDRESSES: AGENT—Alan Iezman, William Morris Agency, 151 El Camino Drive, Beverly Hills, CA 90212. MANAGER—Bill Treusch Associates, 853 Seventh Avenue, Suite 9-A, New York, NY 10019.*

ROBERTS, Tanya   1955-

PERSONAL: Born Tanya Leigh, October 15, 1955, in Bronx, NY; father, a pen salesman; married Barry Roberts (a screenwriter). EDUCATION: Trained for the stage with Uta Hagen and Lee Strasberg.

VOCATION: Actress.

CAREER: PRINCIPAL STAGE APPEARANCES—*Picnic* and *Antigone,* both in New York City; also appeared at the La Mama Experimental Theatre Club, New York City.

PRINCIPAL FILM APPEARANCES—Stewardess, *The Private Files of J. Edgar Hoover*, American International, 1978; Stephanie, *California Dreaming*, American International, 1979; Becky, *Tourist Trap*, Compass/Manson, 1979; Bambi, *Racquet*, Cal-Am, 1979; Julia, *Fingers*, Brut, 1977; Kiri, *The Beastmaster*, Metro-Goldwyn-Mayer/United Artists (MGM/UA), 1982; Isabella, *I Paladini storia d' armi e d' amori* (also known as *Hearts in Armor*), Warner Brothers/APIC, 1983; Stacey Sutton, *A View to a Kill*, MGM/UA, 1984; title role, *Sheena*, Columbia, 1984; Candace Van Der Vegen, *Body Slam*, De Laurentiis Entertainment Group, 1987. Also appeared in *Forced Entry* (also known as *The Last Weekend*), Century International/Two Kodiak, 1975; *Le Armi e gli amori* (also known as *Arms and Loves*), Warner Brothers, 1983; and *Purgatory*, New Star Entertainment, 1989.

PRINCIPAL TELEVISION APPEARANCES—Series: Julie Rogers, *Charlie's Angels*, ABC, 1980-81. Pilots: Officer Britt Blackwell, *Ladies in Blue* (shown as an episode of *Vega$*), ABC, 1980; Velda, *Mickey Spillane's Mike Hammer: Murder Me, Murder You*, CBS, 1983. Movies: Denise, *Zuma Beach*, NBC, 1978; Sally, *Pleasure Cove*, NBC, 1979; Carol, *Waikiki*, ABC, 1980.

RELATED CAREER—Professional model; actress in television commercials.

NON-RELATED CAREER—Dance instructor, Arthur Murray Dance Studio.

ADDRESSES: AGENT—Agency for the Performing Arts, 9000 Sunset Boulevard, Suite 1200, Los Angeles, CA 90069.*

*　　*　　*

ROBERTS, Tony   1939-

PERSONAL: Full name, David Anthony Roberts; born October 22, 1939, in New York, NY; son of Kenneth (an announcer) and Norma (an animator) Roberts; married first wife, December 14, 1969 (divorced, 1975); children: Nicole. EDUCATION: Northwestern University, B.S., 1961; studied acting with Alvina Krause. MILITARY: U.S. Army, 1962.

VOCATION: Actor.

CAREER: BROADWAY DEBUT—(As Anthony Roberts) Air cadet, *Something about a Soldier*, Ambassador Theatre, 1962. LONDON DEBUT—(As Anthony Roberts) Chuck Baxter, *Promises, Promises*, Prince of Wales Theatre, 1969. PRINCIPAL STAGE APPEARANCES—All as Anthony Roberts: Richard Gluck, *Take Her, She's Mine*, Biltmore Theatre, New York City, 1962; Max Bummidge,

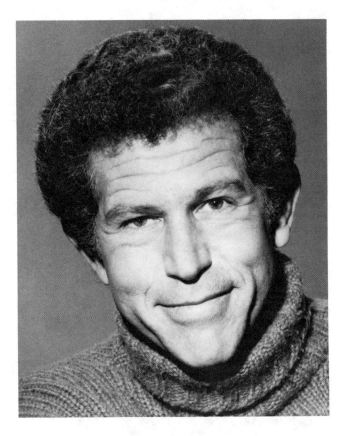

TONY ROBERTS

The Last Analysis, Belasco Theatre, New York City, 1964; Charlie, *Never Too Late,* Playhouse Theatre, New York City, 1964; Paul Bratter, *Barefoot in the Park,* Biltmore Theatre, 1965; Axel Magee, *Don't Drink the Water,* Morosco Theatre, New York City, 1966; Charley Matson, *How Now, Dow Jones,* Lunt-Fontanne Theatre, New York City, 1967; Dick Christie, *Play It Again, Sam,* Broadhurst Theatre, 1969.

(As Anthony Roberts) Chuck Baxter, *Promises, Promises,* Shubert Theatre, New York City, 1971; Joe/Josephine, *Sugar,* Majestic Theatre, 1972; Antonio, *The Tempest,* and Richard, *Darkroom,* both Yale Repertory Theatre, New Haven, CT, 1973; Geoffrey, *Absurd Person Singular,* Kennedy Center for the Performing Arts, Washington, DC, then Music Box Theatre, New York City, both 1974; title role, *Hamlet,* Otterbein University Theatre, Westerville, OH, 1976; Petruchio, *The Taming of the Shrew,* Alliance Theatre, Atlanta, GA, 1978; Mitchell Lavell, *Murder at the Howard Johnson's,* John Golden Theatre, New York City, 1979; Todd, *Losing Time,* Manhattan Theatre Club, New York City, 1979; Vernon Gersch, *They're Playing Our Song,* Imperial Theatre, New York City, 1979; Brian "Sonny" Levine, *The Good Parts,* Astor Place Theatre, New York City, 1982; George, *Doubles,* Second Stage Theatre, then Ritz Theatre, both New York City, 1985; Mortimer Brewster, *Arsenic and Old Lace,* 46th Street Theatre, New York City, 1986; Luther Billis, *South Pacific,* New York City Opera, State Theatre, New York City, 1987. Also appeared in *The Cradle Will Rock,* Theatre Four, New York City, 1964; *Serenading Louie,* Academy Festival Theatre, Lake Forest, IL, 1978; *Let 'em Eat Cake,* Berkshire Theatre Festival, Stockbridge, MA; as Jeff, *Brigadoon,* New York City Opera, State Theatre; and in *Time Framed,* Off-Broadway production.

MAJOR TOURS—As Anthony Roberts: Buddy, *Come Blow Your Horn,* U.S. cities, 1962; Chuck Baxter, *Promises, Promises,* U.S. cities, 1970-71.

FILM DEBUT—Fred Hines, *$1,000,000 Duck,* Buena Vista, 1971. PRINCIPAL FILM APPEARANCES—Andy Hobart, *Star Spangled Girl,* Paramount, 1971; Dick Christie, *Play It Again, Sam,* Paramount, 1972; Bob Blair, *Serpico,* Paramount, 1973; Warren LaSalle, *The Taking of Pelham One, Two, Three,* United Artists, 1974; Alex Fox, *Le Sauvage* (also known as *The Savage* and *Lovers Like Us*), Gaumont, 1975; Rob, *Annie Hall,* United Artists, 1977; Mike Berger, *Just Tell Me What You Want,* Warner Brothers, 1980; Tony, *Stardust Memories,* United Artists, 1980; Dr. Maxwell Jordan, *A Midsummer Night's Sex Comedy,* Warner Brothers, 1982; John Baxter, *Amityville 3-D,* Orion, 1983; David Slattery, *Key Exchange,* Twentieth Century-Fox, 1985; Mickey's ex-partner, *Hannah and Her Sisters,* Orion, 1986; "Silver Dollar" emcee, *Radio Days,* Orion, 1987; Arnold, *Eighteen Again!,* New World, 1988. Also appeared in *Opening Night,* Miracle/Faces Distribution, 1977.

PRINCIPAL TELEVISION APPEARANCES—Series: Lee Pollock, *The Edge of Night,* CBS, 1963-65; Joseph Rosetti, *Rosetti and Ryan,* NBC, 1977; Ted Bolen, *The Four Seasons,* CBS, 1984; Jim Gordon, *The Lucie Arnaz Show,* CBS, 1985; Sloan Thorn, *The Thorns,* ABC, 1988. Pilots: Sergeant Mike Conroy, *Snafu,* NBC, 1976; Joseph Rosetti, *Rosetti and Ryan: Men Who Love Women,* NBC, 1977. Episodic: Doctor, "The Messiah on Mott Street," *Night Gallery* (also known as *Rod Serling's Night Gallery*), NBC; also *Love, American Style,* ABC; *The Defenders,* CBS; *The Trials of O'Brien,* CBS. Movies: Lieutenant Jim Finn, *The Lindbergh Kidnapping Case,* NBC, 1976; Mike Holden, *The Girls in the Office,* ABC, 1979; Michael Boden, *If Things Were Different,* CBS, 1980; Marlowe, *A Question of Honor,* CBS, 1982; Charlie Baumgarten, *Packin' It In,* CBS, 1983; Dr. Jeffrey Newman, *A Different Affair,* CBS, 1987. Specials: *Let's Celebrate,* ABC, 1972; *The Way They Were,* syndicated, 1981; Bernie Pell, "Seize the Day," *Great Performances,* PBS, 1986.

AWARDS: Antoinette Perry Award nomination, Best Actor in a Musical, 1968, for *How Now, Dow Jones;* Antoinette Perry Award nomination, Best Supporting or Featured Actor—Dramatic, 1969, for *Play It Again, Sam;* London Critics Poll Award, Best Actor in a Musical, 1970, for *Promises, Promises.*

MEMBER: Actors' Equity Association (governing council, 1968-74).

SIDELIGHTS: RECREATIONS—Chess, sailing, and photography.

ADDRESSES: AGENT—William Morris Agency, 1350 Avenue of the Americas, New York, NY 10019.*

*   *   *

ROBERTSON, Lainie

VOCATION: Playwright and screenwriter.

CAREER: See *WRITINGS* below.

WRITINGS: STAGE—*Lady Day at Emerson's Bar and Grill,* Alliance Theatre Company, Atlanta, GA, then Vineyard Theatre,

New York City, later Westside Arts Theatre, New York City, all 1986; *Nasty Little Secrets,* Walnut Street Theatre, Philadelphia, PA, 1987. TELEVISION—Episodic: "Journey into Genius," *American Playhouse,* PBS, 1988. Specials: *Diana Ross . . . Red Hot Rhythm and Blues,* 1987.

ADDRESSES: HOME—484 W. 43rd Street, Apartment 9-C, New York, NY 10036. AGENT—Rick Leed, Agency for the Performing Arts, 888 Seventh Avenue, New York, NY 10106.*

*   *   *

ROBINSON, Andrew   1942-

PERSONAL: Born February 14, 1942, in New York, NY. EDUCATION: Graduated from the New School for Social Research; studied acting at the London Academy of Music and Dramatic Arts.

VOCATION: Actor.

CAREER: OFF-BROADWAY DEBUT—*MacBird!,* Village Gate Theatre, 1967. PRINCIPAL STAGE APPEARANCES—Sheriff Tom Sluck, *Futz!,* Theatre De Lys, then Actors Playhouse, both New York City, 1968; Klaub, *The Cannibals,* and Dante, "The Young Master Dante" in *Trainer, Dean, Liepolt, and Company,* both American Place Theatre, New York City, 1968; young man, *Operation Sidewinder,* Vivian Beaumont Theatre, New York City, 1970; Prince Myshkin, *Subject to Fits,* New York Shakespeare Festival (NYSF), Public Theatre, New York City, 1971; Sir William Davison, *Mary Stuart,* Repertory Theatre of Lincoln Center, Vivian Beaumont Theatre, 1971; Kiro, *Narrow Road to the Deep North,* Repertory Theatre of Lincoln Center, Vivian Beaumont Theatre, 1972; Professor Leo Lehrer, *The Genius,* Center Theatre Group, Mark Taper Forum, Los Angeles, CA, 1984; Jack Henry Abbot, *In the Belly of the Beast,* Center Theatre Group, Mark Taper Forum, 1984, then Joyce Theatre, New York City, 1985. Also appeared in *The Death and Life of Jesse James,* New Theatre for Now, Ahmanson Theatre, Los Angeles, 1974; *The Changing Room,* Odyssey Theatre, Los Angeles; *The Bacchae* and *Macbeth,* both Los Angeles Actors Theatre, Los Angeles; *Curse of the Starving Class,* Tiffany Theatre, Los Angeles; *Woyzeck,* La Mama Experimental Theatre Company, New York City; *The Man Who Came to Dinner,* Long Beach Theatre Festival, Long Beach, CA; *Gogol, A Mystery Play,* NYSF, New York City; *The Genius,* Mark Taper Forum; and with the Milwaukee Repertory Theatre, Milwaukee, WI, 1965-66; Playhouse in the Park, Cincinnati, OH, 1966-67; and Trinity Square Repertory Company, Providence, RI, 1966-67.

PRINCIPAL FILM APPEARANCES—Scorpio, *Dirty Harry,* Warner Brothers, 1971; Harman Sullivan, *Charley Varrick,* Universal, 1973; Pat Reaves, *The Drowning Pool,* Warner Brothers, 1975; Coley Phipps, *Mackintosh and T.J.,* Penland, 1975; Dr. Vinton, *Mask,* Universal, 1985; Detective Monte, *Cobra,* Warner Brothers, 1986; Larry Cotton, *Hellraiser,* New World, 1987; Harvey, *Shoot to Kill,* Buena Vista, 1988. Also appeared in *A Woman for All Men,* 1975.

PRINCIPAL TELEVISION APPEARANCES—Series: Frank Ryan, *Ryan's Hope,* ABC. Mini-Series: Reb Rayburne, *Once an Eagle,* NBC, 1976-77; Private Stack, *From Here to Eternity,* NBC, 1979. Pilots: Andy, *The Catcher,* CBS, 1972; Butch Kovack, *The Family Kovack,* CBS, 1974; Willie Norman, *Lanigan's Rabbi,* NBC,

1976; Frank Morrella, *Reward,* ABC, 1980; Derek, *Ladies in Blue,* ABC, 1980; Beau, *Beyond Witch Mountain,* CBS, 1982; Seamus, *Desperate,* ABC, 1987. Episodic: Gregory Waples, "The Trial of Bernhard Goetz," *American Playhouse,* PBS, 1988; also *The Twilight Zone,* CBS, 1985; "Incident at Vichy," *Hollywood Theatre,* PBS; *Cagney and Lacey,* CBS. Movies: Frank Berlin, *Someone I Touched,* ABC, 1975; Dr. Royce, *Not My Kid,* CBS, 1985; Jack Mallard, *The Atlanta Child Murders,* CBS, 1985; title role, *Liberace,* ABC, 1988.

AWARDS: Los Angeles Drama Critics Award, Best Actor, 1984, for *In the Belly of the Beast.*

MEMBER: Founding member, La Mama Plexus Company, New York City.*

*   *   *

ROCHE, Eugene   1928-

PERSONAL: Born September 22, 1928, in Boston, MA; son of Robert F. (in the U.S. Navy) and Mary M. (Finnegan) Roche; married Ann Toni C. Bratman (an actress), April 16, 1982; children: Jamie, Sean, Chad, Tara, Megan, Brogan, Liam, Eamonn, and Caitlin. EDUCATION: Studied speech and drama at Emerson College; trained for the stage at the Actors Workshop, San Francisco, CA. MILITARY: U.S. Army, sergeant.

VOCATION: Actor.

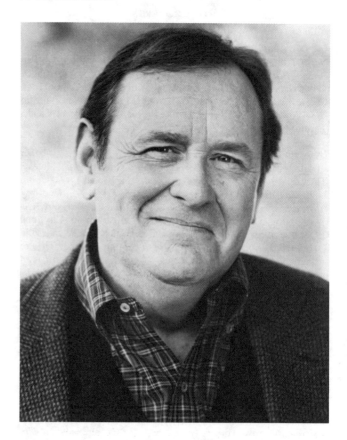

EUGENE ROCHE

CAREER: PRINCIPAL STAGE APPEARANCES—Peter, *Between Two Thieves*, and Father Colley-Mahoney, *Valmouth*, both York Playhouse, New York City, 1960; (as Gene Roche) Mr. Waldo, Mr. Pugh, Dai Bread, and Mog Edwards, *Under Milkwood*, Circle in the Square, New York City, 1961, then 1962; Swedish commander and second soldier, *Mother Courage and Her Children*, Martin Beck Theatre, New York City, 1963; White House butler, French John, Zachary Taylor, and Dr. Grayson, *In the White House*, Henry Miller's Theatre, New York City, 1964; Fred Gorman, *The Secret Life of Walter Mitty*, Players Theatre, New York City, 1964; Joe Thompson, *All in Good Time*, Royale Theatre, New York City, 1965; Morgan O'Shaunnessy, *Laughwind*, Bouwerie Lane Theatre, New York City, 1966; (as Gene Roche) Morden, *Father Uxbridge Wants to Marry*, American Place Theatre, New York City, 1967. Also appeared in *Blood, Sweat, and Stanley Poole*, Morosco Theatre, New York City, 1961; *Great Day in the Morning*, Henry Miller's Theatre, 1962; *The Price*, Morosco Theatre, 1968; and as Vladimir, *Waiting for Godot*, in an Off-Broadway production.

MAJOR TOURS—Insurance agent, *The Time of the Barracudas*, U.S. cities, 1963.

FILM DEBUT—Private detective, *Splendor in the Grass*, Warner Brothers, 1961. PRINCIPAL FILM APPEARANCES—Motorcycle officer, *The Happening*, Columbia, 1967; Anderson, *Cotton Comes to Harlem*, United Artists, 1970; policeman, *They Might Be Giants*, Universal, 1971; Edgar Derby, *Slaughterhouse Five*, Universal, 1972; Reardon, *Newman's Law*, Universal, 1974; Charles Jasper, *W* (also known as *I Want Her Dead*), Cinerama, 1974; Detective Cronyn, *Mr. Rico*, Metro-Goldwyn-Mayer, 1975; Ron Birdwell, *The Late Show*, Warner Brothers, 1977; Ed McGrath, *Corvette Summer* (also known as *The Hot Summer*), United Artists, 1978; Archbishop Thorncrest, *Foul Play*, Paramount, 1978; Charlie Gray, *Oh God! You Devil*, Warner Brothers, 1984.

PRINCIPAL TELEVISION APPEARANCES—Series: McEthany, *Higher and Higher: Attorneys at Law*, CBS, 1968; Frank Flynn, *The Corner Bar*, ABC, 1973; Eddie Egan, *Egan*, ABC, 1973; Harvey Gordon, *Local 306*, NBC, 1976; Attorney Ronald Mallu, *Soap*, ABC, 1978-81; Jimmy Hughes, *Good Time Harry*, NBC, 1980; Bill Parker, *Webster*, ABC, 1984-86; Max Davis, *Take Five*, CBS, 1987; Harry Burns, *Perfect Strangers*, ABC, 1987-88. Pilots: Sergeant Harry Isadore, *The Art of Crime*, NBC, 1975; Daniel Lawrence, *Crime Club*, CBS, 1975; Bob Lattimer, *Mallory: Circumstantial Evidence*, NBC, 1976; Davy Allman, *People Like Us*, NBC, 1976; Schroeder, *Never Con a Killer*, ABC, 1977; District Attorney Patrick Shannon, *Corey: For the People*, NBC, 1977; Judge Crupper, *The New Maverick*, ABC, 1978; Larry Elliott, *Alone at Last*, NBC, 1980; Walter Chester, *Two the Hard Way*, CBS, 1981; Patrick J. Malloy, *Farrell: For the People*, NBC, 1982; Sergeant Khoury, *Cocaine and Blue Eyes*, NBC, 1983; Mitch Mitchell, *Johnny Blue*, CBS, 1983; title role, *The Return of Luther Gillis* (shown as two episodes of *Magnum P.I.*), CBS, 1984.

Episodic: Pinky Peterson, *All in the Family* (two episodes), CBS, 1976; Pinky Peterson, *All in the Family*, CBS, 1978; Jack Sullivan, *Night Court*, NBC, 1985; Joe Murphy, *Hardcastle and McCormick*, ABC, 1985; Billy Simms, *Murder, She Wrote*, CBS, 1986; Clancy, *Highway to Heaven*, NBC, 1986; James Elliott, *Downtown*, CBS, 1986; John B. Lucas, *Hotel*, ABC, 1986; Clifford Tresch, *Mr. President*, Fox, 1987; Greenwood, *Stingray*, NBC, 1986; Phil Kroger, *Hotel*, ABC, 1987; Lieutenant Jarvis, *Murder, She Wrote*, CBS, 1988; also *No Soap, Radio*, ABC, 1982; *Taxi*, ABC, 1982; *Baby Makes Five*, ABC, 1983; *Ironside*, NBC; *The*

Streets of San Francisco, ABC; *Police Woman*, NBC; *Hawaii Five-O*, CBS; *Kojak*, CBS; *Maude*, CBS; *Kaz*, CBS; *Quincy, M.E.*, NBC; *What Really Happened to the Class of 65?*, NBC; *Lou Grant*, CBS; *Mr. Merlin*, CBS; *Airwolf*, CBS. Movies: Emil Birge, *Crawlspace*, CBS, 1972; Mayor Clinton Bickford, *Winter Kill*, ABC, 1974; prosecutor, *The Last Survivors*, NBC, 1975; Sergeant Taplinger, *The Possessed*, NBC, 1977; Matt Andrews, *The Ghost of Flight 401*, NBC, 1978; Lew Beck, *The Child Stealer*, ABC, 1979; Sloane, *Love for Rent*, ABC, 1979; Bishop Milton Wright, *The Winds of Kitty Hawk*, NBC, 1979; Gary Gortmaker, *Rape and Marriage—The Rideout Case*, CBS, 1980; Mr. Craig, *Miracle on Ice*, ABC, 1981; Chief Frank Brockmeyer, *Off-Sides*, NBC, 1984; Sullivan, *Stranded*, NBC, 1986. Specials: Paul, *You Can't Take It with You*, CBS, 1979; Paul, *Princess*, syndicated, 1980; Father Delaney, *The Juggler of Notre Dame*, syndicated, 1982; *Life's Most Embarrassing Moments*, ABC, 1983.

ADDRESSES: AGENT—The Artists Agency, 10000 Santa Monica Boulevard, Los Angeles, CA 90067.

*   *   *

RODDAM, Franc   1946-

PERSONAL: Born April 29, 1946, in Stockton-on-Tees, England; son of Vincent Nicholson and Ellen Maud (Canavan) Roddam; married Carina Mary Cooper (a director; marriage ended); married Barbara Margaret Deehan (a televison producer); children: Annie Canavan, Patrick Michael. EDUCATION: Received degree from the London International Film School, 1971.

VOCATION: Director, screenwriter, and producer.

CAREER: Also see WRITINGS below. PRINCIPAL FILM WORK—Director: *Quadrophenia*, World Northal, 1979; *The Lords of Discipline*, Paramount, 1983; *The Bride*, Columbia, 1985; *Aria* (sequence 7), Virgin Vision, 1987; (also executive producer) *War Party*, Hemdale, 1988.

PRINCIPAL TELEVISION WORK—Series: Creator, *Auf Wiedersehn, Pet*, Central TV, 1984; creator, *Making Out*, BBC, 1987. Specials: Director, *Mini* (documentary), BBC, 1973; director, *The Family* (documentary), BBC, 1974; director, *Dummy*, ATV, 1977; (with Brian Lewis) director, *Catastrophe: Airships* (documentary), syndicated, 1978.

RELATED CAREER—Documentary filmmaker for the BBC.

NON-RELATED CAREER—Copywriter and producer, Ogilvy, Benson, and Mather (an advertising agency).

WRITINGS: FILM—*Quadrophenia*, World Northal, 1979; *Rain Forest*, Twentieth Century-Fox, 1981; *American Dreams*, Paramount, 1983. TELEVISION—Series: *Auf Wiedersehn, Pet*, Central TV, 1984; creator, *Making Out*, BBC, 1987.

AWARDS: Critics award (U.K.), Best Documentary, 1973, for *Mini*; Critics award (U.K.), Best Documentary, 1974, for *The Family*; Prix Italia Drama Prize, 1977, for *Dummy*.

MEMBER: Directors Guild of America, Academy of Motion Picture Arts and Sciences, Association of Cinematograph, Television, and Allied Technicians, Groucho Club.

ADDRESSES: AGENT—Jim Wiatt, International Creative Management, 8899 Beverly Boulevard, Los Angeles, CA 90048.

*   *   *

RODGERS, Mark

VOCATION: Screenwriter and producer.

CAREER: Also see *WRITINGS* below. PRINCIPAL TELEVISION WORK—All as producer, unless indicated. Series: (With James H. Brown) *Joe Forrester*, NBC, 1975-76; (with Brown) *The Quest*, NBC, 1976; (with Charles B. Fitzsimons) *Wonder Woman* (also known as *The New Adventures of Wonder Woman*), CBS, 1977-79; *Operation Runaway*, NBC, 1978; (with Mel Swope) *David Cassidy—Man Undercover*, NBC, 1978-79; *240-Robert*, ABC, 1981; (with Stuart Cohen and John G. Stephens) *The Gangster Chronicles*, NBC, 1981; (with Robert H. Justman) *McClain's Law*, NBC, 1981-82; (with Harker Wade and Andrew Schneider) *Masquerade*, ABC, 1983-84. Pilots: (With Fitzsimons) *Cover Girls*, NBC, 1977; *Uncommon Valor*, CBS, 1983. Episodic: Director, *Jigsaw*, ABC.

WRITINGS: FILM—*Let's Kill Uncle*, Universal, 1966; *Flareup*, Metro-Goldwyn-Mayer, 1969.

TELEVISION—Pilots: (With William Link and Richard Levinson) *Savage*, NBC, 1973; *The Return of Joe Forrester*, NBC, 1975; *Cover Girls*, NBC, 1977; *Uncommon Valor*, CBS, 1983. Episodic: *Eischied*, NBC, 1979; *The Gangster Chronicles*, NBC, 1981; *T.J. Hooker*, ABC, 1982; also *McClain's Law*, NBC; *The F.B.I.*, ABC; *Jigsaw*, ABC; *Wonder Woman* (also known as *The New Adventures of Wonder Woman*), CBS; *Masquerade*, ABC. Movies: *The Forgotten Man*, ABC, 1971; *The Girl on the Late, Late Show*, NBC, 1974; (with Sidney A. Glass) *Detour to Terror*, NBC, 1980; *Women of San Quentin*, NBC, 1983; *The Dirty Dozen: The Deadly Mission*, NBC, 1987; *Police Story: The Freeway Killings*, NBC, 1987; *The Dirty Dozen: The Fatal Mission*, NBC, 1988.*

*   *   *

RODRIGUEZ, Paul

PERSONAL: Born in Mazatlan, Mexico; son of migrant farm workers. EDUCATION: Received A.A. from Long Beach City College; also attended California State University. MILITARY: U.S. Air Force.

VOCATION: Comedian and actor.

CAREER: PRINCIPAL FILM APPEARANCES—Xavier, *D.C. Cab*, Universal, 1983; Hector Rodriguez, *Quicksilver*, Columbia, 1985; Barney Bonnare, *The Whoopee Boys*, Paramount, 1986; Juan, *Miracles*, Orion, 1987; Javier, *Born in East L.A.*, Universal, 1987. Also appeared in and *The Californians* (documentary), Cori, 1984.

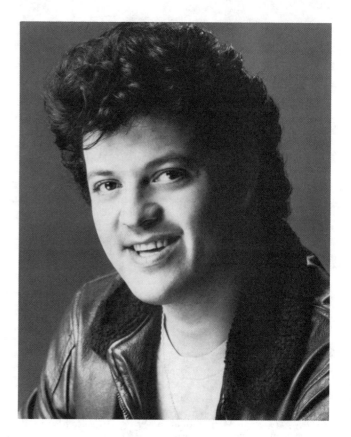

PAUL RODRIGUEZ

PRINCIPAL TELEVISION APPEARANCES—Series: Paul (Pablo) Rivera, *a.k.a. Pablo*, ABC, 1984; Tony Rivera, *Trial and Error*, CBS, 1988; host, *The Newlywed Game Starring Paul Rodriguez*, syndicated, 1988-89. Pilots: Ray Gonzales, *Hardesty House*, ABC, 1986; also *Hardball*, CBS, 1989. Episodic: Ramone, *The Golden Girls*, NBC, 1986; Julio, "Ponce De Leon and the Search for the Fountain of Youth," *Shelley Duvall's Tall Tales and Legends*, Showtime, 1986; host, *The Late Show*, Fox, 1986. Specials: *Disneyland's Summer Vacation Party*, NBC, 1986; *The Noel Edmonds Show*, ABC, 1986; *Comic Relief*, HBO, 1986; human cannonball, "The Big Bang" (also known as "Robert Wuhl's The Big Bang"), *Cinemax Comedy Experiment*, Cinemax, 1986; *Emmanuel Lewis: My Very Own Show*, ABC, 1987; *Paul Rodriguez: I Need the Couch*, HBO, 1987; *Comic Relief II*, HBO, 1987; *The Comedy Store Fifteenth Year Class Reunion*, NBC, 1988; *The American Comedy Awards*, ABC, 1988; "The Twelfth Annual Young Comedians Show," *HBO: On Location*, HBO, 1988; "An All-Star Toast to the Improv," *HBO Comedy Hour*, HBO, 1988; *An All-Star Celebration: The '88 Vote*, ABC, 1988; *The Hollywood Christmas Parade*, syndicated, 1988; *Comic Relief III*, HBO, 1989; also *Paul Rodriguez Live*, HBO.

RELATED CAREER—As a comedian, has appeared in nightclubs and concert halls throughout the United States.

ADDRESSES: AGENT—William Morris Agency, 151 El Camino Drive, Beverly Hills, CA 90212. MANAGER—Jeff Wald, Barris/Guber/Peters, 1990 S. Bundy Drive, Los Angeles, CA 90025. PUBLICIST—Cindy Guagenti, Baker/Winokur/Ryder, 9348 Civic Center Drive, Suite 407, Beverly Hills, CA 90210.

ROGERS, Mimi

PERSONAL: Born January 27, in Coral Gables, FL; married Tom Cruise (an actor).

VOCATION: Actress.

CAREER: FILM DEBUT—Liz, *Blue Skies Again*, SB, 1983. PRINCIPAL FILM APPEARANCES—Audrey, *Gung Ho*, Paramount, 1985; Claire Gregory, *Someone to Watch Over Me*, Columbia, 1987; Alison Parker, *Street Smart*, Cannon, 1987; Hadley, *The Mighty Quinn*, Metro-Goldwyn-Mayer/United Artists, 1989. Also appeared in *Hider in the House*.

PRINCIPAL TELEVISION APPEARANCES—Series: Ellen Slade, *The Rousters*, NBC, 1983-84; Blair Harper Fenton, *Paper Dolls*, ABC, 1984. Pilots: Meg, *Hear No Evil*, CBS, 1982; Nancy Russell, *Embassy*, ABC, 1985. Episodic: *Magnum P.I.*, CBS; *Hart to Hart*, ABC; *Quincy, M.E.*, NBC; *Hill Street Blues*, NBC. Movies: Belinda Wittiker, *Divorce Wars*, ABC, 1982; Charlotte, "You Ruined My Life," *Disney Sunday Movie*, ABC, 1987.

ADDRESSES: AGENT—Paula Wagner, Creative Artists Agency, 1888 Century Park E., Suite 1400, Los Angeles, CA 90067.*

*   *   *

ROOS, Fred   1934-

PERSONAL: Full name, Frederick Ried Roos; born May 22, 1934, in Santa Monica, CA; son of Victor Otto and Florence Mary (Stout) Roos. EDUCATION: University of California, Los Angeles, B.A., 1956. MILITARY: U.S. Army, 1957-59.

VOCATION: Producer.

CAREER: PRINCIPAL FILM WORK—Producer, *Back Door to Hell*, Twentieth Century-Fox, 1964; producer, *Flight to Fury* (also known as *Cordillera*), Twentieth Century-Fox, 1966; casting director, *Five Easy Pieces*, Columbia, 1970; associate producer, *Drive, He Said*, Columbia, 1971; casting director, *The Godfather*, Paramount, 1972; casting supervisor, *American Graffiti*, Universal, 1973; producer (with Francis Ford Coppola), *The Conversation*, Paramount, 1974; producer (with Coppola and Gray Frederickson), *The Godfather, Part II*, Paramount, 1974; producer (with Coppola, Frederickson, and Tom Sternberg), *Apocalypse Now*, United Artists, 1979; producer (with Sternberg), *The Black Stallion*, United Artists, 1979; executive producer, *The Escape Artist*, Warner Brothers, 1981; producer (with Ronald Colby and Don Guest), *Hammett*, Warner Brothers, 1982; producer (with Frederickson and Armyan Bernstein), *One from the Heart*, Columbia, 1982; producer (with Sternberg and Doug Claybourne), *The Black Stallion Returns*, Metro-Goldwyn-Mayer/United Artists, 1983; producer (with Frederickson), *The Outsiders*, Warner Brothers, 1983; producer (with Claybourne), *Rumble Fish*, Universal, 1983; producer (with Robert Evans and Silvio Tabet), *The Cotton Club*, Orion, 1984; producer, *One Magic Christmas*, Buena Vista, 1985; producer, *Seven Minutes in Heaven*, Warner Brothers, 1986; special

consultant, *Peggy Sue Got Married*, Tri-Star, 1986; casting consultant, *Tough Guys Don't Dance*, Cannon, 1987; producer (with Barbet Schroeder and Tom Luddy), *Barfly*, Cannon, 1987; executive producer (with Stan Weston, Jay Emmett, and David Valdes), *Gardens of Stone*, Tri-Star, 1987; producer (with Fred Fuchs), *Tucker: The Man and His Dreams*, Paramount, 1988; producer (with Fuchs), "Life without Zoe" in *New York Stories*, Touchstone, 1989.

RELATED CAREER—Director of documentary films for the Armed Forces Radio and Television Network; agent, MCA, Los Angeles, CA; story editor, Robert Lippert Productions; also casting director.

WRITINGS: FILMS—*Flight to Fury* (also known as *Cordillera*), Twentieth Century-Fox, 1966.

AWARDS: Golden Palm from the Cannes Film Festival and Academy Award nomination, both Best Picture, 1974, for *The Conversation;* Academy Award, Best Picture, 1974, for *The Godfather, Part II;* Golden Palm from the Cannes Film Festival, Academy Award nomination, and British Academy Award nomination, all Best Picture, 1979, for *Apocalypse Now*.

ADDRESSES: OFFICE—2980 Beverly Glen Circle, Los Angeles, CA 90077.*

*   *   *

ROSE, Jack   1911-

PERSONAL: Born November 4, 1911, in Warsaw, Poland; wife's name, Audrey Mary. EDUCATION: Ohio University, B.A., 1934.

VOCATION: Screenwriter and producer.

CAREER: Also see *WRITINGS* below. PRINCIPAL FILM WORK—Producer: *The Seven Little Foys*, Paramount, 1955; *Beau James*, Paramount, 1957; *Houseboat*, Paramount, 1958; *The Five Pennies*, Paramount, 1959; *It Started in Naples*, Paramount, 1960; *On the Double*, Paramount, 1961; *Who's Got the Action?*, Paramount, 1962; *Papa's Delicate Condition*, Paramount, 1963; *Who's Been Sleeping in My Bed?*, Paramount, 1963.

PRINCIPAL TELEVISION WORK—Creator and producer (with Bob Schiller and Bob Weiskopf), *The Good Guys*, CBS, 1968-70.

WRITINGS: FILM—(With Edmund Beloin and Lewis Meltzer) *Ladies' Man*, Paramount, 1947; (with Beloin) *My Favorite Brunette*, Paramount, 1947; (with Beloin) *Road to Rio*, Paramount, 1947; (with Edmund Hartman and Frank Tashlin) *The Paleface*, Paramount, 1948; (with Melville Shavelson) *Always Leave Them Laughing*, Warner Brothers, 1949; (with Beloin and Shavelson) *The Great Lover*, Paramount, 1949; (with Shavelson) *It's a Great Feeling*, Warner Brothers, 1949; (with Shavelson and Hartman) *Sorrowful Jones*, Paramount, 1949; (with Shavelson and Peter Milne) *The Daughter of Rosie O'Grady*, Warner Brothers, 1950; (with Shavelson) *Riding High*, Paramount, 1950; (with Shavelson)

I'll See You in My Dreams, Warner Brothers, 1951; (with Shavelson) *On Moonlight Bay,* Warner Brothers, 1951; (with Shavelson) *Room for One More* (also known as *The Easy Way*), Warner Brothers, 1952; (with Shavelson) *April in Paris,* Warner Brothers, 1953; (with Shavelson) *Trouble Along the Way,* Warner Brothers, 1953; (with Shavelson) *Living It Up,* Paramount, 1954; (with Shavelson) *The Seven Little Foys,* Paramount, 1955; (with Shavelson) *Beau James,* Paramount, 1957; (with Shavelson) *Houseboat,* Paramount, 1958; (with Shavelson) *The Five Pennies,* Paramount, 1959.

(With Shavelson and Suso Cecchi d'Amico) *It Started in Naples,* Paramount, 1960; (with Shavelson) *On the Double,* Paramount, 1961; *Who's Got the Action?,* Paramount, 1962; *Papa's Delicate Condition,* Paramount, 1963; *Who's Been Sleeping in My Bed?,* Paramount, 1963; (with Melvin Frank) *A Touch of Class,* AVCO-Embassy, 1973; (with Frank and Barry Sandler) *The Duchess and the Dirtwater Fox,* Twentieth Century-Fox, 1976; (with Frank) *Lost and Found,* Columbia, 1979; (with Tom Patchett, Jay Tarses, and Jerry Juhl) *The Great Muppet Caper,* Universal, 1981.*

*   *   *

ROSEMONT, Norman   1924-

PERSONAL: Born December 12, 1924, in New York, NY.

VOCATION: Producer.

CAREER: PRINCIPAL FILM WORK—Producer, *Stiletto,* AVCO-Embassy, 1969; producer, *The Count of Monte Cristo,* ITC, 1976.

PRINCIPAL TELEVISION WORK—All as producer, unless indicated. Mini-Series: *Master of the Game,* CBS, 1984. Pilots: *Variety,* ABC, 1974; *Big Bend Country,* CBS, 1981; *Little Lord Fauntleroy,* CBS, 1982; "My Africa" (also known as "Two Worlds"), *CBS Summer Playhouse,* CBS, 1988. Movies: *The Man without a Country,* ABC, 1973; *Miracle on 34th Street,* CBS, 1973; executive producer, *The Red Badge of Courage,* NBC, 1974; *A Tree Grows in Brooklyn,* NBC, 1974; *The Count of Monte Cristo,* NBC, 1975; *The Man in the Iron Mask,* NBC, 1977; *Captains Courageous,* ABC, 1977; *The Four Feathers,* NBC, 1978; *Les Miserables,* CBS, 1978; *All Quiet on the Western Front,* CBS, 1979; *Little Lord Fauntleroy,* CBS, 1980; *A Tale of Two Cities,* CBS, 1980; *Pleasure Palace,* CBS, 1980; *Ivanhoe,* CBS, 1982; *The Hunchback of Notre Dame,* CBS, 1982; *Witness for the Prosecution,* CBS, 1982; *Camille,* CBS, 1984; executive producer, *The Corsican Brothers,* CBS, 1985; executive producer, *The Christmas Gift,* CBS, 1986. Specials: Executive producer, *An Hour with Robert Goulet,* CBS, 1964; executive producer, *Brigadoon,* ABC, 1966; *Carousel,* ABC, 1967; *Kismet,* ABC, 1967; (with Robert Goulet) *Kiss Me Kate,* ABC, 1968; executive producer, *The Mad Mad Mad Mad World of the Super Bowl,* NBC, 1977; "The Court-Martial of George Armstrong Custer," *Hallmark Hall of Fame,* NBC, 1977; executive producer, "The Secret Garden," *Hallmark Hall of Fame,* CBS, 1987; executive producer, "Graham Greene's The Tenth Man," *Hallmark Hall of Fame,* CBS, 1988.

ADDRESSES: OFFICE—Rosemont Productions Ltd., 100 Universal City Plaza, Bungalow 73, Universal City, CA 91608.*

ROSSELLINI, Isabella   1952-

PERSONAL: Born June 18, 1952, in Rome, Italy; daughter of Roberto Rossellini (a director) and Ingrid Bergman (an actress); married Martin Scorsese (a director), September, 1979 (divorced, November, 1982); married Jonathan Wiedemann (divorced); children: Elettra Ingrid (second marriage). EDUCATION: Attended Finch College, 1972, and the New School for Social Research.

VOCATION: Actress.

CAREER: PRINCIPAL FILM APPEARANCES—Sister Pia, *A Matter of Time,* American International, 1976; Eugenia, *Il Prato* (also known as *The Meadow*), SACIS, 1979; Isabella, *Il Pap'occhio* (also known as *In the Pope's Eye*), Titanus, 1980; Darya Greenwood, *White Nights,* Columbia, 1985; Dorothy Vallens, *Blue Velvet,* De Laurentiis Entertainment Group, 1986; Lady Jeanne, *Red Riding Hood,* Cannon, 1987; Marie, *Siesta,* Lorimar, 1987; Madeline, *Tough Guys Don't Dance,* Cannon, 1987; Mademoiselle (Zelly), *Zelly and Me,* Columbia, 1988; Maria Hardy, *Cousins,* Paramount, 1989.

PRINCIPAL TELEVISION APPEARANCES—Series: *The Other Sunday.*

RELATED CAREER—Professional model; interviewer, RAI-TV (Italy).

NON-RELATED CAREER—Teacher of Italian, New School for Social Research, New York City.

ADDRESSES: AGENT—Martha Luttrell, International Creative Management, 8899 Beverly Boulevard, Los Angeles, CA, 90048. PUBLICIST—Marion Billings, M/S Billings, 250 W. 57th Street, New York, NY, 10107.*

*   *   *

ROSSOVICH, Rick   1957-

PERSONAL: Born August 28, 1957, in Palo Alto, CA.

VOCATION: Actor.

CAREER: FILM DEBUT—Marine, *Losin' It,* Lions Gate, 1981. PRINCIPAL FILM APPEARANCES—Pig, *The Lords of Discipline,* Paramount, 1983; Officer Cooley, *Streets of Fire,* Universal/RKO, 1984; Matt, *The Terminator,* Orion, 1984; Bob, *Warning Sign,* Twentieth Century-Fox, 1985; detective, *The Morning After,* Twentieth Century-Fox, 1986; Slider, *Top Gun,* Paramount, 1986; Kurt Klein, *Let's Get Harry,* Tri-Star, 1987; Chris McDonell, *Roxanne,* Columbia, 1987; Derek Clayton, *Spellbinder,* Metro-Goldwyn-Mayer, 1988; Jonathan Dunbar, *Paint It Black,* Vestron, 1989. Also appeared in *Secret Ingredient,* Hemdale, 1988.

PRINCIPAL TELEVISION APPEARANCES—Series: Sergeant Geller, *MacGruder and Loud,* ABC, 1985. Movies: Craig, *Deadly Lessons,* ABC, 1983; Dolph, *Single Bars, Single Women,* ABC, 1984; Roy "Jackjaw" Kelton, *14 Going on 30,* ABC, 1988; also *Girls of Starkwater Hall,* ABC, 1983.

ADDRESSES: AGENT—Agency for the Performing Arts, 9000

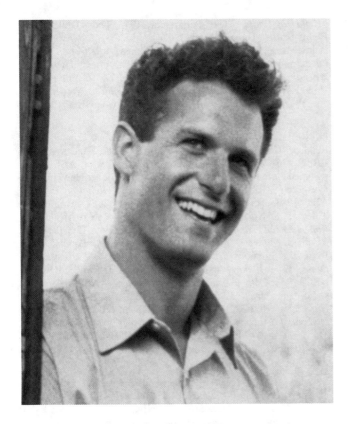

RICK ROSSOVICH

Sunset Boulevard, Suite 1200, Los Angeles, CA 90069. PUBLI-CIST—Jim Dobson and Associates, 1917 1/2 Westwood Boulevard, Suite 2, Los Angeles, CA 90025.

*   *   *

ROTH, Joe

VOCATION: Producer.

CAREER: PRINCIPAL FILM APPEARANCES—*Tunnelvision,* Worldwide, 1976. PRINCIPAL FILM WORK—All as producer, unless indicated: *Tunnelvision,* World-Wide, 1976; executive producer, *Cracking Up,* American International, 1977; *Our Winning Season,* American International, 1978; *Americathon,* United Artists, 1979; *Ladies and Gentlemen, the Fabulous Stains,* Paramount, 1982; *The Final Terror* (also known as *Campsite Massacre, Bump in the Night,* and *The Forest Primeval*), Comworld/Watershed/Roth, 1983; executive producer, *Bachelor Party,* Twentieth Century-Fox, 1983; (with Ivan Bloch) *The Stone Boy,* Twentieth Century-Fox, 1984; (with Harry Ufland) *Moving Violations,* Twentieth Century-Fox, 1985; (with Ufland) *Off Beat,* Silver Screen Partners II, 1986; (with Ufland) and director, *Streets of Gold,* Twentieth Century-Fox, 1986; (with Ufland) *Where the River Runs Black,* Metro-Goldwyn-Mayer/United Artists, 1986; *P.K. and the Kid,* Lorimar, 1987; executive producer and director, *Revenge of the Nerds II: Nerds in Paradise,* Twentieth Century-Fox, 1987; executive producer, *Skin Deep,* Twentieth Century-Fox, 1989.*

RUNYON, Jennifer

VOCATION: Actress.

CAREER: PRINCIPAL FILM APPEARANCES—Nancy, *To All a Goodnight,* Intercontinental, 1983; student, *Ghostbusters,* Columbia, 1984; Heather Merriweather, *Up the Creek,* Orion, 1984; Carole, *The Falcon and the Snowman,* Orion, 1985; Terry, *Flight of the Spruce Goose,* Filmhaus, 1986; Vicky, *The In Crowd* (also known as *Dance Party* and *Bandstand*), Orion, 1987; Robin, *Eighteen Again!,* New World, 1988.

PRINCIPAL TELEVISION APPEARANCES—Series: Gwendolyn Pierce, *Charles in Charge,* CBS, 1984-85; Peg Stratton, *Quantum Leap,* NBC, 1989—; also Sally Frame, *Another World,* NBC. Mini-Series: Marcia Grant, *James A. Michener's ''Space''* (also known as *Space*), CBS, 1985. Pilots: Heather ''Breezy'' Akins, *Six Pack,* NBC, 1983; Christy, *Pros and Cons,* ABC, 1986; J.C. Swift, *Blue de Ville,* NBC, 1986; Amanda Merrick, *The Highwayman,* NBC, 1987. Episodic: Christine, *Magnum, P.I.,* CBS, 1987; Doreen, *Who's the Boss?,* ABC, 1987; Gwen, *The Hogan Family,* NBC, 1988; Karen, *Dear John,* NBC, 1988; Mrs. Roomer, *Empty Nest,* NBC, 1988. Movies: Angel Fisher, *Dreams of Gold: The Mel Fisher Story,* CBS, 1986; Cindy Brady, *A Very Brady Christmas,* CBS, 1988.

ADDRESSES: MANAGER—Monica Dremann and Associates, Los Angeles, CA.*

*   *   *

RUTTAN, Susan

PERSONAL: Born Susan Dunrud in Oregon City, OR; father, a logger; mother, a nurse; married Mel Ruttan (deceased). EDUCATION: Attended the University of California, Santa Cruz.

VOCATION: Actress.

CAREER: PRINCIPAL FILM APPEARANCES—Nurse, *Independence Day,* Warner Brothers, 1983; biker, *Bad Manners* (also known as *Growing Pains*), New World, 1984.

PRINCIPAL TELEVISION APPEARANCES—Series: Roxanne Melman, *L.A. Law,* NBC, 1986—. Pilots: Marge, *After George,* CBS, 1983. Episodic: Marge, *Empire,* CBS, 1984; also Katherine Shub, *Buffalo Bill,* NBC; *Newhart,* CBS; *Night Court,* NBC; *Remington Steele,* NBC; *The Misadventures of Sheriff Lobo* (also known as *Lobo*), NBC. Movies: Woman prude, *Dropout Father,* CBS, 1982; hostess, *The Fighter,* CBS, 1983; Mrs. Estep, *Packin' It In,* CBS, 1983; Portsmouth nurse, *Thursday's Child,* CBS, 1983; Robin, *Second Sight: A Love Story,* CBS, 1984; Margie, *Scorned and Swindled,* CBS, 1984; Judge M. Tyson, *Murder: By Reason of Insanity,* CBS, 1985; Rosemary, *Kicks,* ABC, 1985; Julie Myers, *Do You Remember Love?,* CBS, 1985; Ms. Morgan, *Under the Influence,* CBS, 1986; Mrs. McGwin, *Bay Coven,* NBC, 1987. Specials: *NBC Presents the AFI Comedy Special,* NBC, 1987; *Jay Leno's Family Comedy Special,* NBC, 1987.

RELATED CAREER—Member, Staircase Theatre, Santa Cruz, CA, 1976-77.

NON-RELATED CAREER—Secretary and bar manager.

AWARDS: Emmy Award nomination, Best Supporting Actress, for *L.A. Law.*

ADDRESSES: AGENT—J. Michael Bloom, 9200 Sunset Boulevard, Suite 710, Los Angeles, CA 90069. PUBLICIST—Cynthia Snyder Public Relations, 3518 Cahuenga Boulevard W., Suite 304, Los Angeles, CA 90068.*

*   *   *

RYAN, Mitchell   1928-
(Mitch Ryan)

PERSONAL: Born January 11, 1928, in Cincinnati, OH. MILITARY: U.S. Navy.

VOCATION: Actor.

CAREER: PRINCIPAL STAGE APPEARANCES—(As Mitch Ryan) Clyde Gevedon, *Whisper to Me,* Players Theatre, New York City, 1960; Antonio, *The Tempest,* New York Shakespeare Festival (NYSF), Shakespeare Theatre, New York City, 1962; Agrippa, *Antony and Cleopatra,* Duke Senior, *As You Like It,* and Leontes, *The Winter's Tale,* all NYSF, Delacorte Theatre, New York City, 1963; Iago, *Othello,* NYSF, Delacorte Theatre, 1964, then Martinique Theatre, New York City, 1965; title role, *Baal,* Martinique Theatre, 1965; Tullus Aufidius, *Coriolanus,* NYSF, Delacorte Theatre, 1965; Mike Talman, *Wait until Dark,* Ethel Barrymore Theatre, New York City, 1966; Agamemnon, *Iphigenia in Aulis,* Circle in the Square, New York City, 1967; James Tyrone, Jr., *A Moon for the Misbegotten,* Circle in the Square, 1968; Clint Barlowe, *The Sudden and Accidental Re-Education of Horse Johnson,* Belasco Theatre, New York City, 1968; Jason, *Medea,* Clarence Brown Company, Knoxville, TN, then Cort Theatre, New York City, both 1982. Also appeared with the Arena Stage, Washington, DC, 1969-70.

PRINCIPAL FILM APPEARANCES—(As Mitch Ryan) Shorty Austin, *Monte Walsh,* National General, 1970; Charles Kincaid, *Chandler,* Metro-Goldwyn-Mayer, 1971; Sergeant Martin Flood, *Glory Boy* (also known as *My Old Man's Place* and *The Old Man's Place*), Cinerama, 1971; Lowell, *The Honkers,* United Artists, 1972; Harve Poole, *Electra Glide in Blue,* United Artists, 1973; Waters, *The*

Friends of Eddie Coyle, Paramount, 1973; Dave Drake, *High Plains Drifter,* Universal, 1973; Charlie McCoy, *Magnum Force,* Warner Brothers, 1973; Inspector McKenna, *A Reflection of Fear* (also known as *Labyrinth*), Columbia, 1973; priest, *Two-Minute Warning,* Universal, 1976; Doc Harrison, *The Hunting Party,* United Artists, 1977; the General, *Lethal Weapon,* Warner Brothers, 1987; Drury Campbell, *Winter People,* Columbia, 1989.

PRINCIPAL TELEVISION APPEARANCES—Series: Captain Chase Reddick, *Chase,* NBC, 1973-74; Don Walling, *Executive Suite,* CBS, 1976-77; Dr. Blake Simmons, *Having Babies,* ABC, 1978, renamed *Julie Farr, M.D.,* ABC, 1978-79; Cooper Hawkins, *The Chisholms,* CBS, 1980; Brennan Flannery, *High Performance,* ABC, 1983; also Burke Devlin, *Dark Shadows,* ABC. Mini-Series: Tillet Main, *North and South,* ABC, 1985; Robert McNamara, *Robert Kennedy and His Times,* CBS, 1985. Pilots: Ben, *The Fuzz Brothers,* ABC, 1973; Captain Chase Reddick, *Chase,* NBC, 1973; Dr. Blake Simmons, *Having Babies III,* ABC, 1978; Keyes, *Joe Dancer: The Monkey Mission* (also known as *The Monkey Mission*), NBC, 1981; Colonel Evan Marshall, *Northstar,* ABC, 1986. Episodic: Sam Garrett, *King's Crossing,* ABC, 1982; Edward Wyler, *Hot Pursuit,* NBC, 1984; Bane, *Hell Town,* NBC, 1985; George Deaton, *St. Elsewhere,* NBC, 1987; (as Mitch Ryan) Ernest Lenko, *Murder, She Wrote,* CBS, 1987; Admiral Edgar Sheppard, *Mission: Impossible,* ABC, 1989.

Movies: (As Mitch Ryan) Mr. Pasko, *The Entertainer,* NBC, 1976; Matthew, *Christmas Miracle in Caulfield U.S.A.* (also known as *The Christmas Coal Mine Miracle*), NBC, 1977; (as Mitch Ryan) Jethro Lundy, *Peter Lundy and the Medicine Hat Stallion,* NBC, 1977; (as Mitch Ryan) Ambler Bowman, *Escape from Bogen County,* CBS, 1977; (as Mitch Ryan) Lieutenant Colonel Applegate, *Sergeant Matlovich versus the U.S. Air Force,* NBC, 1978; Jack Fallon, *Flesh and Blood,* CBS, 1979; Silas Creedy, *Angel City,* CBS, 1980; Dr. Ralph B. Allison and narrator, *The Five of Me,* CBS, 1981; Jerry Clements, *The Choice,* CBS, 1981; Hugh Hefner, *Death of a Centerfold: The Dorothy Stratten Story,* NBC, 1981; Slim, *Of Mice and Men,* NBC, 1981; Charlie McCourt, *Kenny Rogers as "The Gambler"—The Adventure Continues,* CBS, 1983; Chief Tom Riordan, *Uncommon Valor,* CBS, 1983; Paul Strombaugh, *Fatal Vision,* NBC, 1984; Captain Malone, *Hostage Flight,* NBC, 1985; Judge Donald Faulkner, *Penalty Phase,* CBS, 1986; Dan Eastman, *Favorite Son,* NBC, 1988; Tom Hale, *The Ryan White Story,* ABC, 1989. Specials: *Medea.**

S

SADLER, Bill 1950-

PERSONAL: Full name, William Sadler; born April 13, 1950, in Buffalo, NY. EDUCATION: Graduated from the State University of New York, Genesee; also attended Cornell University.

VOCATION: Actor.

CAREER: STAGE DEBUT—Title role, Hamlet, Colorado Shakespeare Festival. OFF-BROADWAY DEBUT—Title role, Ivanov, City Playworks, 1975. BROADWAY DEBUT—Sergeant Merwin J. Toomey, Biloxi Blues, Neil Simon Theatre, 1985. PRINCIPAL STAGE APPEARANCES—Ensemble, Henry V and Measure for Measure, both New York Shakespeare Festival (NYSF), Delacorte Theatre, New York City, 1977; editor, bellboy, janitor, body guard, Harry the Horse, priest, soundman, and pirate, New Jerusalem, New York Shakespeare Festival (NYSF), Public Theatre, New York City, 1979; Jimmy, A History of the American Film, Seattle Repertory Theatre, Seattle, WA, 1979; jeweler, Dark Ride, Soho Repertory Theatre, New York City, 1981; Betty and Gerry, Cloud 9, Theatre De Lys (renamed Lucille Lortel Theatre), New York City, 1981; Hector, The Chinese Viewing Pavilion, The Production Company, Actors and Directors Theatre, New York City, 1982; Jasper, boyfriend of Ginger, and friend of Burt, Necessary Ends, NYSF, Public Theatre, 1982; Pete Shotton, Alan Williams, Victor Spinetti, Arthur Janov, and Andy Peebles, Lennon, Entermedia Theatre, New York City, 1982; Sergeant Merwin J. Toomey, Biloxi Blues, Center Theatre Group, Ahmanson Theatre, Los Angeles, CA, 1984. Also appeared in Ramblings and Cracks, both Playwrights Horizons, New York City, 1977; Dial M for Murder, Playwrights Horizons, 1978; Journey's End, Long Wharf Theatre, New Haven, CT, 1978; Time Steps, Playwrights Horizons, 1980; Ladies in Retirement, Royal Poinciana Playhouse, Palm Beach, FL, 1981; as Len Jenkins, Limbo Tales, Off-Broadway production, New York City, 1981; Night Must Fall, Hartman Theatre, Stamford, CT, 1982; Much Ado about Nothing, Yale Repertory Theatre, New Haven, CT, 1982; as Bill Sprightly, A Mad World, My Masters, La Jolla Playhouse, La Jolla, CA; Charley, Charley's Aunt, Academy Festival Theatre; Hamm, Endgame, Florida Studio Theatre; in Hannah, Off Broadway production, New York City; and with the Trinity Square Repertory Company, Providence, RI, 1975-76.

FILM DEBUT—Hotel clerk, Hanky-Panky, Columbia, 1982. PRINCIPAL FILM APPEARANCES—Dickson, Off Beat, Silver Screen Partners II, 1986; Dr. Lynnard Carroll, Project X, Twentieth Century-Fox, 1987.

PRINCIPAL TELEVISION APPEARANCES—Series: Lieutenant Charlie Fontana, Private Eye, NBC, 1987-88. Pilots: Colonel Tom Sturdivant, Cadets (also known as Rotten to the Corps), ABC, 1988; also The Neighborhood, NBC, 1982. Episodic: Rick Dillon,

The Equalizer, CBS, 1986; Richie Epson, In the Heat of the Night (two episodes), NBC, 1988; Ken, Dear John, NBC, 1988; Colonel Fitzpatrick, Murphy Brown, CBS, 1989; Dwight Hooper, Roseanne (two episodes), ABC, 1989; Larry Harbin, Hooperman (two episodes), ABC, 1989; also AfterM*A*S*H, CBS; Newhart, CBS. Movies: Dieter Schmidt, The Great Wallendas, NBC, 1978; Joey, Charlie and the Great Balloon Race, NBC, 1981; Coach Dickey, Unconquered (also known as Invictus), CBS, 1989. Specials: Henry Winkler Meets William Shakespeare, CBS, 1977; also Assaulted Nuts, Cinemax. Also appeared in The Other Side of Victory and The Rocking Chair Rebellion.

AWARDS: Obie Award from the Village Voice and Villager Award, both 1981, for Limbo Tales.

ADDRESSES: AGENT—Abrams Artists and Associates, 9200 Sunset Boulevard, Suite 625, Los Angeles, CA, 90069.*

* * *

SAGET, Bob 1956-

PERSONAL: Full name, Robert Saget; born May 17, 1956, in Philadelphia, PA; son of Benjamin M. (a supermarket executive) and Rosalyn C. (a hospital administrator) Saget; married Sherri K. Kramer (an attorney), May 16, 1983; children: Aubrey Michelle. EDUCATION: Temple University, B.A., film, 1978; graduate work, University of Southern California; trained for the stage with Darryl Hickman, Harvey Lembeck, and Vincent Chase.

VOCATION: Comedian, actor, and writer.

CAREER: Also see WRITINGS below. STAGE DEBUT-Douglas, Audience, Fig Tree Theatre, Hollywood, CA, 1986, for ten performances, PRINCIPAL STAGE WORK-Producer, Audience, Fig Tree Theatre, Hollywood, CA, 1986.

FILM DEBUT—Sportscaster, Full Moon High, Orion, 1979. PRINCIPAL FILM APPEARANCES—Computer voice, Spaced Out, Miramax, 1981; Dr. Joffe, Critical Condition, Paramount, 1987. PRINCIPAL FILM WORK—Producer, director, and editor, Through Adam's Eyes (documentary), 1978.

TELEVISION DEBUT—Make Me Laugh, syndicated, 1980. PRINCIPAL TELEVISION APPEARANCES—Series: Co-host, The Morning Program, CBS, 1987; Danny Tanner, Full House, ABC, 1987—. Pilots: Love, American Style '85, ABC; co-host, Knock-Knock, syndicated; co-host, Surprise, CBS; also Good News/Bad News. Episodic: The Greatest American Hero, ABC, 1984; It's a

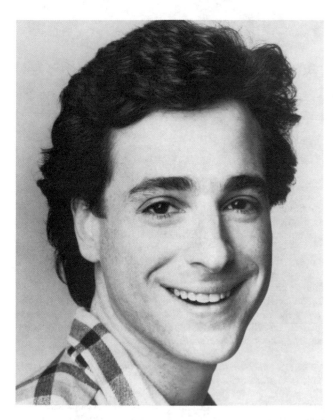

BOB SAGET

Living, ABC, 1985; *Late Night with David Letterman,* NBC, 1988; also *Bosom Buddies,* ABC; *At Ease,* ABC; *The Merv Griffin Show,* syndicated; *The Tonight Show,* NBC. Specials: *Rodney Dangerfield Hosts the Ninth Annual Young Comedians Special,* HBO, 1985; *HBO Young Comedians Special,* HBO, 1986; *A Comedy Celebration: The Comedy and Magic Club's Tenth Anniversary Special,* Showtime, 1989; also *Comedy Tonight,* PBS; *Evening at the Improv,* syndicated; *Comic of the Month,* Showtime; *Comedy Break,* syndicated.

PRINCIPAL TELEVISION WORK—Producer and director of video segments, *The Morning Program,* CBS, 1987.

RELATED CAREER—As a comedian has appeared in nightclubs and concert halls throughout the United States and Canada, 1979—; member of Groundlings (an improvisational comedy troupe).

WRITINGS: FILM—*Through Adam's Eyes* (documentary), 1978; (additional dialogue) *Spaced Out,* Miramax, 1981; *Stepbrothers,* 1985; *Two Orphans* (short film), 1985; *Coffee Shop* (short film), 1986; *Temporary Asylum,* 1988. TELEVISION—*The Morning Program,* CBS, 1987.

AWARDS: Student Academy Award, 1978, for *Through Adam's Eyes.*

MEMBER: Screen Actors Guild, American Federation of Television and Radio Artists, Directors Guild of America, American Society of Composers, Authors, and Publishers.

SIDELIGHTS: FAVORITE ROLES—Dr. Joffe in *Critical Condition* and Danny in *Full House.*

ADDRESSES: AGENT—Leading Artists, 445 N. Bedford Drive, Penthouse, Beverly Hills, CA 90210. MANAGER—The Brillstein Company, 9200 Sunset Boulevard, Suite 428, Los Angeles, CA 90069.

*   *   *

SAHL, Mort   1927-

PERSONAL: Full name, Morton Lyon Sahl; born May 11, 1927, in Montreal, PQ, Canada; son of Harry Sahl; married Sue Babior, June 25, 1955 (divorced, 1957); married China Lee; children: Morton, Jr. EDUCATION: Attended Compton Junior College; received B.S. in city management and engineering from the University of Southern California. MILITARY: U.S. Army Air Forces, private, during World War II.

VOCATION: Comedian, actor, and writer.

CAREER: PRINCIPAL STAGE APPEARANCES—*The Next President* (revue), Bijou Theatre, New York City, 1958; *Mort Sahl on Broadway* (one-man show), Neil Simon Theatre, New York City, 1987.

FILM DEBUT—Danny Krieger, *In Love and War,* Twentieth Century-Fox, 1958. PRINCIPAL FILM APPEARANCES—Crane, *All the Young Men,* Columbia, 1960; Ben Morro, *Johnny Cool,* United Artists, 1963; Dan Ruskin, *Doctor, You've Got to Be Kidding,* Metro-Goldwyn-Mayer (MGM), 1967; Sam Lingonberry, *Don't Make Waves,* MGM, 1967; Uncle Mort, *Nothing Lasts Forever,* Metro-Goldwyn-Mayer/United Artists, 1984. Also appeared in *The Hungry i Reunion* (documentary), 1981.

PRINCIPAL TELEVISION APPEARANCES—Episodic: *The Big Party,* CBS, 1959; *The Jerry Lewis Show,* ABC, 1963; also "Kiss Me Again, Stranger," *Pursuit,* CBS; *The Steve Allen Show,* NBC; *The Jack Paar Show,* NBC; *The Eddie Fisher Show,* NBC; *The Tonight Show,* NBC; *Nightline,* ABC. Pilots: *Comedy News II,* ABC, 1973. Movies: Werner Fink, *Inside the Third Reich,* ABC, 1982. Specials: *The Mort Sahl Special,* NBC, 1960; *Dick Clark's Good Old Days: From Bobby Sox to Bikinis,* NBC, 1977; *All Star Party for Clint Eastwood,* CBS, 1986; *Jonathan Winters: On the Ledge,* Showtime, 1987; *Humor and the Presidency,* HBO, 1987; also *Wide Wide World.*

PRINCIPAL RADIO APPEARANCES—Series: Talk show host, WRC-Radio, Washington, DC, 1978.

RELATED CAREER—As a comedian, has appeared in nightclubs and concert halls throughout the United States; also editor, *Poop from the Group;* and actor in experimental theatre productions.

WRITINGS: Heartland (autobiography), Harcourt, 1976; also writer for magazines in Los Angeles, CA, and San Francisco, CA.

RECORDINGS: ALBUMS—*Sing a Song of Watergate,* GNP Crescendo; has also recorded for Verve Records.

ADDRESSES: HOME—Beverly Hills, CA. AGENT—Norman Brokaw, William Morris Agency, 151 El Camino Drive, Beverly Hills, CA 90212. MANAGER—Stanley Weinstein Arts Management, 210 Rutgers Lane, Parsippany, NJ 07054.*

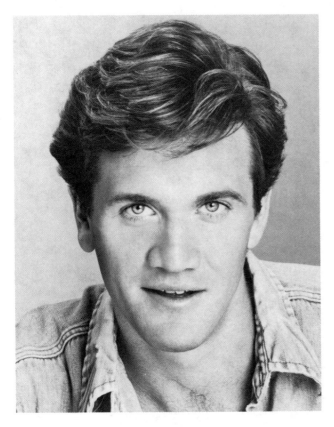

MATT SALINGER

SALINGER, Matt   1960-

PERSONAL: Born February 13, 1960, in Windsor, VT; son of Jerome David (a writer) and Alison Claire (a psychologist; maiden name, Douglas) Salinger; married Betsy Jane Becker (a jewelry manufacturer and designer), May 19, 1985. EDUCATION: Attended Princeton University, 1978-80; Columbia University, B.A., art history, 1983; studied acting with Peggy Feury and at the Royal Academy of Dramatic Arts.

VOCATION: Actor.

CAREER: OFF-BROADWAY DEBUT—Manke, *Drums in the Night,* Horace Mann Theatre, New York City, 1982. BROADWAY DE-BUT—James Bernard, *Dancing in the End Zone,* Ritz Theatre, 1985, for twenty-eight performances. PRINCIPAL STAGE APPEAR-ANCES—Pete, *One Night at Studio,* Zephyr Theatre, Los Angeles, CA, 1984; Charly Bacon, *Charly Bacon and His Family,* John Drew Theatre, East Hampton, NY, 1988. Also appeared in *All God's Children Got Wings,* Horace Mann Theatre, New York City, 1983; *No Exit,* Theatre East, New York City, 1983; and with the Ensemble Studio Theatre, New York City.

FILM DEBUT—Danny Burke, *Revenge of the Nerds,* Twentieth Century-Fox, 1984. PRINCIPAL FILM APPEARANCES—Phillip Aarons, *Power,* Lorimar, 1985; Donald Anderson, *Options,* Vestron, 1989.

TELEVISION DEBUT—Dave Meehan, *One Life to Live,* ABC, 1983. PRINCIPAL TELEVISION APPEARANCES—Pilots: Andrew Jackson, *Rainbow in the Thunder,* NBC, 1988. Movies: Lieutenant

Bryce Parker, *Blood and Orchids,* CBS, 1986; Claude Dallas, Jr., *Manhunt for Claude Dallas,* CBS, 1986; Jack Shoat, *Deadly Deception,* CBS, 1987; James Barrington, *Barrington,* CBS, 1987. Specials: Young Frederick Remington, *West of the Imagination,* PBS, 1985.

MEMBER: Young Artists United (a community service group).

SIDELIGHTS: RECREATIONS—Hiking, skiing, and outdoor activities.

Matt Salinger told *CTFT* that he is active in many environmental and conservation groups.

ADDRESSES: AGENT—Creative Artists Agency, 1888 Century Park E., Suite 1400, Los Angeles, CA 90067.

*   *   *

SALT, Jennifer   1944-

PERSONAL: Born September 4, 1944, in Los Angeles, CA; daughter of Waldo (a screenwriter) and Mary (Davenport) Salt; children: one. EDUCATION: Graduated from the High School of the Performing Arts, New York City; graduated from Sarah Lawrence College.

VOCATION: Actress.

CAREER: PRINCIPAL STAGE APPEARANCES—Gloria, "Water-color" in *Watercolor and Crisscrossing,* American National Thea-tre and Academy Theatre, New York City, 1970; Estelle, *Father's Day,* John Golden Theatre, New York City, 1971. Also appeared in *The Hot l Baltimore,* Center Theatre Group, Mark Taper Forum, Los Angeles, CA, 1973; in *Hasty Heart,* 1981; and in *Diplomacy,* 1982.

PRINCIPAL FILM APPEARANCES—Phoebe, *The Wedding Party,* Ajay, 1969; Annie, *Midnight Cowboy,* United Artists, 1969; Hope, *Brewster McCloud,* Metro-Goldwyn-Mayer, 1970; Judy Bishop, *Hi, Mom!,* Sigma III, 1970; Helen Peret, *The Revolutionary,* United Artists, 1970; Sharon, *Play It Again, Sam,* Paramount, 1972; Grace Collier, *Sisters,* American International, 1973; Maisie, *It's My Turn,* Columbia, 1980. Also appeared in *Murder a la Mod,* Aries Documentaries, 1968.

PRINCIPAL TELEVISION APPEARANCES—Series: Eunice Tate, *Soap,* ABC, 1977-81. Pilots: Laura King, *Old Friends,* ABC, 1984. Episodic: *Family Ties,* NBC. Movies: Diana Boley, *Gar-goyles,* CBS, 1972; Lois, *The Great Niagara,* ABC, 1974; Connie Paxton, *Terror Among Us,* CBS, 1981; Ann Zigo, *Out of the Darkness,* CBS, 1985; Carol Arbiter, *Deadly Care,* CBS, 1987. Specials: *All-Star Family Feud,* ABC, 1978.

RELATED CAREER—Company member, Charles Playhouse, Bos-ton, MA, 1967-68; company member, Hartford Stage Company, Hartford, CT, 1967-68.

NON-RELATED CAREER—Worked in publishing.

AWARDS: Theatre World Award, 1971, for *Father's Day.*

ADDRESSES: AGENT—Artists Agency, 10000 Santa Monica Boulevard, Suite 305, Los Angeles, CA 90067.*

*   *   *

SANTOS, Joe   1931-

PERSONAL: Born June 9, 1931, in Brooklyn, NY; son of Joseph and Rose (Sarno) Minieri; married Mary Montero, March 31, 1958; children: Joseph, Perry. EDUCATION: Attended Fordham University, 1949-50, and Miami University (Ohio), 1950-51. RELIGION: Roman Catholic. MILITARY: U.S. Army, Medical Corps, 1952-54.

VOCATION: Actor.

CAREER: PRINCIPAL FILM APPEARANCES—Truck driver, *My Body Hungers,* Haven International, 1967; Ezmo, *The Gang That Couldn't Shoot Straight,* Metro-Goldwyn-Mayer (MGM), 1971; DiBono, *Panic in Needle Park,* Twentieth Century-Fox, 1971; Reverend, *The Legend of Nigger Charley,* Paramount, 1972; Pascal, *Shaft's Big Score,* MGM, 1972; Spinelli, *Blade,* Pintoff, 1973; Joe Lucci, *The Don Is Dead* (also known as *Beautiful But Deadly*), Universal, 1973; Artie Van, *The Friends of Eddie Coyle,* Paramount, 1973; Lieutenant Promuto, *Shamus,* Columbia, 1973; Frank Gallo, *Zandy's Bride,* Warner Brothers, 1974; Montoya, *Blue Thunder,* Columbia, 1983; Frank, *Fear City,* Chevy Chase Distribution, 1984. Also appeared in *Moonlighting Wives,* Craddock, 1966; and *A Knife for the Ladies,* Bryanston, 1974.

PRINCIPAL TELEVISION APPEARANCES—Series: Detective Dennis Becker, *The Rockford Files,* NBC, 1974-80; Norman Davis, *Me and Maxx,* NBC, 1980; Domingo Rivera, *a.k.a. Pablo,* ABC, 1984; Lieutenant Frank Harper, *Hardcastle and McCormick,* ABC, 1985-86. Pilots: Jabbo, *Nightside,* ABC, 1973; Sergeant Dennis Becker, *The Rockford Files,* NBC, 1974; Lieutenant Vince Promuto, *A Matter of Wife . . . and Death,* NBC, 1976. Episodic: Doug, ''The Library,'' *The Twilight Zone,* CBS, 1986; Jimmy ''The Eraser'' Kendall, *MacGyver,* ABC, 1986 and 1987; Ben Mohammed, *Adderly,* CBS, 1987; Joe Rinaldi, *Murder, She Wrote,* CBS, 1987; Lieutenant Nolan Page, *Magnum P.I.* (four episodes), CBS, 1987 and 1988; Lieutenant Alfano, *Murder, She Wrote,* CBS, 1988; Oscar Carrera, *Miami Vice,* NBC, 1988; also *The Doctors,* NBC. Movies: Sergeant Cruz Segovia, *The Blue Knight,* NBC, 1973; Sergeant Scott, *The Girl on the Late, Late Show,* NBC, 1974; Mr. Layton, *The Hustler of Muscle Beach,* ABC, 1980; Arthur Konigsburg, *Power,* NBC, 1980; Tony, *The Ratings Game,* Movie Channel, 1984; Jake Gilbert, *Deadline: Madrid* (also known as *Deadline*), ABC, 1988.

NON-RELATED CAREER—Construction worker.

ADDRESSES: AGENT—Gores/Fields Agency, 10100 Santa Monica Boulevard, Suite 700, Los Angeles, CA, 90067.*

*   *   *

SAVALAS, Telly   1923-

PERSONAL: Born Aristoteles Savalas, January 21, 1923 (some sources say 1924 or 1926), in Garden City, NY; son of Nicholas

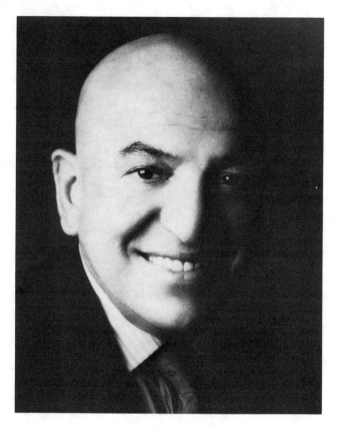

TELLY SAVALAS

Constantine and Christina (Kapsallis) Savalas; married Katherine Nicolaides, 1950 (divorced); married Marilynn Gardner, October 28, 1960 (divorced, 1974); married Sally Adams, 1974 (divorced); married Julie Hovland, December 22, 1984; children: Christina (first marriage); Penelope, Candace (second marriage); Nicholas (third marriage); Christian (fourth marriage). EDUCATION: Received B.S. from Columbia University. RELIGION: Greek Orthodox. MILITARY: U.S. Army.

VOCATION: Actor.

CAREER: PRINCIPAL FILM APPEARANCES—Lieutenant Dawson, *Mad Dog Coll,* Columbia, 1961; Lieutenant Richard Gunnison, *The Young Savages,* United Artists, 1961; Feto Gomez, *Birdman of Alcatraz,* United Artists, 1962; Charles Sievers, *Cape Fear,* Universal, 1962; Dr. Riccio, *The Interns,* Columbia, 1962; Mr. Santangelo, *Johnny Cool,* United Artists, 1963; Dr. Gump, *Love Is a Ball* (also known as *All This and Money Too*), United Artists, 1963; Foots Pulardos, *The Man from the Diners' Club,* Columbia, 1963; harem recruiter, *John Goldfarb, Please Come Home,* Twentieth Century-Fox, 1964; Dr. Riccio, *The New Interns,* Columbia, 1964; Shan, *Genghis Khan* (also known as *Dschingus Khan* and *Dzingis-Kan*), Columbia, 1965; Guffy, *Battle of the Bulge,* Warner Brothers, 1965; Pontius Pilate, *The Greatest Story Ever Told,* United Artists, 1965; Dr. Coburn, *The Slender Thread,* Paramount, 1965; Dagineau, *Beau Geste,* Universal, 1966; Archer Maggott, *The Dirty Dozen,* Metro-Goldwyn-Mayer (MGM), 1967; Count de Franzini, *The Karate Killers,* MGM, 1967; Walter Braddock, *Buona Sera, Mrs. Campbell,* United Artists, 1968; Jim Howie, *The Scalphunters,* United Artists, 1968; Emil Dietrich, *Sol Madrid* (also known as *The Heroin Gang*), MGM, 1968; Lord Bostwick,

The Assassination Bureau, Paramount, 1969; Vince Carden, *Land Raiders* (also known as *Day of the Landgrabbers*), Columbia, 1969; Sergeant Tibbs, *MacKenna's Gold*, Columbia, 1969; Ernst Stavro, *On Her Majesty's Secret Service*, United Artists, 1969.

Big Joe, *Kelly's Heroes*, MGM, 1970; Herbie Hassler, *Sophie's Place* (also known as *Crooks and Coronets*), Warner Brothers/Seven Arts, 1970; Redford, *Clay Pigeon*, MGM, 1971; Captain Sam Surcher, *Pretty Maids All in a Row*, MGM, 1971; Don Carlos, *A Town Called Hell* (also known as *A Town Called Bastard*), Scotia International, 1971; Captain Kazan, *Horror Express* (also known as *Panico en el Transiberia* and *Panic on the Trans-Siberian Express*), Benmar Scotia International, 1972; Weber, *The Family* (also known as *Violent City* and *Citta Violenta*), International Coproductions & EDP Films, released in the United States in 1974; Major Ward, *A Reason to Live, A Reason to Die* (also known as *Una regione per vivere e una per morire* and *Massacre at Fort Holman*), K-Tel, 1974; Franciscus, *Sonny and Jed* (also known as *La banda J&S cronaca criminale del Far West*), Loyola Cinematography/Terra K-Tel, released in the United States in 1974; Harry Morgan, *Inside Out* (also known as *Hitler's Gold* and *The Golden Heist*), Warner Brothers, 1975; Harry Webb, *Killer Force*, American International, 1975; title role, *Pancho Villa*, Scotia International, 1975; Leandro, *House of Exorcism* (also known as *La casa dell' exorcismo* and *Lisa and the Devil*), Peppercorn-Wormser, 1976; Albain, *Capricorn One*, Warner Brothers, 1978; Captain Stefan Svevo, *Beyond the Poseidon Adventure*, Warner Brothers, 1979; Zeno, *Escape to Athena*, Associated Film Distribution, 1979; El Sleezo Tough, *The Muppet Movie*, Associated Film Distriubtors, 1979; Hymie, *Cannonball Run II*, Warner Brothers, 1984; voice of Magmar, *Gobots: Battle of the Rocklords* (animated), Atlantic, 1986. Also appeared in *Redneck*, International Amusements, 1975; *Diamond Mercenaries*, 1975; *Crime Boss*, Cinema Shares International, 1976; as Pete Panakos, *My Palikari*, 1980; Police Lieutenant Thurston, *Fake-Out*, 1982; and as Hallen, *Les Predateurs de la nuit*, 1987.

TELEVISION DEBUT—"Bring Home a Baby," *Armstrong Circle Theatre*, CBS. PRINCIPAL TELEVISION APPEARANCES—Series: Mr. Carver, *Acapulco*, NBC, 1961; Lieutenant Theo Kojak, *Kojak*, CBS, 1973-76. Pilots: Ramon Castillo, *The Watchman* (pilot for a series to be titled *Second Look;* broadcast as an episode of *Kraft Suspense Theatre*), NBC, 1964; Theo Kojak, *Kojak: The Marcus-Nelson Murders* (also known as *Kojak and the Marcus-Nelson Murders*), CBS, 1973; Nick Hellinger, *Hellinger's Law*, CBS, 1981. Episodic: Hendricks, "The Cat and the Canary," *The Dow Hour of Great Mysteries*, NBC, 1960; Lucky Luciano, *Witness*, CBS, 1960; Erich Streator, "Living Doll," *The Twilight Zone*, CBS, 1963; Fleeger, *George Burns Comedy Week*, CBS, 1985; Dimitrious Kousakis, *J.J. Starbuck*, NBC, 1987; Father Joseph Haydn, *The Equalizer*, CBS, 1987; also *The Untouchables*, ABC, 1961; *77 Sunset Strip*, ABC, 1963; *The Fugitive*, ABC, 1965; *Garrison's Gorillas*, ABC, 1967; *Combat*, ABC, 1967; *Alice*, CBS, 1976; *The Dick Powell Show* (also known as *Hollywood Showcase*), NBC; *Naked City*, ABC; *Cain's Hundred*, NBC; *Burke's Law*, ABC.

Movies: Lieutenant Pete Tolstad, *Mongo's Back in Town*, CBS, 1971; Lieutenant Phil Keegan, *Visions . . .* (also known as *Visions of Death*), CBS, 1972; Inspector Joe Brody, *She Cried Murder*, CBS, 1973; Craig Dunleavy, *The French Atlantic Affair*, ABC, 1979; Cretzer, *Alcatraz: The Whole Shocking Story*, NBC, 1980; Phil Drexler, *The Cartier Affair*, NBC, 1984; Theo Kojak, *Kojak: The Belarus File*, CBS, 1985; Cheshire Cat, *Alice in Wonderland*, CBS, 1985; Theo Kojak, *Kojak: The Price of Justice*, CBS, 1987;

Major Wright, *The Dirty Dozen: The Deadly Mission*, NBC, 1987; Major Wright, *The Dirty Dozen: The Fatal Mission*, NBC, 1988. Specials: Decision Maker, *Dinah in Search of the Ideal Man*, NBC, 1973; *Battle of the Network Stars*, ABC, 1976 and 1977; host, *Telly . . . Who Loves Ya, Baby?*, CBS, 1976; *Bob Hope Special: Bob Hope in "Joys,"* NBC, 1976; ringmaster, *Circus of the Stars*, CBS, 1977; co-host, *Windows, Doors, and Keyholes*, NBC, 1978; co-host, *CBS: On the Air*, CBS, 1978; *Dean Martin Celebrity Roast: Frank Sinatra*, NBC, 1978; *I Love You*, NBC, 1978; *Texaco Presents the Bob Hope Comedy Special from Palm Springs*, NBC, 1978; *Variety '77—The Year in Entertainment*, CBS, 1978; *Dom DeLuise and Friends, Part 2*, ABC, 1984; host, *Return to the Titanic . . . Live*, syndicated, 1987; also *The Flintstones Twenty-Fifth Anniversary Celebration*, 1986.

PRINCIPAL RADIO WORK—Series: Producer, *Your Voice of America*, 1955-58.

RELATED CAREER—Assistant director for the Near East, South Asia, and Africa, Information Service of the U.S. Department of State, 1955; senior director, news and special events department, ABC-TV, 1955-58; director, Stamford Playhouse, Stamford, CT, 1958-59; commercial spokesman for the Ford Motor Company.

AWARDS: Academy Award nomination, Best Supporting Actor, 1962, for *Birdman of Alcatraz;* Emmy Award, Best Lead Actor in a Drama Series, 1974, *The [London] Sun* Television Award, Top Actor, 1975, Golden Globe Awards, Best Television Actor—Drama, 1975 and 1976, People's Choice Awards, 1975 and 1976, Peabody Award, and Freedom Foundation Award, all for *Kojak*.

ADDRESSES: OFFICE—333 Universal City Plaza, Universal City, CA 91608. AGENT—Jack Gilardi, International Creative Management, 8899 Beverly Boulevard, Beverly Hills, CA 90048.*

*   *   *

SAVINI, Tom

PERSONAL: Born in Pittsburgh, PA; married Nancy Hare, 1984.

VOCATION: Special effects makeup artist and actor.

CAREER: PRINCIPAL FILM APPEARANCES—Arthur, *Martin*, Libra, 1979; Nicky, *Effects* (also known as *The Manipulator*), International Harmony, 1980; Disco Boy, *Maniac*, Analysis Film Corporation, 1980; Morgan, *Knightriders*, United Film Distribution, 1981; garbage man, *Creepshow*, Warner Brothers, 1982; Jack the Ripper, *The Ripper*, United Home Video, 1986; the creep, *Creepshow 2*, New World, 1987. Also appeared in *Dawn of the Dead*, United Film, 1979.

PRINCIPAL FILM WORK—All as special effects makeup artist: *Deathdream* (also known as *Death of Night, Night Walk*, and *The Veteran*), Europix, 1972; *Dawn of the Dead*, United Film, 1979; *Martin*, Libra, 1979; *Effects* (also known as *The Manipulator*), International Harmony, 1980; *Eyes of a Stranger*, Warner Brothers, 1980; *Friday the 13th*, Paramount, 1980; *The Burning*, Filmways, 1981; (also stunt coordinator) *Maniac*, Analysis Film Distribution, 1981; *The Prowler* (also known as *Rosemary's Killer*), Sandhurst, 1981; *Alone in the Dark*, New Line, 1982; *Creepshow*, Warner Brothers, 1982; *Midnight*, Independent International, 1983; *Friday the 13th—The Final Chapter*, Paramount, 1984; *Day of the Dead*,

United Film, 1985; *The Texas Chainsaw Massacre, Part 2,* Cannon, 1986; also *Nightmares in a Damaged Brain,* 1981.

PRINCIPAL TELEVISION APPEARANCES—Episodic: "Halloween Candy," *Tales from the Darkside,* syndicated.

PRINCIPAL TELEVISION WORK—Episodic: Director, *Tales from the Dark Side,* syndicated.

WRITINGS: *Grande Illusions* (nonfiction), Imagine, 1983, reissued as *Bizarro!,* Harmony Books, 1986; *Grande Illusions, Book II* (nonfiction), Michelucci, 1988.*

*   *   *

SCACCHI, Greta

PERSONAL: Born in England. EDUCATION: Trained for the stage at the Bristol Old Vic Theatre School.

VOCATION: Actress.

CAREER: PRINCIPAL STAGE APPEARANCES—Yelena, *Uncle Vanya,* Vaudeville Theatre, London, 1988; also appeared in productions in Perth, Australia.

FILM DEBUT—Olivia, *Heat and Dust,* Universal, 1983. PRINCIPAL FILM APPEARANCES—Julia Matthews, *Burke and Wills,* Hoyts Edgley, 1985; Terri, *The Coca-Cola Kid,* Film Gallery,

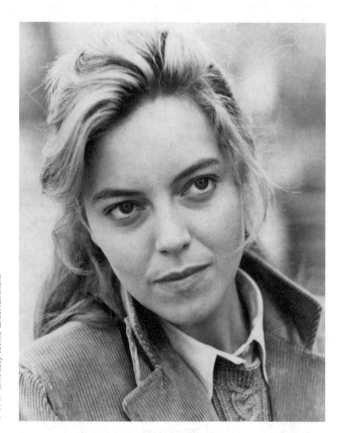

GRETA SCACCHI

© 1987 Embassy Home Entertainment

1985; Nina Beckman, *Defence of the Realm,* Rank/Warner Brothers, 1985; Edna, *Good Morning Babylon* (also known as *Good Morning Babilonia*), Vestron, 1987; Jane Steiner, *A Man in Love* (also known as *Un Homme amoureux*), Cinecom, 1987; Diana, *White Mischief,* Columbia, 1987; Maria and Maria's mother, *Paura e amore* (also known as *Three Sisters*), Erre Produzioni-Reteitalia, 1988; Angela, *La donna della luna* (also known as *Woman in the Moon*), DMV, 1988; Anna Chieri, *Waterfront,* Prism Entertainment, 1988.

PRINCIPAL TELEVISION APPEARANCES—Movies: Marguerite Gautier, *Camille,* CBS, 1984. Specials: Anna-Louise, *Dr. Fischer of Geneva,* BBC, 1983, then *Great Performances,* PBS, 1985; Mouse, "The Ebony Tower," *Great Performances,* PBS, 1987.

NON-RELATED CAREER—Ranch hand.

ADDRESSES: AGENT—Smith-Freedman and Associates, 121 N. San Vicente Boulevard, Beverly Hills, CA 90211.*

*   *   *

SCALIA, Jack   1951-

PERSONAL: Born November, 10, 1951, in Brooklyn, NY; father, a baseball player; married Joan Rankin (a model; divorced); married Karen Baldwin; children: Olivia. EDUCATION: Attended Ottawa University (Kansas). RELIGION: Roman Catholic.

VOCATION: Actor.

CAREER: PRINCIPAL FILM APPEARANCES—Nicky Piacenza, *Fear City,* Chevy Chase Distribution, 1984.

PRINCIPAL TELEVISION APPEARANCES—Series: Nick Corsello, *The Devlin Connection,* NBC, 1982; Blue Stratton, *High Performance,* ABC, 1983; Danny Krucek, *Berrengers,* NBC, 1985; Detective Nick McCarren, *Hollywood Beat,* ABC, 1985; Nicholas Pearce, *Dallas,* CBS, 1987-88; title role, *Wolf,* CBS, 1989—. Mini-Series: Rocco Cipriani, *I'll Take Manhattan,* CBS, 1987. Pilots: Nick Corsello, *The Devlin Connection,* 1982. Episodic: Tony Roselli, *Remington Steele,* NBC, 1987. Movies: Vince Martino, *The Star Maker,* NBC, 1981; Lieutenant Tony Monaco, *Amazons,* ABC, 1984; Jack Hollander, *The Other Lover,* CBS, 1985; O'Shea, *Club Med,* ABC, 1986.

RELATED CAREER—Professional model.

NON-RELATED CAREER—Professional baseball player in the Montreal Expos organization, construction worker, and food packager.

SIDELIGHTS: CTFT learned that Jack Scalia has competed in the Boston and Los Angeles marathons.

ADDRESSES: AGENT—Leigh Brillstein, International Creative Management, 8899 Beverley Boulevard, Los Angeles, CA 90048. PUBLICIST—Jonni Hartman, Slade, Grant, Hartman, and Hartman, 9145 Sunset Boulevard, Suite 218, Los Angeles, CA 90069.*

SCHAFFNER, Franklin J.   1920-

PERSONAL: Full name, Franklin James Schaffner; born May 30, 1920, in Tokyo, Japan; son of Paul Franklin and Sarah (Swords) Schaffner; married Helen Jean Gilchrist, April 17, 1948; children: Jenny, Kate. EDUCATION: Franklin and Marshall College, A.B., 1942; studied law at Columbia University. MILITARY: U.S. Navy, lieutenant, 1942-46.

VOCATION: Director and producer.

CAREER: PRINCIPAL STAGE WORK—Director, *Advise and Consent,* Cort Theatre, New York City, 1960.

PRINCIPAL FILM APPEARANCES—Man at station, *The Double Man,* Warner Brothers, 1967. FIRST FILM WORK—Director, *A Summer World* (unfinished, 1961), Twentieth Century-Fox. PRINCIPAL FILM WORK—Director: *The Stripper* (also known as *Woman of Summer*), Twentieth Century-Fox, 1963; *The Best Man,* United Artists, 1964; *The War Lord,* Universal, 1965; *The Double Man,* Warner Brothers, 1967; *Planet of the Apes,* Twentieth Century-Fox, 1968; *Patton* (also known as *Patton—Lust for Glory* and *Patton: A Salute to a Rebel*), Twentieth Century-Fox, 1970; (also producer) *Nicholas and Alexandra,* Columbia, 1971; (also producer with Robert Dorfman) *Papillon,* Allied Artists, 1973; *Islands in the Stream,* Paramount, 1977; *The Boys from Brazil,* Twentieth Century-Fox, 1978; (also executive producer) *Sphinx,* Warner Brothers, 1981; *Yes, Giorgio,* Metro-Goldwyn-Mayer/United Artists, 1982; *Lionheart,* Orion, 1987; *Welcome Home,* Columbia, 1989. Also assistant director, *March of Time* series.

PRINCIPAL TELEVISION WORK—All as director, unless indicated. Series: *Wesley,* CBS, 1949; (also producer) *Studio One,* CBS, 1948-51 and 1952-56; *Ford Theatre,* CBS, 1951-52; *Person to Person,* CBS, 1956-58; (also producer with Worthington Miner, George Roy Hill, and Fielder Cook) *Kaiser Aluminum Hour,* NBC, 1957-58; *Playhouse 90,* CBS, 1958-60; (also producer) *DuPont Show of the Week,* ABC, 1963-65. Pilots: *One-Eyed Jacks Are Wild* (unaired), 1966. Episodic: "Twelve Angry Men," *Studio One,* CBS, 1954; "The Caine Mutiny Court-Martial," *Ford Star Jubilee,* CBS, 1955; *The Defenders,* CBS. Plays: *The World's Greatest Robbery, The Army Game,* and *The Cruel Day.* Specials: "Broadway," *The Best of Broadway,* CBS, 1955; (also producer) "The Wide Open Door," *ABC Stage '67,* ABC, 1967; also *United Nations Telecast,* 1950; and *Tour of the White House* (documentary), 1962.

RELATED CAREER—Founder and producer (with Worthington Miner, George Roy Hill, and Fielder Cook), Unit Four Production Company, 1955; television counselor to President John F. Kennedy, 1961-63; president, Gilchrist Productions, 1962-68; president, Franklin Schaffner Productions, Beverly Hills, CA, 1969—.

AWARDS: Peabody Award, 1950, for *United Nations Telecast;* Sylvania Award, 1953; Emmy Award, Best Direction, and Sylvania Award, both 1955, for *Twelve Angry Men;* Emmy Award, Best Director (Live Series), 1956, for "The Caine Mutiny Court-Martial," *Ford Star Jubilee;* Variety New York Drama Critics Award, Best Direction, 1961, for *Advise and Consent;* Emmy Award, Outstanding Directorial Achievement in Drama, 1962, for *The Defenders;* American Academy of Television Arts and Sciences Trustee Award, 1962, for *Tour of the White House;* Kalrovy Vary Festival Diploma, 1964, for *The Best Man;* Academy Award, Best Director, and Directors Guild of America Award, both 1970, for *Patton.*

MEMBER: Directors Guild of America (national board of directors, 1960-65, then 1973-74; president, 1987—), National Academy of Television Arts and Sciences, Academy of Motion Pictures Arts and Sciences, Players Club, Phi Beta Kappa, Riviera Tennis Club, Waramaug Country Club, Reform Club.

ADDRESSES: HOME—2159 La Mesa Chene, Santa Monica, CA 90402. OFFICE—Executive Business Management, 132 S. Rodeo, Beverly Hills, CA 90212. AGENT—Jeff Berg, International Creative Management, 8899 Beverly Boulevard, Los Angeles, CA 90048.*

*   *   *

SCHLATTER, George

PERSONAL: Born December 31, in Birmingham, AL; father, a salesman; mother, a violinist; married Jolene Brand (an actress); children: Andrea (A.J.), Maria. EDUCATION: Attended Missouri Valley College and Pepperdine University.

VOCATION: Producer, director, and writer.

CAREER: Also see *WRITINGS* below. PRINCIPAL FILM WORK—Producer and director, *Norman . . . Is That You?,* Metro-Goldwyn-Mayer/United Artists, 1976.

PRINCIPAL TELEVISION APPEARANCES—Series: Host, *George Schlatter's Comedy Club,* syndicated, 1987; host, *George Schlatter's Funny People,* NBC, 1988.

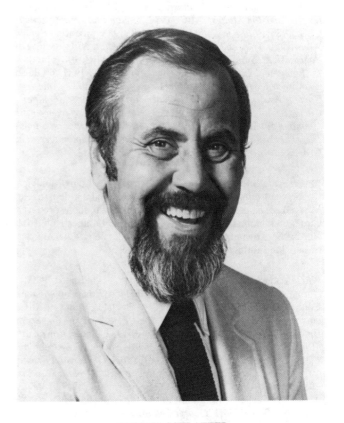

GEORGE SCHLATTER

PRINCIPAL TELEVISION WORK—All as executive producer, unless indicated. Series: Producer, *The Dinah Shore Chevy Show,* NBC, 1962; producer, *The Judy Garland Show,* CBS, 1963-64; producer, *The Steve Lawrence Show,* CBS, 1965; producer, *Rowan and Martin's Laugh-In,* NBC, 1968-73; *Turn-On,* ABC, 1969; producer, *The New Bill Cosby Show,* CBS, 1972-73; *Cher,* CBS, 1975-76; *Laugh-In,* NBC, 1977-78; *Real People,* NBC, 1979-84; *Speak Up America,* NBC, 1980; *Look at Us,* syndicated, 1981; *The Shape of Things,* NBC, 1982; (also director) *George Schlatter's Comedy Club,* syndicated, 1987; (also director) *George Schlatter's Funny People,* NBC, 1988; also producer, *Soul,* NBC. Pilots: Producer, *The Colgate Comedy Hour,* NBC, 1967; producer, *Rowan and Martin's Laugh-In Special,* NBC, 1967; *Arnold's Closet Review,* NBC, 1971; *The Lisa Hartman Show,* ABC, 1979; *Real Kids,* NBC, 1981; *The Best of Times,* ABC, 1981.

Specials: Producer, *Victor Borge's Twentieth Anniversary Show,* CBS, 1961; producer, *NBC Follies of 1965,* NBC, 1964; producer, *Texaco Star Parade,* CBS, 1964; producer, *Texaco Star Parade II,* CBS, 1964; producer, *The Danny Thomas Television Family Reunion,* NBC, 1965; producer and director, *Radio City Music Hall at Christmas Time,* NBC, 1967; producer, *The Tennessee Ernie Ford Special,* CBS, 1967; producer, *The Fabulous Funnies,* NBC, 1968; *One More Time,* ABC, 1968; producer and director, *Diana Ross and the Supremes and the Temptations on Broadway,* NBC, 1969; *The Shape of Things,* CBS, 1973; *One More Time,* CBS, 1974; producer, *Rowan and Martin's Laugh-In Special,* NBC, 1974; producer, *Cher,* CBS, 1975; producer, *Doris Day Today,* CBS, 1975; producer, *John Denver and Friend,* ABC, 1976; producer, *The Great American Laugh-Off,* NBC, 1977; producer, *The Shirley MacLaine Special: Where Do We Go from Here?,* CBS, 1977; *Just for Laughs,* NBC, 1978; producer, *The Goldie Hawn Special,* CBS, 1978; *Cher and Other Fantasies,* NBC, 1979; producer, *John Denver and the Ladies,* ABC, 1979; *Goldie and Liza Together,* CBS, 1980; *Salute to Lady Liberty,* CBS, 1984; producer, *Funny,* ABC, 1986; *The Joe Piscopo New Jersey Special,* ABC, 1986; *Las Vegas: An All Star Seventy-Fifth Anniversary,* ABC, 1987; producer, *Emmanuel Lewis: My Very Own Show,* ABC, 1987; producer and director, *Humor and the Presidency,* HBO, 1987; *American Comedy Awards,* ABC, 1987, 1988, and 1989; *George Schlatter's Comedy Club Special,* ABC, 1989; *Beverly Hills Seventy-Fifth Diamond Jubilee,* NBC, 1989; producer, *Frank, Liza, and Sammy . . . The Ultimate Event,* Showtime, 1989; also producer, *The Grammy Awards Show,* 1964-70.

RELATED CAREER—Singer (as a teenager), St. Louis Municipal Opera, St. Louis, MO; agent with the band and act department, MCA, Los Angeles, CA; general manager and show producer, Ciro's nightclub, Hollywood, CA; producer, Frontier Hotel, Las Vegas, NV; owner, George Schlatter Productions, Los Angeles; owner, the Editing Company, Los Angeles.

WRITINGS: See production details above, unless indicated. FILM— *Norman . . . Is That You?,* 1976; *Fire and Ice* (American version), Concorde/New Horizons/Goldcrest, 1986. TELEVISION—All as co-writer. Series: *Cher,* 1975-76; *Real People,* 1979-84; *Speak Up America,* 1980; *The Shape of Things,* 1982. Pilots: *Rowan and Martin's Laugh-In,* 1967; *Real Kids,* 1981. Specials: *The Fabulous Funnies,* 1968; *Doris Day Today,* 1975; *John Denver and Friend,* 1976; *John Denver and the Ladies,* 1979; *Salute to Lady Liberty,* 1984; *Funny,* 1986; *Humor and the Presidency,* 1987; *Las Vegas: An All Star Seventy-Fifth Anniversary,* 1987; *Emmanuel Lewis: My Very Own Show,* 1987; *George Schlatter's Comedy Club Special,* 1989.

AWARDS: Emmy Award, Outstanding Musical or Variety Program, 1968, for *Rowan and Martin's Laugh-In Special;* Emmy Award, Outstanding Musical or Variety Series, 1969, for *Rowan and Martin's Laugh-In;* also sixteen other Emmy Award nominations; Golden Globe Award; Man of the Year Award from the International Radio and Television Society; Directors Guild Award; received star on Hollywood Walk of Fame, 1989.

SIDELIGHTS: RECREATIONS—Skiing, dirt biking, sailing, racquetball, and scuba diving.

OTHER SOURCES: *Hollywood Reporter,* January 26, 1988.

ADDRESSES: OFFICE—George Schlatter Productions, 8321 Beverly Boulevard, Los Angeles, CA 90048.

*   *   *

SCHNEIDER, Helen

PERSONAL: Born in Brooklyn, NY.

VOCATION: Actress and singer.

CAREER: PRINCIPAL STAGE APPEARANCES—Bebe, *Idiot's Delight,* American National Theatre, Eisenhower Theatre, Washington, DC, 1986; Sally Bowles, *Cabaret,* Theater des Westens, Berlin, West Germany, 1987; ensemble, *Side by Side by Sondheim* (revue), Coconut Grove Playhouse, Miami Beach, FL, 1987.

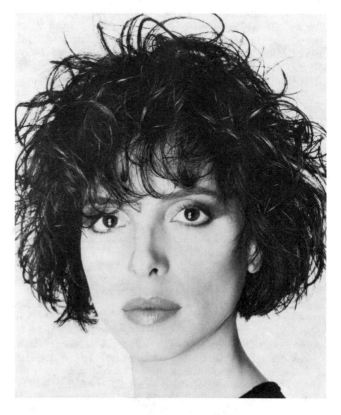

HELEN SCHNEIDER

MAJOR TOURS—*Helen Schneider with the Kick,* European cities.

PRINCIPAL FILM APPEARANCES—Joann Carlino, *Eddie and the Cruisers,* Embassy, 1983.

PRINCIPAL TELEVISION APPEARANCES—Episodic: *All My Children,* ABC. Movies: *Ein Madchen aus New York* (West German television). Specials: *The Helen Schneider and Steve Landesburg Show,* Showtime.

RELATED CAREER—Appeared in cabaret productions, including: *A Flapper's Folly* (one-woman show), Main Stage, Ballroom, New York City, then Cinegrill Theatre, Los Angeles, CA, both 1986; *Schneider Sings the Music of Kurt Weill* (one-woman show), Main Stage, Ballroom, 1988; and (with David Carroll) *Schneider Sings Sondheim,* Main Stage, Ballroom. Also, singer in nightclubs throughout the United States, including Caesars Palace, Las Vegas, NV; MGM Grand Hotel, Las Vegas; Fairmont Hotel, New Orleans, LA; Bottom Line, New York City; and the Roxy, Los Angeles, CA.

RECORDINGS: ALBUMS—*Back on Track,* Columbia, 1988; also *Smuggled Out Alive,* Atlantic; *Breakout,* Warner-Elektra-Asylum; *Exposed,* Warner-Elektra-Asylum/Atlantic; *Schneider with the Kick,* Warner-Elektra-Asylum/Atlantic; *Crazy Lady,* Warner-Elektra-Asylum; *Live in Hamburg,* RCA; *Let It Be Now,* RCA; *So Close,* RCA.

AWARDS: New York Music Award nomination and Manhattan Association of Cabarets Award, both 1987, for *A Flapper's Folly;* also Golden Europa Media Award (West Germany), Performer of the Year; (co-winner) International Artist of the Year from the West German Phono Academy; Singer of the Year Award from *Musik Express* (magazine); Performer of the Year Award from *Musik Markt* (magazine); Carbonelle Award nomination for *Side by Side by Sondheim.*

ADDRESSES: OFFICE—35-64 81st Street, Suite 1-K, Jackson Heights, NY 11372. PUBLICIST—Dale Olson, Dale C. Olson and Associates, 292 S. La Cienega Boulevard, Beverly Hills, CA 90211.

*　　*　　*

SCHREIBER, Avery　1935-

PERSONAL: Full name, Avery Lawrence Schreiber; born April 9, 1935, in Chicago, IL; son of George and Minnie (Shear) Schreiber; married Rochelle Isaacs, December 16, 1962; children: Jenny, Benjamin Joshua. EDUCATION: Received certificate in directing from the Goodman Theatre School, Chicago, IL, 1960. MILITARY: U.S. Army, Special Services-Europe, private, 1951-53.

VOCATION: Actor, comedian, director, and writer.

CAREER: Also see *WRITINGS* below. OFF-BROADWAY DEBUT—Ensemble, *Second City at Square East,* Square East Theatre, 1965. PRINCIPAL STAGE APPEARANCES—Mendl, *Dreyfus in Rehearsal,* Ethel Barrymore Theatre, New York City, 1974; Sammy Samuels, *Comedians,* Mark Taper Forum, Los Angeles, 1977; Boris Adzinidzinadze, *Can-Can,* Minskoff Theatre, New York City, 1981; Schuppanzigh, "The Public Eye" and "Black Comedy" in *Light Comedies,* Center Theatre Group, Ahmanson Theatre, Los Angeles, CA, 1984; Falstaff, *The Merry Wives of Windsor,* Los

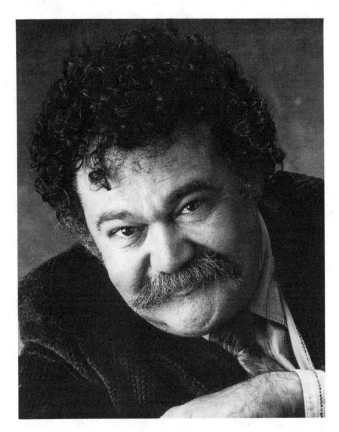

AVERY SCHREIBER

Angeles City College, Los Angeles, 1988; Milton Meltzer, *Welcome to the Club,* Music Box Theatre, New York City, 1989. Also appeared in *Ovid's Metamorphosis,* Ambassador Theatre, New York City, then in Los Angeles, both 1971; as the gravedigger, *Hamlet,* and title role, *Volpone,* both Mark Taper Forum; Tevye, *Fiddler on the Roof,* Pocono Playhouse, Mountainhome, PA; Dracula, *Tired Blood,* Chicago, IL; and in *Conerico Was Here to Stay,* New York City.

PRINCIPAL STAGE WORK—Director, *How To Be a Jewish Mother,* Hudson Theatre, New York City, 1967.

MAJOR TOURS—Hysterium, then Pseudolus, *A Funny Thing Happened on the Way to the Forum,* U.S. cities; also title role, *Wally's Cafe,* dinner theatre productions throughout the U.S. and Canada.

PRINCIPAL FILM APPEARANCES—Sultan, *Don't Drink the Water,* AVCO-Embassy, 1969; Max Jordan, *The Monitors,* Commonwealth United Entertainment, 1969; Polonski, *Swashbuckler* (also known as *The Scarlet Buccaneer*), Universal, 1976; used camel salesman, *The Last Remake of Beau Geste,* Universal, 1977; zoo keeper, *Scavenger Hunt,* Twentieth Century-Fox, 1979; Coach Fyodor Markov, *The Concorde—Airport '79* (also known as *Airport '79* and *Airport '80: The Concorde*), Universal, 1979; Captain Butt, *Galaxina,* Crown International, 1980; theatre manager, *Loose Shoes* (also known as *Coming Attractions*), Atlantic, 1980; Sergeant Maury Rusin, *Silent Scream,* American Cinema Releasing, 1980; Ock, *Caveman,* United Artists, 1981; the Boss, *Deadhead Miles,* filmed in 1970, released by Paramount, 1982; Dr. Stevens, *Jimmy the Kid,* New World, 1982; Constantine Constapopolis,

Hunk, Crown International, 1987. Also appeared in *Southern Double Cross,* 1973; and in *Saturday the 14th Strikes Back,* Concorde, 1988.

PRINCIPAL TELEVISION APPEARANCES—Series: Captain Mancini, *My Mother the Car,* NBC, 1965-66; regular, *Our Place,* CBS, 1967; co-host, *The Burns and Schreiber Comedy Hour,* ABC, 1973; regular, *The Harlem Globetrotters Popcorn Machine,* CBS, 1974-75; regular, *Ben Vereen . . . Comin' at Ya,* NBC, 1975; regular, *Sammy and Company,* syndicated, 1975-77; regular, *Sha Na Na,* syndicated, 1977-78; voice characterization, *Smurfs,* NBC, 1981-89; voice characterization, *Saturday Supercade* (animated), CBS, 1983; voice characterization, *The New Jetsons* (animated), syndicated, 1985; voice characterization, *The Flintstone Kids* (also known as *Captain Caveman and Sons;* animated), ABC, 1986. Mini-Series: *Glory Years,* HBO, 1987. Pilots: Spivak, *Operation Greasepaint,* CBS, 1968; Nicholas Slye, *Escape,* ABC, 1971; co-host, *The Burns and Schreiber Comedy Hour,* ABC, 1973; host, *Avery Schreiber's Time Slot,* syndicated, 1978; Munroe, *Flatbed Annie and Sweetiepie: Lady Truckers,* CBS, 1979; Russian ambassador, *More Wild Wild West,* CBS, 1980; Phil Jenkins, *Fast Food* (also known as *The Comedy Factory*), ABC, 1985.

Episodic: Guest host, *An Evening at the Improv,* syndicated, 1981; Jordan Kerner, *Shadow Chasers* (three episodes), ABC, 1985; Morton Halifax, *Outlaws,* CBS, 1986; Harry Krellman, *The Wizard,* CBS, 1986; also *Masquerade,* PBS, 1971; "Act Break," *The Twilight Zone,* CBS, 1984; *Love, American Style,* ABC; *The Doris Day Show,* CBS; *That Girl,* ABC; *Chico and the Man,* NBC; *The Muppet Show,* syndicated; *Fantasy Island,* ABC; *Love Boat,* ABC; *The New Love, American Style,* ABC; *What a Country,* syndicated; *The Ghost and Mrs. Muir,* ABC; *Down to Earth;* and *Rocky Road.* Movies: Roberto Gazzari, *Second Chance,* ABC, 1972; announcer, *Don't Push, I'll Charge When I'm Ready,* NBC, 1977. Specials: Co-host, *That Was the Year That Was,* ABC, 1972; *The Perry Como Winter Show,* NBC, 1973; co-host, *This Will Be the Year That Will Be,* ABC, 1973; *Fabulous Funnies,* NBC, 1976; *Lindsay Wagner—Another Side of Me,* ABC, 1977; Dosbergen, "The Ascent of Mt. Fuji," *Hollywood Television Theatre,* PBS, 1978; *Dorothy Hamill's Corner of the Sky,* ABC, 1979; *All Commercials—A Steve Martin Special,* NBC, 1980; *M & W: Men and Women,* ABC, 1988; also voice characterization, *Top Cat in Beverly Hills* (animated); *Second City 20th Anniversary Special.*

PRINCIPAL RADIO APPEARANCES—Plays: *God.*

RELATED CAREER—Member, Second City (improvisational comedy troupe), Chicago, IL, 1960-64; member, the Committee (improvisational comedy troupe), San Francisco, CA, 1964, then 1968; director, the Committee, Los Angeles, CA, 1965; as part of the comedy team Burns and Schreiber (with Jack Burns), performed in nightclubs throughout the United States, 1965—; actor in television commercials.

NON-RELATED CAREER—Member, board of education, Los Angeles, CA, 1970—; chairor, Harvest of Wellness Foundation, Palm Springs, CA, 1977.

WRITINGS: TELEVISION—Series: (With Jack Burns) *The Burns and Schreiber Comedy Hour,* ABC, 1973. Movies: Co-writer, *Zero Hour,* ABC, 1967.

AWARDS: Los Angeles Critic's Circle Award, 1971, for *Ovid's Metamorphosis;* Writers Guild Award, 1973, for *The Burns and Schreiber Comedy Hour;* Clio Award, 1977, for Doritos television

commercial; Joseph Jefferson Award nomination, 1979; Outer Critics Circle Award nomination, 1989, for *Welcome to the Club;* also Benny Award for *God.*

MEMBER: Actors' Equity Association, Canadian Actors' Equity Association, Screen Actors Guild, American Federation of Television and Radio Artists (member, national board of directors), American Guild of Variety Artists, Writers Guild of America, Shakespeare Society of America.

ADDRESSES: AGENT—Stone/Manners Agency, 9113 Sunset Boulevard, Los Angeles, CA 90069. OFFICE—Mucci, Weber, and Lagnese, 570 Wilshire Boulevard, Suite 580, Los Angeles, CA 90036.*

      *   *   *

SCHUCK, John   1940-

PERSONAL: Born February 4, 1940, in Boston, MA.

VOCATION: Actor.

CAREER: PRINCIPAL STAGE APPEARANCES—Oliver Warbucks, *Annie,* Alvin Theatre, 1980; Brody, *Detective Story,* Center Theatre Group, Ahmanson Theatre, Los Angeles, CA, 1984. MAJOR TOURS—Oliver Warbucks, *Annie,* U.S. cities.

PRINCIPAL FILM APPEARANCES—Policeman Johnson, *Brewster McCloud,* Metro-Goldwyn-Mayer (MGM), 1970; Painless Pole, *M*A*S*H,* Twentieth Century-Fox, 1970; E.J. Royce, *The Moonshine War,* MGM, 1970; Smalley, *McCabe and Mrs. Miller,* Warner Brothers, 1971; Henry Joe, *Hammersmith Is Out,* Cinerama, 1972; Reardon, *Blade,* Pintoff, 1973; Chicamaw, *Thieves Like Us,* United Artists, 1974; Harvey Logan, *Butch and Sundance: The Early Days,* Twentieth Century-Fox, 1979; Stan, *Just You and Me, Kid,* Columbia, 1979; Sheriff, *Earthbound,* Taft International, 1981; Police Chief Norris, *Finders Keepers,* Warner Brothers, 1984; Klingon ambassador, *Star Trek IV: The Voyage Home,* Paramount, 1986; Atkins, *Outrageous Fortune,* Buena Vista, 1987. Also appeared in *My Mom's a Werewolf,* Crown International, 1988.

PRINCIPAL TELEVISION APPEARANCES—Series: Sergeant Charles Enright, *McMillan and Wife,* NBC, 1971-77; Gregory "Yoyo" Yoyonovich, *Holmes and Yoyo,* ABC, 1976; Sam Alston, *Turnabout,* NBC, 1979; Murray, *The New Odd Couple,* ABC, 1982-83; Herman Munster, *The Munsters Now,* syndicated, 1988—. Mini-Series: Ordell, *Roots,* ABC, 1977. Pilots: Sergeant Enright, *Once Upon a Dead Man,* NBC, 1971; McDaniel, *Hunter,* CBS, 1973; also *Windows, Doors, and Keyholes,* NBC, 1978. Episodic: "Keep Your Guard Up," *The Mary Tyler Moore Show,* CBS, 1970; also *Gunsmoke,* CBS; *NET Playhouse,* NET. Specials: *Battle of the Network Stars,* ABC, 1976; Frankenstein, *The Halloween That Almost Wasn't,* ABC, 1979.

ADDRESSES: AGENT—Contemporary Artists, 132 Lasky Drive, Beverly Hills, CA 90212.*

SCOTT, George C. 1927-

PERSONAL: Full name, George Campbell Scott; born October 18, 1927, in Wise, VA; son of George C. (an executive) and Helena Scott; married Carolyn Hughes (divorced); married Patricia Reed (an actress; divorced); married Colleen Dewhurst (an actress), 1960 (divorced, July, 1965); remarried Colleen Dewhurst, July 4, 1967 (divorced, February 2, 1972); married Trish Van Devere (an actress), September 14, 1972; children: six. EDUCATION: Attended the University of Missouri, 1950. MILITARY: U.S. Marine Corps, 1945-49.

VOCATION: Actor and director.

CAREER: BROADWAY DEBUT—Title role, *Richard III*, New York Shakespeare Festival, Heckscher Theatre, 1957. LONDON DEBUT—Vershinin, *The Three Sisters*, Aldwych Theatre, 1965. PRINCIPAL STAGE APPEARANCES—Jacques, *As You Like It*, New York Shakespeare Festival (NYSF), Heckscher Theatre, New York City, 1958; Lord Wainwright, *Children of Darkness*, Circle in the Square, New York City, 1958; Tydings Glenn, *Comes a Day*, Ambassador Theatre, New York City, 1958; Antony, *Antony and Cleopatra*, NYSF, Heckscher Theatre, New York City, 1959; Lieutenant Colonel N.P. Chipman, *The Andersonville Trial*, Henry Miller's Theatre, New York City, 1959; Dolek Berson, *The Wall*, Billy Rose Theatre, New York City, 1960; title role, *General Seeger*, Lyceum Theatre, New York City, 1962; Shylock, *The Merchant of Venice*, NYSF, Delacorte Theatre, New York City, 1962; Ephraim Cabot, *Desire under the Elms*, Circle in the Square, 1963; Benjamin Hubbard, *The Little Foxes*, Vivian Beaumont Theatre, New York City, 1967; Sam Nash, Jesse Kiplinger, and Roy Hubley, *Plaza Suite*, Plymouth Theatre, New York City, 1968; Michael Astrov, *Uncle Vanya*, Circle in the Square, 1973; Willy Loman, *Death of a Salesman*, Circle in the Square, 1975; Foxwell J. Sly, *Sly Fox*, Broadhurst Theatre, New York City, 1976; Dr. August Browning, *Tricks of the Trade*, Brooks Atkinson Theatre, 1980; Garry Essendine, *Present Laughter*, Circle in the Square, 1982; Henry Finnegan, *The Boys in Autumn*, Circle in the Square, 1986. Also appeared as the in various theatrical companies, 1950-57; as Shylock, *The Merchant of Venice*, Salt Lake City, UT, 1960; and as Chester Norton, *Personal Appearance*, Stephens Playhouse, Columbia, MO.

MAJOR TOURS—Henry II, *The Lion in Winter*, U.S. cities, 1966.

PRINCIPAL STAGE WORK—Producer (with Theodore Mann), *Great Day in the Morning*, Henry Miller's Theatre, New York City, 1962; producer (with Mann) and director, *General Seeger*, Lyceum Theatre, New York City, 1962; director, *Death of a Salesman*, Circle in the Square, New York City, 1975; director, *All God's Chillun Got Wings*, Circle in the Square, 1975; director, *Sly Fox*, Broadhurst Theatre, New York City, 1976; director, *Present Laughter*, Circle in the Square, New York City, 1982; director, *Design for Living*, Circle in the Square, 1984.

FILM DEBUT—Dr. George Grubb, *The Hanging Tree*, Warner Brothers, 1959. PRINCIPAL FILM APPEARANCES—Claude Dancer, *Anatomy of a Murder*, Columbia, 1959; Bert Gordon, *The Hustler*, Twentieth Century-Fox, 1961; Anthony Gethryn, *The List of Adrian Messenger*, Universal, 1963; General "Buck" Turgidson, *Dr. Strangelove, or How I Learned to Stop Worrying and Love the Bomb*, Columbia, 1964; Paolo Maltese, *The Yellow Rolls-Royce*, Metro-Goldwyn-Mayer (MGM), 1964; Abraham, *The Bible . . . In the Beginning*, Twentieth Century-Fox, 1966; Tank Martin, *Not with My Life, You Don't*, Warner Brothers, 1966; Mordecai, *The*

Flim-Flam Man (also known as *One Born Every Minute*), Twentieth Century-Fox, 1967; Archie Bollen, *Petulia*, Warner Brothers, 1968; Jud Barker, *This Savage Land* (also known as *The Road West*), Universal, 1969.

General George S. Patton, Jr., *Patton* (also known as *Patton—Lust for Glory* and *Patton: A Salute to a Rebel*), Twentieth Century-Fox, 1970; Dr. Herbert Bock, *The Hospital*, United Artists, 1971; Edward Rochester, *Jane Eyre*, British Lion, 1971; Harry Garmes, *The Last Run*, MGM, 1971; Justin Playfair/Sherlock Holmes, *They Might Be Giants*, Universal, 1971; Sergeant Kilvinsky, *The New Centurions* (also known as *Precinct 45: Los Angeles Police*), Columbia, 1972; Dan Logan, *Rage*, Warner Brothers, 1972; Dr. Jake Terrell, *The Day of the Dolphin*, AVCO-Embassy, 1973; Noble "Mase" Mason, *Oklahoma Crude*, Columbia, 1973; Walter Ballantine, *Bank Shot*, United Artists, 1974; John, *The Savage Is Loose*, Campbell Devon, 1974; Colonel Ritter, *The Hindenberg*, Universal, 1975; Thomas Hudson, *Islands in the Stream*, Paramount, 1977; Ruffler, *Crossed Swords* (also known as *The Prince and the Pauper*), Warner Brothers, 1978; Gloves Malloy, "Dynamite Hands," and Spats Baxter, "Baxter's Beauties of 1933," in *Movie, Movie*, Warner Brothers, 1978; Jake Van Dorn, *Hardcore* (also known as *The Hardcore Life*), Columbia, 1979; John Russell, *The Changeling*, Associated Film Distributors, 1980; Barney Caine, *The Formula*, MGM, 1980; General Harlan Bache, *Taps*, Twentieth Century-Fox, 1981; Fun Priest, *The Beastmaster*, MGM/United Artists, 1982; John Rainbird, *Firestarter*, Universal, 1984. Also appeared in *Arthur Miller: On Home Ground* (documentary), 1979; *The Indomitable Teddy Roosevelt*, 1984.

PRINCIPAL FILM WORK—Director, *Rage*, Warner Brothers, 1972; producer and director, *The Savage Is Loose*, Universal, 1975.

PRINCIPAL TELEVISION APPEARANCES—Series: Neil Brock, *East Side/West Side*, CBS, 1963-64; President Samuel Arthur Tresch, *Mr. President*, Fox, 1987-88. Mini-Series: Benito Mussolini, *Mussolini: The Untold Story*, NBC, 1985. Episodic: Gardener, "I Haven't Seen Her Lately," *Kraft Mystery Theatre*, NBC, 1958; Juan, "Target for Three," *Playhouse 90*, CBS, 1959; the Devil, "Don Juan in Hell," *Play of the Week*, WNTA, 1960; Karl Anderson, "I Remember a Lemon Tree," *Ben Casey*, ABC, 1961; also "The Empty Chair," *Omnibus*, NBC, 1958; "A Tale of Two Cities," *Dupont Show of the Month*, CBS, 1958; "People Kill People Sometimes," *NBC Sunday Showcase*, NBC, 1959; "A Time for Killing," *Bob Hope Presents the Chrysler Theatre*, NBC, 1965; Jud Barker, *The Road West*, NBC; "Trap for a Stranger," *The U.S. Steel Hour*, CBS; *Armstrong Circle Theatre*, NBC; *Naked City*, ABC; *The Virginian*, NBC; *The Eleventh Hour*, NBC; *Open End*, syndicated; *The Red Skelton Show*, CBS; *Hollywood Squares*, NBC.

Movies: Louis Nizer, *Fear on Trial*, CBS, 1975; Fagin, *Oliver Twist*, CBS, 1982; Burton Allen, *China Rose*, CBS, 1983; Ebenezer Scrooge, *A Christmas Carol*, CBS, 1984; Evan Granger, *Choices*, ABC, 1986; General George S. Patton, Jr., *The Last Days of Patton*, CBS, 1986; August Dupin, *The Murders in the Rue Morgue*, CBS, 1986; Jack Stobbs, *Pals*, CBS, 1987; also Charles Vaughn, Sr., *The Ryan White Story*, ABC, 1989. Specials: Trock, "Winterset," *Hallmark Hall of Fame*, NBC, 1959; Gordon Cross, "The Burning Court," *The Dow Hour of Great Mysteries*, NBC, 1960; police lieutenant, *The Power and the Glory*, CBS, 1961; Lord Henry Wotton, *The Picture of Dorian Gray*, CBS, 1961; John Proctor, *The Crucible*, CBS, 1967; Max Maxwell and N.Y. Rome, *Mirror, Mirror, Off the Wall*, NBC, 1969; Victor, "The Price," *Hallmark Hall of Fame*, NBC, 1971; Edward Rochester, "Jane

Eyre,'' *Hallmark Hall of Fame*, NBC, 1971; narrator, *From Yellowstone to Tomorrow*, NBC, 1972; driver, "The Man Who Got a Ticket," *The Trouble with People*, NBC, 1972; the Beast, "Beauty and the Beast," *Hallmark Hall of Fame*, NBC, 1976; *Bob Hope's All-Star Comedy Birthday Party at West Point*, NBC, 1981; *Happy Birthday, Bob!*, NBC, 1983; *Television Academy Hall of Fame*, Fox, 1987.

PRINCIPAL TELEVISION WORK—Episodic: Director, ''The Andersonville Trial,'' *Hollywood Television Theatre*, PBS, 1970.

RELATED CAREER—Founder (with Theodore Mann), Theatre of Michigan Company, 1961.

NON-RELATED CAREER—Truck driver and bricklayer.

AWARDS: Theatre World Award, 1958, for *Richard III;* Clarence Derwent Award, Most Promising Young Actor, and Vernon Rice Award, Outstanding Contribution to Off-Broadway Theatre, both 1958, for *Children of Darkness;* Obie Award from the *Village Voice*, Best Actor, 1958, for *Richard III, As You Like It*, and *Children of Darkness;* Antoinette Perry Award nomination, Best Supporting or Featured Actor—Dramatic, 1959, for *Comes a Day;* Antoinette Perry Award nomination, Best Actor—Dramatic, 1960, for *The Andersonville Trial;* Academy Award nomination, Best Supporting Actor, 1960, for *Anatomy of a Murder;* Academy Award nomination, Best Supporting Actor, 1962, for *The Hustler;* Emmy Award nomination, 1962, for ''I Remember a Lemon Tree,'' *Ben Casey;* Obie Award, Best Actor, 1963, for *Desire under the Elms;* Emmy Award for directing, 1971, for *The Andersonville Trial;* Emmy Award, Outstanding Single Performance by an Actor in a Leading Role, 1971, for *The Price;*, New York Film Critics Award, Best Actor, 1970, Golden Globe Award, Best Motion Picture Actor—Drama, and Academy Award, Best Actor, both 1971, all for *Patton;* Academy Award nomination, Best Actor, 1972, for *The Hospital;* Antoinette Perry Award nomination, Best Actor—Dramatic, 1974, for *Uncle Vanya;* Emmy Award nomination, Best Actor, 1976, for ''Beauty and the Beast,'' *Hallmark Hall of Fame;* Antoinette Perry Award nomination, Best Actor—Play, 1976, for *Death of a Salesman;* Genie Award from the Academy of Canadian Cinema and Television, Best Foreign Actor, 1980, for *The Changeling;* Emmy Award nomination, Best Actor, 1984, for *A Christmas Carol.*

MEMBER: Actors' Equity Association, Screen Actors Guild, American Federation of Television and Radio Artists, Directors Guild of America, Society of Stage Directors and Choreographers.

ADDRESSES: AGENT—Jane Deacy Agency, Inc., 181 Revolutionary Road, Scarborough, NY 10510. PUBLICIST—Paul Wasserman, Mahoney/Wasserman, 237 Park Avenue, Suite 2116, New York, NY 10017.*

*   *   *

SCOTTI, Vito   1918-

PERSONAL: Born January 26, 1918, in San Francisco, CA.

VOCATION: Actor.

CAREER: PRINCIPAL FILM APPEARANCES—Julio, *Cry of the City*, Twentieth Century-Fox, 1948; track usher, *Criss Cross*,

Universal, 1949; Mexican youth, *Illegal Entry*, Universal, 1949; Estaban, *The Fabulous Senorita*, Republic, 1952; Rama, *The Hindu* (also known as *Sabake*), United Artists, 1953; Sanella, *Conquest of Space*, Paramount, 1955; hotel clerk, *Party Girl*, Metro-Goldwyn-Mayer (MGM), 1958; Simonetti, *Pay or Die*, Allied Artists, 1960; maitre d', *Where the Boys Are*, MGM, 1960; custodian, *The Explosive Generation*, United Artists, 1961; Topage, *Master of the World*, American International, 1961; assistant director, *Two Weeks in Another Town*, MGM, 1962; Major Alfredo Fortuno, *Captain Newman, M.D.*, Universal, 1963; doorman, *Dime with a Halo*, MGM, 1963; neighbor, *The Pleasure Seekers*, Twentieth Century-Fox, 1964; Mexican bandit, *Rio Conchos*, Twentieth Century-Fox, 1964; Andre, *Wild and Wonderful*, Universal, 1964; Italian train engineer, *Von Ryan's Express*, Twentieth Century-Fox, 1965; Michelangelo Vincenti, *Blindfold*, Universal, 1966; Federico, *What Did You Do in the War, Daddy?*, United Artists, 1966; Francois Morel, *The Caper of the Golden Bulls* (also known as *Carnival of Thieves*), Embassy, 1967; Frandisi, *The Perils of Pauline*, Universal, 1967; designer, *Warning Shot*, Paramount, 1967; I. Vittelloni, *Head*, Columbia, 1968; Cook, *How Sweet It Is*, National General, 1968; Colonel Ferrucci, *The Secret War of Harry Frigg*, Universal, 1968; Senor Sanchez, *Cactus Flower*, Columbia, 1969.

Voice of Italian Cat, *The Aristocats* (animated), Buena Vista, 1970; Pepe Galindo, *The Boatniks*, Buena Vista, 1970; Nazorine, *The Godfather*, Paramount, 1972; clown, *Napoleon and Samantha*, Buena Vista, 1972; Meo, *When Legends Die*, Twentieth Century-Fox, 1972; sports fan, *The World's Greatest Athlete*, Buena Vista, 1973; taxi driver, *Herbie Rides Again*, Buena Vista, 1974; Bill, *How to Seduce a Woman*, Cinerama, 1974; Tony, *The Wild McCullochs* (also known as *The McCullochs* and *J.J. McCulloch*), American International, 1975; Italian delegate, *The Nude Bomb* (also know as *The Return of Maxwell Smart*), Universal, 1980; Armando Moccia, *Herbie Goes Bananas*, Buena Vista, 1980; Vittorio, *Chu Chu and the Philly Flash*, Twentieth Century-Fox, 1981; Carl Stromboli, *Stewardess School*, Columbia, 1986. Also appeared in *Stop That Cab*, Lippert, 1951; and *I Wonder Who's Killing Her Now?*, Cinerama Releasing, 1975.

PRINCIPAL TELEVISION APPEARANCES—Series: Nikolai, *Mama Rosa*, ABC, 1950; Rama, *The Buster Brown TV Show with Smilin' Ed McConnell and the Buster Brown Gang*, NBC, 1950-51, then as *Smilin' Ed McConnell and His Gang*, NBC, 1951-55, later renamed *Andy's Gang*, NBC, 1955-58; Luigi Basco, *Life with Luigi*, CBS, 1952-53; Police Captain Gaspar Formento, *The Flying Nun*, ABC, 1968-69; Gino Mancini, *To Rome with Love*, CBS, 1969-71; Mr. Velasquez, *Barefoot in the Park*, ABC, 1970-71. Pilots: Marcello Carbini, *Which Way'd They Go?*, ABC, 1963; Barracutti, *Campo 44*, NBC, 1967; Carlos, *Twice in a Lifetime*, NBC, 1974; ship's captain, *The Big Ripoff*, NBC, 1975; warehouse man, *The Eyes of Texas II*, NBC, 1980; also as Tout, *Knight's Gambit*, NBC. Episodic: Peddler, ''Mr. Bevis,'' *The Twilight Zone*, CBS, 1960; Rudolpho, ''The Gift,'' *The Twilight Zone*, CBS, 1962; Murillos, ''The Gypsies,'' *The Andy Griffith Show*, CBS, 1966; Uncle Aldo, *Who's the Boss?*, ABC, 1985 and 1988; Vicenzo, *The Golden Girls*, NBC, 1988; also ''Give Me Your Walls!,'' *The Dick Van Dyke Show*, CBS, 1963; ''The Penguin's Nest'' and ''The Bird's Last Jest,'' *Batman*, ABC, 1966; as Dr. Boris Balinkoff, *Gilligan's Island*, CBS; Pepe, *The Odd Couple*, ABC; in *The Monkees*, NBC; and in *The Bionic Woman*. Movies: Bill Schuster, *Adventures of the Queen*, CBS, 1975; Vince Bocca, *Blood Feud*, syndicated, 1983. Specials: Mikey, *Halloween with the New Addams Family*, NBC, 1977; *Lindsay Wagner—Another*

Side of Me, ABC, 1977; Marco Roselli, "The Haunting of Harrington House," *CBS Children's Mystery Theatre*, CBS, 1981.

ADDRESSES: MANAGER—Frank Campana Personal Management, 20121 Ventura Boulevard, Suite 343, Woodland Hills, CA 91364.*

* * *

SEAGROVE, Jenny

PERSONAL: Born July 4 in Kuala Lumpur, Malaysia. EDUCATION: Studied acting at the Bristol Old Vic Theatre School.

VOCATION: Actress.

CAREER: STAGE DEBUT—Jan, *Bedroom Farce*, Adeline Genee Theatre, East Grinstead, U.K., 1979, for thirty-two performances. LONDON DEBUT—Title role, *Hedda Gabler*, Upstream Theatre, 1983, for twenty-one performances. PRINCIPAL STAGE APPEARANCES—Title role, *Jane Eyre*, Chichester Festival Theatre, Chichester, U.K., 1986; also appeared in *Rebecca*, Colchester, U.K., 1986.

PRINCIPAL FILM APPEARANCES—Ana, *Moonlighting*, Universal, 1982; Sally, *A Shooting Accident*, Flamingo Films, 1982; Marina, *Local Hero*, Warner Brothers, 1983; Sophie, *Nate and Hayes* (also known as *Savage Islands*), Paramount, 1983; Dr. Sarah King, *Appointment with Death*, Cannon, 1988. Also appeared as Fay Hubbard, *A Chorus of Disapproval*, 1988; as Sally, *A Shocking*

JENNY SEAGROVE

Accident (short film); in *Tattoo*, Hammer Films; and in *To Hell and Back in Time for Breakfast.*

TELEVISION DEBUT—Angela Brack, *The Brack Report*, Thames, 1981. PRINCIPAL TELEVISION APPEARANCES—Mini-Series: Emma Harte, *A Woman of Substance*, syndicated, 1984; Paula Fairlie, *Hold That Dream*, syndicated, 1986. Pilots: Terri McLane, *In Like Flynn*, ABC, 1985. Episodic: Mary Morstan, "The Sign of Four," *The Return of Sherlock Holmes*, Granada, then *Mystery*, PBS, 1988; also "The Killer," *The Hitchhiker*, HBO, 1985. Also appeared as Laura, *The Woman in White*, BBC, 1981, then Entertainment Channel, 1982-83; title role, *Diana*, BBC, 1983; Lucy Walker, *Mountain Men*, BBC, 1985; Melanie, *Magic Moments*, Yorkshire Television, then Showtime, both 1988; Helen, *Some Other Spring*, HTV, 1988; title role, *Lucy Walker*, BBC; Marjorie Anderson, *Soldier Soldier*, Granada; and in *The Betrothed*, RAI-TV.

PRINCIPAL RADIO APPEARANCES—Series: Anna, *Flesh Made Word*, BBC Radio 4, 1988; also Eleanor Harding, *The Warden*, BBC Radio 4. Episodic: "The Attic," *Morning Story*, BBC Radio 4, 1988; "Polo Neck," *Morning Story*, BBC Radio 4, 1988.

AWARDS: Best magazine award, Best Actress, for *Diana.*

SIDELIGHTS: FAVORITE ROLES—Emma in *A Woman of Substance* and Fay in *A Chorus of Disapproval*. RECREATIONS—Gardening, sports, and "the arts in general."

ADDRESSES: AGENT—International Creative Management, 8899 Beverly Boulevard, Los Angeles, CA 90048.

* * *

SELBY, Tony   1938-

PERSONAL: Full name, Anthony Samuel Selby; born February 26, 1938, in London, England; son of Samuel Joseph (a cab driver) and Annie Elizabeth (a waitress; maiden name, Weaver) Selby; married Jacqui Milburn, October 30, 1964 (divorced, 1981); married Gina Sellers (a public relations consultant), November 22, 1986; children: Samantha, Matt (first marriage). EDUCATION: Trained for the stage at the Italia Conti Stage School, 1948-53.

VOCATION: Actor.

CAREER: LONDON DEBUT—Curly, *Peter Pan*, Scala Theatre, 1950, for sixty performances. PRINCIPAL STAGE APPEARANCES—Schol, *The Quare Fellow*, Comedy Theatre, 1956; ensemble, *Living for Pleasure* (revue), Garrick Theatre, London, 1958; ensemble, *On the Avenue* (revue), Globe Theatre, London, 1961; ensemble, *Old Time Music Hall* (revue), Players' Theatre, London, 1964; Fred, *Saved*, Royal Court Theatre, London, 1965; Touchwood Senior, *A Chaste Maid in Cheapside*, Royal Court Theatre, 1966; Christopher Budgett, *Sometime Never*, Fortune Theatre, London, 1969; Ken, *Enemy*, Saville Theatre, London, 1969; Eric, *Friday*, Theatre Upstairs, London, 1971; Carter, *Flashpoint*, May Fair Theatre, London, 1977, then New End Theatre, London, 1978; Cullin, *Tishoo*, Wyndham's Theatre, London, 1979; Straker, *Man and Superman*, Cambridge Theatre, London, 1983; Troughton, *Run for Your Wife*, Princess Alexander Theatre, Toronto, ON, Canada, then Criterion Theatre, London, both 1984; Ron, *The Light Rough*, Hampstead Theatre Club, London, 1986.

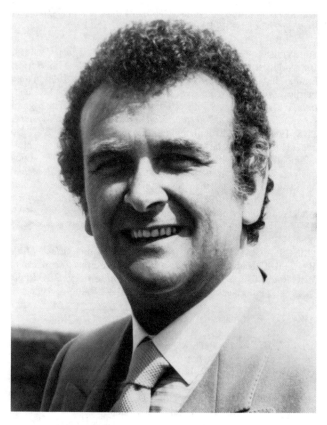

TONY SELBY

MAJOR TOURS—Troughton, *Run for Your Wife,* Australian cities, 1985.

PRINCIPAL FILM APPEARANCES—Marsh, *Press for Time,* Rank, 1966; Salter, *The Conqueror Worm* (also known as *Edgar Allan Poe's Conqueror Worm* and *Witchfinder General*), American International, 1968; cameraman, *The High Commissioner* (also known as *Nobody Runs Forever*), Cinerama, 1968; pub customer, *Poor Cow,* National General, 1968; Ted, *Before Winter Comes,* Columbia, 1969; taxi driver, *In Search of Gregory* (also known as *Alla ricerca di Gregory*), Universal, 1970; Duncan, *Villain,* Metro-Goldwyn-Mayer, 1971. Also appeared in *Alfie,* Paramount, 1966; *Adolf Hitler: My Part in His Downfall,* United Artists, 1973; and *Nobody Ordered Love,* 1973.

TELEVISION DEBUT—Porky, *Mencius Was a Bad Boy,* BBC-1, 1950. PRINCIPAL TELEVISION APPEARANCES—Series: Sabalom Glitz, *Dr. Who,* BBC, 1986-87. Mini-Series: Terry, *Hideaway,* BBC-1, 1986. Specials: Title role, "Toad of Toad Hall," *Musical in 3-2-1,* Yorkshire Television, 1986; Sergeant Barney, "The Secret Garden," *Hallmark Hall of Fame,* CBS, 1987; messenger, *The Theban Plays,* BBC, then PBS, 1988. Also appeared in *Silent Song, Get Some In, A Touch of the Tiny Hacketts,* and *Minder.*

AWARDS: Best Actor of the Series Award from the Dr. Who Appreciation Society, 1987, for *Dr. Who.*

MEMBER: Lord's Taverners, Showbiz XI.

SIDELIGHTS: RECREATIONS—Playing in charity soccer and cricket matches; swimming with his children.

Tony Selby told *CTFT* that he began his performing career "by blacking-up as Al Jolson and singing around the hospitals in London for badly wounded soldiers at the end of the second World War. [I] wanted to perform on the stage from the time I was eight years old and always have."

ADDRESSES: AGENT—Morris Aza, Aza Artistes, 652 Finchley Road, London NW11 7NT, England.

*   *   *

SHAFFER, Paul   1949-

PERSONAL: Born November 28, 1949, in Thunder Bay, ON, Canada; father, an attorney. EDUCATION: Received a degree in sociology from the University of Toronto. RELIGION: Jewish.

VOCATION: Musician, composer, writer, bandleader, and actor.

CAREER: Also see *WRITINGS* below. PRINCIPAL STAGE APPEARANCES—Don Kirshner, *Gilda: Live from New York,* Winter Garden Theatre, New York City, 1979; Phil Spector, *Leader of the Pack,* Bottom Line, New York City, 1984.

PRINCIPAL STAGE WORK—Pianist, *The Magic Show,* Cort Theatre, New York City, 1974; keyboardist, *Gilda: Live from New York,* Winter Garden Theatre, New York City, 1979; keyboardist, *Leader of the Pack,* Bottom Line, New York City, 1984; also musical director, *Godspell,* Toronto, ON, Canada, 1972.

PRINCIPAL FILM APPEARANCES—Artie Fufkin, *This Is Spinal Tap,* Embassy, 1984; voice of Optilow, *Light Years* (animated), Miramax Films, 1988; street musician, *Scrooged,* Paramount, 1988; also appeared in *Gilda Live,* 1980.

PRINCIPAL FILM WORK—Music supervisor, *Mr. Mike's Mondo Video,* 1979.

PRINCIPAL TELEVISION APPEARANCES—Series: Paul, *A Year at the Top,* CBS, 1977; musician and performer, *Saturday Night Live,* NBC, 1978-80; bandleader and performer, *Late Night with David Letterman,* NBC, 1982—. Pilots: Lionel, *Hereafter,* NBC, 1975. Specials: *Steve Martin's Best Show Ever,* NBC, 1981; *Late Night Film Festival,* NBC, 1985; *David Letterman's Second Annual Holiday Film Festival,* NBC, 1986; *Don Johnson's Heartbeat,* HBO, 1987; *Late Night with David Letterman Fifth Anniversary Show,* NBC, 1987; *Viva Shaf Vegas,* Cinemax, 1987; *Comic Relief,* HBO, 1987; *David Letterman's Old-Fashioned Christmas,* NBC, 1987; *Late Night with David Letterman Sixth Anniversary Show,* NBC, 1988; *Late Night with David Letterman Seventh Anniversary Show,* NBC, 1989; also *Fats Domino and Friends,* 1986; *The Beach Boys: 25 Years Together,* 1987; *Ashford and Simpson: Going Home,* 1988.

PRINCIPAL TELEVISION WORK—Series: Music director, *Late Night with David Letterman,* NBC, 1982—. Specials: Music director, *Late Night with David Letterman Fifth Anniversary Show,* NBC, 1987; executive producer, *Viva Shaf Vegas,* Cinemax, 1987; music director, *David Letterman's Old-Fashioned Christmas,* NBC, 1987; music director, *Late Night with David Letterman Sixth Anniversary Show,* NBC, 1988; music director, *Late Night with David Letterman Seventh Anniversary Show,* NBC, 1989; also music director, *Fats Domino and Friends,* 1986.

PRINCIPAL RADIO APPEARANCES—Musician, *The National Lampoon Radio Hour;* also host of a monthly program from the Hard Rock Cafe, New York City.

RELATED CAREER—Musician in rock and roll band, the Fabulous Fugitives, Ontario, 1964-68; organizer, Paul Shaffer Celebrity Seder, New York City; bandleader for the Blues Brothers (musical group featuring John Belushi and Dan Aykroyd); studio musician for various recording artists.

WRITINGS: FILM—(With Gilda Radner) *Gilda Live,* 1980. TELEVISION—Specials: *Viva Shaf Vegas,* Cinemax, 1987. OTHER—Songs: (With Gilda Radner) "Gimme Mick" and "Honey (Touch Me with My Clothes On)," both 1979; (with Paul Jabarra) "It's Raining Men," 1981; (with Billy Crystal) "You Look Mahvelous," 1985.

ADDRESSES: OFFICE—*Late Night with David Letterman,* NBC, 30 Rockefeller Plaza, New York, NY 10112.*

*   *   *

SHAVER, Helen   1952-

PERSONAL: Born February 24, 1952, in St. Thomas, ON, Canada; moved to Los Angeles, CA, in 1978. EDUCATION: Studied acting at the Banff School of Fine Arts, Banff, AB, Canada.

VOCATION: Actress.

CAREER: PRINCIPAL STAGE APPEARANCES—Julia, *Ghost on Fire,* La Jolla Playhouse, La Jolla, CA, 1985; also appeared in *Tamara,* Los Angeles, CA, 1984.

PRINCIPAL FILM APPEARANCES—Paula Lissitzen, *Shoot,* AVCO-Embassy, 1976; girl, *The Supreme Kid,* Cinepix, 1976; Jo, *Outrageous!,* Cinema V, 1977; pickup, *High Ballin',* American International, 1978; Ann MacDonald, *In Praise of Older Women,* AVCO-Embassy, 1978; Betty, *Starship Invasions* (also known as *Alien Encounter, War of the Aliens,* and *Winged Serpent*), Warner Brothers, 1978; Carolyn, *The Amityville Horror,* American International, 1979; Ruth Thompson, *Who Has Seen the Wind?,* Cinema World, 1980; Rhonda, *Gas,* Paramount, 1981; Catherine, *Harry Tracy—Desperado* (also known as *Harry Tracy*), Quartet, 1982; Virginia Tremayne, *The Osterman Weekend,* Twentieth Century-Fox, 1983; Claire Lewis, *Best Defense,* Paramount, 1984; Vivian Bell, *Desert Hearts,* Samuel Goldwyn, 1985; Janelle, *The Color of Money,* Touchstone, 1986; Linda, *Lost!,* Simcom-Norstar, 1986; Jessica Halliday, *The Believers,* Orion, 1987; voice of Littlefoot's mother, *The Land Before Time* (animated), Universal, 1988. Also appeared in *Walking after Midnight,* Kay Film, 1988; and in *Bethune* and *The Making of a Hero.*

PRINCIPAL TELEVISION APPEARANCES—Series: Dr. Liz Warren, *Search and Rescue: The Alpha Team,* NBC, 1977-1978; Libby Chapin, *United States,* NBC, 1980; title role, *Jessica Novak,* CBS, 1981. Episodic: Teresa, *Hill Street Blues,* NBC; also "Mirror Mirror," *Steven Spielberg's Amazing Stories,* NBC; *Philip Marlowe, Private Eye,* HBO. Movies: Patty, *Lovey: A Circle of Children, Part II,* CBS, 1978; Susan Frazer, *Between Two Brothers,* CBS, 1982; Valery Weaver, *The Park Is Mine,* HBO, 1985; Sally Robinson, *Many Happy Returns,* CBS, 1986. Specials: "The

Emissary," *Ray Bradbury Theatre III,* First Choice (Canada), 1988.

AWARDS: Genie Award, 1979, for *In Praise of Older Women;* Bronze Leopard Award from the Locarno Film Festival, 1985, for *Desert Hearts;* also Genie Award nomination, Best Supporting Actress, for *Who Has Seen the Wind?.*

ADDRESSES: MANAGER—Barbara Gale, Litke/Gale & Associates, 10390 Santa Monica Boulevard, Suite 300, Los Angeles, CA 90025.*

*   *   *

SHEFFER, Craig   1960-

PERSONAL: Born April 23, 1960, in York, PA; father, a prison guard and scriptwriter; mother, a worker in a nursing home. EDUCATION: Studied drama at East Stroudsberg College.

VOCATION: Actor.

CAREER: PRINCIPAL STAGE APPEARANCES—Alan, *Torch Song Trilogy,* Little Theatre, New York City, 1983; Billy Dukes, *Punchy,* Westside Mainstage Theatre, New York City, 1983; Larkin, *Fresh Horses,* WPA Theatre, New York City, 1986. Also appeared in productions of *Death of a Salesman, The Tempest, The American Dream,* and *The Glass Menagerie.*

PRINCIPAL FILM APPEARANCES—Byron Douglas, *That Was Then . . . This Is Now,* Paramount, 1985; Frankie, *Voyage of the Rock Aliens,* Prism Entertainment, 1985; Joe Fisk, *Fire with Fire,* Paramount, 1986; Hardy Jenns, *Some Kind of Wonderful,* Paramount, 1987; Eddie McGuinn, *Split Decisions,* New Century/Vista, 1989.

PRINCIPAL TELEVISION APPEARANCES—Series: Brian Chadway, *The Hamptons,* ABC, 1983; also Ian, *One Life to Live,* ABC. Movies: *Babycakes,* CBS, 1989.

RELATED CAREER—Actor in television commercials; co-founder, Desert Wind Films.

NON-RELATED CAREER—Waiter and busboy; also valet to Count Basie.

MEMBER: SANE (formerly National Committee for a Sane Nuclear Policy).

SIDELIGHTS: RECREATIONS—Motorcycle riding, rodeos, boxing, writing, and playing guitar and harmonica.

ADDRESSES: AGENT—J. Michael Bloom, 9200 Sunset Boulevard, Suite 710, Los Angeles, CA 90069.*

*   *   *

SHEPHERD, Cybill   1950-

PERSONAL: Born February 18, 1950, in Memphis, TN; daughter of William Jennings and Patty Shobe (Micci) Shepherd; married

David Ford, November 19, 1978 (divorced); married Bruce Oppenheim, March 1, 1987; children: Clementine (first marriage); Molly Ariel and Cyrus Zachariah (twins; second marriage). EDUCATION: Attended Hunter College, 1969; College of New Rochelle, 1970; New York University, 1971; University of Southern California, 1972; and New York University, 1973.

VOCATION: Actress.

CAREER: PRINCIPAL STAGE APPEARANCES—*A Shot in the Dark,* 1977; *Picnic,* 1980; *Vanities,* 1982.

FILM DEBUT—Jacy Farrow, *The Last Picture Show,* Columbia, 1971. PRINCIPAL FILM APPEARANCES—Kelly Corcoran, *The Heartbreak Kid,* Twentieth Century-Fox, 1972; Annie P. "Daisy" Miller, *Daisy Miller,* Paramount, 1974; Brooke Carter, *At Long Last Love,* Twentieth Century-Fox, 1975; Mary Jane, *Special Delivery,* American International, 1976; Betsy, *Taxi Driver,* Columbia, 1976; Debbie Luckman, *Silver Bears,* Columbia, 1978; Amanda Kelly, *The Lady Vanishes,* Rank/Group 1, 1980; daughter, *The Return* (also known as *The Alien's Return*), Greydon Clark, 1980; Corinne Jeffries, *Chances Are,* Tri-Star, 1989.

PRINCIPAL TELEVISION APPEARANCES—Series: Colleen Champion, *The Yellow Rose,* NBC, 1983-84; Maddie Hayes, *Moonlighting,* ABC, 1985—. Mini-Series: Eula Varner, *The Long Hot Summer,* NBC, 1985. Movies: Julie, *A Guide for the Married Woman,* ABC, 1978; Elaine, *Secrets of a Married Man,* NBC, 1984; Vicki Orloff, *Seduced,* CBS, 1985. Specials: *Elvis Memories,* syndicated, 1985; *ABC All-Star Spectacular,* ABC, 1985; *The Barbara Walters Special,* ABC, 1985; *Superstars and Their Moms,* ABC, 1987.

RELATED CAREER—Fashion model.

RECORDINGS: ALBUMS—*Cybill Does It to Cole Porter,* Paramount, 1974; also *Cybill and Stan Getz,* 1977; and *Vanilla with Phineas Newborn, Jr.,* 1978.

AWARDS: Golden Globe Award, Best Actress in a Comedy Series, 1987, for *Moonlighting.*

ADDRESSES: AGENT—David Shapira and Associates, 15301 Ventura Boulevard, Suite 345, Sherman Oaks, CA 91403.*

*　　*　　*

SHULL, Richard B.　1929-

PERSONAL: Full name, Richard Bruce Shull; born February 24, 1929, in Evanston, IL; son of Ulysses Homer (a manufacturing executive) and Zana Marie (a court stenographer; maiden name, Brown) Shull; married Margaret Ann Haddy, July 14, 1951 (divorced, 1956); married Peggy Joan Barringer, June 9, 1957 (divorced, 1967); married Marilyn Sandra Swartz, July 6, 1969 (divorced, 1984). EDUCATION: State University of Iowa, B.A., drama, 1950. POLITICS: Populist. RELIGION: Pantheist. MILITARY: U.S. Army, 1950-53.

VOCATION: Actor.

CAREER: OFF-BROADWAY DEBUT—*Coriolanus,* Phoenix Theatre, 1953. BROADWAY DEBUT—*Black-Eyed Susan,* Playhouse

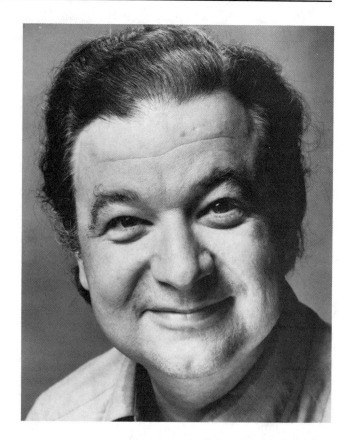

RICHARD B. SHULL

Theatre, 1954. PRINCIPAL STAGE APPEARANCES—Maxie and Sandow the Great, *Minnie's Boys,* Imperial Theatre, New York City, 1970; Minguet, *Goodtime Charley,* Palace Theatre, New York City, 1975; Stephano, *The Tempest,* Mark Taper Forum, Los Angeles, CA, 1979; E.M. Frimbo, *Frimbo,* Grand Central Terminal, Tracks 39-42, New York City, 1980; Gregor Yousekevitch, *Fools,* Eugene O'Neill Theatre, New York City, 1981; Lew, *Oh, Brother!,* American National Theatre and Academy Theatre, New York City, 1981; Father Donnally and doctor, *The Marriage of Bette and Boo,* New York Shakespeare Festival, Public Theatre, New York City, 1985; Sheriff Hartman, *The Front Page,* Vivian Beaumont Theatre, New York City, 1986; Monsieur de la Corniche, *Opera Comique,* Eisenhower Theatre, Kennedy Center for the Performing Arts, Washington, DC, 1986. Also appeared in *Each in His Own Way,* New York City, 1950; *Red Roses for Me,* Booth Theatre, New York City, 1955; *Wake Up Darling,* Ethel Barrymore Theatre, New York City, 1956; *Purple Dust,* Cherry Lane Theatre, New York City, 1957; *I Knock at the Door,* Belasco Theatre, New York City, 1957; *Pictures in the Hallway,* Playhouse Theatre, New York City, 1958; *Have I Got a Girl for You,* Music Box Theatre, New York City, 1963; *Journey to the Day,* Theatre De Lys, New York City, 1963; *Mr. Ferris and the Model,* Warner Playhouse, Hollywood, CA, 1967; *The American Hamburger League,* New Theatre, New York City, 1969; as Ephraim Cabot, *Desire under the Elms,* New York City, 1982; in *Fade the Game,* New York City, 1984; and in productions of *The Petrified Forest, The Contrast, Luv, Ring 'round the Moon, High Tor,* and *The Odd Couple.*

PRINCIPAL STAGE WORK—All as stage manager: *Coriolanus,* Phoenix Theatre, New York City, 1953; *Black-Eyed Susan,* Playhouse Theatre, New York City, 1954; *Red Roses for Me,* Booth

Theatre, New York City, 1955; *Wake Up Darling,* Ethel Barrymore Theatre, New York City, 1956; *Purple Dust,* Cherry Lane Theatre, New York City, 1957; *I Knock at the Door,* Belasco Theatre, New York City, 1957; *Pictures in the Hallway,* Playhouse Theatre, 1958; *Night of Stars,* Madison Square Garden, New York City, 1960; *Journey to the Day,* Theatre De Lys, New York City, 1963; *Mr. Ferris and the Model,* Warner Playhouse, Hollywood, CA, 1967.

FILM DEBUT—Werner, *The Anderson Tapes,* Columbia, 1971. PRINCIPAL FILM APPEARANCES—Sugarman, *Klute,* Warner Brothers, 1971; Harris, *B.S. I Love You,* Motion Pictures International, 1971; Clarence Fitch, *Such Good Friends,* Paramount, 1971; Secretary of Health, *Hail* (also known as *Hail to the Chief* and *Washington, B.C.*), Cine-Globe, 1973; Harry Moss, *Slither,* Metro-Goldwyn-Mayer, 1973; Dr. Ken Daniels, *SSSSSSSS* (also known as *SSSSnake*), Universal, 1973; Omar Baradinsky, *Born to Kill* (also known as *Cockfighter*), New World, 1975; chief detective, *The Fortune,* Columbia, 1975; stout crook, *Hearts of the West* (also known as *Hollywood Cowboy*), Metro-Goldwyn-Mayer/United Artists (MGM/UA), 1975; Vernon Prizer, *The Black Bird,* Columbia, 1975; Emery Bush, *The Big Bus,* Paramount, 1976; Clyde Hardiman, *The Pack* (also known as *The Long Dark Night*), Warner Brothers, 1977; Taylor, *Dreamer,* Twentieth Century-Fox, 1979; Jethro, *Wholly Moses,* Columbia, 1980; factory boss, *Heartbeeps,* Universal, 1981; Dr. Fessner, *Lovesick,* Warner Brothers, 1983; Eddie, *Spring Break,* Columbia, 1983; Shepard Plotkin, *Garbo Talks,* MGM/UA, 1984; Dr. Ross, *Splash,* Buena Vista, 1984; Jess Keller, *Unfaithfully Yours,* Twentieth Century-Fox, 1984; also Rojax, *Seize the Day,* 1986.

PRINCIPAL FILM WORK—Art director, *Tears Are for Tomorrow,* 1960.

PRINCIPAL TELEVISION APPEARANCES—Series: Howard Tolbrook, *Diana,* NBC, 1973-74; Detective Alexander Holmes, *Holmes and Yoyo,* ABC, 1976. Mini-Series: Davey's father, *Studs Lonigan,* NBC, 1979. Pilots: Uncle Jack, *Say Uncle,* NBC, 1978; Blake Simmons, *Sutter's Bay,* CBS, 1983. Episodic: Police Lieutenant Wilbur Gillis, *Hart to Hart,* ABC, 1978 and 1979; Seymour Bindle, *Blacke's Magic,* NBC, 1986; also *Your Hit Parade,* NBC, 1950; *Robert Montgomery Presents,* NBC, 1950; *Ironside,* NBC, 1975; *Good Times,* CBS, 1975; *The Rockford Files,* NBC, 1978; *Lou Grant,* CBS, 1979 and 1980; *The Ropers,* ABC, 1980; *Alice,* CBS, 1980; *Nurse,* CBS, 1981; *Love, American Style,* ABC. Movies: Joseph Ervin, *Ziegfeld: The Man and His Women,* NBC, 1978; publicist, *Will There Really Be a Morning?,* CBS, 1983. Also appeared in *The Boy Who Loved Trolls,* 1984; *Keeping the Faith,* 1984; and as Doc Clinton, *Slickers,* 1987.

RELATED CAREER—Executive assistant producer, Gordon W. Pollack Productions, 1953-56; stage manager, Hyde Park Playhouse, Hyde Park, NY, 1954-55; production manager, Kaufman Auditorium, New York City, 1956; general manager, Music Circle Theatre, Detroit, MI, 1957; production supervisor, Ford Motor Company American Road Show, 1959; production manager, Dana Productions, Inc. (a film production company), 1959-60; director, Lake Luzerne Playhouse, Luzerne, PA, 1962 and 1964; director, Showboat Dinner Theatre, Pinellas Park, FL, 1968-69; also program director, Armed Forces Radio Network station GYPSY.

WRITINGS: FILM—*Aroused,* 1964; *Pamela, Pamela You Are,* 1967; also *The Abortion.*

AWARDS: Scarlet Mask Award from the State University of Iowa,

1949; Antoinette Perry Award nomination, Best Supporting or Featured Actor in a Musical, 1975, for *Goodtime Charley;* Obie Award from the *Village Voice,* 1985, for *The Marriage of Bette and Boo.*

MEMBER: Actors' Equity Association (founding member of the editorial board, member of the consulting review committee, 1975), Screen Actors Guild, Academy of Motion Pictures Arts and Sciences, American Federation of Television and Radio Artists, Episcopal Actors Guild (life member), Actors Fund (life member), Friars Club, Players Club, Lambs Club (life member), University Club (New York City), Dutch Treat Club, Sons of the Revolution, General Society of Colonial Wars, Veteran Corps of Artillery (council member), General Society of the War of 1812 (vice-president, New York State society), Colonial Order of the Acorn, Sons of Union Veterans of the Civil War (treasurer, Tilden Camp), First Families of Ohio, Orders and Medals Society of America, Society of Independent Pioneers, Pioneer Association of the State of Washington, Sons of American Colonists (governor, New York chapter), Pennsylvania-German Society, Chemists Club of New York, Squadron A Club.

SIDELIGHTS: RECREATIONS—Antique autos, railroading, and animal protection.

ADDRESSES: OFFICE—130 W. 42nd Street, Suite 2400, New York, NY 10036. AGENT—The Gersh Agency, 222 N. Canon Drive, Beverly Hills, CA 90210.

*   *   *

SIERRA, Gregory

VOCATION: Actor.

CAREER: PRINCIPAL FILM APPEARANCES—Gorilla sergeant, *Beneath the Planet of the Apes,* Twentieth Century-Fox, 1970; Garcia, *Getting Straight,* Columbia, 1970; Chamaco, *Red Sky at Morning,* Universal, 1971; one-eyed thief, *The Culpepper Cattle Company,* Twentieth Century-Fox, 1972; Jurado, *The Wrath of God,* Metro-Goldwyn-Mayer, 1972; Antonio, *Papillon,* Allied Artists, 1973; Dynamite, *The Thief Who Came to Dinner,* Warner Brothers, 1973; Carlos, *The Towering Inferno,* Twentieth Century-Fox/Warner Brothers, 1974; Jesus Gonzales, *Mean Dog Blues,* American International, 1978; the Count, *The Prisoner of Zenda,* Universal, 1979; Alphonso, *Let's Get Harry,* Tri-Star, 1987; Captain Sanchez, *The Trouble with Spies,* DeLaurentiis Entertainment Group/HBO Productions, 1987; also appeared in *The Clones,* Filmmakers International, 1973.

PRINCIPAL TELEVISION APPEARANCES—Series: Julio Fuentes, *Sanford and Son,* NBC, 1972-75; Detective Sergeant Chano Amenguale, *Barney Miller,* ABC, 1975-76; Dr. Antonio "Tony" Menzies, *A.E.S. Hudson Street,* ABC, 1978; Carlos "El Puerco" Valdez, *Soap,* ABC, 1980-81; Commandante Paco Pico, *Zorro and Son,* CBS, 1983. Pilots: Deputy, *McCloud: Who Killed Miss U.S.A.?* (also known as *Portrait of a Dead Girl*), NBC, 1970; Renaldo, *Where's the Fire?,* ABC, 1975; Officer Mike Rodriguez, *Farrell: For the People,* NBC, 1982; George Callender, *Uncommon Valor,* CBS, 1983; Delgado, *Command 5,* ABC, 1985; Tony Mendosa, *Stingray,* NBC, 1985; also *Something Is Out There,* NBC, 1988. Episodic: "Archie Is Branded," *All in the Family,* CBS, 1973; also Lieutenant Lou Rodriguez, *Miami Vice,* NBC; and

Columbo, NBC; *Police Story*, NBC. Movies: Police sergeant, *Weekend of Terror*, ABC, 1970; Omar Welk, *The Night They Took Miss Beautiful*, NBC, 1977; Fabricio, *Evening in Byzantium*, syndicated, 1978; Dr. Galfas, *Three Hundred Miles for Stephanie*, NBC, 1981; Silvera, *Kenny Rogers as "The Gambler"—The Legend Continues*, CBS, 1983; Diego Ramirez, *The Night the Bridge Fell Down*, NBC, 1983; the Dancer, *Her Secret Life*, ABC, 1987. Specials: *Loser Take All*, HBO.

ADDRESSES: MANAGER—Jerry Levy, Associated Management Company, 9200 Sunset Boulevard, Suite 808, Los Angeles, CA 90069.*

*   *   *

SILVA, Trinidad   1950-1988

PERSONAL: Full name, Trinidad Silva, Jr.; born in 1950 in Mission, TX; died in a traffic accident, July 31, 1988, in Whittier, CA; children: one son.

VOCATION: Actor.

CAREER: PRINCIPAL STAGE APPEARANCES—*Hijos*, in Los Angeles.

PRINCIPAL FILM APPEARANCES—Joe, *Alambrista!*, Filmhaus, 1977; Dagger, *Walk Proud* (also known as *Gang*), Universal, 1979; punk, *The Jerk*, Universal, 1979; first Latino, *Second Thoughts*, Universal, 1983; Ramo, *Crackers*, Universal, 1984; Monty, *El Norte*, Cinecom/Island Alive, 1984; Chito, *Jocks* (also known as *Road Trip*), Crown, 1987; Tito, *The Night Before*, King's Road, 1988; Frog, *Colors*, Orion, 1988; Milagro townsperson, *The Milagro Beanfield War*, Universal, 1988.

PRINCIPAL TELEVISION APPEARANCES—Series: Jesus Martinez, *Hill Street Blues*, NBC, 1981-88. Mini-Series: Benny, *Maximum Security*, HBO, 1985. Pilots: Eddie Fuentes, *Home Free*, NBC, 1988. Episodic: Juan, *Stir Crazy*, CBS, 1986; Hector Rivas, *Hunter*, NBC, 1986; also *Barney Miller*, ABC, 1981. Specials: Joe, "*Alambrista!*," *Visions*, PBS, 1977; Basilio Garcia, "*Stones for Ibarra*," *Hallmark Hall of Fame*, CBS, 1988.

OBITUARIES AND OTHER SOURCES: Variety, August 3, 1988.*

*   *   *

SILVERMAN, Fred   1937-

PERSONAL: Born September, 1937, in New York, NY; married Cathy Kihn; children: Melissa, William. EDUCATION: Attended Syracuse University; received M.A. in television and theatre arts from Ohio State University.

VOCATION: Producer and television executive.

CAREER: PRINCIPAL TELEVISION APPEARANCES—Specials: *ABC's Silver Anniversary Celebration—25 and Still the One*, ABC, 1978.

PRINCIPAL TELEVISION WORK—All as executive producer, un-

less indicated. Series: (With David DePatie) *Pandamonium* (animated), CBS, 1982-83; (with DePatie) *Meatballs and Spaghetti* (animated), CBS, 1982-83; producer, *Thicke of the Night*, syndicated, 1983-84; (with Gordon Farr; also producer) *We Got It Made*, NBC, 1983-84, then syndicated, 1987-88; (with E.V. DiMissa, Jr.) *The Love Report*, ABC, 1984; (with Yutaka Fujioka) *Mighty Orbots* (animated), ABC, 1984; *Morningstar/Eveningstar*, CBS, 1986; (with Dean Hargrove) *Matlock*, NBC, 1986—; (with Hargrove) *Jake and the Fatman*, CBS, 1987—; (with Juanita Bartlett) *In the Heat of the Night*, NBC, 1988—; (with Marty Cohan and Blake Hunter) *One of the Boys*, NBC, 1989; *The Father Dowling Mysteries*, NBC, 1989—; also *The Time of Their Lives*, 1987. Pilots: (With Tony Cacciotti) *Farrell for the People*, NBC, 1982; (with George Reeves) *Big John*, NBC, 1983; *The Love Report*, ABC, 1984; *Fatal Confession: A Father Dowling Mystery*, NBC, 1987; (with Bartlett) *In the Heat of the Night*, NBC, 1988; also *2 1/2 Dads*, 1986; *Honeymoon Hotel*, 1987.

Movies: *Great Day*, CBS, 1983; (with Hargrove) *Perry Mason Returns*, NBC, 1985; (with Hargrove) *Diary of a Perfect Murder*, NBC, 1986; (with Hargrove) *Perry Mason: The Case of the Notorious Nun*, NBC, 1986; (with Hargrove) *Perry Mason: The Case of the Shooting Star*, NBC, 1986; (with Hargrove) *Perry Mason: The Case of the Lost Love*, NBC, 1987; (with Hargrove) *Perry Mason: The Case of the Murdered Madam*, NBC, 1987; (with Hargrove) *Perry Mason: The Case of the Scandalous Scoundrel*, NBC, 1987; (with Hargrove) *Perry Mason: The Case of the Sinister Spirit*, NBC, 1987; (with Hargrove) *Perry Mason: The Case of the Avenging Ace*, NBC, 1988; (with Hargrove) *Perry Mason: The Case of the Lady in the Lake*, NBC, 1988; (with Hargrove) *Perry Mason: The Case of the Lethal Lesson*, NBC, 1989; (with Hargrove) *Perry Mason: The Case of the Musical Murder*, NBC, 1989; *She Knows Too Much*, NBC, 1989.

RELATED CAREER—Director of daytime programming, CBS, 1963; vice-president of programming, CBS, 1970-75; president, ABC Entertainment, 1975-78; president and chief executive officer, NBC, 1978-81; founder and president, Fred Silverman Company (a film and television production company), Los Angeles, CA, 1982—; also worked at television stations WGN-TV, Chicago, IL, and WPIX-TV, New York City.

ADDRESSES: HOMES—New York, NY; Beverly Hills, CA. OFFICE—Fred Silverman Company, 12400 Wilshire Boulevard, Suite 920, Los Angeles, CA 90025.*

*   *   *

SILVESTRI, Alan

PERSONAL: EDUCATION: Attended Berklee College of Music.

VOCATION: Composer.

CAREER: Also see *WRITINGS* below. PRINCIPAL FILM WORK— Song producer, "Take Me/I'll Follow," *Mac and Me*, Orion, 1988. RELATED CAREER—Guitar player, Wayne Cochran Band, Las Vegas, NV.

WRITINGS: All as film score composer. FILM—(With Bradford Craig) *The Doberman Gang*, Dimension, 1972; *The Amazing Dobermans*, Golden, 1976; *Las Vegas Lady*, Crown International, 1976; *America: From Hitler to M-X* (documentary), Parallel Films/

Outer Cinema, 1982; *Romancing the Stone*, Twentieth Century-Fox, 1984; *Par ou t'es rentre? On t'as vu sortir* (also known as *How'd You Get In? We Didn't See You Go Out*) Carthago, 1984; *Back to the Future*, Universal, 1985; *Cat's Eye* (also known as *Stephen King's "Cat's Eye"*), Metro-Goldwyn-Mayer/United Artists (MGM/UA), 1985; *Fandango*, Warner Brothers, 1985; *Summer Rental*, Paramount, 1985; *American Anthem*, Columbia, 1986; *The Clan of the Cave Bear*, Warner Brothers, 1986; *The Delta Force*, Cannon, 1986; *Flight of the Navigator*, Buena Vista, 1986; *No Mercy*, Tri-Star, 1986; *Critical Condition*, Paramount, 1987; *Outrageous Fortune*, Buena Vista, 1987; *Overboard*, MGM/UA, 1987; *Predator*, Twentieth Century-Fox, 1987; *Who Framed Roger Rabbit?*, Buena Vista, 1988; *My Stepmother Is an Alien*, Columbia, 1988; *Mac and Me*, Orion, 1988; *She's Out of Control* (also known as *Daddy's Little Girl*), Weintraub Entertainment Group, 1989.

TELEVISION—Series: *CHiPs*, NBC, 1978-83; *Manimal*, NBC, 1983. Pilots: *Mitchell and Woods*, NBC, 1981. Specials: *Roger Rabbit and the Secrets of Toontown*, CBS, 1988.*

*   *   *

SIMPSON, O.J.   1947-

PERSONAL: Full name, Orenthal James Simpson; born July 9, 1947, in San Francisco, CA; son of Jimmie (a bank custodian and chef) and Eunice (a hospital administrator; maiden name, Durton) Simpson; married Marguerite Whitley, June 24, 1967 (divorced, 1980); married Nicole Brown, 1985; children: Aaren (deceased), Arnelle, Jason (first marriage); Sydney (second marriage). EDUCATION: Attended San Francisco City College, 1965-67; University of Southern California, B.A., 1969.

VOCATION: Actor, producer, and sports commentator.

CAREER: PRINCIPAL FILM APPEARANCES—Garth, *The Klansman*, Paramount, 1974; Security Chief Jernigan, *The Towering Inferno*, Twentieth Century-Fox/Warner Brothers, 1974; "Bopper" Alexander, *Killer Force* (also known as *The Diamond Mercenaries*), American International, 1975; Father Haley, *The Cassandra Crossing*, AVCO-Embassy, 1977; Navy Commander John Walker, *Capricorn One*, Warner Brothers, 1978; Catlett, *Firepower*, Associated Film Distribution, 1979; Tucker, *Hambone and Hillie*, New World, 1984; Nordberg, *The Naked Gun—From the Files of Police Squad!*, Paramount, 1988.

PRINCIPAL TELEVISION APPEARANCES—Series: Announcer, *Monday Night Football*, ABC, 1983-86; T.D. Parker, *First and Ten*, HBO, 1986-88; also commentator, *Wide World of Sports*, ABC. Mini-Series: Kadi Touray, *Roots*, ABC, 1977. Pilots: Mike Brennen, *Cocaine and Blue Eyes*, NBC, 1983. Episodic: *Cade's County*, CBS; *Owen Marshall, Counselor at Law*, ABC. Movies: Woodrow York, *A Killing Affair*, CBS, 1977; Joe Gallagher, *Goldie and the Boxer*, NBC, 1979; Lee Hayes, *Detour to Terror*, NBC, 1980; as himself, *The Golden Moment—An Olympic Love Story*, NBC, 1980; Joe Gallagher, *Goldie and the Boxer Go to Hollywood*, NBC, 1981; Coach Seaver, "Student Exchange" (also known as "Foreign Exchange"), Disney Sunday Movie, ABC, 1987. Specials: Host, *The Heisman Trophy Awards Special*, CBS, 1977; *Celebrity Challenge of the Sexes*, CBS, 1977; *Dick Clark's Good Ol' Days: From Bobby Sox to Bikinis*, NBC, 1977; *Superstars Competition*, ABC, 1975; color commentator, *Summer Olympics*, ABC, 1976;

color commentator, *Rose Bowl*, ABC, 1979 and 1980; *Bob Hope's Stand Up and Cheer for the National Football League's Sixtieth Year*, NBC, 1981; special events commentator, *Summer Olympic Sports*, ABC, 1984; *Whatta Year . . . 1986*, ABC, 1986; *The Special Olympics Opening Ceremonies*, ABC, 1987; *Circus of the Stars*, CBS, 1988; *America's Tribute to Bob Hope*, NBC, 1988.

PRINCIPAL TELEVISION WORK—All as executive producer. Pilots: *High Five*, NBC, 1982; *Cocaine and Blue Eyes*, NBC, 1983. Movies: *Goldie and the Boxer*, NBC, 1979; *Detour to Terror*, NBC, 1980; *Goldie and the Boxer Go to Hollywood*, NBC, 1981.

RELATED CAREER—Commentator, ABC Sports, 1969-77, then NBC-TV Sports, 1978-82; commercial spokesman, Hertz Rent-a-Car, 1978—; executive producer, Orenthal Productions, 1978—.

NON-RELATED CAREER—Professional football player with the Buffalo Bills, 1969-78, then San Francisco Forty-Niners, 1978-79.

WRITINGS: (With Pete Axthelm) *O.J.: The Education of a Rich Rookie* (autobiography), Macmillan, 1970.

AWARDS: All-American collegiate football player, 1965-68; named Outstanding Player, 1967 Rose Bowl; Walter Camp Memorial Trophy, Maxwell Memorial Trophy, Heisman Trophy, and UPI and AP College Athlete of the Year, all 1968; *Sport* (magazine) Man of the Year, 1969; ABC Sports College Player of the Decade, 1970; named to American Football Conference All-Star team, 1970, and to Pro Bowl teams, 1972-76; American Football Conference Most Valuable Player, 1972, 1973, 1975; National Football League, Most Valuable Player, 1973; Hickok Belt for Professional Athlete of the Year, 1973; National Football League Player of the Decade, 1979; inducted into the College Football Hall of Fame, 1983; inducted into the Professional Football Hall of Fame, 1985.

ADDRESSES: OFFICE—O.J. Simpson Enterprises, 11661 San Vicente Boulevard, Suite 632, Los Angeles, CA 90049.*

*   *   *

SINDEN, Donald   1923-

PERSONAL: Born October 9, 1923, in Plymouth, England; son of Alfred Edward and Mabel Agnes (Fuller) Sinden; married Diana Mahony (an actress), May 3, 1948; children: Jeremy, Marc. EDUCATION: Trained for the stage at the Webber-Douglas School of Dramatic Art, 1944.

VOCATION: Actor and writer.

CAREER: STAGE DEBUT—Dudley, *George and Margaret*, Theatre Royal, Brighton, U.K., 1942. LONDON DEBUT—Romeo, *Romeo and Juliet*, His Majesty's Theatre, 1947. BROADWAY DEBUT—Sir William Harcourt Courtly, *London Assurance*, Palace Theatre, 1974. PRINCIPAL STAGE APPEARANCES—Dumain, *Love's Labour's Lost*, Arviragus, *Cymbeline*, and Pride, *Dr. Faustus*, all Shakespeare Memorial Theatre Company, Shakespeare Memorial Theatre, Stratford-on-Avon, U.K., 1945; Paris, *Romeo and Juliet*, Adrian, *The Tempest*, Aumerle, *Richard II*, and Lorenzo, *The Merchant of Venice*, all Shakespeare Memorial Theatre Company, Shakespeare Memorial Theatre, 1947; Aumerle, *Richard II*, His

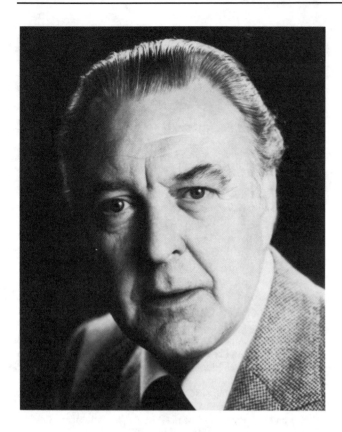

DONALD SINDEN

Majesty's Theatre, London, 1947; Rosencrantz, *Hamlet,* Bristol Old Vic Company, St. James's Theatre, London, 1948; Sebastian, *Twelfth Night,* and Envy and the Scholar, *Dr. Faustus,* both New Theatre, London, 1948; Arthur Townsend, *The Heiress,* Haymarket Theatre, London, 1949; Manuel Del Vega, *Red Letter Day,* Garrick Theatre, London, 1952; Mervyn Browne, *Odd Man In,* St. Martin's Theatre, London, 1957; Bob Brewster, *Who's Your Father?,* Cambridge Theatre, London, 1958; Frank Marescaud, *All in the Family,* Strand Theatre, London, 1959.

Brian Curtis, *Joie de Vivre,* Queen's Theatre, London, 1960; Captain Hook and Mr. Darling, *Peter Pan,* Scala Theatre, London, 1960; title role, *JB,* Phoenix Theatre, London, 1961; Edward Bromley, *Guilty Party,* St. Martin's Theatre, 1961; Sebastian, *The Tempest,* Royal Shakespeare Company (RSC), Royal Shakespeare Theatre, Stratford-on-Avon, U.K., 1963; Solinus, *The Comedy of Errors,* RSC, Royal Shakespeare Theatre, then Aldwych Theatre, London, both 1963; Richard Plantaganet, "Henry VI" and "Edward IV" in *The Wars of the Roses,* RSC, Royal Shakespeare Theatre, then Aldwych Theatre, 1964, later Royal Shakespeare Theatre, 1964; Mr. Price, *Eh?,* RSC, Aldwych Theatre, 1964; Robert Danvers, *There's a Girl in My Soup,* Globe Theatre, London, 1966; Lord Foppington, *The Relapse,* RSC, Aldwych Theatre, 1967; Gilbert Bodley, *Not Now, Darling,* Strand Theatre, London, 1968; Malvolio, *Twelfth Night,* and title role, *Henry VIII,* both RSC, Royal Shakespeare Theatre, 1969, then Aldwych Theatre, 1970; Sir William Harcourt Courtly, *London Assurance,* RSC, Aldwych Theatre, 1970, then New Theatre, 1972; Baron Scarpia, "Before Dawn," and Sebastian Crutwell, "After Lydia," in *In Praise of Love,* Duchess Theatre, London, 1973; Dr. Stockmann, *An Enemy of the People,* Chichester Festival Theatre, Chichester, U.K., 1975; Arthur Wicksteed, *Habeas Corpus,* Martin Beck

Theatre, New York City, 1975; Benedick, *Much Ado about Nothing,* and title role, *King Lear,* both RSC, Royal Shakespeare Theatre, then Aldwych Theatre, 1977; Arthur Pullen, *Shut Your Eyes and Think of England,* Apollo Theatre, London, 1977; title role, *Othello,* RSC, Royal Shakespeare Theatre, 1979. Also appeared in *The Lady's Not for Burning, The Good Natured Man, The Merry Wives of Windsor,* and *Puss in Boots,* all with the Bristol Old Vic Company, Bristol, U.K., 1950; *King Lear, Henry VIII, Othello, The Scarlet Pimpernel,* and *Oscar Wilde,* all London productions; with Mobile Entertainments Southern Area, for four years; and with the Leicester Repertory Company, Leicester, U.K., 1945.

PRINCIPAL STAGE WORK—Director, *Relatively Speaking,* U.K. cities, 1968.

MAJOR TOURS—George Bernard Shaw, *Dear Liar,* and Willie, *Happy Days,* both British Council for the Arts, South American cities, 1965; Malvolio, *Twelfth Night,* Japanese and Australian cities, 1970; Sir William Harcourt Courtly, *London Assurance,* U.S. cities, 1974; also *The Normandy Story,* Mobile Entertainments Southern Area, in French, Belgian, German, Indian, and Burmese cities, 1944-45; and in *Shakespearean Recital,* U.K. cities, 1946-47.

FILM DEBUT—*The Girl in the Painting* (also known as *Portrait from Life*), Universal, 1948. PRINCIPAL FILM APPEARANCES—Lockhart, *The Cruel Sea,* General Film Distributors, 1953; Donald Nordley, *Mogambo,* Metro-Goldwyn-Mayer, 1953; Jim Carver, *A Day to Remember,* General Film Distributors, 1953; Benskin, *Doctor in the House,* General Film Distributors, 1954; Jeff Saunders, *Mad about Men,* General Film Distributors, 1954; Lieutenant Sylvester Green, *You Know What Sailors Are,* United Artists, 1954; Tom Drummond, *Simba,* Lippert, 1955; Ewart Gray, *The Beachcomber,* United Artists, 1955; Alan Hartley, *Josephine and Men,* British Lion, 1955; Lieutenant Tom Corbett, *Above Us the Waves,* Republic, 1956; Charles Holland, *The Black Tent,* Rank, 1956; Wade, *Eyewitness,* Rank, 1956; Geoffrey Levett, *Tiger in the Smoke,* Rank, 1956; Peter Weston, *An Alligator Named Daisy,* Rank, 1957; Benskin, *Doctor at Large,* Rank, 1957; Hugh Mander, *Mad Little Island* (also known as *Rockets Galore*), Rank, 1958.

Shawe-Wilson, *The Captain's Table,* Rank, 1960; Inspector John Mannering, *The Siege of Sidney Street* (also known as *The Siege of Hell Street*), United Producers, 1960; Ian Richards, *Twice Around the Daffodils,* Anglo Amalgamated, 1962; Philip Bellamy, *Mix Me a Person,* British Lion, 1962; Lieutenant Gordon Brown, *Operation Bullshine,* Seven Arts/Manhattan Films International, 1963; Pelham Butterworth, *Your Money or Your Wife,* Ellis, 1965; prison governor, *Decline and Fall . . . of a Bird Watcher* (also known as *Decline and Fall*), Twentieth Century-Fox, 1969; Gerald Draycott, *Villain,* MGM, 1971; Mallinson, *The Day of the Jackal,* Universal, 1973; Mr. Carr and Boyd, *The National Health, or Nurse Norton's Affair,* Columbia, 1973; Sir Anthony Ross, *The Island at the Top of the World,* Buena Vista, 1974; General Armstrong, *That Lucky Touch,* Allied Artists, 1975. Also appeared in *Rentadick,* Virgin, 1972.

TELEVISION DEBUT—Inspector Quill, *Bullet in the Ballet,* BBC, 1948. PRINCIPAL TELEVISION APPEARANCES—Series: Philip Glover, *Father, Dear Father,* 1977; Simon Peel, *Never the Twain,* PBS, 1987; also *Our Man at St. Mark's, Two's Company, The Organisation, Seven Days in the Life of Andrew Pelham, Discovering English Churches.* Mini-Series: *Playing Shakespeare,* London Weekend Television, then PBS, 1983. Episodic: The Colonel, "Many Happy Returns," *The Prisoner,* CBS, 1968. Movies: *Road to Rome, Dinner with the Family, Odd Man In, Love from Italy, The Frog, The Glove, The Mystery of Edwin Drood, The Happy Ones, The Red House, Blackmail, A Bachelor Gray, The Wind in the Tall Paper Chimney, A Woman Above Reproach, Call My Bluff, Relatively Speaking, The 19th Hole, The Assyrian Rejuvenator, The Confederacy of Wives,* and *Tell It to the Chancellor.* Plays: *The Comedy of Errors, The Wars of the Roses, The Rivals,* and *All's Well That Ends Well.*

RELATED CAREER—Vice-president, London Appreciation Society, 1960; associate artist, Royal Shakespeare Company, 1967—; president, Federation of Playgoers' Societies, 1968—; member, Arts Council Drama Panel, 1973-77; president, British Theatre Museum Association, 1973—; council member, London Academy of Music and Dramatic Arts, 1975—; member, Arts Council, 1982—; president, Royal General Theatrical Fund, 1982—; fellow, Royal Society of Arts; advisory council member, Victoria and Albert Museum.

WRITINGS: A Touch of the Memoirs (autobiography), Hodder and Stoughton, 1982; *Laughter in the Second Act* (autobiography), Hodder and Stoughton, 1985; editor, *The Everyman Book of Theatrical Anecdotes,* Dent, 1986.

AWARDS: Antoinette Perry Award nomination, Best Actor in a Play, 1976, for *Habeas Corpus;* Knight Commander of the British Empire, 1979.

MEMBER: British Actors' Equity Association (council member, 1966-75), Garrick Club (trustee), Beefsteak Club, Marylebone Cricket Club.

SIDELIGHTS: RECREATIONS—Theatrical history, London, architecture, ecclesiology.

Donald Sinden told *CTFT* that he became an actor because, "I couldn't think of a more attractive way to earn a living."

ADDRESSES: HOME—60 Temple Fortune Lane, London NW11, England. AGENT—Michael Whitehall, 125 Gloucester Road, London SW7, England.

*   *   *

SLATER, Helen 1963-

PERSONAL: Full name, Helen Rachel Slater; born December 15, 1963; daughter of Gerald (a television executive) and Alice Joan (a lawyer; maiden name, Chrin) Slater. EDUCATION: Attended the High School of the Performing Arts; trained for the stage with Gary Austin, Bill Esper, Sandra Seacat, Merry Conway, and at Shakespeare and Company. POLITICS: Democrat. RELIGION: Jewish.

VOCATION: Actress.

CAREER: STAGE DEBUT—Tina, *Responsible Parties,* Vineyard Theatre, New York City, 1985. PRINCIPAL STAGE APPEARANCES—Nicole, "Almost Romance" in *Festival of One-Act Comedies,* Manhattan Punch Line, New York City, 1987.

FILM DEBUT—Linda Lee/title role, *Supergirl,* Tri-Star, 1984. PRINCIPAL FILM APPEARANCES—Title role, *The Legend of Billie Jean,* Tri-Star, 1985; Sandy Kessler, *Ruthless People,* Touchstone,

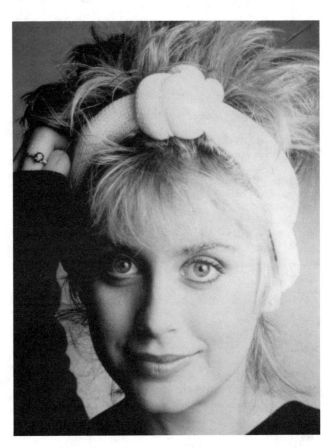

HELEN SLATER

1986; Christy Wills, *The Secret of My Success,* Universal, 1987; Hattie, *Sticky Fingers,* Spectrafilm, 1988; Alexandra Page, *Happy Together,* Apollo, 1989.

PRINCIPAL TELEVISION APPEARANCES—Specials: Amy Watson, "Amy and the Angel," *ABC Afterschool Special,* ABC, 1982.

RELATED CAREER—Co-founder, Naked Angels (a theatre company), New York City; composer of piano music.

ADDRESSES: AGENT—Toni Howard, William Morris Agency, 151 El Camino Drive, Beverly Hills, CA 90210.

*   *   *

SMIAR, Brian 1937-

PERSONAL: Born August 27, 1937, in Cleveland, OH. EDUCATION: Graduated from Kent State University; also attended Emerson College.

VOCATION: Actor.

CAREER: OFF-BROADWAY DEBUT—*Edmond,* Provincetown Playhouse, 1982. PRINCIPAL STAGE APPEARANCES—Man's voice and chief, "Sonata," and Jack, "True to Life," in *The Young Playwrights Festival,* Playwrights Horizons, New York City, 1985; jailor and old shepherd, *The Winter's Tale,* Symphony Space, New

York City, 1985; Gerald, *Self Defense*, Long Wharf Theatre, New Haven, CT, 1986. Also appeared in *The Miracle Worker*, Merrimack Regional Theatre, Lowell, MA, 1981; and in *3 x 3*, Off-Broadway production.

PRINCIPAL STAGE WORK—Director, *Of Mice and Men*, Merrimack Regional Theatre, Lowell, MA, 1983.

PRINCIPAL TELEVISION APPEARANCES—Series: Nelson Kruger, *The "Slap" Maxwell Story*, ABC, 1987-88. Episodic: Gus, "The Great American Fourth of July and Other Disasters," *American Playhouse*, PBS, 1982; General Dean Cunliffe, *China Beach* (two episodes), ABC, 1988. Movies: *The Murder of Mary Phagan*, NBC, 1988.

ADDRESSES: AGENT—Patricia Woo Agency, 156 Fifth Avenue, Suite 3417, New York, NY 10010.*

*   *   *

SMINKEY, Tom

PERSONAL: Full name, Thomas Sminkey; son of Herbert and Ellen (Robbins) Sminkey; married Victoria Hall (a ballet dancer), October 19, 1980. EDUCATION: Attended Nassau Community College and the University of Alabama.

VOCATION: Actor and playwright.

CAREER: STAGE DEBUT—Hamlet, *Rosencrantz and Guildenstern Are Dead*, Nassau Repertory Theatre, Long Island, NY. PRINCIPAL STAGE APPEARANCES—Mike, "The Love Course" in *Two One-Act Plays*, Equity Library Theatre, New York Public Library at Lincoln Center, New York City, 1973; Mickey, *All God's Chillun' Got Wings*, Circle in the Square, New York City, 1975; Guildford Dudley, *The Chronicle of Nine*, WPA Theatre, New York City, 1976; cop in drag, *Ho Ho Ho*, Cape Playhouse, Dennis, MA, then Berkshire Playhouse, Stockbridge, MA, both 1977; Doro, *Each in His Own Way*, Classic Theatre, Caras Nuevas Theatre, New York City, 1977; T'ien-ming, *Fanshen*, Soho Repertory Theatre, New York City, 1983; Stanley Kowalski, *A Streetcar Named Desire*, and townsperson, *The Devil's Disciple*, both Circle in the Square, 1988. Also appeared in *Knickerbocker Holiday*, Octagon: The American Musical Theatre Company, Bert Wheeler Theatre, New York City, 1974; *The Last War*, Actors' Alliance, Provincetown Playhouse, New York City, 1977; *Richard II*, American Musical and Dramatic Academy (AMDA), AMDA Studio One Theatre, New York City, 1978; *Freshwater* and *An Evening in Bloomsbury*, both Gene Frankel Theatre, New York City, 1978; and as Mack, *The Second Shepherd's Play*, Herbert Berghof Studios, New York City.

FILM DEBUT—Shawn, *American Moments*, 1976. PRINCIPAL FILM APPEARANCES—Park ranger, *Nasty Habits*, Scotia International, 1976.

RELATED CAREER—Artistic director, New York Actors Co-Op, New York City; substitute acting teacher, Nassau Community College, Garden City, NY.

WRITINGS: STAGE—*Fine Tuning*, 1986.

MEMBER: Catholic Big Brothers.

ADDRESSES: HOME—59 W. 74th Street, New York, NY 10023.

*   *   *

SMITH, Bubba   1945-

PERSONAL: Full name, Charles Aaron Smith; born February 28, 1945, in Orange, Texas.

VOCATION: Actor.

CAREER: PRINCIPAL FILM APPEARANCES—Arnold, *Stoker Ace*, Warner Brothers/Universal, 1983; Moses Hightower, *Police Academy*, Warner Brothers, 1984; Moses Hightower, *Police Academy 2: Their First Assignment*, Warner Brothers, 1985; Johnson, *Black Moon Rising*, New World, 1986; Sergeant Hightower, *Police Academy 3: Back in Training*, Warner Brothers, 1986; Hightower, *Police Academy 4: Citizens on Patrol*, Warner Brothers, 1987; Benny Avalon, *The Wild Pair* (also known as *Devil's Odds*), Trans World Entertainment, 1987; Hightower, *Police Academy 5: Assignment Miami Beach*, Warner Brothers, 1988; Hightower, *Police Academy 6: City Under Siege*, Warner Brothers, 1989.

PRINCIPAL TELEVISION APPEARANCES—Series: Puddin, *Semi-Tough*, ABC, 1980; Robin, *Open All Night*, ABC, 1981-82; Lyman "Bubba" Kelsey, *Blue Thunder*, ABC, 1984; Beau, *Half Nelson*, NBC, 1985. Pilots: Puddin, *Semi-Tough*, ABC, 1980; Big Foot, *Joe Dancer: The Big Black Pill*, NBC, 1981. Episodic: "Tony's Comeback," *Taxi*, ABC, 1982. Movies: Jacobs, *Fighting Back*, ABC, 1980; Moses, *Superdome*, ABC, 1978. Specials: *Kraft Salutes Super Night at the Super Bowl*, NBC, 1987; *The Mother-Daughter Pageant*, syndicated, 1989; also *All-American Sports Nuts*, 1988.

RELATED CAREER—Actor in television commercials.

NON-RELATED CAREER—Professional football player with the Baltimore Colts, Oakland Raiders, and Houston Oilers.*

*   *   *

SMITH, Cotter   1949-

PERSONAL: Full name, Joseph Cotter Smith; born May 29, 1949, in Washington, DC; son of John Lewis, Jr. (a federal judge) and Madeline (Cotter) Smith. EDUCATION: Trinity College, B.A., literature, 1972; trained for the stage at the Actors Studio and with Stella Adler and Milton Katselas.

VOCATION: Actor.

CAREER: STAGE DEBUT—James, *The Collection*, Woods Hole Theatre Festival, Woods Hole, MA, 1974. OFF-BROADWAY DEBUT—Morris, *The Blood Knot*, Roundabout Theatre, 1980, for one hundred performances. PRINCIPAL STAGE APPEARANCES—Lieutenant Byrd, *A Soldier's Play*, Negro Ensemble Company, Theatre Four, New York City, 1981, then Center Theatre Group, Mark Taper Forum, Los Angeles, CA, 1982; Jack, *The Death of a Miner*, Portland Stage Company, Portland, ME, then American

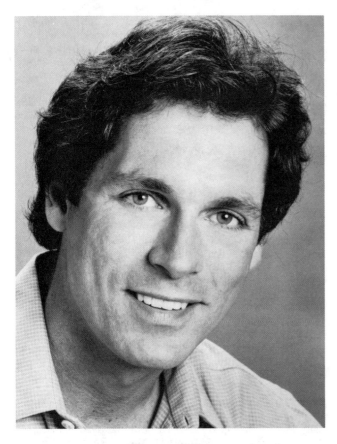

COTTER SMITH

Place Theatre, New York City, both 1982; Mercutio, *Romeo and Juliet,* Skylight Theatre, Los Angeles, 1984; Pinder, *El Salvador,* Circle Repertory Company, New York City, 1987; Charles, "Borderline," and psychiatrist, "Keepin' an Eye on Looie," both in *Borderlines,* Circle Repertory Company, 1988. Also appeared as the understudy for the role of Avery Graham, *Particular Friendships,* Astor Place Theatre, New York City, 1981; as Victor/Tony, *The Last Carnival,* Trinidad, West Indies, 1982; in *Borderline,* Los Angeles, 1985; and in *A Soldier's Play,* Edinburgh Festival, Edinburgh, Scotland, and Charles Theatre, Boston, MA.

FILM DEBUT—*Lady Beware,* Scotti Brothers, 1987.

TELEVISION DEBUT—Robert Kennedy, *Blood Feud,* syndicated, 1983. PRINCIPAL TELEVISION APPEARANCES—Mini-Series: Frank, *Mistral's Daughter,* CBS, 1984. Episodic: *Hill Street Blues,* NBC, 1983; *St. Elsewhere,* NBC, 1983; *Cagney and Lacey,* CBS, 1985; *Murder, She Wrote,* CBS, 1986. Movies: Ned Holcomb, *A Bunny's Tale,* ABC, 1985; Lieutenant Hugo, *The Rape of Richard Beck,* ABC, 1985.

RELATED CAREER—Member, Circle Repertory Company.

AWARDS: Los Angeles Drama Critics Circle Award nomination, 1985, for *Borderlines; Drama-Logue* awards, 1985, for *Borderlines* and *Romeo and Juliet;* named one of the Outstanding Young Men of America, 1982.

MEMBER: Actors' Equity Association, Screen Actors Guild, American Federation of Television and Radio Artists.

ADDRESSES: AGENT—Writers and Artists Agency, 70 W. 36th Street, New York, NY 10018.

*   *   *

SMITH, Derek   1927-

PERSONAL: Born June 15, 1927, in London, England; son of Wilfred James (a surveyor) and Constance Alice (Betambeau) Smith; married Lilian Box (a librarian), January 2, 1963; children: Bill, Jenny. EDUCATION: Trained for the stage at the Royal Academy of Dramatic Art, 1958-60; studied acting with Ilan Reichel at the Actors Centre, London, and singing with Christopher Littlewood.

VOCATION: Actor and singer.

CAREER: STAGE DEBUT—Baron Hardup, *Cinderella* (pantomime), Capitol Theatre, St. Austell, U.K., 1956. LONDON DEBUT—Medvedenko, *The Seagull,* Old Vic Theatre Company, Old Vic Theatre, 1960. PRINCIPAL STAGE APPEARANCES—Medvedenko, *The Seagull,* Old Vic Theatre Company, Edinburgh Festival, Edinburgh, Scotland, 1960; chorus, *Romeo and Juliet,* Egeus, *A Midsummer Night's Dream,* and Fabian, *Twelfth Night,* all Old Vic Theatre Company, Old Vic Theatre, London, 1960; Pierre Bezhukov, *War and Peace,* Bristol Old Vic Theatre, Bristol, U.K., 1961, then Old Vic Theatre, later Phoenix Theatre, London, both 1962; title role, *Fiorello!,* Bristol Old Vic Theatre, then Piccadilly Theatre, London, both 1962; Stephano, *The Tempest,* Pinch, *The Comedy of Errors,* and Talbot and Jack Cade, *The Wars of the Roses,* all Royal Shakespeare Company (RSC), Royal Shakespeare Theatre, Stratford-on-Avon, U.K., 1963; Professor, *Incident at Vichy,* Phoenix Theatre, 1966; Carol Newquist, *Little Murders,* RSC, Aldwych Theatre, London, 1967; title role, *Toad of Toad Hall,* Fortune Theatre, London, 1967; Casca, *Julius Caesar,* and Caius, *The Merry Wives of Windsor,* both RSC, Royal Shakespeare Theatre, then Aldwych Theatre, both 1968; President, *Indians,* and Bull, *The Relapse,* both RSC, Aldwych Theatre, 1968; Autolycus, *The Winter's Tale,* Simonides, *Pericles,* Guardiano, *Women Beware Women,* and Caius, *The Merry Wives of Windsor,* all RSC, 1969.

Meddle, *London Assurance,* and Bishop Gardiner, *Henry VIII,* both RSC, Aldwych Theatre, 1970; title role, *Toad of Toad Hall,* Duke of York's Theatre, London, 1971; Chief of Police, *The Feydeau Farce Festival of 1909,* Greenwich Theatre, London, 1972; Meddle, *London Assurance,* Albery Theatre, London, 1972; Touchstone, *As You Like It,* Holofernes, *Love's Labour's Lost,* and Baptista, *The Taming of the Shrew,* all RSC, Royal Shakespeare Theatre, 1973; title role, *Toad of Toad Hall,* RSC, Other Place Theatre, Stratford-on-Avon, 1973; Fluther Good, *The Plough and the Stars,* Manitoba Theatre Center, Winnipeg, MB, Canada, 1974; Caius, *The Merry Wives of Windsor,* and Archbishop of Canterbury and Gower, *Henry V,* both RSC, Royal Shakespeare Theatre, 1975; Scheidecker, *Lenz,* Hampstead Theatre Club, London, 1976; Joe Diamonds, *Fire Angel,* Her Majesty's Theatre, London, 1977; Herr Schultz, *Cabaret,* Crucible Theatre, Sheffield, U.K., 1977.

Director, *Yes and No,* and Colonel Fenwick, *For Whom the Bell Chimes,* both Haymarket Theatre, Leicester, U.K., 1980; Cess, *Going Native,* Leeds Playhouse, Leeds, U.K., 1981; Polonius, *Hamlet,* Royal Exchange Theatre, Manchester, U.K., then Barbican Theatre, London, both 1984; Bottom, *A Midsummer Night's Dream,* Ludlow Festival, Ludlow, U.K., 1984; Chief of Police, *Big in*

Brazil, Old Vic Theatre, 1984; Monsieur Boniface, *Hotel Paradiso,* Swan Theatre, Worcester, U.K., 1985; Headmaster, *Gotcha!,* Liverpool Playhouse, Liverpool, U.K., 1986; Harold Twine, *Rookery Nook,* Shaftesbury Theatre, London, 1986; Marius, *Court in the Act,* Phoenix Theatre, 1987. Also appeared as Caspar Darde, *Captain Carvallo,* Theatre Clwyd, 1988; and in *Mouth Organ,* RSC, Other Place Theatre, 1975.

MAJOR TOURS—Baron Hardup, *Cinderella* (pantomime), U.K. cities, 1956; Boss Mangan, *Heartbreak House,* and Burgess, *Candida,* both Birmingham Repertory Company, European cities, 1965; Autolycus, *The Winter's Tale,* and Caius, *The Merry Wives of Windsor,* both RSC, Japanese cities, 1970; Autolycus, *The Winter's Tale,* Australian cities, 1970; Polonius, *Hamlet,* Royal Exchange Theatre Company, U.K. cities, 1984.

FILM DEBUT—Harold, *Alfie Darling,* EMI, 1975. PRINCIPAL FILM APPEARANCES—Television executive, *Who Is Killing the Great Chefs of Europe?* (also known as *Someone Is Killing the Great Chefs of Europe* and *Too Many Chefs*), Warner Brothers, 1978. Also appeared in *Return Journey,* Concord Films Council, 1981; and in the title role, *The Recluse,* 1982.

TELEVISION DEBUT—Barrister, *Baccarat Scandal,* Granada, 1960. PRINCIPAL TELEVISION APPEARANCES—Series: Polteed, *The Forsyte Saga,* PBS; also Norman, *The Guardians.* Mini-Series: "Reilly, Ace of Spies," *Mystery,* PBS, 1984; also as King Leopold, "Lillie," *Masterpiece Theatre,* PBS; in "The Duchess of Duke Street," *Masterpiece Theatre,* PBS; "Rumpole of the Bailey," *Mystery,* PBS. Episodic: Baverstock, *The Carnation Killers,* ATV, then *Thriller,* ABC, 1973; inspector, *Screamer,* ATV, then *Thriller,* ABC, 1974; Punk, *The Equalizer,* CBS, 1986; also *Coronation Street,* syndicated, 1972; *The Adventures of Black Beauty,* London Weekend Television, then syndicated, 1972; *Target,* Entertainment Channel, 1982; *Bergerac,* Entertainment Channel, 1982; *Play for Today.* Movies: Marc Gales, *Internal Affairs,* CBS, 1988. Specials: Mr. Maraczek, *She Loves Me,* BBC, then PBS, 1979. Also appeared as Luzhin, *Crime and Punishment;* Gepetto, *Pinocchio;* Noah, *The Chester Mystery Plays;* Mr. Grimwig, *The Further Adventure of Oliver Twist;* Abbot Napp, *Garden of Inheritance;* Norman, *Heart Attack Hotel;* and in *Singles, Gentle Touch, Jemima Shore, The Professionals, Z Cars, Emergency Ward 10,* and *Squirrels.*

PRINCIPAL TELEVISION WORK—Series: Executive producer, *Celebrity Cooks,* syndicated, 1978.

PRINCIPAL RADIO APPEARANCES—Plays: Autolycus, *The Winter's Tale;* title role, *Toad of Toad Hall;* Samuel Pepys, *Such Men Are Dangerous;* Willie Wonka, *Charlie and the Chocolate Factory;* Mr. York, *Shirley.*

RELATED CAREER—Member, Radio Repertory, 1959-60; associate artist, Royal Shakespeare Company, 1969—; member, Actors Centre, London.

WRITINGS: STAGE—Co-writer, *Mouth Organ,* Royal Shakespeare Company, Other Place Theatre, Stratford-on-Avon, U.K., 1975.

AWARDS: Bancroft Gold Medal from the Royal Academy of Dramatic Art.

MEMBER: British Actors' Equity Association.

SIDELIGHTS: FAVORITE ROLES—Autolycus in *The Winter's Tale,* Harold Twine in *Rookery Nook,* Pierre Bezhukov in *War and Peace,* Holofernes in *Love's Labour's Lost,* and Bottom in *A Midsummer Night's Dream.* RECREATIONS—Going to the theatre and to the cinema.

ADDRESSES: HOME—63 Elstree Road, Bushey Heath, Hertfordshire WD2 3QX, England. AGENT—Michelle Braidman, 10-11 Lower John Street, London W1R 3PE, England.

*   *   *

SMITH, Jaclyn   1947-

PERSONAL: Born October 26, 1947, in Houston, TX; daughter of Jack and Margaret Ellen Smith; married Dennis Cole (divorced, 1981); married third husband, Tony Richmond, August 4, 1981; children: Gaston Anthony, Spencer Margaret. EDUCATION: Attended Trinity University.

VOCATION: Actress.

CAREER: PRINCIPAL STAGE APPEARANCES—Appeared in regional theatre productions of *West Side Story, Gentlemen Prefer Blondes, Bye Bye Birdie,* and *Peg.*

PRINCIPAL FILM APPEARANCES—A model, *Goodbye Columbus,* Paramount, 1969; Belinda, *The Adventurers,* Paramount, 1970; Sally Frannie Tatum, *Bootleggers* (also known as *Bootlegger's Angel*), Howco International, 1974; Maggie Rogers and Brooke Ashley, *Deja Vu,* Cannon, 1985.

PRINCIPAL TELEVISION APPEARANCES—Series: Kelly Garrett, *Charlie's Angels,* ABC, 1976-81. Mini-Series: Sally Fairfax, *George Washington,* CBS, 1984; Mary Ashley, *Sidney Sheldon's Windmills of the Gods,* CBS, 1988; Marie St. Jacques, *The Bourne Identity,* ABC, 1988. Pilots: Alice, *Switch,* CBS, 1975; Susan Cole, *Fools, Females, and Fun: Is There a Doctor in the House?,* NBC, 1974; Kelly Garrett, *Charlie's Angels,* ABC, 1976; also *Probe* (also known as *Search*), NBC, 1972. Episodic: *Get Christy Love,* ABC; *McCloud,* NBC; *The Rookies,* ABC; *Love Boat,* ABC; *Switch,* CBS; *The World of Disney,* ABC. Movies: Maggie Bowman, *Escape from Bogen County,* CBS, 1977; Elena Schneider, *The Users,* ABC, 1978; title role, *Jacqueline Bouvier Kennedy,* ABC, 1981; Jennifer Parker, *Rage of Angels,* NBC, 1983; Claudia Baldwin, *The Night They Saved Christmas,* ABC, 1984; Julie Ross-Gardner, *Sentimental Journey,* CBS, 1984; title role, *Florence Nightingale,* NBC, 1985; Jennifer Parker, *Rage of Angels: The Story Continues,* NBC, 1986; also *Nightkill,* 1980; *My Angry Son,* CBS. Specials: *Battle of the Network Stars,* ABC, 1977; co-host, *The Mad Mad Mad Mad World of the Super Bowl,* NBC, 1977; *ABC's Silver Anniversary Celebration—25 and Still the One,* ABC, 1978; *Magic with the Stars,* NBC, 1982; *Lifetime Salutes Mom,* Lifetime, 1987; *Happy Birthday Hollywood,* ABC, 1987; *Sea World's All-Star Lone Star Celebration,* CBS, 1988; also *Texas 150: A Celebration Special,* 1986; and *Kraft All-Star Salute to Ford's Theatre,* 1986.

RELATED CAREER—Professional model.

WRITINGS: *The Jaclyn Smith Beauty Book,* Simon & Schuster, 1985.

MEMBER: American Federation of Television and Radio Artists.

ADDRESSES: AGENT—William Morris Agency, 151 El Camino Drive, Beverly Hills, CA 90212. PUBLICIST—Jerry Pam, Guttman & Pam, 8500 Wilshire Boulevard, Suite 801, Beverly Hills, CA 90211.*

*   *   *

SMITH, Lane

PERSONAL: Born April 29, in Memphis, TN. EDUCATION: Attended the Carnegie Institute of Technology; trained for the stage with Lee Strasberg at the Actors Studio, 1965. MILITARY: U.S. Army.

VOCATION: Actor.

CAREER: OFF-BROADWAY DEBUT—*Leave It to Jane,* Sheridan Square Playhouse, 1959. PRINCIPAL STAGE APPEARANCES—Lieutenant Addy, *Borak,* Martinique Theatre, New York City, 1960; Max, *Children in the Rain,* Cherry Lane Theatre, New York City, 1970; Stephen, *The Nest,* Mercury Theatre, New York City, 1970; the Captain, *Pinkville,* Theatre at St. Clement's Church, New York City, 1971; Randle Patrick McMurphy, *One Flew Over the Cuckoo's Nest,* Mercer-Hansbury Theatre, New York City, 1971; Mr. Hum, *A Break in the Skin,* Actors Studio Theatre, New York City, 1973; Lon Tanner, *The Emperor of Late Night Radio,* and Leroy Hollingsworth, *Barbary Shore,* both New York Shakespeare Festival, Public Theatre, New York City, 1974; P. Sigmund Furth, *The Leaf People,* Booth Theatre, New York City, 1975; Joe, "Dialogue for Two Men," Harley Ffaulkes, "Midwestern Music," and Byron, "The Love Death," all in *Love Death Plays of William Inge (Part One),* Billy Rose Theatre, New York City, 1975; Scott, *Jack Gelber's New Play: Rehearsal,* American Place Theatre, New York City, 1976; Jack Kerouac, *Visions of Kerouac,* New Dramatists, then Lion Theatre, both New York City, 1976; Harold, *Orphans,* Matrix Theatre, Los Angeles, CA, 1984; James Lingk, *Glengarry Glen Ross,* John Golden Theatre, New York City, 1984. Also appeared at the Center Stage Theatre, Baltimore, MD, 1972; in *Billy Irish,* Manhattan Theatre Club, New York City, 1977; and as Adolph Hitler, *Brechtesgarten,* in New York City.

PRINCIPAL FILM APPEARANCES—Rick Penny, *The Last American Hero* (also known as *Hard Driver*), Twentieth Century-Fox, 1973; Ted Ronan, *Man on a Swing,* Paramount, 1974; Leroy, *Rooster Cogburn,* Universal, 1975; Robert McDonough, *Network,* Metro-Goldwyn-Mayer/United Artists (MGM/UA), 1976; Officer Mackie, *The Bad News Bears in Breaking Training,* Paramount, 1977; Roy Walsh, *Between the Lines,* Midwest, 1977; Clarence Hill, *Blue Collar,* Universal, 1978; Captain Blake, *On the Yard,* Midwest, 1978; Sloan, *Over the Edge,* Orion/Warner Brothers, 1979; Brag, *Honeysuckle Rose* (also known as *On the Road Again*), Warner Brothers, 1980; preacher, *On the Nickel,* Rose's Park, 1980; Don, *Resurrection,* Universal, 1980; Tug Barnes, *Prince of the City,* Warner Brothers, 1981; Dr. Symington, *Frances,* Universal, 1982; Albert Denby, *Places in the Heart,* Tri-Star, 1984; Commander Markel, *Purple Hearts,* Warner Brothers, 1984; Mayor Bates, *Red Dawn,* MGM/UA, 1984; Britton, *Native Son,* Cinecom, 1986; Claude, *Weeds,* De Laurentiis Entertainment Group, 1987; Ethan Sharpe, *Prison,* Empire, 1988. Also appeared in *Maidstone,* Supreme Mix, 1970; and *Soggy Bottom, U.S.A.,* Gaylord, 1982.

PRINCIPAL TELEVISION APPEARANCES—Series: Nathan Bates, *V,* NBC, 1984-85; Dr. Robert Moffitt, *Kay O'Brien,* CBS, 1986. Mini-Series: Hoss Spence, *Chiefs,* CBS, 1983; Warden Brannigan, *If Tomorrow Comes,* CBS, 1986. Pilots: Lieutenant Frank Medley, *The Big Easy,* NBC, 1982. Episodic: Mr. Shortley, "The Displaced Person," *The American Short Story,* PBS, 1977; Captain Milton Treadwell, *Hollywood Beat,* ABC, 1985; Dr. Joseph K. Fitzgerald, "Profile in Silver," *The Twilight Zone,* CBS, 1986; Robert Warren, *Alfred Hitchcock Presents,* NBC, 1986; Dr. Caruso, *Amazing Stories,* NBC, 1986; Sonny Mims, *In the Heat of the Night,* NBC, 1988; Movies: Bob Hartman, *A Death in Canaan,* CBS, 1978; John Carlson, *Disaster on the Coastliner,* ABC, 1979; Jack Collins, *The Solitary Man,* CBS, 1979; Brian, *City in Fear,* ABC, 1980; Randolph Dukane, *The Georgia Peaches,* CBS, 1980; Fred Turner, *Gideon's Trumpet,* CBS, 1980; Don Payer, *Mark, I Love You,* CBS, 1980; Sergeant William Holgren, *A Rumor of War,* CBS, 1980; Harless Hocker, *Dark Night of the Scarecrow,* CBS, 1981; Clarence Blake, *Thou Shalt Not Kill,* NBC, 1982; Tom Keating, *Prime Suspect,* CBS, 1982; Morton Sanders, *Special Bulletin,* NBC, 1983; Officer Dealy, *Something About Amelia,* ABC, 1984; Anson Whitfield, *Bridge Across Time,* NBC, 1985; Captain Max Rosenberg, *Beverly Hills Cowgirl Blues,* CBS, 1985; Colonel King, *Dress Gray,* NBC, 1986; Sam Gavin, *A Place to Call Home,* CBS, 1987; Dr. Butler, *Killer Instinct* (also known as *Over the Edge*), NBC, 1988; also *Crash,* ABC, 1978. Specials: Mr. Addams, *The Member of the Wedding,* NBC, 1982.

AWARDS: Drama Desk Award for *Glengarry Glen Ross.*

ADDRESSES: AGENT—Harris and Goldberg, 2121 Avenue of the Stars, Suite 950, Los Angeles, CA 90067.*

*   *   *

SMITH, Martha

PERSONAL: Born October 16 in Cleveland, OH; daughter of Robert Jeffrey (a sales engineer) and Elsie Marie (Dayhoff) Smith; married Noel Blanc, July 15, 1977 (divorced, February, 1986); married Dean Glasse (an electronics designer), 1988. EDUCATION: Attended Michigan State University; studied acting with Peggy Feury.

VOCATION: Actress.

CAREER: STAGE DEBUT—Kathy, *Vanities,* Beverly Hills Playhouse, Beverly Hills, CA, 1980, for twenty-five performances. PRINCIPAL STAGE APPEARANCES—Jenny, *Almost Perfect,* Burt Reynolds Dinner Theatre, Jupiter, FL, 1987. PRINCIPAL STAGE WORK—Producer, *Vanities,* Beverly Hills Playhouse, 1980.

FILM DEBUT—*Winds of Autumn,* Charles B. Pierce Productions, 1976. PRINCIPAL FILM APPEARANCES—Babs Jansen, *National Lampoon's Animal House,* Universal, 1978; also appeared as Hedwig, *The Blood Link,* 1981; and Major Benpole, *Ridiculous War* (also known as *Abenko*), 1982.

TELEVISION DEBUT—*Quincy, M.E.,* NBC, 1976. PRINCIPAL TELEVISION APPEARANCES—Series: Doctor Sandy Horton, *Days of Our Lives,* NBC, 1982-83; Francine Desmond, *Scarecrow and Mrs. King,* CBS, 1983-87. Pilots: Maggie "Ivory" David, *Ebony,*

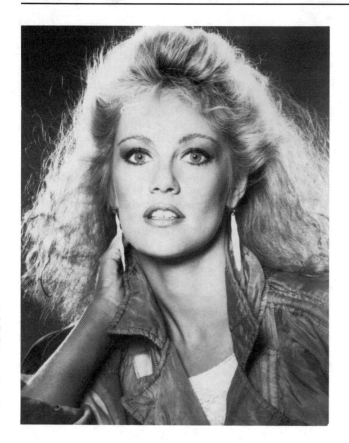

MARTHA SMITH

Ivory, and Jade, CBS, 1979; Susan Hamilton, *Alex and the Dober-man Gang,* NBC, 1980; Monica Hill, *Hard Knocks,* ABC, 1981. Episodic: *Charlie's Angels,* ABC, 1976; *Switch,* CBS, 1976; *The Nancy Walker Show,* ABC, 1976; *The Dukes of Hazzard,* CBS, 1981; *Fantasy Island,* ABC, 1981; *Happy Days,* ABC, 1981; *Taxi,* ABC, 1981; *Dallas,* CBS, 1982; *Love, Sidney,* NBC, 1982; *The New Love, American Style,* ABC, 1986; *Hotel,* ABC, 1986; *Life-styles of the Rich and Famous,* syndicated, 1986; *The New Mike Hammer,* CBS, 1986; also *$25,000 Pyramid,* ABC; and *$100,000 Pyramid,* syndicated. Movies: Kelly, *When the Whistle Blows,* ABC, 1980; also *How the West Was Won,* ABC, 1978. Specials: *Battle of the Network Stars,* ABC, 1983; *New Year's Cotton Bowl Parade,* CBS, 1985; *Thanksgiving Day Parade,* CBS, 1986; also *Coca-Cola 100 Year Anniversary Parade,* 1986.

RELATED CAREER—Fashion model.

NON-RELATED CAREER—Founder, Tickled Pink, Inc. (a greeting card company).

MEMBER: Actors' Equity Association, Screen Actors Guild, American Federation of Television and Radio Artists, National Academy of Television Arts and Sciences, Writers Guild of America-West.

SIDELIGHTS: RECREATIONS—Hiking, tennis, travel, and "raising raccoons."

ADDRESSES: AGENT—Paul Kohner Agency, Inc., 9169 Sunset Boulevard, Los Angeles, CA 90069.

SMITH, Rex   1956-

PERSONAL: Born September 19, 1956, in Jacksonville, FL.

VOCATION: Actor and singer.

CAREER: BROADWAY DEBUT—*Grease,* Royale Theatre, 1978. PRINCIPAL STAGE APPEARANCES—Frederic, *The Pirates of Penzance,* New York Shakespeare Festival, Delacorte Theatre, New York City, 1980, then Uris Theatre, New York City, 1981; Spangler, *The Human Comedy,* Royale Theatre, New York City, 1984; Tony, *West Side Story,* Opera House, Kennedy Center for the Performing Arts, Washington, DC, 1985; Stuart, *Brownstone,* Roundabout Theatre, New York City, 1986. Also appeared in *Baby,* Theatre Under the Stars, Houston, TX, 1988.

MAJOR TOURS—Danny Zuko, *Grease,* U.S. cities, 1979.

PRINCIPAL FILM APPEARANCES—Frederic, *The Pirates of Penzance,* Universal, 1983; Rick Peterson, *Ballerina and the Blues,* Karl/Lorimar Home Video/Astral, 1988. Also appeared in *Headin' for Broadway,* Twentieth Century-Fox, 1980; *No Dead Heroes,* Cineventures/Maharaj/Miller, 1987.

TELEVISION DEBUT—Michael Syke, *Sooner or Later,* NBC, 1979. PRINCIPAL TELEVISION APPEARANCES—Series: Host, *Solid Gold,* syndicated, 1982-83; Officer Jesse Mach/title role, *Street Hawk,* ABC, 1985. Pilots: Ben Berlin, *Dear Penelope and Peter* (broadcast as an episode of *The New Love, American Style*), ABC, 1986. Episodic: Stew Bennett, *Murder, She Wrote,* CBS, 1986; Jake Bodine, *Houston Knights,* CBS, 1987; Jerry Wickes, *Cagney and Lacey,* CBS, 1988. Specials: *How to Be a Man,* CBS, 1985; *We the People 200: The Constitutional Gala,* CBS, 1987; *Broadway Sings: The Music of Jule Styne,* PBS, 1987; *Kennedy Center Honors: A Celebration of the Performing Arts,* CBS, 1988.

WRITINGS: FILM—Lyricist, *Ballerina and the Blues,* Karl/Lorimar Home Video/Astral, 1988.

RECORDINGS: ALBUMS—*Sooner or Later,* Columbia, 1979. SINGLES—"You Take My Breath Away," Columbia, 1979.

AWARDS: Theatre World Award, 1981, for *The Pirates of Penzance.*

ADDRESSES: MANAGER—Joanna Kinkaid, Kinkaid Management, 36 Navy Street, Suite 2, Venice, CA 90291.*

*   *   *

SMITHERS, Jan   1949-

PERSONAL: Born July 3, 1949, in North Hollywood, CA; married James Brolin (an actor), November 28, 1987; children: one daughter. EDUCATION: Attended the California Institute of Art.

VOCATION: Actress.

CAREER: PRINCIPAL FILM APPEARANCES—Devola, *Where the Lilies Bloom,* United Artists, 1974; Cathy Wakefield, *Our Winning Season,* American International, 1978; Dr. Lisa Rayon, *Mr. Nice Guy,* Shapiro Entertainment, 1987.

PRINCIPAL TELEVISION APPEARANCES—Series: Bailey Quarters, *WKRP in Cincinnati*, CBS, 1978-82. Pilots: Carol Clark, *The Love Tapes*, ABC, 1980. Episodic: Barrie Shepherd, "The Columnist," *Comedy Factory*, ABC, 1985; Janice Copland, *Hotel*, ABC, 1986; also *Love Story*, NBC, 1973. Specials: *Battle of the Network Stars*, ABC, 1979.

ADDRESSES: PUBLICIST—Lippin Group Public Relations, 8124 W. Third Street, Suite 204, Los Angeles, CA 90048.*

*   *   *

SOFAER, Abraham   1896-1988

PERSONAL: Born October 1, 1896, in Rangoon, Burma; died of congestive heart failure, January 21, 1988, in Woodland Hills, CA; son of Isaac and Rahma (Solomon) Sofaer; married Psyche Angela Christian; children: one son, four daughters.

VOCATION: Actor.

CAREER: STAGE DEBUT—*The Merchant of Venice*, Charles Doran Shakespeare Company, Palace Theatre, Newark-on-Trent, U.K., 1921. LONDON DEBUT—Bishop of Avila and other roles, *Gloriana*, Little Theatre, 1925. BROADWAY DEBUT—Isaac Cohen, *The Matriarch*, Longacre Theatre, 1930. PRINCIPAL STAGE APPEARANCES—Claude Montague, *Scotch Mist*, St. Martin's Theatre, London, 1926; Zasha, *The Mountain*, Shaftesbury Theatre, London, 1926; Bazilio, *The Marriage of Figaro*, Court Theatre, London, 1926; Comte de Sallaz, *Israel*, Everyman Theatre, Liverpool, U.K., 1927; the Arab, *The Beetle*, Strand Theatre, London, 1928; the Pack Pedlar, *Black Velvet*, Arts Theatre, London, 1929; Odderitto, *The Man in Dress Clothes*, Lyceum Theatre, London, 1929; Professor Fell, *Before Midnight*, Little Theatre, London, 1929; Isaac Cohen, *The Matriarch*, Royalty Theatre, London, 1929.

Feste, *Twelfth Night*, and Claudius, *Hamlet*, both Embassy Theatre, London, 1930; Abraham Kaplan, *Street Scene*, Globe Theatre, London, 1930; Ali and Ben Hussein, *If*, Arts Theatre, 1931; Piderit, *Twelve Thousand*, and Count Mario Grazia, *The Mask and the Face*, both Embassy Theatre, 1931; Leone, *Volpone*, and Leonti Levine, *The Bear Dances*, both Garrick Theatre, London, 1932; Brutus, *Julius Caesar*, His Majesty's Theatre, London, 1932; Biron, *Love's Labour's Lost*, Westminster Theatre, London, 1932; Chief Rabbi Forbach, *Miracle at Verdun*, Comedy Theatre, London, 1932; Dr. Zodiac, *He Wanted Adventure*, Saville Theatre, London, 1933; Rufus Sonnenberg, *Success Story*, Fulham Theatre, then Cambridge Theatre, both London, 1934; the Messenger, *Antony and Cleopatra*, Bolingbroke, *Richard II*, Don Pedro, *Much Ado about Nothing*, Bishop of Beauvais, *Saint Joan*, Gremio, *The Taming of the Shrew*, title role, *Othello*, Theseus, *Hippolytus*, title role, *Henry IV, Part II*, and Claudius, *Hamlet*, all Old Vic Company, Sadler's Wells Theatre, London, 1934-35; Count de Reinach, *The Great Experiment*, St. Martin's Theatre, 1936; title role, *Professor Bernhardi*, Embassy Theatre, then Phoenix Theatre, London, both 1936; Disraeli, *Victoria Regina*, Broadhurst Theatre, New York City, 1936, then Martin Beck Theatre, New York City, 1938; Shylock, *The Merchant of Venice*, Shubert Theatre, Chicago, IL, 1938; Jonah Goodman, *The Gentle People*, Strand Theatre, 1939.

King of France, *King John*, and Jason, *Medea*, both Old Vic Company, New Theatre, London, 1941; Ross, *Macbeth*, Piccadilly

Theatre, London, 1942; title role, *Othello*, and Leontes, *The Winter's Tale*, both Shakespeare Memorial Company, Shakespeare Memorial Theatre, Stratford-on-Avon, U.K., 1942; Master Absolon Beyer, *The Witch*, Arts Theatre, 1944; Claudius, *Hamlet*, Haymarket Theatre, London, 1945; Rabbi, *Skipper Next to God*, Embassy Theatre, 1945; Nils Krogstad, *A Doll's House*, Winter Garden Theatre, London, 1946; Ernesti, *The Silver Trumpets*, New Lindsey Theatre, London, 1946; Edward Max, *Native Son*, Boltons Theatre, London, 1948; Kurt Auerbach, *The Least of These*, Strand Theatre, 1948; Evangelist, *The Pilgrim's Progress*, Covent Garden Theatre, London, 1948; Svengali, *Trilby*, Bedford Theatre, London, 1950; Samson, *Samson Agonistes*, St. Martin-in-the-Fields, London, 1951; Zeus, *The Flies*, Group Theatre Company, New Theatre, 1951. Also appeared with the Charles Doran Shakespeare Company, 1921-23; as Vasco, *Command Performance*, 1933; and in *In the Matter of J. Robert Oppenheimer*, Mark Taper Forum, Los Angeles, CA, 1967.

PRINCIPAL STAGE WORK—Director, *The Merchant of Venice*, Shubert Theatre, Chicago, IL, 1938.

MAJOR TOURS—Rajah of Rukh, *The Green Goddess*, U.K. cities, 1925; Leon, *Dawn*, U.K. cities, 1927; Doctor Chan Fu, *The Silent House*, U.K. cities, 1928; De Levis, *Loyalties*, U.K. cities, 1929; Hector Frome, *Justice*, U.K. cities, 1929; Disraeli, *Victoria Regina*, U.S. cities, 1937; Macduff, *Macbeth*, U.K. cities, 1940; King of France, *King John*, Old Vic Company, U.K. cities, 1941; Doctor Gortler, *I Have Been Here Before*, U.K. cities, 1944. Also appeared on tours of U.K. cities with Harold V. Neilson's Company for four years, performing nearly one hundred Shakespearean roles including the title role, *Othello*, Shylock, *The Merchant of Venice*, Brutus, *Julius Caesar*, and Malvolio, *Twelfth Night*.

PRINCIPAL FILM APPEARANCES—Dubois, *The Dreyfus Case* (also known as *Dreyfus*), Columbia, 1931; Fahmy, *The House Opposite*, Pathe, 1931; Mahmed Pasha, *Stamboul*, Paramount, 1931; Lieutenant Joseph, *The Flying Squad*, British Lion, 1932; Ali Ben Achmed, *Insult*, Paramount, 1932; Mehett Salos, *The Flag Lieutenant*, Gaumont, 1932; Baki, *Ask Beccles*, Paramount, 1933; Myers, *High Finance*, Warner Brothers/First National, 1933; holy man, *Karma*, India and British Film, 1933; Mr. Beal, *Little Miss Nobody*, Warner Brothers, 1933; Ali, *Trouble*, United Artists, 1933; Don Pablo y Gonzales, *The Admiral's Secret*, RKO, 1934; Skelton, *Oh, No Doctor!*, Metro-Goldwyn-Mayer (MGM), 1934; street bookseller, *The Private Life of Don Juan* (also known as *Don Juan*), United Artists, 1934; *Nell Gwyn*, United Artists, 1935; Zapportas, *The Wandering Jew*, Olympic, 1935; Doctor Menasseh, *Rembrandt*, United Artists, 1935; the Jew, *Things to Come*, United Artists, 1936; Ali, *Crooks Tour*, Anglo American, 1940; Heini Meyer, *A Voice in the Night* (also known as *Freedom Radio*), Columbia, 1941; the Judge, *Stairway to Heaven* (also known as *A Matter of Life and Death*), Universal, 1946; French judge, *Dual Alibi*, British National, 1947; Disraeli, *Ghosts of Berkeley Square*, British National, 1947; Doctor Kohima, *Calling Paul Temple*, Nettleford, 1948; Luis de Santangel, *Christopher Columbus*, Universal, 1949.

Commandant, *Cairo Road*, Associated British Films/Pathe, 1950; judge, *Pandora and the Flying Dutchman*, MGM, 1951; Paul, *Quo Vadis*, MGM, 1951; Chancellor, *Judgment Deferred*, Associated British Films, 1952; Fatumak, *His Majesty O'Keefe*, Warner Brothers, 1953; Incacha, *The Naked Jungle*, Paramount, 1953; Appuhamy, *Elephant Walk*, Paramount, 1954; Surabhai, *Bhowani Junction*, MGM, 1956; Don Carlos, *The First Texan*, Allied Artists, 1956; Tutush, *Omar Khayyam*, Paramount, 1957; Indian, *Out of the*

Clouds, Rank, 1957; Hassim, *The Sad Sack*, Paramount, 1957; Indian chief, *The Story of Mankind*, Warner Brothers, 1957; abbot, *Taras Bulba*, United Artists, 1962; Calgo, *Captain Sinbad*, MGM, 1963; Professor Pietro Baglioni, "Rappaccini's Daughter" in *Twice Told Tales* (also known as *Nathaniel Hawthorne's "Twice Told Tales"*), United Artists, 1963; Joseph of Arimathaea, *The Greatest Story Ever Told*, United Artists, 1965; Doctor Von Steiner, *Journey to the Center of Time*, American General Pictures/Western International, 1967; swami, *Head*, Columbia, 1968; proprietor, *Justine*, Twentieth Century-Fox, 1969; Pablo Rojas, *Che!*, Twentieth Century-Fox, 1969; White Buffalo, *Chisum*, Warner Brothers, 1970. Also appeared in *King of Kings*, MGM, 1961.

PRINCIPAL TELEVISION APPEARANCES—Episodic: Dr. Stillman, "The Mighty Casey," *The Twilight Zone*, CBS, 1960; Thasian, "Charlie X," *Star Trek*, NBC, 1966; also "Revenge of the Gods," *The Time Tunnel*, ABC, 1966; "The Flaming Planet," *Lost in Space*, CBS, 1968.

NON-RELATED CAREER—Schoolmaster in Rangoon and London.

MEMBER: Green Room Club (London).

OBITUARIES AND OTHER SOURCES: Variety, February 3, 1988.*

*   *   *

SOTO, Rosana
   See DeSOTO, Rosana

*   *   *

SOUTHERN, Terry   1926-
   (Maxwell Kenton—a joint pseudonym)

PERSONAL: Born May 1, 1926, in Alvarado, TX; son of Terry M. (a pharmacist) and Helen (Simonds) Southern; married Carol Kauffman, July 14, 1958; children: Nile (son). EDUCATION: Attended Southern Methodist University and University of Chicago; Northwestern University, B.A., 1948; also attended the Sorbonne, Paris, 1948-50. MILITARY: U.S. Army, 1943-45.

VOCATION: Writer.

CAREER: See *WRITINGS* below. RELATED CAREER—Advisory editor, *Best American Short Stories, 1955-56* (short story collection).

WRITINGS: FILM—(With Stanley Kubrick and Peter George) *Dr. Strangelove, or How I Learned to Stop Worrying and Love the Bomb*, Columbia, 1964; (with Ring Lardner, Jr.) *The Cincinnati Kid*, Metro-Goldwyn-Mayer (MGM), 1965; (with Christopher Isherwood) *The Loved One*, MGM, 1965; (with Brian Degas, Claude Brule, Jean-Claude Forest, Clement Biddle Wood, Tudor Gates, Vittorio Bonicelli, and Roger Vadim) *Barbarella* (also known as *Barbarella, Queen of the Galaxy*), Paramount, 1968; (with Peter Fonda and Dennis Hopper) *Easy Rider*, Columbia, 1969, published by New American Library, 1969; (with Aram Avakian) *The End of the Road*, Allied Artists, 1969; (with Joseph McGrath, Peter Sellers, Graham Chapman, and John Cleese) *The Magic Christian*, Commonwealth United, 1970. Also (with David

Burnett) *Candy Kisses*, 1955; and *The Private War of Welsey Fickett*.

OTHER—*Flash and Filigree* (fiction), Coward McCann, 1958; (with Mason Hoffenberg under the joint pseudonym Maxwell Kenton) *Candy* (fiction), Olympia Press (Paris), 1959, then (under the names Terry Southern and Mason Hoffenberg) Putnam, 1964, later Penguin, 1985; *The Magic Christian* (fiction), Random House, 1960, then Penguin, 1985; (editor, with Alexander Trocchi and R. Seaver) *Writers in Revolt* (anthology), Frederick Fell, 1963; *The Journal of "The Loved One": The Production Log of a Motion Picture* (nonfiction), Random House, 1965; *Red Dirt Marijuana and Other Tastes* (short story collection), New American Library, 1967; *Blue Movie* (fiction), World Publishing, 1970, then New American Library, 1985. Also contributor to *Evergreen Review, Paris Review, Esquire, Harper's Bazaar, Encounter, Argosy, Nugget, London Magazine, Playboy, New York Times, Nation*, and other publications.

AWARDS: British Screen Writers Award, 1964, for *Dr. Strangelove, or How I Learned to Stop Worrying and Love the Bomb*; Academy Award nomination, Best Screenplay, 1970, for *Easy Rider*.

SIDELIGHTS: RECREATIONS—Animals and hunting.

ADDRESSES: HOME—R.F.D., East Canaan, CT 06024. AGENT—Sterling Lord Agency, One Madison Avenue, New York, NY 10001.*

*   *   *

SPELVIN, George, Jr.
   See DOUGLAS, Kirk

*   *   *

STANDING, John   1934-

PERSONAL: Born John Leon, August 16, 1934, in London, England; son of Sir Ronald George (a stock broker) and Dorothy Katherine (an actress; maiden name, Standing; professional name, Kay Hammond) Leon; married Jill Melford (divorced, 1972); married Sarah Kate Forbes (a writer), April 7, 1984; children: Alexander, India, Archie. POLITICS: Liberal. RELIGION: Church of England. MILITARY: British Army, Kings Royal Rifle Corps, second lieutenant.

VOCATION: Actor.

CAREER: STAGE DEBUT—Various roles, *Titus Andronicus*, Shakespeare Memorial Theatre Company, Sarah Bernhardt Theatre, Paris, France. LONDON DEBUT—Mr. Charlton, *The Darling Buds of May*, Saville Theatre, 1959. BROADWAY DEBUT—Elyot Chase, *Private Lives*, 76th Street Theatre, 1975. PRINCIPAL STAGE APPEARANCES—Andrew Rankin, *The Irregular Verb to Love*, Criterion Theatre, London, 1961; title role, *Norman*, Duchess Theatre, London, 1962; ensemble, *So Much to Remember* (revue), Vaudeville Theatre, London, 1963; Clive Winton, *See How They Run*,

Vaudeville Theatre, 1964; Sir John Melvil, *The Clandestine Marriage*, Lennox, *Macbeth*, Yepihodov, *The Cherry Orchard*, and Mendigales, *The Fighting Cock*, all Chichester Festival Theatre, Chichester, U.K., 1966; Mendigales, *The Fighting Cock*, Duke of York's Theatre, London, 1966; George Smerdon, *The Farmer's Wife*, Aimwell, *The Beaux' Stratagem*, and Emile Tavernier, *An Italian Straw Hat*, all Chichester Festival Theatre, 1967; Algernon Moncrieff, *The Importance of Being Earnest*, and Hugo and Frederick, *Ring 'round the Moon*, both Haymarket Theatre, London, 1968; Lorn Mason, *Girlfriend*, Apollo Theatre, London, 1970; Dapper, *The Alchemist*, and Bluntschli, *Arms and the Man*, both Chichester Festival Theatre, 1970; Clive Popkiss, *Popkiss*, Globe Theatre, London, 1972; Chap, *A Sense of Detachment*, Royal Court Theatre, London, 1972; Elyot Chase, *Private Lives*, Queen's Theatre, London, 1973; Dauphin, *Saint Joan*, Oxford Festival, Oxford, U.K., 1974; George, *Jingo*, Royal Shakespeare Company, Aldwych Theatre, London, 1975; Dr. Watson, *Dead-Eyed Dicks*, Gaiety Theatre, Dublin, Ireland, 1976; Freddy Malone, *Plunder*, and Dr. Paramore, *The Philanderer*, both National Theatre Company, Lyttleton Theatre, London, 1978; Benedict, *Close of Play*, National Theatre Company, Lyttleton Theatre, 1979. Also appeared with the Bristol Old Vic Theatre Company, Bristol, U.K., 1960.

PRINCIPAL FILM APPEARANCES—Hubert Shannon, *A Pair of Briefs*, Davis, 1963; Humphrey, *The Swingin' Maiden* (also known as *The Iron Maiden*), Columbia, 1963; Arthur, *Young and Willing* (also known as *The Wild and the Willing* and *The Young and the Willing*), Universal, 1964; Captain Daven, *King Rat*, Columbia, 1965; Mark Von Sturm, *The Psychopath*, Paramount, 1966; Julius P. Haversack, *Walk, Don't Run*, Columbia, 1966; Leo Winston, *Torture Garden*, Columbia, 1968; Roger, *Thank You All Very Much* (also known as *A Touch of Love*), Columbia, 1969; Gordon, *X, Y, and Zee* (also known as *Zee and Co.*), Columbia, 1972; Bernie, *All the Right Noises*, Twentieth Century-Fox, 1973; Father Philip Verecker, *The Eagle Has Landed*, Columbia, 1976; Fairbrother, *The Class of Miss MacMichael*, Brut, 1978; Jason Mountolive, *The Legacy* (also known as *The Legacy of Maggie Walsh*), Universal, 1979; Fox, *The Elephant Man*, Paramount, 1980; Finley, *The Sea Wolves*, Paramount, 1981; Captain Sholto Savory, *Privates on Parade*, Handmade Films, 1982; Earl Harry, *Invitation to the Wedding*, New Realm, 1985; Michael D'Branin, *Nightflyers*, Vista/New Century, 1987. Also appeared in *Captain Stirrick*, 1982.

PRINCIPAL TELEVISION APPEARANCES—Series: Edward Wingate, *Lime Street*, ABC, 1985-86. Mini-Series: Sam Collins, *Tinker, Tailor, Soldier, Spy*, PBS, 1980; Sir George, *Sidney Sheldon's Windmills of the Gods*, CBS, 1988; also "The First Churchills," *Masterpiece Theatre*, PBS, 1971. Episodic: Vernon Bennett, *Hotel*, ABC, 1987; Arthur Constable, *Murder, She Wrote*, CBS, 1987; Ian Ludlow, *Murphy's Law*, ABC, 1989; *Visitors*, BBC, 1987; *Hunter*, NBC, 1988. Movies: Duke of Windsor, *To Catch a King*, HBO, 1984. Specials: *Flapjack Floozie*, HBO, 1988; also Colonel Pickering, *Pygmalion*, 1983; *Our Planet Tonight*, 1987.

AWARDS: Olivier Award nomination, Best Actor, 1979, for *Close of Play*.

SIDELIGHTS: FAVORITE ROLES—Algernon Moncrieff in *The Importance of Being Earnest*. RECREATIONS—Painting.

ADDRESSES: AGENT—Agency for the Performing Arts, 9000 Sunset Boulevard, Los Angeles, CA 90069.

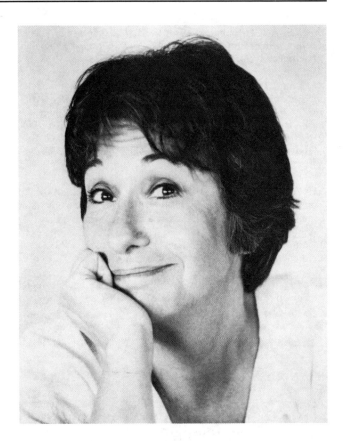

FLORENCE STANLEY

STANLEY, Florence

PERSONAL: Born July 1 in Chicago, IL; daughter of Jack and Hanna (Weil) Schwartz; married Martin Newman. EDUCATION: Graduated from Northwestern University.

VOCATION: Actress and director.

CAREER: OFF-BROADWAY DEBUT—Mother, *Machinal*, Gate Theatre, 1960. BROADWAY DEBUT—*The Glass Menagerie*, Brooks Atkinson Theatre, 1965. PRINCIPAL STAGE APPEARANCES—Clytemnestra, *Electra*, Delacorte Theatre, New York City, 1964; Yente, *Fiddler on the Roof*, Imperial Theatre, New York City, 1965; Pearl, *The Prisoner of Second Avenue*, Eugene O'Neill Theatre, New York City, 1971; Bertha Gale, *The Secret Affairs of Mildred Wild*, Ambassador Theatre, New York City, 1972; housemother, *A Safe Place*, New Dramatists, New York City, 1974; Yenchna, *Fools*, Eugene O'Neill Theatre, 1981; Nurse, *Romeo and Juliet*, Seattle Repertory Theatre, Seattle, WA, 1982; Thelma Cates, *'night Mother*, Syracuse Stage, Syracuse, NY, 1984; Bella, *What's Wrong with This Picture?*, Manhattan Theatre Club, New York City, 1985; Emma Bovary, *It's Only a Play*, Manhattan Theatre Club, 1986; Leah, *Reunion*, Center Stage, Baltimore, MD, 1986. Also appeared in *The Palace of Amateurs*, Plaza Theatre, Dallas, TX, 1983.

PRINCIPAL STAGE WORK—Director, *Delmore*, Jewish Repertory Theatre, New York City, 1982.

PRINCIPAL FILM APPEARANCES—Ella Friedenberg, *Up the Down Staircase*, Warner Brothers, 1967; club woman, *The Day of the*

Dolphin, AVCO-Embassy, 1973; Pearl, *The Prisoner of Second Avenue,* Warner Brothers, 1975; landlady, *The Fortune,* Columbia, 1975; ticket agent, *Outrageous Fortune,* Buena Vista, 1987.

PRINCIPAL TELEVISION APPEARANCES—Series: Aunt Josephine, *Joe and Sons,* CBS, 1975-76; Bernice Fish, *Barney Miller,* ABC, 1975-77; Bernice Fish, *Fish,* ABC, 1977-78; Judge Wilbur, *My Two Dads,* NBC, 1987—. Pilots: Marjorie Waller, *Sonny Boy,* CBS, 1974. Movies: Adele, *Mickey and Nora,* CBS, 1987. Specials: *ABC's Silver Anniversary Celebration—25 and Still the One,* ABC, 1978.

RELATED CAREER—Guest artist, Sundance Institute Playwrights Conference, Salt Lake City, UT, 1985; actress in television commercials.

MEMBER: Actors' Equity Association, Screen Actors Guild, American Federation of Television and Radio Artists.

ADDRESSES: AGENT—Artists Agency, 10000 Santa Monica Boulevard, Suite 305, Los Angeles, CA 90067.

*   *   *

STANLEY, Gordon   1951-

PERSONAL: Born December 20, 1951, in Boston, MA; son of Malcolm McClain (a medical research scientist) and Edith (a medical research scientist; maiden name, Dumoff) Stanley; married Renee Lutz (a stage manager), May 18, 1980. EDUCATION: Brown University, A.B., 1973; Temple University, M.F.A., 1976; studied singing with Mark Peason and Ellen Repp.

VOCATION: Actor.

CAREER: STAGE DEBUT—First murderer, *Richard III,* Court Theatre, Chicago, IL, 1969. OFF-BROADWAY DEBUT—*Lyrical and Satirical,* Joseph Jefferson Theatre, 1977, for fourteen performances. BROADWAY DEBUT—Fleming, *Onward Victoria,* Martin Beck Theatre, 1980, for one performance. PRINCIPAL STAGE APPEARANCES—First voice, *Under Milkwood,* Court Theatre, Chicago, IL, 1970; Puck, *A Midsummer Night's Dream* (opera), Curtis Opera Theatre, Chicago, 1976; various roles, *Bullshot Crummond,* Grendel's Lair Dinner Theatre, Philadelphia, PA, 1977; Charlie, *Allegro,* Equity Library Theatre, New York City, 1978; Mr. Snow, *Carousel,* Coachlight Theatre, Warehouse Point, CT, 1980; Motel, *Fiddler on the Roof,* Artpark Theatre, Lewiston, NY, 1981; Mr. Erlanson, *A Little Night Music,* York Players Company (later York Theatre Company), Church of the Heavenly Rest, New York City, 1981; Sid el Kar, *The Desert Song,* Light Opera of Manhattan, New York City, 1981; Rodney, *Two on the Isles,* Actors' Holiday, New York City, 1981; Jacob, *Joseph and the Amazing Technicolor Dreamcoat,* Entermedia Theatre, New York City, 1981, then Royale Theatre, New York City, 1982; Freddy, *My Fair Lady,* Theatre of the Stars, Atlanta, GA, 1983; Courtice Pounds, *Sullivan and Gilbert,* Stage Arts Theatre Company, Actors Outlet, New York City, 1984; Cecil, *Elizabeth and Essex,* York Theatre Company, Chancel of the Heavenly Rest, New York City, 1984; Fingers, *Red, Hot, and Blue!,* Equity Library Theatre, 1984; Wesley, *Mrs. Farmer's Daughter,* American Musical Theatre Festival, Philadelphia, 1984.

Peleg and Captain of the *Rachael, Moby Dick* (opera), York Theatre

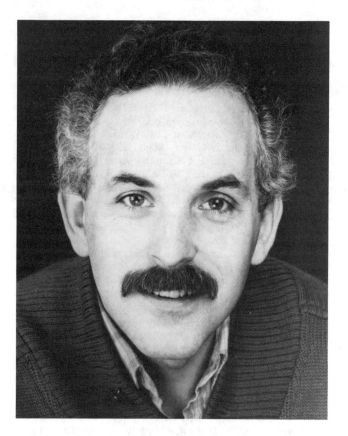

GORDON STANLEY

Company, Paul Mazur Theatre, New York City, 1986; Signor Bocciarelli, *Into the Light,* Neil Simon Theatre, New York City, 1986; Padre, *Man of La Mancha,* Theatre Virginia, Richmond, VA, 1986; Salisbury, *King John,* Riverside Shakespeare Company, New York City, 1986; Doctor, *A Good Life,* Kennedy Center for the Performing Arts, Washington, DC, 1986; Victor, *Private Lives,* South Jersey Regional Theatre, Somers Point, NJ, 1987; Elihu Root, *Teddy and Alice,* Minskoff Theatre, New York City, 1987; Ulysses, *Bertha, the Sewing Machine Girl,* Merrimack Regional Theatre, Lowell, MA, 1988; Bill, *Johnny Pye and the Foolkiller,* Lamb's Theatre, New York City, 1988. Also appeared as Allan Felix, *Play It Again, Sam,* Benvolio, *Romeo and Juliet,* second gangster, *Kiss Me, Kate,* and Boss Mangan, *Heartbreak House,* all Weathervane Theatre, 1971; Doc, *The Tooth of Crime,* Off-Broadway production, 1979; Cecil, *Elizabeth and Essex,* Off-Broadway production, 1980; Morris, *1776,* Carter-Barron Theatre, 1980; Leo, *Transatlantic* (opera), Encompass the Music Theatre, 1981; in *Joseph and the Amazing Technicolor Dreamcoat,* Paper Mill Playhouse, Millburn, NJ, 1984; as an understudy in the ensemble, *Diamonds* (revue), Circle in the Square Downtown, New York City, 1984; and member of ensemble, *Who Does She Think She Is?* (revue), Off-Broadway production, 1987.

MAJOR TOURS—Harold Ickes, *Annie,* U.S. cities, 1978.

RELATED CAREER—Guest artist, Curtis Institute of Music, Philadelphia, PA, 1976; president, Shaker Barn Theatre Inc., New Lebanon, NY, 1980—; guest artist and teacher, Centenary College, Hackettstown, NJ, 1983.

AWARDS: Design demonstration grant from the National Endowment for the Arts, 1981, for the Shaker Barn Theatre.

MEMBER: Actors' Equity Association, Screen Actors Guild, National Trust for Historic Preservation.

ADDRESSES: OFFICE—305 W. 45th Street, Apartment 6-A, New York, NY 10036. AGENTS—Donna Massetti and Julie Lord, Monty Silver Agency, 200 W. 57th Street, New York, NY 10019.

*   *   *

STAPLETON, Jean   1923-

PERSONAL: Born Jeanne Murray, January 19, 1923, in New York, NY; daughter of Joseph E. (a billboard advertising salesman) and Marie (a singer; maiden name, Stapleton) Murray; married William H. Putch (a theatre producer and director), October 26, 1957 (died, 1983); children: John, Pamela. EDUCATION: Attended Hunter College; trained for the stage with Carli Laklan at the American Apprentice Theatre, with Jane Rose and William Hansen at the American Actors Company, with Joseph Anthony and Peter Frye at the American Theatre Wing and with Harold Clurman.

VOCATION: Actress.

CAREER: BROADWAY DEBUT—Inez, *In the Summer House,* Playhouse Theatre, 1953. PRINCIPAL STAGE APPEARANCES—Mrs. Watty, *The Corn Is Green,* Equity Library Theatre, New York

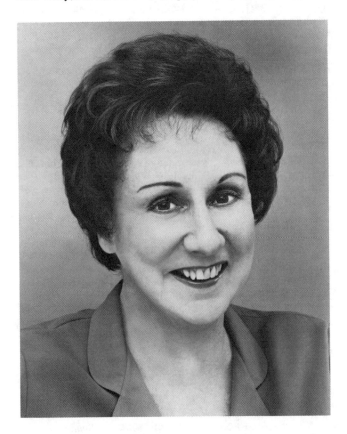

JEAN STAPLETON

City, 1948; Mother, *American Gothic,* Circle in the Square, New York City, 1953; Sister, *Damn Yankees,* 46th Street Theatre, New York City, 1955; Sue, *Bells Are Ringing,* Shubert Theatre, New York City, 1956; Swart Petry, *A Swim in the Sea,* Walnut Street Theatre, Philadelphia, PA, 1958; Maisie Madigan, *Juno,* Winter Garden Theatre, New York City, 1959; Mrs. Ochs, *Rhinoceros,* Longacre Theatre, New York City, 1961; Mrs. Strakosh, *Funny Girl,* Winter Garden Theatre, 1964; wardrobe mistress, *Parade of Stars Playing the Palace,* Palace Theatre, New York City, 1983; Old Woman, *Candide,* Baltimore Opera Company, Baltimore, MD, 1984; Abby Brewster, *Arsenic and Old Lace,* 46th Street Theatre, 1986; Julia Child, *Bon Appetit,* Terrace Theatre, Kennedy Center for the Performing Arts, Washington, DC, 1989. Also appeared at the Peterborough Playhouse, Peterborough, NH, 1941; Chase Barn Playhouse, Whitefield, NH, 1947-48; Pocono Playhouse, Mountainhome, PA, 1951-53; in *A Soft Touch,* Coconut Grove Playhouse, Miami, FL, 1957; *The Time of the Cuckoo,* Center Theatre Group, Ahmanson Theatre, Los Angeles, CA, 1974; *The Late Christopher Bean,* Kennedy Center for the Performing Arts, 1983; *The Show-Off,* Syracuse Stage, Syracuse, NY, 1983, then Paper Mill Playhouse, Millburn, NJ, 1984; and *The Italian Lesson,* Baltimore Opera Company, 1985.

With the Totem Pole Playhouse, Fayetteville, PA: Woody, *Goodbye, My Fancy,* Miss Cooper, *Separate Tables,* Mother, *Charm,* Grace, *Bus Stop,* and Madame St. Pe, *The Waltz of the Toreadors,* all 1958; Sally Adams, *Call Me Madam,* 1959; Laura Partridge, *The Solid Gold Cadillac,* 1960; Mrs. Keller, *The Miracle Worker,* Emma, *Apple in the Attic,* ensemble, *A Thurber Carnival* (revue), title role, *Everybody Loves Opal,* and Aunt Eller, *Oklahoma!,* all 1962; Mrs. Baker, *Come Blow Your Horn,* Mrs. Spofford, *Gentleman Prefer Blondes,* and Nannie, *All for Mary,* all 1963; Brewster, *A Rainy Day in Newark,* Rosemary, *Picnic,* Annabelle, *George Washington Slept Here,* Mrs. Walworth, *Speaking of Murder,* Mrs. Pearce, *My Fair Lady,* Mrs. Yoder, *Papa Is All,* and Mother Abbess, *The Sound of Music,* all 1964; Anna Leonowens, *The King and I,* Bloody Mary, *South Pacific,* Lottie, *The Dark at the Top of the Stairs,* Miss Skillon, *See How They Run,* Veta Louise, *Harvey,* Abby Brewster, *Arsenic and Old Lace,* Grace Kimbrough, *Never Too Late,* Mother, *Enter Laughing,* and Anne Michaelson, *Take Her, She's Mine,* all 1965; Miss Holroyd, *Bell, Book, and Candle,* Mrs. Deazy, *Jenny Kissed Me,* Aunt Kate Barnaby, *How Far Is the Barn?,* Nettie Fowler, *Carousel,* and Dorothy, *Any Wednesday,* all 1966; Dolly Gallagher Levi, *Hello Dolly!,* 1971; Mrs. Baer, *Butterflies Are Free,* Lola, *Come Back, Little Sheba,* and title role, *Everybody Loves Opal,* all 1972; title role, *The Secret Affairs of Mildred Wild,* 1975; title role, *Daisy Mayme,* 1978; Miss Marple, *A Murder Is Announced,* 1979; Miss Marple, *Murder at the Vicarage,* and Aunt Eller, *Oklahoma!,* both 1981. Also appeared in *Southwest Corner,* 1971; *The Time of the Cuckoo,* 1973; *Lullaby* and *The Vinegar Tree,* both 1974; *Hay Fever* and *The Late Christopher Bean,* both 1976; *The Reluctant Debutante* and *The Show-Off,* both 1977; *The Great Sebastian's* and *Little Mary Sunshine,* both 1978; *Papa Is All,* 1979; *The Curious Savage* and *Butterfly Days,* both 1981; *The Corn Is Green,* 1982; and *Ernest in Love,* 1983.

MAJOR TOURS—Mrs. Watty, *The Corn Is Green,* U.S. cities, 1948-49; Myrtle Mae, *Harvey,* U.S. cities, 1948-49 and 1949-50; Mrs. Coffman, *Come Back, Little Sheba,* U.S. cities, 1950-51; Mrs. Ochs, *Rhinoceros,* U.S. cities, 1961; Aary, *Morning's at Seven,* U.S. cities, 1976; title role *Daisy Mayme,* U.S. cities, 1979-80; Abby Brewster, *Arsenic and Old Lace,* U.S. cities, 1987; also *The Show-Off* and *Clara's Play,* both U.S. cities, 1983.

FILM DEBUT—Sister, *Damn Yankees* (also known as *What Lola*

Wants), Warner Brothers, 1958. PRINCIPAL FILM APPEARANCES— Sue, *Bells Are Ringing,* Metro-Goldwyn-Mayer, 1960; Shirley Johnson, *Something Wild,* United Artists, 1961; Sadie Finch, *Up the Down Staircase,* Warner Brothers, 1967; Mrs. Wrappler, *Cold Turkey,* United Artists, 1971; Goldfarb's secretary, *Klute,* Warner Brothers, 1971; Mrs. Price, *The Buddy System,* Twentieth Century-Fox, 1984.

PRINCIPAL TELEVISION APPEARANCES—Series: Gwen, *Woman with a Past,* CBS, 1954; Edith Bunker, *All in the Family,* CBS, 1971-80. Episodic: Emily Farnsworth, *Scarecrow and Mrs. King,* CBS, 1983; widow, *The Love Boat,* ABC, 1986; also Ogress, "Jack and the Beanstalk," and Fairy Godmother, "Cinderella," *Faerie Tale Theatre,* Showtime; *Camera Three,* CBS; *Danger,* CBS; *Studio One,* CBS; *Philco Television Playhouse,* NBC; *Omnibus,* CBS; *Today Is Ours,* NBC; *Naked City,* ABC; *Armstrong Circle Theatre,* NBC; *The Defenders,* CBS; *The Nurses,* CBS; *Eleventh Hour,* NBC; *Dr. Kildare,* NBC; *Dennis the Menace,* CBS; *The Jackie Gleason Show,* CBS; *Car 54, Where Are You?,* NBC; *True Story,* NBC; *The Patty Duke Show,* ABC; *Laugh-In,* NBC; *The Sonny and Cher Show,* CBS; *The Mike Douglas Show,* ABC; *The Carol Burnett Show,* CBS.

Movies: Mrs. DeCamp, *Tail Gunner Joe,* NBC, 1977; Aunt Mary Dobkin, *Aunt Mary,* CBS, 1979; Isabel Cooper, *Isabel's Choice,* CBS, 1981; Betty Eaton, *Angel Dusted,* NBC, 1981; Eleanor Roosevelt, *Eleanor, First Lady of the World,* CBS, 1982; Irene Wallin, *A Matter of Sex,* NBC, 1984; Ariadne Oliver, *Agatha Christie's "Dead Man's Folly,"* CBS, 1986. Specials: *Circus of the Stars,* CBS, 1977; *CBS: On the Air,* CBS, 1978; *The Stars Salute Israel at Thirty,* ABC, 1978; *Good Evening, Captain,* CBS, 1981; *Marlo Thomas in Acts of Love—And Other Comedies,* ABC, 1973; Penny Sycamore, *You Can't Take It with You,* CBS, 1979; Helen, "Grown Ups," *Broadway on Showtime,* Showtime, 1985, then *Great Performances,* PBS, 1986; *We the People,* CBS, 1986; Josephine, *Tender Places,* syndicated, 1987. Also appeared as Mrs. Tweed, *Something's Afoot.*

RELATED CAREER—Singer with the Robert Shaw Chorale in the production *Double Dozen Double Damask Dinner Napkins* on a tour of women's clubs, 1940.

NON-RELATED CAREER—U.S. Commissioner to the International Women's Year Commission and National Conference of Women, 1977; honorary board member, Center for Women in the Performing Arts, Emerson College, Boston, MA; president, advisory board, Women's Research and Institute, Washington, DC; board member, Eleanor Roosevelt's Val-Kill, Hyde Park, NY; board member, Wonder Woman Foundation, New York City; also worked as a secretary.

AWARDS: Golden Globe Awards and Emmy Awards, Outstanding Actress in a Leading Role in a Comedy Series, 1971, 1972, and 1978, all for *All in the Family;* Golden Globe Award, 1973, for *All in the Family;* honored by the National Commission of Working Women, 1981, for *Isabel's Choice;* Emmy Award nomination, Outstanding Lead Actress, 1982, for *Eleanor, First Lady of the World.* Honorary degrees: Emerson College, L.H.D.; also from Hood College, Frederick, MD, and Monmouth College, West Long Branch, NJ.

MEMBER: Actors' Equity Association (council member, 1958-63), Screen Actors Guild, American Federation of Television and Radio Artists.

SIDELIGHTS: RECREATIONS—Swimming, singing, and reading.

ADDRESSES: AGENT—Bauman, Hiller, and Strain, 9220 Sunset Boulevard, Suite 202, Los Angeles, CA 90069.*

*   *   *

STARR, Ringo   1940-

PERSONAL: Born Richard Starkey, July 7, 1940, in Liverpool, England; son of Richard (a house painter) and Elsie (a barmaid; maiden name, Cleave) Starkey; married Maureen Cox, February 11, 1965 (divorced, 1975); married Barbara Bach (an actress), April 27, 1981; children: Zak, Jason, Lee.

VOCATION: Singer, musician, and actor.

CAREER: FILM DEBUT—As himself, *A Hard Day's Night,* United Artists, 1964. PRINCIPAL FILM APPEARANCES—As himself, *Help!,* United Artists, 1965; as himself, *Yellow Submarine,* United Artists, 1968; Emmanuel, *Candy,* Cinerama, 1968; Youngman Grand, *The Magic Christian,* Commonwealth, 1970; as himself, *Let It Be,* United Artists, 1970; Larry the Dwarf, *200 Motels,* United Artists, 1971; Candy, *Blindman,* Twentieth Century-Fox, 1972; Merlin the Magician, *Son of Dracula* (also known as *Young Dracula*), Apple, 1974; Mike, *That'll Be the Day,* EMI, 1974; Pope, *Lisztomania,* Warner Brothers, 1975; Laslo Karolny, *Sextette,* Crown International, 1978; as himself, *The Last Waltz* (concert film), United Artists, 1978; as himself, *The Kids Are Alright,* New World, 1979; Atouk, *Caveman,* United Artists, 1981; as himself, *Give My Regards to Broad Street,* Twentieth Century-Fox, 1984; as himself, *Water,* Rank, 1985. Also appeared in *Born to Boogie,* 1974; *Ringo Stars,* 1976; *The Cooler,* 1982; and *Walking after Midnight,* Kay Film, 1988.

PRINCIPAL FILM WORK—Producer, *Son of Dracula,* Apple, 1974; also producer and director, *Born to Boogie,* 1974.

PRINCIPAL TELEVISION APPPEARANCES—Series: Mr. Conductor, *Shining Time Station,* PBS, 1989—. Mini-Series: Robin Valerian, *Princess Daisy,* NBC, 1983. Episodic: *The Jack Paar Show,* NBC, 1964; *The Ed Sullivan Show,* CBS, 1964, then 1965; *The David Frost Show,* syndicated, 1968. Movies: As himself, *Magical Mystery Tour,* BBC, 1967; voice of Dad/narrator, *The Point* (animated), ABC, 1971; Mock Turtle, *Alice in Wonderland,* CBS, 1985. Specials: As himself and Ognir Rrats, *Ringo,* NBC, 1978.

RECORDINGS: SINGLES—"Beaucoups of Blues," Apple, 1970; "It Don't Come Easy," Apple, 1971; "Back off Boogaloo," Apple, 1972; "Photograph," Apple, 1973; "You're Sixteen," Apple, 1974; "Oh My My," Apple, 1974; "Only You," Apple, 1974; "No No Song," Apple, 1975; "It's All Down to Goodnight Vienna," Apple, 1975; "A Dose of Rock 'n' Roll," Atlantic, 1976; "Hey Baby," Atlantic, 1977.

ALBUMS—*Sentimental Journey,* Apple, 1969; *Beaucoups of Blues,* Apple, 1970; *Ringo,* Apple, 1973; *Goodnight Vienna,* Apple, 1975; *Blast from Your Past,* Capitol, 1975; *Rotogravure,* Atlantic, 1976; *Ringo the 4th,* Atlantic, 1977; *Old Wave,* RCA, 1985.

With the Beatles: *Please, Please Me,* EMI, 1963; *With the Beatles,* EMI, 1963; *A Hard Day's Night,* EMI, 1964; *The Beatles for Sale,* EMI, 1965; *Help!,* EMI, 1965; *Rubber Soul,* EMI, 1966; *Revolver,*

EMI, 1966; *Sergeant Pepper's Lonely Hearts Club Band*, EMI, 1967; *Magical Mystery Tour*, EMI, 1967; *Yellow Submarine*, Apple, 1968; *The Beatles* (also known as *The White Album*), Apple, 1968; *Abbey Road*, Apple, 1969; *Let It Be*, Apple, 1970.

AWARDS: Order of the British Empire, 1966; as a member of the Beatles received numerous Grammy awards and inducted into the Rock and Roll Hall of Fame, 1988.

ADDRESSES: MANAGER—Bruce Grakal, Management III, 4570 Encino Avenue, Encino, CA 90069.*

*   *   *

STEENBURGEN, Mary   1953-

PERSONAL: Surname is pronounced "Steen-berjen"; born in 1953 in Newport, AR; father, a railroad conductor; married Malcolm MacDowell (an actor), 1980 (separated); children: Lilly Amanda, Charlie. EDUCATION: Attended Hendrix College; studied acting with Sanford Meisner at the Neighborhood Playhouse, New York City, 1972.

VOCATION: Actress.

CAREER: PRINCIPAL STAGE APPEARANCES—*Holiday*, Old Vic Theatre, London, 1987.

FILM DEBUT—Julia Tate, *Goin' South*, Paramount, 1978. PRINCIPAL FILM APPEARANCES—Amy Robbins, *Time After Time*, Warner Brothers/Orion, 1979; Lynda Dummar, *Melvin and Howard*, Universal, 1980; Mother, *Ragtime*, Paramount, 1981; Adrian, *A Midsummer Night's Sex Comedy*, Warner Brothers, 1982; Marjorie Kinnan Rawlings, *Cross Creek*, Universal, 1983; Phoebe, *Romantic Comedy*, Metro-Goldwyn-Mayer/United Artists (MGM/UA), 1983; Ginny Grainger, *One Magic Christmas*, Buena Vista, 1985; Kate McGovern, *Dead of Winter*, MGM/UA, 1987; young Sarah, *The Whales of August*, Island Alive, 1987; Rose Pickett, *End of the Line*, Orion, 1988. Also appeared in *Sanford Meisner—The Theatre's Best Kept Secret* (documentary), 1984.

PRINCIPAL FILM WORK—Executive producer, *End of the Line*, Orion, 1988.

PRINCIPAL TELEVISION APPEARANCES—Mini-Series: Nicole Warren Diver, *Tender Is the Night*, Showtime, 1985. Movies: Miep Gies, *The Attic: The Hiding of Anne Frank*, CBS, 1988. Episodic: "Little Red Riding Hood," *Faerie Tale Theatre*, Showtime.

RELATED CAREER—Member of an improvisational comedy troupe.

NON-RELATED CAREER—Waitress.

AWARDS: New York Film Critics Award, 1980, and Academy Award, 1981, both Best Supporting Actress, for *Melvin and Howard*.

ADDRESSES: AGENT—Martha Luttrell, Creative Artists Agency, 1888 Century Park E., 14th Floor, Los Angeles, CA 90067.*

STEINBERG, David   1942-

PERSONAL: Born August 9, 1942, in Winnipeg, MB, Canada; son of Jacob and Ruth Steinberg; wife's name, Judy; children: Sasha, Rebecca. EDUCATION: University of Chicago, M.A., English literature, 1962; also attended Hebrew Theological College.

VOCATION: Comedian, actor, director, and writer.

CAREER: Also see *WRITINGS* below. PRINCIPAL STAGE APPEARANCES—Ensemble, *The Return of the Second City in "20,000 Frozen Grenadiers,"* Square East Theatre, New York City, 1966; ensemble, *The Mad Show*, New Theatre, New York City, 1966; Kenny Newquist, *Little Murders*, Broadhurst Theatre, New York City, 1967; Seymour Levin, *Carry Me Back to Morningside Heights*, John Golden Theatre, New York City, 1968.

MAJOR TOURS—*From the Second City*, U.S cities, 1965.

PRINCIPAL FILM APPEARANCES—The Rat, *Fearless Frank* (also known as *Frank's Greatest Adventure*), American International, 1967; photographer, *The Lost Man*, Universal, 1969; Marty Lieberman, *The End*, United Artists, 1978; Harris Soane, *Something Short of Paradise*, American International, 1979; Meegosh, *Willow*, Metro-Goldwyn-Mayer/United Artists, 1988.

PRINCIPAL FILM WORK—Director: *The End*, United Artists, 1978; *Paternity*, Paramount, 1981; *Going Berserk*, Universal, 1983.

PRINCIPAL TELEVISION APPEARANCES—Series: Host, *The Music Scene*, ABC, 1969-70; host, *The David Steinberg Show*, CBS, 1972; host, *The Noonday Show*, NBC, 1975. Pilots: Host, *Out of Our Minds*, syndicated, 1984; host, *Just for Laughs*, CBS (Canada), 1987. Episodic: *The Tonight Show*, NBC, 1969—; also *The Smothers Brothers Comedy Hour*, CBS. Specials: *The Return of the Smothers Brothers*, NBC, 1970; *The George Segal Show*, NBC, 1974; *The Marx Brothers in a Nutshell*, PBS, 1982; voice of casting director, *Billy Crystal: A Comic's Line*, HBO, 1984; host, "Just for Laughs II," *Showtime Comedy Spotlight*, Showtime, 1987; also *Second City: Twenty-Five Years in Revue*.

PRINCIPAL TELEVISION WORK—All as director, unless indicated. Pilots: *Man about Town*, ABC, 1986; *One Big Family*, syndicated, 1986; *Baby on Board*, CBS, 1988. Episodic: *Newhart*, CBS, 1982—; "The Uncle Devil Show," *The Twilight Zone*, CBS, 1985; "Casey at the Bat," *Shelley Duvall's Tall Tales and Legends*, Showtime, 1986; *The Golden Girls*, NBC, 1986; *Designing Women*, CBS, 1987; *The Popcorn Kid*, CBS, 1987; *Duet*, Fox, 1987; *Family Man*, ABC, 1988; *Annie McGuire*, CBS, 1988; *Eisenhower and Lutz*, CBS, 1988.

Specials: All as executive producer. *The Young Comedians All-Star Reunion*, HBO, 1986; "Robin Williams—An Evening at the Met," *On Location*, HBO, 1986; *Michael Davis—The Life of the Party*, Cinemax, 1986; "Billy Crystal—Don't Get Me Started," *On Location*, HBO, 1986; "The Eleventh Annual Young Comedians Show," *On Location*, HBO, 1987; "Women of the Night," *On Location*, HBO, 1987; "Women of the Night II," *On Location*, HBO, 1988; "The Twelfth Annual Young Comedians Show," *On Location*, HBO, 1988; "An Evening with Sammy Davis, Jr. and Jerry Lewis," *HBO Comedy Hour*, HBO, 1988.

RELATED CAREER—Member, Second City (improvisational comedy troupe), Chicago, IL; director of television commercials for Pizza Hut, NCR, and Jell-O.

WRITINGS: FILM—(With Dana Olsen) *Going Berserk,* Universal, 1983. TELEVISION—Series: *The Music Scene,* ABC, 1969-70; (co-writer) *The Noonday Show,* NBC, 1975. Specials: (With Tom Smothers) *The Return of the Smothers Brothers,* NBC, 1970; *Michael Davis—The Life of the Party,* Cinemax, 1986.

RECORDINGS: David Steinberg Disguised as a Normal Person.

AWARDS: (With Roseanne Barr) Clio Award, 1987, for Pizza Hut commercial.

ADDRESSES: AGENT—Mark Teitelbaum, William Morris Agency, 151 El Camino Drive, Beverly Hills, CA 90212.*

*   *   *

STERLING, Jan   1923-
(Jane Sterling)

PERSONAL: Born Jane Sterling Adriance, April 3, 1923, in New York, NY; daughter of William Allen Adriance; married John Merivale (divorced); married Paul Douglas (an actor), May 12, 1950 (died, 1959); children: one son. EDUCATION: Trained for the stage at the Fay Compton Dramatic School.

VOCATION: Actress.

CAREER: BROADWAY DEBUT—(As Jane Sterling) Chris Faringdon, *Bachelor Born,* Morosco Theatre, 1938. PRINCIPAL STAGE APPEARANCES—(As Jane Sterling) Nancy Holmes, *When We Are Married,* Lyceum Theatre, New York City, 1939; (as Jane Sterling) Judith Weaver, *Grey Farm,* Hudson Theatre, New York City, 1940; (as Jane Sterling) Florrie, *Panama Hattie,* 46th Street Theatre, New York City, 1941; (as Jane Sterling) Margaret Stanley, *This Rock,* Longacre Theatre, New York City, 1943; (as Jane Sterling) Jan Lupton, *Over 21,* Music Box Theatre, New York City, 1944; Edith Bowsmith, *The Rugged Path,* Plymouth Theatre, New York City, 1945; Zelda Rainier, *Dunnigan's Daughter,* John Golden Theatre, New York City, 1945; Janet Alexander, *This, Too, Shall Pass,* Belasco Theatre, New York City, 1946; Daphne Stillington, *Present Laughter,* Plymouth Theatre, 1946; Karen Norwood, *Two Blind Mice,* Cort Theatre, New York City, 1949; Billie Dawn, *Born Yesterday,* Lyceum Theatre, 1949; Mary Murray, *Small War on Murray Hill,* Ethel Barrymore Theatre, New York City, 1957; Ann, *The Perfect Setup,* Cort Theatre, 1962; Madelaine Robbins, *Once for the Asking,* Booth Theatre, New York City, 1963; Terry, "The River," and Mary, "Mary Agnes Is Thirty-Five," in *Friday Night* (double-bill), Pocket Theatre, New York City, 1965; Mollie Malloy, *The Front Page,* Ethel Barrymore Theatre, 1970; Lola, *Come Back, Little Sheba,* Queens Playhouse, Flushing, NY, then Studio Arena Theatre, Buffalo, NY, both 1974; Mary, *The November People,* Billy Rose Theatre, New York City, 1978. Also appeared in *The Three Sisters,* Ethel Barrymore Theatre, 1942; *The Spider's Web,* Chicago, IL, 1958; with the New Theatre for Now Workshop, Mark Taper Forum, Los Angeles, CA, 1969; and in *Hot l Baltimore,* Royal Alexandra Theatre, Toronto, ON, Canada, 1975.

MAJOR TOURS—Billie Dawn, *Born Yesterday,* U.S. cities, 1947;

Mary, *John Loves Mary,* U.S. cities, 1948; Nell Nash, *The Gazebo,* U.S. cities, 1959; Sophie, Baroness Lemberg, *White Lies,* and Clea, *Black Comedy,* both U.S. cities, 1969; also in *Butterflies Are Free,* U.S. cities, 1971-72.

FILM DEBUT—Stella McGuire, *Johnny Belinda,* Warner Brothers, 1948. PRINCIPAL FILM APPEARANCES—Smoochie, *Caged,* Warner Brothers, 1950; Vivian Heldon, *Mystery Street,* Metro-Goldwyn-Mayer (MGM), 1950; Rita Rossini, *The Skipper Surprised His Wife,* MGM, 1950; Marge Wrighter, *Union Station,* Paramount, 1950; Dodie, *Appointment with Danger,* Paramount, 1951; Lorraine, *The Big Carnival* (also known as *Ace in the Hole* and *The Human Interest Story*), Paramount, 1951; Betsy, *The Mating Season,* Paramount, 1951; Polly Sickles, *Rhubarb,* Paramount, 1951; Sonya Baratow, *Flesh and Fury,* Universal, 1952; Dixie Delmar, *Sky Full of Moon,* MGM, 1952; Denny, *Pony Express,* Paramount, 1953; Dottie, *Split Second,* RKO, 1953; Rose Slater, *The Vanquished,* Paramount, 1953; Nicky, *Alaska Seas,* Paramount, 1954; Sally McKee, *The High and the Mighty,* Warner Brothers, 1954; Mary, *The Human Jungle,* Allied Artists, 1954; Frieda, *Return from the Sea,* Allied Artists, 1954; Amy Rawlinson, *Female on the Beach,* Universal, 1955; Nelly Bain, *Man with the Gun* (also known as *The Trouble Shooter* and *Man without a Gun*), United Artists, 1955; Brenda Martin, *Women's Prison,* Columbia, 1955; Beth Willis, *The Harder They Fall,* Columbia, 1956; Julia, *1984,* Columbia, 1956; Madge Pitts, *Slaughter on Tenth Avenue,* Universal, 1957; Lily Frayne, *The Female Animal,* Universal, 1958; Arlene Williams, *High School Confidential* (also known as *The Young Hellions*), MGM, 1958; Celeste Saunders, *Kathy O,* Universal, 1958; Sandra Slide, *Love in a Goldfish Bowl,* Paramount, 1961; Muriel Purvis, *The Incident,* Twentieth Century-Fox, 1967; Gloria Patton, *The Angry Breed,* Commonwealth United, 1969; Louise Baxter, *The Minx,* Cambist, 1969; Christine Snow, *First Monday in October,* Paramount, 1981. Also appeared in *Sammy Somebody,* 1976.

PRINCIPAL TELEVISION APPEARANCES—Series: Title role, *Publicity Girl,* syndicated, 1956; panelist, *You're in the Picture,* CBS, 1961; panelist, *Made in America,* CBS, 1964; also *The Guiding Light,* CBS, 1969-70. Mini-Series: Lou Hoover, *Backstairs at the White House,* NBC, 1979. Pilots: Selena Royce, *Luxury Liner* (broadcast as an episode of *The Dick Powell Show*), NBC, 1963; Gloria Miles, *At Your Service,* CBS, 1964; Mrs. Fontreil, *Having Babies,* ABC, 1976. Episodic: Barbara Howland, *Baby Boom,* NBC, 1988; also "The Book Overdue," *Medallion Theatre,* CBS, 1954; "Trip around the Block," *Ford Theatre,* NBC, 1954; *Rheingold Theatre,* NBC, 1955; *Lux Video Theatre,* NBC, 1956 and 1957; "Requiem for a Heavyweight," *Playhouse 90,* CBS, 1956; *Climax!,* CBS, 1956 and 1957; "Clipper Ship," *Playhouse 90,* CBS, 1957; *Kraft Theatre,* NBC, 1958; *Alfred Hitchcock Presents,* CBS, 1958 and 1962; *Wagon Train,* NBC, 1959 and 1961; *Alcoa Theatre,* NBC, 1960; *The Untouchables,* ABC, 1960; *Bonanza,* NBC, 1960; *General Electric Theatre,* CBS, 1960; *Naked City,* ABC, 1961; *The Dick Powell Theatre,* NBC, 1961; *Burke's Law,* ABC, 1963 and 1965; *Mannix,* CBS, 1968; *The Name of the Game,* NBC, 1969; *Medical Center,* CBS, 1971; also "Stand-In for Murder," *Lux Playhouse,* CBS. Movies: Letty Fairlain, *My Kidnapper, My Love,* NBC, 1980; Ray's mother, *Dangerous Company,* CBS, 1982.

AWARDS: Academy Award nomination, Best Supporting Actress, 1954, for *The High and the Mighty.*

MEMBER: Actors' Equity Association, Screen Actors Guild, American Federation of Television and Radio Artists.*

STERLING, Jane
  See STERLING, Jan

*   *   *

STERN, Daniel   1957-

PERSONAL: Born August 28, 1957, in Bethesda, MD.

VOCATION: Actor.

CAREER: PRINCIPAL STAGE APPEARANCES—Leo, *Lost and Found*, Ensemble Studio Theatre, New York City, 1979; the Reporter, *How I Got That Story*, Second Stage Theatre, New York City, 1980; Lee, *True West*, Cherry Lane Theatre, New York City, 1982. Also appeared in *Frankie and Annie*, Manhattan Theatre Club, New York City, 1978; *The Old Glory*, American Place Theatre, New York City; *Apparitions*, New York City; *Almost Men*, *Pastorale*, and *The Undefeated Rumba Champs*, all Off-Broadway productions.

PRINCIPAL FILM APPEARANCES—Student, *Starting Over*, Paramount, 1979; Cyril, *Breaking Away*, Twentieth Century-Fox, 1979; Cooperman, *It's My Turn*, Columbia, 1980; Hare Krishna, *One-Trick Pony*, Warner Brothers, 1980; actor, *Stardust Memories*, United Artists, 1980; crazy kid, *A Small Circle of Friends*, United Artists, 1980; Spanky, *Honky Tonk Freeway*, Universal, 1981; Laurence "Shrevie" Schreiber, *Diner*, Metro-Goldwyn-Mayer/United Artists (MGM/UA), 1982; Jim, *I'm Dancing as Fast as I Can*, Paramount, 1982; Lymangood, *Blue Thunder*, Columbia, 1983; Neil Allan, *Get Crazy*, Embassy, 1983; Reverend, *C.H.U.D.*, New World, 1984; Dusty, *Hannah and Her Sisters*, Orion, 1985; Michael Fine, *Key Exchange*, Twentieth Century-Fox, 1985; Joel Keefer, *The Boss' Wife*, Tri-Star, 1986; Jimmy, *Born in East L.A.*, Universal, 1987; Hal Petersham, *D.O.A.*, Buena Vista, 1988; Herbie Platt, *The Milagro Beanfield War*, Universal, 1988; Sixpack, *Leviathan*, MGM/UA, 1989.

TELEVISION DEBUT—*Vegetable Soup*. PRINCIPAL TELEVISION APPEARANCES—Series: Joey Nathan, *Hometown*, CBS, 1985; narrator (Kevin as an adult), *The Wonder Years*, ABC, 1988—. Pilots: Leon, *Man About Town*, ABC, 1986. Movies: Micah, *Samson and Delilah*, ABC, 1984; David Garfield, *Weekend War*, ABC, 1988. Specials: *Day-to-Day Affairs*, HBO, 1985.

PRINCIPAL TELEVISION WORK—Episodic: Director, *The Wonder Years*, ABC, 1989.

ADDRESSES: AGENTS—Nicole David and Cynthia Wolferson, Triad Artists, 10100 Santa Monica Boulevard, Suite 1600, Los Angeles, CA 90067.*

*   *   *

STEVENS, Craig   1918-

PERSONAL: Born Gail Shekles, July 8, 1918, in Liberty, MO; married Alexis Smith (an actress), 1944. EDUCATION: Attended the University of Kansas; studied acting at the Pasadena Playhouse.

VOCATION: Actor.

CAREER: BROADWAY DEBUT—Fred Gaily, *Here's Love*, Shubert Theatre, 1963. PRINCIPAL STAGE APPEARANCES—Appeared in productions of *King of Hearts*, *Plain and Fancy*, *Critic's Choice*, and *Mary, Mary*.

MAJOR TOURS—Julian, *Cactus Flower*, U.S. cities, 1958.

PRINCIPAL FILM APPEARANCES—Senate reporter, *Mr. Smith Goes to Washington*, Columbia, 1939; Robert Struck, *The Body Disappears*, Warner Brothers, 1941; John Thomas Anthony, *Dive Bomber*, Warner Brothers/First National, 1941; Alfred King, Jr., *Law of the Tropics*, Warner Brothers, 1941; Chuck Evans, *Steel against the Sky*, Warner Brothers, 1941; Peter Thorne, *The Hidden Hand*, Warner Brothers, 1942; Carl Becker, *Secret Enemies*, Warner Brothers, 1942; Ward Prescott, *Spy Ship*, Warner Brothers, 1942; Tom, *The Doughgirls*, Warner Brothers, 1944; as himself, *Hollywood Canteen*, Warner Brothers, 1944; Danny Williams, *Since You Went Away*, United Artists, 1944; Ed Rector, *God Is My Co-Pilot*, Warner Brothers, 1945; Jack Leslie, *Roughly Speaking*, Warner Brothers, 1945; Major Bruce, *Too Young to Know*, Warner Brothers, 1945; Monte Loeffler, *Humoresque*, Warner Brothers, 1946; Johnson, *The Man I Love*, Warner Brothers, 1946; Willard, *Love and Learn*, Warner Brothers, 1947; Carter Andrews, *That Way with Women*, Warner Brothers, 1947; Danvers, *The Lady Takes a Sailor*, Warner Brothers, 1949; Tony, *Night unto Night*, Warner Brothers, 1949.

Rick Martin, *Blues Busters*, Monogram, 1950; Ken Paine, *Where the Sidewalk Ends*, Twentieth Century-Fox, 1950; Braxton Summers, *Drums in the Deep South*, RKO, 1951; Stuart Grumbly, *Katie Did It*, Universal, 1951; Cyril Guthrie, *The Lady from Texas*, Universal, 1951; Mike Carr, *Phone Call from a Stranger*, Twentieth Century-Fox, 1952; Steve O'Malley, *Murder without Tears*, Allied Artists, 1953; Bruce Adams, *Abbott and Costello Meet Dr. Jekyll and Mr. Hyde*, Universal, 1954; Phil Barton, *The French Line*, RKO, 1954; Rene LaFarge, *Duel on the Mississippi*, Columbia, 1955; Colonel Joe Parkman, *The Deadly Mantis* (also known as *The Incredible Praying Mantis*), Universal, 1957; Abe Carbo, *Buchanan Rides Alone*, Columbia, 1958; Peter Gunn, *Gunn*, Paramount, 1967; Manston, *The Limbo Line*, London Independent Producers, 1969; Willard Gaylin, *S.O.B.*, Paramount, 1981; Carter, *The Trout* (also known as *La Truite*), Triumph, 1982. Also appeared in *Affectionately Yours*, Warner Brothers, 1941.

PRINCIPAL TELEVISION APPEARANCES—Series: Title role, *Peter Gunn*, NBC, 1958-60, then ABC, 1960-61; Michael Strait, *Man of the World*, ATV, then syndicated, 1962; Mike Bell, *Mr. Broadway*, CBS, 1964; Walter Carlson, *The Invisible Man*, NBC, 1975-76; Craig Stewart, *Dallas*, CBS, 1981. Mini-Series: Asher Berg, *Rich Man, Poor Man*, ABC, 1976. Pilots: Chief Joe Slattery, *Mighty O*, CBS, 1962; Walt Randolph, *The Best Years*, NBC, 1969; Whitman, *McCloud: Who Killed Miss U.S.A.?* (also known as *Portrait of a Dead Girl*), NBC, 1970; Charles Corman, *Female Instinct*, NBC, 1972; Nick Charles, *Nick and Nora*, ABC, 1975; Marcus Cabot, *The Cabot Connection*, CBS, 1977; Robert Grant, *The Love Boat II*, ABC, 1977; Hank Rogers, *The Eyes of Texas II*, NBC, 1980; John Travis, *The Home Front*, CBS, 1980; Cyrus Hampton, *Condor*, ABC, 1986.

Episodic: Amelia's brother-in-law, *Hotel*, ABC, 1985; Ames Caulfield, *Murder, She Wrote*, CBS, 1986; Admiral Andrews, *Supercarrier*, ABC, 1988; also *Ghost Story*, NBC, 1972; "The Villa," *The Love Boat*, ABC, 1985; as George Pfister, *Happy Days*, ABC; in *Studio '57* (also known as *Heinz Studio '57*), Dumont; *Jane Wyman Presents the Fireside Theatre*, NBC; *The*

Loretta Young Theatre, NBC; *Matinee Theatre*, NBC; *On Trial* (also known as *The Joseph Cotton Show*), CBS; *Pepsi-Cola Playhouse*, ABC; *Schlitz Playhouse of Stars*, CBS; *Undercurrent*, CBS; *The Millionaire*, CBS; *The Bold Ones*, NBC; *The Name of the Game*, NBC; *The Chevy Show*, NBC; *Four Star Playhouse*, CBS; *The Dinah Shore Show*, NBC; *Gruen Playhouse*, Dumont; *The Tennessee Ernie Ford Show* (also known as *The Ford Show*), NBC; *Ford Television Theatre*; *Lux Video Theatre*; *Summer on Ice*. Movies: Dr. Stuart Reynolds, *The Elevator*, ABC, 1974; Rudolf Van Bohlen, *Killer Bees*, ABC, 1974; Bill McClure, *Secrets of Three Hungry Wives*, NBC, 1978; Frank Poston, *Marcus Welby, M.D.—A Holiday Affair* (also known as *Dr. Marchus Welby in Paris*), ABC, 1988. Specials: *NBC's Sixtieth Anniversary Celebration*, NBC, 1986.

ADDRESSES: AGENT—Contemporary Artists, 132 Lasky Drive, Beverly Hills, CA 90212.*

*   *   *

STEVENS, Stella   1938-

PERSONAL: Born Estelle Caro Eggleston, October 1, 1938, in Yazoo City, MS; daughter of Thomas Ellett and Dovey Estelle (Caro) Eggleston; married Noble Herman Stephens, September 1, 1954; children: Herman Andrew. EDUCATION: Attended Memphis State University.

VOCATION: Actress and director.

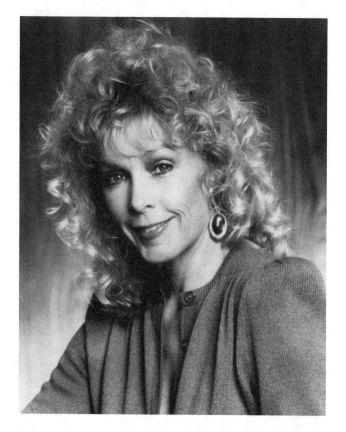

STELLA STEVENS

CAREER: PRINCIPAL FILM APPEARANCES—Chorine, *Say One for Me*, Twentieth Century-Fox, 1959; Chorine, *The Blue Angel*, Twentieth Century-Fox, 1959; Appassionata Von Climax, *Li'l Abner*, Paramount, 1960; Nina Jameson, *Man-Trap* (also known as *Man in Hiding*), Paramount, 1961; Robin Gantner, *Girls! Girls! Girls!*, Paramount, 1962; Jess Polanski, *Too Late Blues*, Paramount, 1962; Dolly Daley, *The Courtship of Eddie's Father*, Metro-Goldwyn-Mayer (MGM), 1963; Stella Purdy, *The Nutty Professor*, Paramount, 1963; Martha Lou, *Advance to the Rear* (also known as *Company of Cowards?*), MGM, 1964; Violet Lawson, *The Secret of My Success*, MGM, 1965; Joaney Adamic, *Synanon* (also known as *Get Off My Back*), Columbia, 1965; Perla, *Rage*, Columbia, 1966; Gail Hendricks, *The Silencers*, Columbia, 1966; Carol Corman, *How to Save a Marriage—And Ruin Your Life* (also known as *Band of Gold*), Columbia, 1968; Stacey Woodward, *Sol Madrid* (also known as *The Heroin Gang*), MGM, 1968; Sister George, *Where Angels Go . . . Trouble Follows*, Columbia, 1968; Ellen Hardy, *The Mad Room*, Columbia, 1969.

Hildy, *The Ballad of Cable Hogue*, Warner Brothers, 1970; Alvira, *A Town Called Hell* (also known as *A Town Called Bastard*), Scotia International, 1971; Ann Cooper, *Slaughter*, American International, 1972; Yvonne Kellerman, *Stand Up and Be Counted*, Columbia, 1972; Linda Rogo, *The Poseidon Adventure*, Twentieth Century-Fox, 1973; Karen, *Arnold*, Cinerama, 1973; Dragon Lady, *Cleopatra Jones and the Casino of Gold*, Warner Brothers, 1975; Lucky, *Las Vegas Lady*, Crown International, 1976; Marty Reeves, *Nickelodeon*, Columbia, 1976; Amelia Crusoe, *The Manitou*, AVCO-Embassy, 1978; Captain Taylor, *Chained Heat*, Jensen Farley, 1983; Marg Graves, *Wacko*, Greydon Clark, 1984; Nicki Dixon, *The Longshot*, Orion, 1986; Margo Crane, *The Monster in the Closet*, Troma, 1987. Also appeared in *Adventures beyond Belief*, Sony Video Software, 1988; *Beverly Hills Mom*, 1989.

PRINCIPAL FILM WORK—Director: *The American Heroine* (documentary), Stellar Films, 1983; *The Ranch*, Westsky Entertainment, 1988.

TELEVISION DEBUT—Laura, *Johnny Ringo*, ABC, 1962. PRINCIPAL TELEVISION APPEARANCES—Series: Lute Mae Sanders, *Flamingo Road*, NBC, 1981-82. Pilots: Marcia, *The New, Original Wonder Woman*, ABC, 1975; Martha McVea, *Charlie Cobb: Nice Night for a Hanging*, NBC, 1977; Leonara Klopman, *The New Love Boat* (also known as *The Love Boat III*), ABC, 1977; Stella Stafford, *Kiss Me, Kill Me*, CBS, 1977; Virna Stewart, *The Jordan Chance*, CBS, 1978; Dr. Fleming, *Hart to Hart*, ABC, 1979; Lute Mae Sanders, *Flamingo Road*, NBC, 1980; Sheriff Nellie Wilder, *No Man's Land*, NBC, 1984; Loretta Kimbell, *Neat and Tidy*, syndicated, 1986. Episodic: Laura Jericho, "The Graduation Dress," *General Electric Theatre*, CBS, 1964; Lovi Alberti, "The Great Alberti," *General Electric Theatre*, CBS, 1965; Jane Hancock, *Ben Casey* (five episodes), ABC, 1965; Ellen, "Craig's Will," *Alfred Hitchcock Presents*, NBC, 1965; Lally Vanderpost, *Magnum, P.I.*, CBS, 1986; Mimi Carteret, "Tales from the Hollywood Hills: A Table at Ciro's," *Great Performances*, PBS, 1987; also *Ghost Story*, NBC, 1972.

Movies: Elizabeth Chapel, *In Broad Daylight*, ABC, 1971; Sheila Chilko, *Climb an Angry Mountain*, NBC, 1972; Linda Reston, *Linda*, ABC, 1973; Kate Barker, *The Day the Earth Moved*, ABC, 1974; Gold Dust, *Honky Tonk*, NBC, 1974; Lola Watkins, *Wanted: The Sundance Woman* (also known as *Mrs. Sundance Rides Again*, ABC, 1976; Kate Malloy, *The Night They Took Miss Beautiful*, NBC, 1977; Stella Chernak, *Murder in Peyton Place*, NBC, 1977; Marilyn Magnesun, *Cruise into Terror*, ABC, 1978; Louise Crawford, *The French Atlantic Affair,* ABC, 1979; Edyth, *Friendships, Secrets, and Lies,* NBC, 1979; Deidra Price, *Make Me an Offer,* ABC, 1980; Sherry Malik, *Children of Divorce,* NBC, 1980; Carolyn Moore, *Twirl,* NBC, 1981; Lieutenant Janet Alexander, *Women of San Quentin,* NBC, 1983; Katherine Lundquist, *Amazons,* ABC, 1984; Della Valance/Deb Potts, *A Masterpiece of Murder,* NBC, 1986; Joey Day, *Man against the Mob,* NBC, 1988; Katherine St. Urban, *Fatal Confessions: A Father Dowling Mystery,* NBC, 1988. Specials: *The Bob Hope Show,* NBC, 1968; *Nashville Remembers Elvis on His Birthday,* NBC, 1978; *Bob Hope's All-Star Look at TV's Prime Time Wars,* NBC, 1980; *Bob Hope's Women I Love—Beautiful but Funny,* NBC, 1982; judge, *1989 Miss U.S.A. Pageant,* CBS, 1989.

RELATED CAREER—Model, author, artist, and songwriter.

ADDRESSES: OFFICE—Stellavisions, 6520 Selma Avenue, Suite 649, Hollywood, CA 90028. AGENTS—Jim Cota and Michael Livingston, The Artists Agency, 10000 Santa Monica Boulevard, Suite 305, Beverly Hills, CA 90067.

*   *   *

STEWART, Catherine Mary

PERSONAL: Born April 22, in Edmonton, AB, Canada; father, a biology professor; mother, a physiology teaching assistant; married John Findlater (an actor and photographer), 1983.

VOCATION: Actress.

CAREER: FILM DEBUT—Bibi, *The Apple* (also known as *Star-Rock*), Cannon Releasing, 1980. PRINCIPAL FILM APPEARANCES—London salesgirl, *Nighthawks,* Universal, 1981; Maggie Gordon, *The Last Starfighter,* Universal, 1984; Regina, *Night of the Comet,* Atlantic, 1984; Bunny, *Mischief,* Twentieth Century-Fox, 1984; Jessie, *Dudes,* New Century/Vista, 1987; Miranda Dorlac, *Nightflyers,* New Century/Vista, 1987; Debi DiAngelo, *Scenes from the Goldmine,* Hemdale Releasing, 1987; Angie, *World Gone Wild,* Lorimar/Media Home Entertainment, 1988.

PRINCIPAL TELEVISION APPEARANCES—Series: Kayla Brady, *Days of Our Lives,* NBC. Mini-Series: Angel Hudson, *Hollywood Wives,* ABC, 1985; young Helene, *Sins,* CBS, 1986. Pilots: Angela Taylor, *The Annihilator,* NBC, 1986. Movies: Carol, *A Killer in the Family,* ABC, 1983; Lisa Nolen, *With Intent to Kill,* CBS, 1984; Betsy, *Midas Valley,* ABC, 1985; Merissa Winfield, *Murder by the Book,* CBS, 1987; Nancy Oakes DeMarigny, *Passion and Paradise,* ABC, 1989.

RELATED CAREER—Performed with a professional dance company, Middle Eastern and European cities.

ADDRESSES: AGENT—The Gage Group, 9229 Sunset Boulevard, Suite 306, Los Angeles, CA 90069.*

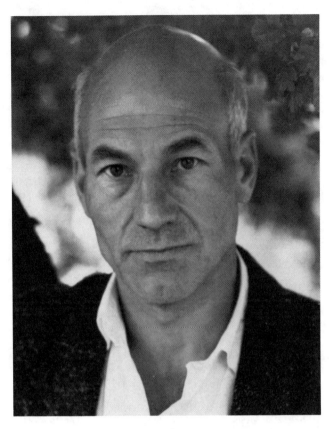

PATRICK STEWART

STEWART, Patrick   1940-

PERSONAL: Born July 13, 1940, in Mirfield, England; son of Alfred (a professional soldier) and Gladys (a weaver; maiden name, Barraclough) Stewart; married Sheila Falconer (a choreographer), March 3, 1966; children: Sophie Alexandra Falconer, Daniel Freedom. EDUCATION: Trained for the stage at the Bristol Old Vic Theatre School.

VOCATION: Actor and writer.

CAREER: Also see *WRITINGS* below. STAGE DEBUT—Morgan, *Treasure Island,* Lincoln Repertory Company, Theatre Royal, Lincoln, U.K., 1959. LONDON DEBUT—Second witness, *The Investigation,* Royal Shakespeare Company, Aldwych Theatre, 1966. BROADWAY DEBUT—Snout, *A Midsummer Night's Dream,* Billy Rose Theatre, 1971. PRINCIPAL STAGE APPEARANCES—Title role, *Henry V,* and Aston, *The Caretaker,* both Manchester Library Theatre, Manchester, U.K., 1963; Alexander Grant, *Body and Soul,* Palace Theatre, Watford, U.K., 1983; King David, then title role, *Yonadab,* National Theatre, London, 1985; George, *Who's Afraid of Virginia Woolf?,* Young Vic Theatre, London, 1987. Also appeared as Goldberg, *The Birthday Party,* title role, *Galileo,* and Shylock, *The Merchant of Venice;* and in repertory at the Playhouse Theatre, Sheffield, U.K., 1959-61, Liverpool Playhouse, Liverpool, U.K., 1963-64, and with the Bristol Old Vic Theatre Company, Bristol, U.K., 1965.

With the Royal Shakespeare Company (RSC): Sir Walter Blunt, *Henry IV, Part One,* Mowbray, *Henry IV, Part Two,* First Player and Player King, *Hamlet,* second witness, *The Investigation,* Dauphin, *Henry V,* and Hippolito, *The Revenger's Tragedy,* all Stratford-on-Avon, U.K., 1966; Duke Senior, *As You Like It,* Grumio, *The Taming of the Shrew,* and Worthy, *The Relapse,* all Stratford-on-Avon, then Aldwych Theatre, London, both 1967; Cornwall, *King Lear,* Touchstone, *As You Like It,* Hector, *Troilus and Cressida,* and Borachio, *Much Ado about Nothing,* all Stratford-on-Avon, then Aldwych Theatre, 1968; Teddy Foran, *The Silver Tassie,* Hippolito, *The Revenger's Tragedy,* Hector, *Troilus and Cressida,* and Leatherhead, *Bartholomew Fayre,* all Aldwych Theatre, 1969; Edward IV, *Richard III,* title role, *King John,* and Stephano, *The Tempest,* all Stratford-on-Avon, 1970; Launce, *The Two Gentlemen of Verona,* Stratford-on-Avon, then Aldwych Theatre, both 1970; Snout, *A Midsummer Night's Dream,* Roger, *The Balcony,* and Mikhail Skrobotov, *Enemies,* all Aldwych Theatre, 1971; Kabac, *Occupations,* The Place Theatre, London, 1971; Aufidius, *Coriolanus,* and Bassianus, *Titus Andronicus,* both Stratford-on-Avon, 1972; Cassius, *Julius Caesar,* and Enobarbus, *Antony and Cleopatra,* both Stratford-on-Avon, 1972, then Aldwych Theatre, 1973; Aaron, *Titus Andronicus,* Aldwych Theatre, 1973; Astrov, *Uncle Vanya,* Other Place Theatre, Stratford-on-Avon, 1974; Eilert Lovborg, *Hedda Gabler,* Aldwych Theatre, 1975; Larry Slade, *The Iceman Cometh,* Aldwych Theatre, 1976; Oberon, *A Midsummer Night's Dream,* Royal Shakespeare Theatre, Stratford-on-Avon, then Aldwych Theatre, both 1977; doctor, *Every Good Boy Deserves Favour,* Royal Festival Hall, London, 1977; Knatchbull, *That Good Between Us,* Shakespeare, *Bingo,* and Basho, *The Bundle,* all Warehouse Theatre, London, 1977; Enobarbus, *Antony and Cleopatra,* Royal Shakespeare Theatre, 1978, then Aldwych Theatre, 1979; Shylock, *The Merchant of Venice,* and Theseus, *Hippolytus,* both Other Place Theatre, 1978, then Warehouse Theatre, 1979; Colonel Guieson, *The Biko Inquest,* Other Place Theatre, 1979; Viktor Myshlaevsky, *The White Guard,* Aldwych Theatre, 1979; Leontes, *The Winter's Tale,* title role, *Titus Andronicus,* and Sir Eglamour, *The Two Gentlemen of Verona,* all Stratford-on-Avon, 1981, then London, 1982; title role, *Henry IV, Part One* and *Part Two,* Barbican Theatre, London, 1982-83.

MAJOR TOURS—Duke de Gire, *Lady of the Camelias,* second officer, *Twelfth Night,* and cafe customer, *Duel of Angels,* all Old Vic Theatre Company, Australian, New Zealand, and South American cities, 1961-62; Duke Senior, *As You Like It,* Grumio, *The Taming of the Shrew,* and Worthy, *The Relapse,* all RSC, U.S. cities, 1967-68; Cornwall, *King Lear,* Touchstone, *As You Like It,* Borachio, *Much Ado about Nothing,* and Hector, *Troilus and Cressida,* all RSC, U.S. cities, 1968-69; Eilert Lovborg, *Hedda Gabler,* RSC, U.S., Canadian, and Australian cities, 1975.

PRINCIPAL FILM APPEARANCES—McCann, *Hennessy,* American International, 1975; Eilert Lovborg, *Hedda,* Brut, 1975; Leondegrance, *Excalibur,* Warner Brothers, 1981; voice of Major, *The Plague Dogs* (animated), United International, 1982; Mr. Duffner, *Uindii* (also known as *Races*), Toho-Toha, 1984; Gurney Halek, *Dune,* Universal, 1984; Dr. Armstrong, *Lifeforce,* Tri-Star, 1985; Colonel Watson, *Code Name: Emerald,* Metro-Goldwyn-Mayer/United Artists, 1985; Russian general, *Wild Geese II,* Allied Artists, 1985; Dr. Mackie, *The Doctor and the Devils,* Twentieth Century-Fox, 1985; Henry Grey, Duke of Suffolk, *Lady Jane,* Paramount, 1986.

PRINCIPAL TELEVISION APPEARANCES—Series: The Inventor, *Eleventh Hour,* BBC, 1975; Doctor Edward Roebuck, *Maybury,* BBC, 1980; Captain Jean-Luc Picard, *Star Trek: The Next Genera-*

tion, syndicated, 1987—. Mini-Series: Sejanus, *I, Claudius,* BBC, 1976, then *Masterpiece Theatre,* PBS, 1977; Karla, *Tinker, Tailor, Soldier, Spy,* BBC and PBS, both 1979; Karla, *Smiley's People,* BBC, then syndicated, both 1982; also *Playing Shakespeare,* London Weekend Television (LWT), then PBS, 1983. Episodic: Narrator, "Great Plains Massacre" and "Reflections on a River," *Horizon,* BBC; narrator, "Henry VII," *Timewatch,* BBC; narrator, *The Making of Modern London: London at War,* LWT. Movies: Wilkins, *Little Lord Fauntleroy,* CBS, 1980; Party Secretary Gomulka, *Pope John Paul II,* CBS, 1984. Plays: Enobarbus, *Antony and Cleopatra,* ATV, 1973, then PBS, 1975; title role, *Oedipus Rex,* BBC, 1976; Jean, *Miss Julie,* BBC, 1977; Claudius, *Hamlet,* BBC and PBS, both 1980; Reverend Anthony Anderson, *The Devil's Disciple,* BBC, 1986. Also appeared as Lenin, *Fall of Eagles,* BBC, 1973; Anton, *The Artist's Story,* BBC, 1973; Gurvich, *The Love Girl and the Innocent,* BBC, 1973; Joseph Conrad, *Conrad,* BBC, 1974; Father, *Joby,* Yorkshire Television, 1974; Attlee, *A Walk with Destiny,* BBC, 1974; Guthrum, *Alfred the Great,* BBC, 1974; John Thornton, *North and South,* BBC, 1975; Largo Caballero, *The Madness,* BBC, 1976; Milos, *When the Actors Come,* BBC, 1978; Sergey Tolstoy, *Tolstoy: A Question of Faith,* BBC, 1979; Doctor Knox, *The Anatomist,* BBC, 1980; Signor Carini, *The Holy Experiment,* BBC, 1984; Salieri, *The Mozart Inquest,* BBC, 1985.

PRINCIPAL RADIO APPEARANCES—Plays: Mr. Peachum, *The Beggar's Opera;* Ludovico Notta, *Naked;* Caliban, *The Tempest;* Creon, *Oedipus Rex, Oedipus at Colonus,* and *Antigone;* Bernard Thorpe, *Mrs. Moffat, Mrs. Moffat;* the Doctor, *A Country Doctor's Notebook;* John Dundas Cochran, *Explorers Extraordinary;* Hillary Hawkins, *Bluey;* Edward, *Myths and Legacies.*

RELATED CAREER—Associate artist, Royal Shakespeare Company, 1967—; joint artistic director, Alliance for Creative Theatre, Education, and Research (ACTER) Shakespeare Company; associate director, ACTER, University of California, Santa Barbara; acting teacher.

NON-RELATED CAREER—Journalist and furniture salesman.

WRITINGS: STAGE—(Adaptor, with Michael Glenny) *The Procurator* (based on *The Master and Margharita* by M. Bulgakov). RADIO—(Adaptor) *A Country Doctor's Notebook* and (adaptor) *A Christmas Carol.* OTHER—*Wooing, Wedding and Repenting* (a Shakespeare anthology); "Shylock," *Players of Shakespeare,* Cambridge University Press; "Titus Andronicus," *Prefaces to Shakespeare,* BBC Publications.

AWARDS: Olivier Award, Best Supporting Actor, 1979, for *Antony and Cleopatra;* Olivier Award nomination, Best Actor, 1979, for *The Merchant of Venice;* London Fringe Award, Best Actor, 1987, for *Who's Afraid of Virginia Woolf?*

MEMBER: British Association of Film and Television Arts.

SIDELIGHTS: RECREATIONS—Cinema; fell-walking.

ADDRESSES: AGENTS—Duncan Heath Associates, Paramount House, 162 Wardour Street, London W1, England; International Creative Management, 8899 Beverly Boulevard, Los Angeles, CA 90048.

STING 1951-

PERSONAL: Full name, Gordon Matthew Sumner; born October 2, 1951, in Newcastle-on-Tyne, England; son of Ernest Matthew (a milkman) and Audrey (a hairdresser; maiden name, Cowell) Sumner; married Frances Eleanor Tomelty, May 1, 1976 (divorced, March, 1984); children: Joseph, Katherine; also two children with actress Trudie Styler. EDUCATION: Graduated from Warwick University.

VOCATION: Singer, actor, and songwriter.

CAREER: PRINCIPAL FILM APPEARANCES—Ace Face, *Quadrophenia,* World Northal, 1979; Just Like Eddie, *Radio On,* Unifilm, 1980; Martin Taylor, *Brimstone and Treacle,* United Artists, 1982; Feyd-Rautha, *Dune,* Universal, 1984; Victor Frankenstein, *The Bride,* Columbia, 1985; as himself, *Bring on the Night* (concert film), Goldwyn/A&M, 1985; Mick, *Plenty,* Twentieth Century-Fox, 1985; Daniel, *Julia and Julia,* Cinecom, 1987; Finney, *Stormy Monday,* Atlantic, 1988; heroic officer, *The Adventures of Baron Munchausen,* Columbia, 1988. Also appeared in (with the Police) *The Secret Policeman's Other Ball* (concert film), 1982; (with the Police) *Urgh! A Music War* (concert film); and *The Police—Synchronicity Concert Film.*

PRINCIPAL TELEVISION APPEARANCES—Episodic: *Saturday Night Live,* NBC, 1987; *Top of the Pops,* CBS, 1987. Specials: *The Prince's Trust All-Star Rock Concert,* HBO, 1986; *Rolling Stone Magazine's 20 Years of Rock 'n' Roll,* ABC, 1987; "Human Rights Now Tour," *HBO World Stage,* HBO, 1988; "Sting in Tokyo," *HBO World Stage,* HBO, 1989. Also appeared as an angel, *Artemus 81,* BBC.

RELATED CAREER—Singer, bass player, and songwriter with the Police; actor in British television commercials.

NON-RELATED CAREER—School teacher, Newcastle-on-Tyne, U.K., 1975-77.

RECORDINGS: All released on A&M Records, unless indicated. ALBUMS—(Contributor; also with the Police) *Brimstone and Treacle* (original soundtrack), 1982; *The Dream of The Blue Turtles,* 1985; *Bring on the Night,* 1985; *Nothing Like the Sun,* 1987.

With the Police: *Outlandos d'Amour,* 1977; *Reggatta De Blanc,* 1979; *Zenyatta Mondatta,* 1980; *Ghost in the Machine,* 1981; (contributor) *Party, Party* (original soundtrack), 1982; *Synchronicity,* 1983; *Every Breath You Take: The Singles* (compilation), 1986; also (contributor) *The Secret Policeman's Other Ball,* 1982.

AWARDS: (With the Police) Grammy Awards, 1980, 1981, and 1983; Grammy Award, 1987.

MEMBER: Performing Rights Society.

ADDRESSES: OFFICES—IRL, Bugle House, 21-A Noel Street, London W1, England; Frontier Booking International, 1776 Broadway, New York, NY 10019. AGENT—Hildy Gottlieb, International Creative Management, 8899 Beverly Boulevard, Los Angeles, CA 90048.*

STOCKWELL, John 1961-

PERSONAL: Born John Samuels IV, March 25, 1961, in Galveston, TX; son of John Samuels III (an attorney). EDUCATION: Received degree in visual and environmental studies from Harvard University; studied acting at the Royal Academy of Dramatic Art and with Hal Asprey at the Actors Workshop, New York University School of the Arts; studied voice technique with Marv Duff at the National Theatre, London.

VOCATION: Actor, screenwriter, and director.

CAREER: Also see *WRITINGS* below. PRINCIPAL STAGE APPEARANCES—Lobo, *Camino Real,* Williamstown Theatre Festival, Williamstown, MA; also appeared in *The Merry Wives of Windsor* and *Macbeth,* both Houston Shakespeare Festival, Houston, TX; *Spring's Awakening,* Brighton Festival, Brighton, U.K.; *Three Boys,* Playwrights Horizons, New York City; as Hal, *Loot;* and in *Ah, Wilderness!.*

FILM DEBUT—Jim Sterling, *So Fine,* Warner Brothers, 1981. PRINCIPAL FILM APPEARANCES—Dennis Guilder, *Christine,* Columbia, 1983; Keith Livingston, *Eddie and the Cruisers,* Embassy, 1983; Spider, *Losin' It,* Embassy, 1983; Leland ("Lee"), *City Limits,* Atlantic, 1985; Michael Harlan, *My Science Project,* Buena Vista, 1985; Randy McDevitt, *Dangerously Close,* Cannon, 1986; Phillip Marlowe, *Radioactive Dreams,* De Laurentiis Entertainment Group, 1986; Cougar, *Top Gun,* Paramount, 1986.

PRINCIPAL FILM WORK—Director (with Scott Fields), *Under Cover,* Cannon, 1987.

PRINCIPAL TELEVISION APPEARANCES—Series: *The Guiding Light,* CBS. Mini-Series: Billy Hazard, *North and South,* ABC, 1985. Pilots: Mick, *Too Good to Be True,* ABC, 1983. Episodic: Gilmore, *Miami Vice,* NBC, 1986. Movies: Scott Massey, *Quarterback Princess,* CBS, 1983; Brad Sedgwick, *Billionaire Boys Club,* NBC, 1987. Specials: Maxwell Fletcher, "A Family Tree," *Trying Times,* PBS, 1987.

RELATED CAREER—Rhythym guitarist and lead singer, the Brood (a New York City-based rock group).

WRITINGS: FILM—(With Scott Fields and Marty Ross) *Dangerously Close,* Cannon, 1986; (with Fields) *Under Cover,* Cannon, 1987.

ADDRESSES: AGENT—John Kimble, Triad Artists, 10100 Santa Monica Boulevard, 16th Floor, Los Angeles, CA 90067.*

*   *   *

STONE, Sharon

PERSONAL: Born c. 1958, in Meadville, PA. EDUCATION: Studied English and drama at Edinboro State University.

VOCATION: Actress.

CAREER: FILM DEBUT—Pretty girl on train, *Stardust Memories,* United Artists, 1980. PRINCIPAL FILM APPEARANCES—Lana, *Deadly Blessing,* United Artists, 1981; Blake Chandler, *Irreconcilable Differences,* Warner Brothers, 1984; Jesse Huston, *King*

Solomon's Mines, Cannon, 1985; Jesse Huston, *Allan Quatermain and the Lost City of Gold,* Cannon, 1986; Cathy Conners, *Cold Steel,* Cintel, 1987; Claire Mattson, *Police Academy 4: Citizens on Patrol,* Warner Brothers, 1987; Patrice Dellaplane, *Action Jackson,* Lorimar, 1988; Sara Toscani, *Above the Law,* Warner Brothers, 1988. Also appeared in *Les Uns et les autres* (also known as *Bolero*), Double 13, 1982; in *Personal Choice,* 1989; and in *Blood and Sand.*

PRINCIPAL TELEVISION APPEARANCES—Series: Cathy St. Marie, *Bay City Blues,* NBC, 1983. Mini-Series: Janice Henry, *War and Remembrance,* ABC, 1988. Pilots: Detective Dani Starr, *Hollywood Starr* (broadcast as an episode of *T.J. Hooker*), ABC, 1985; Ashley Hamilton Ryan, *Mr. and Mrs. Ryan,* ABC, 1986; Alex Neil, *Badlands 2005* (also known as *Badlands*), ABC, 1988. Episodic: *Magnum P.I.,* CBS. Movies: Lynette, *Not Just Another Affair,* CBS, 1982; Cassie Bascomb, *Calendar Girl Murders,* ABC, 1984; Sarah Shipman, *The Vegas Strip Wars,* NBC, 1984; Casey Cantrell, *Tears in the Rain* (also known as *Harlequin Romance Movie*), Showtime, 1988.

RELATED CAREER—Contestant, Miss Pennsylvania beauty pageant; professional model; actress in television commercials.

ADDRESSES: AGENT—Paula Wagner, Creative Artists Agency, 1888 Century Park E., Suite 1400, Los Angeles, CA 90067.*

*   *   *

STRAIGHT, Beatrice   1918-

PERSONAL: Full name, Beatrice Whitney Straight; born August 2, 1918, in Old Westbury, NY; daughter of Willard Dickerman (a career U.S. Army officer, businessman, and diplomat) and Dorothy Payne (Whitney) Straight; married Peter Cookson (a producer, actor, and writer), June 2, 1949; children: Gary, Tony. EDUCATION: Trained for the stage with Michael Chekhov at the Michael Chekhov Theatre Studio and with Tamara Daykarhanova.

VOCATION: Actress, producer, and director.

CAREER: BROADWAY DEBUT—A spinning girl, *Bitter Oleander,* Lyceum Theatre, 1935. PRINCIPAL STAGE APPEARANCES—Viola, *Twelfth Night,* and Goneril, *King Lear,* both Dartington Hall Players, Ridgefield, CT, 1939; Lisa, *The Possessed,* Lyceum Theatre, New York City, 1939; Viola, *Twelfth Night,* St. James Theatre, New York City, 1941; Angela, *Land of Fame,* Belasco Theatre, New York City, 1943; Felina, *The Wanhope Building,* Princess Theatre, New York City, 1947; Emily Dickinson, *Eastward in Eden,* Royale Theatre, New York City, 1947; Lady Macduff, *Macbeth,* National Theatre, New York City, 1948; Catherine Sloper, *The Heiress,* Biltmore Theatre, New York City, 1948; Miss Giddens, *The Innocents,* Playhouse Theatre, New York City, 1950; Nell Valentine, *The Grand Tour,* Martin Beck Theatre, New York City, 1951; Hesione Hushabye, *Heartbreak House,* Brattle Theatre, Cambridge, MA, 1952; Elizabeth Proctor, *The Crucible,* Martin Beck Theatre, 1953; Christine Collinger, *Sing Me No Lullaby,* Phoenix Theatre, New York City, 1954; Marie Chassaigne, *The River Line,* Carnegie Hall Playhouse, New York City, 1957.

Title role, *Phedre,* Greenwich Mews Theatre, New York City, 1966; Blanche du Bois, *A Streetcar Named Desire,* Berkshire Theatre Festival, Stockbridge, MA, 1967; Mrs. Toothe, *Everything*

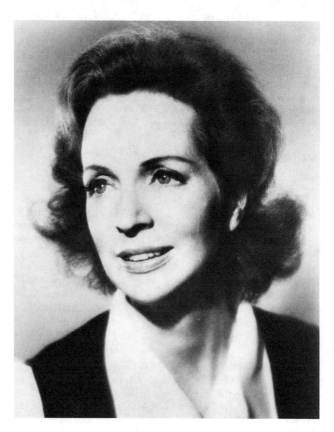

BEATRICE STRAIGHT

in the Garden, Plymouth Theatre, New York City, 1967; the Mother, *The Palace at 4 A.M.,* John Drew Theatre, Easthampton, NY, 1972; Helene Alving, *Ghosts,* Roundabout Theatre, New York City, 1973; Kate Keller, *All My Sons,* Roundabout Theatre, 1974; Gertrude, *Hamlet,* Circle Repertory Company, New York City, 1979. Also appeared with the Long Island Festival Repertory Company, Long Island, NY, 1968; and as Kate, *Old Times,* Lake Forest, IL, 1977.

PRINCIPAL STAGE WORK—Producer, *Pygmalion,* Ethel Barrymore Theatre, New York City, 1945; producer, *Playboy of the Western World,* Booth Theatre, New York City, 1946; producer, *Henry IV, Parts I and II, Uncle Vanya,* and a double bill of *Oedipus* and *The Critic,* all Old Vic Theatre Company, Century Theatre, New York City, 1946; director, *Who Am I?,* Young World Foundation Theatre Company, New York City, 1971-73.

MAJOR TOURS—Catherine Sloper, *The Heiress,* U.S. cities, 1948; title role, *Phedre,* U.K. cities, 1966-67; Blanche du Bois, *A Streetcar Named Desire,* U.S. cities, 1969-70; also *The Right Honourable Gentleman,* U.S. cities, 1971.

PRINCIPAL FILM APPEARANCES—Mrs. Fortness, *Phone Call from a Stranger,* Twentieth Century-Fox, 1952; Nancy Staples, *Patterns,* United Artists, 1956; Theorai, *The Silken Affair,* RKO, 1957; Mother Christophe, *The Nun's Story,* Warner Brothers, 1959; Mrs. Burns, *The Young Lovers,* Metro-Goldwyn-Mayer, 1964; Louise Schumacher, *Network,* United Artists, 1977; Kate Erling, *Bloodline,* Paramount, 1979; Marion, *The Promise,* Univeral, 1979; Kay Neeley, *The Formula,* United Artists, 1980; Rose, *Endless Love,* Universal, 1981; Dr. Lesh, *Poltergeist,* Metro-

Goldwyn-Mayer/United Artists, 1983; Ruth, *Two of a Kind,* Twentieth Century-Fox, 1983; Claire Hastings, *Power,* Twentieth Century-Fox, 1986.

PRINCIPAL TELEVISION APPEARANCES—Series: Mrs. Hacker, *Beacon Hill,* CBS, 1975; Louisa Beauchamp, *King's Crossing,* ABC, 1982; also Mrs. Phillips, *Love of Life,* CBS. Mini-Series: Alice Dain Leggett, *The Dain Curse,* CBS, 1978; Rose Kennedy, *Robert Kennedy and His Times,* CBS, 1985. Pilots: Joanna Sanford, *World of Darkness,* CBS, 1977. Episodic: Queen Mother, *Wonder Woman,* CBS, 1977; also *Cosmopolitan Theatre,* DuMont, 1951; *The Inner Sanctum,* syndicated, 1954; *Love Story,* DuMont, 1954; ''Where Have You Been, Lord Randall, My Son?,'' *Eleventh Hour,* NBC, 1963; *Mission: Impossible,* CBS, 1966; *Felony Squad,* ABC, 1967; *Matt Lincoln,* ABC, 1970; *Morningstar/Eveningstar,* CBS, 1986; *Playhouse 90,* CBS; *Kraft Television Theatre,* NBC; *Studio One,* CBS; *Ben Casey,* ABC; *Dr. Kildare,* NBC; *The Nurses,* CBS; *Lamp unto My Feet,* CBS; *St. Elsewhere,* NBC; ''The Princess and the Pea,'' *Faerie Tale Theatre,* Showtime; *Jack and Mike,* ABC. Movies: Beatrice Richmond, *Killer on Board,* NBC, 1977; Marion Creighton, *Chiller,* CBS, 1985; Margaret Sloan, *Under Siege,* NBC, 1986; also *Run Till You Fall,* CBS. Specials: Mrs. Crampfurl, ''The Borrowers,'' *Hallmark Hall of Fame,* NBC, 1973; also ''The Magnificent Failure,'' *Hallmark Hall of Fame,* NBC, 1952.

RELATED CAREER—Founding director, Theatre, Inc., New York City, 1945; acting teacher, Michael Chekhov Studio, New York City, 1982—; also director, Young World Foundation, New York City.

AWARDS: Antoinette Perry Award, Best Actress in a Play, 1953, for *The Crucible;* Academy Award, Best Supporting Actress, 1976, for *Network;* Emmy Award nomination, Best Supporting Actress, 1978, for *The Dain Curse.*

MEMBER: Actors' Equity Association, Screen Actors Guild, American Federation of Television and Radio Artists.

SIDELIGHTS: RECREATIONS—Painting.

ADDRESSES: AGENT—STE Representation, 888 Seventh Avenue, New York, NY 10019. PUBLICIST—Gertrude Brooks, 333 W. 56th Street, New York, NY 10019.

*   *   *

STRASSMAN, Marcia   1948-

PERSONAL: Born April 28, 1948, in New York, NY.

VOCATION: Actress.

CAREER: PRINCIPAL FILM APPEARANCES—Kristine, *Changes,* Cinerama, 1969; Maria, *Soup for One,* Warner Brothers, 1982; Rose Stiller, *The Aviator,* Metro-Goldwyn-Mayer/United Artists, 1984.

PRINCIPAL TELEVISION APPEARANCES—Series: Nurse Margie Cutler, *M*A*S*H,* CBS, 1972-1973; Julie Kotter, *Welcome Back, Kotter,* ABC, 1975-79; Carol Younger, *Good Time Harry,* CBS, 1980. Pilots: Kentucky Smith, *Brenda Starr,* NBC, 1976; Pat MacFarland, *The Love Boat II,* ABC, 1977; Officer Jenny Palermo,

The Nightingales, NBC, 1979; Sandy Goldberg, *Wednesday Night Out,* NBC, 1972; Dr. Eve Sheridan, *E/R,* CBS, 1984. Episodic: *Fantasy Island,* ABC. Movies: Nancy, *Journey from Darkness,* NBC, 1975; Lenina Disney, *Brave New World,* NBC, 1980; Pam Ferguson, *Once Upon a Family,* CBS, 1980; also *Haunted by Her Past,* NBC, 1987. Specials: Julie Kotter, *Sweathog Back-to-School Special,* ABC, 1977; also *ABC's Silver Anniversary Celebration—25 and Still the One,* ABC, 1978.

ADDRESSES: AGENT—The Gage Group, 9229 Sunset Boulevard, Suite 306, Los Angeles, CA 90069.*

*   *   *

STREISAND, Barbra   1942-

PERSONAL: Born Barbara Joan Streisand, April 24, 1942, in Brooklyn, NY; daughter of Emanuel (an English teacher) and Diana (a school clerk; maiden name, Rosen) Streisand; married Elliott Gould (an actor), March 21, 1963 (divorced, 1971); children: Jason Emanuel.

VOCATION: Actress, singer, director, producer, and writer.

CAREER: STAGE DEBUT—Ensemble, *Another Evening with Harry Stoones* (revue), Gramercy Arts Theatre, New York City, 1961. BROADWAY DEBUT—Miss Marmelstein, *I Can Get It for You Wholesale,* Shubert Theatre, 1962. LONDON DEBUT—Fanny Brice, *Funny Girl,* Prince of Wales Theatre, 1966. PRINCIPAL STAGE APPEARANCES—Fanny Brice, *Funny Girl,* Winter Garden Theatre, New York City, 1964.

FILM DEBUT—Fanny Brice, *Funny Girl,* Columbia, 1968. PRINCIPAL FILM APPEARANCES—Dolly Levi, *Hello Dolly!,* Twentieth Century-Fox, 1969; Daisy Gamble, *On a Clear Day You Can See Forever,* Paramount, 1970; Doris, *The Owl and the Pussycat,* Columbia, 1970; Margaret Reynolds, *Up the Sandbox,* National General, 1972; Judy Maxwell, *What's Up, Doc?,* Warner Brothers, 1972; Katie Morosky, *The Way We Were,* Columbia, 1973; Henrietta, *For Pete's Sake* (also known as *July Pork Bellies*), Columbia, 1974; Fanny Brice, *Funny Lady,* Columbia, 1975; Esther Hoffman, *A Star Is Born,* Warner Brothers, 1976; Hillary Kramer, *The Main Event,* Warner Brothers, 1979; Cheryl Gibbons, *All Night Long,* Universal, 1981; title role, *Yentl,* Metro-Goldwyn-Mayer/United Artists, 1983; Claudia Draper, *Nuts,* Warner Brothers, 1987.

PRINCIPAL FILM WORK—Producer (with Jon Peters), *The Main Event,* Warner Brothers, 1979; producer (with Rusty Lemorande) and director, *Yentl,* Metro-Goldwyn-Mayer/United Artists, 1983; producer, *Nuts,* Warner Brothers, 1987.

PRINCIPAL TELEVISION APPEARANCES—Episodic: *PM East,* WNEW (New York City), 1961; *The Jack Paar Show,* NBC, 1961; *The Joe Franklin Show,* syndicated, 1961; *The Ed Sullivan Show,* CBS, 1962 and 1963; *The Dinah Shore Show,* NBC, 1962; *The Judy Garland Show,* CBS, 1963; *The Keefe Brasselle Show,* CBS, 1963; *The Bob Hope Show,* NBC, 1963; also *The Tonight Show,* NBC; *The Garry Moore Show,* CBS. Specials: *My Name Is Barbra,* CBS, 1965; *Color Me Barbra,* CBS, 1966; *The Belle of 14th Street,* CBS, 1967; *Barbra Streisand: A Happening in Central Park,* CBS, 1968; *Barbra S—and Other Musical Instruments,* CBS, 1973; *From Funny Girl to Funny Lady,* ABC, 1974; *The Stars Salute Israel at 30,* ABC, 1978; *The Entertainer of the Year Awards,* CBS, 1978;

The Barbara Walters Special, ABC, 1985; *Barbra Streisand: One Voice,* HBO, 1986; *Funny, You Don't Look 200,* CBS, 1987.

PRINCIPAL TELEVISION WORK—Executive producer, *Barbra Streisand: One Voice,* HBO, 1986.

RELATED CAREER—Singer in nightclubs throughout the United States, including: Bon Soir, Blue Angel, and Basin Street East, all New York City, hungry i, San Francisco, CA, Coconut Grove, Los Angeles, CA, and Riviera Hotel, Las Vegas, NV, all during the early 1960s; performed in concerts including those with Sammy Davis, Jr., Hollywood Bowl, Hollywood, CA, 1963, and in Central Park, New York City, 1968; founder (with Paul Newman, Sidney Poitier, Steve McQueen, and Dustin Hoffman), First Artists Productions, 1969.

WRITINGS: FILM—(With Jack Rosenthal) *Yentl,* Metro-Goldwyn-Mayer/United Artists, 1983. TELEVISION—Specials: *Barbra Streisand: One Voice,* HBO, 1986. OTHER—(With Paul Williams) "Evergreen" (song), 1976.

RECORDINGS: ALBUMS—*Pins and Needles,* Columbia, 1962; *I Can Get It for You Wholesale* (original cast recording), Columbia, 1962; *The Barbra Streisand Album,* Columbia, 1963; *The Second Barbra Streisand Album,* Columbia, 1963; *Funny Girl* (original cast recording), Capitol, 1964; *Barbra Streisand: The Third Album,* Columbia, 1964; *People,* Columbia, 1964; *My Name Is Barbra,* Columbia, 1965; *Color Me Barbra,* Columbia, 1966; *Je m'appelle Barbra,* 1966; *Harold Arlen and Barbra Streisand—Harold Sings Arlen (with Friend),* Columbia, 1966; *Simply Streisand,* Columbia, 1967; *A Christmas Album,* Columbia, 1967; *A Happening in Central Park,* Columbia, 1968; *What about Today?,* Columbia, 1969; *On a Clear Day You Can See Forever* (original soundtrack), Columbia, 1970; *Barbra Streisand's Greatest Hits,* Columbia, 1970; *Stoney End,* Columbia, 1971; *Barbra Joan Streisand,* Columbia, 1972; *Barbra Streisand Live Concert at the Forum,* Columbia, 1972; *Barbra Streisand and Other Musical Instruments,* Columbia, 1973; *The Way We Were,* Columbia, 1974; *Lazy Afternoon,* Columbia, 1975; (with Kris Kristofferson) *A Star Is Born* (original soundtrack), Columbia, 1976; *Classical Barbra,* Columbia, 1977; *Barbra Streisand—Superman,* Columbia, 1977; *The Stars Salute Israel at 30,* Columbia, 1978; *Wet,* Columbia, 1979; *Songbird,* Columbia, 1980; (with Barry Gibb) *Guilty,* Columbia, 1980; *Butterfly,* Columbia, 1981; *Yentl* (original soundtrack), Columbia, 1983; *Barbra Streisand's Greatest Hits, Volume 2,* Columbia, 1983; *Emotion,* Columbia, 1984; *The Broadway Album,* Columbia, 1986; *Barbra Streisand—One Voice,* Columbia, 1986; *Till I Loved You,* Columbia, 1988. Also *Memories,* Columbia.

VIDEOS—*Barbra Streisand: Putting It Together—The Making of "The Broadway Album,"* CBS/Fox, 1986.

AWARDS: Antoinette Perry Award nomination, Best Supporting or Featured Actress in a Musical, *Variety* New York Drama Critics Poll Award (co-winner), both 1962, and *Cue* magazine Entertainer of the Year Award, 1963, all for *I Can Get It for You Wholesale;* Emmy Award nomination, 1963, for *The Judy Garland Show;* Grammy Awards, Best Album and Best Female Performer of the Year, both 1963, for *The Barbra Streisand Album;* Antoinette Perry Award nomination, Best Actress in a Musical Comedy, 1964, for *Funny Girl;* Grammy Award, Best Female Pop Vocalist, 1964; Emmy Award, Outstanding Individual Achievement in Entertainment, 1965, for *My Name Is Barbra;* Grammy Award, Best Female Vocalist, 1965; London Critics' Musical Award, 1966; Academy Award and Golden Globe Award, both Best Actress, 1969, for

Funny Girl; Antoinette Perry Award, Special Award, 1970; (with Paul Williams) Academy Award, Best Song, 1976, and Grammy Award nomination, Best Song Writer, 1977, both for "Evergreen"; Georgie Award from the American Guild of Variety Artists, 1977; Grammy Award, Best Female Vocalist, 1978; Grammy Award, Best Pop Vocal Performance—Female, 1987, for *The Broadway Album;* Golden Globe Award nomination, Best Actress in a Drama, 1988, for *Nuts;* ShoWest Star of the Decade, 1988.

OTHER SOURCES: *Barbra: The First Decade—The Films and Career of Barbra Streisand,* by James Spada, Lyle Stuart, 1974; *Streisand: The Woman and the Legend,* by James Spada and Christopher Nickens, revised and updated edition, Pocket Books, 1983; *Barbra Streisand: The Woman, the Myth, the Music,* by Shaun Considine, Delacorte, 1985; *Barbra: The Second Decade—The Films and Career of Barbra Streisand,* by Karen Swenson, Lyle Stuart, 1985.

ADDRESSES: AGENT—Creative Artists Agency, 1888 Century Park E., Suite 1400, Los Angeles, CA 90067.*

*   *   *

STRITCH, Elaine   1926-

PERSONAL: Born February 2, 1926, in Detroit, MI; daughter of George Joseph (a rubber company executive) and Mildred (Jobe) Stritch; married John M. Bay (an actor), February 2, 1973 (died, 1982). EDUCATION: Trained for the stage with Erwin Piscator at the Dramatic Workshop of the New School for Social Research, 1944; studied singing with Burt Knapp, 1948-88.

VOCATION: Actress and singer.

CAREER: STAGE DEBUT—Tiger and cow, *Bobino* (children's show), New School for Social Research, Adelphi Theatre, New York City, 1944. BROADWAY DEBUT—Pamela Brewster, *Loco,* Biltmore Theatre, 1946. LONDON DEBUT—Mimi Paragon, *Sail Away!,* Savoy Theatre, 1962. PRINCIPAL STAGE APPEARANCES—Parlor maid, *The Private Life of the Master Race,* Theatre of All Nations, City College of New York Auditorium, New York City, 1945; Betty Lord, *Woman Bites Dog,* Walnut Street Theatre, Philadelphia, PA, 1946; Lady Sybil, *What Every Woman Knows,* Westport Country Playhouse, Westport, CT, 1946; Miss Crowder, *Made in Heaven,* Henry Miller's Theatre, New York City, 1946; Roberts, *Three Indelicate Ladies,* Shubert Theatre, New Haven, CT, 1947; ensemble, *The Shape of Things* (revue), John Drew Theatre, Easthampton, NY, 1947; Regina Giddens, *The Little Foxes,* Rooftop Theatre, New York City, 1947; ensemble, *Angel in the Wings* (revue), Coronet Theatre, New York City, 1947; Dallas Smith, *Texas Li'l Darlin',* Westport Country Playhouse, 1949; June Farrell, *Yes, M'Lord,* Booth Theatre, New York City, 1949.

Melba Snyder, *Pal Joey,* Broadhurst Theatre, New York City, 1952; Carol Frazer, *Once Married, Twice Shy,* Westport Country Playhouse, 1953; title role, *Panama Hattie,* Iroquois Amphitheatre, Louisville, KY, 1954; Peggy Porterfield, *On Your Toes,* 46th Street Theatre, New York City, 1954; Grace, *Bus Stop,* Music Box Theatre, New York City, 1955; Gertrude Muldoon, *The Sin of Pat Muldoon,* Cort Theatre, New York City, 1957; Maggie Harris, *Goldilocks,* Lunt-Fontanne Theatre, New York City, 1958; Leona Samish, *The Time of the Cuckoo,* Hunterdon Hills Playhouse, Jutland, NJ, 1959; Mimi Paragon, *Sail Away!,* Broadhurst Theatre,

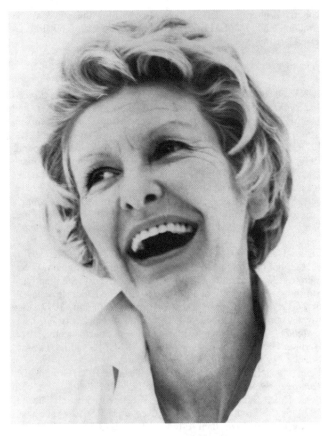

ELAINE STRITCH

1961; Martha, *Who's Afraid of Virginia Woolf?*, Billy Rose Theatre, New York City, 1962; Babylove Dallas, *The Grass Harp*, Trinity Square Repertory Company, Providence, RI, 1966; Ruth, *Wonderful Town*, City Center Theatre, New York City, 1967; Amanda Prynne, *Private Lives*, Theatre De Lys, New York City, 1968; Joanne, *Company*, Alvin Theatre, New York City, 1970, then Her Majesty's Theatre, London, 1972; Leona Dawson, *Small Craft Warnings*, Hampstead Theatre Club, then Comedy Theatre, both London, 1973; Evy Meara, *The Gingerbread Lady*, Phoenix Theatre, London, 1974; Madeleine Bernard, *Dancing in the End Zone*, Coconut Grove Playhouse, Coconut Grove, FL, 1983. Also appeared in *Suite in Two Keys*, Paper Mill Playhouse, Millburn, NJ, 1982; *"Follies" in Concert*, Avery Fisher Hall, New York City, 1982.

MAJOR TOURS—Sally Adams, *Call Me Madam*, U.S. cities, 1952-53; Stella, *The Time of the Barracudas*, U.S. cities, 1963; Martha, *Who's Afraid of Virginia Woolf?*, U.S. cities, 1965 and 1966; Anna Leonowens, *The King and I*, 1965; Dorothy Cleves, *Any Wednesday*, U.S. cities, 1967; Vera Charles, *Mame*, U.S. cities, 1968; title role, *Mame*, U.S. cities, 1969; Joanne, *Company*, U.S. cities, 1971.

PRINCIPAL FILM APPEARANCES—Phyllis Rycker, *The Scarlet Hour*, Paramount, 1956; Ruby LaSalle, *Three Violent People*, Paramount, 1956; Helen Ferguson, *A Farewell to Arms*, Twentieth Century-Fox, 1957; Liz Baker, *The Perfect Furlough* (also known as *Strictly for Pleasure*), Universal, 1958; Billie, *Who Killed Teddy Bear?*, Magna, 1965; tough lady, *The Sidelong Glances of a Pigeon Kicker* (also known as *Pigeons*), Metro-Goldwyn-Mayer/Plaza,

1970; nurse, *The Spiral Staircase*, Warner Brothers, 1975; Helen Weiner/Molly Langham, *Providence*, Cinema V, 1977; Diane Frazier, *September*, Orion, 1987; Ruby, *Cocoon: The Return*, Twentieth Century-Fox, 1988. Also appeared in *Kiss Her Goodbye*, 1959.

TELEVISION DEBUT—Mrs. Payne, *The Growing Paynes*, Dumont, 1949. PRINCIPAL TELEVISION APPEARANCES—Series: Regular, *Pantomime Quiz*, CBS, 1953, then Dumont, 1953-54, later ABC, 1955; Ruth Sherwood, *My Sister Eileen*, CBS, 1960-61; Miss G., *The Trials of O'Brien*, CBS, 1965-66; Sydney Brewer, *The Ellen Burstyn Show*, ABC, 1986-87; also *Two's Company*, British television, 1975-76 and 1979; and a British version of the U.S. series *Maude*. Mini-Series: Regular, *Song by Song*, PBS, 1975. Pilots: Ruth Sherwood, *You Should Meet My Sister* (broadcast as an episode of *Goodyear Theater*), NBC, 1960; also *The Mourner* (broadcast as an episode of *The Powder Room*), NBC, 1971. Episodic: Franny Tattinger, *Tattingers*, NBC, 1988; also *The Motorola Television Hour*, CBS, 1954; *Mr. Peepers*, NBC, 1955; Anna, "The Wedding," *Esso Repertory Theatre*, 1965; *Tales of the Unexpected*, NBC, 1977; "The Red Mill" and "Red Peppers," both *Studio One*, CBS; *Climax!*, CBS; *Alcoa Hour*, NBC; *The Ed Sullivan Show*, CBS; *The Milton Berle Show*, NBC; *The Nurses*, CBS; *The Honeymooners*, CBS; *Shades of Greene*, PBS; *Wagon Train*. Movies: Lily Pepper, "Red Pepper," *Three in One*, NBC, 1960; Maxine, *Stranded*, NBC, 1986. Specials: Carmenita, *Full Moon over Brooklyn*, NBC, 1960; *Original Cast Album: Company*, ABC, 1970; *Sylvia Fine Kaye's Musical Comedy Tonight III*, PBS, 1985; "Follies in Concert," *Great Performances*, PBS, 1986; also *Kennedy Center Tonight*. Also appeared in *Washington Square*, NBC; and *Polyanna*.

PRINCIPAL RADIO APPEARANCES—Episodic: *Inner Sanctum*, *Young Widder Brown*, and *Real Life Stories*.

WRITINGS: TELEVISION—Episodic: British version of the U.S. series *Maude*. OTHER—*Am I Blue?: Living with Diabetes and, Dammit, Having Fun* (nonfiction), Evans, 1984.

MEMBER: Actors' Equity Association, Screen Actors Guild, American Guild of Variety Artists, American Federation of Television and Radio Artists.

SIDELIGHTS: FAVORITE ROLES—Grace in *Bus Stop*, Martha in *Who's Afraid of Virginia Woolf?*, and Melba in *Pal Joey*. RECREATIONS—People.

ADDRESSES: AGENT—Michael Whitehall, Ltd., 125 Gloucester Road, London SWT 4TE, England.

*   *   *

STRUTHERS, Sally   1948-

PERSONAL: Full name, Sally Ann Struthers; born July 28, 1948, in Portland, OR; daughter of Robert Alden and Margaret Caroline (Jernes) Struthers; married William Rader (a psychiatrist; divorced); children: Samantha. EDUCATION: Trained for the stage at the Pasadena Playhouse, 1967.

VOCATION: Actress.

CAREER: BROADWAY DEBUT—Janet, *Wally's Cafe*, Brooks

Atkinson Theatre, 1981. PRINCIPAL STAGE APPEARANCES—Florence Unger, *The Odd Couple,* Center Theatre Group, Ahmanson Theatre, Los Angeles, CA, then Broadhurst Theatre, New York City, both 1985.

PRINCIPAL FILM APPEARANCES—(As Sally Ann Struthers) Betty, *Five Easy Pieces,* Columbia, 1970; (as Sally Ann Struthers) world's number one fan, *The Phynx,* Warner Brothers, 1970; Fran Clinton, *The Getaway,* National General, 1972. Also appeared in *Charlotte,* Gamma III, 1975.

PRINCIPAL TELEVISION APPEARANCES—Series: Regular, *The Summer Brothers Smothers Show,* ABC, 1970; regular, *The Tim Conway Comedy Hour,* CBS, 1970; voice of Pebbles Flintstone, *Pebbles and Bamm Bamm* (animated), CBS, 1971-72; Gloria Bunker Stivic, *All in the Family,* CBS, 1971-78; Gloria Bunker Stivic, *Gloria,* CBS, 1982-83; Marsha McMurray Shrimpton, *Nine to Five,* syndicated, 1986-88. Pilots: *The Teller and the Tales,* syndicated, 1985. Episodic: *Sweethearts,* syndicated, 1988. Movies: Sara Moore, *Aloha Means Goodbye,* CBS, 1974; Helen Klaben, *Hey, I'm Alive!,* ABC, 1975; Bess Houdini, *The Great Houdini,* ABC, 1976; Janis Halston, *Intimate Strangers,* ABC, 1977; Kathy Eaton, *My Husband Is Missing,* NBC, 1978; Jenny Corelli, *And Your Name Is Jonah,* CBS, 1979; Emily Cates, *A Gun in the House,* CBS, 1981; Tiger Lily, *Alice in Wonderland,* CBS, 1985. Specials: *The Bob Hope Show,* NBC, 1971; *Christmas with the Bing Crosbys,* NBC, 1972; *The Perry Como Winter Show,* CBS, 1973; *Hotel 90,* CBS, 1973; co-host, *The Leningrad Ice Show,* CBS, 1978; *The Stars Salute Israel at Thirty,* ABC, 1978; *Bob Hope's Women I Love—Beautiful but Funny,* NBC, 1982; *Secret World of the Very Young,* CBS, 1984; voice of Poison Ivy, *The Charmkins,* syndicated, 1985; *Lifetime Salutes Mom,* Lifetime, 1987; *This Is Your Life,* NBC, 1987; *Hollywood Women,* syndicated, 1988.

RELATED CAREER—Singer with the Spike Jones, Jr. band; actress in television commercials.

NON-RELATED CAREER—Board of directors, Christian Children's Fund, 1976—.

AWARDS: Emmy Award, Outstanding Performance by an Actress in a Supporting Role in a Comedy, 1972, for *All in the Family;* Emmy Award, Outstanding Supporting Actress in a Comedy Series for a Continuing or Single Performance in a Regular Series, 1979, for *All in the Family.*

ADDRESSES: AGENT—Sandy Bresler, Bresler-Kelly and Associates, 15760 Ventura Boulevard, Suite 1730, Encino, CA 91436.*

*   *   *

SU, Louis
See KAUFMAN, Lloyd

*   *   *

SUCHET, David   1946-

PERSONAL: Surname is pronounced "Soo-*shay*"; born May 2, 1946, in London, England; son of Jack (a doctor) and Joan Jarche Suchet; married Sheila Ferris (an actress), June 31, 1976; children:

Robert, Katherine. EDUCATION: Trained for the stage at the London Academy of Music and Dramatic Arts, 1966-69. RELIGION: Christian.

VOCATION: Actor.

CAREER: PRINCIPAL STAGE APPEARANCES—Tybalt, *Romeo and Juliet,* messenger, *Richard II,* Orlando, *As You Like It,* and Tranio, *The Taming of the Shrew,* all Royal Shakespeare Company (RSC), Royal Shakespeare Theatre, Stratford-on-Avon, U.K., 1973; Zamislov, *Summerfolk,* RSC, Aldwych Theatre, London, 1974; Wilmer, *Comrades,* and the Fool, *Lear,* both RSC, Place Theatre, London, 1974; Pisanio, *Cymbeline,* RSC, Royal Shakespeare Theatre, then Aldwych Theatre, London, both 1974; Hubert, *King John,* and Ferdinand, King of Navarre, *Love's Labour's Lost,* both RSC, Aldwych Theatre, 1975; the Fool, *Lear,* Zamislov, *Summerfolk,* and Ferdinand, King of Navarre, *Love's Labour's Lost,* all RSC, Brooklyn Academy of Music, Brooklyn, NY, 1975; Lucio, *Measure for Measure,* and Thomas Gilthead, *The Devil Is an Ass,* both Birmingham Repertory Theatre, Birmingham, U.K., then Lyttleton Theatre, London, 1977; Grigory Stephanovich Smirnov, "The Bear," and Posdnyshev, "The Kreutzer Sonata," in *The Kreutzer Sonata,* Theatre Upstairs, London, 1977, then Royal Court Theatre, London, 1978; Tsaravitch and Georg Wochner, *Laughter!,* English Stage Company, Royal Court Theatre, 1978; Herman Glogauer, *Once in a Lifetime,* RSC, Piccadilly Theatre, London, 1978; Caliban, *The Tempest,* and Shylock, *Merchant of Venice,* both RSC, Royal Shakespeare Theatre, 1978; Grumio, *The Taming of the Shrew,* and Sir Nathaniel, *Love's Labour's Lost,* both RSC, Royal Shakespeare Theatre, 1978, then Aldwych Theatre, 1979; Sextus Pompey, *Antony and Cleopatra,* RSC, Royal Shakespeare Theatre, 1978, then Aldwych Theatre, 1979; Angelo, *Measure for Measure,* RSC, Aldwych Theatre, 1979; Joe Green, *Separation,* Hampstead Theatre Club, then Comedy Theatre, both London, 1987. Also appeared in *This Story of Yours,* Hampstead Theatre Club; *Every Good Boy Deserves Favour,* Barbican Concert Hall, London; as Achilles, *Troilus and Cressida,* and as Bolingbroke, *Richard II,* both RSC.

MAJOR TOURS—With the Royal Shakespeare Company, U.S. cities, 1975, and Israeli and European cities.

FILM DEBUT—Barsad, *Tale of Two Cities,* Norman Rosemont, 1978. PRINCIPAL FILM APPEARANCES—Gustav Klimt, *Schiele in Prison,* Concord Films Council, 1980; Corbett, *The Missionary,* Columbia, 1982; Laurenti P. Beria, *Red Monarch,* Goldcrest, 1983; Inspector Stagnos, *Trenchcoat,* Buena Vista, 1983; Buller/Prince Max Von Hesse, *Greystoke: The Legend of Tarzan, Lord of the Apes,* Warner Brothers, 1984; Mesterbein, *The Little Drummer Girl,* Warner Brothers, 1984; Alex Okana, *The Falcon and the Snowman,* Orion, 1985; Steven Dyer, *The Song for Europe* (also known as *Cry for Justice*), Channel Four, 1985; defense minister, *Iron Eagle,* Tri-Star, 1986; Stephen Dyer, *Crime of Honor,* Academy Home Entertainment, 1987; Jacques Lafleur, *Harry and the Hendersons,* Universal, 1987; Muller, *A World Apart,* Atlantic, 1988; the Bishop, *Popielusko* (also known as *To Kill a Priest*), Columbia, 1988. Also appeared as Wil, *Why the Whales Came,* Signet Films; and in *Stress,* 1986.

TELEVISION DEBUT—Edward Teller, *Oppenheimer,* BBC, 1978, then *American Playhouse,* PBS, 1982. PRINCIPAL TELEVISION APPEARANCES—Mini-Series: D'Usseau, *Master of the Game,* CBS, 1984; Tsientsin, *Reilly—Ace of Spies,* Euston, then *Mystery,* PBS, 1984; title role, *Blott on the Landscape,* BBC, then Arts and Entertainment, 1986; T.J. O'Connor, *Cause Celebre,* Anglia TV, then *Mystery*, PBS, 1988; Inspector Poirot, *Hercule Poirot's Casebook*, ITV, 1989; *Playing Shakespeare*, London Weekend Television, then PBS, 1983. Episodic: Colin, "The Muse," *Oxbridge Blues*, BBC, then Arts and Entertainment, 1986, later PBS, 1988. Movies: Barsad, *A Tale of Two Cities*, CBS, 1980; Trouillefou, *The Hunchback of Notre Dame*, CBS, 1982; Inspector Japp, *Agatha Christie's "Thirteen at Dinner,"* CBS, 1985; Matvei, *Gulag*, HBO, 1985; Dino Grandi, *Mussolini: The Untold Story*, NBC, 1985; William L. Shirer, *Murrow*, HBO, 1986; Jonathan Gault, *The Last Innocent Man*, HBO, 1987. Specials: Herman Glogauer, *Once in a Lifetime*, BBC, then *Great Performances*, PBS, 1988. Also appeared as Howard Bollsover, *Saigon—The Last Days*, BBC; Freud, *The Life of Freud*, BBC; Yves Drouard, *Time to Die*, Anglia TV; Leopold Bloom, *Ulysses*, LWT; *Being Normal*, BBC; *Kings and Castles*, Thames.

PRINCIPAL RADIO APPEARANCES—Plays: Shylock, *The Merchant of Venice*, World Radio Service; also *Never Been Kissed in the Same Place Twice, Ironhand, Gorky on Tolstoy, The Kreutzer Sonata, Memoirs of Lorenzo Da Ponte, Barn's People—Peace of Westphalia, First Night Impressions, The Shout, Right Ho Jeeves: Rosenburg in the Trenches, Gorky on Chekhov, Debussy, Richard II*, and *No One Knows Why*, all BBC.

RELATED CAREER—Visiting professor of theatre, University of Nebraska; council member, London Academy of Music and Dramatic Arts.

WRITINGS: Essays on acting the roles of Shylock, Caliban, and Iago, *Players of Shakespeare*.

AWARDS: Evening Standard Award nomination, Best Actor, 1978, for *Merchant of Venice;* Best Radio Actor, 1979, for *The Kreutzer Sonata;* Society of West End Theatres Award nomination, Best Supporting Actor, 1980, for *Once in a Lifetime;* Society of West End Theatres Award, 1981, for *The Merchant of Venice;* Marseilles Film Festival Award, Best Actor, 1983, for *Red Monarch;* Craft Award from the British Industry and Scientific Film Association, 1986, for *Stress;* Royal Television Society Performance Awards, all as Best Actor, 1986, for *The Life of Freud, Blott on the Landscape*, and *The Song for Europe;* British Academy of Film and Television Award nomination, Best Actor in a Supporting Role, 1989, for *A World Apart*.

MEMBER: British Actors' Equity Association, Screen Actors Guild, Savile Club.

SIDELIGHTS: RECREATIONS—Playing the clarinet and drums, horseback riding, photography.

ADDRESSES: AGENTS—Harris and Goldberg, 2121 Avenue of the Stars, Suite 950, Los Angeles, CA 90067; Brunskill Management, Ltd., Suite 8, 169 Queens Gate, London SW7 5EH, England.

*　　*　　*

SVENSON, Bo　1941-

PERSONAL: Born February 13, 1941, in Goteborg, Sweden; came to the United States in 1958; son of Birger Ragnar and Lola Iris Viola (Johansson) Svenson; married Lise Hartmann-Berg, December 30, 1966; children: Pia, Maja. EDUCATION: Attended the

University of Meiji, 1960-63, and the University of California, Los Angeles, 1970-74. MILITARY: U.S. Marine Corps, 1959-65.

VOCATION: Actor.

CAREER: PRINCIPAL FILM APPEARANCES—Jack Twyman, *Maurie* (also known as *Big Mo*), National General, 1973; Axel Olsson, *The Great Waldo Pepper*, Universal, 1975; Buford Pusser, *Walking Tall, Part II*, American International, 1975; Michael McBain, *Breaking Point*, Twentieth Century-Fox, 1976; Jack Murdock, *Special Delivery*, American International, 1976; Buford Pusser, *Final Chapter—Walking Tall*, American International, 1977; Jo Bob Priddy, *North Dallas Forty*, Paramount, 1979; Major Carter, *Virus* (also known as *Fukkatsu No Hi*), Media, 1980; Lieutenant Yeager, *Counterfeit Commandos* (also known as *Inglorius Bastards*), Aquarius, 1981; cop, *Deadly Impact*, Vestron, 1983; Kor, *Wizards of the Lost Kingdom*, New Horizons/Concorde/Cinema Group, 1985; captain, *Choke Canyon*, UFDC, 1986; sheriff, *Manhunt*, Goldwyn, 1986; Captain Campbell, *The Delta Force*, Cannon, 1986; Roy Jennings, *Heartbreak Ridge*, Warner Brothers, 1986; Sheriff Bill Cook, *Thunder Warrior* (also known as *Thunder*), Trans World Entertainment, 1986; Sheriff Roger, *Thunder Warrior II*, Trans World, 1987; Colonel Slater, *White Phantom*, Spectrum, 1987; Captain Robertson, *Deep Space*, Trans World Entertainment, 1988. Also appeared in *Our Man in Mecca*, 1977; *Son of the Sheik*, 1978; *Butcher, Baker (Nightmare Maker)* (also known as *Nightmare Maker*), International Films, 1982; *Portrait of a Hitman*, 1984; and *Mania*, Eurocine, 1988.

PRINCIPAL TELEVISION APPEARANCES—Series: Big Swede, *Here Come the Brides* ABC, 1968-70; Sheriff Buford Pusser, *Walking Tall*, NBC, 1981. Pilots: Jay Appleby, *Hitched*, NBC, 1973; Lee Driscoll, *Target Risk*, NBC, 1975; Earl Hewitt, *I Do, I Don't*, ABC, 1983. Episodic: Milovan Drumm, "Lost Treasure," *Suspense Playhouse*, CBS, 1971; Earl Verrick, *The Fall Guy*, ABC, 1985; Karl Anderson, *Murder, She Wrote*, CBS, 1988. Movies: Raeder, *The Bravos*, ABC, 1972; the Monster, *Frankenstein*, ABC, 1973; Sam, *You'll Never See Me Again*, ABC, 1973; Gar Seberg, *Snowbeast*, NBC, 1977; Tom Jensen, *Gold of the Amazon Women*, NBC, 1979; Bo, *Jealousy*, ABC, 1984; Maurice Fontenac, *The Dirty Dozen: The Deadly Mission*, NBC, 1987. Specials: *Battle of the Network Stars*, ABC, 1978; *U.S. Against the World II*, ABC, 1978; *Celebrity Daredevils*, ABC, 1983.

NON-RELATED CAREER—Far East Heavyweight Division Judo Champion (third degree black belt), 1961; professional hockey player; race car driver.

ADDRESSES: AGENT—Agency for the Performing Arts, 9000 Sunset Boulevard, Suite 1200, Los Angeles, CA 90069. OFFICE—Sy Litvinoff, 10351 Santa Monica Boulevard, Suite 211, Los Angeles, CA 90025.*

*　　*　　*

SWENSON, Inga　1934-

PERSONAL: Born December 19, 1934 (some sources say 1932), in Omaha, NE; daughter of A.C.R. (an attorney) and Geneva (Seeger) Swenson; married Lowell M. Harris (an actor and singer), February 21, 1953; children: two sons. EDUCATION: Trained for the stage with Alvina Krause at Northwestern University, 1950-54, with Uta

Hagen and Herbert Berghof at the Herbert Berghof Studios, 1954, and with Lee Strasberg at the Actors Studio, 1958.

VOCATION: Actress and singer.

CAREER: STAGE DEBUT—Maid, *Peg O' My Heart*, Berkshire Playhouse, Stockbridge, MA, 1949. BROADWAY DEBUT—Singer, *New Faces of '56* (revue), Ethel Barrymore Theatre, 1956. LONDON DEBUT—Lizzie Currie, *110 in the Shade*, Palace Theatre, 1967. PRINCIPAL STAGE APPEARANCES—Princess Alexandria, *The Swan*, Minnie Fay, *The Merchant of Yonkers*, singer, *Sing Out, Sweet Land*, and extra, *Othello*, all Playhouse Theatre, Eaglesmere, PA, 1952; Aunt Anna Rose, *Treasure Hunt*, Monica, *The Medium*, Lucy, *The Telephone*, Dunyasha, *The Cherry Orchard*, Alizon Elliot, *The Lady's Not for Burning*, and Isabelle, *Ring' round the Moon*, all Playhouse Theatre, 1953; Georgie Elgin, *The Country Girl*, Celia Copplestone, *The Cocktail Party*, Mrs. Larue, *Mrs. McThing*, Countess Aurelia, *The Madwoman of Chaillot*, and Angelique, *The Imaginary Invalid*, all Playhouse Theatre, 1954; Olivia, *Twelfth Night*, Shakespearewrights, Jan Hus Playhouse, New York City, 1954; Princess Charlotte, *The First Gentleman*, Belasco Theatre, New York City, 1957; Madge, *Picnic*, and Amy Kittridge, *A Swim in the Sea*, both Royal Poinciana Playhouse, Palm Beach, FL, 1958; Ophelia, *Hamlet*, Helena, *A Midsummer Night's Dream*, and Perdita, *The Winter's Tale*, all American Shakespeare Festival, Stratford, CT, 1958; Amy Kittridge, *A Swim in the Sea*, Walnut Street Theatre, Philadelphia, PA, 1958; Juliet, *Romeo and Juliet*, American Shakespeare Festival, 1959.

Solveig, *Peer Gynt*, Phoenix Theatre, New York City, 1960; Julie Jordan, *Carousel*, Melody Top Theatre, Hillside, IL, 1962; Gillian, *Bell, Book, and Candle*, Kiamesha Playhouse, Kiamesha Lake, NY, 1962; Desdemona, *Othello*, Arena Stage, Washington, DC, 1963; Magnolia, *Show Boat*, Kenley Players, Warren, OH, then Columbus, OH, both 1963; Lizzie Currie, *110 in the Shade*, Broadhurst Theatre, New York City, 1963; Irene Adler, *Baker Street*, Broadway Theatre, New York City, 1965; title role, *Mary Stuart*, Parker Playhouse, Ft. Lauderdale, FL, 1967; Eliza Doolittle, *My Fair Lady*, City Center Light Opera Company, City Center Theatre, New York City, 1968; Lady Alice More, *A Man for All Seasons*, Center Theatre Group, Ahmanson Theatre, Los Angeles, CA, 1979. Also appeared in *The Crucible*, Center Theatre Group, Ahmanson Theatre, 1972; and in *The Four Poster*, New Stage Theatre, Jackson, MS, 1979.

MAJOR TOURS—Marie Louise, *My Three Angels*, U.S. cities, 1957; Julie Jordan, *Carousel*, U.S. cities, 1960; Lizzie Currie, *110 in the Shade*, U.S. cities, 1963-64.

PRINCIPAL FILM APPEARANCES—Ellen Anderson, *Advise and Consent*, Columbia, 1962; Kate Keller, *The Miracle Worker*, United Artists, 1962; Sister Monica, *Lipstick*, Paramount, 1976; Mrs. Craddock, *The Betsy*, Allied Artists, 1978.

TELEVISION DEBUT—Singer, *Chrysler Special*, CBC (Canadian television), 1957. PRINCIPAL TELEVISION APPEARANCES—Series: Gretchen Kraus, *Benson*, ABC, 1979-86. Mini-Series: Amelia Foster, *Testimony of Two Men*, syndicated, 1977; Maude Hazard, *North and South*, ABC, 1985; Maude Hazard, *North and South, Book II*, ABC, 1986. Episodic: Liza, "The Best Wine," *Goodyear Playhouse*, NBC, 1957; Marjorie, "The World of Nick Adams," *Seven Lively Arts*, CBS, 1957; Maria, "Heart of Darkness," and Milly Theale, "Wings of the Dove," both *Playhouse 90*, CBS, 1958; Vera, "Goodbye, but It Doesn't Go Away," *U.S. Steel Hour*, CBS, 1958; Rose Maylie, "Oliver Twist," *Dupont*

Show of the Month, CBS, 1959; Lady Jane, "Victoria Regina," *Hallmark Hall of Fame*, NBC, 1961; Inger, "Inger, My Love," *Bonanza*, NBC, 1962; Sonya Green, *Hotel*, ABC, 1988; Holly, *The Golden Girls*, NBC, 1989; Madelyn Stone, *Newhart*, CBS, 1989; also *The Defenders*, CBS, 1961 and 1962; *Dr. Kildare*, NBC, 1962; *Bonanza*, NBC, 1963; *The Nurses*, CBS, 1963; *American Musical Theatre*, CBS, 1964; *The Tonight Show*, NBC, 1964; "My Father and My Mother," *CBS Playhouse*, CBS, 1968; *Medical Center*, CBS, 1970 and 1971; "The Tape Recorder," *NET Playhouse*, PBS, 1970; Ingrid, *Soap*, ABC.

Movies: Ilyana Kovalefskii, *Earth II*, ABC, 1971; Nora Bayes, *Ziegfeld: The Man and His Women*, NBC, 1978; Matty Kline, *Bay Coven*, NBC, 1987; Marilyn Broadshaw Reagan, *Nutcracker: Money, Madness, and Murder*, NBC, 1987. Specials: Lavinia, *Androcles and the Lion*, NBC, 1967; Mrs. Trimble, "My Dear Uncle Sherlock," *ABC Short Story Specials*, ABC, 1977; Mrs. Marston, "The Terrible Secret," *ABC Afterschool Special*, ABC, 1979. Also appeared as Kate, *The Gay Deceivers*, CBC, 1956.

RELATED CAREER—Singer and dancer in cabaret production *Come As You Are*, Versailles Club, New York City, 1955; singer in cabaret production *Brothers and Sisters*, New York City, 1975; appeared as a soloist with the Boston Symphony Orchestra and with the Omaha Symphony.

AWARDS: Aegis Theatre Award, 1956, for *New Faces of '56;* Theatre World Award, Outer Critics Circle Award, and *Variety* New York Drama Critics Poll Award, all 1957, for *The First Gentleman;* Outer Critics Circle Award and Antoinette Perry Award nomination, Best Actress in a Musical, both 1964, for *110 in the Shade;* Antoinette Perry Award nomination, Best Actress in a Musical, 1965, for *Baker Street.*

MEMBER: Actors' Equity Association, American Federation of Television and Radio Artists, Screen Actors Guild, American Guild of Variety Artists.

SIDELIGHTS: FAVORITE ROLES—Lizzie Currie in *110 in the Shade.* RECREATIONS—Reading and music.

ADDRESSES: HOME—48 Paloma Avenue, Venice, CA 90291.*

       *   *   *

SWERLING, Jo, Jr.   1931-

PERSONAL: Born June 18, 1931, in Los Angeles, CA; son of Jo (a writer) and Florence (Manson) Swerling; children: Timothy David, Tanya Manson. EDUCATION: Attended the University of California, Los Angeles, 1948-51; California Maritime Academy, 1951-54. MILITARY: U.S. Navy, lieutenant j.g., 1954-56.

VOCATION: Producer and screenwriter.

CAREER: Also see WRITINGS below. PRINCIPAL FILM WORK—Executive producer, *The November Man*, 1976.

PRINCIPAL TELEVISION WORK—Series: Producer (with Paul Freeman), *Run For Your Life*, NBC, 1965-68; producer (with Roy Huggins), *The Outsider*, NBC, 1968-69; producer (with Steve Helpern), *The Lawyers*, NBC, 1969-72; executive producer (with Huggins), *Alias Smith and Jones*, ABC, 1971-73; producer (with

David J. O'Connor), *Cool Million*, NBC, 1972-73; associate executive producer (with Stephen J. Cannell), *Toma*, ABC, 1973-74; supervising producer, *The Rockford Files*, NBC, 1974-80; producer, *Baretta*, ABC, 1975-78; supervising producer and executive producer, *City of Angels*, NBC, 1976; supervising producer, *Lobo*, NBC, 1980-81; executive producer (with Frank Lupo) and supervising producer, *The Greatest American Hero*, ABC, 1981-83; supervising producer (with John Ashley and Lupo), *The Quest*, ABC, 1982; supervising producer, *The A-Team*, NBC, 1983-87; supervising producer, *Hardcastle and McCormick*, ABC, 1983; supervising producer, *The Rousters*, NBC, 1983-84; supervising producer (with Cannell and Lupo), *Riptide*, NBC, 1983-86; supervising producer, *Hunter*, NBC, 1984—; supervising producer, *Stingray*, NBC, 1985; supervising producer, *J.J. Starbuck*, NBC, 1987-88; supervising producer, *21 Jump Street*, Fox, 1987—; supervising producer, *Wiseguy*, CBS, 1987—; supervising producer, *Sonny Spoon*, NBC, 1988; supervising producer, *UNSUB*, NBC, 1989; also associate producer, then producer, *Kraft Suspense Theatre*, NBC; production coordinator, *The Restless Gun*, NBC; production coordinator, *Markham*, CBS; production coordinator, *M Squad*, NBC; production coordinator, *Cimarron City*, NBC; production coordinator, *Suspicion*, NBC; production coordinator, *Thriller*, NBC; production coordinator, *The 87th Precinct*, NBC; production coordinator, *Alcoa Premiere*, ABC; production coordinator, *Wagon Train*. Mini-Series: Producer, *Captains and the Kings*, NBC, 1976; producer, *Aspen*, NBC, 1977; executive producer and co-director, *The Last Convertible*, NBC, 1979.

Pilots: Producer, *The Green Felt Jungle*, NBC, 1965; producer, *Rapture at Two-Forty* (broadcast as an episode of *Kraft Suspense Theater*), NBC, 1965; producer (with Huggins), *The Outsider*, NBC, 1967; producer, *The Sound of Anger*, NBC, 1968; producer, *The Lonely Profession*, NBC, 1969; producer, *The Whole World Is Watching*, NBC, 1969; producer, *Sam Hill: Who Killed the Mysterious Mr. Foster?*, NBC, 1971; executive producer, *Jigsaw* (also known as *Man on the Move*), ABC, 1972; producer, *Toma*, ABC, 1973; associate executive producer, *The Rockford Files*, NBC, 1974; executive producer, *Target Risk*, NBC, 1975; executive producer, *Hazard's People*, CBS, 1976; producer, *The 3000 Mile Chase*, NBC, 1977; producer, *The Jordan Chance*, CBS, 1978; producer, *Pirate's Key*, CBS, 1979; supervising producer, *The A-Team*, NBC, 1983; supervising producer, *Hardcastle and McCormick*, ABC, 1983; supervising producer, *The Rousters*, NBC, 1983; supervising producer (with Cannell and Lupo), *Riptide*, NBC, 1983; supervising producer, *Four Eyes*, NBC, 1984; supervising producer, *Hunter*, NBC, 1984; supervising producer, *21 Jump Street*, Fox, 1987; supervising producer, *Wiseguy*, CBS, 1987; supervising producer, *J.J. Starbuck*, NBC, 1987; supervising producer, *Stingray*, NBC, 1985; supervising producer, *Brothers-in-Law*, ABC, 1985; supervising producer, *The Last Precinct*, NBC, 1986; supervising producer, *Sonny Spoon*, NBC, 1988; also supervising producer, *Sirens*, 1987. Episodic: Producer, *The Bob Hope Chrysler Theater*, NBC. Movies: Producer, *Drive Hard, Drive Fast*, NBC, 1973; producer, *Do You Take This Stranger?*, NBC, 1971; producer, *How to Steal an Airplane*, NBC, 1972; producer, *The Story of Pretty Boy Floyd*, ABC, 1974; producer, *This Is the West That Was*, NBC, 1974; executive producer, *The Invasion of Johnson County*, NBC, 1976; also supervising producer, *Destination: America*, 1987.

RELATED CAREER—Senior vice-president, Stephen J. Cannell Productions, Hollywood, CA; industry advisory committee member, screenwriting department, University of Southern California, Los Angeles, CA; president and executive producer, Public Arts Productions (a television production company).

NON-RELATED CAREER—Planning commissioner, Hidden Hills, CA, 1973-80.

WRITINGS: TELEVISION—Pilots: (With Heywood Gould and Roy Huggins) *Hazard's People*, CBS, 1976. Episodic: *The A-Team*, NBC, 1983; *Sonny Spoon*, NBC, 1988; also *Run for Your Life*, NBC; *The Lawyers*, NBC; *The Rockford Files*, NBC.

AWARDS: Emmy Award nomination, Best Dramatic Series, 1976, for *Baretta;* Emmy Award nomination and Golden Globe Award nomination, both Best Limited Series, 1977, for *Captains and the Kings;* also two Emmy Award nominations, both Best Dramatic Series, for *Run for Your Life*. Military honors: China Service Medal from the U.S. Navy.

MEMBER: Writers Guild of America, Directors Guild of America, Screen Actors Guild, Academy of Television Arts and Sciences.

ADDRESSES: OFFICE—Stephen J. Cannell Productions, 7083 Hollywood Boulevard, Los Angeles, CA 90028.

*   *   *

SWIFT, Clive   1936-

PERSONAL: Full name, Clive Walter Swift; born February 9, 1936, in Liverpool, England; son of Abram Sampson and Lily Rebecca (Greenman) Swift; married Margaret Drabble (a writer), June, 1960 (divorced, 1975); children: Adam Richard George, Rebecca Margaret, Joseph. EDUCATION: Attended Clifton College and Caius College, Cambridge University.

VOCATION: Actor and writer.

CAREER: Also see *WRITINGS* below. STAGE DEBUT—Dr. Bushtact, *Take the Fool Away*, Nottingham Playhouse, Nottingham, U.K., 1959. PRINCIPAL STAGE APPEARANCES—Elvet Cross, *The Big Breaker*, Prospect Theatre Company, Belgrade Theatre, Coventry, U.K., 1965; Henry Straker, *Man and Superman*, Arts Theatre, then Vaudeville Theatre later Garrick Theatre, all London, 1965; Canton, *The Clandestine Marriage*, and Michepain, *The Fighting Cock*, both Chichester Festival Theatre, Chichester, U.K., 1966; Winston, *The Young Churchill*, Phoenix Theatre, Leicester, U.K., then Duchess Theatre, London, both 1969; Bob Acres, *The Rivals*, Chichester Festival Theatre, 1971; Lapinet, *Dear Antoine*, Chichester Festival Theatre, then Piccadilly Theatre, London, both 1971; Robert, *The Two of Me*, Jeannetta Cochrane Theatre, London, 1975; the chairman, *Dirty Linen*, Arts Theatre, London, 1976; Hudson, *Inadmissible Evidence*, Royal Court Theatre, London, 1978; Baron Hardup, *Cinderella*, Royal Exchange Theatre, Manchester, U.K., 1978; James Turney, *All Together Now*, Haymarket Theatre, Leicester, U.K., 1979. Also appeared as Cloten, *Cymbeline*, Pompey, *Measure for Measure*, Fluellen, *Henry V*, Falstaff, *The Merry Wives of Windsor*, Parolles, *All's Well That Ends Well*, porter, *Macbeth*, Oswald, *King Lear*, Inspector Voss, *The Physicists*, and sewerman, *The Devils*, all with the Royal Shakespeare Company, 1960-68; in the title role, *King Lear*, New Victoria Theatre, Stoke-on-Trent, U.K.; in *The Sisterhood*, New End Theatre, London; *An Enemy of the People*, Young Vic Theatre, then Playhouse Theatre, both London; *The Potsdam Quartet*, Lyric Hammersmith Theatre, London; *Roll on Four O'Clock*, Lyric Hammersmith Theatre, then Palace Theatre, London; *Messiah*, Aldwych Theatre, London; *The Genius*, Royal Court Theatre; *The*

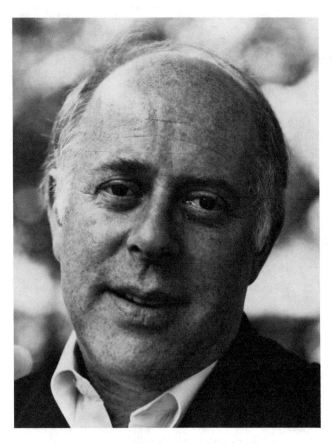

CLIVE SWIFT

Trial of Queen Caroline, English Chamber Theatre, Malvern Festival; *The Tempest, The Poacher's Tale, Richard III, Ivanov*, and *The Oz Obscenity Trial*, all Prospect Theatre Company; and in *Four Quartets* (recital), Manchester, Gorzedale, and Cheltenham Theatre Festivals, all U.K.

PRINCIPAL STAGE WORK—Director, *The Wild Goose Chase* and *The Lower Depths*, both London Academy of Music and Dramatic Arts, London, 1970; producer, *The Two of Me*, Jeannetta Cochrane Theatre, 1975.

MAJOR TOURS—Caliban, *The Tempest*, and Isaac Hooker, *The Gamecock*, Prospect Theatre Company, U.K. cities, 1966; also appeared in *The Hollow Crown*, Royal Shakespeare Company, U.S. cities, 1975; and *The Apple Cart*, U.K. cities.

PRINCIPAL FILM APPEARANCES—Duffle, *Having a Wild Weekend* (also known as *Catch Us If You Can*), Warner Brothers, 1965; Snug, *A Midsummer Night's Dream*, Eagle, 1969; Johnny Porter, *Frenzy*, Universal, 1972; Inspector Richardson, *Deathline* (also known as *Raw Meat*), American International, 1973; Massey, *Man at the Top*, Anglo-EMI, 1973; Ash, *The National Health, or Nurse Norton's Affair*, Columbia, 1973; Reverend Pottock, *The Sailor's Return*, Osprey, 1978; D.G. Rossetti, *News from Nowhere*, Concord Film Council, 1978; Mr. Chubb, *The Great Train Robbery* (also known as *The First Great Train Robbery*), United Artists, 1979; Ector, *Excalibur*, Warner Brothers, 1981; magistrate, *Memed My Hawk*, Focus, 1984; Major Callendar, *A Passage to India*, Columbia, 1984. Also appeared in *The Brides of Fu Manchu*, Anglo-Amalgamated/Seven Arts, 1966; *Machines for the Sup-*

pression of Time, Concord Film Council, 1980; *A Fine and Private Place*, Associated British; and *The Voyage of the Ark*, Alister Hallum.

PRINCIPAL TELEVISION APPEARANCES—Mini-Series: Alec Pimkin, *First Among Equals*, Granada, 1985, then PBS, 1987; Dr. Bartlett, "The Silent World of Nicholas Quinn," *Inspector Morse*, Zenith Productions, 1986, then *Mystery*, PBS, 1988; R.P. Croom Johnson, *Cause Celebre*, Anglia Television, 1987, then *Mystery*, PBS, 1988; also *Barchester Chronicles*, BBC, 1982; "Winston Churchill—The Wilderness Years," Southern Television, then *Masterpiece Theatre*, PBS. Episodic: *Omnibus*, BBC, 1976; *Play for Today*, BBC, 1976; *Playhouse*, BBC, 1977; *Play of the Week*, BBC, 1977; *Bless Me Father*, London Weekend Television (LWT), 1978; *Play of the Week* (two episodes), BBC, 1979; *The Book Programme*, BBC, 1980; *Dr. Who—Revelations of the Dalecks*, BBC, 1984; *A Very Peculiar Practice*, BBC, 1987; *Armchair Theatre*, ABC (U.K.); *Misfit, Number Five*, ATV; *The Frighteners, Number Five*, LWT; *Horizon*, BBC; *Playhouse*, BBC; *Play for Today*, BBC. Plays: Thomas Percy, Earl of Worcester, *Henry IV, Part One*, BBC, 1978, then *The Shakespeare Plays*, PBS, 1980; also *Romeo and Juliet*, Thames, 1976; *The Potsdam Quartet*, BBC, 1980; *Pericles*, BBC, 1983; "King Lear," *South Bank Show*, LWT, 1986; *Roll on Four O'Clock*, Granada. Specials: Ellis, "Pack of Lies," *Hallmark Hall of Fame*, CBS, 1987.

Also appeared in *New Horizons*, BBC, 1975; *The Brothers*, BBC, 1976; *Beasts*, ATV, 1976; *Ogden Nash*, BBC, 1976; *The Game*, BBC, 1976; *Goodbye America*, BBC, 1976; *Queen Victoria's Scandals*, Granada, 1976; *The Trial and Death of Jesus*, BBC, 1977; *Jackanory Playhouse*, BBC, 1977; *Send in the Girls*, Granada, 1977; *1990*, BBC, 1977; *Hazell and the Baker Street Sleuth*, Thames, 1978; *Shadows*, Thames, 1978; *A Horseman Riding By*, BBC, 1978; *A Family Affair*, BBC, 1979; *A Case of Spirits*, Granada, 1979; *In Loving Memory*, Yorkshire Television (YTV), 1979; *The Casebook of Dr. Jekyll*, BBC, 1979; *The Nesbitts Are Coming*, YTV, 1979; *Yours Sincerely*, BBC, 1980; *The British in Germany*, BBC, 1980; *Stranger in Town*, Anglia Television, 1981; *Funeral Director*, BBC, 1981; *Lucky Jim*, BBC, 1981; *The Gentle Touch*, LWT, 1982; *Portrait of Newton*, Central Television (CTV), 1982; *Martin Luther*, BBC, 1983; *Pickwick Papers*, BBC, 1984; *Motive for Murder: Such Sweet Thunder*, BBC, 1984; *The Shakespeare Project*, BBC, 1985; *Black Silk*, BBC, 1985; *What Mad Pursuit*, BBC, 1985; *Journey's End*, BBC, 1988; *The Coffin*, Granada, 1988; *Hard Cases*, CTV, 1988; *Echoes*, BBC, 1988; *Laura and Disorder*, BBC, 1988; *Minder*, Euston Films, 1988; *Gentlemen and Players*, TVS, 1988; *Court Martial*, BBC; *Love Story*, ATV; *Compact*, BBC; *The Company of Eight*, BBC; *Bury the Dead*, BBC; *Knock on Any Door*, ATV; *Tempo*, ABC (U.K.); *Public Eye*, ABC (U.K.); *The East End Three*, BBC; *The Movies*, BBC; *Birthday*, BBC; *The Expert*, BBC; *Canterbury Tales*, BBC; *Mad Jack*, BBC; *Ryan International*, BBC; *Waugh on Crime*, BBC; *The Stalls of Barchester*, BBC; *Can You Prove That*, BBC; *The Liver Birds*, BBC; *The Moon Shines Bright on Charlie Chaplin*, BBC; *A Warning to the Curious—Clive Swift, Esq.*, BBC; *Dead of Night*, BBC; *Villains*, LWT; *The Pearcross Girls*, BBC; *South Riding*, YTV; *Clayhanger*, ATV; *Willow Cabins*, YTV; *Whodunnit?*, Thames; *The Exorcist*; and *Home Movies*.

RELATED CAREER—Teacher and director, Royal Academy of Dramatic Art and London Academy of Music and Dramatic Arts, 1970—; co-founder and secretary, Actors' Centre, 1979—.

WRITINGS: STAGE—(Adaptor) *The Lower Depths*, London Academy of Music and Dramatic Arts, 1970; co-devisor, *All Together*

Now, Haymarket Theatre, 1979. OTHER—*The Job of Acting,* Harrap, 1976, revised 1985; *The Performing World of the Actor,* Hamish Hamilton, 1981.

SIDELIGHTS: RECREATIONS—Music and sports.

ADDRESSES: AGENT—Prestige Talent Agency, Bugle House, 21-A Noel Street, London W1V 3PD, England.

T

TALBOT, Lyle 1902-

PERSONAL: Born Lysle Henderson, February 8, 1902 (some sources say 1904), in Pittsburgh, PA; son of J. Edward (an actor) and Florence (an actress; maiden name, Talbot) Henderson; married Margaret Abbot (an actress), June 19, 1947; children: two sons, two daughters. EDUCATION: Attended the University of Nebraska, 1918. MILITARY: U.S. Army Air Corps, Special Services, staff sergeant, during World War II.

VOCATION: Actor and director.

CAREER: STAGE DEBUT—With MacKnight the Hypnotist, 1921. PRINCIPAL STAGE APPEARANCES—Don Stackhouse, *Separate Rooms,* Maxine Elliott's Theatre, New York City, 1940; Dawson and Kennedy, *The Legend of Lou,* Cass Theatre, Detroit, MI, 1946; also appeared in *South Pacific,* State Theatre, New York City, 1969; as the Villain, *St. Elmo,* Whetten Repertory Company, in Colorado; and in summer theatre productions throughout the United States.

MAJOR TOURS—Krogstad, *A Doll's House,* U.S. cities, 1945; Felix Unger, *The Odd Couple,* U.S. cities, 1966-67; also with the Chase-Lister Repertory Company, U.S. cities, 1923-25; in *Never Too Late,* U.S. cities, 1966; *There's a Girl in My Soup,* U.S. cities.

FILM DEBUT—Eddie Shaw, *Love Is a Racket,* Warner Brothers/ First National, 1932. PRINCIPAL FILM APPEARANCES—Sully, *Big City Blues,* Warner Brothers, 1932; Dr. Cromwell, *Klondike,* Monogram, 1932; editor, *Miss Pinkerton,* First National, 1932; Ed Fields, *The Purchase Price,* Warner Brothers, 1932; Brice, *Stranger in Town,* Warner Brothers, 1932; Phil Winston, *The Thirteenth Guest* (also known as *Lady Beware*), Monogram, 1932; Mike Loftus, *Three on a Match,* Warner Brothers/First National, 1932; Jerry Gregory, *Unholy Love,* Hollywood, 1932; Buck Weaver, *College Coach* (also known as *Football Coach*), Warner Brothers, 1933; Raymond Fox, *Girl Missing,* Warner Brothers, 1933; Bob Jones, *Havana Widows,* Warner Brothers/First National, 1933; Don, *Ladies They Talk About* (also known as *Women in Prison*), Warner Brothers, 1933; Doc Woods, *The Life of Jimmy Dolan* (also known as *The Kid's Last Fight*), Warner Brothers, 1933; Don Andrews, *Mary Stevens, M.D.,* Warner Brothers, 1933; Tony Gage, *No More Orchids,* Columbia, 1933; Danny Drew, *She Had to Say Yes,* Warner Brothers/First National, 1933; Ted Rand, *A Shriek in the Night,* Allied Pictures, 1933; Bud, *20,000 Years in Sing Sing,* Warner Brothers, 1933; Geoffrey Waring, *42nd Street,* Warner Brothers, 1933; Spencer Carleton, *Fog over Frisco,* Warner Brothers, 1934; Jeff, *Heat Lightning,* Warner Brothers, 1934; Neil, *A Lady Lost* (also known as *Courageous*), Warner Brothers, 1934; Dr. Gregory Burton, *Mandalay,* Warner Brothers, 1934; Bob Halsey, *Murder in the Clouds,* Warner Brothers/First National,

1934; Bill Houston, *One Night of Love,* Columbia, 1934; Dr. Connolly, *Registered Nurse,* Warner Brothers/First National, 1934; Leland, *The Dragon Murder Case,* Warner Brothers, 1934; Dr. Goodman, *Return of the Terror,* Warner Brothers/First National, 1934.

Lucky Lorimer, *Broadway Hostess,* Warner Brothers, 1935; Dr. Doray, *The Case of the Lucky Legs,* Warner Brothers, 1935; Ted Lacey, *Chinatown Squad,* Universal, 1935; Charley Barnes, *It Happened in New York,* Universal, 1935; Jim, *Oil for the Lamps of China,* Warner Brothers/First National, 1935; Rolfe Brent, *Our Little Girl,* Twentieth Century-Fox, 1935; Slattery, *Page Miss Glory,* Warner Brothers, 1935; Wallace Storm, *Red Hot Tires* (also known as *Racing Luck*), Warner Brothers, 1935; Deke Lonergan, *While the Patient Slept,* Warner Brothers/First National, 1935; Lacy, *Boulder Dam,* Warner Brothers, 1936; Francis X. Harrigan, *Go West, Young Man,* Paramount, 1936; Frank Gordon, *The Law in Her Hands,* Warner Brothers/First National, 1936; Dr. Allen Carick, *Murder by an Aristocrat,* Warner Brothers/First National, 1936; Bob Carey, *The Singing Kid,* Warner Brothers/First National, 1936; Fred Dennis, *Trapped by Television,* Columbia, 1936; Bill Peck, *Affairs of Cappy Ricks,* Republic, 1937; Crane, *Mind Your Own Business,* Paramount, 1937; Bob Benton, *Second Honeymoon,* Twentieth Century-Fox, 1937; Jimmy, *The Three Legionnaires* (also known as *Three Crazy Legionnaires*), General, 1937; Dave Tolliver, *Westbound Limited,* Universal, 1937; Tom Connors, *What Price Vengeance?,* Rialto, 1937; Matt Collins, *The Arkansas Traveler,* Paramount, 1938; Hugo, *Call of the Yukon,* Republic, 1938; Phillip Reeves, *Change of Heart,* Twentieth Century-Fox, 1938; Henry, *Gateway,* Twentieth Century-Fox, 1938; Eastman, *I Stand Accused,* Republic, 1938; Singer Martin, *One Wild Night,* Republic, 1938; Jack Scott, *Forged Passport,* Republic, 1939; Willie Hogger, *Second Fiddle,* Twentieth Century-Fox, 1939; Marty Collins, *They Asked for It,* Universal, 1939; Lieutenant Bob Bennett, *Torture Ship,* Producers Distributors Corporation, 1939.

Paul Hunter, *He Married His Wife,* Twentieth Century-Fox, 1940; Ross Waring, *Parole Fixer,* Paramount, 1940; Reddy, *Mexican Spitfire's Elephant,* RKO, 1942; Joe, *A Night for Crime,* Producers Distributors Corporation, 1942; Steve, *She's in the Army,* Monogram, 1942; Captain Robert Owen, *They Raid by Night,* Producers Distributors Corporation, 1942; George Dickson, *Man of Courage,* Producers Distributors Corporation, 1943; George Kent, *Are These Our Parents?,* Monogram, 1944; Tex, *The Falcon Out West,* RKO, 1944; Yellow Gloves Weldon, *Gambler's Choice,* Paramount, 1944; Jim Davis, *One Body Too Many,* Paramount, 1944; Randall, *Sensations of 1945* (also known as *Sensations*), United Artists, 1944; Bill Hollister, *Trail to Gunsight,* Universal, 1944; Sergeant Gelsey, *Up in Arms,* RKO, 1944; Tony Sardell, *Dixie Jamboree,* Producers Releasing Corporation, 1945; Lucky Dorgan, *Gun Town,* Universal, 1946; Duell Renslow, *Murder Is My Business,* Producers Releasing Corporation, 1946; King Blaine, *Song of Arizona,* Republic, 1946; Inspector Malloy, *Strange Impersonation,* Republic, 1946; Charles Johnson, *Danger Street,* Paramount, 1947; Morello, *The Devil's Cargo,* Film Classics, 1948; Fred Muller, *Appointment with Murder,* Film Classics, 1948; detective, *Highway 13,* Screen Guild, 1948; Henderson, *Joe Palooka in Winner Take All,* Monogram, 1948; Andy Barrett, *Sky Dragon,* Monogram, 1949; Blinky Harris, *Fighting Fools,* Monogram, 1949; Lieutenant Muldoon, *Joe Palooka in the Big Fight,* Monogram, 1949; Captain Duncan, *The Mutineers* (also known as *Pirate Ship*), Columbia, 1949; police commissioner, *Parole, Inc.,* Eagle-Lion, 1949; Garvey Yager, *Quick on the Trigger,* Columbia, 1949; radio announcer, *Ringside,* Screen Guild, 1949; doctor, *Shep Comes Home,* Screen Guild, 1949; Nick, *Thunder in the Pines,* Screen Guild, 1949; Captain Hayes, *Wild Weed* (also known as *She Should 'a Said No* and *Devil's Weed*), Eureka, 1949.

First logger, *Big Timber,* Monogram, 1950; Captain McLane, *Border Rangers,* Lippert, 1950; Marshall, *Cherokee Uprising,* Monogram, 1950; contractor, *Everybody's Dancin',* Lippert, 1950; Johnson, *Federal Man,* Eagle-Lion, 1950; Fred Burns, *The Jackpot,* Twentieth Century-Fox, 1950; Bruce McDermott, *Lucky Losers,* Monogram, 1950; Mr. Boyer, *One Too Many* (also known as *Killer with a Label*), Hallmark, 1950; Augustus King, *Revenue Agent,* Columbia, 1950; guard, *Triple Trouble,* Monogram, 1950; doctor, *Abilene Trail,* Monogram, 1951; Teasdale, *Blue Blood,* Monogram, 1951; Sheriff Ed Lowery, *Colorado Ambush,* Monogram, 1951; Lieutenant Grayson, *Fingerprints Don't Lie,* Lippert, 1951; Grant, *Fury of the Congo,* Columbia, 1951; physician, *Hurricane Island,* Columbia, 1951; Dr. Mitchell Heller, *Jungle Manhunt,* Columbia, 1951; Lieutenant McLaughlin, *Mask of the Dragon,* Lippert, 1951; Major Green, *Purple Heart Diary* (also known as *No Time for Tears*), Columbia, 1951; detective, *The Scarf,* United Artists, 1951; Gilroy, *African Treasure* (also known as *Bomba and the African Treasure*), Monogram, 1952; Walter Fleming, *Desperadoes Outpost,* Republic, 1952; Big Jim, *Feudin' Fools,* Monogram, 1952; Taggert, *The Gold Raiders,* United Artists, 1952; Collins, *Kansas Territory,* Monogram, 1952; Doc Lockwood, *The Old West,* Columbia, 1952; Judge Dixon, *Outlaw Women,* Lippert, 1952; Williams, *Sea Tiger,* Monogram, 1952; Hamilton, *Texas City,* Monogram, 1952; Colonel Loring, *Untamed Women,* United Artists, 1952; radio director, *With a Song in My Heart,* Twentieth Century-Fox, 1952; Colonel Blair, *Clipped Wings,* Allied Artists, 1953; Major Curwin, *Down among the Sheltering Palms,* Twentieth Century-Fox, 1953; Police Inspector Warren, *Glen or Glenda* (also known as *I Led Two Lives, I Changed My Sex, He or She,* and *The Transvestite*), Paramount, 1953; telegraph operator, *Star of Texas,* Allied Artists, 1953; Weber, *Tumbleweed,* Universal, 1953; Rocky, *White Lightning,* Monogram, 1953; stage manager, *There's No Business Like Show Business,* Twentieth Century-Fox, 1954; admiral, *Tobor the Great,* Republic, 1954.

Cy Bowman, *Jail Busters,* Allied Artists, 1955; Woodruff, *Sudden Danger,* Allied Artists, 1955; Tony Fuller, *Calling Homicide,* Allied Artists, 1956; narrator, *The Mesa of Lost Women* (also known as *Lost Women* and *Lost Women of Zarpa*), A.J. Frances White/Joy Houck, 1956; Harry Connors, *The Great Man,* Universal, 1957; William Remington Kane, *High School Confidential* (also known as *The Young Hellions*), Metro-Goldwyn-Mayer, 1958; Van Richards, *The Hot Angel,* Paramount, 1958; Leonardo, *The Notorious Mr. Monks,* Republic, 1958; Chief Jensen, *City of Fear,* Columbia, 1959; General Roberts, *Plan 9 from Outer Space* (also known as *Grave Robbers from Outer Space*), Distributors Corporation of America, 1959; Mr. Brimmer, *Sunrise at Campobello,*

Warner Brothers, 1960. Also appeared in *A Miracle on Main Street,* Columbia, 1940; *The Vicious Circle* (also known as *The Circle*), 1948; *Mississippi Rhythm,* Monogram, 1949; *The Dalton's Women,* Howco, 1950; *Oklahoma Justice,* Monogram, 1951; *Texas Lawmen* (also known as *Lone Star Lawman*), Monogram, 1951; *Captain Kidd and the Slave Girl,* United Artists, 1954; *Jail Bait* (also known as *Hidden Face*), Howco, 1954; *The Steel Cage,* United Artists, 1954.

PRINCIPAL TELEVISION APPEARANCES—Series: Paul Fonda, *The Bob Cummings Show* (also known as *Love That Bob*), NBC, 1955, then CBS, 1955-57, later NBC, 1957-59; Joe Randolph, *The Adventures of Ozzie and Harriet,* ABC, 1956-66; Lieutenant Choates, *Ben Jerrod,* NBC, 1963. Episodic: Baylor, *Commando Cody,* NBC, 1955; Ralph, *Who's the Boss?,* ABC, 1986; Fletcher, *Alfred Hitchcock Presents,* NBC, 1986; also "Myrt and Marge," *Summer Theatre,* ABC, 1953; *Newhart,* CBS, 1987; as George Wilson, *The Lone Ranger,* ABC; *Pursuit,* CBS; *Climax!,* CBS; *Lux Video Theatre,* NBC; *Matinee Theatre,* NBC; *Arrest and Trial,* ABC; *The Burns and Allen Show,* NBC; *The Lucy Show,* CBS; *The Red Skelton Show,* CBS; *Wagon Train,* NBC; *The Danny Thomas Show,* ABC; *77 Sunset Strip,* ABC; *Revlon Mirror Theatre;* and as Mr. Dennison, *Leave It to Beaver.* Specials: *Howdy,* ABC, 1970; narrator, *World without Walls: Beryl Markham's African Memoir* (documentary), PBS, 1986.

RELATED CAREER—Owner and director of a theatre stock company, Lyceum Theatre, Memphis, TN, 1929—.

AWARDS: Screen Actors Guild Gold Life Membership Card, 1960; honorary mayor, Studio City, CA.

MEMBER: Screen Actors Guild (co-founder and board member), Actors' Equity Association, American Federation of Television and Radio Artists (board member), Masonic Lodge (Shriner), Lambs Club, Masquers, American Legion.

ADDRESSES: HOME—3942 Goodland Avenue, Studio City, CA 91604.*

*   *   *

TANDY, Jessica   1909-

PERSONAL: Born June 7, 1909, in London, England; naturalized U.S. citizen, 1954; daughter of Harry and Jessie Helen (Horspool) Tandy; married Jack Hawkins (an actor), 1932 (divorced, 1940); married Hume Cronyn (an actor), September 27, 1942; children: Susan (first marriage); Christopher, Tandy (second marriage). EDUCATION: Trained for the stage at the Ben Greet Academy of Acting, London, 1924-27.

VOCATION: Actress.

CAREER: STAGE DEBUT—Sara Manderson, *The Manderson Girls,* Playroom Six, London, 1927. BROADWAY DEBUT—Toni Rakonitz, *The Matriarch,* Longacre Theatre, 1930. PRINCIPAL STAGE APPEARANCES—Gladys, *The Comedy of Good and Evil,* and Ginevra, *Alice Sit-by-the Fire,* both Birmingham Repertory Company, Birmingham, U.K., 1928; Lena Jackson, *The Rumour,* Court Theatre, London, 1929; typist, *The Theatre of Life,* Arts Theatre, London, 1929; Maggie, *Water,* Little Theatre, London, 1929; Aude, *The Unknown Warrior,* Haymarket Theatre, London,

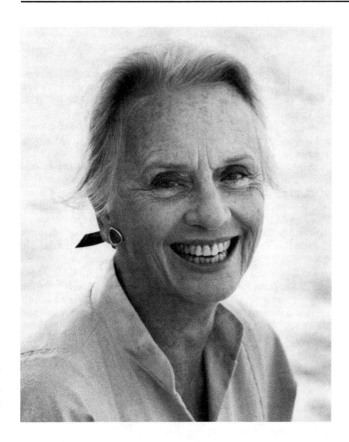

Photography by Zoe Dominic

JESSICA TANDY

1929; Olivia, *Twelfth Night,* Oxford University Dramatic Society, Oxford, U.K., 1930; Cynthia Perry, *The Last Enemy,* Shubert Theatre, New York City, 1930; Fay, *The Man Who Pays the Piper,* St. Martin's Theatre, London, 1931; Audrey, *Autumn Crocus,* Lyric Theatre, London, 1931; Ruth Blair, *Port Said,* Wyndham's Theatre, London, 1931; Anna, *Musical Chairs,* Arts Theatre, 1931; Carlotta, *Mutual Benefit,* St. Martin's Theatre, 1932; Manuela, *Children in Uniform,* Duchess Theatre, London, 1932; Alicia Audley, *Lady Audley's Secret,* Arts Theatre, 1933; Marikke, *Midsummer Fires,* Embassy Theatre, London, 1933; Titania, *A Midsummer Night's Dream,* Open Air Theatre, London, 1933; Betty, *Ten Minute Alibi,* Haymarket Theatre, 1933; Rosamund, *Birthday,* Cambridge Festival Theatre, Cambridge, U.K., 1934; Viola, *Twelfth Night,* and Anne Page, *The Merry Wives of Windsor,* Hippodrome Theatre, Manchester, U.K., 1934; Eva Whiston, *Line Engaged,* Duke of York's Theatre, London, 1934; Ophelia, *Hamlet,* New Theatre, London, 1934; Ada, *Noah,* New Theatre, 1935; Anna Penn, *Anthony and Anna,* Whitehall Theatre, London, 1935; Marie Rose, *The Ante-Room,* Queens Theatre, London, 1936; Jacqueline, *French without Tears,* Criterion Theatre, London, 1936; Pamela March, *Honour Thy Father,* Arts Theatre, 1936; Viola and Sebastian, *Twelfth Night,* and Katherine, *Henry V,* both Old Vic Theatre, London, 1937; Ellen Murray, *Yes, My Darling Daughter,* St. James's Theatre, London, 1937; Kay, *Time and the Conways,* Ritz Theatre, New York City, 1938; Nora Fintry, *The White Steed,* Cort Theatre, New York City, 1939; Viola, *Twelfth Night,* Open Air Theatre, 1939.

Deaconess, *Geneva,* Henry Miller's Theatre, New York City, 1940; Cordelia, *King Lear,* and Miranda, *The Tempest,* both Old Vic Theatre, 1940; Dr. Mary Murray, *Jupiter Laughs,* Biltmore

Theatre, New York City, 1940; Abigail Hill, *Anne of England,* St. James Theatre, New York City, 1941; Cattrin, *Yesterday's Magic,* Guild Theatre, New York City, 1942; Lucretia Collins, *Portrait of a Madonna,* Las Palmas Theatre, Los Angeles, CA, 1946; Blanche du Bois, *A Streetcar Named Desire,* Ethel Barrymore Theatre, New York City, 1947; title role, *Hilda Crane,* Coronet Theatre, New York City, 1950; Agnes, *The Fourposter,* Ethel Barrymore Theatre, 1951; Mary Doyle, *Madam Will You Walk,* Phoenix Theatre, New York City, 1953; Agnes, *The Fourposter,* City Center Theatre, New York City, 1955; Mary Honey, *The Honeys,* Longacre Theatre, 1955; Frances Farrar, *A Day by the Sea,* American National Theatre and Academy Theatre, New York City, 1955; Martha Walling, *The Man in the Dog Suit,* Coronet Theatre, 1958; Lucretia Collins, "Portrait of a Madonna," Innocent Bystander, "A Pound on Demand," and Angela Nightingale, "Bedtime Story" in *Triple Play* (triple-bill), Playhouse Theatre, New York City, 1959; Louise Harrington, *Five Finger Exercise,* Music Box Theatre, New York City, 1959.

Lady Macbeth, *Macbeth,* and Cassandra, *Troilus and Cressida,* both American Shakespeare Festival, Stratford, CT, 1961; Edith Maitland, *Big Fish, Little Fish,* Duke of York's Theatre, 1962; Gertrude, *Hamlet,* Olga, *The Three Sisters,* and Linda Loman, *Death of a Salesman,* all Tyrone Guthrie Theatre, Minneapolis, MN, 1963; Fraulein Doktor Mathilde von Zahnd, *The Physicists,* Martin Beck Theatre, New York City, 1964; Lady Wishfort, *The Way of the World,* Madame Ranevskaya, *The Cherry Orchard,* and Mother-in-Law, *The Caucasian Chalk Circle,* all Tyrone Guthrie Theatre, 1965; Agnes, *A Delicate Balance,* Martin Beck Theatre, 1966; Froisine, *The Miser,* Mark Taper Forum, Los Angeles, 1968; Hesione Hushabye, *Heartbreak House,* Shaw Festival, Niagara-on-the-Lake, ON, Canada, 1968; Pamela Pew-Pickett, *Tchin-Tchin,* Ivanhoe Theatre, Chicago, IL, 1969; Marguerite Gautier, *Camino Real,* Vivian Beaumont Theatre, New York City, 1970; Marjorie, *Home,* Morosco Theatre, New York City, 1970; Wife, *All Over,* Martin Beck Theatre, 1971; Winnie, *Happy Days,* and the Mouth, *Not I,* both Samuel Beckett Festival, Forum Theatre, New York City, 1972; Anna-Mary Conklin, "Come into the Garden, Maud," and Hilde Latymer, "A Song at Twilight," in *Noel Coward in Two Keys* (double-bill), Ethel Barrymore Theatre, 1974; Lady Wishfort, *The Way of the World,* Hippolyta and Titania, *A Midsummer Night's Dream,* and title role, *Eve,* all Stratford Shakespearean Festival, Stratford, ON, Canada, 1976; Mary Tyrone, *Long Day's Journey into Night,* Theatre London, London, ON, Canada, 1977; Fonsia Dorsey, *The Gin Game,* Long Wharf Theatre, New Haven, CT, then John Golden Theatre, New York City, both 1977.

Annie Nations, *Foxfire,* and Mary Tyrone, *Long Day's Journey into Night,* both Stratford Shakespearean Festival, 1980; Mother, *Rose,* Cort Theatre, 1981; Annie Nations, *Foxfire,* Tyrone Guthrie Theatre, 1981, then Ethel Barrymore Theatre, 1982, later Ahmanson Theatre, Los Angeles, 1985; Amanda Wingfield, *The Glass Menagerie,* Eugene O'Neill Theatre, New York City, 1984; Charlotte, *Salonika,* New York Shakespeare Festival, Public Theatre, New York City, 1985; Elizabeth Milne, *The Petition,* John Golden Theatre, 1986. Also appeared in *Below the Surface,* Repertory Players, London, 1932; *Juarez and Maximilian,* Phoenix Theatre, London, 1932; *Troilus and Cressida, See Naples and Die, The Witch, Rose without a Thorn, The Inspector General,* and *The Servant of Two Masters,* all Cambridge Festival Theatre, 1932; *The Romantic Young Lady,* Fulham Shilling Theatre, London, 1934; *Now I Lay Me Down to Sleep,* Stanford University, Palo Alto, CA, 1949; *The Little Blue Light,* Brattle Theatre, Cambridge, MA, 1950; *Hear America Speaking* (readings), the White House, Washington, DC, 1965; and *Many Faces of Love* (readings), Theatre London, 1976.

MAJOR TOURS—Lydia Blake, *Yellow Sands,* U.K. cities, 1928; Martha Walling, *The Man in the Dog Suit,* U.S. cities, 1957; Mrs. Morgan, ''I Spy,'' Innocent Bystander, ''A Pound on Demand,'' and Angela Nightingale, ''Bedtime Story'' in *Triple Play* (triple-bill), U.S. cities, 1958; Louise Harrington, *Five Finger Exercise,* U.S. cities, 1960; Agnes, *A Delicate Balance,* U.S. cities, 1967; the Mouth, *Not I,* U.S. cities, 1973; Anna-Mary Conklin, ''Come into the Garden, Maud,'' and Hilde Latymer, ''A Song at Twilight,'' in *Noel Coward in Two Keys* (double-bill), U.S. cities, 1975; Fonsia Dorsey, *The Gin Game,* U.S. cities, also Toronto, ON, Canada, London, England, and Soviet cities, 1978-79. Also toured in *Charles the King, Geneva,* and *Tobias and the Angel,* Canadian cities, 1939; *Face to Face* (concert readings), U.S. cities, 1954; *Promenade All,* U.S. cities, 1972-73; and *Many Faces of Love,* U.S. cities, 1974-75.

FILM DEBUT—Maid, *Indiscretions of Eve,* Wardour, 1932. PRINCIPAL FILM APPEARANCES—Ann Osborne, *Murder in the Family,* Twentieth Century-Fox, 1938; Liesel Roeder, *The Seventh Cross,* Metro-Goldwyn-Mayer (MGM), 1944; Louise Kane, *The Valley of Decision,* MGM, 1945; Peggy O'Malley, *Dragonwyck,* Twentieth Century-Fox, 1946; Kate Leckie, *The Green Years,* MGM, 1946; Nan Britton, *Forever Amber,* Twentieth Century-Fox, 1947; Janet Spence, *A Woman's Vengeance,* Universal, 1947; Catherine Lawrence, *September Affair,* Paramount, 1950; Frau Rommel, *The Desert Fox* (also known as *Rommel—Desert Fox*), Twentieth Century-Fox, 1951; Myra Butler, *The Light in the Forest,* Buena Vista, 1958; Mrs. Adams, *Adventures of a Young Man* (also known as *Hemingway's Adventures of a Young Man*), Twentieth Century-Fox, 1962; Lydia Brenner, *The Birds,* Universal, 1963; Edna Shaft, *Butley,* American Film Theatre, 1974; Carol, *Honky Tonk Freeway,* Universal/AFD, 1981; Eleanor McCullen, *Best Friends,* Warner Brothers, 1982; Grace Rice, *Still of the Night,* MGM/United Artists, 1982; Mrs. Fields, *The World According to Garp,* Warner Brothers, 1982; Miss Birdseye, *The Bostonians,* Almi, 1984; Alma Finley, *Cocoon,* Twentieth Century-Fox, 1985; Faye Riley, **batteries not included,* Universal, 1987; Miss Venable, *The House on Carroll Street,* Orion, 1988; Alma Finley, *Cocoon: The Return,* Twentieth Century-Fox, 1988. Also appeared as herself, *The Thrill of Genius* (also known as *Hitchcock, Il brivido del genio;* documentary), 1985.

PRINCIPAL TELEVISION APPEARANCES—Series: Liz Marriott, *The Marriage,* NBC, 1954. Episodic: Lucretia Collins, ''Portrait of a Madonna,'' *Actors Studio,* ABC, 1948; also *Masterpiece Playhouse,* NBC, 1950; ''The Fallen Idol,'' *Dupont Show of the Month,* NBC, 1959; *The Alfred Hitchcock Hour,* CBS; *The Somerset Maugham TV Theater,* NBC; *Omnibus,* CBS; *Studio One,* CBS. Specials: Agnes, *The Fourposter,* NBC, 1955; Blanche Stroeve, *The Moon and Sixpence,* NBC, 1959; Annie Nations, ''Foxfire,'' *Hallmark Hall of Fame,* CBS, 1987; as herself, *Onstage: 25 Years at the Guthrie,* syndicated, 1988; also *Christmas' til Closing,* NBC, 1955; *Tennessee Williams' South,* CBC (Canadian television), 1973; *Many Faces of Love,* CBC, 1977; Fonsia Dorsey, *The Gin Game,* 1979.

PRINCIPAL RADIO APPEARANCES—Series: *The Marriage,* 1953-54.

RELATED CAREER—Dramatic advisor, Goddard Neighborhood Center, New York City, 1948.

RECORDINGS: ALBUMS—Volumnia, *Coriolanus;* Amanda Wingfield, *The Glass Menagerie;* also *The Wind and the Willows.*

AWARDS: Antoinette Perry Award, Best Actress in a Play, and Twelfth Night Club Award, both 1948, for *A Streetcar Named Desire;* (with Hume Cronyn) Comedia Matinee Club Award, 1952, for *The Fourposter;* Delia Austrian Award from the New York Drama League, 1960, for *Five Finger Exercise;* Obie Awards from the *Village Voice,* Outstanding Achievement in the Off-Broadway Theatre and Distinguished Performance, both 1973, for *Not I;* Drama Desk Award, 1973, for *Happy Days* and *Not I;* Brandeis University Creative Arts Award, Theatre Arts Medal for a Lifetime of Distinguished Achievement, 1978; Antoinette Perry Award, Best Actress in a Play, Drama Desk Award, Outstanding Actress, Los Angeles Critics Award, Sarah Siddons Award, and National Press Club Award, all 1979, for *The Gin Game;* inducted in the Theatre Hall of Fame in recognition of outstanding contributions to the American theatre, 1979; Antoinette Perry Award, Best Actress in a Play, Drama Desk Award, and Outer Circle Critics Award, all 1983, for *Foxfire;* Common Wealth Award, 1983, for Distinguished Service in Dramatic Arts; Antoinette Perry Award nomination, Best Actress in a Play, 1986, for *The Petition;* Kennedy Center Honors, 1986; Alley Theatre Award, 1987, for Significant Contributions to the Theatre Arts; Academy of Science Fiction, Fantasy, and Horror Films Award, Best Actress, 1987, for **batteries not included;* (with Hume Cronyn) Franklin Haven Sargent Award from the American Academy of Dramatic Arts, 1988, for Outstanding Quality of Acting; Emmy Award, Best Dramatic Actress in a Television Special, 1988, for ''Foxfire,'' *Hallmark Hall of Fame.* Honorary degrees: LL.D., University of Western Ontario, 1974; L.H.D., Fordham University, 1985.

MEMBER: Actors' Equity Association, Screen Actors Guild, American Federation of Television and Radio Artists, Cosmopolitan Club.

ADDRESSES: OFFICE—63-23 Carlton Street, Rego Park, NY 11374. AGENT—International Creative Management, 40 W. 57th Street, New York, NY 10019.

*   *   *

TAVERNIER, Bertrand   1941-

PERSONAL: Born April 25, 1941, in Lyon, France; son of Rene (a writer and publicist) and Genevieve (Dumond) Tavernier; married Colo (a screenwriter; divorced); children: Nils, Tiffany. EDUCATION: Attended the Sorbonne; also studied law for two years.

VOCATION: Screenwriter and director.

CAREER: Also see WRITINGS below. PRINCIPAL FILM WORK—Director: ''Une Chance explosive'' in *La Chance et l'amour,* Rome-Paris Films/ROTOR Film, 1964; ''Baiser de Judas'' in *Les Baisers,* Rome-Paris Films/Flora Films, 1965; *L'Horloger de Saint-Paul,* Lira Films, 1974, released in the United States as *The Clockmaker,* Joseph Green Pictures, 1976; *Que la fete commence . . . ,* Fildebroc, 1975, released in the United States as *Let Joy Reign Supreme,* Specialty Films, 1977; *Le Juge et l'assassin,* Lira Films, 1976, released in the United States as *The Judge and the Assassin,* Libra Films, 1982; *Des Enfants gates,* Gaumont/Sara/Films 66/ Little Bear, 1977, released in the United States as *Spoiled Children,* Corinth, 1981.

Death Watch (also known as *La Morte en direct* and *The Continuous Katherine Mortenhoe*), Selta/Sara/Little Bear/FR-3/Gaumont, 1980, released in the United States by Quartet Films, 1982; (also producer) *Une Semaine de vacances*, Sara Films/Little Bear Productions, 1980, released in the United States as *A Week's Brief Vacation*, Biograph International, 1982; *Coup de torchon*, Films de la Tour/Little Bear Productions, 1982, released in the United States as *Clean Slate*, Biograph International/Quartet Films/Frank Moreno Company, 1982; (with Robert Parrish) *Mississippi Blues*, Odessa/Little Bear Productions, 1983; *Un Dimanche a la campagne*, Sara Films/Little Bear Productions, 1984, released in the United States as *A Sunday in the Country*, Metro-Goldwyn-Mayer/United Artists Classics, 1984; *Round Midnight* (also known as *Autour de minuit*), Warner Brothers, 1986; *La Passion Beatrice*, 1986, released in the United States as *The Passion of Beatrice*, Samuel Goldwyn, 1988. Also producer, *La Question*, 1976; producer, *Rue du pied de Grue*, 1979; producer, *La Trace* (also known as *The Trace*), 1983; director (with Parrish), *October Country*, Odessa/Little Bear Productions.

RELATED CAREER—Assistant to film director Jean-Pierre Melville, 1961; press agent for film producer Georges de Beauregard; freelance press agent (with Pierre Rissient), 1965-1972; assisted with and appeared in *Hotel Terminus: Klaus Barbie, His Life and Times*, 1988; president, Lumiere Institute.

WRITINGS: See production details above, unless indicated. FILMS—"Une Chance explosive" in *La Chance et l'amour*, 1964; "Baiser de Judas" in *Les Baisers*, 1965; (with Jean Aurenche and Pierre Bost) *L'Horloger de Saint-Paul*, 1974; *Que la fete commence . . .*, 1975; (with Aurenche) *Le Juge et l'assassin*, 1976; (with Charlotte Dubreuil and Christine Pascal) *Des Enfants gates*, 1977; (with David Rayfiel) *Death Watch*, 1980; (with Colo Tavernier and Marie-Francoise Hans) *Une Semaine de vacances*, 1980; (with Aurenche) *Coup de torchon*, 1982; *Mississippi Blues*, 1983; (with C. Tavernier) *Un Dimanche a la campagne*, 1984; (with Rayfiel) *Round Midnight*, 1986; (with Laurent Heynemann and Phillippe Boucher) *Les Mois d'Avril sont meurtriers* (also known as *April Is a Deadly Month*), Sara Films/CDF, 1987. Also (co-writer) *Coplan ouvre le feu a Mexico*, 1967; *Capitaine Singrid*, 1968; *La Trace*, 1983; and *October Country*.

OTHER—(With Jean-Pierre Coursodon) *Trente ans de cinema Americaine* (title means *Thirty Years of American Cinema*; nonfiction), Editions C.I.B., 1970. Also contributor to the periodicals *Cahiers du cinema* and *Positif*.

AWARDS: Prix Louis Delluc, Silver Bear from the Berlin Film Festival, and Nugo from the Chicago Film Festival, all 1974, for *L'Horloger de Saint-Paul;* Cesar Awards from the French Academy of Motion Pictures, Best Director and (with Jean Aurenche) Best Original Screenplay, both 1975, for *Que la fete commence . . .;* (with Aurenche) Cesar Award, Best Original Screenplay, 1976, for *Le Juge et l'assassin;* Prix Unifrance and Golden Asteroide, both for *Death Watch;* Academy Award nomination, Best Foreign Film, and Cesar Award nomination, both for *Coup de torchon;* Cannes Film Festival Award, Best Director, New York Film Critics Circle Award, Best Foreign Film, National Board of Review Award, Best Foreign Film, and Cesar Award, Best Screenplay, 1984, all for *Un Dimanche a la campagne;* Italian Critic's Award and Prix de l'Office Catholique, both for *Round Midnight*.

MEMBER: French Directors Guild (past president), Society of Dramatic Authors and Composers (vice-president).

OTHER SOURCES: Contemporary Authors, Volume 123, Gale, 1988.

ADDRESSES: OFFICE—AB Films, 51 rue de la Fontaine au Roy, 75011 Paris, France.

*   *   *

TAYLOR, Clarice   1927-

PERSONAL: Born September 20, 1927, in Buckingham County, VA; daughter of Leon B. and Ophelia (Booker) Taylor; married Claude Banks, Jr. (divorced). EDUCATION: Attended Columbia University; trained for the stage at the American Negro Theatre, the Harlem YMCA theatre group, the New Theatre School, and the Negro Ensemble Company.

VOCATION: Actress.

CAREER: OFF-BROADWAY DEBUT—Sophie Slow, *On Strivers' Row*, American Negro Theatre Playhouse, 1942. LONDON DEBUT—*Song of the Lusitanian Bogey*, Negro Ensemble Company, Aldwych Theatre, 1969. PRINCIPAL STAGE APPEARANCES—Ann Drake, *Home Is the Hunter*, American Negro Theatre Playhouse, New York City, 1945; Sister Maloney, *The Peacemaker*, American Negro Theatre Playhouse, 1946; Willetta, *Trouble in Mind*, Committee for the Negro in the Arts, Greenwich Mews Theatre, New York City, 1955; Naomi, *Nat Turner*, Casa Galacia, New York City, 1960; Emma Leech, *Summer of the Seventeenth Doll*, Sarumi, *Kongi's Harvest*, Annie, *Daddy Goodness*, and Reba, *God Is a (Guess What?)*, all Negro Ensemble Company, St. Mark's Playhouse, New York City, 1968; Mrs. Rogers, "String," and Mrs. Grace Love, "Contribution," in *An Evening of One Acts*, and village woman, *Man Better Man*, both Negro Ensemble Company, St. Mark's Playhouse, 1969; Reba, *God Is a (Guess What?)*, Negro Ensemble Company, Teatro Pariola, Rome, Italy, 1969.

Clubwoman, *Day of Absence*, Negro Ensemble Company, St. Mark's Playhouse, 1970; Mrs. Brooks, *Five on the Black Hand Side*, American Place Theatre, Theatre at St. Clement's Church, New York City, 1970; Dolly Mae Anderson, *Rosalee Pritchett*, and Weedy, *The Sty of the Blind Pig*, both Negro Ensemble Company, St. Mark's Playhouse, 1971; Mamma, *The Duplex*, Forum Theatre, New York City, 1972; Fanny Johnson, *Wedding Band*, Public Theatre, New York City, 1972; Weedy, *The Sty of the Blind Pig*, Negro Ensemble Company, Kammerspiele Theatre, Munich, West Germany, 1972; Addaperle, *The Wiz*, Majestic Theatre, New York City, 1975; Moms Mabley, *Moms*, Hudson Guild Theatre, New York City, 1987. Also appeared in *Juno and the Paycock*, *John Henry*, and *Hits, Bits, and Skits*, all American Negro Theatre Playhouse, 1942; *Rain*, American Negro Theatre Playhouse, 1948; *Simple Speaks His Mind, A Medal for Willie*, and *Gold through the Trees*, all Committee for the Negro in the Arts, 1948; *In Splendid Error* and *Major Barbara*, both Greenwich Mews Theatre, 1954; *The Twisting Road*, Greenwich Mews Theatre, 1957; *The Egg and I*, Greenwich Mews Theatre, 1958; *The Doctor in Spite of Himself*, street theatre production, 1958; *Song of the Lusitanian Bogey*, Negro Ensemble Company, Teatro Pariola, 1969; *Akokawe (Initiation)*, Negro Ensemble Company, St. Mark's Playhouse, 1970.

PRINCIPAL STAGE WORK—Director, *Gold through the Trees*,

Committee for the Negro in the Arts, New York City, 1948; co-director, *Trouble in Mind*, Greenwich Mews Theatre, New York City, 1955.

MAJOR TOURS—*To Be Young, Gifted, and Black*, U.S. cities, 1972.

PRINCIPAL FILM APPEARANCES—Rose Landis, *Change of Mind*, Cinerama, 1969; Minnie, *Tell Me That You Love Me, Junie Moon*, Paramount, 1970; Birdie, *Play Misty for Me*, Universal, 1971; Mrs. McKay, *Such Good Friends*, Paramount, 1971; Mrs. Brooks, *Five on the Black Hand Side*, United Artists, 1973; Lu, *Nothing Lasts Forever*, Metro-Goldwyn-Mayer/United Artists, 1984. Also appeared in *Willie Dynamite*, Universal, 1974.

PRINCIPAL TELEVISION APPEARANCES—Series: Nurse Bailey, *Nurse*, CBS, 1981; Anna Huxtable, *The Cosby Show*, NBC, 1984—. Pilots: Millie, *Salt and Pepe*, CBS, 1975; Velma Williams, *High Five*, NBC, 1982. Episodic: *Ironside*, NBC; *Owen Marshall, Counselor at Law*, ABC; *The Doctors*, NBC; *Sanford and Son*, NBC; *Lady Blue*, ABC. Movies: Lovey, *Beulah Land*, NBC, 1980. Specials: *Wedding Band*, *A Friend to Freedom*, and *Light in the Southern Sky*.

RELATED CAREER—Co-founder, American Negro Theatre Playhouse, New York City, 1940.

ADDRESSES: AGENT—The Gersh Agency, 222 N. Canon Drive, Suite 202, Beverly Hills, CA 90210.*

*   *   *

TAYLOR, Elizabeth   1932-

PERSONAL: Full name, Elizabeth Rosemond Taylor; born February 27, 1932, in London, England; daughter of Francis (an art dealer and historian) and Sara (an actress; maiden name, Southern) Taylor; married Conrad Nicholas Hilton, Jr., May 6, 1950 (divorced, 1951); married Michael Wilding (an actor), 1952 (divorced, 1957); married Michael Todd (a producer), February 2, 1957 (died, March, 1958); married Eddie Fisher (a singer and actor), 1959 (divorced, 1964); married Richard Burton (an actor), March 15, 1964 (divorced, 1974); remarried Richard Burton, October 10, 1975 (divorced, 1976); married William John Warner (a politician), 1976 (divorced, 1982); children: Michael, Christopher (second marriage); Elizabeth Frances (third marriage); Liza (fifth marriage; adopted).

VOCATION: Actress and producer.

CAREER: BROADWAY DEBUT-Regina Giddens, *The Little Foxes*, Martin Beck Theatre, 1981. LONDON DEBUT—Regina Giddens, *The Little Foxes*, 1982. PRINCIPAL STAGE APPEARANCES—Regina Giddens, *The Little Foxes*, Center Theatre Group, Ahmanson Theatre, Los Angeles, CA, 1981; Amanda Prynne, *Private Lives*, Lunt-Fontanne Theatre, New York City, 1983.

PRINCIPAL STAGE WORK—Producer (with Zev Bufman as the Elizabeth Group), *Private Lives* and *The Corn Is Green*, both Lunt-Fontanne Theatre, New York City, 1983.

FILM DEBUT—Gloria Twine, *There's One Born Every Minute*,

Universal, 1942. PRINCIPAL FILM APPEARANCES—Priscilla, *Lassie, Come Home*, Metro-Goldwyn-Mayer (MGM), 1943; Helen Burns, *Jane Eyre*, Twentieth Century-Fox, 1944; Velvet Brown, *National Velvet*, MGM, 1944; Betsy at age ten, *The White Cliffs of Dover*, MGM, 1944; Kathie Merrick, *Courage of Lassie* (also known as *Blue Sierra*), MGM, 1946; Cynthia Bishop, *Cynthia* (also known as *The Rich, Full Life*), MGM, 1947; Mary Skinner, *Life with Father*, Warner Brothers, 1947; Carol Pringle, *A Date with Judy*, MGM, 1948; Susan Packett, *Julia Misbehaves*, MGM, 1948; Melinda Greyton, *Conspirator*, MGM, 1949; Amy March, *Little Women*, MGM, 1949; Mary Belney, *The Big Hangover*, MGM, 1950; Kay Banks, *Father of the Bride*, MGM, 1950; Kay Dunstan, *Father's Little Dividend*, MGM, 1951; as herself, *Callaway Went Thataway* (also known as *The Star Said No*), MGM, 1951; woman in crowd, *Quo Vadis*, MGM, 1951; Angela Vickers, *A Place in the Sun*, Paramount, 1951; Rebecca, *Ivanhoe*, MGM, 1952; Anastacia Macaboy, *Love Is Better Than Ever* (also known as *The Light Fantastic*), MGM, 1952; Jean Latimer, *The Girl Who Had Everything*, MGM, 1953; Lady Patricia, *Beau Brummell*, MGM, 1954; Ruth Wiley, *Elephant Walk*, Paramount, 1954; Helen Ellswirth, *The Last Time I Saw Paris*, MGM, 1954; Louise Durant, *Rhapsody*, MGM, 1954; Leslie Lynnton Benedict, *Giant*, Warner Brothers, 1956; Susanna Drake, *Raintree County*, MGM, 1957; Maggie Pollitt, *Cat on a Hot Tin Roof*, MGM, 1958; Catherine Holly, *Suddenly, Last Summer*, Columbia, 1959.

Gloria Wandrous, *Butterfield 8*, MGM, 1960; Sally Kennedy, *Scent of Mystery* (also known as *Holiday in Spain*), Michael Todd, Jr., 1960; title role, *Cleopatra*, Twentieth Century-Fox, 1963; Frances Andros, *The V.I.P.s*, MGM, 1963; Laura Reynolds, *The Sandpiper*, MGM, 1965; Martha, *Who's Afraid of Virginia Woolf?*, Warner Brothers, 1966; Martha Pineda, *The Comedians*, MGM, 1967; Helen of Troy, *Doctor Faustus*, Columbia, 1967; Leonora Penderton, *Reflections in a Golden Eye*, Warner Brothers, 1967; Katharina, *The Taming of the Shrew*, Columbia, 1967; Flora "Sissy" Goforth, *Boom!*, Universal, 1968; Leonora, *Secret Ceremony*, Universal, 1968; masked courtesan, *Anne of the Thousand Days*, Universal, 1969; Fran Walker, *The Only Game in Town*, Twentieth Century-Fox, 1970; Jimmie Jean Jackson, *Hammersmith Is Out*, Cinerama, 1972; Zee Blakeley, *X, Y, and Zee* (also known as *Zee & Co.*), Columbia, 1972; Ellen Wheeler, *Night Watch*, AVCO-Embassy, 1973; Rosie Probert, *Under Milkwood*, Altura Films International, 1973; narrator, *That's Entertainment*, MGM, 1974; Barbara Sawyer, *Ash Wednesday*, Paramount, 1974; Lise, *The Driver's Seat* (also known as *Identikit*), AVCO-Embassy, 1975; Mother, Light, Witch, and Maternal Love, *The Blue Bird*, Twentieth Century-Fox, 1976; Desiree Armfeldt, *A Little Night Music*, New World Cinema, 1977; Lola Comante, *Winter Kills*, AVCO-Embassy, 1979; Marina Rudd, *The Mirror Crack'd*, Associated Film Distribution, 1980; narrator, *Genocide* (documentary), Simon Wiesenthal Center, 1981; as herself, *George Stevens: A Filmmaker's Journey* (documentary), Castle Hill, 1984; Nadia Bulichoff, *Il Giovane Toscanini* (also known as *Young Toscanini* and *Toscanini*), Italian International/Union Generale Cinematographique/Carthago, 1988. Also appeared in *It's Showtime* (documentary), United Artists, 1975.

PRINCIPAL FILM WORK—Producer (with Richard Burton and Franco Zeffirelli), *The Taming of the Shrew*, Columbia, 1967.

PRINCIPAL TELEVISION APPEARANCES—Mini-Series: Madame Conti, *North and South*, ABC, 1985. Episodic: Helena Cassadine, *General Hospital*, ABC, 1981; charwoman, *All My Children*, ABC, 1983; also *The Lucy Show*, CBS, 1971; *Hotel*, ABC, 1984;

Hour Magazine, syndicated, 1986; *Hollywood and the Stars*, NBC; *The David Frost Show*, syndicated. Movies: Jane Reynolds, *Divorce His/Divorce Hers*, ABC, 1973; Edra Vilnofsky, *Victory at Entebbe*, ABC, 1976; Deborah Shapiro, *Between Friends*, HBO, 1983; Louella Parsons, *Malice in Wonderland*, CBS, 1985; Marguerite Sydney, *There Must Be a Pony*, ABC, 1986; title role, *Poker Alice*, CBS, 1987. Specials: Host, *Elizabeth Taylor in London*, CBS, 1963; Dr. Emily Loomis, "Return Engagement," *The Hallmark Hall of Fame*, NBC, 1978; *General Electric's All-Star Anniversary*, ABC, 1978; *Happy Birthday, Bob*, NBC, 1978; *Bob Hope's Stand Up and Cheer for the National Football League's Sixtieth Year*, NBC, 1981; *Bob Hope's Women I Love—Beautiful but Funny*, NBC, 1982; *Bob Hope's Star-Studded Spoof of the New TV Season—G-Rated—With Glamour, Glitter, and Gags*, NBC, 1982; *The Fiftieth Presidential Inaugural Gala*, ABC, 1985; *An All-Star Celebration Honoring Martin Luther King, Jr.*, NBC, 1986; *Bob Hope's High-Flying Birthday*, NBC, 1986; *Liberty Weekend*, ABC, 1986; *The Spencer Tracy Legacy: A Tribute by Katharine Hepburn*, PBS, 1986; *The Barbara Walters Special*, ABC, 1987; "Natalie Wood," *Crazy about the Movies*, Cinemax, 1987; *AIDS: The Global Explosion*, syndicated, 1988; *America's All-Star Tribute to Elizabeth Taylor* (also known as *America's Hope Award*), ABC, 1989.

RELATED CAREER—Founder and producer (with Zev Bufman), the Elizabeth Group (a theatrical production company).

NON-RELATED CAREER—Contributor and fundraiser, Israel War Victims' Fund, Chaim Sheba Hospital, 1976; founder, Ben Gurion University-Elizabeth Taylor Fund for Children of the Negev, 1982; national chairor, American Foundation for AIDS Research, 1985—; fundraiser Variety Clubs International for hospital children's wings; fundraiser and contributor, Botswana Clinics, Africa.

WRITINGS: Elizabeth Taylor Takes Off on Weight Gain, Weight Loss, Self-Esteem, and Self-Image, Putnam Publishing Group, 1988; also *World Enough and Time* (poetry), 1964; *Elizabeth Taylor—Her Own Story* (autobiography), 1965; and (with Richard Burton) *Nibbles and Me.*

AWARDS: Academy Award nomination, Best Actress, 1957, for *Raintree County;* Academy Award nomination, Best Actress, 1958, for *Cat on a Hot Tin Roof;* Academy Award nomination, Best Actress, 1959, and Golden Globe Award, Best Motion Picture Actress—Drama, 1960, both for *Suddenly, Last Summer;* Academy Award, Best Actress, 1960, for *Butterfield 8;* Academy Award and British Academy Award, both Best Actress, 1966, for *Who's Afraid of Virginia Woolf?* Silver Bear Award from the Berlin Film Festival, Best Actress, 1972, for *Hammersmith Is Out;* Hasty Pudding Woman of the Year Award from the Harvard Hasty Pudding Theatricals, 1977; Theatre World Special Award and Antoinette Perry Award nomination, Best Actress in a Play, both 1981, for *The Little Foxes;* Cecil B. De Mille Award from the Hollywood Foreign Press Association, 1985; Golden Apple Star of the Year Award from the Hollywood Women's Press Club, 1985; Commander des arts et des lettres (France), 1985; French Legion of Honor, 1987; Onassis Prize for Man and Science, 1988, for work against AIDS.

ADDRESSES: AGENT—Chen Sam and Associates, Inc., 315 E. 72nd Street, New York, NY 10021.*

TAYLOR, Holland   1943-

PERSONAL: Born January 14, 1943, in Philadelphia, PA. EDUCATION: Graduated from Bennington College.

VOCATION: Actress.

CAREER: BROADWAY DEBUT—A townsperson, *The Devils*, Broadway Theatre, 1965. OFF-BROADWAY DEBUT—Irene, *The Poker Session*, Martinique Theatre, 1967. PRINCIPAL STAGE APPEARANCES—Anne Butley, *Butley*, Morosco Theatre, New York City, 1972; Minerva, "Boo Hoo" in *Three One Act Plays by Philip Magdalany*, Playwrights Horizons, West Side YWCA-Clark Center, New York City, 1972; Kim and Colonel Howard, *Fashion*, McAlpin Rooftop Theatre, New York City, 1974; Amanda Williams, *We Interrupt This Program . . .*, Ambassador Theatre, New York City, 1975; Barbara, *Children*, Manhattan Theatre Club, New York City, 1976; Cynthia Morse, *Something Old, Something New*, Morosco Theatre, 1977; Bess Dischinger, *Breakfast with Les and Bess*, Hudson Guild Theatre, then Lambs Theatre, both New York City, 1983; Hedda Holloway, *Moose Murders*, Eugene O'Neill Theatre, New York City, 1983; Lois, *The Perfect Party*, Playwrights Horizons, New York City, 1986; Nina, *The Cocktail Hour*, Old Globe Theatre, San Diego, CA, then Promenade Theatre, New York City, both 1988. Also appeared in *The David Show*, Players Theatre, New York City, 1968; *Tonight in Living Color*, Actors Playhouse, New York City, 1969; *Colette*, Ellen Stewart Theatre, New York City, 1970; *The Philanthropist*, Washington Theatre Club, Washington, DC, 1971; and in *Nightlight*, Off-Broadway production.

PRINCIPAL FILM APPEARANCES—TV interviewer, *The Next Man*, Allied Artists, 1976; Gloria, *Romancing the Stone*, Twentieth Century-Fox, 1984; Gloria, *The Jewel of the Nile*, Twentieth Century-Fox, 1985; Mrs. Fanshaw, *Key Exchange*, Twentieth Century-Fox, 1985; Sarah Briggs, *She's Having a Baby*, Paramount, 1988.

PRINCIPAL TELEVISION APPEARANCES—Series: Marilyn Gardiner, *Beacon Hill*, CBS, 1975; Ruth Dunbar, *Bosom Buddies*, ABC, 1980-82; Zena Hunnicutt, *Me and Mom*, ABC, 1985; Nurse Ina Duckett, *Harry*, ABC, 1987; also Denise Cavanaugh, *The Edge of Night*, ABC; and *Somerset*, NBC. Episodic: Ernestine King, "Tales from the Hollywood Hills: Natica Jackson," *Great Performances*, PBS, 1987; also Ruth Taylor, *Silver Spoons*, NBC. Movies: Dottie Birmingham, *I Was a Mail Order Bride*, CBS, 1982; Mrs. Shand Kydd, *The Royal Romance of Charles and Diana*, CBS, 1982; Paula Gordon, *Perry Mason Returns*, NBC, 1985; also *The Saint*, CBS, 1987.

ADDRESSES: AGENT—Bob Gersh, The Gersh Agency, 222 N. Canon Drive, Suite 202, Beverly Hills, CA 90210.*

*   *   *

TEAGUE, Lewis   1941-

PERSONAL: Born in 1941. EDUCATION: Attended New York University.

VOCATION: Director and film editor.

CAREER: PRINCIPAL FILM APPEARANCES—*The Hard Road*,

Four Star-Excelsior, 1970. PRINCIPAL FILM WORK—Director (with Howard Freen), *Dirty O'Neil,* American International, 1974; editor (with Antranig Mahakian), *Summer Run,* Lighthouse, 1974; editor, *Forgotten Island of Santosha* (documentary), Santosha Productions, 1974; editor, *Born to Kill* (also known as *Cockfighter*), New World, 1975; second unit director and editor, *Death Race 2000,* New World, 1975; editor (with Allan Holzman), *Crazy Mama,* New World, 1975; second unit director, *Thunder and Lightning,* Twentieth Century-Fox, 1977; avalanche sequence director and editor, *Avalanche,* New World, 1978; director and editor (with Larry Bock and Ron Medico), *The Lady in Red* (also known as *Guns, Sin, and Bathtub Gin*), New World, 1979; second unit director, *Fast Charlie . . . The Moonbeam Rider* (also known as *Fast Charlie and the Moonbeam*), Universal, 1979; director, *Alligator,* Group 1, 1980; second unit director, *The Big Red One,* United Artists, 1980; director, *Death Vengeance,* EMI, 1982; director, *Fighting Back,* Paramount, 1982; director, *Cujo,* Warner Brothers, 1983; director, *Cat's Eye* (also known as *Stephen King's Cat's Eye*), Metro-Goldwyn-Mayer/United Artists, 1985; director, *The Jewel of the Nile,* Twentieth Century-Fox, 1985.

PRINCIPAL TELEVISION WORK—All as director. Pilots: *Ladies in Blue,* ABC, 1980. Episodic: *Riker,* CBS, 1981; also *Barnaby Jones,* CBS; *A Man Called Sloan,* NBC; *Vega$,* ABC; *Alfred Hitchcock Presents;* and *Daredevils.*

ADDRESSES: AGENT—Phil Gersh, The Gersh Agency, 222 N. Canon Drive, Suite 202, Beverly Hills, CA 90210.*

*   *   *

TER-ARUTUNIAN, Rouben   1920-

PERSONAL: Surname is pronounced "Terr-ah-*roo-too*-ne-ahn"; born July 24, 1920, in Tiflis, U.S.S.R.; immigrated to the United States in 1951; naturalized U.S. citizen, 1957; son of Guegam (an attorney) and Anaida (Seylanian) Ter-Arutunian. EDUCATION: Attended Friedrich-Wilhelm University, Berlin, 1941-42, the University of Vienna, 1944-45, and Ecole des Beaux-Arts, Paris, 1947-50.

VOCATION: Set and costume designer.

CAREER: FIRST STAGE WORK—Costume designer, Berlin Staatsopr, Berlin, Germany, 1941. PRINCIPAL STAGE WORK—Costume designer, *The Bartered Bride* (opera), Dresden Volks Oper, Dresden Opera House, Dresden, Germany, 1942; costume designer, *Getanzte Malerei,* Vera Mahlke Ballet Company, Dresden and Berlin, 1942; costume designer, *Salome,* Vienna Volks Oper, Vienna Opera House, Austria, 1944; set and costume designer, *Concerto* (ballet), Opera Comique, Paris, France, 1950; set and costume designer, *Bluebeard Castle* (opera) and *L'Heure Espagnole* (opera), both New York City Opera Company, City Center Theatre, New York City, 1952; *La Cenerentola* (opera), *The Trial* (opera), and *Hansel and Gretel* (opera), all New York City Opera Company, City Center Theatre, 1953; set and costume designer, *Souvenirs* (ballet), New York City Ballet, City Center Theatre, 1955; set and costume designer, *King John* and *Measure for Measure,* both American Shakespeare Festival, Stratford, CT, 1956, then Phoenix Theatre, New York City, 1957; set and costume designer, *Othello* and *Much Ado about Nothing,* and set designer, *The Merchant of Venice,* all American Shakespeare Festival, 1957; set and costume designer, *New Girl in Town,* 46th Street Theatre, New York City,

1957; set designer, *Who Was That Lady I Saw You With?,* Martin Beck Theatre, New York City, 1958; set designer, *At the Grand,* Los Angeles Civic Light Opera Association, Philharmonic Auditorium, Los Angeles, CA, then Curran Theatre, San Francisco, CA, both 1958; set and costume designer, *The Seven Deadly Sins* (ballet), New York City Ballet, City Center Theatre, 1958; set and costume designer, *Masque of the Wild Man* and *The Scarf,* both John Butler Dance Theatre, Festival of Two Worlds, Spoleto, Italy, 1958; set designer, *Maria Golovin* (opera), World's Fair, Brussels, Belgium, 1958, then Martin Beck Theatre, New York City, 1958, later La Scala, Milan, Italy, 1958, and City Center Theatre, 1959; set and costume designer, *Redhead,* 46th Street Theatre, 1959; set and costume designer, *The Scarf* and *The Devil and Daniel Webster,* all New York City Opera Company, City Center Theatre, 1959.

Set designer, *Advise and Consent,* Cort Theatre, New York City, 1960; set and costume designer, *Twelfth Night* and *Antony and Cleopatra,* both American Shakespeare Festival, 1960; set and costume designer, *Donnybrook!,* 46th Street Theatre, 1961; set and costume designer, *Il trittico* (opera), New York City Opera Company, City Center Theatre, 1961; costume designer, *Blood Moon* (opera), War Memorial Opera House, San Francisco, CA, 1961; set designer, *The Merry Widow* (operetta), Los Angeles Civic Light Opera Association, Philharmonic Auditorium, 1961; set designer, *Martha Graham's "Visionary Recital,"* retitled *Samson Agonistes,* Martha Graham Company, 54th Street Theatre, New York City, 1961; set and costume designer, *A Passage to India,* Ambassador Theatre, New York City, 1962; set designer, *The Umbrella,* New Locust Theatre, Philadelphia, PA, 1962; set and costume designer, *Swan Lake* (ballet), San Francisco Ballet, San Francisco, 1962; set and costume designer, *Hot Spot,* Majestic Theatre, New York City, 1963; set and costume designer, "Save Me a Place at Forest Lawn" and "The Last Minstrel" in *Two by Lorees Yerby* (double-bill), Pocket Theatre, New York City, 1963; set and costume designer, *Arturo Ui,* Lunt-Fontanne Theatre, New York City, 1963; set and costume designer, *Orpheus and Eurydice* (opera), Hamburg State Opera, Hamburg, West Germany, 1963; set and costume designer, *The Play of Herod,* the Cloisters, New York City, 1963; set and costume designer, *Souvenirs* (ballet), Cologne Opera House, Cologne, West Germany, 1963; set and costume designer, *The Milk Train Doesn't Stop Here Any More,* Brooks Atkinson Theatre, New York City, 1964; set designer, *The Deputy,* Brooks Atkinson Theatre, 1964; set designer, *The Merry Widow* (operetta), New York Opera Company, State Theater, New York City, 1964; set and costume designer, *Swan Lake* (ballet), and set designer, *Ballet Imperial* (ballet), and *The Nutcracker* (ballet), all New York City Ballet, State Theatre, 1964.

Set and costume designer, *Sargasso* (ballet), American Ballet Theatre, Metropolitan Opera House, New York City, 1965; set and costume designer, *Harlequinade* (ballet), New York City Ballet, State Theatre, 1965; set and costume designer, *Lucifer* (ballet), San Francisco Ballet, 1965; set designer, *The Nutcracker* (ballet), Cologne Opera House, Cologne, West Germany, 1965; set designer, *The Devils,* Broadway Theatre, New York City, 1965; set and costume designer, *Ivanov,* Shubert Theatre, New York City, 1966; set and costume designer, *Eh?,* Circle in the Square, New York City, 1966; set and costume designer, *Ricercare* (ballet), American Ballet Theatre, Metropolitan Opera House, 1966; production designer, *The Party on Greenwich Avenue,* Cherry Lane Theatre, New York City, 1967; set and costume designer, *Macbeth,* American Shakespeare Festival, 1967; set designer, *Exit, the King,* Lyceum Theatre, New York City, 1968; set designer, *I'm Solomon,* Mark Hellinger Theatre, New York City, 1968; set and costume designer, *Madame Butterfly* (opera), and set designer, *The Bassarids* (opera), Santa Fe Opera, Santa Fe, NM, 1968; set and costume designer, *Requiem Canticle* (ballet), New York City Ballet, State Theatre, 1968; set designer, *Ballet Imperial* (ballet), Berlin Deutsche Opera, Berlin, West Germany, 1969; set and costume designer, *Souvenirs* (ballet), Theater an der Wien, Vienna, Austria, then Harkness Ballet, Monte Carlo, both 1969; production designer, *The Devils of Loundun* (opera), Santa Fe Opera, 1969; production designer, *The Dozens*, Booth Theatre, New York City, 1969; set designer, *Promenade*, Promenade Theatre, New York City, 1969; set designer, *Harbinger*, Festival of Two Worlds, 1969; set and costume designer, *Transitions* (ballet), Cologne Opera House, 1969.

Set and costume designer, *The Minotaur* (ballet), Boston Ballet, Boston, MA, 1970; set and costume designer, *The Unicorn, the Gorgon, and the Manticore* (ballet), Festival of Two Worlds, 1970; set and costume designer, *All Over*, Martin Beck Theatre, New York City, 1971; set and costume designer, *Chronochromie* (ballet), Hamburg State Opera, Hamburg, West Germany, 1971; set amd costume designer, *Liebelei*, Akademie Theatre, Vienna, 1972; set and costume *The Unicorn, the Gorgon, and the Manticore* (ballet), Cincinnati Symphony and Ballet, Cincinnati, OH, 1972; set and costume designer, *Concerto for Piano and Wind, The Song of the Nightingale, Chorale Variations—Von Himmel Hoch,* and *Symphony of Psalms,* all Stravinsky Festival, New York City Ballet, State Theatre, 1972; set and costume designer, *Laborintus* (ballet), Royal Ballet, Royal Opera House, London, 1972; set and costume desinger, *Pierrot Lunaire* (ballet), Bavarian State Opera Ballet, Munich, West Germany, 1972; set and costume designer, *Symphony in Three Movements, Cortege Hongrois,* and *An Evening's Waltzes,* all New York City Ballet, State Theatre, 1973; set and costume designer, *Remembrances* (ballet), Joffrey Ballet, City Center Theatre, 1973; set and costume designer, *Voluntaries* (ballet), Stuttgart Ballet, Stuttgart, West Germany, 1973; set and costume designer, *Celebration* (ballet) and *The Art of the Pas-de-Deux* (ballet), both Festival of Two Worlds, 1973; set and costume designer, *Pelleas and Melisande* (ballet), La Scala, then Teatre La Fenice, Venice, Italy, both 1973; set and costume designer, *Variations pour une porte et un soupir* (ballet) and *Coppelia* (ballet), both New York City Ballet, State Theatre, 1974; set and costume designer, *La Sonnambula*, San Francisco Ballet, 1974.

Set designer, *Goodtime Charley*, Palace Theatre, New York City, 1975; set and costume designer, *Days in the Trees* and *The Lady from the Sea*, both Circle in the Square, 1976; set designer, *Union Jack* (ballet), New York City Ballet, State Theatre, 1976; set designer, *Vienna Waltzes*, New York City Ballet, State Theatre, 1977; set designer, *The Lady from Dubuque*, Morosco Theatre, New York City, 1980; set designer, *Goodbye Fidel*, Ambassador Theatre, New York Cty, 1980; set designer, *Davidsbundlertanz* (ballet), New York City Ballet, State Theatre, 1980; set designer, *Adagio Lamentoso* (ballet), New York City Ballet, State Theatre, 1981; set and costume designer, *Noah and the Flood* (ballet), New York City Ballet, State Theatre, 1982; set designer, *Romantic Pieces*, San Francisco Ballet, 1983; set and costume designer, *Ballet Imperial* (ballet), American Ballet Theatre, Chicago, IL, then New York City, 1988.

Also set and costume designer, unless indicated: *Fibres*, Paul Taylor Dance Company, 1960; *Pierrot Lunaire*, 1962; *Time Out of Mind*, Joffrey Ballet, 1963; *Pierrot Luniare*, Netherlands Dance Theatre, 1964; *Field Mass*, Netherlands Dance Theatre, 1965; *Nine Dances with Music By Corelli*, Paul Taylor Dance Company, 1965; *Ivanov*, London, 1965; set designer, *Villon*, Pennsylvania Ballet,

1966; *Medea*, Rome, Italy, 1966; production designer, *Pierrot Lunaire* and *Ricercare*, both Ballet Rambert, 1967; *Gala Dix*, Pennsylvania Ballet, 1967; *Firebird, After Eden,* and *A Season in Hell,* all Harkness Ballet, 1967; *Ceremony*, Pennsylvania Ballet, 1968; *Pierrot Lunaire*, Royal Danish Ballet, 1968; *A Time of Snow*, Martha Graham Company, 1968; *Villon*, 1969; *Ricercare*, Royal Swedish Ballet, 1970; *Souvenirs* (ballet), Malmo, Sweden, 1970; *According to Eve*, Alvin Ailey American Dance Theatre, 1972; *Black Angel*, Pennsylvania Ballet, 1973; *Voluntaries* (ballet), National Ballet of Canada, 1973; set designer, *The Relativity of Icarus*, 1974; *The Mooche*, Alvin Ailey American Dance Theatre 1975; *Pas de Duke*, Alvin Ailey American Dance Theatre, 1976; *Sphinx* (ballet), 1977; set designer, *As You Like It*, Long Beach, CA, 1979; *Sphinx* (ballet), National Ballet of Canada, 1983; set designer, *Components* (ballet), National Ballet of Canada, 1984; *Pulcinella*, 1984; set designer, *Die Liebe der Danae* (opera), Santa Fe Opera; *Voluntaries* (ballet), Royal Ballet, Royal Danish Ballet, Paris Opera Ballet, and American Ballet Theatre.

MAJOR TOURS—Set and costume designer, *Redhead*, U.S. cities, 1960; set and costume designer, *Pelleas and Melisande* (ballet), European cities, 1966.

PRINCIPAL FILM WORK—Production and costume designer, *The Loved One*, Metro-Goldwyn-Mayer, 1965; production and set designer, *Such Good Friends*, Paramount, 1971.

PRINCIPAL TELEVISION APPEARANCES—Specials: *Rouben Ter-Arutunian—The Art of Stage Design*, PBS. PRINCIPAL TELEVISION WORK—Series: Set designer, *The Bert Parks Show*, CBS, 1951; set designer, *This Is Show Business*, CBS, 1951; set designer, *The Toast of the Town*, CBS, 1952; set designer, *Studio One*, CBS, 1951-53; set and costume designer, *The Bell Telephone Hour*, NBC, 1958. Episodic: Set designer, "Reunion in Vienna," *Producer's Showcase*, NBC, 1955; set and costume designer, "The Art of the Prima Donna," *Bell Telephone Hour*, NBC, 1966. Specials: Costume and set designer, "The Abduction from the Seraglio," *NBC Opera*, NBC, 1954; set and costume designer, "The Would-Be Gentleman" and "Ariadne auf Naxos," both *NBC Opera*, NBC, 1955; set and costume designer, "The Magic Flute," *NBC Opera*, NBC, 1956; set designer, "Maria Golovin," *NBC Opera*, NBC, 1959; set and costume designer, *Antigone*, NBC, 1956; set and costume designer, "The Taming of the Shrew," *Hallmark Hall of Fame*, NBC, 1956; set and costume designer, "Twelfth Night," *Hallmark Hall of Fame*, NBC, 1957; set and costume designer, "The Tempest," *Hallmark Hall of Fame*, NBC, 1959; set and costume designer, *Swing into Spring*, CBS, 1958; set designer, *A Musical Bouquet for Maurice Chevalier*, CBS, 1960; set and costume designer, *Noah and the Flood*, CBS, 1962; set designer, *Marlene Dietrich: I Wish You Love*, CBS, 1973; set and costume designer, "Rachel, La Cubana," *NET Opera Theatre*, PBS, 1973.

RELATED CAREER—Designer of scenery, costumes, and club interiors, U.S. Third Army Special Services, Germany, 1945-47; staff designer, CBS, 1951-53; staff designer, ABC, 1953; staff designer, NBC, 1954-57; designed permanent stages for the American Shakespeare Festival and Academy, Stratford, CT, 1956, then 1960.

AWARDS: Emmy Award, Best Art Direction, 1957, for "Twelfth Night," *Hallmark Hall of Fame;* Outer Critics Circle Award, Best Scenic Design, 1958, for *Who Was That Lady I Saw You With?;* Antoinette Perry Award, Best Costume Design, 1959, for *Redhead*.

MEMBER: United Scenic Artists.

SIDELIGHTS: Rouben Ter-Arutunian's designs can be found among the collections of the Museum of Modern Art and the Library and Museum of the Performing Arts, both in New York City, in the Theatre Collection of Harvard University, Cambridge, MA, and in the Victoria and Albert Museum, London.

ADDRESSES: HOME—360 E. 55th Street, New York, NY 10022.

*   *   *

TEWKESBURY, Joan   1936-

PERSONAL: Born April 8, 1936, in Redlands, CA; daughter of Walter S. (an office machine repairman) and Frances M. (a registered nurse; maiden name, Stevenson) Tewkesbury; married Robert F. Maguire III, November 30, 1960 (divorced, January, 1973); children: Robin Tewkesbury, Peter Harlan. EDUCATION: Attended Mt. San Antonio Junior College, 1956-58; studied drama at the University of Southern California, 1958-60; also attended the American School of Dance, 1947-54.

VOCATION: Screenwriter, director, actress, dancer, and choreographer.

CAREER: Also see *WRITINGS* below. PRINCIPAL STAGE APPEARANCES—Dancer, *Peter Pan,* Winter Garden Theatre, New York City, 1954, then Los Angeles, CA, 1955.

PRINCIPAL STAGE WORK—Director, *Cowboy Jack Street,* Perry Street Theatre, New York City, 1977.

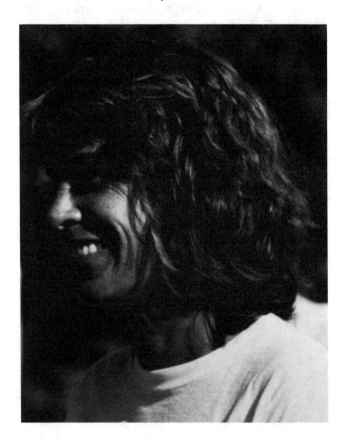

JOAN TEWKESBURY

PRINCIPAL FILM APPEARANCES—Dancer, *The Unfinished Dance,* Metro-Goldwyn-Mayer, 1946; woman in elevator, *Man's Favorite Sport (?),* Universal, 1964; lady in train, *Thieves Like Us,* United Artists, 1974.

PRINCIPAL FILM WORK—Script supervisor, *McCabe & Mrs. Miller,* Warner Brothers, 1971; director, *Old Boyfriends,* AVCO-Embassy, 1979; also director, *Hampstead Center* (documentary), 1976; director, *Angel's Dance Card,* 1988.

PRINCIPAL TELEVISION APPEARANCES—Specials: Ostrich, *Peter Pan,* NBC, 1955. PRINCIPAL TELEVISION WORK—Pilots: Co-executive producer and director, *Elysian Fields,* 1988. Episodic: Director, *Alfred Hitchcock Presents,* NBC, 1986. Movies: Director, *The Tenth Month,* CBS, 1979; director, *The Acorn People,* NBC, 1981.

RELATED CAREER—Director and choreographer of theatre productions, Los Angeles, CA, 1956-64; dance teacher, Mt. San Antonio Junior College, Walnut, CA, 1956-58; choreographer for film productions, 1958-70; dance teacher, American School of Dance, 1959-69; dance and drama teacher, Immaculate Heart College, Los Angeles, 1960-63; choreographer, director, and actress, University of Southern California Repertory Company, 1965-68; dance and drama teacher, University of Southern California, Los Angeles, 1966-69; actress, director, and choreographer, Edinburgh Festival, Edinburgh, Scotland, 1968-70; screenwriting teacher, University of California, Los Angeles, 1986; also dancer in nightclubs.

WRITINGS: STAGE—*Cowboy Jack Street,* Perry Street Theatre, New York City, 1977. FILM—(With Calder Willingham and Robert Altman) *Thieves Like Us,* United Artists, 1974; *Nashville,* Paramount, 1975, published by Bantam, 1976; (with Paul Schrader) *Old Boyfriends,* AVCO-Embassy, 1979; *A Night in Heaven,* Twentieth Century-Fox, 1983; also *The Hampstead Center* (documentary), 1976; *Angel's Dance Card,* 1988; *American Desire.* TELEVISION—Pilots: *Elysian Fields,* 1988. Episodic: *Alfred Hitchcock Presents,* NBC, 1986. Movies: *The Tenth Month,* CBS, 1979; *The Acorn People,* NBC, 1981.

AWARDS: Los Angeles Critics Award, Best Screenplay, 1975, for *Nashville.*

MEMBER: Writers Guild of America, Directors Guild of America, Actors' Equity Association, Screen Actors Guild, American Civil Liberties Union, National Abortion Rights Action League, California Abortion Rights Action League.

ADDRESSES: AGENT—Jane Sindell, Creative Artists Agency, 1888 Century Park E., Suite 1400, Los Angeles, CA 90067.*

*   *   *

THIBEAU, Jack

VOCATION: Actor and screenwriter.

CAREER: Also see *WRITINGS* below. PRINCIPAL FILM APPEARANCES—Clarence Anglin, *Escape from Alcatraz,* Paramount, 1979; aide to Stilwell, *1941,* Universal, 1979; soldier in trench, *Apocalypse Now,* United Artists, 1979; man in bar, *Ms. 45* (also known as *Angel of Vengeance*), Rochelle, 1981; conventioneer,

Honky Tonk Freeway, Universal/Associated Film Distribution, 1981; Coach Jackson, *Tex,* Buena Vista, 1982; detective, *48 Hours,* Paramount, 1982; Kruger, *Sudden Impact,* Warner Brothers, 1983; garage soldier, *City Heat,* Warner Brothers, 1984; Pisarczyk, *Warning Sign,* Twentieth Century-Fox, 1985; Trooper Prestone, *The Hitcher,* Tri-Star, 1986; McCaskey, *Lethal Weapon,* Warner Brothers, 1987; Detective Kotterwell, *Action Jackson,* Lorimar, 1988.

PRINCIPAL TELEVISION APPEARANCES—Mini-Series: Clyde Tolson, *Robert Kennedy and His Times,* CBS, 1985; Captain Penscott, *James A. Michener's "Space"* (also known as *Space*), CBS, 1985; Mr. Morgan, *North and South, Book II,* ABC, 1986. Episodic: Bronson, "Man from the South," *Alfred Hitchcock Presents,* NBC, 1985; John Kogan, *Sledge Hammer!,* ABC, 1986; tough guy, *Amazing Stories,* NBC, 1986; Coark, *Hard Copy* (two episodes), CBS, 1987; Tommy O'Keefe, *Matlock,* NBC, 1987. Movies: Stanton, *Blood Feud,* syndicated, 1983; Zero McKenzie, *Streets of Justice,* NBC, 1985; Donny, *Kids Don't Tell,* CBS, 1985; Mike Carver, *Love Lives On,* ABC, 1985.

WRITINGS: FILM—(With Christopher Crowe) *Off Limits,* Twentieth Century-Fox, 1988.*

*   *   *

THOMAS, Betty   1948-

PERSONAL: Born Betty Thomas Nienhauser, July 27, 1948, in St. Louis, MO. EDUCATION: Received B.F.A. from the University of Ohio.

VOCATION: Actress.

CAREER: PRINCIPAL FILM APPEARANCES—Waitress, *Jackson County Jail,* New World, 1976; also appeared in *The Last Affair,* Chelex, 1976; *Tunnelvision,* Worldwide, 1976; *Used Cars,* Columbia, 1980; *Homework,* Jensen Farley, 1982.

PRINCIPAL TELEVISION APPEARANCES—Series: Sergeant Lucy Bates, *Hill Street Blues,* NBC, 1981-87; also regular, *The Fun Factory,* 1976. Pilots: *Home Again,* ABC, 1988. Episodic: *SCTV Network 90,* NBC, 1984. Movies: Katherine, *Outside Chance,* CBS, 1978; Maxine Pearce, *Nashville Grab,* NBC, 1981; Maude, *When Your Lover Leaves,* NBC, 1983; Angela Brannon, *Prison for Children,* CBS, 1987. Specials: *Circus of the Stars,* CBS, 1982; *Battle of the Network Stars,* ABC, 1982 and 1983; also *The Gift of Love,* 1985.

RELATED CAREER—Member of Second City (an improvisational comedy troupe), Chicago, IL, 1974; actress in television commercials.

NON-RELATED CAREER—School teacher.

AWARDS: Emmy Award nominations, Outstanding Supporting Actress in a Drama Series, 1981, 1982, and 1983, and Emmy Award, Outstanding Supporting Actress in a Drama Series, 1985, all for *Hill Street Blues.*

ADDRESSES: AGENT—Nancy Geller, International Creative Management, 8899 Beverly Boulevard, Los Angeles, CA 90048.*

THOMAS, Heather   1957-

PERSONAL: Born September 8, 1957, in Greenwich, CT; father, a university administrator; mother, a public school special education administrator. EDUCATION: University of California, Los Angeles, B.A., motion picture and television production, 1980.

VOCATION: Actress.

CAREER: PRINCIPAL FILM APPEARANCES—Jane, *Zapped!,* Embassy, 1982; Teri Marshall, *Cyclone,* Cinetel, 1987; Merryl Davis, *Death Stone,* CCC, 1987.

PRINCIPAL TELEVISION APPEARANCES—Series: Sandi, *Co-ed Fever,* CBS, 1979; Jody Banks, *The Fall Guy,* ABC, 1981-86. Mini-Series: Evangeline Cote, *Ford: The Man and the Machine,* syndicated, 1987. Pilots: Sandi, *Co-ed Fever,* CBS, 1979; Detective Caroline Capoty, *The Eyes of Texas II,* NBC, 1980; Jody Banks, *How Do I Kill a Thief—Let Me Count the Ways,* ABC, 1982. Episodic: Andrea Morris, "A Blinding Fear," *The New Mike Hammer,* CBS, 1987. Movies: Marilyn Monroe, *Hoover versus the Kennedys: The Second Civil War,* syndicated, 1987; Lieutenant Carol Campbell, *The Dirty Dozen: The Fatal Mission,* NBC, 1988. Specials: *Battle of the Network Stars,* ABC, 1982 and 1983; host, *The Funniest Joke I Ever Heard,* ABC, 1984; *The Magic of David Copperfield,* CBS, 1984; host, *Miss Teen USA,* CBS, 1984.

SIDELIGHTS: RECREATIONS—Collecting antique circus posters, Balinese carvings, and teddy bears; shooting 8mm films.

ADDRESSES: MANAGER—Sandy Littman, Mickelson/Littman Management, 1707 Clearview Drive, Beverly Hills, CA 90210.*

*   *   *

THOMAS, Richard   1951-

PERSONAL: Full name, Richard Earl Thomas; born June 13, 1951, in New York, NY; son of Richard S. (a ballet instructor) and Barbara (a ballet dancer and instructor; maiden name, Fallis) Thomas; married Alma Gonzales (a former teacher and welfare worker), February 14, 1975; children: Barbara Ayala, Gwyneth Gonzales, Pilar Alma (triplets), Richard Francisco. EDUCATION: Attended Columbia University. RELIGION: Christian.

VOCATION: Actor.

CAREER: STAGE DEBUT—Singer, *Damn Yankees,* Sacandaga Garden Theatre, Sacandaga Park, NY, 1957. BROADWAY DEBUT—John Roosevelt, *Sunrise at Campobello,* Booth Theatre, 1958. PRINCIPAL STAGE APPEARANCES—Gordon Evans (as a child), *Strange Interlude,* Hudson Theatre, New York City, 1963; Edward, Prince of Wales, *King Richard III,* American Shakespeare Festival, Stratford, CT, 1964; Eric, *The Playroom,* Brooks Atkinson Theatre, New York City, 1965; Richard, Duke of York, *King Richard III,* New York Shakespeare Festival, Delacorte Theatre, New York City, 1966; Roger, *Everything in the Garden,* Plymouth Theatre, New York City, 1967; Kenneth Talley, Jr., *Fifth of July,* New Apollo Theatre, New York City, 1981; Treplev, *The Sea Gull,* Circle Repertory Company, American Place Theatre, New York City, 1983; Edmund Dantes/title role, *The Count of Monte Cristo,* Eisenhower Theatre, Kennedy Center for the Performing Arts, Washington, DC, 1985; title role, *Citizen Tom Paine,* Eisenhower

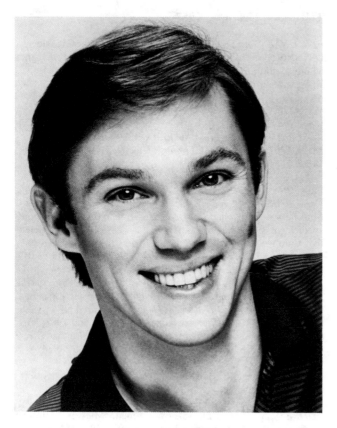

RICHARD THOMAS

Theatre, Kennedy Center for the Performing Arts, 1986; Hildy Johnson, *The Front Page,* Vivian Beaumont Theatre, New York City, 1986. Also appeared in *The Member of the Wedding,* Equity Library Theatre, New York City, 1959; *Saint Joan,* Center Theatre Group, Ahmanson Theatre, Los Angeles, CA, 1974; *Merton of the Movies,* Center Theatre Group, Ahmanson Theatre, 1977; *Hamlet* and *Peer Gynt,* both Hartford Stage Company, Hartford, CT; and *Arms and the Man* and *Streamers,* both in Los Angeles.

MAJOR TOURS—Ken Harrison, *Whose Life Is It Anyway?,* U.S. cities, 1980.

FILM DEBUT—Charley, *Winning,* Universal, 1969. PRINCIPAL FILM APPEARANCES—Peter, *Last Summer,* Allied Artists, 1969; Josh Arnold, *Red Sky at Morning,* Universal, 1971; Billy Roy, *The Todd Killings* (also known as *A Dangerous Friend* and *Skipper*), National General, 1971; Harley MacIntosh, *Cactus in the Snow,* General Film Corporation, 1972; Kenny, *You'll Like My Mother,* Universal, 1972; Jimmy J., *9/30/55,* Universal, 1977; Shad, *Battle beyond the Stars,* New World, 1980; Leo, *Bloody Kids,* Palace/ British Film Institute, 1983. Also appeared in *Beyond Reasonable Doubt,* Satori Releasing Entertainment, 1980.

PRINCIPAL TELEVISION APPEARANCES—Series: Assistant, *1, 2, 3, Go!,* NBC, 1961-62; John Boy Walton, *The Waltons,* CBS, 1972-77; also Chris Austen, *A Time for Us,* ABC; Tom Hughes, *As the World Turns,* CBS. Mini-Series: Jim Warner, *Roots: The Next Generations,* ABC, 1979. Pilots: John Boy Walton, *The Homecoming—A Christmas Story,* CBS, 1971. Episodic: *Way Out,* CBS, 1961; *Great Ghost Tales,* NBC, 1961; "The Sins of the Fathers," *Rod Serling's Night Gallery* (also known as *Night Gallery*), NBC,

1971; *Our World,* ABC, 1986; also *Love, American Style,* ABC; *Medical Center,* CBS; *Marcus Welby, M.D.,* ABC; *The F.B.I.,* ABC; *Bonanza,* NBC; *From These Roots.* Movies: Henry Fleming, *The Red Badge of Courage,* NBC, 1974; Cadet James Pelosi, *The Silence,* NBC, 1975; Michael Carboni, *Getting Married,* CBS, 1978; Andrew Madison, *No Other Love,* CBS, 1979; Paul Baumer, *All Quiet on the Western Front,* CBS, 1979; David Benjamin, *To Find My Son,* CBS, 1980; Sandy Mueller, *Berlin Tunnel 21,* CBS, 1981; Bill Richmond, *Johnny Belinda,* CBS, 1982; Will Mossop, *Hobson's Choice,* CBS, 1983; title role, *Living Proof: The Hank Williams, Jr. Story,* NBC, 1983; Henry Durie, *The Master of Ballantrae,* CBS, 1984; Marty Campbell, *Final Jeopardy,* NBC, 1985; Greg Madison, *Go toward the Light* (also known as *Toward the Light*), CBS, 1988; Reverend Bobby Joe Stuckey, *Glory! Glory!,* HBO, 1989.

Specials: Gangster, "The Filling Station," *Sunday in Town,* NBC, 1954; Ivor, "A Doll's House," *Hallmark Hall of Fame,* NBC, 1959; Paul Bratter, *Barefoot in the Park,* HBO, 1982; Ken Talley, Jr., *Fifth of July,* Showtime, 1982; host, *Un Ballo in Maschera* (also known as *A Masked Ball*), PBS, 1987; Jonathan Smith, *The Blessings of Liberty,* ABC, 1987; host and narrator, *Scenes from La Boheme: A Pavarotti Celebration,* PBS, 1988; host, *A Grand Night: The Performing Arts Salute Public Television,* PBS, 1988; also "A Christmas Tree," *Hallmark Hall of Fame,* NBC, 1959; *The Bobby Van and Elaine Joyce Show,* CBS, 1973; *Miss Teenage America Pageant,* NBC, 1977; *CBS: On the Air,* CBS, 1978; *Pavarotti and Friends,* ABC, 1982; *Broadway Plays Washington! Kennedy Center Tonight,* PBS, 1982; also host, *H.M.S. Pinafore,* 1973; *The American Film Institute Salute to Lillian Gish,* 1984.

PRINCIPAL TELEVISION WORK—Episodic: Director, *The Waltons,* CBS. Movies: Executive producer, *Living Proof: The Hank Williams, Jr. Story,* NBC, 1983.

RELATED CAREER—Owner, Melpomene Productions.

NON-RELATED CAREER—National chairor, Better Hearing Institute, 1987—.

WRITINGS: *Poems by Richard Thomas,* Avon, 1974; *In the Moment,* Avon, 1979; also *Glass.*

AWARDS: Emmy Award, Outstanding Continued Performance by an Actor in a Leading Role—Drama Series, 1973, for *The Waltons; Motion Picture and TV/Radio Daily* Most Promising New Male Star of the Season, 1973; Friends of Robert Frost Award.

ADDRESSES: AGENT—John Gaines, Agency for the Performing Arts, 9000 Sunset Boulevard, Suite 1200, Los Angeles, CA 90069. PUBLICIST—Gary Springer, Springer Associates, 130 E. 67th Street, New York, NY 10021.

*   *   *

THOMPSON, Brian

PERSONAL: Born Brian Ellensberg in Washington; son of two teachers; married Isabelle Mastorakis (executive vice-president of Omega Entertainment); children: Jordan. EDUCATION: Received B.S. in business management from Central Washington University; received M.F.A. in drama from the University of California, Irvine.

VOCATION: Actor.

CAREER: PRINCIPAL STAGE APPEARANCES—Van Der Vane, *Red Square,* Seattle Repertory Theatre, Seattle, WA, 1987; also appeared in *Hobson's Choice,* Intiman Theatre Company, Seattle, WA, 1984; in regional productions of *The King and I, Oliver!, Sweeney Todd,* and *Pippin;* and with the Berkeley Repertory Theatre, Berkeley, CA, 1983-85.

PRINCIPAL FILM APPEARANCES—A punk, *The Terminator,* Orion, 1984; German's friend, *Three Amigos!,* Orion, 1986; night slasher, *Cobra,* Warner Brothers, 1986; James, *You Talkin' to Me?,* Metro-Goldwyn-Mayer/United Artists, 1987; Danny, *Catch the Heat* (also known as *Feel the Heat*), Trans World, 1987; Clint Jensen, *Commando Squad,* Trans World, 1987; Bozworth, *Fright Night, Part II,* New Century/Vista, 1988; Powerlifter, *Miracle Mile,* Hemdale Releasing, 1988; Trent Porter, *Alien Nation,* Twentieth Century-Fox, 1988; Kenny Hamilton, *Pass the Ammo,* New Century, 1988.

PRINCIPAL TELEVISION APPEARANCES—Series: Nicholas Remy, *Werewolf,* Fox, 1988. Episodic: Gibbens, *George Burns Comedy Week,* CBS, 1985; Brian Hopkins, *Falcon Crest* (three episodes), CBS, 1987; Eddie Ringermann, *Something Is Out There,* NBC, 1988; also *Knight Rider,* NBC; *Hardcastle and McCormick,* ABC; *Moonlighting,* ABC. Movies: Lieutenant Harrison, *Fatal Vision,* NBC, 1984. Specials: *River Journeys* (documentary), PBS, 1985.

RELATED CAREER—Actor, Universal Studio Tours.*

*   *   *

THOMPSON, Jack   1940-

PERSONAL: Born John Payne, August 31, 1940, in Sydney, Australia. EDUCATION: Attended Queensland University.

VOCATION: Actor.

CAREER: PRINCIPAL FILM APPEARANCES—Dick, *Outback,* United Artists, 1971; Ken, "The Family Man," *Libido,* Metro-Goldwyn-Mayer/BEF, 1973; Tony "Jock" Petersen, *Petersen* (also known as *"Jock" Petersen*), AVCO-Embassy, 1974; title role, *Scobie Malone,* Cemp/Regent, 1975; Foley, *Sunday Too Far Away,* South Australian, 1975; Ted, *Caddie,* Atlantic, 1976; Detective Manwaring, *Mad Dog Morgan* (also know as *Mad Dog*), BEF, 1976; Simon Morris, *The Journalist,* FJ/New South Wales/FJF Promoters/Edgecliff, 1979; Major J.F. Thomas, *Breaker Morant,* New World, 1980; Reverend Neville, *The Chant of Jimmie Blacksmith,* New Yorker, 1980; Laurie Holden, *The Club,* Roadshow, 1980; Ross Daley, *The Earthling,* Filmways/Roadshow, 1980; Stanley Graham, *Bad Blood,* Rank Film Distributors, 1982; Clancy, *The Man from Snowy River,* Twentieth Century-Fox, 1983; Group Captain Hicksley-Ellis, *Merry Christmas, Mr. Lawrence,* Universal, 1983; Robert O'Hara Burke, *Burke and Wills,* Hemdale, 1985; Hawkwood, *Flesh and Blood,* Riverside, 1985; Trebilcock, *Ground Zero,* Hoyts, 1987; Maxey Woodbury, *Waterfront,* Prism Entertainment, 1988. Also appeared in *Wake in Fright.*

PRINCIPAL TELEVISION APPEARANCES—Movies: Ariel, *A Woman Called Golda,* syndicated, 1982; Robert Crosbie, *The Letter,* ABC, 1982; Nick Stenning, *The Last Frontier,* CBS, 1986; Aubrey Dubose, *Kojak: The Price of Justice* (also known as *Kojak: The*

Investigation), CBS, 1987; Tom Campbell Black, *Beryl Markham: A Shadow on the Sun* (also known as *Shadow on the Sun: The Life of Beryl Markham* and *The Beryl Markham Story*), CBS, 1988; Jake LaFontaine, *Trouble in Paradise,* CBS, 1989. Also appeared in a soap opera for Australian television.

AWARDS: Australian award for *Breaker Morant.*

ADDRESSES: AGENT—Smith-Freedman and Associates, 121 N. San Vicente Boulevard, Beverly Hills, CA 90211.*

*   *   *

THOMPSON, Robert   1937-

PERSONAL: Born May 31, 1937, in Palmyra, NY; son of Roger (a farmer) and Gladys (Smith) Thompson; married Helen M. Miller, August 31, 1957 (divorced, 1976); children: Mark, Peter, Patrick. EDUCATION: Ithaca College, B.S., radio and television, 1960; University of California, Los Angeles, M.F.A., directing, 1961.

VOCATION: Producer, director, and writer.

CAREER: Also see *WRITINGS* below. PRINCIPAL FILM WORK—Producer (with Roderick Paul), *The Paper Chase,* Twentieth Century-Fox, 1973.

PRINCIPAL TELEVISION WORK—Series: Executive producer, *The Paper Chase,* CBS, 1978-79. Pilots: Producer (with Roderick Paul), *Lanigan's Rabbi,* NBC, 1976. Episodic: Director, *Chicago Story,* NBC, 1982; director, *The Renegades,* ABC, 1983; also director, *Dynasty,* ABC; director, *The Greatest American Hero,* ABC; director, *Hill Street Blues,* NBC; director, *Magnum, P.I.,* CBS; director, *The Paper Chase,* CBS; director, *Seven Brides for Seven Brothers,* CBS; director, *Fantasy Island,* ABC; director, *Dallas,* CBS; director, *Fame* director, *The New F.B.I.* Movies: Producer (with Paul), *The Mark of Zorro,* ABC, 1974; director and (with Clyde Phillips) producer, *Bud and Lou,* NBC, 1978; executive producer, *The $5.20 an Hour Dream,* CBS, 1980; producer (with Paul), *Love Lives On,* ABC, 1985; executive producer, *Broken Vows,* CBS, 1987; also director, *Words By Heart,* PBS. Specials: Director, *ABC Afterschool Special,* ABC; director, *ABC Playbreak,* ABC. Also directed *California Fever,* 1980.

RELATED CAREER—Head of talent department, in charge of signing contract players, Universal Studios, Hollywood, CA, 1961-68; head of talent department, Cinema Center Films, CBS, Los Angeles, CA, 1968-72; president, Thompson-Paul Productions, Inc., 1974—; founder, Group Three Management; worked in local radio and television, Ithaca, NY; lecturer, Northwestern University, University of Texas, Austin, University of Southern California, and Southern Methodist University.

WRITINGS: STAGE—*The Preparation, It Is Only a Game,* and *Goodbye My Son,* all one-act plays. FILM—Co-writer, *Leavin' Venus,* Apollo; co-writer, *Heaven Only Knows.* TELEVISION—Episodic: Co-writer, *Trapper John, M.D.,* CBS.

MEMBER: Directors Guild of America.

SIDELIGHTS: RECREATIONS—Racquetball, tennis, weightlifting, reading, movies, and skiing.

ADDRESSES: HOME—4536 Mary Ellen Avenue, Sherman Oaks, CA 91423. AGENT—Shapiro-Lichtman, 8827 Beverly Boulevard, Los Angeles, CA 90048.

*　　*　　*

TIGHE, Kevin 1944-

PERSONAL: Born August 13, 1944, in Los Angeles, CA. EDUCATION: Graduated from the University of Southern California.

VOCATION: Actor and playwright.

CAREER: BROADWAY DEBUT—Peter Carlson, *Open Admissions,* Music Box Theatre, 1983, for seventeen performances. PRINCIPAL STAGE APPEARANCES—Henry, *Design for Living,* Center Theatre Group, Ahmanson Theatre, Los Angeles, CA, 1970; Frank Reid, *The Ballad of Soapy Smith,* Seattle Repertory Theatre, Seattle, WA, 1983, then New York Shakespeare Festival, Public Theatre, New York City, 1984. Also appeared in *The Night of the Iguana,* McCarter Theatre Company, Princeton, NJ, 1982; and with the Arena Stage, Washington, DC, 1983 and 1987.

PRINCIPAL STAGE WORK—Director, *Homegirl,* Seattle Repertory Theatre, Seattle, WA, 1986.

PRINCIPAL FILM APPEARANCES—Hickey, *Matewan,* Cinecom, 1987; Sport Sullivan, *Eight Men Out,* Orion, 1988; Lyman, *K-9,* Universal, 1989; Tilghman, *Roadhouse,* Metro-Goldwyn-Mayer/ United Artists, 1989. Also appeared in *Most Deadly Passage,* 1978.

PRINCIPAL TELEVISION APPEARANCES—Series: Roy DeSoto, *Emergency!,* NBC, 1972-77; voice of Roy DeSoto, *Emergency Plus Four* (animated), NBC, 1973-76. Pilots: Inspector John Fernack, "The Saint," *CBS Summer Playhouse,* CBS, 1987. Movies: Thomas Jefferson, *The Rebels,* syndicated, 1979. Specials: *Battle of the Network Stars,* ABC, 1976.

PRINCIPAL TELEVISION WORK—Episodic: Director, *Emergency!,* NBC.

WRITINGS: STAGE—*Homegirl,* Seattle Repertory Theatre, Seattle, WA, 1986.

ADDRESSES: AGENT—Bauman, Hiller & Strain, 9220 Sunset Boulevard, Suite 202, Los Angeles, CA 90069.*

*　　*　　*

TILLY, Meg

PERSONAL: Born in California; raised in Victoria, BC, Canada.

VOCATION: Actress.

CAREER: FILM DEBUT—*Fame,* United Artists, 1980. PRINCIPAL FILM APPEARANCES—Jamie Collins, *Tex,* Buena Vista, 1982; Julie, *One Dark Night,* Com World, 1983; Chloe, *The Big Chill,* Columbia, 1983; Mary, *Psycho II,* Universal, 1983; Jennifer,

Impulse, Twentieth Century-Fox, 1984; Sister Agnes, *Agnes of God,* Columbia, 1985; Rachel Wareham, *Off Beat,* Buena Vista, 1986; Olivia Lawrence, *Masquerade,* Metro-Goldwyn-Mayer/ United Artists, 1988. Also appeared as Karin Foster, *The Girl on a Swing,* 1988; and in *Rest in Peace.*

PRINCIPAL TELEVISION APPEARANCES—Episodic: *Hill Street Blues,* NBC. Specials: Dorie, "The Trouble with Grandpa," *ABC Afterschool Special,* ABC, 1981.

RELATED CAREER—Appeared in community theatre productions in Canada.

AWARDS: Academy Award nomination, Best Supporting Actress, 1986, for *Agnes of God.*

ADDRESSES: AGENT—Nicole David, Triad Artists, 10100 Santa Monica Boulevard, 16th Floor, Los Angeles, CA 90067.*

*　　*　　*

TOBACK, James 1944-

PERSONAL: Born November 23, 1944, in New York, NY; son of Irwin Lionel (a stockbroker) and Selma (Levy) Toback; married Consuelo Sarah Churchill Rusell, April 26, 1968 (divorced). EDUCATION: Harvard University, A.B., 1966; Columbia University, M.A., 1967.

VOCATION: Writer, director, and producer.

CAREER: Also see *WRITINGS* below. PRINCIPAL FILM APPEARANCES—Leo Boscovitch, *Exposed,* Metro-Goldwyn-Mayer/ United Artists (MGM/UA), 1983. PRINCIPAL FILM WORK— Director, *Fingers,* Brut, 1978; producer and director, *Love and Money,* Paramount, 1982; producer and director, *Exposed,* MGM/ UA, 1983; director, *The Pick-Up Artist,* Twentieth Century-Fox, 1987.

RELATED CAREER—English instructor, City University of New York; sports columnist, *Lifestyle* (magazine); film critic, *Dissent* (magazine); contributing editor, *Sport* (magazine).

WRITINGS: FILM—*The Gambler,* Paramount, 1974; *Fingers,* Brut, 1978; *Love and Money,* Paramount, 1982; *Exposed,* Metro-Goldwyn-Mayer/United Artists, 1983; *The Pick-Up Artist,* Twentieth Century-Fox, 1987. OTHER—*Jim: The Author's Self-Centered Memoir on the Great Jim Brown* (biography), Doubleday, 1971. Also contributor to *Esquire, Sport, Village Voice, Harper's,* and *Commentary.*

MEMBER: Harvard Club.

ADDRESSES: AGENT—Jeff Berg, International Creative Management, 8899 Beverly Boulevard, Los Angeles, CA 90048.*

TOGURI, David

PERSONAL: Born in Vancouver, BC, Canada. EDUCATION: Attended Ryerson Institute of Technology; trained for the stage with Boris Volkoff.

VOCATION: Director, choreographer, and dancer.

CAREER: LONDON DEBUT—Head waiter and principal dancer, *Flower Drum Song,* Palace Theatre, 1960. PRINCIPAL STAGE APPEARANCES—Dancer, *The Sammy Davis, Jr. Show,* Prince of Wales Theatre, London, 1961; dancer, *Six of One* (revue), Adelphi Theatre, London, 1963; dancer, *Chaganog* (revue), Edinburgh Festival, Edinburgh, Scotland, then Vaudeville Theatre, London, both 1964, later St. Martin's Theatre, London, 1965; John Sasaki, *Charlie Girl,* Adelphi Theatre, 1965.

PRINCIPAL STAGE WORK—Assistant director, *Hair,* Shaftesbury Theatre, London, 1968; director (with Robin Phillips), *The Comedy of Errors* and *Two Gentlemen of Verona,* both Stratford Shakespeare Festival, Stratford, ON, Canada, 1975; director, *The Servant of Two Masters,* Nottingham Playhouse, Nottingham, U.K., 1976; director, *Phantomet,* and choreographer, *I Love My Wife,* both Nye Theatre, Oslo, Norway, 1978; choreographer, *As You Like It,* Burgtheatre, Vienna, Austria, 1979; director, *Bloody Mary,* National Theatre, Oslo, 1979; choreographer, *Masquerade,* National Theatre, Oslo, 1980; choreographer, *Shadowplay,* King's Head Theatre, London, 1980; choreographer, *Censored Scenes from King Kong,* Princess Theatre, New York City, 1980; choreographer, *Guys and Dolls,* National Theatre, London, 1982; choreographer, *Falstaff* (opera), Covent Garden Opera House, London, 1982; director, *Robin Hood,* Young Vic Theatre, London, 1982; director, *Camino Real,* National Theatre, Oslo, 1982; director, *Little Shop of Horrors,* Stavanger Theatre, Stavanger, Norway, 1983; director, *John, Paul, George, Ringo, and Bert,* Young Vic Theatre, 1983; choreographer, *Strider, Little Hotel,* and *Rough Crossing,* all National Theatre, London, 1984.

Choreographer, *Jumpers,* Aldwych Theatre, London, 1985; choreographer, *Khovancina* (opera), Metropolitan Opera House, New York City, 1985; choreographer, *Futurists,* National Theatre, London, 1986; choreographer, *Wonderful Town,* Queen's Theatre, London, 1986; choreographer, *High Society,* Victoria Palace Theatre, London, 1986; choreographer, *Oberon,* Edinburgh Festival, Edinburgh, Scotland, 1986; choreographer, *The Pied Piper* and *American Clock,* both National Theatre, London, 1987; choreographer, *Pacific Overtures* (opera), English National Opera Company, Covent Garden Opera House, 1987; choreographer, *Parsifal* (opera), Covent Garden Opera House, 1988; choreographer, *'Tis Pity She's a Whore,* National Theatre, London, 1988; director, *Mack and Mabel in Concert,* Drury Lane Theatre, London, 1988. Also choreographer, *What a Way to Run a Revolution,* London, 1971; choreographer, *The Island of the Mighty,* London, 1972; choreographer, *Zorba,* London, 1973; choreographer, *The Marquis of Keith,* London, 1974; co-director, *Cole,* London, 1974; director, *Farjeon Reviewed,* London, 1975; co-director and choreographer, *I Gotta Shoe,* London, 1976; choreographer, *Censored Scenes from King Kong,* London, 1977; choreographer, *Saratoga,* London, 1978; choreographer, *As You Like It, Romeo and Juliet,* and *Timon of Athens,* all Royal Shakespeare Company (RSC), 1980; choreographer, *A Midsummer Night's Dream* and *A Doll's House,* both RSC, 1981; choreographer, *Women Beware Women,* Genoa, Italy, 1981; choreographer, *The Tempest,* RSC, 1982; and director, *Guys and Dolls* and *Kiss Me Kate,* both Northcott Theatre, Exeter, U.K.

MAJOR TOURS—Director, *Hair,* U.K. and Scottish cities, 1970; choreographer, *The Rocky Horror Show,* U.S. cities, 1980; director, *The Rocky Horror Show,* Australian cities, 1981; director, *Guys and Dolls,* Australian cities, 1986.

PRINCIPAL FILM APPEARANCES—Kideki Ikada, *Welcome to the Club,* Twentieth Century-Fox, 1971. PRINCIPAL FILM WORK—Choreographer: *The Devil's Bride* (also known as *The Devil Rides Out*), Twentieth Century-Fox, 1968; *The Rocky Horror Picture Show,* Twentieth Century-Fox, 1975; *Give My Regards to Broad Street,* Twentieth Century-Fox, 1984; *Absolute Beginners,* Orion, 1986; also *Alice,* 1979.

PRINCIPAL TELEVISION WORK—All as choreographer. Series: *Rock Follies, Good Companions, Upline,* and *The Little Matchgirl.*

AWARDS: Olivier Award from the Society of West End Theatres, Best Choreography, 1982, for *Guys and Dolls;* Green Room Award, Best Director of a Musical, 1986, for *Guys and Dolls.*

ADDRESSES: OFFICE—56-A Finborough Road, London SW10, England. AGENT—William Morris Agency, 147 Wardour Street, London W1, England.

*　　*　　*

TONG, Jacqueline   1950-

PERSONAL: Born February 21, 1950, in Bristol, England; daughter of Stephen Edward (an architect) and Joan Doreen (Connabeer) Tong; married Gordon Robert Nicholas (a lecturer in modern languages), May 28, 1983. EDUCATION: Trained for the stage at Rose Bruford College. RELIGION: Church of England.

VOCATION: Actress.

CAREER: STAGE DEBUT—Jacqueline, *French without Tears,* Bristol Old Vic Theatre, Bristol, U.K. LONDON DEBUT—Irene, *The Dresser,* Queen's Theatre, 1980, for three hundred and four performances. PRINCIPAL STAGE APPEARANCES—Perdita, *The Winter's Tale,* Royal Exchange Theatre, Manchester, U.K., 1978; Valerie, *To Come Home to This,* Royal Court Theatre, London, 1981; Julia, *The Man Who Fell in Love with His Wife,* Lyric Hammersmith Theatre, London, 1985; Armande/Martine, *The Sisterhood,* New End Theatre, London, 1987.

MAJOR TOURS—Perdita, *The Winter's Tale,* European cities, 1978; also in *Alfie,* U.K. cities, 1976.

TELEVISION DEBUT—Anna, *Voyage in the Dark,* London Weekend Television, 1973. PRINCIPAL TELEVISION APPEARANCES—Series: Daisy, *Upstairs, Downstairs,* London Weekend Television, 1973-75. Also Louisa, *Hard Times,* Granada, then PBS, 1977; Sonia, *Heart of the Country,* BBC, 1986; and in *The Virtuoso,* Thames, 1975; *Spearhead,* Southern Television, 1978; *The One and Only Dixie,* Thames, 1979; *Ladies,* BBC, 1979; *Under the Skin,* BBC, 1981; *Out of Step,* BBC, 1981; *Bazaar and Rummage,* BBC, 1982; and *The Climber,* BBC, 1983.

AWARDS: Emmy Award nomination, 1977, for *Upstairs, Downstairs.*

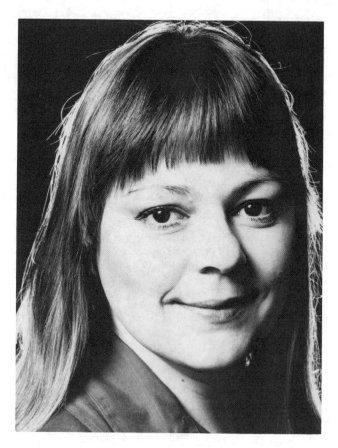

JACQUELINE TONG

ADDRESSES: AGENT—Kate Feast, 43-A Princess Road, London NW1, England.

*   *   *

TRACY, John   1938-

PERSONAL: Born January 11, 1938, in Des Moines, IA. EDUCATION: Attended the University of Iowa; studied acting with Lee Strasberg.

VOCATION: Actor and director.

CAREER: STAGE DEBUT—*Telemachus Clay,* Writers Stage Theatre, New York City, 1963.

PRINCIPAL FILM APPEARANCES—Alan, *The Drifter,* Surfilms, 1966; Tony, *Mister Buddwing* (also known as *Woman without a Face*), Metro-Goldwyn-Mayer, 1966; man, *Dirty Harry,* Warner Brothers, 1971.

PRINCIPAL TELEVISION WORK—All as director. Pilots: *Scalpels,* NBC, 1980; *I Love Her Anyway!,* ABC, 1981; *Irene,* NBC, 1981. Episodic: *The New Mickey Mouse Club,* syndicated, 1977; *The Electric Company,* PBS, 1977; *Out of the Blue,* ABC, 1979; *Makin' It,* ABC, 1979; *Ladies' Man,* CBS, 1980-81; *It's a Living,* ABC, 1981; *Maggie,* ABC, 1981-82; *The New Odd Couple,* ABC, 1982-83; *It's Not Easy,* ABC, 1983; *Spencer,* NBC, 1984-85; *Growing*

Pains, ABC, 1985—; *Head of the Class,* ABC, 1986—; *Roomies,* NBC, 1987; *My Two Dads,* NBC, 1987—; *Just the Ten of Us,* ABC, 1988—; also *Angie,* ABC; *Joanie Loves Chachi,* ABC; *Bosom Buddies,* ABC. Specials: ''Mobile Maidens,'' *The Winners,* PBS, 1977.

AWARDS: Theatre World Award, 1963, for *Telemachus Clay.**

*   *   *

TRUDEAU, Garry   1948-

PERSONAL: Full name, Garretson Beekman Trudeau; born in 1948 in New York, NY; married Jane Pauley (a television journalist), June 14, 1980; children: Rachel, Richard. EDUCATION: Graduated from Yale University, 1970; received M.F.A. from Yale University.

VOCATION: Cartoonist and writer.

CAREER: Also see *WRITINGS* below. PRINCIPAL TELEVISION WORK—Specials: Director and producer (with John Hubley and Faith Hubley), *A Doonesbury Special* (animated), NBC, 1977.

RELATED CAREER—Cartoonist; creator of *Doonesbury* cartoon strip, syndicated by Universal Press Syndicate, 1970—; editor, Cartoons for New Children series, Sheed Publishing; operator of a graphics studio, New Haven, CT.

WRITINGS: STAGE—(Book and lyrics) *Doonesbury,* Biltmore Theatre, New York City, 1983, then U.S. cities, 1984, published by Holt, 1984; (lyrics) *Rap Master Ronnie,* Village Gate Theatre Upstairs, New York City, 1984, published by Lord John, 1986. TELEVISION—Series: *Tanner '88: The Dark Horse,* HBO, 1988. Specials: *A Doonesbury Special* (animated), NBC, 1977.

OTHER—*Doonesbury,* American Heritage Press, 1971; *Still a Few Bugs in the System,* Holt, 1972 (sections published as *Even Revolutionaries Like Chocolate Chip Cookies* and *Just a French Major from the Bronx,* both Popular Library, 1974); *The President Is a Lot Smarter Than You Think,* Holt, 1973; *But This War Had Such Promise,* Holt, 1973 (sections published as *Bravo for Life's Little Ironies,* Popular Library, 1975); *Doonesbury: The Original Yale Cartoons,* Sheed, 1973; *Call Me When You Find America,* Holt, 1973; (with Nicholas von Hoffman) *The Fireside Watergate,* Sheed, 1973; *Joanie,* Sheed, 1974; *Don't Ever Change, Boopsie,* Popular Library, 1974; *Guilty, Guilty, Guilty!,* Holt, 1974.

The Doonesbury Chronicles, Holt, 1975; *Dare to Be Great, Ms. Caucus,* Holt, 1975; *What Do We Have for the Witnesses, Johnnie?,* Holt, 1975; *We'll Take It from Here, Sarge,* Sheed, 1975; *I Have No Son,* Popular Library, 1975; *Wouldn't a Gremlin Have Been More Sensible?,* Holt, 1975; (with von Hoffman) *Tales from the Margaret Mead Taproom: The Compleat Gonzo Governorship of Doonesbury's Uncle Duke,* Sheed, 1976; ''Speaking of Inalienable Rights, Amy. . .'',* Holt, 1976; *You're Never Too Old for Nuts and Berries,* Holt, 1976; *An Especially Tricky People,* Holt, 1977; (with David Levinthal) *Hitler Moves East: A Graphic Chronicle, 1941-43,* Sheed, 1977; *As the Kid Goes for Broke,* Holt, 1977; *Stalking the Perfect Tan,* Holt, 1978; *Doonesbury's Greatest Hits,* Holt, 1978; *Any Grooming Hints for Your Fans, Rollie?,* Holt, 1978; *We're Not Out of the Woods Yet,* Holt, 1979; *But the Pension Fund Was Just Sitting There,* Holt, 1979.

And That's My Final Offer!, Holt, 1980; *A Tad Overweight, but Violet Eyes to Die For*, Holt, 1980; *Guess Who, Fish-Face!*, Fawcett, 1981; (with von Hoffman) *The People's Doonesbury: Notes from Underfoot*, Holt, 1981; *In Search of Reagan's Brain*, Holt, 1981; *He's Never Heard of You, Either*, Holt, 1981; *Do All Birders Have Bedroom Eyes, Dear?*, Fawcett, 1981; *Ask for May, Settle for June*, Holt, 1982; *Gotta Run, My Government Is Collapsing*, Fawcett, 1982; *Unfortunately She Was Also Wired for Sound*, Holt, 1982; *We Who Are About to Fry, Salute You: Selected Cartoons from "In Search of Reagan's Brain," Volume I*, Fawcett, 1982; *Is This Your First Purge, Miss?: Selected Cartoons from "In Search of Reagan's Brain," Volume II*, Fawcett, 1982; *You Give Great Meeting, Sid*, Holt, 1983; *The Wreck of the Rusty Nail*, Holt, 1983; *It's Supposed to Be Yellow, Pinhead: Selected Cartoons from "Ask for May, Settle for June," Volume I*, Fawcett, 1983; *The Thrill Is Gone, Bernie*, Fawcett, 1983; *Sir, I'm Worried about Your Mood Swings*, Fawcett, 1984; *Confirmed Bachelors Are Just So Fascinating*, Fawcett, 1984; *Dressed for Failure, I See*, Fawcett, 1984.

That's Doctor Sinatra, You Little Bimbo!, Holt, 1986; (with others) *Comic Relief: Drawings from the Cartoonists' Thanksgiving Day Hunger Project*, Holt, 1986; *Death of a Party Animal*, Holt, 1986; *Calling Dr. Whoopee*, Holt, 1987; *Downtown Doonesbury*, Holt, 1987; *Doonesbury Deluxe: Selected Glances Askance*, Holt, 1987; *We're Eating More Beets!*, Holt, 1988; *Talking about My G-G-Generation*, Holt, 1988. Also *Doonesbury Dossier: The Reagan Years*, Holt; and *Check Your Egos at the Door*, Holt.

AWARDS: Pulitzer Prize for Editorial Cartooning, 1975, for *Doonesbury;* Academy Award nomination, Best Animated Short, 1977, for *A Doonesbury Special.*

ADDRESSES: OFFICE—Universal Press Syndicate, 4400 Johnson Drive, Fairway, KS 66205.*

*   *   *

TUCCI, Michael   1950-

PERSONAL: Born April 15, 1950 (some sources say 1946), in New York, NY; son of Nicholas (a business executive) and Minerva D. (LaRosa) Tucci; married Kathleen Mary Gately (a network executive), April 30, 1983; children: one. EDUCATION: C.W. Post College, B.A., 1968; Brooklyn Law School, J.D., 1971; studied acting at the American Place Theatre with Mira Rostova, Wynn Handman, and Howard Fine; studied voice with Lee and Sally Sweetland.

VOCATION: Actor.

CAREER: OFF-BROADWAY DEBUT—Herbie, *Godspell*, 1973. BROADWAY DEBUT—Sonny, *Grease*, Royale Theatre, 1975. PRINCIPAL STAGE APPEARANCES—*Theatre Songs by Maltby and Shire*, Manhattan Theatre Club, New York City, 1976; *Hold Me!*, American Place Theatre, New York City, 1977; *Kid Twist*, Mark Taper Forum, Los Angeles, CA, 1978; also *The Boys from Syracuse*, Los Angeles, 1987; *The Wizard of Oz*, Los Angeles, 1988; and *American Mosaic*, Mark Taper Forum.

MAJOR TOURS—Chico Marx, *Minnie's Boys*, U.S. cities; also *Grease*, U.S. cities; *Godspell*, U.S. cities; *Turn to the Right*, U.S. cities.

PRINCIPAL FILM APPEARANCES—Lou, *The Night They Robbed Big Bertha's*, Scotia American, 1975; Sonny, *Grease*, Paramount, 1978; Harry Cimoli, *Sunnyside*, American International, 1979; Arnie, *Lunch Wagon* (also known as *Lunch Wagon Girls* and *Come 'n Get It*), Bordeaux, 1981.

PRINCIPAL TELEVISION APPEARANCES—Series: Dr. Charlie Nichols, *Trapper John, M.D.*, CBS, 1980-84; Gerald Golden, *The Paper Chase: The Second Year*, Showtime, 1983; also Pete, *It's Gary Shandling's Show*, Showtime. Pilots: Teddy Serrano, *Friends*, CBS, 1978; Armando, *The Rainbow Girl*, NBC, 1982. Episodic: *Barney Miller*, ABC, 1976 and 1978; *People's Court*, ABC, 1980; also Phil Goldenstein, *On Our Own*, CBS. Movies: Captain Claude Eatherly, *Enola Gay*, NBC, 1980. Specials: Chico Marx, *Groucho in Revue*, HBO.

NON-RELATED CAREER—Lawyer.

WRITINGS: STAGE—(With Joe Mantegna) *Leonardo.*

AWARDS: Drama-Logue Awards for acting, 1978, for *Kid Twist*, 1987, for *The Boys from Syracuse*, and 1988, for *The Wizard of Oz.*

ADDRESSES: HOME—2535 Kenilworth Avenue, Los Angeles, CA 90039. AGENT—Pat Quinn, International Creative Management, 8899 Beverly Boulevard, Los Angeles, CA 90048.

*   *   *

TUNE, Tommy   1939-

PERSONAL: Full name, Thomas James Tune; born February 28, 1939, in Wichita Falls, TX; son of Jim P. (an oil rig worker and horse trainer) and Eva Mae (Clark) Tune. EDUCATION: Attended Lon Morris Junior College, 1958-59; University of Texas, Austin, B.F.A., 1962; graduate work, University of Houston, 1962-63.

VOCATION: Director, choreographer, dancer, and actor.

CAREER: BROADWAY DEBUT—Chorus, *Baker Street*, Broadway Theatre, 1965. PRINCIPAL STAGE APPEARANCES—Tommy, *A Joyful Noise*, Mark Hellinger Theatre, New York City, 1966; David, *Seesaw*, Uris Theatre, New York City, 1973; Captain Billy Buck Chandler, *My One and Only*, St. James Theatre, New York City, 1983; also appeared in *How Now Dow Jones*, Lunt-Fontanne Theatre, New York City, 1967.

PRINCIPAL STAGE WORK—Director, *The Club*, Circle in the Square Downtown, New York City, 1976; director, *Sunset*, Studio Arena, Buffalo, NY, 1977; director (with Peter Masterson) and choreographer, *The Best Little Whorehouse in Texas*, Entermedia Theatre, New York City, 1978, then 46th Street Theatre, New York City, 1979; choreographer, *Double Feature*, Long Wharf Theatre, New Haven, CT, 1979; director and choreographer, *A Day in Hollywood/A Night in the Ukraine*, John Golden Theatre, New York City, 1980; director, *Cloud 9*, Theatre De Lys, New York City, 1981; director and choreographer, *Nine*, 46th Street Theatre, 1982; director and choreographer (both with Thommie Walsh), *My One and Only*, St. James Theatre, New York City, 1983; director, *Stepping Out*, John Golden Theatre, 1987.

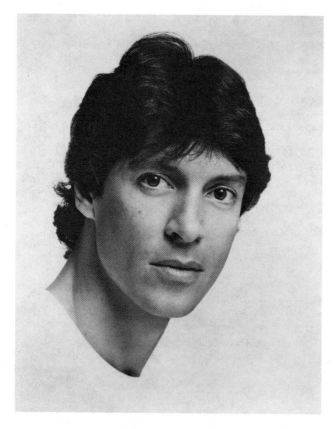

TOMMY TUNE

MAJOR TOURS—Choreographer, *Canterbury Tales*, U.S. cities, 1969; David, *Seesaw*, U.S. cities, 1974; director (with Peter Masterson) and choreographer, *The Best Little Whorehouse in Texas*, U.S. cities, 1979; Captain Billy Buck Chandler (also director and choreographer with Thommie Walsh), *My One and Only*, U.S. cities, 1985-86; director and choreographer, *Nine*, U.S. cities, 1984.

PRINCIPAL FILM APPEARANCES—Ambrose Kemper, *Hello, Dolly!*, Twentieth Century-Fox, 1969; Tommy, *The Boy Friend*, Metro-Goldwyn-Mayer, 1971.

PRINCIPAL TELEVISION APPEARANCES—Series: Regular, *Dean Martin Presents the Golddiggers*, NBC, 1969-70. Specials: *Irving Berlin's 100th Birthday Salute*, CBS, 1988.

AWARDS: Antoinette Perry Award, Best Supporting or Featured Actor in a Musical, 1974, for *Seesaw;* Obie Award from the *Village Voice*, 1977, for *The Club;* Antoinette Perry Award nominations, Best Director of a Musical (with Peter Masterson) and Best Choreography, and Drama Desk Award, Best Director of a Musical (with Masterson), all 1979, for *The Best Little Whorehouse in Texas;* Drama Desk Awards, Best Musical Staging and Best Choreography, Antoinette Perry Award, Best Choreography, and Antoinette Perry Award nomination, Best Director of a Musical, all 1980, for *A Day in Hollywood/A Night in the Ukraine;* Drama Desk Award, Best Director, and Obie Award, Distinguished Direction, both 1982, for *Cloud Nine;* Drama Desk Award and Antoinette Perry Award, both Best Director of a Musical, and Antoinette Perry Award nomination, Best Choreography, all 1982, for *Nine;* Antoinette Perry Awards, Best Actor in a Musical and Best Choreogra-

phy (with Thommie Walsh), Antoinette Perry Award nomination, Best Musical Director (with Walsh), and Drama Desk Award, Outstanding Choreography (with Walsh), all 1983, for *My One and Only;* Dance Magazine Award, 1984.

MEMBER: Directors Guild of America, Society of Stage Directors and Choreographers, Actors' Equity Association.

SIDELIGHTS: FAVORITE ROLE—Captain Billy Buck Chandler in *My One and Only*.

ADDRESSES: OFFICE—Towerhouse Productions, Inc., 890 Broadway, New York, NY 10003. AGENT—International Creative Management, 40 W. 57th Street, New York, NY 10019.*

                              *   *   *

TUSHINGHAM, Rita   1942-

PERSONAL: Born March 14, 1942, in Liverpool, England; daughter of John and Enid Ellen (Lott) Tushingham; married Terence William Bicknell (divorced); married Ouasama Rawi. EDUCATION: Trained for the stage at the Liverpool Playhouse.

VOCATION: Actress.

CAREER: LONDON DEBUT—Madwoman, *The Changeling*, Royal Court Theatre, 1961. PRINCIPAL STAGE APPEARANCES—Waitress, *The Kitchen*, Royal Court Theatre, London, 1961; Hermia, *A*

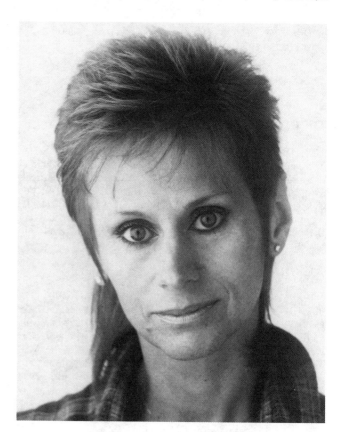

RITA TUSHINGHAM

Midsummer Night's Dream, Maria, *Twelfth Night,* and Nancy, *The Knack,* all Royal Court Theatre, 1962; Daisy Wink, *The Give-Away,* Garrick Theatre, London, 1969; Lorna, *Lorna and Ted,* Greenwich Theatre, London, 1970; Bernadette Soubirous, *Mistress of Novices,* Piccadilly Theatre, London, 1973.

FILM DEBUT—Jo, *A Taste of Honey,* Continental Distributing, 1962. PRINCIPAL FILM APPEARANCES—Kate Brady, *The Girl with Green Eyes,* Lopert, 1964; Catherine, *A Place to Go,* British Lion, 1964; girl, *Dr. Zhivago,* Metro-Goldwyn-Mayer, 1965; Dot, *The Leather Boys,* Allied Artists, 1965; Nancy Jones, *The Knack . . . And How to Get It* (also known as *The Knack*), Lopert, 1965; Brenda, *Smashing Time,* Paramount, 1967; Eve, *The Trap* (also known as *L'Aventure sauvage*), Continental Distributing, 1967; Bridget, *Diamonds for Breakfast,* Paramount, 1968; Penelope, *The Bedsitting Room,* United Artists, 1969; Jenny, *The Guru,* Twentieth Century-Fox, 1969; Brenda Thompson, *Straight on 'till Morning,* International Co-Productions, 1974; Janice, *The Human Factor,* Bryanston, 1975; Lea, *Rachel's Man,* Hemdale Releasing, 1975; Martha Gude, *Mysteries,* Cine-Vog, 1979; Kate, *Spaghetti House,* Titanus/SACIS/Axon Video, 1982; Jean, *Flying,* Golden Communications, 1986; Eunice Parchman, *A Judgement in Stone* (also known as *The Housekeeper*), Norstar, 1986; Mrs. Deakin, *Resurrected* (also known as *Resurrection*), Hobo Film Enterprises, 1989. Also appeared in *Ragazzo di borgata* (also known as *Slum*

Boy), RPA International, 1976; and in *The Black Journal, The Incredible Mrs. Chadwick, Situation, Instant Coffee, Felix Krull, Lady Killers, Seeing Red,* and *Bread, Butter, and Jam.*

PRINCIPAL TELEVISION APPEARANCES—Series: *Bread,* BBC, 1989; also *No Strings.* Movies: Margaret Sheen, *Green Eyes,* ABC, 1977. Specials: Mrs. Prysselius, ''Pippi Longstocking,'' *ABC Weekend Specials,* ABC, 1985. Plays: *Dante and Beatrice in Liverpool,* 1989.

AWARDS: Variety Club of Great Britain Award and British Film and Television Society Award, both Most Promising Newcomer, 1961, Best Actress Award from the Cannes Film Festival, 1962, New York Film Critics Award, Best Actress, and Golden Globe Award, Most Promising Newcomer, both 1963, all for *A Taste of Honey;* also Variety Club of Great Britain Award, Best Actress, 1964; Silver Goddess Award from the Mexico Film Festival, Best Foreign Actress, 1965; Czechoslovak Film Critics Award, Best Actress, 1966; Variety Club of Great Britain Award, BBC-TV Personality of the Year, 1988.

SIDELIGHTS: RECREATIONS—Cooking.

ADDRESSES: AGENT—International Creative Management, 388 Oxford Street, London W1N 9HE, England.

V

VACCARO, Brenda 1939-

PERSONAL: Full name, Brenda Buell Vaccaro; born November 18, 1939, in Brooklyn, NY; daughter of Mario A. (a restaurateur) and Christine M. (Pavia) Vaccaro; married Martin Fried (a stage manager; divorced); married William Bishop, 1977 (divorced); married Charles Cannizzaro (divorced, 1981); married Guy P. Hector (a restaurateur). EDUCATION: Trained for the stage at the Neighborhood Playhouse, 1958-60, and with David Pressman. POLITICS: Democrat. RELIGION: Roman Catholic.

VOCATION: Actress.

CAREER: STAGE DEBUT—Angelina, *The Willow Tree,* Margo Jones Theatre, Dallas, TX, 1951. BROADWAY DEBUT—Gloria Gulock, *Everybody Loves Opal,* Longacre Theatre, 1961. PRINCIPAL STAGE APPEARANCES—Miss Novick, *Tunnel of Love,*

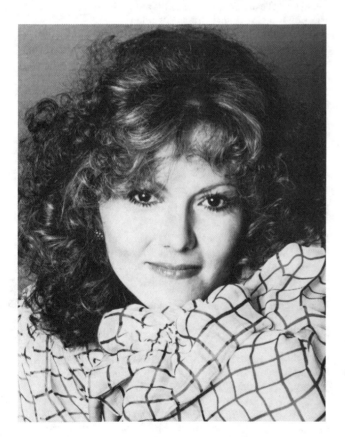

BRENDA VACCARO

Westbury Music Fair, Westbury, NY, 1962; Laura Howard, *The Affair,* Henry Miller's Theatre, New York City, 1962; Melissa Peabody, *Children from Their Games,* Morosco Theatre, New York City, 1963; Toni, *Cactus Flower,* Royale Theatre, New York City, 1965; Reedy Harris, *The Natural Look,* Longacre Theatre, New York City, 1967; Cynthia, *How Now, Dow Jones,* Lunt-Fontanne Theatre, New York City, 1967; Nancy Scott, *The Goodbye People,* Ethel Barrymore Theatre, New York City, 1968; Louise, *Father's Day,* John Golden Theatre, New York City, 1971; Olive Madison, *The Odd Couple,* Broadhurst Theatre, New York City, 1985.

MAJOR TOURS—Miss Novick, *Tunnel of Love,* U.S. cities, 1962.

FILM DEBUT—Molly Hirsch, *Where It's At,* United Artists, 1969. PRINCIPAL FILM APPEARANCES—Shirley, *Midnight Cowboy,* United Artists, 1969; Jody Burrows, *I Love My Wife,* Universal, 1970; Jenny, *Going Home,* Metro-Goldwyn-Mayer, 1971; Vanetta, *Summertree,* Columbia, 1971; Linda, *Once Is Not Enough* (also known as *Jacqueline Susann's "Once Is Not Enough"*), Paramount, 1975; Eve Clayton, *Airport '77,* Universal, 1977; Diane, *The House by the Lake* (also known as *Death Weekend*), American International, 1977; Kay Brubaker, *Capricorn One,* Warner Brothers, 1978; Grace Wolf, *Fast Charlie . . . The Moonbeam Rider* (also known as *Fast Charlie and the Moonbeam*), Universal, 1979; Monica Gilbert, *The First Deadly Sin,* Filmways, 1980; Florinda, *Zorro, the Gay Blade,* Twentieth Century-Fox, 1981; Bianca, *Supergirl,* Tri-Star, 1984; Dolores, *Water,* Rank/Atlantic Releasing, 1985; Betty, *Heart of Midnight,* Samuel Goldwyn, 1988; Bunny, *Cookie,* Warner Brothers, 1989. Also appeared in *Chanel Solitaire,* United Film Distribution, 1981; and *Death on Safari,* 1988.

PRINCIPAL TELEVISION APPEARANCES—Series: Sara Yarnell, *Sara,* CBS, 1976; Detective Sergeant Kate Hudson, *Dear Detective,* CBS, 1979; Julia Blake, *Paper Dolls,* ABC, 1984. Pilots: Jenny Penny, *My Lucky Penny,* CBS, 1966; Lucille Sand, *Travis Logan, D.A.,* CBS, 1971; Brenda Brooks, *The Big Ripoff,* NBC, 1975; Maxine, "Changing Patterns," *CBS Summer Playhouse,* CBS, 1987. Episodic: Felicia Sartene, *The Greatest Show on Earth,* ABC, 1963; Mimi Harcourt, *Murder, She Wrote,* CBS, 1988; also *The Fugitive,* ABC, 1963; *The Defenders,* CBS, 1964 and 1965; *The Doctors and the Nurses,* CBS, 1965; *Coronet Blue,* CBS, 1967; *The F.B.I.,* ABC, 1969; *The Psychiatrist,* NBC, 1971; *The Name of the Game,* NBC, 1971; *Marcus Welby, M.D.,* ABC, 1972; *Banacek,* NBC, 1972; *McCloud,* NBC, 1972; *The Helen Reddy Show,* NBC, 1973; *McCoy,* NBC, 1976; *The Streets of San Francisco,* ABC, 1976.

Movies: Shirley Campbell, *What's a Nice Girl Like You. . .?,* ABC, 1971; Dr. Carol Gillman, *Sunshine,* CBS, 1973; Rosalie

Bonanno, *Honor Thy Father,* CBS, 1973; Jane Briggs, *Guyana Tragedy: The Story of Jim Jones,* CBS, 1980; Lillian Jacobs, *A Long Way Home,* ABC, 1981; Marion Galucci, *The Pride of Jesse Hallam,* CBS, 1981; Dolores Baker, *The Star Maker,* NBC, 1981; Helen Adams, *Deceptions,* NBC, 1985; also *The Trial of Julius and Ethel Rosenberg,* ABC, 1974. Specials: *The Shape of Things,* CBS, 1973; *That Was the Year That Was,* NBC, 1976; *Oscar Presents John Wayne and the War Movies,* ABC, 1977; *Celebrity Challenge of the Sexes,* CBS, 1977; *The Fourth Annual International Circus Festival of Monte Carlo,* CBS, 1978; voice of Tillie, *Nestor, the Long-Eared Christmas Donkey* (animated), ABC, 1978; *The Paul Lynde Comedy Hour,* ABC, 1978; *Battle of the Network Stars,* ABC, 1984; *Supergirl: The Making of the Movie,* ABC, 1985; *Hollywood Women,* syndicated, 1988.

RELATED CAREER—Professional model; actress in television commercials.

NON-RELATED CAREER—Waitress.

AWARDS: Theatre World Award, 1962, for *Everybody Loves Opal;* Antoinette Perry Award nomination, Best Supporting or Featured Actress in a Drama, 1965, for *Cactus Flower;* Antoinette Perry Award nomination, Best Actress in a Musical, 1968, for *How Now, Dow Jones;* Antoinette Perry Award nomination, Best Actress—Dramatic, 1969, for *The Goodbye People;* Emmy Award, Best Supporting Actress in a Variety Program, 1974, for *The Shape of Things;* Academy Award nomination and Golden Globe Award, both Best Supporting Actress, 1975, for *Once Is Not Enough;* also Emmy Award nomination, Best Dramatic Actress, for *Sara;* and two Hollywood Press Association Award nominations.

MEMBER: Actors' Equity Association, Screen Actors Guild, American Federation of Television and Radio Artists.

ADDRESSES: AGENT—Susan Smith, Smith-Freedman and Associates, 121 N. San Vicente Boulevard, Beverly Hills, CA 90211. PUBLICIST—Joni Hartman, Slade, Grant, Hartman, and Hartman, 9145 Sunset Boulevard, Suite 218, Los Angeles, CA 90069.

*   *   *

VAN ARK, Joan   1948-

PERSONAL: Born June 16, 1948 (some sources say 1943 or 1946), in New York, NY; daughter of Carroll (in public relations) and Dorothy Jean (a writer; maiden name, Hemenway) Van Ark; married John Marsillo (a news reporter), February 1, 1966; children: Vanessa Jean. EDUCATION: Attended Yale University. RELIGION: Presbyterian.

VOCATION: Actress.

CAREER: PRINCIPAL STAGE APPEARANCES—Corie Bratter, *Barefoot in the Park,* Biltmore Theatre, New York City, 1965; Agnes, *The School for Wives,* Lyceum Theatre, New York City, 1971; Silia Gala, *The Rules of the Game,* New Phoenix Repertory Company, Helen Hayes Theatre, New York City, 1974. Also appeared in *Chemin de Fer,* New Theatre for Now, Los Angeles, CA, 1969; *In a Fine Castle,* New Theatre for Now, 1971; in productions of *Cyrano de Bergerac* and *Ring Round the Moon;* at the Tyrone Guthrie Theatre, Minneapolis, MN; and at the Arena Stage, Washington, DC.

MAJOR TOURS—Corie Bratter, *Barefoot in the Park,* U.S. cities, 1965.

PRINCIPAL FILM APPEARANCES—Karen Crockett, *Frogs,* American International, 1972.

PRINCIPAL TELEVISION APPEARANCES—Series: Nurse Annie Carlisle, *Temperatures Rising,* ABC, 1972-73; Dee Dee Baldwin, *We've Got Each Other,* CBS, 1977-78; voice of Manta, "Manta and Moray, Monarchs of the Deep," *Tarzan and the Super Seven* (animated), CBS, 1978-80; Valene Ewing, *Dallas,* CBS, 1978-81; voices of Jessica Drew and Spider-Woman, *Spider-Woman* (animated), ABC, 1979-80; Valene Ewing, *Knots Landing,* CBS, 1979—; voice of Moray, "Manta and Moray, Monarchs of the Deep," *Batman and the Super Seven* (animated), NBC, 1980-81; voice characterizations, *Thundarr the Barbarian* (animated), ABC, 1980-82; also voice characterizations, *Heathcliff and Dingbat* (animated). Mini-Series: Jane Robson, *Testimony of Two Men,* syndicated, 1977. Pilots: Alicia Dodd, *The Judge and Jake Wyler,* NBC, 1972; Nina, *Big Rose,* CBS, 1974; Shirley, *Shell Game,* CBS, 1975. Episodic: "Radar's Report," *M*A*S*H,* CBS, 1973; *Quark,* NBC, 1978; *The Pat Sajak Show,* CBS, 1989; also as Marian Gerard, *Rhoda,* CBS; Haven Grant, *Vega$,* ABC; in *Night Gallery,* NBC; *The F.B.I.,* ABC; *The Girl with Something Extra,* NBC. Movies: Frankie Banks, *The Last Dinosaur,* ABC, 1977; Marie Rivers, *Red Flag: The Ultimate Game,* CBS, 1981; Brenda Allen, *Shakedown on the Sunset Strip,* CBS, 1988; Claire, *My First Love,* ABC, 1988. Specials: *Celebrity Challenge of the Sexes,* CBS, 1980; *Battle of the Network Stars,* ABC, 1980, 1982, and 1983.

AWARDS: Theatre World Award, 1971, for *The School for Wives;* also Los Angeles Drama Critics Award, 1973.

MEMBER: Actors' Equity Assocation, Screen Actors Guild, American Federation of Television and Radio Artists, San Fernando Valley Track Club.

ADDRESSES: OFFICE—c/o Addis, 8444 Wilshire Boulevard, Los Angeles, CA 90048. AGENT—William Morris Agency, 151 El Camino Drive, Beverly Hills, CA 90212.

*   *   *

VAN PEEBLES, Melvin   1932-

PERSONAL: Born August 21, 1932, in Chicago, IL; children: Mario. EDUCATION: Ohio Wesleyan University, B.A., 1953; also attended West Virginia State College. MILITARY: U.S. Air Force, navigator and bombardier.

VOCATION: Writer, composer, producer, director, and actor.

CAREER: Also see *WRITINGS* below. PRINCIPAL STAGE APPEARANCES—*Out There by Your Lonesome* (one-man show), Philharmonic Hall, New York City, 1973; *Don't Play Us Cheap,* Shubert Theatre, Chicago, IL, 1975; *Waltz of the Stork,* Century Theatre, New York City, 1982.

PRINCIPAL STAGE WORK—Producer and director, *Don't Play Us Cheap,* Ethel Barrymore Theatre, New York City, 1972; producer and director, *Waltz of the Stork,* Century Theatre, New York City,

1982; director, *Champeeen!,* New Federal Theatre, Harry DeJur Playhouse, New York City, 1983.

MAJOR TOURS—*Out There by Your Lonesome* (one-man show), U.S. cities, 1973; also appeared in *The Hostage* with the Dutch National Theatre.

PRINCIPAL FILM APPEARANCES—Sweetback, *Sweet Sweetback's Baadasssss Song,* Cinemation, 1971; Jake, *Jaws: The Revenge,* Universal, 1987; Wino Bob, *O.C. and Stiggs,* Metro-Goldwyn-Mayer/United Artists, 1987; also appeared in *America,* ASA, 1986.

PRINCIPAL FILM WORK—Director: *The Story of a Three Day Pass* (also known as *La Permission*), Sigma III, 1968; (also music director) *Watermelon Man,* Columbia, 1970; (also producer and editor) *Sweet Sweetback's Baadasssss Song,* Cinemation, 1971; (also producer and editor) *Identity Crisis,* Block and Chip, 1989. Also director, *Don't Play Us Cheap,* 1973.

PRINCIPAL TELEVISION APPEARANCES—Episodic: Hawk, "Taking Care of Terrific," *Wonderworks,* PBS, 1988; Mel, *Sonny Spoon* (four episodes), NBC, 1988. Movies: Walter Moon and Silkie Porter, *The Sophisticated Gents,* NBC, 1981.

PRINCIPAL TELEVISION WORK—Movies: Associate producer, *The Sophisticated Gents,* NBC, 1981.

RELATED CAREER—Appeared in a cabaret production, Bottom Line, New York City, 1974; appeared in nightclubs and cabarets in France; avant-garde filmmaker in France, created such short films as *Sunlight* and *Three Pick Up Men for Herrick,* both released by Cinema 16.

NON-RELATED CAREER—Cable car gripman, San Francisco, CA.

WRITINGS: STAGE—Also composer and lyricist, unless indicated: *Harlem Party,* first produced in Belgium, 1964, then as *Don't Play Us Cheap,* Ethel Barrymore Theatre, 1972; *Ain't Supposed to Die a Natural Death,* Ethel Barrymore Theatre, New York City, 1971, published by Bantam, 1973; *Out There by Your Lonesome* (one-man show), Phiharmonic Hall, New York City, 1973; (book only) *Reggae,* Biltmore Theatre, New York City, 1980; *Waltz of the Stork,* Century Theatre, New York City, 1982; *Champeeen!,* New Federal Theatre, Harry DeJur Playhouse, New York City, 1983; also music and comedy material for cabaret productions.

FILM—(Also composer with Mickey Baker) *The Story of a Three Day Pass,* Sigma III, 1968; (composer) *Watermelon Man,* Columbia, 1970; (also composer) *Sweet Sweetback's Baadasssss Song,* Cinemation, 1971, published by Lancer Books, 1971; (also composer and lyricist) *Don't Play Us Cheap,* 1973; (with Kenneth Vose, Lawrence Dukore, and Leon Capetanos) *Greased Lightning,* Warner Brothers, 1977; *Identity Crisis,* Block and Chip, 1989.

TELEVISION—Pilots: (Also composer of title song) *Just an Old Sweet Song,* CBS, 1976, published by Ballantine, 1976; *Down Home,* CBS, 1978. Movies: (Also composer) *The Sophisticated Gents,* NBC, 1981. Specials: "The Day They Came to Arrest the Book," *CBS Schoolbreak Special,* CBS, 1987.

OTHER—*Un ours pour le F.B.I.* (novel), Buchet-Chastel, 1964, translated as *A Bear for the F.B.I.,* Trident, 1968; *Un Americain en enfer* (novel), Editions Denoel, 1965, translated as *The True American: A Folk Fable,* Doubleday, 1976; *Le Chinois du XIV* (short stories), Le Gadenet, 1966; *La Fete a Harlem* (novel adapted from his play *Harlem Party*), J. Martineau, 1967, translated as *Don't Play Us Cheap: A Harlem Party,* Bantam, 1973; *The Big Heart* (photo essay), 1967; *La Permission,* J. Martineau, 1967; *The Making of Sweet Sweetback's Baadasssss Song* (nonfiction), Lancer Books, 1972.

RECORDINGS: ALBUMS—*As Serious as a Heart Attack,* A&M, 1971; *What the . . . You Mean I Can't Sing,* A&M, 1974; also *Br'er Soul,* 1969; *Ain't Supposed to Die a Natural Death.*

AWARDS: First Prize from the Belgian Festival for *Don't Play Us Cheap.*

MEMBER: Directors Guild of America, French Directors Guild.

ADDRESSES: OFFICE—Ballantine Books, 201 E. 50th Street, New York, NY 10022.*

                    *   *   *

VENNERA, Chick

PERSONAL: Born Francis Vennera, March 27, in Herkimer, NY; son of Frank (a musician) and Victoria (Guido) Vennera; married Suzanne Messbauer (a clothing designer), April 9, 1983; children: Nicole. EDUCATION: Trained for the stage at the Pasadena Playhouse and with Milton Katselas at the Actors Lab. MILITARY: U.S. Army, Signal Corps, Special Services.

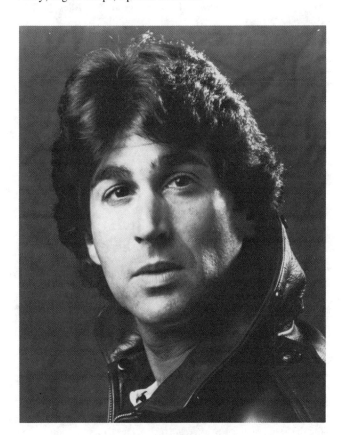

CHICK VENNERA

VOCATION: Actor, screenwriter, and composer.

CAREER: BROADWAY DEBUT—Sonny, *Grease,* Royale Theatre, New York City, 1976. OFF-BROADWAY DEBUT—Angel Quiton, *Jockeys,* Promenade Theatre, New York City, 1977, for fifty performances. PRINCIPAL STAGE APPEARANCES—Appeared in productions of *The Tigers, Dark of the Moon,* and *The Rose Tattoo,* all in Los Angeles, CA.

MAJOR TOURS—Sonny, *Grease,* U.S. and Canadian cities, 1973-75.

FILM DEBUT—Marv Gomez, *Thank God It's Friday,* Columbia, 1978. PRINCIPAL FILM APPEARANCES—Sergeant Danny Ruffelo, *Yanks,* Universal, 1979; Tony, *High Risk,* American Cinema, 1981; Pepper Zombie, *Hysterical,* American Cinema, 1981; Ness, *Boarding School,* Trankis, 1985; Tony, *Kidnapped,* Hickmar, 1986; Joe Mondragon, *The Milagro Beanfield War,* Universal, 1988; Nuzo, *Last Rites,* Metro-Goldwyn-Mayer, 1988; also appeared in *Free Ride.*

TELEVISION DEBUT—Episodic: Ruffian, *Lucas Tanner,* NBC. PRINCIPAL TELEVISION APPEARANCES—Series: Luis, *Baretta,* ABC, 1976; Raoul, *Hail to the Chief,* ABC, 1985; also voice of Sammy the Rat, *Foofer* (animated), NBC. Mini-Series: *Arthur Hailey's "The Moneychangers"* (also known as *The Moneychangers*), NBC, 1976; *Once an Eagle,* NBC, 1976-77. Pilots: Costigan, *Vega$,* ABC, 1978; Private Joseph Battaglia, *G.I.'s,* CBS, 1980. Episodic: Stack, *Hollywood Beat,* ABC, 1985; Hector Rivera, *Night Court,* NBC, 1986; Spider, *Diff'rent Strokes,* ABC, 1986; also Costigan, *Vega$,* ABC; *T.J. Hooker,* ABC. Movies: Luis, *Billy: Portrait of Street Kid,* CBS, 1977; Frankie, *A Bunny's Tale,* ABC, 1985.

RELATED CAREER—Saxophone player and singer in a nightclub band, New York City; appeared as Goofy, *Disney on Parade;* commercial voiceover performer.

NON-RELATED CAREER—Telephone salesman; delivered flowers.

WRITINGS: TELEVISION—Episodic: (Also composer) *Vega$,* ABC.

AWARDS: Theatre World Award, 1977, for *Jockeys.*

MEMBER: Academy of Motion Picture Arts and Sciences, Nosotros.

SIDELIGHTS: RECREATIONS—Golf.

ADDRESSES: OFFICE—P.O. Box 415, Burbank, CA 91503. AGENTS—Dick Berman, Jerome Zeitman, and Larry Becsey, The Agency, 10351 Santa Monica Boulevard, Suite 2111, Los Angeles, CA 90025. PUBLICIST—Richard Grant and Associates, 8500 Wilshire Boulevard, Suite 520, Beverly Hills, CA 90211.

*   *   *

VERNON, John   1932-

PERSONAL: Born Adolphus Vernon Agopsowicz, February 24, 1932, in Regina, SK, Canada; children: Kate. EDUCATION: Trained for the stage at the Royal Academy of Dramatic Arts and at the Banff School of Fine Arts.

VOCATION: Actor.

CAREER: PRINCIPAL STAGE APPEARANCES—Farm hand, *The Merry Wives of Windsor,* Stratford Shakespearean Festival, Stratford, ON, Canada, 1956; Charles, *As You Like It,* and second senator, *Othello,* both Stratford Shakespearean Festival, 1959; Montague, *Romeo and Juliet,* and Duke of Austria, *King John,* both Stratford Shakespearean Festival, 1960; Titus Laritius and Volscian officer, *Coriolanus,* and Duke of Suffolk, *Henry VIII,* both Stratford Shakespearean Festival, 1961; Curtis, *The Taming of the Shrew,* Ross, *Macbeth,* and musketeer, *Cyrano de Bergerac,* all Stratford Shakespearean Festival, 1962; Achilles, *Troilus and Cressida,* New York Shakespeare Festival, Delacorte Theatre, New York City, 1965; Hernando de Soto, *The Royal Hunt of the Sun,* American National Theatre and Academy Theatre, New York City, 1965. Also appeared in *Henry V,* Stratford Shakespearean Festival, 1956.

PRINCIPAL FILM APPEARANCES—Lot supervisor, *Nobody Waved Goodbye,* Cinema V, 1965; Mal Reese, *Point Blank,* Metro-Goldwyn-Mayer (MGM), 1967; Nessim, *Justine,* Twentieth Century-Fox, 1969; Hacker, *Tell Them Willie Boy Is Here,* Universal, 1969; Rico Parra, *Topaz,* Universal, 1969; Mayor, *Dirty Harry,* Warner Brothers, 1971; Timothy X. Nolan, *One More Train to Rob,* Universal, 1971; Maynard Boyle, *Charley Varrick,* Universal, 1973; Vyland, *Fear Is the Key,* Paramount, 1973; McKee, *The Black Windmill,* Universal, 1974; Arnie Felson, *W* (also known as *I Want Her Dead*), Cinerama, 1974; Mr. Kapital, *Sweet Movie,* CFDC, 1974; Larkin, *Brannigan,* United Artists, 1975; Fletcher, *The Outlaw Josey Wales,* Warner Brothers, 1976; Ben Kincaid, *Angela,* Montreal Travel Company, 1977; Luis Carreras, *Golden Rendezvous,* Golden Rendezvous, 1977; Boulder Allin, *Journey,* EPQH, 1977; Emanuele, *A Special Day* (also known as *Una giornata speciale, Una giornata particolare,* and *The Great Day*), Cinema V, 1977; Pomeroy, "Hollywood, 1936" in *The Uncanny,* Rank, 1977; Dean Vernon Wormer, *National Lampoon's Animal House,* Universal, 1978.

Jim, *Fantastica,* Gaumont, 1980; Prindle, *Herbie Goes Bananas,* Buena Vista, 1980; voice of alien, *Heavy Metal* (animated), Columbia, 1981; Malone, *The Kinky Coaches and the Pom-Pom Pussycats,* Summa Vista, 1981; Dr. Stone, *Airplane II: The Sequel,* Paramount, 1982; Warden Backman, *Chained Heat,* Jensen Farley, 1983; Jonathan Stryker, *Curtains,* Jensen Farley, 1983; Vito, *Jungle Warriors,* Aquarius, 1984; Principal Underwood, *Savage Streets,* Motion Picture Marketing, 1984; Big Mac, *Doin' Time,* Warner Brothers, 1985; Chief Ferret, *Fraternity Vacation,* New World, 1985; Roger Levering, *Blue Monkey* (also known as *Green Monkey*), Spectrafilm, 1987; Sherman Krader, *Ernest Goes to Camp,* Buena Vista, 1987; Adam Beardsley, *Nightstick* (also known as *Calhoun*), Production Distribution, 1987; Karrothers, *Double Exposure,* United Film Distribution, 1987; Elmer Sinclair, *Dixie Lanes,* Miramax, 1988; Mitchell, *Deadly Stranger,* Manson International, 1988; Officer Mooney, *Killer Klowns from Outer Space,* Trans World, 1988; Mr. Big, *I'm Gonna Git You Sucka,* Metro-Goldwyn-Mayer/United Artists, 1988. Also appeared in *Crunch,* 1975; and in *Office Party,* Miramax, 1988.

PRINCIPAL TELEVISION APPEARANCES—Series: Dean Vernon Wormer, *Delta House,* ABC, 1979; General Hannibal Stryker, *Hail to the Chief,* ABC, 1985; voice of Wildfire, *Wildfire* (animated), CBS, 1986-87. Mini-Series: Secretary of State Seward, *The Blue and the Gray,* CBS, 1982. Pilots: Charles Walding, *Escape,* ABC, 1971; Inspector Duprez, *Cool Million* (also known as *Mask of Marcella*), NBC, 1972; David Hunter/Praetorius, *Hunter,* CBS,

1973; Geoffrey Darro, *The Questor Tapes*, NBC, 1974; Robin Templar, *The Barbary Coast*, ABC, 1975; Sheriff Turner, *The Imposter*, NBC, 1975; Harry Paine, *Matt Helm*, ABC, 1975; Charles Forsythe, *The Swiss Family Robinson*, ABC, 1975. Episodic: Dave Ryerson, *MacGyver*, ABC, 1985; Henry Hayward, *Murder, She Wrote*, CBS, 1985; Claude Watkins, *Knight Rider*, NBC, 1986; Gus Cavalaris, *Tough Cookies*, CBS, 1986; Mayor Flambo, *Sledge Hammer!*, ABC, 1986; the Principal, "Fuzzbucket," *Disney Sunday Movie*, ABC, 1986; Donald Jordan, *Scarecrow and Mrs. King*, CBS, 1987; Number One, *The New Adventures of Beans Baxter*, Fox, 1987. Movies: Leo D'Agosta, *Trial Run*, NBC, 1969; Nick Rubanos, *The Virginia Hill Story*, NBC, 1974; David Richardson, *Mousey* (also known as *Cat and Mouse*), ABC, 1974; Dr. Orrin Helgerson, *Mary Jane Harper Cried Last Night*, CBS, 1977; Jonathan Pritts, *Louis L'Amour's "The Sacketts,"* (also known as *The Sacketts*), NBC, 1979; General Karlheinz von Loenig, *The Blood of Others*, HBO, 1984.*

*   *   *

VICKERY, John   1951-

PERSONAL: Born in 1951 in Alameda, CA. EDUCATION: Attended the University of California, Berkeley, and the University of California, Davis.

VOCATION: Actor.

CAREER: PRINCIPAL STAGE APPEARANCES—Malcolm, *Macbeth*, Vivian Beaumont Theatre, New York City, 1981; Reverend Rushbrooke, *A Call from the East*, Manhattan Theatre Club, New York City, 1981; Henry, Prince of Wales, *Henry IV, Part One*, New York Shakespeare Festival (NYSF), Delacorte Theatre, New York City, 1981; Edward "Ned" Sheldon, *Ned and Jack*, Little Theatre, New York City, 1981; Victor Salt, *Eminent Domain*, Circle in the Square, New York City, 1982; Charles Lutwidge Dodgson/Lewis Carroll, *Looking-Glass*, Entermedia Theatre, New York City, 1982; Manfred von Richthofen, the Red Dragon, *The Death of von Richthofen as Witnessed from Earth*, NYSF, Public Theatre, New York City, 1982; Ian, *The Vampires*, Astor Place Theatre, New York City, 1984; Henry, *The Real Thing*, Plymouth Theatre, New York City, 1984; Henry David Thoreau and George Armstrong Custer, *Romance Language*, Mark Taper Forum, Los Angeles, CA, 1986; Marcus Brutus, *Julius Caesar*, National Shakespeare Festival, Old Globe Theatre, San Diego, CA, 1987; Stephen Britter, *Made in Bangkok*, Mark Taper Forum, 1988. Also appeared with the California Actors Theatre, Los Gatos, CA, 1976; and in *Richard II*, Yale Repertory Theatre, New Haven, CT, 1984.

PRINCIPAL FILM APPEARANCES—Detective, *Out of Bounds*, Columbia, 1986; hotel.manager, *Big Business*, Buena Vista, 1988; also appeared in *Game Show Models*, 1977.

PRINCIPAL TELEVISION APPEARANCES—Movies: Pastor, *Promised a Miracle*, CBS, 1988.

ADDRESSES: AGENT—J. Michael Bloom, 233 Park Avenue South, New York, NY 10003.*

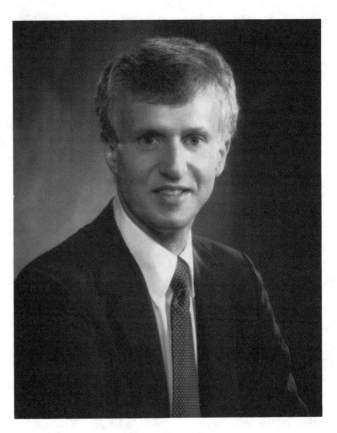

Photography by Bachrach

THOMAS VIERTEL

VIERTEL, Thomas   1941-

PERSONAL: Born November 3, 1941, in New York, NY; son of Joseph M. (a novelist) and Janet (a photographer; maiden name, Man) Viertel; married Toni Wurzburg, April 10, 1965; children: Jessica, Joel. EDUCATION: Harvard University, B.A., 1963.

VOCATION: Producer.

CAREER: FIRST STAGE WORK—Producer (with Steven Baruch and Jeffrey Joseph as Ivy Properties and with Richard Frankel), *Penn and Teller*, Westside Arts Theatre Downstairs, New York City, 1985, for six hundred forty-one performances. PRINCIPAL STAGE WORK—Producer (with Steven Baruch, Richard Frankel, and Jeffrey Joseph), *Sills and Company*, Lambs Theatre, then Actors Playhouse, both New York City, 1986; (with Baruch and Frankel) *Driving Miss Daisy*, John Houseman Theatre, New York City, 1987; producer (with Baruch and Frankel) *Frankie and Johnny in the Clair de Lune*, Westside Arts Theatre, New York City, 1987; (with Baruch and Frankel) *Penn and Teller on Broadway*, Ritz Theatre, New York City, 1988; producer (with Baruch and Frankel) *The Cocktail Hour*, Promenade Theatre, New York City, 1988; producer (with Baruch and Frankel), *Love Letters*, Promenade Theatre, 1989.

MAJOR TOURS—Co-producer, *Driving Miss Daisy*, U.S. cities, 1988; producer, *Penn and Teller*, U.S. cities, 1988.

RELATED CAREER—Board chairor, Ivy Properties (production company with Steven Baruch and Jeffrey Joseph), 1979—.

NON-RELATED CAREER—Board chairor, Council for Owner Occupied Housing, 1986—.

ADDRESSES: OFFICE—180 S. Broadway, White Plains, NY 10605.

* * *

VOIGHT, Jon 1938-

PERSONAL: Born December 29, 1938, in Yonkers, NY; son of Elmer (a professional golf player) and Barbara (Camp) Voight; married Lauri Peters (an actress), 1962 (divorced, 1967); married Marcheline Bertrand, December 12, 1971 (divorced); children: James Haven, Angelina Jolie. EDUCATION: Catholic University, B.F.A., 1960; trained for the stage with Sanford Meisner at the Neighborhood Playhouse, 1960-64, and with Samantha Harper.

VOCATION: Actor, producer, and screenwriter.

CAREER: Also see WRITINGS below. STAGE DEBUT—O Oysters Revue, Village Gate Theatre, New York City, 1961. PRINCIPAL STAGE APPEARANCES—Rolf Gruber, The Sound of Music, Lunt-Fontanne Theatre, New York City, 1961; Rodolpho, A View from the Bridge, Sheridan Square Playhouse, New York City, 1965; Romeo, Romeo and Juliet, Ariel, The Tempest, and Thurio, Two Gentlemen of Verona, all National Shakespeare Festival, Old Globe Theatre, San Diego, CA, 1966; Steve, That Summer—That Fall, Helen Hayes Theatre, New York City, 1967; Stanley Kowalski, A Streetcar Named Desire, Center Theatre Group, Ahmanson Theatre, Los Angeles, CA, then Studio Arena, Buffalo, NY, both 1973; title role, Hamlet, Levin Theater, Rutgers University, New Brunswick, NJ, 1976; also appeared in The Dwarfs, Theatre Company of Boston, Boston, MA, 1967; and in two seasons of summer theatre productions at Winooski, VT.

PRINCIPAL STAGE WORK—Co-producer, The Hashish Club, Bijou Theatre, New York City, 1975.

FILM DEBUT—Frank and False Frank, Fearless Frank (also known as Frank's Greatest Adventure), American International, 1967.

PRINCIPAL FILM APPEARANCES—Curly Bill Brocius, Hour of the Gun, United Artists, 1967; Joe Buck, Midnight Cowboy, United Artists, 1969; Russ, Out of It, United Artists, 1969; Milo Minderbinder, Catch-22, Filmways, 1970; A, The Revolutionary, United Artists, 1970; Ed Gentry, Deliverance, Warner Brothers, 1972; Vic Bealer, The All-American Boy, Warner Brothers, 1973; Pat Conroy, Conrack, Twentieth Century-Fox, 1974; Peter Miller, The Odessa File, Columbia, 1974; Walter Tschantz, End of the Game (also known as Getting Away with Murder, Murder on the Bridge, and Der Richter und sein Henker), Twentieth Century-Fox, 1976; Luke Martin, Coming Home, United Artists, 1978; Billy, The Champ, Metro-Goldwyn-Mayer/United Artists, 1979; Alex Kovac, Lookin' to Get Out, Paramount, 1982; J.P. Tannen, Table for Five, Warner Brothers, 1983; as himself, Sanford Meisner—The Theatre's Best Kept Secret (documentary), Columbia, 1984; Manny, Runaway Train, Cannon, 1985; Jack, Desert Bloom, Columbia, 1986.

PRINCIPAL FILM WORK—Producer: Lookin' to Get Out, Paramount, 1982; Table for Five, Warner Brothers, 1983.

PRINCIPAL TELEVISION APPEARANCES—Episodic: Cimarron Strip, CBS; Gunsmoke, CBS. Specials: The Barbour Report, ABC, 1986; Welcome Home, HBO, 1987; Unauthorized Biography: Jane Fonda, syndicated, 1988.

WRITINGS: FILM—(With Al Schwartz) Lookin' to Get Out, Paramount, 1982.

AWARDS: Theatre World Award, 1967, for That Summer—That Fall; Academy Award nomination, New York Film Critics Award, and Los Angeles Film Critics Award, all Best Actor, and British Academy Award, Most Promising Newcomer to Leading Film Roles, all 1969, for Midnight Cowboy; Academy Award, Golden Globe Award, Cannes International Film Festival Award, New York Film Critics Award, and Los Angeles Film Critics Award, all Best Actor, 1978, for Coming Home; Golden Globe Award, Best Actor, 1979, for The Champ; Academy Award nomination, Best Actor, and London Film Critics Award nomination, both 1986, for Runaway Train.

ADDRESSES: AGENT—Ron Meyer, Creative Artists Agency, 1888 Century Park E., Suite 1400, Los Angeles, CA 90067.*

W

WAGGONER, Lyle 1935-

PERSONAL: Full name, Lyle Wesley Waggoner; born April 13, 1935, in Kansas City, KS; son of Myron and Marie Waggoner; married Sharon Adele Kennedy, September 17, 1960; children: Jason Kennedy, Beau Justin. EDUCATION: Attended Washington University. MILITARY: U.S. Army, 1954-56.

VOCATION: Actor.

CAREER: PRINCIPAL STAGE APPEARANCES—Appeared in productions of *Teahouse of the August Moon, Born Yesterday,* and *Boeing, Boeing.*

MAJOR TOURS—*Li'l Abner.*

PRINCIPAL FILM APPEARANCES—Deputy, *Swamp Country,* Patrick/Sandy, 1966; Angelo, *The Catalina Caper,* Crown International, 1967; Chief Boyardie, *Surf II* (also known as *Surf II—The End of the Trilogy*), International Film Marketing, 1984. Also appeared in *Women of the Prehistoric Planet,* Real Art, 1966; *Journey to the Center of Time,* American General/Western International, 1967; *Love Me Deadly,* Cinema National, 1972.

PRINCIPAL TELEVISION APPEARANCES—Series: Regular, *The Carol Burnett Show,* CBS, 1967-74; host, *It's Your Bet,* syndicated, 1969; regular, *The Jimmie Rodgers Show,* CBS, 1969; regular, *Dinah's Place,* NBC, 1970-74; Major Steve Trevor, *Wonder Woman,* ABC, 1976-77, then as Steve Trevor, Jr., *The New Adventures of Wonder Woman,* CBS, 1977-79. Pilots: Cameo, *Hellzapoppin',* ABC, 1972; Barry Michaels, *The Barbara Eden Show,* ABC, 1973; Sam, *Letters from Three Lovers,* ABC, 1973; Major Steve Trevor, *The New, Original Wonder Woman,* ABC, 1975; Roger, *The Love Boat II,* ABC, 1977; Terry Anderson, *The Gossip Columnist,* syndicated, 1980; Kenny Bing, *The Ugily Family,* ABC, 1980; Rodney West, *Two the Hard Way,* CBS, 1981; Hampton Fraser, *Bulba,* ABC, 1981. Episodic: Dex Falcon, *Hardcastle and McCormick,* ABC, 1986; Don Manning, *Simon and Simon,* CBS, 1986; Leo Raffle, *The New Mike Hammer,* CBS, 1986. Movies: Wilbur Stokes, *Gridlock* (also known as *The Great American Traffic Jam*), NBC, 1980. Specials: *Mitzi and a Hundred Guys,* CBS, 1975; *Battle of the Network Stars,* ABC, 1977.

RELATED CAREER—With Metro-Goldwyn-Mayer Talent Program, 1964, and Twentieth Century-Fox Talent School, 1966; founder of sales-promotion company, 1965; actor in television commercials.

NON-RELATED CAREER—Salesman.*

WAHL, Ken 1957-

PERSONAL: Born in 1957 in Chicago, IL; father, an auto mechanic; married Corinne Alphen (an actress), 1984; children: Raymond.

VOCATION: Actor.

CAREER: FILM DEBUT—Richie Gennaro, *The Wanderers,* Orion, 1979. PRINCIPAL FILM APPEARANCES—Andy Corelli, *Fort Apache, the Bronx,* Twentieth Century-Fox, 1981; Willie Broadax, *Jinxed!,* Metro-Goldwyn-Mayer/United Artists, 1982; title role, *The Soldier* (also known as *Codename: The Soldier*), Embassy, 1982; Don Jardian, *Purple Hearts,* Warner Brothers, 1984; Barney Whitaker, *Race for the Yankee Zephyr* (also known as *Treasure of the Yankee Zephyr*), Hemdale/Film Ventures, 1984; Jack Corbett, *Omega Syndrome,* New World, 1987. Also appeared as Charlie McClain, *Back in the U.S.A.*

TELEVISION DEBUT—Anthony Valentine, *The Dirty Dozen: The Next Mission,* NBC, 1985. PRINCIPAL TELEVISION APPEARANCES—Series: Ken Sisko, *Double Dare,* CBS, 1985; Vinnie Terranova, *Wiseguy,* CBS, 1987—. Pilots: Rick Benson, *Gladiator,* ABC, 1986.

NON-RELATED CAREER—Auto mechanic.

ADDRESSES: AGENT—Toni Howard, William Morris Agency, 151 El Camino Drive, Beverly Hills, CA 90212.*

*　　*　　*

WALKER, Jimmie 1947-

PERSONAL: Full name, James Carter Walker; born June 25, 1947 (some sources say 1948 or 1949), in Bronx, NY.

VOCATION: Comedian and actor.

CAREER: PRINCIPAL FILM APPEARANCES—Bootney Farnsworth, *Let's Do It Again,* Warner Brothers, 1975; Umbuto, *Rabbit Test,* AVCO-Embassy,, 1978; Boise Girard, *The Concorde—Airport '79* (also known as *Airport '79* and *Airport '80: The Concorde*), Universal, 1979; windshield wiper man, *Airplane!,* Paramount, 1980; Shaker, *Doin' Time,* Warner Brothers, 1985; porno shop clerk, *Kidnapped,* Hickmar Productions, 1987; Mozambo, *My African Adventure,* Cannon, 1987; also appeared in *Water,* Rank, 1985; and in *Deadly Serious.*

TELEVISION DEBUT—*The Jack Paar Show,* NBC. PRINCIPAL

TELEVISION APPEARANCES—Series: James "J.J." Evans, Jr., *Good Times*, CBS, 1974-79; Rodney Washington, *B.A.D. Cats*, ABC, 1980; Sergeant Val Valentine, *At Ease*, ABC, 1983; Sonny Barnes, *Bustin' Loose*, syndicated, 1987; also host, *Matchmaker*, 1987. Pilots: Card player, *The Jerk, Too*, NBC, 1984. Episodic: *The Gladys Knight and the Pips Show*, NBC, 1975; *The New Celebrity Bowling*, syndicated, 1987; also *The Tonight Show*, NBC; *The Mac Davis Show*, NBC; *Donny and Marie*, ABC; *Cher*, CBS; *The John Davidson Show*, NBC; *The Merv Griffin Show*, syndicated; *Dinah*, syndicated; *The Mike Douglas Show*, syndicated; *The Hollywood Squares*, syndicated; *Celebrity Sweepstakes*, syndicated; *The Match Game*, syndicated. Movies: Morris Bird III, *The Greatest Thing That Almost Happened*, CBS, 1977; as himself, *Telethon*, ABC, 1977; Parks, *Murder Can Hurt You!*, ABC, 1977. Specials: *The Rowan and Martin Laugh-In Special*, NBC, 1974; *Perry Como's Summer of '74*, CBS, 1974; *Cotton Club '75*, NBC, 1974; *The Mad, Mad, Mad, Mad World of the Super Bowl*, NBC, 1974; *Battle of the Network Stars*, ABC, 1976, 1977, and 1978; *The Dean Martin Celebrity Roast: Dan Haggerty*, NBC, 1977; *General Electric's All Star Anniversary*, ABC, 1978; *The Dean Martin Celebrity Roast: Betty White*, NBC, 1978; *The Osmond Brothers Special*, ABC, 1978; *U.S. against the World II*, ABC, 1978; *Cinderella at the Palace* (also known as *Las Vegas Palace of Stars*), CBS, 1979; *The Comedy Store Fifteenth Year Class Reunion*, NBC, 1988; also *An Evening of Comedy with Jimmie Walker and Friends*, 1988; *Jimmie Walker and Friends II*, 1989.

RELATED CAREER—As a comedian, has performed in nightclubs and concert halls throughout the United States; also disc jockey and radio engineer.

NON-RELATED CAREER—Honorary chairman, Los Angeles Free Clinic, Los Angeles, CA, 1977.

RECORDINGS: ALBUMS—*Dyn-o-mite*, Buddah Records.

AWARDS: Named Most Popular TV Performer by *Family Circle* (magazine), 1975; also named Comedian of the Decade by *Time* (magazine).

SIDELIGHTS: Early in his career as a stand-up comic, Jimmie Walker entertained studio audiences on the set of the CBS television series *Carlucci's Department*.

ADDRESSES: OFFICE—General Management Corporation, 9000 Sunset Boulevard, Suite 400, Los Angeles, CA 90069.*

*   *   *

WALKER, Kathryn

PERSONAL: Born January 9, in Philadelphia, PA; married James Taylor (a musician). EDUCATION: Graduated from Wells College; also attended Harvard University; trained for the stage London Academy of Music and Dramatic Art.

VOCATION: Actress.

CAREER: OFF-BROADWAY DEBUT—Ann, *Slag*, New York Shakespeare Festival, Public Theatre, 1971. BROADWAY DEBUT—*The Good Doctor*, Eugene O'Neill Theatre, 1973. PRINCIPAL STAGE APPEARANCES—Mrs. Sally Cary Fairfax, *Sally, George, and Martha*, American National Theatre and Academy,

Theatre De Lys, New York City, 1971; Norma Elliot, *Alpha Beta*, Eastside Playhouse, New York City, 1973; Margaret, *Mourning Pictures*, Lyceum Theatre, New York City, 1974; Jill McDill, *Kid Champion*, New York Shakespeare Festival (NYSF), Public Theatre, New York City, 1974; Mrs. Mary Law Robarts, *Rebel Women*, NYSF, Public Theatre, 1976; Sara Melody, *A Touch of the Poet*, Helen Hayes Theatre, New York City, 1977; Sybil Chase, *Private Lives*, Lunt-Fontanne Theatre, New York City, 1983; Anna Petrovna, *Wild Honey*, Virginia Theatre, New York City, 1986. Also appeared in *The Night of the Tribades*, McCarter Theatre Company, Princeton, NJ, 1976; and with the McCarter Theatre Company, 1969-70.

PRINCIPAL FILM APPEARANCES—Maggie, *Blade*, Pintoff, 1973; Anita McCambridge, *Slap Shot*, Universal, 1977; Carpel's receptionist, *Girlfriends*, Warner Brothers, 1978; Madeleine Philips, *Rich Kids*, United Artists, 1979; Enid Keese, *Neighbors*, Columbia, 1981; Ellen Lamb, *D.A.R.Y.L.*, Paramount, 1985; Lily Boyd, *Bullseye*, Cinema Group, 1986; Kathryn, *Dangerous Game*, Quantum, 1988. Also appeared in *Too Far to Go*, Zoetrope, 1982; *In Our Hands*, Almi Classics, 1984.

PRINCIPAL TELEVISION APPEARANCES—Series: Fawn Lassiter, *Beacon Hill*, CBS, 1975; also Barbara Weaver, *Another World*, NBC; Emily Hunter, *Search for Tomorrow*. Mini-Series: Abigail Adams, *The Adams Chronicles*, PBS, 1976. Pilots: Miss Thompson, *The House without a Christmas Tree*, CBS, 1972; Helen, "When Widows Weep," *Light's Out*, NBC, 1972; Hilda Kemper, *Rx for the Defense*, ABC, 1973; Miss Thompson, *The Thanksgiving Treasure*, CBS, 1973; Claire Braden, *Private Sessions*, NBC, 1985. Movies: Kate Wright, *The Winds of Kitty Hawk*, NBC, 1978; Marion Sales, *Too Far to Go*, NBC, 1979; Anna, *F.D.R.—The Last Year*, NBC, 1980; Louisa King, *Family Reunion*, NBC, 1981; Dr. Linda McFarland, *A Whale for the Killing*, ABC, 1981; Susan Myles, *Special Bulletin*, NBC, 1983; Sarah, *Mrs. Delafield Wants to Marry*, CBS, 1986; Marie St. Clair, *Uncle Tom's Cabin*, Showtime, 1987; Sally Slaton, *The Murder of Mary Phagan*, NBC, 1988. Specials: Susan, *Mandy's Grandmother*, syndicated, 1980; *Private Contentment*, PBS, 1982; narrator, *Paul Gauguin: The Savage Dream* (documentary), PBS, 1989. Also appeared in *O Youth and Beauty*.

AWARDS: Emmy Award, Outstanding Lead Actress in a Single Performance, 1976, for *The Adams Chronicles*.

ADDRESSES: AGENTS—Sheila Robinson and Paul Martino, International Creative Management, 8899 Beverly Boulevard, Los Angeles, CA 90048.*

*   *   *

WALLACE, Lee   1930-

PERSONAL: Born Leo Melis, July 15, 1930, in Brooklyn, NY; son of Eddie and Celia (Gross) Melis; married Marilyn Chris (an actress), December 14, 1974; children: Paul Christopoulos. EDUCATION: Attended New York University; trained for the stage with Michael Howard. RELIGION: Jewish. MILITARY: U.S. Army, 1951-53.

VOCATION: Actor.

CAREER: STAGE DEBUT—Young man, *A Flag Is Born*, Joan of

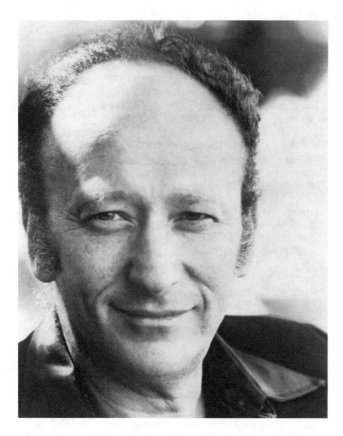

LEE WALLACE

Arc Theatre, New York City, 1949. OFF-BROADWAY DEBUT—Pandalevski and Bizimionkov, *The Journey of the Fifth Horse*, American Place Theatre, New York City, 1966. BROADWAY DEBUT—Ted, "Eli, the Fanatic" in *Unlikely Heroes*, Plymouth Theatre, 1970. PRINCIPAL STAGE APPEARANCES—Siward, *Macbeth*, New York Shakespeare Festival (NYSF), Mobile Theatre, New York City, 1966; Vershinin, *The Three Sisters*, Long Wharf Theatre, New Haven, CT, 1968; Gabe, *Saturday Night*, Sheridan Square Playhouse, New York City, 1968; Mike, *A Teaspoon Every Four Hours*, American National Theatre and Academy Theatre, New York City, 1969; Sergeant Brisbey, *The Basic Training of Pavlo Hummel*, NYSF, Public Theatre, New York City, 1971; Hickey, *The Iceman Cometh*, Long Wharf Theatre, 1971; Roy Wild, *The Secret Affairs of Mildred Wild*, Ambassador Theatre, New York City, 1972; Jake, *Molly*, Alvin Theatre, New York City, 1973; Inspector for the Ministry of Religious Affairs, *Zalman, or the Madness of God*, Lyceum Theatre, New York City, 1976; Irving Buxbaum, *Some of My Best Friends*, Longacre Theatre, New York City, 1977; Niall Scringeour, *Curtains*, T. Screiber Theatre, New York City, 1977.

Henry Leider, *Elephants*, Jewish Repertory Theatre, New York City, 1982; Morris, *Goodnight, Grandpa*, Entermedia Theatre, New York City, 1983; Harry, *Grind*, Mark Hellinger Theatre, New York City, 1985; Phil Lehman, *Self Defense*, Long Wharf Theatre, 1987. Also appeared in *The Shepherd of Avenue B*, Fortune Theatre, New York City, 1970; *Uncle Vanya*, Yale Repertory Theatre, New Haven, CT, 1981; *Booth Is Back in Town*, Forum Theatre, New York City; *Awake and Sing!* and *An Evening with Garcia Lorca*, both Off-Broadway productions; title role, *In the Matter of J. Robert Oppenheimer*, Atlanta Municipal Theatre,

Atlanta, GA; Orgon, *Tartuffe*, American Conservatory Theatre, San Francisco, CA; Lopahin, *The Cherry Orchard*, Williamstown Theatre Festival, Williamstown, MA; *The Servant of Two Masters*, *Death of a Salesman*, and *Antigone*, all American Conservatory Theatre; Max, *The Homecoming*, Gregory Solomon, *The Price*, Sade, *Marat/Sade*, Henry II, *Lion in Winter*, John Cleary, *The Subject Was Roses*, Dunois, *Saint Joan*, and Pat, *The Hostage*, all regional theatre productions.

PRINCIPAL STAGE WORK—Director, *Uncle Vanya*, T. Schreiber Studio, New York City, 1974.

MAJOR TOURS—*Irene*, U.S. cities; *Laugh a Little, Cry a Little*, U.S. cities.

PRINCIPAL FILM APPEARANCES—Nate Goldfarb, *Klute*, Warner Brothers, 1971; Dr. Strauss, *The Hot Rock* (also known as *How to Steal a Diamond in Four Easy Lessons*), Twentieth Century-Fox, 1972; the Mayor, *The Taking of Pelham One, Two, Three*, United Artists, 1974; Mr. Knowlton, *The Happy Hooker*, Cannon, 1975; Harry, *Thieves*, Paramount, 1977; Mr. Waxman, *Private Benjamin*, Warner Brothers, 1980; Oskar Kohn, *War and Love*, Cannon, 1985; Dr. Herbert A. Morrison, *Nuts*, Warner Brothers, 1987. Also appeared in *The Children's War*.

PRINCIPAL TELEVISION APPEARANCES—Mini-Series: "Concealed Enemies," *American Playhouse*, PBS, 1984. Pilots: Anesthesiologist, *A Doctor's Story*, NBC, 1984. Episodic: Whitney, *The Equalizer*, CBS, 1986; manager, *Kate and Allie*, CBS, 1987; also "Blessings," *Visions*, PBS; *Lou Grant*, CBS; *Kojak*, CBS. Movies: Dr. Chisholm, *Long Journey Back*, ABC, 1978; Sam Blumenkrantz, *And Baby Makes Six*, NBC, 1979; Hoskins, *The Child Stealer*, ABC, 1979; Samuel Goldwyn, *Moviola: This Year's Blonde*, NBC, 1980; Sam Blumenkrantz, *Baby Comes Home*, CBS, 1980; Dr. Jules Farber, *World War III*, NBC, 1982; Chief Barnes, *Kojak: The Price of Justice*, CBS, 1987. Specials: *Journey of the Fifth Horse*, WNET.

RELATED CAREER—Acting teacher and coach, 1978—.

MEMBER: Actors' Equity Association, Screen Actors Guild, American Federation of Television and Radio Artists.

ADDRESSES: HOME—175 Riverside Drive, New York, NY 10024. AGENT—Monty Silver Agency, 200 W. 57th Street, New York, NY 10019.

*   *   *

WALLACH, Eli   1915-

PERSONAL: Born December 7, 1915, in Brooklyn, NY; son of Abraham and Bertha (Schorr) Wallach; married Anne Jackson (an actress), March 5, 1948; children: Peter Douglas, Roberta Lee, and Katherine Beatrice. EDUCATION: University of Texas, B.A., 1936; City College of New York, M.S., education, 1938; trained for the stage at the Neighborhood Playhouse, 1938-40, and with Lee Strasberg at the Actors Studio. MILITARY: U.S. Army, Medical Corps, captain, during World War II.

VOCATION: Actor.

CAREER: BROADWAY DEBUT—Crew chief, *Skydrift*, Belasco

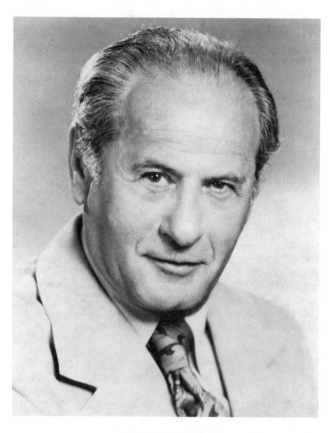

ELI WALLACH

Theatre, 1945. LONDON DEBUT—Sakini, *The Teahouse of the August Moon*, Her Majesty's Theatre, 1954. PRINCIPAL STAGE APPEARANCES—Title role, *Liliom*, Curtain Club, University of Texas, Austin, TX, 1936; Cromwell, *Henry VIII*, American Repertory Theatre, International Theatre, New York City, 1946; Busch, *Yellow Jack*, and Two of Spades and Leg of Mutton, *Alice in Wonderland*, both American Repertory Theatre, International Theatre, 1947; Diomedes, *Antony and Cleopatra*, Martin Beck Theatre, New York City, 1947; Stefanowski, *Mister Roberts*, Alvin Theatre, New York City, 1949; Alvarro Mangiacavallo, *The Rose Tattoo*, Martin Beck Theatre, 1951; Kilroy, *Camino Real*, National Theatre, New York City, 1953; Dickson, *Scarecrow*, Theatre De Lys, New York City, 1953; Julien, *Mademoiselle Colombe*, Longacre Theatre, New York City, 1954; Sakini, *The Teahouse of the August Moon*, Martin Beck Theatre, 1955; Bill Walker, *Major Barbara*, Martin Beck Theatre, 1956; Old Man, "The Chairs" in *The Chairs [and] The Lesson* (double-bill), Phoenix Theatre, New York City, 1958; Willie, *The Cold Wind and the Warm*, Morosco Theatre, New York City, 1958.

Berenger, *Rhinoceros*, Longacre Theatre, 1961; Ben, "The Tiger," and Paul XXX, "The Typists," in *The Tiger [and] The Typists* (double-bill), Orpheum Theatre, New York City, 1963, then Globe Theatre, London, 1964; Milt Manville, *Luv*, Booth Theatre, New York City, 1964; Charles Dyer, *Staircase*, Biltmore Theatre, New York City, 1968; Ollie H. and Wesley, *Promenade All!*, Alvin Theatre, 1972; General St. Pe, *The Waltz of the Toreadors*, Circle in the Square, New York City, then Eisenhower Theatre, Kennedy Center for the Performing Arts, Washington, DC, 1973; Peppino, *Saturday, Sunday, Monday*, Martin Beck Theatre, 1974; Arthur Canfield, *The Sponsor*, Peachtree Play-

house, Atlanta, GA, 1975; Colin, *Absent Friends*, Long Wharf Theatre, New Haven, CT, then Eisenhower Theatre, Kennedy Center for the Performing Arts, later Royal Alexandra Theatre, Toronto, ON, Canada, all 1977; Mr. Frank, *The Diary of Anne Frank*, Theatre Four, New York City, 1978; Alexander, *Every Good Boy Deserves Favour*, Metropolitan Opera House, New York City, then Concert Hall, Kennedy Center for the Performing Arts, both 1979.

Leon Rose, "A Need for Brussels Sprouts," and Gus Frazier, "A Need for Less Expertise," in *Twice around the Park* (double-bill), Syracuse Stage, Syracuse, NY, 1981, then Cort Theatre, New York City, 1982, later Edinburgh Festival, Edinburgh, Scotland, 1984; Stephan, *The Nest of the Woodgrouse*, New York Shakespeare Festival (NYSF), Public Theatre, New York City, 1984; Monsieur Paul Vigneron, *Opera Comique*, Eisenhower Theatre, Kennedy Center for the Performing Arts, 1987; David Cole, *Cafe Crown*, NYSF, Public Theatre, 1988, then Brooks Atkinson Theatre, New York City, 1989. Also appeared in *The Bo Tree*, Locust Valley, NY, 1939; *Androcles and the Lion*, American Repertory Theatre, International Theatre, 1947; *The Neighborhood Playhouse at Fifty: A Celebration*, Shubert Theatre, New York City, 1978; *Flowering Peach*, in Florida, 1986; *This Property Is Condemned*, Equity Library Theatre, New York City.

MAJOR TOURS—Alvarro Mangiacavallo, *The Rose Tattoo*, U.S. cities, 1951; Sakini, *The Teahouse of the August Moon*, U.S. cities, 1956; Ben, "The Tiger," and Paul XXX, "The Typists," in *The Tiger [and] The Typists* (double-bill), U.S. cities, 1966; Ollie H. and Wesley, *Promenade All!*, U.S. cities, 1971; General St. Pe, *Waltz of the Toreadors*, U.S. cities, 1973-74; Colin, *Absent Friends*, U.S. cities, 1977; Alexander, *Every Good Boy Deserves Favour*, U.S. cities, 1979.

FILM DEBUT—Silva Vacarro, *Baby Doll*, Warner Brothers, 1956. PRINCIPAL FILM APPEARANCES—Dancer, *The Lineup*, Columbia, 1958; Calvera, *The Magnificent Seven*, United Artists, 1960; Poncho, *Seven Thieves*, Twentieth Century-Fox, 1960; Guido, *The Misfits*, United Artists, 1961; John, *Adventures of a Young Man* (also known as *Hemingway's Adventures of a Young Man*), Twentieth Century-Fox, 1962; Charlie Gant, *How the West Was Won*, Cinerama, 1962; Sergeant Craig, *The Victors*, Columbia, 1963; Warren Stone, *Act One*, Warner Brothers, 1964; Rodriguez Valdez, *Kisses for My President* (also known as *Kisses for the President*), Warner Brothers, 1964; Stratos, *The Moon-Spinners*, Buena Vista, 1964; Shah of Khwarezm, *Genghis Khan* (also known as *Dschingis Khan* and *Dzingis-Kan*), Columbia, 1965; the General, *Lord Jim*, Columbia, 1965; David Leland, *How to Steal a Million*, Twentieth Century-Fox, 1966; Locarno, *The Poppy Is Also a Flower*, Comet, 1966; Tuco, *The Good, the Bad, and the Ugly* (also known as *Il buono, il brutto, il cattivo*), United Artists, 1967; Ben Harris, *The Tiger Makes Out*, Columbia, 1967; Harry Hunter, *How to Save a Marriage . . . and Ruin Your Life* (also known as *Band of Gold*), Columbia, 1968; Tennessee Fredericks, *A Lovely Way to Die* (also known as *A Lovely Way to Go*), Universal, 1968; Cacopoulos, *Revenge at El Paso* (also known as *Il quattro dell'ave Maria* and *Ace High*), Paramount, 1969; Scannapieco, *The Brain* (also known as *Le Cerveau*), Paramount, 1969; Ben Baker, *MacKenna's Gold*, Columbia, 1969.

Napoleon Bonaparte, *The Adventures of Gerard*, United Artists, 1970; store clerk, *The Angel Levine*, United Artists, 1970; Arthur Mason, *The People Next Door*, AVCO-Embassy, 1970; Mario Gambretti, *Zigzag* (also known as *False Witness*), Metro-Goldwyn-Mayer, 1970; Kifke, *Romance of a Horse Thief*, Allied Artists,

1971; Forshay, *Cinderella Liberty,* Twentieth Century-Fox, 1973; Don Vittorio, *Crazy Joe,* Columbia, 1974; Black, *Il bianco, il giallo, il nero* (also known as *Samurai* and *White, Yellow, Black*), CIDIF, 1975; Ras, *Attenti al buffone!* (also known as *Eye of the Cat*), Medusa Distribuzione, 1975; Monsignor, *Nasty Habits,* Brut, 1976; Benjamin Franklin, *Independence* (short film), Twentieth Century-Fox, 1976; Adam Coffin, *The Deep,* Columbia, 1977; General Tom Reser, *The Domino Principle* (also known as *The Domino Killings*), AVCO-Embassy, 1977; Gatz, *The Sentinel,* Universal, 1977; Rabbi Gold, *Girlfriends,* Warner Brothers, 1978; Vince Marlowe, "Dynamite Hands," and Pop, "Baxter's Beauties of 1933," *Movie Movie,* Warner Brothers, 1978; man in oil, *Circle of Iron* (also known as *The Silent Flute*), AVCO-Embassy, 1979; Sal Hyman, *Firepower,* Associated Film Distribution, 1979; Joe Diamond, *Winter Kills,* AVCO-Embassy, 1979.

Ritchie Blumenthal, *The Hunter,* Paramount, 1980; as himself, *Acting: Lee Strasberg and the Actors Studio* (documentary), Davada Enterprises, 1981; Leporello, *The Salamander,* ITC, 1983; Sam Orowitz, *Sam's Son,* Invictus, 1984; as himself, *Sanford Meisner—The Theatre's Best Kept Secret* (documentary), Columbia, 1984; Leon B. Little, *Tough Guys,* Buena Vista, 1986; as himself, *Hello Actors Studio* (documentary), Actors Studio, 1987; Dr. Herbert A. Morrison, *Nuts,* Warner Brothers, 1987. Also appeared as cabdriver, *New York City—The Most* (documentary), 1968; in *Don't Turn the Other Cheek* (also known as *Viva la muerte . . . tua* and *The Killer from Yuma*), International Amusement Corporation, 1974; narrator, *L'Chaim—To Life!,* 1974; *Stateline Motel* (also known as *Last Chance for a Born Loser, L'ultima chance,* and *Last Chance Motel*), International Cinefilm-NMD, 1976; detective, *E tanta paura,* 1976; *Twenty Shades of Pink,* 1977; *Squadra antimafia* (also known as *Little Italy*), 1978; "The Sahara Forest" and "Climbed up the Ladder and Had Her" in *Funny,* Associates and Ferren, 1988.

PRINCIPAL TELEVISION APPEARANCES—Series: Vincent Danzig, *Our Family Honor,* ABC, 1985-86. Mini-Series: Gus Farber, *Seventh Avenue,* NBC, 1977; Hernando DeTalavera, *Christopher Columbus,* CBS, 1985. Pilots: Joe Verga, *Embassy,* ABC, 1985. Episodic: Mr. Freeze, "Ice Spy" and "The Duo Defy," *Batman,* ABC, 1967; Tim Charles, *Highway to Heaven,* NBC, 1986; Gene Malloy, *Highway to Heaven,* NBC, 1987; Salvatore Gambini, *Murder, She Wrote,* CBS, 1988; also "The Baby," *Philco Playhouse,* NBC, 1953; "Shadow of the Champ," *Philco Playhouse,* NBC, 1955; "The Outsiders," *Philco Playhouse,* NBC, 1955; "Albert Anastasia," *Climax!,* CBS, 1958; "The Plot to Kill Stalin," *Playhouse 90,* CBS, 1958; "For Whom the Bell Tolls," *Playhouse 90,* CBS, 1959; "Hope Is the Thing with Feathers," *Robert Herridge Theatre,* CBS, 1960; "Tomorrow the Man," *Dick Powell Theatre,* NBC, 1962; "The Typists," *Hollywood Television Theatre,* PBS, 1971; *Alcoa/Goodyear Theater,* NBC; *Dupont Show of the Month;* CBS; *The Kaiser Aluminum Hour,* NBC; *Light's Out,* NBC; *Suspicion,* NBC; *Studio One,* CBS; *Kojak,* CBS; *The Web.*

Movies: Dr. Frank Enari, *A Cold Night's Death,* ABC, 1973; DeWitt Foster, *Indict and Convict,* ABC, 1974; Ben Ezra, *Harold Robbins' "The Pirate,"* CBS, 1978; Olan Vacio, *Fugitive Family,* CBS, 1980; Sal Galucci, *The Pride of Jesse Hallam,* CBS, 1981; Bert Silverman, *Skokie,* CBS, 1981; Mauritzi Apt, *The Wall,* CBS, 1982; Uncle Vern Damico, *The Executioner's Song,* NBC, 1982; Dr. William Hitzig, *Anatomy of an Illness,* CBS, 1984; Dr. Huffman, *Murder: By Reason of Insanity,* CBS, 1985; Norman Voss, *Something in Common,* CBS, 1986; Yacov, *The Impossible Spy,* HBO, 1987. Specials: Dauphin, "The Lark," *Hallmark Hall of Fame,*

NBC, 1957; Happy Locarno, *The Poppy Is Also a Flower* (also known as *Poppies Are Also Flowers*), ABC, 1966; "Paradise Lost," *Great Performances,* PBS, 1974; *Kennedy Center Honors: A Celebration of the Performing Arts,* CBS, 1984; *The ABC All-Star Spectacular,* ABC, 1985; Mr. Prince, *Rocket to the Moon,* PBS, 1986; *We the People 200: The Constitutional Gala,* CBS, 1987; host and narrator, *Hollywood's Favorite Heavy: Businessmen on Primetime TV,* PBS, 1987; narrator, *It's Up to Us: The Giraffe Project* (documentary), PBS, 1988; Ira Abrams, "A Matter of Conscience" (also known as "Silent Witness"), *CBS Schoolbreak Special,* CBS, 1989.

RELATED CAREER—Actor in radio plays, WLID-Radio, Brooklyn, NY, 1936-38; original member, Actors Studio, New York City, 1947—, then vice-president, 1980-81; member and director, Neighborhood Playhouse School Theatre.

NON-RELATED CAREER—Playground director, camp counselor, and hospital registrar.

AWARDS: Antoinette Perry Award, *Variety* New York Drama Critics Poll, Donaldson Award, and Theatre World Award, all 1951, for *The Rose Tattoo;* British Academy Award, Most Outstanding Newcomer to Film, 1956, for *Baby Doll;* Emmy Award, 1966, for *The Poppy Is Also a Flower;* inducted into the Theatre Hall of Fame, 1988. Honorary degrees: Emerson College, Boston, MA.

MEMBER: Actors' Equity Association, Screen Actors Guild, American Federation of Television and Radio Artists.

SIDELIGHTS: FAVORITE ROLES—Kilroy in *Camino Real,* and Alvarro Mangiacavallo in *The Rose Tattoo.* RECREATIONS—Woodworking, collecting antiques, collecting clocks, tennis, baseball, architecture, photography, watercoloring, and swimming.

ADDRESSES: AGENT—International Creative Management, 8899 Beverly Boulevard, Los Angeles, CA 90048.

*   *   *

WALSH, M. Emmet   1935-

PERSONAL: Full name, Michael Emmet Walsh; born March 22, 1935, in Ogdensburg, NY; son of Harry Maurice, Sr. (with the U.S. Customs Service) and Agnes Kathrine (Sullivan) Walsh. EDUCATION: Clarkson College, B.B.A., 1958; trained for the stage at the American Academy of Dramatic Arts, 1959-61.

VOCATION: Actor.

CAREER: PRINCIPAL STAGE APPEARANCES—Citizen of Boston, "My Kinsman Major Molineux," and American sailor, "Benito Cereno," in *The Old Glory* (double-bill), American Place Theatre, New York City, 1964; Bill Leap, *The Death of the Well-Loved Boy,* St. Mark's Playhouse, New York City, 1967; Ringo, *Does a Tiger Wear a Necktie?,* Belasco Theatre, New York City, 1969; George Sikowski, *That Championship Season,* Booth Theatre, New York City, 1973; also appeared in *Shepards of the Shelf,* Blackfriars Theatre, New York City, 1961; *The Outside Man,* American Place Theatre, 1964; *Three from Column "A",* Theatre 73, New York City, 1968; *Are You Now or Have You Ever Been?,* Ford's Theatre, Washington, DC, and Los Angeles, CA, both 1975; with College

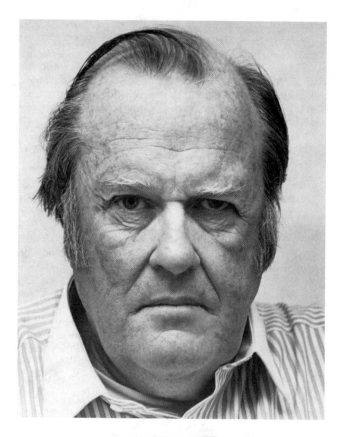

M. EMMET WALSH

Theatre, American Academy of Dramatic Arts, 1954-61; Bucks County Playhouse, New Hope, PA, 1962; Brattleboro Summer Theatre, Brattleboro, VT, 1963; Caravan Theatre, Dorset, CT, 1964; Theatre of the Living Arts, Philadelphia, PA, 1965; Studio Arena Theatre, Buffalo, NY, 1966; Long Wharf Theatre, New Haven, CT, 1967; Berkshire Theatre Festival, Stockbridge, MA, 1967-70; Vermont Summer Theatre Festival, Johnson, VT, 1974; and with the Santa Barbara Theatre Festival, Santa Barbara, CA, 1985.

PRINCIPAL STAGE WORK—Production assistant, *The Beauty Part*, Music Box Theatre, New York City, 1962.

PRINCIPAL FILM APPEARANCES—Group W sergeant, *Alice's Restaurant*, United Artists, 1969; shotgun guard, *Little Big Man*, National General, 1970; Warden Brodski, *The Traveling Executioner*, Metro-Goldwyn-Mayer (MGM), 1970; Art, *Cold Turkey*, United Artists, 1971; aide, *Escape from the Planet of the Apes*, Twentieth Century-Fox, 1971; sanitation man, *They Might Be Giants*, Universal, 1971; Mr. Wendell, *Get to Know Your Rabbit*, Warner Brothers, 1972; arresting officer, *What's Up, Doc?*, Warner Brothers, 1972; barber, *Kid Blue*, Twentieth Century-Fox, 1973; Gallagher, *Serpico*, Paramount, 1973; Las Vegas gambler, *The Gambler*, Paramount, 1974; Harold, *At Long Last Love*, Twentieth Century-Fox, 1975; bus driver, *Mikey and Nicky*, Paramount, 1976; "Father" Logan, *Nickelodeon*, Columbia, 1976; Dr. Williams, *Airport '77*, Universal, 1977; Dickie Dunn, *Slap Shot*, Universal, 1977; Earl Frank, *Straight Time*, Warner Brothers, 1978; Wally Cantrell, *The Fish That Saved Pittsburgh*, United Artists, 1979; madman, *The Jerk*, Universal, 1979.

C.P. Woodward, *Brubaker*, Twentieth Century-Fox, 1980; swim coach, *Ordinary People*, Paramount, 1980; MCPO Vinnie Giordino, *Raise the Titanic*, Associated Film Distributors, 1980; Arthur, *Back Roads*, Warner Brothers, 1981; speaker at the Liberal Club, *Reds*, Paramount, 1981; Captain Bryant, *Blade Runner*, Warner Brothers, 1982; Mack, *Cannery Row*, Metro-Goldwyn-Mayer/United Artists (MGM/UA), 1982; Fritz, *The Escape Artist*, Warner Brothers, 1982; Sergeant Sanger, *Fast-Walking*, Pickman, 1982; Walt Yarborough, *Silkwood*, Twentieth Century-Fox, 1983; Private Detective Visser, *Blood Simple*, Circle, 1984; Dr. Dolan, *Fletch*, Universal, 1984; Mr. Clark, *Grandview, U.S.A.*, Warner Brothers, 1984; Tuck, *Missing in Action*, Cannon, 1984; Burns, *The Pope of Greenwich Village*, MGM/UA, 1984; Colonel Crouse, *Raw Courage* (also known as *Courage*), New World, 1984; Simon Reynolds, *Scandalous*, Orion, 1984.

Coach Turnbull, *Back to School*, Orion, 1986; Charlie, *The Best of Times*, Universal, 1986; Harv, *Critters*, New Line/Smart Egg, 1986; Coes, *Wildcats*, Warner Brothers, 1986; George Henderson, Sr., *Harry and the Hendersons*, Universal, 1987; Captain Haun, *No Man's Land*, Orion, 1987; machine shop worker, *Raising Arizona*, Twentieth Century-Fox, 1987; governor, *The Milagro Beanfield War*, Universal, 1988; Detweiler, *War Party*, Hemdale, 1988; Chief Dibner, *Sunset*, Tri-Star, 1988; Richard Dirks, *Clean and Sober*, Warner Brothers, 1988; Miller, *The Mighty Quinn*, MGM/UA, 1989; Dewey Ferguson, *Red Scorpion*, Shapiro Glickenhaus Entertainment, 1989. Also appeared in *Midnight Cowboy*, United Artists, 1969; *Stiletto*, AVCO-Embassy, 1969; *End of the Road*, Allied Artists, 1970; *Loving*, Columbia, 1970; *The Prisoner of Second Avenue*, Warner Brothers, 1975; *Bound for Glory*, United Artists, 1976; *Chattahoochee*, RCA/Columbia International, 1989; *Sundown*, Vestron, 1989; *Catch Me If You Can*, Forum Home Video, 1989; *Thunderground*, Shapiro Glickenhaus, 1989.

PRINCIPAL TELEVISION APPEARANCES—Series: Alex Lembeck, *The Sandy Duncan Show*, CBS, 1972; Captain Gorcey, *Dear Detective*, CBS, 1979; Ned Platt, *UNSUB*, NBC, 1989. Mini-Series: Sheriff Horace Quinn, *John Steinbeck's "East of Eden,"* ABC, 1981; also *The French Atlantic Affair*, ABC, 1979. Pilots: Mr. Wallace, *Doctor Dan*, CBS, 1974; Lieutenant Jack Doyle, *Crime Club*, CBS, 1975; Moran, *Skag*, NBC, 1980; Mr. Graebner, *Hellinger's Law*, CBS, 1981; Joe Kirby, *Night Partners*, CBS, 1983; Warden MacDonald, *The Outlaws*, ABC, 1984; Samuel Lynn, *You Are the Jury*, NBC, 1984; Bear Werner, *The City*, ABC, 1986. Episodic: Gabe, *Nichols*, NBC, 1971; Arthur Kingston, *The Don Rickles Show*, CBS, 1972; Police Chief Demsey, *Amy Prentiss*, NBC, 1974; Man, "Dealer's Choice," *The Twilight Zone*, CBS, 1985; Grampa Norman, *Amazing Stories*, NBC, 1986; also *Men at Law*, CBS, 1971; *Kate McShane*, CBS, 1975; *The Cop and the Kid*, NBC, 1976; *Joe and Sons*, CBS, 1976; *The Nancy Walker Show*, ABC, 1976; *Gibbsville*, NBC, 1976; *Julia*, NBC; *Arnie*, CBS; *The Jimmy Stewart Show*, NBC; *Bonanza*, NBC; *AfterMash*, CBS; *Starsky and Hutch*, ABC; *Mary Hartman, Mary Hartman*, syndicated; *The Texas Wheelers*, ABC; *The Rockford Files*, NBC; *All in the Family*, CBS; *The Bob Newhart Show*, CBS; *Ironside*, NBC; *The Waltons*, CBS; *Little House on the Prairie*, NBC; *Baretta*, ABC; *N.Y.P.D.*, ABC; *McMillan and Wife*, NBC; *The Hitchhiker*, HBO; *Love of Life*; *The Doctors*; *Prudential's "On Stage"*; *Brahmins*; *Mississippi*; *The Tony Randall Show*; and *Vanishing America*.

Movies: Mr. Peterson, *Sarah T.—Portrait of a Teenage Alcoholic*, NBC, 1975; Irvine, *The Invasion of Johnson County*, NBC, 1976; Sheriff Sweeney, *Red Alert*, CBS, 1977; Whitley, *Superdome*, ABC, 1978; McCartney, *A Question of Guilt*, CBS, 1978; DeFranco,

No Other Love, CBS, 1979; legion commander, *The Gift,* CBS, 1979; Sheldon Lewis, *City in Fear,* ABC, 1980; Harold Patton, *High Noon, Part II: The Return of Will Kane,* CBS, 1980; Detective Sam Davies, *The Deliberate Stranger,* NBC, 1986; Sarge, *Resting Place,* CBS, 1986; Mayor, *The Right of the People,* ABC, 1986; General Presser, *Hero in the Family,* ABC, 1986; Don Nichols, *The Abduction of Kari Swenson,* NBC, 1987; Vern Humphrey, *Murder Ordained,* CBS, 1987; Detective Mulligan, *Broken Vows* (also known as *Where the Dark Streets Go* and *Hennessey*), NBC, 1987; Hardy, *Brotherhood of the Rose,* NBC, 1989; also *The Law,* NBC, 1974; *Panic on Page One,* ABC, 1974; *Mrs. R.'s Daughter,* NBC, 1979. Specials: Joe Lemke, ''The Woman Who Willed a Miracle,'' *ABC Afterschool Special,* ABC, 1983; Rocco, ''Con Sawyer and Hucklemary Finn,'' *ABC Weekend Special,* ABC, 1985.

RELATED CAREER—Artist in residence, University of Kentucky, Lexington, KY, 1966; artist in residence, University of Tulsa, Tulsa, OK, 1983.

AWARDS: IFPW Spirit Award, Best Actor, for *Blood Simple.*

MEMBER: Actors' Equity Association, Screen Actors Guild, American Federation of Radio and Television Artists, Academy of Motion Picture Arts and Sciences, Academy of Television Arts and Sciences, Players Club.

ADDRESSES: AGENT—The Gersh Agency, 222 N. Canon Drive, Suite 202, Beverly Hills, CA 90210.

*   *   *

WALTER, Jessica   1944-

PERSONAL: Born January 31, 1944 (some sources say 1940), in New York, NY; daughter of David (a musician) and Esther (a teacher; maiden name, Groisser) Walter; married Ross Bowman, March 27, 1966 (divorced, 1978); married Ron Leibman (an actor), June 26, 1983; children: Brooke (first marriage). EDUCATION: Trained for the stage at the Neighborhood Playhouse and the Bucks County Playhouse.

VOCATION: Actress.

CAREER: STAGE DEBUT—Kid sister, *Middle of the Night,* Bucks County Playhouse, New Hope, PA, 1958. BROADWAY DEBUT— Liz, *Advise and Consent,* Cort Theatre, 1961. PRINCIPAL STAGE APPEARANCES—Cigarette girl, *Nightlife,* Brooks Atkinson Theatre, New York City, 1962; Clarice and Ada, *Photofinish,* Brooks Atkinson Theatre, 1963; mistress, *A Severed Head,* Royale Theatre, New York City, 1964; Rosalind Gambol, *Fighting International Fat,* Playwrights Horizons, New York City, 1985; Claire Ganz, *Rumors,* Broadhurst Theatre, New York City, 1988; also appeared in *The Women,* Repertory Theatre of New Orleans, New Orleans, LA, 1970; *Tartuffe,* Los Angeles Theatre Center, Los Angeles, CA, 1986; and in *The Murder of Me,* New York City.

MAJOR TOURS—*Tartuffe,* U.S. cities, 1986.

FILM DEBUT—Laura, *Lilith,* Columbia, 1964. PRINCIPAL FILM APPEARANCES—Pat, *Grand Prix,* Metro-Goldwyn-Mayer, 1966; Libby MacAusland, *The Group,* United Artists, 1966; Inez Braverman, *Bye Bye Braverman,* Warner Brothers, 1968; Julie Catlan, *Number One* (also known as *The Pro*), United Artists,

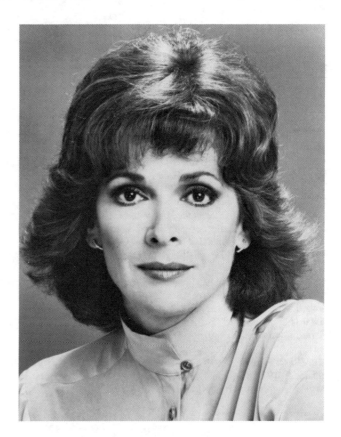

JESSICA WALTER

1969; Evelyn Draper, *Play Misty for Me,* Universal, 1971; Fiona, *Going Ape!,* Paramount, 1981; Celia Berryman, *Spring Fever,* Com-World, 1983; Phyllis Brody, *The Flamingo Kid,* Twentieth Century-Fox, 1984; Kay Mart, *Tapeheads,* De Laurentiis Entertainment Group, 1988.

PRINCIPAL TELEVISION APPEARANCES—Series: Julie Morano, *Love of Life,* CBS, 1962-65; Phyllis Koster, *For the People,* CBS, 1965; title role, *Amy Prentiss,* NBC, 1974-75; Joan Hamlyn, *All That Glitters,* syndicated, 1977; Ava Marshall, *Bare Essence,* NBC, 1983; voice of Diabolyn, *Wildfire* (animated), CBS, 1986-87; Connie Lo Verde, *Aaron's Way,* NBC, 1988. Mini-Series: Ursula, *Arthur Hailey's ''Wheels''* (also known as *Wheels*), NBC, 1978; Maggie McGregor, *Scruples,* ABC, 1981. Pilots: Vivien Scott, *Pursue and Destroy,* ABC, 1966; Janet Braddock, *The Immortal,* ABC, 1969; Jane Antrim, *They Call It Murder,* NBC, 1971; Sally McNamara, *Having Babies,* ABC, 1976; Morgan LeFay, *Dr. Strange,* CBS, 1978; Astrid Carlisle, *The Return of Marcus Welby, M.D.,* ABC, 1984; Jessica Craigmont, *T.L.C.,* NBC, 1984; Connie Lo Verde, *Aaron's Way,* NBC, 1988.

Episodic: Melanie McIntyre, *Trapper John, M.D.,* CBS, 1979 and 1985; Claudia Bradford, *Three's a Crowd,* ABC, 1984; Joyce Holleran, *Murder, She Wrote,* CBS, 1985; Irene Fitzgerald, *Hotel,* ABC, 1986; Joan Fulton, *Murder, She Wrote,* CBS, 1986; Joan Fulton, *Magnum, P.I.,* CBS, 1986; interior design editor, *J.J. Starbuck,* NBC, 1988; also Janet Braddock, *The Immortal,* ABC; Valerie, *Mission: Impossible,* CBS; *The F.B.I.,* ABC; *Cannon,* CBS; *Medical Center,* CBS; *Mannix,* CBS; *Barnaby Jones,* CBS; *Hawaii Five-O,* CBS; *Ironside,* NBC; *Route 66,* CBS; *East Side/*

West Side, CBS; *Flipper,* NBC; *The Streets of San Francisco,* ABC.

Movies: Jessica Carson, *Three's a Crowd,* ABC, 1969; Dee Dee, *Women in Chains,* ABC, 1972; Fredrica Morgan, *Home for the Holidays,* ABC, 1972; Louise Damon, *Hurricane,* ABC, 1974; Nomi Haroun, *Victory at Entebbe,* ABC, 1976; Louise Carmino, *Black Market Baby* (also known as *Don't Steal My Baby*), ABC, 1977; Christina Wood, *Secrets of Three Hungry Wives,* NBC, 1978; Megan, *Wild and Wooly,* ABC, 1978; Nicole DeCamp, *Vampire,* ABC, 1979; Irene Barton, *She's Dressed to Kill* (also known as *Someone's Killing the World's Greatest Models*), NBC, 1979; Pat Brooks, *Miracle on Ice,* ABC, 1981; Roz Richardson, *Thursday's Child,* CBS, 1983; Gertrude Simon, *The Execution,* NBC, 1985; Francesca DeLorca, *Killer in the Mirror,* NBC, 1986; Ms. Shields, *Jenny's Song,* syndicated, 1988. Specials: Lois Lane, *Kiss Me, Kate,* ABC, 1968; Anna II, "The Prison Game," *Visions,* PBS, 1977; *Day-to-Day Affairs,* HBO, 1985; Dr. Stein, "Just a Regular Kid: An AIDS Story," *ABC Afterschool Special,* ABC, 1987.

AWARDS: Clarence Derwent Award, 1963, for *Photofinish;* Emmy Award, Outstanding Lead Actress, 1975, for *Amy Prentiss;* Emmy Award nomination, 1976, for *The Streets of San Francisco;* Emmy Award nomination, 1980, for *Trapper John, M.D.* .

MEMBER: Screen Actors Guild (board member, 1973—; vice-president, 1975-83), American Federation of Television and Radio Artists, Actors' Equity Association.

ADDRESSES: AGENT—Bob Gersh, The Gersh Agency, 222 N. Canon Drive, Beverly Hills, CA 90210.*

*   *   *

WALTERS, Julie   1950-

PERSONAL: Born February 22, 1950, in Birmingham, England.

VOCATION: Actress.

CAREER: STAGE DEBUT—*The Taming of the Shrew,* Liverpool, U.K. LONDON DEBUT—Irene Tinsley, *Funny Peculiar,* Mermaid Theatre, 1976. PRINCIPAL STAGE APPEARANCES—Irene Tinsley, *Funny Peculiar,* Garrick Theatre, London, 1976; Vera, *Breezeblock Park,* Mermaid Theatre, then Whitehall Theatre, both London, 1977; Irene Goodnight, *Flaming Bodies,* ICA Theatre, London, 1979. Also appeared as Rita, *Educating Rita,* Royal Shakespeare Company, London; and in productions of *Jumpers* and *Fool for Love.*

PRINCIPAL FILM APPEARANCES—Rita, *Educating Rita,* Columbia, 1983; voice of the Dormouse, *Dreamchild,* Universal, 1985; Fran, *She'll Be Wearing Pink Pajamas,* Film Four, 1985; Jacqueline Spong, *Car Trouble,* Columbia/EMI/Warner Brothers, 1986; Christine Painter, *Personal Services,* Vestron, 1987; Elsie Orton, *Prick Up Your Ears,* Samuel Goldwyn, 1987; June Edwards, *Buster,* Tri-Star, 1988.

PRINCIPAL TELEVISION APPEARANCES—Series: *Wood and Walters* and *The Secret Diary of Adrian Mole.* Also appeared in *Nearly a Happy Ending, Living Together, Happy Since I Met You, Say Something Happened, Intensive Care, The Boys from Black*

Stuff, Family Man, Unfair Exchanges, and *Victoria Wood as Seen on TV.*

AWARDS: British Academy Award, 1983, Academy Award nomination, 1984, Golden Globe Award, and Variety Club Award, all Best Actress, for *Educating Rita;* British Academy of Film and Television Arts Award, Best Actress, 1988, for *Personal Services.*

ADDRESSES: AGENT—Saraband Associates, 265 Liverpool Road, London N1, England.*

*   *   *

WARFIELD, Marsha   1955-

PERSONAL: Born March 5, 1955, in Chicago, IL.

VOCATION: Actress and comedienne.

CAREER: PRINCIPAL FILM APPEARANCES—Ophelia, *D.C. Cab,* Universal, 1983; second inmate, *A Fistful of Chopsticks* (also known as *They Call Me Bruce*), Film Ventures International, 1983; homeroom teacher, *Mask,* Universal, 1986; Officer White, *The Whoopee Boys,* Paramount, 1986; also appeared in *I Be Done Been Was Is* (documentary), Cinema of Women, 1983; *Caddyshack II,* Warner Brothers, 1988; and *Gidget Goes to Harlem.*

PRINCIPAL TELEVISION APPEARANCES—Series: Regular, *The Richard Pryor Show,* NBC, 1977; Mama Max, *Riptide,* NBC, 1983; Roz Russell, *Night Court,* NBC, 1986—. Pilots: Cleo, *Anything for Love,* NBC, 1985. Episodic: *The Jim Nabors Show,* syndicated, 1978; *The Late Show,* Fox, 1986. Movies: Lela Boland, *The Marva Collins Story,* CBS, 1981. Specials: *That Thing on ABC,* ABC, 1978; *Teddy Pendergrass in Concert,* HBO, 1982; *The Noel Edmonds Show,* ABC, 1986; *Harry Anderson's Sideshow,* NBC, 1987; *The Nineteenth Annual NAACP Image Awards,* NBC, 1987; *Comic Relief,* HBO, 1987; *Just for Laughs,* Showtime, 1987; "Uptown Comedy Express," *On Location,* HBO, 1987; *Motown Merry Christmas,* NBC, 1987; *The Thirteenth Annual Circus of the Stars,* CBS, 1988; *The Tenth Annual Black Achievement Awards,* syndicated, 1989; also *The Mac Davis Special,* NBC.

RELATED CAREER—As a stand-up comedienne, has appeared in comedy clubs throughout the United States, 1976—.

AWARDS: Winner, San Francisco National Stand-Up Comedy Competition, 1979; winner, National Stand-Up Comedy Competition, 1979.

ADDRESSES: AGENT—Fred Amsel, Fred Amsel and Associates, 6310 San Vicente Boulevard, Suite 407, Los Angeles, CA 90048. PUBLICIST—The Brokaw Company, 9255 Sunset Boulevard, Suite 706, Los Angeles, CA 90069.*

*   *   *

WARREN, Michael   1946-

PERSONAL: Born March 5, 1946, in South Bend, IN; wife's name, Susie; children: Koa, Cash. EDUCATION: Received B.A. in theater arts from the University of California, Los Angeles.

VOCATION: Actor.

CAREER: PRINCIPAL STAGE APPEARANCES—*A Flea in Her Ear,* Meadow Brook Theatre, Rochester, MI, 1986.

PRINCIPAL FILM APPEARANCES—Easly, *Drive, He Said,* Columbia, 1971; Roy, *Butterflies Are Free,* Columbia, 1972; Andy, *Cleopatra Jones,* Warner Brothers, 1973; Norman Chambers, *Norman . . . Is That You?,* Metro-Goldwyn-Mayer/United Artists, 1976; Preacher, *Fast Break,* Columbia, 1979; Ace, *Dreamaniac* (video), Infinity, 1987.

PRINCIPAL TELEVISION APPEARANCES—Series: Ranger P.J. Lewis, *Sierra,* NBC, 1974; Willie Miller, *Paris,* CBS, 1979-80; Officer Bobby Hill, *Hill Street Blues,* NBC, 1981-87. Pilots: Michael Davis, *Home Free,* NBC, 1988; Ben Masters, *A Little Bit Strange,* NBC, 1989; also *Most Wanted,* ABC, 1976. Episodic: Mitchell Evans, *227,* NBC, 1987; Matthew Pogue, *In the Heat of the Night,* NBC, 1988; widower, *L.A. Law,* NBC, 1989; also guest host, *Friday Night Videos,* NBC; Detective Marshall, *Joe Forrester,* NBC; in *Adam-12,* NBC; *Marcus Welby, M.D.,* ABC; *The Mod Squad,* ABC; *The White Shadow,* CBS; *Police Story,* NBC; *Days of Our Lives,* NBC. Movies: Rennie Stuart, *The Child Saver,* NBC, 1988. Specials: *Battle of the Network Stars,* ABC, 1981 and 1982; *Just a Little More Love,* NBC, 1984.

PRINCIPAL TELEVISION WORK—Pilots: Producer (with Kevin Inch), *Home Free,* NBC, 1988.

RELATED CAREER—Basketball technical advisor, *Drive, He Said,* Columbia, 1971.

AWARDS: Emmy Award nomination for *Hill Street Blues.*

SIDELIGHTS: While attending the University of California, Los Angeles, Michael Warren was an All-American basketball player for the national champion Bruins.

ADDRESSES: AGENT—Sandy Bresler, Bresler/Kelly and Associates, 15760 Ventura Boulevard, Suite 1730, Encino, CA 91436.*

*   *   *

WASS, Ted   1952-

PERSONAL: Born October 27, 1952, in Lakewood, OH. EDUCATION: Studied acting at the Goodman School, Chicago, IL.

VOCATION: Actor.

CAREER: OFF-BROADWAY DEBUT—*Columbus,* 1975. BROADWAY DEBUT—*Grease,* Royale Theatre, 1976. PRINCIPAL STAGE APPEARANCES—Vernon Gersch, *They're Playing Our Song,* Imperial Theatre, New York City, 1981.

PRINCIPAL FILM APPEARANCES—Clifton Sleigh, *Curse of the Pink Panther,* Metro-Goldwyn-Mayer/United Artists, 1983; Bobby Shelton, *Oh God! You Devil,* Warner Brothers, 1984; Vic Casey, *Sheena,* Columbia, 1984; Stump, *The Longshot,* Orion, 1986.

PRINCIPAL TELEVISION APPEARANCES—Series: Danny Dallas, *Soap,* ABC, 1977-81. Pilots: Corporal Tillingham, *Handle with*

Care, CBS, 1977; Simon, *The 13th Day: The Story of Esther,* ABC, 1979. Movies: Vinnie, *The Triangle Factory Fire Scandal,* NBC, 1979; Robert Fitzgerald, *I Was a Mail Order Bride,* CBS, 1982; David Mitchell, *Baby Sister,* ABC, 1983; Greg Murchison, *Sins of the Father,* NBC, 1985; Elliot Taffle, *Triplecross,* ABC, 1986; Paul Sheridan, *Sunday Drive,* ABC, 1986; Harry, *The Canterville Ghost,* syndicated, 1986; Mickey, *Mickey and Nora,* CBS, 1987. Specials: *ABC's Silver Anniversary Celebration—25 and Still the One,* ABC, 1978.

ADDRESSES: AGENT—Bob Gersh, The Gersh Agency, 222 Canon Drive, Suite 202, Beverly Hills, CA 90210.*

*   *   *

WASSER, Jane   1957-

PERSONAL: Born July 5, 1957, in Santa Monica, CA; daughter of Dewey (an auditor) and Julie (a secretary; maiden name, Terlesky) Wasser. EDUCATION: Received B.A., music, Trenton State College; studied voice with Bill Schuman.

VOCATION: Actress and singer.

CAREER: PRINCIPAL STAGE APPEARANCES—Princess Olga, *Carnival,* All Soul's Hall, New York City, 1981; semi-Barbarian, *The Apple Tree,* York Theatre Company, New York City, 1987; Thea, *Fiorello!,* Equity Library Theatre, New York City, 1988. Also appeared as Fay Doring, *The King's Men,* Carter Theatre,

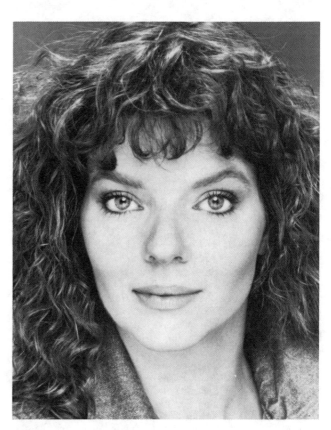

JANE WASSER

433

New York City; Mary Catherine, *Eat the Clock,* 78th Street Theatre Lab, New York City; Abigail Adams, *1776,* and Guenevere, *Camelot,* both Cooperstown Theatre Festival, Cooperstown, NY; in *Leave It to Jane,* New Amsterdam Theatre Company, Town Hall Theatre, New York City; *The Little Rascals,* Goodspeed Opera House, East Haddam, CT; *My Fair Lady,* Darien Dinner Theatre, Darien, CT; *Evita,* An Evening Dinner Theatre, Elmsford, NY; ensemble, *By George* (revue), Cohoes Music Hall, Cohoes, NY; as Marta, *Company,* and Agnes, *I Do! I Do!,* both Music Theatre North; Sonia, *They're Playing Our Song,* and ensemble, *Side by Side by Sondheim,* both Candlewood Playhouse; Catherine, *Pippin,* McAteers Dinner Theatre; Prudie, *Pumpboys and Dinettes,* Gateway Playhouse; Grace, *Annie,* Diamond Horseshoe Dinner Theatre; Emma Goldman, *Tintypes,* Shawnee Playhouse.

MAJOR TOURS—Moorish dancer, *Man of La Mancha,* U.S. cities.

PRINCIPAL FILM APPEARANCES—*If We Knew Then* and *The Baby Sitter.*

PRINCIPAL TELEVISION APPEARANCES—Episodic: *Another World,* NBC.

RELATED CAREER—Performer in *That's Entertainment* for the Holland American Cruise Lines and in *Broadway Tonight,* a production staged at various resorts in the Catskills, New York.

MEMBER: Actors' Equity Association, Screen Actors Guild.

ADDRESSES: HOME—New York, NY.

*   *   *

WATKIN, David   1925-

PERSONAL: Born March 23, 1925; son of John Wilfrid (a lawyer) and Beatrice Lynda (Dadswell) Watkin.

VOCATION: Cinematographer.

CAREER: PRINCIPAL FILM WORK—Cinematographer: *The Knack . . . And How to Get It* (also known as *The Knack*), Lopert, 1965; *Help!,* United Artists, 1965; *Mademoiselle,* United Artists, 1966; *The Persecution and Assassination of Jean-Paul Marat as Performed by the Inmates of the Asylum of Charenton under the Direction of the Marquis de Sade* (also known as *Marat/Sade*), United Artists, 1967; *How I Won the War,* United Artists, 1967; *The Charge of the Light Brigade,* United Artists, 1968; *The Bed Sitting Room,* United Artists, 1969; *Catch-22,* Filmways, 1970; *The Devils,* Warner Brothers, 1971; *The Boy Friend,* Metro-Goldwyn-Mayer, 1971; *A Delicate Balance,* American Film Theatre, 1973; *Yellow Dog,* Akari, 1973; *The Homecoming,* American Film Theatre, 1973; *The Three Musketeers,* Twentieth Century-Fox, 1974; *The Four Musketeers* (also known as *The Revenge of Milady*), Twentieth Century-Fox, 1975; *Mahogany,* Paramount, 1975; *Robin and Marian,* Columbia, 1976; *To the Devil, a Daughter,* EMI, 1976; *Joseph Andrews,* Paramount, 1976; *Hanover Street,* Columbia, 1979; *That Summer,* Columbia, 1979; *Cuba,* United Artists, 1979; *Endless Love,* Universal, 1981; *Chariots of Fire,* Twentieth Century-Fox/Warner Brothers, 1981; *Yentl,* Metro-Goldwyn-Mayer/United Artists (MGM/UA), 1983; *The Hotel New Hampshire,* Orion, 1984; *White Nights,* Columbia, 1985; *Out of Africa,* Universal, 1985; *Return to Oz,* Buena Vista,

1985; *Journey to the Center of the Earth,* Cannon Releasing, 1986; *Sky Bandits,* Galaxy International, 1986; *Moonstruck,* MGM/UA, 1987; *Last Rites,* MGM/UA, 1988; *Masquerade,* MGM/UA, 1988; *The Good Mother,* Buena Vista/Warner Brothers, 1988.

PRINCIPAL TELEVISION WORK—Mini-Series: Cinematographer, *Jesus of Nazareth,* NBC, 1977. Movies: Cinematographer, *Murder by Moonlight,* CBS, 1989.

AWARDS: Academy Award, British Academy of Film and Television Arts Award, and New York Film Critics Circle Award, all Best Cinematography, 1986, for *Out of Africa.*

ADDRESSES: HOME—6 Sussex Mews, Brighton, England.

*   *   *

WAYNE, David   1914-

PERSONAL: Born Wayne James McMeekan, January 30, 1914, in Traverse City, MI; son of David (in sales) and Helen (Mason) McMeekan; married Jane Gordon Trix, December 21, 1941; children: one son, two daughters. EDUCATION: Attended Western Michigan University, 1931-33. MILITARY: American Field Service, lieutenant, Libya and Egypt, 1941-43; U.S. Army, first lieutenant, 1944-46.

VOCATION: Actor.

CAREER: STAGE DEBUT—Touchstone, *As You Like It,* Eldred Players, Globe Shakespearean Theatre, Cleveland, OH, 1936. BROADWAY DEBUT—*Escape This Night,* 44th Street Theatre, 1938. PRINCIPAL STAGE APPEARANCES—Harvey Bodine, *Dance Night,* Belasco Theatre, New York City, 1938; Karl Gunther, *The American Way,* Center Theatre, New York City, 1939; Jimmy Hanley, *Scene of the Crime,* Fulton Theatre, New York City, 1940; Nish, *The Merry Widow,* Majestic Theatre, New York City, 1943; Jonathan's conscience, *Peepshow,* Fulton Theatre, 1944; Mr. Meachem, *Park Avenue,* Shubert Theatre, New York City, 1946; Og, *Finian's Rainbow,* 46th Street Theatre, New York City, 1947; Ensign Pulver, *Mr. Roberts,* Alvin Theatre, New York City, 1948; Sakini, *The Teahouse of the August Moon,* Martin Beck Theatre, New York City, 1953; Uncle Daniel Ponder, *The Ponder Heart,* Music Box Theatre, New York City, 1956; Mr. Finnegan, *The Loud Red Patrick,* Ambassador Theatre, New York City, 1956; Jack Jordan, *Say, Darling,* American National Theatre and Academy (ANTA) Theatre, New York City, 1958.

George Kimball, *Send Me No Flowers,* Brooks Atkinson Theatre, New York City, 1960; Sonny Stone, *Venus at Large,* Morosco Theatre, New York City, 1962; Private Meek, *Too True to Be Good,* 54th Street Theatre, New York City, 1963; Bellac, *Apollo and Miss Agnes,* State Fair, Dallas, TX, 1963; the Chairman, *After the Fall,* Kublai, the Great Khan, *Marco Millions,* Brock Dunnaway, *But for Whom Charlie,* and Von Berg, *Incident at Vichy,* all Lincoln Center Repertory Company, ANTA-Washington Square Theatre, New York City, 1964; Ezra Baxter, *The Yearling,* Alvin Theatre, 1965; Captain Andy, *Show Boat,* State Theatre, New York City, 1966; Dr. Jack Kingsley, *The Impossible Years,* Playhouse in the Park, Philadelphia, PA, 1966, then Royal Poinciana Playhouse, Palm Beach, FL, 1967; Grandpere Brounard, *The Happy Time,* Broadway Theatre, New York City, 1968; H.L. Mencken, *An Unpleasant Evening with H.L. Mencken* (one-man show), Ford's

Theatre, Washington, DC, 1972; Charlie Beddoes, *Halloween,* Bucks County Playhouse, New Hope, PA, 1972. Also appeared in summer theatre productions at the Chase Barn Theatre, Whitefield, NH, 1938; and as Felix, *Marcus in the High Grass,* summer theatre production, 1959.

MAJOR TOURS—Michael, *The Male Animal,* U.S. cities, 1939; Juniper, *Juniper and the Pagans,* U.S. cities, 1959; also appeared with Tatterman Marionettes, U.S. cities, 1936-37.

PRINCIPAL STAGE WORK—Co-producer, *The Loud Red Patrick,* Ambassador Theatre, New York City, 1956.

FILM DEBUT—Gus O'Toole, *Portrait of Jennie* (also known as *Jennie* and *Tidal Wave*), Selznick International, 1949. PRINCIPAL FILM APPEARANCES—Kip Lurie, *Adam's Rib,* Metro-Goldwyn-Mayer (MGM), 1949; Walter Pringle, *My Blue Heaven,* Twentieth Century-Fox, 1950; Arthur Colner Maxwell, *The Reformer and the Redhead,* MGM, 1950; Carl Granger, *Stella,* Twentieth Century-Fox, 1950; Joe, *As Young as You Feel,* Twentieth Century-Fox, 1951; Martin Harrow, *M,* Columbia, 1951; Joe, *Up Front,* Universal, 1951; Ed McCoy, *The I Don't Care Girl,* Twentieth Century-Fox, 1952; Horace, "The Cop and the Anthem" in *O. Henry's Full House* (also known as *Full House*), Twentieth Century-Fox, 1952; Ben Halper, *Wait 'til the Sun Shines, Nellie,* Twentieth Century-Fox, 1952; Jeff Norris, *We're Not Married,* Twentieth Century-Fox, 1952; Don Ross, *With a Song in My Heart,* Twentieth Century-Fox, 1952; Lieutenant Carl Schmidt, *Down among the Sheltering Palms,* Twentieth Century-Fox, 1953; Freddie Denmark, *How to Marry a Millionaire,* Twentieth Century-Fox, 1953; Sol Hurok, *Tonight We Sing,* Twentieth Century-Fox, 1953; Dugboat Walker, *Hell and High Water,* Twentieth Century-Fox, 1954; Joe McCall, *The Tender Trap,* MGM, 1955; Tracy Powell, *The Naked Hills,* Allied Artists, 1956; Dolan, *The Sad Sack,* Paramount, 1957; Ralph White, *The Three Faces of Eve,* Twentieth Century-Fox, 1957; Woodrow Wilson Thrasher, *The Last Angry Man,* Columbia, 1959; Samuel Brennan, *The Big Gamble,* Twentieth Century-Fox, 1961; narrator, *The African Elephant* (documentary), National General, 1971; Dr. Dutton, *The Andromeda Strain,* Universal, 1971; Bensinger, *The Front Page,* Universal, 1974; Duke, *Huckleberry Finn,* United Artists, 1974; Colonel T.T. Clydesdale, *The Apple Dumpling Gang,* Buena Vista, 1975; Pop Morgan, *The Prize Fighter,* New World, 1979; Stapleton, *Finders Keepers,* Warner Brothers, 1984; Dub Daniels, *The Survivalist,* Skouras, 1987.

TELEVISION DEBUT—*The Thousand Dollar Bill,* ABC, 1948. PRINCIPAL TELEVISION APPEARANCES—Series: Norby, *Pearson Norby,* NBC, 1955; Charles Dutton, *The Good Life,* NBC, 1971-72; Inspector Richard Queen, *The Adventures of Ellery Queen,* NBC, 1975-76; Willard "Digger" Barnes, *Dallas,* CBS, 1978; Dr. Amos Weatherby, *House Calls,* CBS, 1979-82. Mini-Series: Colonel Terwilliger, *Once an Eagle,* NBC, 1976-77; Dr. Moe Sinden, *Loose Change* (also known as *Those Restless Years*), NBC, 1978. Pilots: Willis Reynolds, *Junior Miss,* CBS, 1957; George Holloway, *Holloway's Daughter* (broadcast as an episode of *The Bob Hope Chrysler Theatre*), NBC, 1966; Charles Dutton, *The Good Life,* NBC, 1971; Armand Faber, *The Catcher,* NBC, 1972; Inspector Richard Queen, *Ellery Queen: Too Many Suspects,* NBC, 1975; Dr. Amos Rheams, *Lassie: The New Beginning,* ABC, 1978.

Episodic: Mad Hatter, "The Thirteenth Hat" and "Batman Stands

Pat," *Batman,* ABC, 1966; Mad Hatter, "The Contaminated Cowl" and "The Mad Hatter Runs Afoul," *Batman,* ABC, 1967; also *NBC Repertory Theatre,* NBC, 1949; *Studio One,* CBS, 1950; "Escape Clause," *Twilight Zone,* CBS, 1959; *The Bing Crosby Show,* ABC, 1964; *Mr. Broadway,* CBS, 1964; *Burke's Law,* ABC, 1964; *The Trailmaster,* ABC, 1964-65; *Wendy and Me,* ABC, 1964-65; *The Twilight Zone,* CBS, 1965; *Alumni Fun,* CBS, 1965; *The Legend of Mark Twain,* ABC, 1967; *The American Sportsman,* ABC, 1967; *Barney Miller,* ABC, 1975; as James Lawrence, *Family,* ABC; Bill Houston, *Matt Houston,* ABC; Stanley Riverside, Sr., *Trapper John, M.D.,* CBS; in *Sam Benedict,* NBC; *Naked City,* ABC; *The World of Disney,* NBC; *CBS Playhouse,* CBS; *Matt Lincoln,* ABC; *The Name of the Game,* NBC; *Men at Law,* CBS; *Route 66,* CBS; *Cade's County,* CBS; *The Streets of San Francisco,* ABC; *Eye on New York,* WCBS; *Omnibus,* CBS; *Eight Is Enough,* ABC; *Alfred Hitchcock Presents.*

Movies: Maynard Richards, *The F.B.I. Story: The F.B.I. versus Alvin Karpis, Public Enemy Number One* (also known as *The F.B.I. Story—Alvin Karpis*), CBS, 1974; Nate Redstone, *In the Glitter Palace,* NBC, 1977; O. Henry and narrator, *The Gift of Love,* ABC, 1978; Mickey Mills, *Murder at the Mardi Gras,* CBS, 1978; Ben Nayfak, *The Girls in the Office,* ABC, 1979; Merrivale, *An American Christmas Carol,* ABC, 1979; Amos, *Poker Alice,* CBS, 1987. Specials: Sea captain, *Great Catherine,* NBC, 1948; emcee, *The Judy Garland Show,* NBC, 1955; Harlequin (narrator), *Sleeping Beauty,* NBC, 1955; Egbert Floud, *Ruggles of Red Gap,* NBC, 1957; Biff Grimes, *The Strawberry Blonde,* NBC, 1959; Sakini, *The Teahouse of the August Moon,* NBC, 1962; *The Lincoln Center Day Special,* CBS, 1964; Father Firenzuola, "Lamp at Midnight," *Hallmark Hall of Fame,* NBC, 1966; Dr. Sedgwick, *It's a Bird, It's a Plane, It's Superman,* ABC, 1975; Arthur Lee, *The Statesman,* CBS, 1975; also *Arsenic and Old Lace,* ABC; and the Devil, *The Devil and Daniel Webster.*

NON-RELATED CAREER—Statistician.

RECORDINGS: ALBUMS—*Finian's Rainbow* (original cast recording), Columbia, 1947; *Show Boat* (cast recording), RCA 1966; *The Happy Time* (original cast recording), RCA, 1968.

AWARDS: Antoinette Perry Award, Best Supporting or Featured Actor, and Theatre World Award, both 1947, Drama Guild Award and Comoedia Club Award, both 1948, all for *Finian's Rainbow;* Antoinette Perry Award, Best Actor—Dramatic, Drama Guild Award, Comoedia Club Award, and Barter Theatre Award, all 1954, for *The Teahouse of the August Moon;* Antoinette Perry Award nomination, Best Actor in a Musical, 1968, for *The Happy Time.*

MEMBER: Actors' Equity Association (council member, 1948 and 1957), American Federation of Television and Radio Artists, Screen Actors Guild, Players Club, Lambs Club, Friars Club, Weston Gun Club.

SIDELIGHTS: RECREATIONS—Fishing, hunting, swimming, horses, boating, and golf.

ADDRESSES: AGENT—Gary Rado, International Creative Management, 8899 Beverly Boulevard, Los Angeles, CA 90048.*

WEATHERS, Carl

PERSONAL: Born January 14, c. 1947, in New Orleans, LA.

VOCATION: Actor.

CAREER: PRINCIPAL STAGE APPEARANCES—*Nevis Mountain Dew,* Los Angeles Actors' Theatre, Los Angeles, CA, 1981.

PRINCIPAL FILM APPEARANCES—Hambone, *Bucktown,* American International, 1975; Apollo Creed, *Rocky,* United Artists, 1976; military policeman, *Close Encounters of the Third Kind,* Columbia, 1977; Dreamer Tatum, *Semi-Tough,* United Artists, 1977; Weaver, *Force 10 from Navarone,* American International, 1978; Apollo Creed, *Rocky II,* United Artists, 1979; Sundog, *Death Hunt,* Twentieth Century-Fox, 1981; Apollo Creed, *Rocky III,* Metro-Goldwyn-Mayer/United Artists (MGM/UA), 1982; Apollo Creed, *Rocky IV,* MGM/UA, 1985; Dillon, *Predator,* Twentieth Century-Fox, 1987; Jericho Jackson, *Action Jackson,* Lorimar, 1988. Also appeared in *Friday Foster,* American International, 1975.

PRINCIPAL TELEVISION APPEARANCES—Series: Title role, *Fortune Dane,* ABC, 1986. Pilots: Lieutenant Harry Braker, *Braker,* ABC, 1985. Movies: Bateman Hooks, *The Hostage Heart,* CBS, 1977; Eric, *The Bermuda Depths,* ABC, 1978; Cullen Monroe, *The Defiant Ones,* ABC, 1986.

PRINCIPAL TELEVISION WORK—(With Robert Urich) Producer, *The Defiant Ones,* ABC, 1986.

RELATED CAREER—Founder, Stormy Weathers Productions.

NON-RELATED CAREER—Professional football player with the Oakland Raiders.

ADDRESSES: OFFICE—Stormy Weathers Productions, 10202 W. Washington Boulevard, Culver City, CA 90232.*

*   *   *

WEBBER, Robert   1924-1989

PERSONAL: Full name, Robert L. Webber; born October 14, 1924, in Santa Ana, CA; died of Lou Gehrig's disease, May 17, 1989, in Malibu, CA; son of Robert (a merchant seaman) and Alice Webber; married Miranda Jones, October 1, 1953 (divorced, July, 1958); married Del Mertens, April 23, 1972. EDUCATION: Attended Compton Junior College, 1946. MILITARY: U.S. Marine Corps, 1943-45.

VOCATION: Actor.

CAREER: STAGE DEBUT—Wint Selby, *Ah, Wilderness!,* Lake Whalom Playhouse, Fitchburg, MA, 1947. BROADWAY DEBUT—Marine sergeant, *Two Blind Mice,* Cort Theatre, 1949. PRINCIPAL STAGE APPEARANCES—Matt Cole, *Goodbye, My Fancy,* Morosco Theatre, New York City, 1949; Perry Stewart, *The Royal Family,* City Center Theatre, New York City, 1951; Irvin Blanchard, *No Time for Sergeants,* Alvin Theatre, New York City, 1955; David Cutrere, *Orpheus Descending,* Martin Beck Theatre, New York City, 1957; Harry Bohlan, *Fair Game,* Longacre Theatre, New York City, 1957; Chick Clark, *Wonderful Town,* World's Fair,

Brussels, Belgium, 1958; Ricky Powers, *A Loss of Roses,* Eugene O'Neill Theatre, New York City, 1959; George Haverstick, *Period of Adjustment,* Helen Hayes Theatre, New York City, 1960.

MAJOR TOURS—Matt Cole, *Goodbye, My Fancy,* U.S. cities, 1949.

FILM DEBUT—William B. Phillips, *Highway 301,* Warner Brothers, 1950. PRINCIPAL FILM APPEARANCES—Juror, *Twelve Angry Men,* United Artists, 1957; Sergeant McGrath, *The Nun and the Sergeant,* United Artists, 1962; Ricky Powers, *The Stripper* (also known as *Woman of Summer*), Twentieth Century-Fox, 1963; "Mr. Smith," *Hysteria,* Metro-Goldwyn-Mayer (MGM), 1965; Ward Hendricks, *The Sandpiper,* MGM, 1965; Dom Guardiano, *The Third Day,* Warner Brothers, 1965; Milo Stewart, *Dead Heat on a Merry-Go-Round,* Columbia, 1966; Dwight Troy, *Harper* (also known as *The Moving Target*), Warner Brothers, 1966; Sam Gunther, *The Silencers,* Columbia, 1966; General Denton, *The Dirty Dozen,* MGM, 1967; Rod Prescott, *Don't Make Waves,* MGM, 1967; Clint Harris, *The Hired Killer* (also known as *Tecnica di un omicidio* and *Technique d'un meurtre*), Paramount, 1967; Ravaggi, *Manon 70,* Valoria, 1968; Bob Rogers, *The Big Bounce,* Warner Brothers/Seven Arts, 1969.

Dixon, *The Great White Hope,* Twentieth Century-Fox, 1970; rich man, *Macedoine,* CineTel, 1970; Sappensly, *Bring Me the Head of Alfredo Garcia,* United Artists, 1974; attorney, *$ (Dollars)* (also known as *The Heist*), Columbia, 1971; narrator, *Pacific Challenge* (documentary), Concord Film Council, 1973; Rear Admiral Frank J. "Jack" Fletcher, *Midway* (also known as *The Battle of Midway*), Universal, 1976; Howard Jameson, *Madame Claude,* Columbia/Warner Brothers/Orphee Art, 1977; Le Cadre Americain, *L'Imprecateur* (also known as *The Accuser* and *Der Anklager*), Exportation Francaise Cinematographique/Parafrance, 1977; Deputy Chief Riggs, *The Choirboys,* Universal, 1977; Mike Marsh, *Casey's Shadow,* Columbia, 1978; Philippe Douvier, *Revenge of the Pink Panther,* United Artists, 1978; Hugh, *10,* Warner Brothers, 1979; Charley, *Courage Fuyons* (also known as *Courage, Let's Run for It*), Gaumont International/Curzon Film Distributors, 1979; Colonel Clay Thornbush, *Private Benjamin,* Warner Brothers, 1980; Henry Morrison, "The French Method," *Sunday Lovers,* United Artists, 1980; Ben Coogan, *S.O.B.,* Paramount, 1981; Harvey, *Wrong Is Right* (also known as *The Man with the Deadly Lens*), Columbia, 1982; General Potter, *The Final Option* (also known as *Who Dares Wins*), MGM, 1983; Robert McCann, *Wild Geese II,* Universal, 1985; Francis MacMillan, *Nuts,* Warner Brothers, 1987. Also appeared in *Tous vedettes* (also known as *All Stars*), Gaumont International, 1980.

PRINCIPAL TELEVISION APPEARANCES—Series: Alexander Hayes, *Moonlighting* (recurring role), ABC, 1986-88; also Philip Caprice, *The Edge of Night,* CBS. Mini-Series: District Attorney John Hackson DeWitt, *Harold Robbins' "79 Park Avenue"* (also known as *79 Park Avenue*), NBC, 1977. Pilots: Richard Meredith, *Cutter,* NBC, 1972; Carl Vincent, *Hawkins on Murder,* CBS, 1973; Charles Egan, *Judgement Day,* NBC, 1981; J. Woodrow Norton, *Shooting Stars,* ABC, 1983; Will Blackfield, *No Man's Land,* NBC, 1984; Colonel Harper, *In Like Flynn,* ABC, 1985; Jerry Patten, *The Ladies,* NBC, 1987; Commissioner Eastabrook, *Something Is Out There* (also known as *Invader*), NBC, 1988. Episodic: Ikar (human form), "Keeper of the Purple Twilight," *The Outer Limits,* ABC, 1964; also *Eye Witness,* NBC, 1953; "The Captain's Guests, *One Step Beyond,* ABC, 1959; *Playhouse 90,* CBS; *Studio One,* CBS; *Kraft Television Theatre,* NBC; *Robert Montgomery Presents,* NBC; *The Dick Powell Theatre,* NBC; *The Defenders,*

CBS; *Ben Casey*, ABC; *The Nurses*, CBS; *The Greatest Show on Earth*, ABC; *Naked City*, ABC; *Route 66*, CBS; *McCloud*, NBC; *Ironside*, NBC; *Cannon*, CBS; *The Bold Ones*, NBC; *Mannix*, CBS; *The Champions*, NBC; *The Streets of San Francisco*, ABC; *Kojak*, CBS; *Barnaby Jones*, CBS; *Quincy*, NBC; *Banacek*, NBC; *The Rockford Files*, NBC; *Alfred Hitchcock Presents*, CBS; *Espionage*, NBC.

Movies: Dorsey, *Hauser's Memory*, NBC, 1970; Karel Kessler, *The Movie Murderer*, NBC, 1970; James Calendar, *Thief*, ABC, 1971; Edward Norton, *Double Indemnity*, ABC, 1973; Dr. Eric Stoneman, *Murder or Mercy*, ABC, 1974; Hugh Webster, *Death Stalk*, NBC, 1975; Ralph Salkin, *The Streets of L.A.*, CBS, 1979; Ed Lemmons, *The Two Lives of Carol Letner*, CBS, 1981; Wally Dawson, *Not Just Another Affair*, CBS, 1982; Dr. Cole, *Don't Go to Sleep*, ABC, 1982; Felix Duncan, *Starflight: The Plane That Couldn't Land* (also know as *Starflight One*), ABC, 1983; Hugh Gibley, *Getting Physical*, CBS, 1984; Calvin Lantz, *Assassin*, CBS, 1986. Specials: Dawes, *Full Moon over Brooklyn*, NBC, 1960; Andre Latour, "The Paradine Case," *Theater '62*, NBC, 1962.

MEMBER: Actors' Equity Association, Screen Actors Guild, American Federation of Television and Radio Artists.

OBITUARIES AND OTHER SOURCES: [New York] *Daily News*, May 21, 1989; *New York Times*, May 20, 1989; *Variety*, May 24-30, 1989.*

*   *   *

WEDGEWORTH, Ann   1935-

PERSONAL: Born January 21, 1935, in Abilene, TX; married Rip Torn (an actor), January 15, 1955 (divorced, June, 1961); married Ernest Martin; children: Danae (first marriage); Dianna (second marriage). EDUCATION: Received B.A. in drama from Southern Methodist University; also attended the University of Texas.

VOCATION: Actress.

CAREER: PRINCIPAL STAGE APPEARANCES—Abigail Williams, *The Crucible*, Martinique Theatre, New York City, 1958; Julie Martin, *Make a Million*, Playhouse Theatre, then Morosco Theatre, both New York City, 1959; Nettie-Jo, *The Days and Nights of Beebee Fenstermaker*, Sheridan Square Playhouse, New York City, 1962; Jo Britten, *Blues for Mister Charlie*, American National Theatre and Academy Theatre, New York City, 1964; Pamela, *The Last Analysis*, Belasco Theatre, New York City, 1964; Rachel, *Ludlow Fair*, Theatre East, New York City, 1966; Molly, "Line" in *Acrobats and Line*, Theatre De Lys, New York City, 1971; Nancy, *Thieves*, Broadhurst Theatre, New York City, 1974; Norma Dodd, *The Dream*, Forrest Theatre, Philadelphia, PA, 1977; Faye Medwick, *Chapter Two*, Imperial Theatre, New York City, 1977; Harley, *Elba*, Manhattan Theatre Club, New York City, 1983; Meg, *A Lie of the Mind*, Promenade Theatre, New York City, 1985. Also appeared in *Chaparral*, Sheridan Square Playhouse, 1958; *Period of Adjustment*, Helen Hayes Theatre, New York City, 1960; *The Honest-to-God Shnozzola*, Gramercy Arts Theatre, New York City, 1969; and *Copperhead*, Pennsylvania Stage Company, Allentown, PA, 1983.

MAJOR TOURS—*The Sign in Sidney Brustein's Window*, U.S. cities; *Kennedy's Children*, U.S. cities.

PRINCIPAL FILM APPEARANCES—Margie, *Andy*, Universal, 1965; Katie, *Bang the Drum Slowly*, Paramount, 1973; Frenchy, *Scarecrow*, Warner Brothers, 1973; Sally, *Law and Disorder*, Columbia, 1974; Kit Loring, *The Catamount Killing*, Hallmark, 1975; Marie, *Birch Interval*, Gamma III, 1976; Pearlie Craigle, *One Summer Love* (also known as *Dragonfly*), American International, 1976; Joyce Rissley/"Dallas Angel," *Citizens Band* (also known as *Handle with Care*), Paramount, 1977; Nancy, *Thieves*, Paramount, 1977; Joan Cummings, *No Small Affair*, Columbia, 1984; Dolores, *My Science Project*, Buena Vista, 1985; Hilda Hensley, *Sweet Dreams*, Tri-Star, 1985; Jo, *The Men's Club*, Atlantic, 1986; Annette Shea, *Made in Heaven*, Lorimar, 1987; Claudine, *A Tiger's Tale*, Atlantic, 1987; Amy, *Far North*, Alive, 1988. Also appeared in *Soggy Bottom U.S.A.*, Gaylord, 1982.

PRINCIPAL TELEVISION APPEARANCES—Series: Lahoma Lucas, *Somerset*, NBC, 1970; Lana Shields, *Three's Company*, ABC, 1979-80; Bootsie Weschester, *Filthy Rich*, CBS, 1982-83; also Lahoma Vane, *Another World*, NBC; *The Edge of Night*. Pilots: Polly, *Sylvan in Paradise*, NBC, 1986. Episodic: *All That Glitters*, syndicated, 1977; also *The Defenders*, CBS; *Bronk*, CBS. Movies: Danielle, *The War Between the Tates*, NBC, 1977; Mayo Methot, *Bogie*, CBS, 1980; Aunt Betty, *Elvis and the Beauty Queen*, NBC, 1981; Rosie, *Killjoy*, CBS, 1981; Eve Whitcomb, *Right to Kill?*, ABC, 1985; Susan Berger, *A Stranger Waits*, CBS, 1987.

AWARDS: Antoinette Perry Award, Best Featured Actress in a Play, 1977, for *Chapter Two;* National Society of Film Critics Award, 1977, for *Citizens Band.*

ADDRESSES: AGENT—Camden Artists, 2121 Avenue of the Stars, Suite 410, Los Angeles, CA 90067.*

*   *   *

WEIL, Samuel
See KAUFMAN, Lloyd

*   *   *

WEINTRAUB, Jerry   1937-

PERSONAL: Born September 26, 1937, in Brooklyn, NY; father, a gem salesman; mother's name, Rose Weintraub; married second wife, Jane Morgan (a singer), 1965; children: Michael (first marriage); Julie Caroline, Jamie Cee, Jody Christine (second marriage; adopted).

VOCATION: Producer, personal manager, agent, and promoter.

CAREER: PRINCIPAL FILM WORK—All as producer, unless indicated: Executive producer, *Nashville*, Paramount, 1975; *Oh, God!*, Warner Brothers, 1977; *9/30/55*, Universal, 1977; *Cruising*, United Artists, 1980; (with Leonard Goldberg) *All Night Long*, Universal, 1981; *Diner*, Metro-Goldwyn-Mayer/United Artists, 1982; *The Karate Kid*, Columbia, 1984; *The Karate Kid, Part II*, Columbia, 1986; *Happy New Year*, Columbia, 1987.

PRINCIPAL TELEVISION WORK—All as executive producer. Series: *Szysznyk*, CBS, 1977-78; (with Leonard Goldberg) *When the Whistle Blows*, ABC, 1980. Pilots: *Father, O Father*, ABC, 1977; (with Norman Lear) *King of the Road*, CBS, 1978; (with Goldberg) *Blue Jeans*, ABC, 1980; (with Barry Levinson) *Diner*, CBS, 1983; *Poor Richard*, CBS, 1984. Movies: (With Lee Majors) *The Cowboy and the Ballerina*, CBS, 1984. Specials: *Sinatra—The Main Event*, ABC, 1974; *The John Denver Special*, ABC, 1974; *John Denver Rocky Mountain Christmas*, ABC, 1975; *An Evening with John Denver*, ABC, 1975; *The Carpenters*, ABC, 1976; *The Dorothy Hamill Special*, ABC, 1976; *The John Denver Special*, ABC, 1976; *John Denver and Friend*, ABC, 1976; *The Carpenters at Christmas*, ABC, 1977; *The Dorothy Hamill Winter Carnival Special*, ABC, 1977; *John Denver—Thank God I'm a Country Boy*, ABC, 1977; *The Neil Diamond Special*, NBC, 1977; *Neil Diamond Special: I'm Glad You're Here with Me Tonight*, NBC, 1977; *The Starland Vocal Band*, CBS, 1977; *The Carpenters . . . Space Encounters*, ABC, 1978; *Pat Boone and Family*, ABC, 1978; (with Roone Arledge) *Alaska: The American Child*, ABC, 1978; *Dorothy Hamill Presents Winners*, ABC, 1978; *Dorothy Hamill's Corner of the Sky*, ABC, 1979; *John Denver and the Ladies*, ABC, 1979; *The Pat Boone and Family Easter Special*, ABC, 1979; *The Carpenters—Music, Music, Music*, ABC, 1980; *The Jimmy McNichol Special*, CBS, 1980; *Two of a Kind: George Burns and John Denver* (also known as *John Denver with His Special Guest George Burns: Two of a Kind*), ABC, 1981.

RELATED CAREER—Talent agent, MCA, during the 1950s; personal manager for Jack Paar, the Four Seasons, and Jane Morgan, 1960; co-founder, Jerry Weintraub/Armand Hammer Productions, 1982—; co-owner of six Broadway theatres with the Nederlander Organization, New York City, 1984; chairman and chief executive officer, United Artists Corporation, 1985-86; founder and president, Weintraub Entertainment Group, 1987—; owner and chairman, Management Three; founder and co-owner (with Donald Ohlmeyer) Intercontinental Broadcasting Systems, Inc. (television production company); personal manager, business agent, and concert promoter for musical acts including Elvis Presley, Frank Sinatra, Wayne Newton, John Davidson, John Denver, Neil Diamond, Bob Dylan, and the Moody Blues.

NON-RELATED CAREER—Board member, St. John's Hospital, Santa Monica, CA.

AWARDS: Emmy Award, Outstanding Special—Comedy- Variety or Music, 1975, for *An Evening with John Denver;* Irvin Feld Humanitarian Award from the National Conference of Christians and Jews, 1985.

MEMBER: Variety Club International.

ADDRESSES: OFFICE—Management Three, 4570 Encino Avenue, Encino, CA 91316.*

         *   *   *

WEIS, Don   1922-

PERSONAL: Born May 13, 1922, in Milwaukee, WI. EDUCATION: Attended the University of Southern California.

VOCATION: Director and producer.

CAREER: PRINCIPAL FILM WORK—All as director, unless indicated: Dialogue director, *Body and Soul* (also known as *An Affair of the Heart*), United Artists, 1947; (with Abraham Polonsky) *Force of Evil*, Metro-Goldwyn-Mayer (MGM), 1948; dialogue director, *The Red Pony*, Republic, 1949; dialogue director, *Champion*, United Artists, 1949; dialogue director, *Home of the Brave*, United Artists, 1949; dialogue director, *The Men* (also known as *Battle Stripe*), United Artists, 1950; *Bannerline*, MGM, 1951; *It's a Big Country*, MGM, 1951; *Just This Once*, MGM, 1952; *You for Me*, MGM, 1952; *The Affairs of Dobie Gillis*, MGM, 1953; *Half a Hero*, MGM, 1953; *I Love Melvin*, MGM, 1953; *Remains to Be Seen*, MGM, 1953; *A Slight Case of Larceny*, MGM, 1953; *Adventures of Hajji Baba*, Twentieth Century-Fox, 1954; *Ride the High Iron*, Columbia, 1956; *The Gene Krupa Story* (also known as *Drum Crazy*), Columbia, 1959; *Critic's Choice*, Warner Brothers, 1963; *Looking for Love*, MGM, 1964; *Pajama Party*, American International, 1964; *Ghost in the Invisible Bikini*, American International, 1966; *King's Pirate*, Universal, 1967; *Did You Hear the One about the Traveling Saleslady?*, Universal, 1968; *Zero to Sixty* (also known as *Repo*), First Artists, 1978.

PRINCIPAL TELEVISION WORK—All as director. Series: *Dear Phoebe*, NBC, 1954-55; (with Stanley Z. Cherry) *McKeever and the Colonel*, NBC, 1962-63. Pilots: *Skip Taylor*, syndicated, 1953; *Papa Said No*, CBS, 1958; *Secrets of the Old Bailey*, CBS, 1958; *Head of the Family* (broadcast as an episode of *Comedy Spot*), CBS, 1960; *Lollipop Louie*, ABC, 1963; *Off We Go*, CBS, 1966; *Riddle at 24,000*, NBC, 1974; *Flo's Place*, NBC, 1976; *The Millionaire*, CBS, 1978; *The Dooley Brothers*, CBS, 1979; *Quick and Quiet*, CBS, 1981; *Hard Knocks*, ABC, 1981.

Episodic: "The Joker Is Wild" and "Batman Gets Riled," *Batman*, ABC, 1966; "Hot off the Griddle" and "The Cat and the Fiddle," *Batman*, ABC, 1967; *Paris 7000*, ABC, 1970; *M*A*S*H*, CBS, 1972-78; "The Vampire," "The Werewolf," "Fire-Fall," and "The Trevi Collection," *Kolchak: The Night Stalker*, ABC, 1974; *Planet of the Apes*, CBS, 1974; *Matt Helm*, ABC, 1975; *Spencer's Pilots*, CBS, 1976; *The Andros Targets*, CBS, 1977; *The San Pedro Beach Bums*, ABC, 1977; *Kingston: Confidential*, NBC, 1977; *Delta House*, ABC, 1979; *The Six O'Clock Follies*, NBC, 1980; *Lottery!*, ABC, 1983; *Eye to Eye*, ABC, 1985; *MacGyver*, ABC, 1985; *Crazy Like a Fox*, CBS, 1985; *The New Mike Hammer* (two episodes), CBS, 1986; *Remington Steele*, NBC, 1986; *Buck James*, ABC, 1987; *Hill Street Blues*, NBC, 1987; *The Wizard*, CBS, 1987; *Simon and Simon*, CBS, 1988; *Murphy's Law*, ABC, 1988 and 1989; also *Starsky and Hutch*, ABC; *T.J. Hooker*, ABC; *The Bob Hope Chrysler Theater*, NBC; *Burke's Law*, ABC; *Casablanca*, ABC; *Checkmate*, CBS; *It Takes a Thief*, ABC; *The Patty Duke Show*, ABC; *Roll Out!*, CBS; *The Survivors* (also known as *Harold Robbins' "The Survivors"*), ABC; *The Virginian*, NBC; *The Barbary Coast*, ABC; *Baretta*, ABC; *Bring 'em Back Alive*, CBS; *Cagney and Lacey*, CBS; *Charlie's Angels*, ABC; *CHiPs*, NBC; *Code Red*, ABC; (also producer) *Fantasy Island*, ABC; *Flamingo Road*, NBC; *Happy Days*, ABC; *Harry O*, ABC; *Hawaii Five-O*, CBS; *Ironside*, NBC; *The Love Boat*, ABC; *Mannix*, CBS; *Bronk*, CBS; *Petrocelli*, NBC; *The Magician*, NBC; *The Courtship of Eddie's Father*, ABC; *Wagon Train; Alfred Hitchcock Presents; The Jack Benny Program; Command Performance*. Movies: *The Longest Hundred Miles*, NBC, 1967; *Now You See It, Now You Don't*, NBC, 1968; *The Munsters' Revenge*, NBC, 1981.

AWARDS: Screen Directors Guild Award, Best Director, 1956 and 1958, both for *Dear Phoebe*.*

WEITZ, Bruce   1943-

PERSONAL: Full name, Bruce Peter Weitz; born May 27, 1943, in Norwalk, CT; son of Alvin Weitz (a liquor store owner) and Sybil Weitz Rubel; married second wife, Cecilia Hart (an actress), 1973 (divorced, 1980). EDUCATION: Carnegie Institute of Technology, B.A., 1964, M.F.A., 1966.

VOCATION: Actor.

CAREER: PRINCIPAL STAGE APPEARANCES—Polo Pope, *A Hatful of Rain,* Equity Library Theatre, Master Theatre, New York City, 1970; Roland, *The Conditioning of Charlie One,* Playwrights Horizons, New York City, 1973; Sam, *Creeps,* Playhouse Two Theatre, New York City, 1973; Johnny, *Frankie and Johnny in the Claire de Lune,* Westside Arts Theatre, New York City, 1988. Also appeared in *Oh, What a Lovely War!,* Long Wharf Theatre, New Haven, CT, 1966; *In the Matter of J. Robert Oppenheimer,* Goodman Theatre Center, Chicago, IL, 1972; *Death of a Salesman, The Basic Training of Pavlo Hummel,* and *Norman, Is That You?,* all in New York City; with the Long Wharf Repertory Theatre, New Haven, CT, 1967; Tyrone Guthrie Theatre, Minneapolis, MN, 1967-69; Arena Stage, Washington, DC, 1971-72; the Actors Theatre of Louisville, Louisville, KY, 1971-73; and in thirteen New York Shakespeare Festival productions, Delacorte Theatre, New York City, 1976-80.

PRINCIPAL TELEVISION APPEARANCES—Series: Detective Mick Belker, *Hill Street Blues,* NBC, 1981-87; Jake McCasky, *Mama's Boy,* NBC, 1987. Pilots: Sergeant Mike Pirelli, *Every Stray Dog and Kid,* NBC, 1981; Dr. Matt Jennings, *Catalina C-Lab,* NBC, 1982; Mick Belker, *Hill Street Blues,* NBC, 1981. Episodic: *Quincy, M.E.,* NBC; *Happy Days,* ABC; *Lou Grant,* CBS; *The Rockford Files,* NBC; *The White Shadow,* CBS. Movies: Paul Snider, *Death of a Centerfold: The Dorothy Stratten Story,* NBC, 1981; Bob Cousins, *A Reason to Live,* NBC, 1985; Martini, *If It's Tuesday, It Still Must Be Belgium,* NBC, 1987; Rick Whitehead, *Baby M,* ABC, 1988. Specials: "Henry Winkler Meets William Shakespeare," *CBS Festival of Lively Arts for Young People,* CBS, 1977; *Battle of the Network Stars,* ABC, 1982 and 1983; *Celebrity Daredevils,* ABC, 1983; *The Chemical People* (documentary), PBS, 1983; *The Stuntman Awards,* syndicated, 1986; host, *Man and the Animals* (documentary), PBS, 1987; *Macy's Thanksgiving Day Parade,* NBC, 1987.

NON-RELATED CAREER—Restaurant manager on Formentera (a Spanish island), 1966.

AWARDS: Emmy Award nominations, Outstanding Supporting Actor in a Drama Series, 1981, 1982, and 1983, and Emmy Award, Outstanding Supporting Actor in a Drama Series, 1984, all for *Hill Street Blues.*

MEMBER: Parent Teacher Association.

SIDELIGHTS: RECREATIONS—Golf, racquetball, weaving, cooking, and reading.

ADDRESSES: AGENT—William Morris Agency, 151 El Camino Boulevard, Beverly Hills, CA 90212. PUBLICIST—Nancy Paul, Richard Grant and Associates, 8500 Wilshire Boulevard, Suite 520, Beverly Hills, CA 90211.*

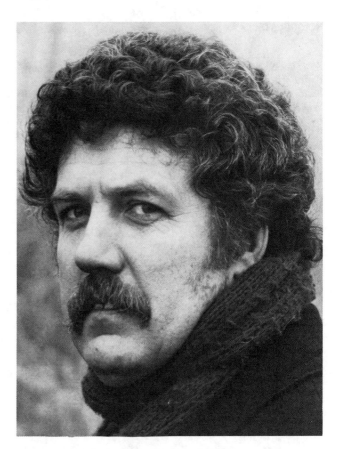

COLIN WELLAND

WELLAND, Colin   1934-

PERSONAL: Born Colin Williams, July 4, 1934, in Liverpool, England; son of John Arthur and Norah Williams; married Patricia Sweeney, 1962; children: one son, three daughters. EDUCATION: Attended Bretton Hall College and Goldsmith's College.

VOCATION: Writer and actor.

CAREER: Also see *WRITINGS* below. PRINCIPAL STAGE APPEARANCES—Tony Weston, *Say Goodnight to Grandma,* Manchester Forum Theatre, Manchester, U.K., 1972, then St. Martin's Theatre, London, 1973; also appeared with the Manchester Library Theatre, Manchester, U.K., 1962-64; in *Waiting for Godot,* National Theatre, London, 1988; and in *The Churchill Play,* Royal Shakespeare Company, London, 1989.

PRINCIPAL FILM APPEARANCES—Mr. Farthing, *Kes,* United Artists, 1970; Reverend Hood, *Straw Dogs,* Cinerama, 1971; Tom Binney, *Villain,* EMI/Metro-Goldwyn-Mayer, 1971; Chadwick, *Sweeney,* EMI, 1977.

TELEVISION DEBUT—Defendant, *The Verdict Is Yours.* PRINCIPAL TELEVISION APPEARANCES—Series: *Z Cars.* Also appeared in *Blue Remembered Hills, United Kingdom,* and *The Trial of Klaus Barbie.*

RELATED CAREER—Television newscaster, Manchester, U.K.; stage director; sports commentator and journalist.

NON-RELATED CAREER—Art teacher, 1958-62; also English teacher.

WRITINGS: STAGE—*Say Goodnight to Grandma,* Manchester Forum Theatre, 1972, then St. Martin's Theatre, 1973; *Roll on Four O'Clock,* Palace Theatre, London, 1981. FILM—(With Walter Bernstein) *Yanks,* Universal, 1979; *Chariots of Fire,* Warner Brothers, 1981; *Twice in a Lifetime,* Yorkin, 1987. TELEVISION—Series: *The Wild West Show,* 1975. Plays: *Bangelstein's Boys,* 1968; *Slattery's Mounted Foot,* 1970; (with William Gaunt and Janet Key) *The Catherine Wheel,* 1970; *The Hallelujah Handshake,* 1970; *Say Goodnight to Your Grandma,* 1970; *A Roomful of Holes,* 1971, published by Davis-Poynter, 1971; *Roll on Four O'Clock,* 1971; *Jack Point,* 1973; *Kisses at Fifty,* 1973, published in *The Television Play,* 1976; *Leeds—United!,* 1974; *Your Man from Six Counties,* 1976; *Bank Holiday,* 1977.

AWARDS: British Academy of Film and Television Arts Award, Best Supporting Actor, 1970, for *Kes;* British Academy of Film and Television Arts Award, Best Script, 1970; Writers Guild Awards, 1970, 1973, and 1974; Broadcasting Press Guild Award, 1973; Academy Award, Best Original Screenplay, 1981, for *Chariots of Fire.*

MEMBER: Fulham Rugby League Club (director).

SIDELIGHTS: RECREATIONS—Cricket and watching rugby and soccer films.

ADDRESSES: AGENT—Anthony Jones, A.D. Peters Ltd., 10 Buckingham Street, London WC2N 6BU, England.

*   *   *

WELLER, Peter   1947-

PERSONAL: Born June 24, 1947, in Stevens Point, WI; father, a career army pilot and lawyer. EDUCATION: Attended North Texas State University; trained for the stage at the American Academy of Dramatic Arts with Uta Hagen and at the Actors Studio with Lee Strasberg.

VOCATION: Actor.

CAREER: BROADWAY DEBUT—*Sticks and Bones,* John Golden Theatre, 1972. PRINCIPAL STAGE APPEARANCES—Russian sergeant, *Full Circle,* American National Theatre and Academy (ANTA) Theatre, New York City, 1973; Lennox, *Macbeth,* New York Shakespeare Festival (NYSF), Mitzi E. Newhouse Theatre, New York City, 1974; Alan Seymour, *Summer Brave,* ANTA Theatre, 1975; Lieutenant Henry Hitchcock, *Rebel Women,* NYSF, Public Theatre, New York City, 1976; Billy, *Streamers,* NYSF, Mitzi E. Newhouse Theatre, 1976; Cliff, *The Woolgatherer,* Circle Repertory Theatre, New York City, 1980; Nick, *The Woods,* Second Stage Theatre, New York City, 1982. Also appeared in *The Merchant of Venice,* Repertory Theatre of Lincoln Center, Vivian Beaumont Theatre, New York City, 1973; *Burning Bright,* New Dramatists, New York City, 1977; *Cat on a Hot Tin Roof,* Long Wharf Theatre, New Haven, CT, 1984; and in *Children* and *Serenading Louie,* both Off-Broadway productions.

PRINCIPAL FILM APPEARANCES—Joe LeFors, *Butch and Sundance: The Early Days,* Twentieth Century-Fox, 1979; Steven Routledge,

Just Tell Me What You Want, Warner Brothers, 1980; Frank Henderson, *Shoot the Moon,* Metro-Goldwyn-Mayer/United Artists (MGM/UA), 1982; Bart Hughes, *Of Unknown Origin,* Warner Brothers, 1983; title role, *The Adventures of Buckaroo Banzai: Across the Eighth Dimension,* Twentieth Century-Fox, 1984; Sam, *Firstborn,* Paramount, 1984; Alex J. Murphy/title role, *Robocop,* Orion, 1987; Baston Morris, *A Killing Affair* (also known as *Monday, Tuesday, Wednesday*), Hemdale, 1988; Roland Dalton, *Shakedown,* Universal, 1988; Juan Pablo Castel, *El Tunel* (also known as *The Tunnel*), Interaccess Film, 1988; Beck, *Leviathan,* MGM/UA, 1989. Also appeared in *My Sister's Keeper,* Interpictures Releasing, 1986; and in *Vera.*

PRINCIPAL TELEVISION APPEARANCES—Episodic: Soldier, ''The Dancing Princess,'' *Faerie Tale Theatre,* Showtime, 1987; also *Lou Grant,* CBS. Movies: Lieutenant Fellows, *The Man without a Country,* ABC, 1973; Red Sash, *The Silence,* NBC, 1975; Deke Cullover, *Kentucky Woman,* CBS, 1983; Joe Farley, *Two Kinds of Love,* CBS, 1983; Rad Hungate, *Apology,* HBO, 1986. Also appeared in *Exit 10* and *Earring.*

RELATED CAREER—Member of the Actors Studio, New York City.

NON-RELATED CAREER—Co-owner (with Treat Williams) of a restaurant in New York City.

SIDELIGHTS: RECREATIONS—Playing the trumpet and running.

CTFT has learned that Peter Weller has competed in the New York City Marathon.

ADDRESSES: AGENT—Rick Nicita, Creative Artists Agency, 1888 Century Park E., Suite 1400, Los Angeles, CA 90067.*

*   *   *

WELSH, Kenneth

PERSONAL: Born in Canada; father, a worker for the Canadian National Railway; married Donna Haley (an actress; divorced). EDUCATION: University of Alberta, Edmonton.

VOCATION: Actor.

CAREER: PRINCIPAL STAGE APPEARANCES—Sir Thomas Grey, citizen, and attendant, *Henry V,* first murderer and captain to Talbot, *Henry VI,* and guard and courtier, *Twelfth Night,* all Stratford Shakespearean Festival, Festival Theatre, Stratford, ON, Canada, 1966; Lord Hastings, *Richard III,* Fenton, *The Merry Wives of Windsor,* and Octavius Caesar, *Antony and Cleopatra,* all Stratford Shakespearean Festival, Festival Theatre, 1967; MacDuff, *Macbeth,* Stratford Shakespearean Festival, Festival Theatre, 1971; Sir Oliver Martext, *As You Like It,* Edgar, *King Lear,* and Alessandro de Medici, *Lorenzaccio,* all Stratford Shakespearean Festival, Festival Theatre, 1972; Orlando, *As You Like It,* American Shakespeare Theatre, Stratford, CT, 1976; Dave, *Treats,* Hudson Guild Theatre, New York City, 1977; Charlie Evans, *One Crack Out,* Marymount Manhattan Theatre, New York City, 1978; Taylor, *Curse of the Starving Class,* Public Theatre, New York City, 1978; Ivan Kusmich Shpyokin (the Postmaster), *The Inspector General,* Circle in the Square, New York City, 1978; Philip Hill, *Whose Life Is It, Anyway?,* Trafalgar Theatre, New York City, 1979.

Title role, *Cyrano de Bergerac,* Goodman Theatre, Chicago, IL, 1980; Police Inspector, Georges, and the Physiotherapist, *Piaf,* Plymouth Theatre, New York City, 1981; Max, *The Real Thing,* Plymouth Theatre, 1984; Virginia's father and Leonard Woolf, *Virginia,* Public Theatre, 1985; Martin Heyman, *Social Security,* Ethel Barrymore Theatre, New York City, 1986; Johnny, *Frankie and Johnny in the Clair de Lune,* Manhattan Theatre Club, New York City, 1986; John Honeyman, *A Walk in the Woods,* Yale Repertory Theatre, New Haven, CT, 1987. Also appeared in *Hamlet,* Stratford Shakespearean Festival, Festival Theatre, 1969; *Much Ado about Nothing,* Stratford Shakespearean Festival, Festival Theatre, 1971; *Arturo Ui,* 1975; with the McCarter Theatre Company, Princeton, NJ, 1977; in *Mary Barnes,* Long Wharf Theatre, New Haven, CT, 1980; and in *Standup Shakespeare,* Theatre 890, New York City, 1987.

PRINCIPAL STAGE WORK—Director, *Under Milkwood,* Tyrone Guthrie Theatre, Minneapolis, MN; also director with the Denver Center Theatre Company, Denver, CO, 1981.

PRINCIPAL FILM APPEARANCES—Dr. Webber, *Double Negative,* Quadrant, 1980; Sergeant Wheeler, *Phobia,* Paramount, 1980; James, *Of Unknown Origin,* Warner Brothers, 1983; Harrison, *Covergirl* (also known as *Dreamworld*), New World, 1984; Doctor, *Falling in Love,* Paramount, 1984; Reginald "Reno" Coltchinsky, *Reno and the Doc,* New World, 1984; Joe McKenzie, *Perfect,* Columbia, 1985; Dr. Appel, *Heartburn,* Paramount, 1986; Jim, *Lost!,* Norstar, 1986; David Sutton, *Loyalties,* Norstar, 1986; radio voice, *Radio Days,* Orion, 1987. Also appeared in *Love and Larceny,* 1983.

PRINCIPAL TELEVISION APPEARANCES—Mini-Series: Sir James Munro, *Empire, Inc.,* Canadian television, 1984. Episodic: Charles Surface, "The School for Scandal," *Great Performances,* PBS, 1975; Jack, "Acts of Terror," *Twilight Zone,* syndicated, 1988. Movies: Richard Miller, *A Stranger Waits,* CBS, 1987; also *The Murder of Mary Phagan,* NBC, 1988. Specials: Georges, *Piaf,* Entertainment Channel, 1982.

WRITINGS: STAGE—(With Ray Leslee) *Standup Shakespeare,* Theatre 890, New York City, 1987.

AWARDS: Joseph Jefferson Award for *Arturo Ui,* 1975; Association of Canadian Television and Radio Artists Award, 1984, for *Empire, Inc.**

* * *

WENDT, George 1948-

PERSONAL: Born October 17, 1948, in Chicago, IL; married Bernadette Birkitt (an actress); children: three sons, one daughter. EDUCATION: Received degree in economics from Rockhurst College, 1971.

VOCATION: Actor.

CAREER: PRINCIPAL STAGE APPEARANCES—*Super Sunday* and *Tom Jones,* both Williamstown Theatre Festival, Williamstown, MA, 1988.

PRINCIPAL FILM APPEARANCES—Student, *Somewhere in Time,* Universal, 1980; engineer, *My Bodyguard,* Twentieth Century-Fox, 1980; agent at counter, *Airplane II: The Sequel,* Paramount, 1982; Charlie Prince, *Dreamscape,* Twentieth Century-Fox, 1984; Fat Sam, *Fletch,* Universal, 1984; Jake, *No Small Affair,* Columbia, 1984; Marty Morrison, *Thief of Hearts,* Paramount, 1984; Buster, *Gung Ho,* Paramount, 1986; Harold Gorton, *House,* New World, 1986; Witten, *Never Say Die,* Kings Road International, 1988; Chet Butler, *Plain Clothes* (also known as *Glory Day*), Paramount, 1988. Also appeared in *Jekyll and Hyde . . . Together Again,* Paramount, 1982; and *The Woman in Red,* Orion, 1984.

PRINCIPAL TELEVISION APPEARANCES— Series: Gus Bertoia, *Making the Grade,* CBS, 1982; Norm Peterson, *Cheers,* NBC, 1982—. Pilots: *Nothing but Comedy,* NBC. Episodic: Barney Slessinger, "The World Next Door," *The Twilight Zone,* CBS, 1985; Norm Peterson, *The Tortellis,* NBC, 1987; Stan, *Day by Day,* NBC, 1989; also *Taxi,* ABC, 1981; *American Dream,* ABC, 1981; *M*A*S*H,* CBS, 1982; *Alice,* CBS; *Soap,* ABC; *Hart to Hart,* ABC. Movies: Mr. Sweeney, *The Ratings Game,* Movie Channel, 1984. Specials: Voice of Raoul, *Garfield on the Town* (animated), CBS, 1983; voice of second ranger, *Garfield in the Rough* (animated), CBS, 1984; voice of Johnnie Throat, *The Romance of Betty Boop* (animated), CBS, 1985; *The Second City Twenty-Fifth Anniversary Special,* HBO, 1985; *Comic Relief,* HBO, 1986; *King Orange Jamboree Parade,* NBC, 1988; *Improv Tonight,* syndicated, 1988; *Mickey's Sixtieth Birthday Special* (also known as *The Magical World of Disney*), NBC, 1988.

RELATED CAREER—Member, Second City (an improvisational comedy troupe), Chicago, IL, for six years; actor in television commercials.

NON-RELATED CAREER—Construction worker.

SIDELIGHTS: RECREATIONS—Baseball, football, and basketball.

ADDRESSES: AGENTS—Lou Pitt and Nancy Josephson, International Creative Management, 8899 Beverly Boulevard, Los Angeles, CA 90048. MANAGER—Bernie Brillstein, Brillstein Company, 9200 Sunset Boulevard, Suite 428, Los Angeles, CA 90069.*

* * *

WESKER, Arnold 1932-

PERSONAL: Born May 24, 1932, in London, England; son of Joseph (a tailor's machinist) and Leah (a tailor's machinist and cook; maiden name, Perlmutter) Wesker; married Doreen Cecile Bicker, November 14, 1958; children: Lindsay Joe, Tanya Jo, Daniel. EDUCATION: Attended the London School of Film Technique, 1955-56. POLITICS: Humanist. RELIGION: Jewish. MILITARY: Royal Air Force, 1950-52.

VOCATION: Writer and director.

CAREER: Also see *WRITINGS* below. PRINCIPAL STAGE WORK— Director: *The Friends,* Roundhouse Theatre, London, and in Stockholm, Sweden, both 1970; *Love Letters on Blue Paper,* National Theatre, London, 1978, then Oslo, Norway, 1980; *Yardsale,* Royal Shakespeare Company, Stratford-on-Avon, U.K., 1985; *Yardsale* and *Whatever Happened to Betty Lemon,* both Lyric Hammersmith Theatre, London, 1987; also *The Four Seasons,* Havana, Cuba, 1968; *The Old Ones,* Munich, West Germany, 1973; *Their Very Own and Golden City,* Aarhaus, Denmark, 1974; *The Merchant,* in

Canada, 1980; *The Entertainer,* Theatre Clwyd, Wales, 1983; and *Annie Wobbler,* Birmingham, U.K., and London, both 1984.

RELATED CAREER—Co-founder and artistic director, Centre 42, Ltd., London, 1961-70; chairman, International Theatre Institute (British section); co-president, International Playwrights Committee of the International Theatre Institute.

NON-RELATED CAREER—Carpenter's helper, bookseller's assistant, plumber's assistant, seed sorter, kitchen porter, and pastry cook in London, Norwich, U.K., and Paris, France, 1954-58.

WRITINGS: STAGE—*Chicken Soup with Barley,* Belgrade Theatre, Coventry, U.K., then Royal Court Theatre, London, both 1958, later Cleveland, OH, 1962, published in *New English Dramatists,* Penguin, 1959, in *The Wesker Trilogy,* Jonathan Cape, 1960, then Random House, 1961, published separately by Evans, 1961, and in *The Plays of Arnold Wesker,* Volume I, Harper, 1976; *Roots,* Belgrade Theatre, then Royal Court Theatre, both 1959, later Duke of York's Theatre, London, then Mayfair Theatre, New York City, both 1961, published by Penguin, 1959, then in *The Wesker Trilogy,* 1960, later in *The Plays of Arnold Wesker,* Volume I, 1976; *The Kitchen,* Royal Court Theatre, 1959, published in *New English Dramatists 2,* Penguin, 1960, expanded version produced at Royal Court Theatre, 1961, then New Theatre Workshop and New 81st Street Theatre, both New York City, 1966, published by Jonathan Cape, 1961, then Random House, 1962, later in *Three Plays,* Penguin, 1976, and in *The Plays of Arnold Wesker,* Volume I, 1976; *I'm Talking about Jerusalem,* Belgrade Theatre, then Royal Court Theatre, both 1960, published by Penguin, 1960, then in *The Wesker Trilogy,* 1960, later in *The Plays of Arnold Wesker,* Volume I, 1976; *Chips with Everything,* Royal Court Theatre, then Vaudeville Theatre, London, both 1962, later Plymouth Theatre, New York City, 1963, published by Jonathan Cape, 1962, then Random House, 1963, later in *The Plays of Arnold Wesker,* Volume I, 1976; *The Nottingham Captain: A Moral for Narrator, Voices, and Orchestra,* Centre 42 Festival, Wellingborough, U.K., 1962, published in *Six Sundays in January,* Jonathan Cape, 1971; *Their Very Own and Golden City,* Belgium National Theatre, Brussels, Belgium, 1964, then Royal Court Theatre, 1966, published by Jonathan Cape, 1966, then in *Three Plays,* 1976; later in *The Plays of Arnold Wesker,* Volume II, Harper, 1977.

The Four Seasons, Belgrade Theatre, then Saville Theatre, London, both 1965, later Theatre Four, New York City, 1968, published by Jonathan Cape, 1966, then in *Three Plays,* 1976, later in *The Plays of Arnold Wesker,* Volume II, 1977; *The Friends,* Stadsteater Theatre, Stockholm, Sweden, then Roundhouse Theatre, London, both 1970, published by Jonathan Cape, 1970, then in *The Plays of Arnold Wesker,* Volume II, 1977; *The Old Ones,* Royal Court Theatre, 1972, then Lambs Theatre, New York City, 1974, published by Jonathan Cape, 1973, then in *The Plays of Arnold Wesker,* Volume II, 1977; *The Wedding Feast,* Stadsteater Theatre, 1974, then Leeds Playhouse, Leeds, U.K., 1977, published by Jonathan Cape, 1973, then in *The Journalists, The Wedding Feast, The Merchant,* Penguin, 1980; *The Journalists,* Jackson's Lane Community Theatre, London, 1975, then Criterion Theatre, Coventry, 1977, published by Writer and Readers Publishing Cooperative, 1975, then in *The Journalists, The Wedding Feast, The Merchant,* 1980; *The Merchant,* Royal Dramatenteater, Stockholm, 1976, then Plymouth Theatre, New York City, 1977, later Birmingham Repertory Theatre, Birmingham, U.K., 1978, published in *The Journalists, The Wedding Feast, The Merchant,* 1980, then separately by Methuen, 1983; *Love Letters on Blue Paper,* Cottseloe Theatre, London, then Syracuse Stage, Syracuse,

NY, both 1978, later Folger Theatre, Washington, DC, 1980, published by Writer and Readers Publishing Cooperative, 1978.

Caritas, Cottesloe Theatre, 1981, published by Jonathan Cape, 1981; *Mothers: Four Protraits,* Mitzukoshi Theatre, Tokyo, Japan, 1982, published by Jonathan Cape, 1982; *Annie Wobbler,* Birmingham Repertory Theatre, 1983, then Westbeth Theatre Center, New York City, 1986. Also *Fatlips,* first produced in 1980; *Cinders,* first produced in 1983; *Sullied Hand,* first produced in Edinburgh, Scotland, 1984; *Yardsale,* first produced in Edinburgh, 1985, then London, 1987, published in *Plays International,* 1987; *One More Ride on the Merry-Go-Round,* first produced in Leicester, U.K., 1985; *Whatever Happened to Betty Lemon,* first produced in Paris, France, 1986, then London, 1987, published in *Plays International,* 1987; *When God Wanted a Son,* first produced in 1986; *Badenheim 1939,* first produced in 1987; *Shoeshine,* first produced in 1987; *Little Old Lady,* first produced in 1987; *Lady Othello,* first produced in 1987.

FILM—*The Kitchen,* Kingsley International, 1962; also *I'm Talking about Jerusalem,* 1979; *Lady Othello,* 1980.

TELEVISION—Episodic: "Menace," *First Night,* BBC, 1963, published in *Six Sundays in January,* Jonathan Cape, 1971, then in *The Plays of Arnold Wesker,* Harper, 1977. Plays: *Love Letters on Blue Paper,* BBC, 1976. Also *Breakfast,* 1981; *Thieves in the Night,* 1984-85.

RADIO—Plays: *Annie, Anna, Annabella,* 1983; *Yardsale,* 1984; *Bluey,* 1985.

OTHER—*Labour and the Arts II, or What, Then, Is to Be Done?,* Gemini, 1960; *The Modern Playwright, or "O Mother, Is It Worth It?"* Gemini, 1960; (introduction) *The Serving Boy,* by Roger Frith, Colchester, 1968; *Fears of Fragmentation* (essays), Jonathan Cape, 1970; *Six Sundays in January* (short stories), Jonathan Cape, 1971; *Say Goodbye, You May Never See Them Again: Scenes from Two East-End Backgrounds,* Jonathan Cape, 1974; *Love Letters on Blue Paper* (short stories), Jonathan Cape, 1974, then Harper, 1975, later Penguin, 1980; *Words as Definitions of Experience* (essays), Writers and Readers Publishing Cooperative, 1976; *Journey into Journalism: A Very Personal Account in Four Parts* (essays), Writers and Readers Publishing Cooperative, 1977; *Fatlips: A Story for Children,* Harper, 1978; *Said the Old Man to the Young Man: Three Stories* (short stories), Jonathan Cape, 1978.

AWARDS: Arts Council of Great Britain grant, 1958; Arts Council Bursary Award, *Evening Standard* Award, Most Promising British Playwright, 1959, and Encyclopaedia Britannica Award, 1960, all for *Chicken Soup with Barley; Variety* London Critics Poll, Best Play of the Year, 1963, for *Chips with Everything;* Premio Marzotto Drama Award, Best Unpublished Play, 1964, for *Their Very Own and Golden City;* Public and Critic's Gold Medal Award, 1973, for *The Kitchen;* Best Foreign Play Award (Spain), 1979.

SIDELIGHTS: RECREATIONS—Listening to records.

ADDRESSES: HOME—27 Bishops Road, London N6 4HR, England. AGENT—Nathan Joseph, NJ Media Enterprises, Ltd., 10 Clorane Gardens, London NW3 7PR, England.

WESTENBERG, Robert 1953-

PERSONAL: Born October 26, 1953, in Miami Beach, FL. EDU-CATION: Graduated from the University of California, Fresno; studied acting with the American Conservatory Theatre, San Francisco, CA, 1979-80.

VOCATION: Actor.

CAREER: OFF-BROADWAY DEBUT—Vintner and Sir Richard Vernon, *Henry IV, Part One,* New York Shakespeare Festival, Delacorte Theatre, 1981. PRINCIPAL STAGE APPEARANCES—R. Raymond Barker and Manfred, *The Death of Von Richthofen as Witnessed from Earth,* New York Shakespeare Festival (NYSF), Public Theatre, New York City, 1982; Laertes, *Hamlet,* NYSF, Public Theatre, 1983; Niko, *Zorba,* Broadway Theatre, New York City, 1983; soldier and Alex, then Georges Seurat, *Sunday in the Park with George,* Booth Theatre, New York City, 1984; John Proctor, *The Crucible,* Arena Stage, Washington, DC, 1987, then Jerusalem, Israel; Cinderella's Prince and the Wolf, *Into the Woods,* Martin Beck Theatre, New York City, 1987. Also appeared at the Arena Stage, 1985-86.

MAJOR TOURS—Niko, *Zorba,* U.S. cities, 1983.

PRINCIPAL TELEVISION APPEARANCES—Specials: Soldier and Alex, *Sunday in the Park with George,* PBS, 1986.

RELATED CAREER—Company member, American Conservatory Theatre, San Francisco, CA, 1979-80; member, Arena Acting Company, Arena Stage, Washington, DC, 1980-81, then 1986-87.

AWARDS: Theatre World Award, 1984, for *Zorba;* Drama Desk Award and Antoinette Perry Award nomination, both Best Featured Actor in a Musical, 1988, for *Into the Woods.**

*   *   *

WEXLER, Haskell 1926-

PERSONAL: Born in 1926 in Chicago, IL; son of Simon Wexler; married Nancy Ashenhurst (divorced); married Marian Witt (divorced); children: two (first marriage); Mark (second marriage). EDUCATION: Graduated from the University of Chicago.

VOCATION: Cinematographer, director, producer, and writer.

CAREER: Also see *WRITINGS* below. PRINCIPAL FILM APPEARANCES—*Underground* (documentary), New Yorker, 1976. FIRST FILM WORK—Cinematographer, *Stakeout on Dope Street* (uncredited), Warner Brothers, 1958. PRINCIPAL FILM WORK—All as cinematographer, unless indicated: Second unit photographer, *Picnic,* Columbia, 1955; *Five Bold Women,* Citation, 1959; (with Jack Couffer and Helen Levitt) *The Savage Eye,* Trans-Lux, 1960; *Studs Lonigan,* United Artists, 1960; (with Jack Marta) *Angel Baby,* Allied Artists, 1961; *The Hoodlum Priest,* United Artists, 1961; *America, America* (also known as *The Anatolian Smile*), Warner Brothers, 1963; *A Face in the Rain,* Embassy, 1963; *Lonnie,* Futuramic, 1963; *The Best Man,* United Artists, 1964; (also producer, with John Calley) *The Loved One,* Metro-Goldwyn-Mayer (MGM), 1965; (also director and producer) *The Bus* (documentary), Harrison Pictures, 1965; (with Harry Stradling) *Who's Afraid of Virginia Woolf?,* Warner Brothers, 1966; *In the Heat of the Night,* United Artists, 1967; *The Thomas Crown Affair* (also known as *Thomas Crown and Company* and *The Crown Caper*), United Artists, 1968; (also producer, with Jerrold Wexler, and director) *Medium Cool,* Paramount, 1969.

Interviews with My Lai Veterans (documentary short film), Laser, 1970; (with others) *Gimme Shelter,* Cinema V, 1970; (also co-producer and co-director) *Brazil: A Report on Torture* (documentary), New Yorker, 1971; *The Trial of the Catonsville Nine,* Melville, 1972; consultant, *American Graffiti,* Universal, 1973; *Introduction to the Enemy* (documentary), IPC, 1974; (with William Fraker and Bill Butler) *One Flew Over the Cuckoo's Nest,* United Artists, 1975; *Bound for Glory,* United Artists, 1976; (also co-producer and co-director) *Underground* (documentary), New Yorker, 1976; *Coming Home,* United Artists, 1978; additional photography, *Days of Heaven,* Paramount, 1978; *CIA: Case Officer* (documentary short film), Institute for Policy Studies, 1978; additional photography, *The Rose,* Twentieth Century-Fox, 1979; (also documentary footage director) *No Nukes,* Warner Brothers, 1980; *Second-Hand Hearts* (also known as *Hamsters of Happiness*), Paramount, 1981; *Lookin' to Get Out,* Paramount, 1982; *Richard Pryor Live on the Sunset Strip,* Columbia, 1982; additional photography, *The Black Stallion Returns,* Metro-Goldwyn-Mayer/United Artists, 1983; *The Man Who Loved Women,* Columbia, 1983; director, *Latino,* Cinecom, 1985; *Three for the Road,* New Century/Vista, 1987; *Matewan,* Cinecom, 1987; *Colors,* Orion, 1988; *Three Fugitives,* Buena Vista/Warner Brothers, 1989. Also cinematographer and director, *The Living City* (short film), 1955; cinematographer, *Jangadero,* 1961; cinematographer, *T for Tumbleweed* (short film), 1962; cinematographer, co-producer, and co-director, *Interview with President Allende* (documentary), 1971; cinematographer, *Target Nicaragua: Inside a Secret War* (documentary), 1983; and cinematographer, director, and producer, *Bus II* (documentary), 1983.

PRINCIPAL TELEVISION WORK—Movies: Special photography, *The Kid from Nowhere,* NBC, 1982.

RELATED CAREER—Cinematographer of educational and industrial films for ten years; founder (with Conrad Hall), Wexler-Hall, Inc. (a television commercial production company), during the mid-1970s.

NON-RELATED CAREER—Merchant seaman for four years.

WRITINGS: FILM—*The Bus* (documentary), Harrison Pictures, 1965; *Medium Cool,* Paramount, 1969; (with others) *Introduction to the Enemy* (documentary), IPC, 1974; (with others) *Underground* (documentary), New Yorker, 1976; *Latino,* Cinecom, 1985.

AWARDS: Academy Award, Best Cinematography (Black and White), 1966, for *Who's Afraid of Virginia Woolf?;* Academy Award nomination, Best Cinematography, 1975, for *One Flew Over the Cuckoo's Nest;* Academy Award, Best Cinematography, 1976, for *Bound for Glory;* American Society of Cinematographers Award nomination, Outstanding Achievement in Cinematography for a 1987 Feature Film, and Academy Award nomination, Best Cinematography, 1988, both for *Matewan.*

ADDRESSES: OFFICE—3659 Las Flores Canyon Road, Malibu, CA 90265.*

PRINCIPAL TELEVISION APPEARANCES—Series: Mr. Baxter, *The Guiding Light.*

RELATED CAREER—Board of directors, Vietnam Veterans Ensemble Theatre Company; actor in industrial films and commercials.

NON-RELATED CAREER—Consultant, National Executive Service Corps.

AWARDS: Military honors: Pacific Theater Ribbon and two Battle Stars.

MEMBER: Princeton Club (vice president and house committee chairor, 1986—), Canterbury Choral Society (president, 1980-81).

SIDELIGHTS: FAVORITE ROLES—Ambassador Wade in *The Killing Fields* and Dr. Abel in *Hannah and Her Sisters.*

ADDRESSES: OFFICE—One Gracie Terrace, Apartment 4-F, New York, NY 10028. AGENT—The Gersh Agency, 130 W. 42nd Street, New York, NY 10036.

*   *   *

WHITEMORE, Hugh   1936-

PERSONAL: Born June 16, 1936, in Tunbridge Wells, England; married Jill Brooke, 1961 (divorced); married Sheila Lemon, 1976; children: one son (second marriage). EDUCATION: Attended the Royal Academy of Dramatic Art, 1956-57.

VOCATION: Writer.

WRITINGS: STAGE—*Stevie: A Play from the Life and Work of Stevie Smith,* first produced in Richmond, U.K., then Vaudeville Theatre, London, both 1977, later Manhattan Theatre Club, New York City, 1979, published by Samuel French, Inc., 1977, then Limelight, 1984; *Pack of Lies,* first produced in Brighton, U.K., then Lyric Theatre, London, both 1983, later Royale Theatre, New York City, 1985, published by Amber Lane Press, 1983, then Applause, 1986; *Breaking the Code,* Haymarket Theatre, London, 1986, then Eisenhower Theatre, Kennedy Center for the Performing Arts, Washington, DC, later Neil Simon Theatre, New York City, both 1987, published by Amber Lane Press, 1987; *Best of Friends,* Apollo Theatre, London, 1988.

FILM—(With Jane Gaskell) *All Neat in Black Stockings,* Warner Brothers/Pathe, 1969; (with Ivan Foxwell and Alan Hackney) *Decline and Fall . . . of a Bird Watcher* (also known as *Decline and Fall*), Twentieth Century-Fox, 1969; (with John Junkin) *Man at the Top,* Anglo-EMI, 1973; *All Creatures Great and Small,* EMI, 1975; (with Alfred Hayes and Alexi Kapler) *The Blue Bird,* Twentieth Century-Fox, 1976; *Stevie,* First Artists, 1978; *The Return of the Soldier,* Twentieth Century-Fox, 1983; *84 Charing Cross Road,* Columbia, 1987.

TELEVISION—Series: *All for Love.* Mini-Series: (With Douglas Livingstone, Alan Plater, and Ken Taylor) *Shoulder to Shoulder,* BBC, then *Masterpiece Theatre,* PBS, 1975; *Moll Flanders,* BBC, 1975, then PBS, 1980; *Rebecca,* BBC, 1979, then *Mystery!,* PBS, 1980; ''Concealed Enemies,'' *American Playhouse,* PBS, 1984; *My Cousin Rachel,* BBC, then *Mystery!,* PBS, 1985. Episodic:

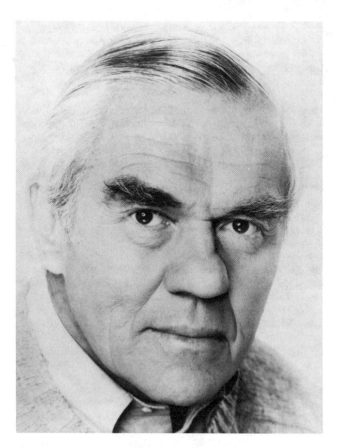

IRA WHEELER

WHEELER, Ira   1920-

PERSONAL: Born November 9, 1920, in New York, NY; son of Ira B. (an executive) and Helen (Muir) Wheeler; married Grace Elizabeth Tufts, November 1, 1942 (divorced, 1968); married Mary Walker Tison (an executive recruiter), April 25, 1981; children: Dorothy T., Ann D., Timothy M. EDUCATION: Princeton University, B.A., 1942; studied acting with Anthony Mannino at Drama Tree, and with Tony Barr. POLITICS: Democrat. RELIGION: Protestant. MILITARY: U.S. Coast Guard, lieutenant, 1942-46.

VOCATION: Actor.

CAREER: PRINCIPAL STAGE APPEARANCES—Grumio, *The Taming of the Shrew,* New Canaan Town Players, New Canaan, CT; also usher, *Trial by Jury,* chorus member, *Yeoman of the Guard,* chorus member, *Patience,* and chorus member, *The Sorcerer,* all Blue Hill Troupe, Ltd.

FILM DEBUT—Bill Whitelaw, *Rollover,* Warner Brothers, 1981. PRINCIPAL FILM APPEARANCES—Ambassador Wade, *The Killing Fields,* Warner Brothers, 1984; Dr. Abel, *Hannah and Her Sisters,* Orion, 1986; Dr. Monroe, *Radio Days,* Orion, 1987; Roland Owens, *The Secret of My Success,* Universal, 1987; Jay Raines, *September,* Orion, 1987; newscaster, *Wall Street,* Twentieth Century-Fox, 1987; Mr. Bates, *New York Stories,* Touchstone, 1989; also appeared in *Swimming to Cambodia,* Cinecom, 1989; and as Charles Fairchild, *Masquerade,* Metro-Goldwyn-Mayer.

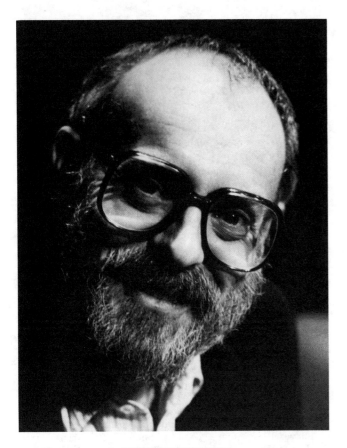

HUGH WHITEMORE

"Act of Betrayal," *Play for Today*, BBC, 1971; "Breeze Anstey," *Country Matters*, 1972; "Horrible Conspiracies," *Elizabeth R*, published in *Elizabeth R*, Elek, 1972; also *The Wednesday Play*, *Armchair Theatre*, and *Play of the Month*. Movies: *The Adventures of Don Quixote*, CBS, 1973; *All Creatures Great and Small*, NBC, 1975.

Plays: *The Full Chatter*, 1963; *Dan, Dan the Charity Man*, 1965; *Angus Slowly Sinking*, 1965; *The Regulator*, 1965; *Application Form*, 1965; *Mrs. Bixby and the Colonel's Coat*, 1965; *Macready's Gala*, 1966; *Final Demand*, 1966; *Girl of My Dreams*, 1966; *Frankenstein Mark II*, 1966; *Amerika*, 1966; *What's Wrong with Humpty Dumpty?*, 1967; *Party Games*, 1968; *The Last of the Big Spenders*, 1968; *Hello, Good Evening, and Welcome*, 1968; *Mr. Guppy's Tale*, 1969; *Unexpectedly Vacant*, 1970; *The King and His Keeper*, 1970; *Killing Time*, 1970; *Cider with Rosie*, 1971; *An Object of Affection*, 1971; *The Strange Shapes of Reality*, 1972; *The Serpent and the Comforter*, 1972; *At the Villa Pandora*, 1972; *Eric*, 1972; *Disappearing Trick*, 1972; *Good at Games*, 1972; *Bedtime*, 1972; *Intruders*, 1972; *Deliver Us from Evil*, 1973; *The Pearcross Girls*, 1973; *A Thinking Man as Hero*, 1973; *Death Waltz*, 1974; *Outrage*, 1974; *David Copperfield*, 1974; *Trilby*, 1975; *Goodbye*, 1975; *84 Charing Cross Road*, 1975; (with Brian Clark and Clive Exton) *The Eleventh Hour*, 1975; (with David Edgar and Robert Muller) *Censors*, 1975; *Brensham People*, 1976; *William Wilson*, 1976; *Moths*, 1977; *Exiles*, 1977; *Dummy*, 1977; *Mrs. Ainsworth*, 1978; *Losing Her*, 1978; *Contract*, 1981; *A Dedicated Man*, 1982; *I Remember Nelson*, 1982; *A Bit of Singing and Dancing*, 1982; *Lovers of Their Time*, 1982; *Down at the Hydro*, 1983; *The Boy in the Bush*, 1984.

RELATED CAREER—Former drama critic, *Harpers* and *Queen* magazines.

AWARDS: Emmy Award, 1970, for "Horrible Conspiracies," *Elizabeth R;* Writers Guild Award, 1971, for *Cider with Rosie;* Writers Guild Award, 1972, for *Country Matters;* RAI Prize, 1979, for *Dummy;* Prix Italia, 1979; Neil Simon Jury Award and Emmy Award, Best Mini-Series, both 1984, for *Concealed Enemies;* Society of the West End Theatre Award nomination for *Pack of Lies;* British Academy of Film and Television Arts Award nomination for *84 Charing Cross Road*.

ADDRESSES: OFFICE—Hugh Whitemore, Ltd., 170 Finchley Road, London NW3 6BP, England. AGENTS—Judy Daish Associates, 83 Eastbourne Mews, London W2 6LQ, England; Phyllis Wender, Rosenstone and Wender, 3 E. 48th Street, 4th Floor, New York, NY 10017.

*   *   *

WHITFORD, Bradley

PERSONAL: EDUCATION: Graduated from Wesleyan University; trained for the stage at the Juilliard Theatre Center.

VOCATION: Actor.

CAREER: PRINCIPAL STAGE APPEARANCES—Wesley, *Curse of the Starving Class*, Promenade Theatre, New York City, 1985; Claudio, *Measure for Measure*, Mitzi E. Newhouse Theatre, New York City, 1989. Also appeared as Oberon and Theseus, *A Midsummer Night's Dream*, Hartford Stage Company, Hartford, CT; Richmond, *Richard III*, Tyrone Guthrie Theatre, Minneapolis, MN; Paris, *Romeo and Juliet*, and Kyle, *Human Gravity*, both in New York City.

PRINCIPAL FILM APPEARANCES—Terry Reilly, *Doorman*, Manley Productions, 1986; Mike Tedwell, *Adventures in Babysitting*, Buena Vista, 1987; Roger, *Revenge of the Nerds II: Nerds in Paradise*, Twentieth Century-Fox, 1987.

PRINCIPAL TELEVISION APPEARANCES—Pilots: Leon Trepper, *C.A.T. Squad*, NBC, 1986. Episodic: Dillart, *The Equalizer*, CBS, 1985; also *The Guiding Light*, CBS; *All My Children*, ABC; *Tales from the Darkside*, syndicated. Movies: Jack Ford, *The Betty Ford Story*, ABC, 1987.

ADDRESSES: AGENT—Triad Artists Agency, 10100 Santa Monica Boulevard, 16th Floor, Los Angeles, CA 90067.*

*   *   *

WHITMORE, James   1921-

PERSONAL: Full name, James Allen Whitmore, Jr.; born October 1, 1921, in White Plains, NY; son of James Allen and Florence Belle (Crane) Whitmore; married Audra Lindley (an actress), 1971 (divorced, 1978); married Nancy Mygatt, March 24, 1978 (divorced); children: James, Steven, Daniel. EDUCATION: Yale University, B.A., 1942; trained for the stage at the American Theatre

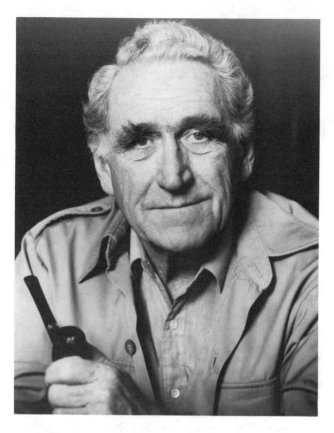

JAMES WHITMORE

Wing School, 1947. MILITARY: U.S. Marine Corps Reserves, 1942-46.

VOCATION: Actor.

CAREER: STAGE DEBUT—Appeared with the Players, Peterboro, NH, 1947. BROADWAY DEBUT—Sergeant Harold Evans, *Command Decision,* Fulton Theatre, 1947. PRINCIPAL STAGE APPEARANCES—Title role, *Peer Gynt,* University of California, Los Angeles, Los Angeles, CA, 1953; Barney, *Summer of the Seventeenth Doll,* Bucks County Playhouse, New Hope, PA, 1958; Tom Willard, *Winesburg, Ohio,* National Theatre, New York City, 1958; narrator, *Under Milk Wood,* University of California, Los Angeles, 1959; title role, *Brand,* Fresno State College, Fresno, CA, 1961; title role, *Gideon,* Playhouse on the Mall, Paramus, NJ, 1963; Emanuel Bloch, *Inquest,* Music Box Theatre, New York City, 1970; title role, *Will Rogers' USA* (one-man show), Ford's Theatre, Washington, DC, 1970, then Helen Hayes Theatre, New York City, 1974; President Harry S. Truman, *Give 'em Hell Harry!* (one-man show), Ford's Theatre, 1975; Theodore Roosevelt, *Bully* (one-man show), 46th Street Theatre, New York City, then Tyrone Guthrie Theatre, Minneapolis, MN, both 1977; title role, *Will Rogers' USA* (one-man show), Ford's Theatre, 1978; the Colonel, *Almost an Eagle,* Longacre Theatre, New York City, 1982; Don, *Elba,* Manhattan Theatre Club, New York City, 1983; Will Rogers, *Parade of Stars Playing the Palace,* Palace Theatre, New York City, 1983; Henry Pulaski, *Handy Dandy,* Syracuse Stage, Syracuse, NY, and John Drew Theatre, East Hampton, NY, both 1985; title role, *Will Rogers' USA* (one-man show), Ford's Theatre, 1984; He, *The Eighties,* George Street Playhouse, New Brunswick, NJ, 1989. Also appeared as Starbuck, *The Rainmaker,* La Jolla,

CA, 1954; Mr. Antrobus, *The Skin of Our Teeth,* 1957; and in *The Magnificent Yankee,* Eisenhower Theatre, Kennedy Center for the Performing Arts, Washington, DC, 1976.

MAJOR TOURS—Title role, *Will Rogers' USA* (one-man show), U.S. cities, 1970-72, 1974, and 1977; President Harry S. Truman, *Give 'em Hell, Harry!* (one-man show), U.S. cities, 1975; Theodore Roosevelt, *Bully* (one-man show), U.S. cities, 1977.

FILM DEBUT—Kinnie, *Battleground,* Metro-Goldwyn-Mayer, 1949. PRINCIPAL FILM APPEARANCES—George Pappas, *The Undercover Man,* Columbia, 1949; Gus Ninissi, *The Asphalt Jungle,* Metro-Goldwyn-Mayer (MGM), 1950; John J. Malone, *Mrs. O'Malley and Mr. Malone,* MGM, 1950; Joe Smith, *The Next Voice You Hear,* MGM, 1950; Clint Priest, *The Outriders,* MGM, 1950; Vincent Maran, *Please Believe Me,* MGM, 1950; Mr. Stacey, *It's a Big Country,* MGM, 1951; narrator, *The Red Badge of Courage,* MGM, 1951; Lou, *Shadow in the Sky,* MGM, 1951; Sergeant Batterson, *Because You're Mine,* MGM, 1952; Major Uanna, *Above and Beyond,* MGM, 1953; Fetcher, *All the Brothers Were Valiant,* MGM, 1953; Charles "Chico" Menlow, *The Girl Who Had Everything,* MGM, 1953; Remlick, *The Great Diamond Robbery,* MGM, 1953; Slug, *Kiss Me Kate,* MGM, 1953; Sergeant Elliott, *The Command,* Warner Brothers, 1954; Sergeant Ben Peterson, *Them!,* Warner Brothers, 1954; Gus, *The Last Frontier* (also known as *Savage Wilderness*), Columbia, 1955; Ty Whitman, *The McConnell Story* (also known as *Tiger in the Sky*), Warner Brothers, 1955; Carnes, *Oklahoma!,* Magna Theatres, 1955; Sergeant Mac, *Battle Cry,* Warner Brothers, 1955; Ben Wagner, *Crime in the Streets,* Allied Artists, 1956; Lou Sherwood, *The Eddy Duchin Story,* Columbia, 1956; Rudy Krist, *The Young Don't Cry,* Columbia, 1957; Commander Meredith, *The Deep Six,* Warner Brothers, 1958; Ed Henderson, *The Restless Years* (also known as *The Wonderful Years*), Universal, 1958; Monk Johnson, *Face of Fire,* Allied Artists, 1959.

Harry Powell, *Who Was That Lady?,* Columbia, 1960; John Finley Horton, *Black Like Me,* Continental, 1964; Trent, *Chuka,* Paramount, 1967; Captain Shipley, *Waterhole No. 3,* Paramount, 1967; Chief Inspector Charles Kane, *Madigan,* Universal, 1968; Captain Mike Riley, *Nobody's Perfect,* Universal, 1968; President of the Assembly, *Planet of the Apes,* Twentieth Century-Fox, 1968; Herb Sutro, *The Split,* MGM, 1968; Levi Morgan, *Guns of the Magnificent Seven,* United Artists, 1969; Admiral William F. Halsey, *Tora! Tora! Tora!,* Twentieth Century-Fox, 1970; Joshua Everett, *Chato's Land,* United Artists, 1972; Philip Tenhausen, *The Harrad Experiment,* Cinerama, 1973; Grandpa, *Where the Red Fern Grows,* Doty-Dayton, 1974; Harry S. Truman, *Give 'em Hell, Harry,* Theatre Television, 1975; priest, *The Serpent's Egg* (also known as *Das Schlangenei*), Paramount, 1977; Jupiter, *The Hills Have Eyes,* Vanguard, 1978; Theodore Roosevelt, *Bully,* Emerson, 1978; Dr. Sanford Ferguson, *The First Deadly Sin,* Filmways, 1980; voice of Mark Twain, *The Adventures of Mark Twain* (also known as *Mark Twain*), Harbour Towns, 1985; Judge Stanley Murdoch, *Nuts,* Warner Brothers, 1987. Also appeared in *Across the Wide Missouri,* MGM, 1951.

PRINCIPAL TELEVISION APPEARANCES—Series: Abraham Lincoln Jones, *The Law and Mr. Jones,* ABC, 1960-62; host and narrator, *Survival,* syndicated, 1964; Professor John Woodruff, *My Friend Tony,* NBC, 1969; Dr. Vincent Campanelli, *Temperatures Rising,* ABC, 1972-73; host, *Comeback,* syndicated, 1979. Mini-Series: George Wheeler, *The Word,* CBS, 1978; Clifford Casey, *Celebrity,* NBC, 1984; host, *West of the Imagination,* PBS, 1986; President Dan Baker, *Favorite Son,* NBC, 1988. Pilots: Joel

Begley, "Checkmate," *Zane Grey Theatre* (also known as *Dick Powell's Zane Grey Theatre*), CBS, 1959. Episodic: William Benteen, "On Thursday We Leave for Home," *The Twilight Zone,* CBS, 1963; Scrooge, *George Burns Comedy Week,* CBS, 1985; Ben Wilkerson, *Riptide,* NBC, 1985; Joe Keller, "All My Sons," *American Playhouse,* PBS, 1987; also *Panic!,* NBC, 1957; *Alcoa Premiere,* ABC; *The Desilu Playhouse,* CBS; *Playhouse 90,* CBS; *Kraft Television Theatre,* NBC; *Cowboy in Africa,* ABC.

Movies: Overman, *The Challenge,* ABC, 1970; Frank Phillips, *If Tomorrow Comes,* ABC, 1971; General Oliver O. Howard, *I Will Fight No More Forever,* ABC, 1975; Dwight Hamilton, *Mark, I Love You,* CBS, 1980; Hugh Borski, *Rage,* NBC, 1980; Lester Babbitt, *Glory! Glory!,* HBO, 1989. Specials: Title role, *Will Rogers' USA,* CBS, 1972; *Celebration: The American Spirit,* ABC, 1976; *General Electric's All-Star Anniversary,* ABC, 1978; *A Celebration at Ford's Theatre,* NBC, 1978; narrator, "Love Those Trains," *National Geographic Special,* PBS, 1984; narrator, "Chesapeake Borne," *National Geographic Special,* PBS, 1986.

AWARDS: Comedy Award from the American Academy of Humor, 1947; Antoinette Perry Award and Theatre World Award, both 1948, for *Command Decision;* Academy Award nomination, Best Supporting Actor, 1949, for *Battleground;* Academy Award nomination, Best Actor, 1975, for *Give 'em Hell, Harry.*

MEMBER: Actors' Equity Association, American Federation of Television and Radio Artists, Screen Actors Guild.

ADDRESSES: AGENT—Abrams, Rubaloff, and Lawrence, 8075 W. Third Street, Suite 303, Los Angeles, CA 90048.*

*   *   *

WICKES, Mary

PERSONAL: Born Mary Isabella Wickenhauser, June 13, in St. Louis, MO; daughter of Frank August (a banker) and Mary Isabella (a civic leader; maiden name, Shannon) Wickenhauser. EDUCATION: Received B.A. from Washington University; graduate work, theatre arts, University of California, Los Angeles. RELIGION: Episcopalian.

VOCATION: Actress and teacher.

CAREER: STAGE DEBUT—With the Berkshire Playhouse, Stockbridge, MA, 1934. BROADWAY DEBUT—Understudy for the role of Lucy Gurget, *The Farmer Takes a Wife,* 46th Street Theatre, 1934. PRINCIPAL STAGE APPEARANCES—Mary McCune (Little Mary), *Stage Door,* Music Box Theatre, New York City, 1936; Mildred, *Spring Dance,* Empire Theatre, New York City, 1936; Annie, *Father Malachy's Miracle,* Guild Theatre, New York City, 1937; Christine, *Danton's Death,* Mercury Theatre, New York City, 1938; Miss Preen, *The Man Who Came to Dinner,* Music Box Theatre, 1939; Annabelle Fuller, *George Washington Slept Here,* Bucks County Playhouse, New Hope, PA, 1941; Nancy Parker, *Jackpot,* Alvin Theatre, New York City, 1944; Amelia, *Dark Hammock,* Forrest Theatre, New York City, 1944; Miss Hebe, *Hollywood Pinafore,* Alvin Theatre, 1945; Nina Stover, *Apple of His Eye,* Biltmore Theatre, New York City, 1946; title role, *Elizabeth the Queen,* Berkshire Playhouse, Stockbridge, MA, 1946; Mrs. Betty Nelson, *Park Avenue,* Shubert Theatre, New

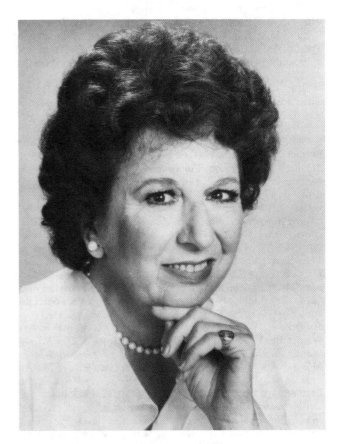

MARY WICKES

York City, 1946; Esther Murray, *Town House,* National Theatre, New York City, 1948.

Mrs. Noah, *The Mystery Cycle,* American Conservatory Theatre, San Francisco, CA, 1972; Penny, *You Can't Take It with You,* and Goody Nurse, *The Crucible,* both American Conservatory Theatre, 1973; Juno, *Juno and the Paycock,* Center Theatre Group, Mark Taper Forum, Los Angeles, CA, 1974; Aunt Eller, *Oklahoma!,* Palace Theatre, New York City, then Kennedy Center for the Performing Arts, Washington, DC, both 1979; Mistress Quickly, *Henry IV, Part I,* American Shakespeare Festival, Stratford, CT, 1982; Rosemary, *The Palace of Amateurs,* Berkshire Theatre Festival, 1982; Willie, *Detective Story,* Center Theatre Group, Ahmanson Theatre, Los Angeles, 1983, then Auditorium, Denver, CO, 1984; Stella, *Light Up the Sky,* Coconut Grove Playhouse, Coconut Grove, FL, 1983; Betty Meeks, *The Foreigner,* Alliance Theatre Company, Atlanta, GA, 1986. Also appeared in *Biography,* Berkshire Playhouse, 1934; *One Good Year,* Lyceum Theatre, New York City, 1935; *Swing Your Lady,* Booth Theatre, New York City, 1937; *Hitch Your Wagon,* 48th Street Theatre, New York City, 1937; *Too Much Johnson,* 1938; *Stars in Your Eyes,* Majestic Theatre, New York City, 1939; *Hey Day,* Shubert Theatre, New Haven, CT, 1947; as Amanda Wingfield, *The Glass Menagerie,* Washington University, St. Louis, MO; Lady Jane, *Patience,* Eulalie McKechnie Shinn, *The Music Man,* Parthy Ann, *Show Boat,* and Clothilde, *The New Moon,* all St. Louis Municipal Opera, St. Louis; Lady Bracknell, *The Importance of Being Earnest,* College of William and Mary, Williamsburg, VA; *Wonderful Town,* Los Angeles Civic Light Opera, Dorothy Chandler Pavilion, Los Angeles; in one-woman show, Geary Theatre, San Francisco;

with the St. Louis Little Theatre, St. Louis; Cape Playhouse, Dennis, MA; Houston Music Theatre, Houston, TX; Starlight Theatre; Arthur Casey Stock Company; Woodstock Playhouse; and in more than eighty productions with the Berkshire Playhouse.

MAJOR TOURS—Nancy Parker, *Jackpot,* U.S. cities, 1941; Madame Arcati, *Blithe Spirit,* U.S. cities, 1966; Aunt Eller, *Oklahoma!,* U.S. cities, 1979.

FILM DEBUT—Miss Preen, *The Man Who Came to Dinner,* Warner Brothers, 1942. PRINCIPAL FILM APPEARANCES—Sarah Miller, *Blondie's Blessed Event,* Columbia, 1942; Mamie, *The Mayor of 44th Street,* RKO, 1942; Dora Pickford, *Now, Voyager,* Warner Brothers, 1942; Bonnie-Belle Schlopkiss, *Private Buckaroo,* Universal, 1942; Juliet Collins, *Who Done It?,* Universal, 1942; Emmy, *Happy Land,* Twentieth Century-Fox, 1943; Sandy, *Higher and Higher,* RKO, 1943; Mike Tracy, *How's About It?,* Universal, 1943; Agnes Willoughby, *My Kingdom for a Cook,* Columbia, 1943; Susie Dugan, *Rhythm of the Islands,* Universal, 1943; Clara, *The Decision of Christopher Blake,* Warner Brothers, 1948; Rosemary McNally, *June Bride,* Warner Brothers, 1948; Stella, *Anna Lucasta,* Columbia, 1949; Professor Whitman, *The Petty Girl* (also known as *Girl of the Year*), Columbia, 1950; Anna, *I'll See You in My Dreams,* Warner Brothers, 1951; Stella, *On Moonlight Bay,* Warner Brothers, 1951; Mrs. Foster, *The Story of Will Rogers,* Warner Brothers, 1952; Mrs. Gilpin, *Young Man with Ideas,* Metro-Goldwyn-Mayer (MGM), 1952; Emma Glavey, *The Actress,* MGM, 1953; Stella, *By the Light of the Silvery Moon,* Warner Brothers, 1953; Mrs. Watts, *Half a Hero,* MGM, 1953; Bessie Mae Curtis, *Destry,* Universal, 1954; Miss Wetter, *Ma and Pa Kettle at Home,* Universal, 1954; Emma, *White Christmas,* Paramount, 1954; Miss Ellwood, *Good Morning, Miss Dove,* Twentieth Century-Fox, 1955; Miss Mayberry, *Dance with Me, Henry,* United Artists, 1956; Janie, *Don't Go Near the Water,* MGM, 1957; Matilda Runyon, *It Happened to Jane* (also known as *Twinkle and Shine*), Columbia, 1959.

Mrs. Hefner, *Cimarron,* MGM, 1960; Marie Grieux, *The Sins of Rachel Cade* (also known as *Rachel Cade*), Warner Brothers, 1960; voice characterization, *One Hundred and One Dalmations* (animated), Buena Vista, 1961; Mrs. Squires, *The Music Man,* Warner Brothers, 1962; Miss Fox, *Dear Heart,* Warner Brothers, 1964; Mrs. Llewelyn, *Fate Is the Hunter,* Twentieth Century-Fox, 1964; Harold's secretary, *How to Murder Your Wife,* United Artists, 1965; Sister Clarissa, *The Trouble with Angels,* Columbia, 1966; Gloria Tritt, *The Spirit Is Willing,* Paramount, 1967; Sister Clarissa, *Where Angeles Go . . . Trouble Follows,* Columbia, 1968; clerk, *Napoleon and Samantha,* Buena Vista, 1972; Miss Wigginton, *Snowball Express,* Buena Vista, 1972; Margaret, *Touched by Love* (also known as *To Elvis, with Love*), Columbia, 1980. Also appeared in *Who's Minding the Store?,* Paramount, 1963.

TELEVISION DEBUT—Title role, "Mary Poppins," *Studio One,* CBS, 1946. PRINCIPAL TELEVISION APPEARANCES—Series: Regular, *Inside U.S.A. with Chevrolet,* CBS, 1949-50; Miss Wickes (the housekeeper), *The Peter Lind Hayes Show* (also known as *The Peter and Mary Show*), NBC, 1950; Martha (the maid), *Bonino,* NBC, 1953; Alice, *The Halls of Ivy,* CBS, 1954-55; Miss Esther Cathcart, *Dennis the Menace,* CBS, 1959-61; Maxfield, *The Gertrude Berg Show* (also known as *Mrs. G. Goes to College*), CBS, 1961-62; Melba Chegley, *Julia,* NBC, 1968-71; Zelda Marshall, *Sigmund and the Sea Monsters,* NBC, 1973; Beatrice Tully, *Doc,* 1975-76; Marie, *Father Dowling Mysteries,* NBC, 1989—. Pilots: Mrs. Medford, *The Monk,* ABC, 1969; Ma, *Ma and Pa,* CBS, 1974.

Episodic: Katie, "Annette," *The Mickey Mouse Club,* ABC, 1958; Alva Crane, *Murder, She Wrote,* CBS, 1985; Mrs. Umney, "The Canterville Ghost," *Wonderworks,* PBS, 1985; Mrs. Greyson, "Almost Partners," *Wonderworks,* PBS, 1987; Minnie, *Highway to Heaven,* NBC, 1988; also "U.F.O." *Kolchak: The Night Stalker,* ABC, 1974; "House Arrest," *M*A*S*H,* CBS, 1975; Jo Ballard, *The Jimmy Stewart Show,* NBC; plant lady, *Sesame Street,* PBS; *I Love Lucy,* CBS; *Playhouse 90,* CBS; *The Lucy Show,* CBS; *Here's Lucy,* CBS; *The Love Boat,* ABC; *The Waltons,* CBS; *Trapper John, M.D.,* CBS; *Matt Houston,* ABC; *Punky Brewster,* NBC; Elizabeth O'Neal, *Make Room for Daddy; Alfred Hitchcock Presents.* Movies: Eunice, *Willa,* CBS, 1979; Henrietta Sawyer, *The Christmas Gift,* CBS, 1986; Marie, *Fatal Confession: A Father Dowling Mystery,* NBC, 1987. Specials: Lizzie, *Time Out for Ginger,* CBS, 1955; *The Lucille Ball Special,* CBS, 1977; Miss Preen, "The Man Who Came to Dinner," *Hallmark Hall of Fame,* NBC, 1972; Ms. Crandall, "First the Egg," *ABC Afterschool Special,* ABC, 1985; Agatha Megpeace, *ALF Loves a Mystery,* NBC, 1987. Also appeared in *The Catbird Seat,* NBC.

PRINCIPAL RADIO APPEARANCES—Irma Barker, *Lorenzo Jones,* NBC.

RELATED CAREER—Teacher of acting and comedy seminars at Washington University, St. Louis, MO, College of William and Mary, Williamsburg, VA, and the American Conservatory Theatre, San Francisco, CA.

NON-RELATED CAREER—Chairor, National Crippled Children's Society, 1969; board of directors, Medical Auxiliary Center for Health Sciences, University of California, Los Angeles, 1977—; board of directors, Los Angeles Oncologic Institute, 1987—; member, Cancer Research Associates; auxiliary, Hospital of the Good Samaritan.

AWARDS: Emmy Award nomination, Best Supporting Actress in a Series, 1962, for *Mrs. G. Goes to College;* Outstanding Actress Award from the St. Louis Variety Clubs, 1967; Emmy Award nomination, 1975, for *M*A*S*H;* elected to the St. Louis Municipal Opera House Hall of Fame, 1987; awards for volunteer work from the Hospital of the Good Samaritan, University of California, Los Angeles, and the University of Southern California School of Medicine; Masons Humanitarian Award; Brass Tack Award from the St. Louis Junior Chamber of Commerce; Missouri Society for Crippled Children Award; Outstanding St. Louisan Award from the St. Louis *Globe-Democrat;* Missouri Woman of Achievement Award. Honorary degrees: Doctor of Arts, Washington University, St. Louis, MO, 1969.

MEMBER: Actors' Equity Association, American Federation of Television and Radio Artists, Screen Actors Guild, Academy of Motion Picture Arts and Sciences, National Academy of Television Arts and Sciences, Phi Mu.

ADDRESSES: AGENT—Artists Agency, 10000 Santa Monica Boulevard, Los Angeles, CA 90067.*

        *   *   *

WILDER, Gene   1935-

PERSONAL: Born Jerome Silberman, June 11, 1935, in Milwaukee, WI; son of William J. (an importer) and Jeanne (Baer)

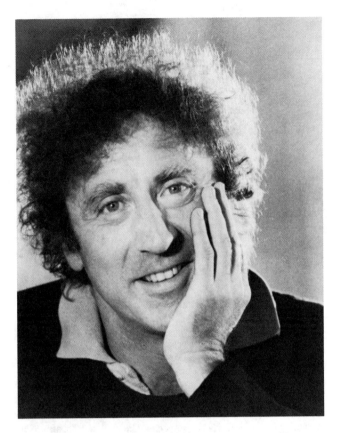

GENE WILDER

Silberman; married Mary Joan Schutz, October 27, 1967 (divorced, 1974); married Gilda Radner (an actress and comedienne) 1984 (died, May 20, 1989); children: Katharine Anastasia. EDUCATION: University of Iowa, B.A., 1955; studied acting with Herman Gottlieb, 1946-51, at the Bristol Old Vic Theatre School, 1955-56, at the Herbert Berghof Studio, 1957-59, and at the Actors Studio. MILITARY: U.S. Army, 1956-58.

VOCATION: Actor, director, producer, and screenwriter.

CAREER: Also see *WRITINGS* below. STAGE DEBUT—Balthazar, *Romeo and Juliet,* Milwaukee Playhouse, Milwaukee, WI, 1948. OFF-BROADWAY DEBUT—Frankie Bryant, *Roots,* Mayfair Theatre, 1961. PRINCIPAL STAGE APPEARANCES—Rosen, *The Late Christopher Bean,* Reginald Goode Theatre, Poughkeepsie, NY, 1949; Vernon, *Summer and Smoke,* Mansky, *The Play's the Thing,* and Mr. Weatherbee, *Arsenic and Old Lace,* all Tower Ranch Tenthouse Theatre, Eagle River, WI, 1951; Howard, *Death of a Salesman,* Ed, *Come Back, Little Sheba,* and the Principal, *The Happy Time,* all Tower Ranch Tenthouse Theatre, 1952; Andrew, *All the Way Home,* Playhouse-in-the-Park, Philadelphia, PA, 1961; hotel valet, *The Complaisant Lover,* Ethel Barrymore Theatre, New York City, 1961; the Captain, *Mother Courage and Her Children,* Martin Beck Theatre, New York City, 1963; Billie Bibbit, *One Flew over the Cuckoo's Nest,* Cort Theatre, New York City, 1963; Smiley, *Dynamite Tonight,* York Theatre, New York City, 1964; various roles, *The White House,* Henry Miller's Theatre, New York City, 1964; Harry Berlin, *Luv,* Royal Poinciana Playhouse, Palm Beach, FL, then Booth Theatre, New York City, both 1966. Also appeared in *The Cat and the Canary,* Reginald Goode Theatre, 1949; *The Drunkard,* Tower Ranch Tenthouse

Theatre, 1951; and in *Twelfth Night* and *Macbeth,* both Cambridge Drama Festival, Cambridge, MA, 1959.

MAJOR TOURS—Hotel valet, *The Complaisant Lover,* U.S. cities, 1962; Julius Sagamore, *The Millionairess,* Theatre Guild, U.S. cities, 1963; various roles, *The White House,* U.S. cities, 1964.

PRINCIPAL STAGE WORK—Fencing choreographer, *Twelfth Night* and *Macbeth,* both Cambridge Drama Festival, 1959.

FILM DEBUT—Eugene Grizzard, *Bonnie and Clyde,* Warner Brothers, 1967. PRINCIPAL FILM APPEARANCES—Leo Bloom, *The Producers,* Embassy, 1967; title role, *Quackser Fortune Has a Cousin in the Bronx* (also known as *Fun Loving*), UMC, 1970; Claude Coupe and Philippe DeSisi, *Start the Revolution without Me,* Warner Brothers, 1970; title role, *Willy Wonka and the Chocolate Factory,* Paramount, 1971; Dr. Ross, *Everything You Always Wanted to Know about Sex** (**but were afraid to ask*), United Artists, 1972; Jim, *Blazing Saddles,* Warner Brothers, 1974; the Fox, *The Little Prince,* Paramount, 1974; Stanley, *Rhinoceros,* American Film Theatre, 1974; Dr. Frederick Frankenstein, *Young Frankenstein,* Twentieth Century-Fox, 1974; Sigerson Holmes, *The Adventures of Sherlock Holmes' Smarter Brother,* Twentieth Century-Fox, 1975; George Caldwell, *Silver Streak,* Twentieth Century-Fox, 1976; Rudy Hickman/"Valentine," *The World's Greatest Lover,* Twentieth Century-Fox, 1977; Avram Belinsky, *The Frisco Kid* (also known as *No Knife*), Warner Brothers, 1979; Skip Donahue, *Stir Crazy,* Columbia, 1980; title role, "Skippy" in *Sunday Lovers,* United Artists, 1980; Michael Jordon, *Hanky Panky,* Columbia, 1982; Theodore Pierce, *The Woman in Red,* Orion, 1984; Larry Abbot, *Haunted Honeymoon,* Orion, 1986; as himself, *Hello Actors Studio* (documentary), Actors Studio, 1987; Dave, *See No Evil, Hear No Evil,* Tri-Star, 1989.

PRINCIPAL FILM WORK—Director: *The Adventures of Sherlock Holmes' Smarter Brother,* Twentieth Century-Fox, 1975; (also producer) *The World's Greatest Lover,* Twentieth Century-Fox, 1977; "Skippy" in *Sunday Lovers,* United Artists, 1980; *The Woman in Red,* Orion, 1984; (also producer) *Haunted Honeymoon,* Orion, 1986.

PRINCIPAL TELEVISION APPEARANCES—Episodic: Happy Penny, "Wingless Victory," *Play of the Week,* WNTA, 1961; Muller, "The Sound of Hunting," the Reporter, "Windfall," and Wilson, "The Interrogators," all *Dupont Show of the Week,* NBC, 1962; German voice, *The Twentieth Century,* CBS, 1962; head waiter, "Reunion with Death," *The Defenders,* CBS, 1962; Yonkel, "Home for Passover," *Eternal Light,* NBC, 1966; also *Armstrong Circle Theatre,* CBS, 1962. Movies: Harry Evers, *Thursday's Game,* ABC, 1974. Specials: Bernard, *Death of a Salesman,* CBS, 1966; Ernie, "The Office Sharers," *The Trouble with People,* NBC, 1972; *Marlo Thomas in Acts of Love—And Other Comedies,* ABC, 1973; *Annie and the Hoods,* ABC, 1974; *Baryshnikov in Hollywood,* CBS, 1982. Also appeared in *The Scarecrow,* 1972.

RELATED CAREER—Member, Actors Studio, New York City, 1961—.

NON-RELATED CAREER—Chauffeur, toy salesman, and fencing instructor.

WRITINGS: See production details above. FILM—(With Mel Brooks) *Young Frankenstein,* 1974; *The Adventures of Sherlock Holmes' Smarter Brother,* 1975; *The World's Greatest Lover,* 1977; "Skippy" in *Sunday Lovers,* 1980; (also song writer) *The*

Woman in Red, 1984; (with Terence Marsh) *Haunted Honeymoon,* 1986; (with Earl Barret, Arne Sultan, Eliot Wald, and Andrew Kurtzman) *See No Evil, Hear No Evil,* 1989.

AWARDS: Clarence Derwent Award, 1962, for *The Complaisant Lover;* Academy Award nomination, Best Supporting Actor, 1968, for *The Producers;* Academy Award nomination (with Mel Brooks), Best Screenplay Adapted from Other Material, 1974, for *Young Frankenstein.*

MEMBER: Actors' Equity Association, American Federation of Television and Radio Artists.

SIDELIGHTS: RECREATIONS—Tennis, fencing, and bridge.

ADDRESSES: OFFICE—9350 Wilshire Boulevard, Suite 400, Beverly Hills, CA 90212.

*   *   *

WILLARD, Fred   1939-

PERSONAL: Born September 18, 1939, in Shaker Heights, OH. EDUCATION: Graduated from the Virginia Military Institute.

VOCATION: Actor.

CAREER: PRINCIPAL THEATRE APPEARANCES—*The Return of the Second City in "20,000 Frozen Grenadiers,"* Square East Theatre, New York City, 1966; *Arf,* Stage 73, New York City, 1969; *Little Murders,* Circle in the Square, New York City, 1969.

PRINCIPAL FILM APPEARANCES—Gas station attendant, *The Model Shop,* Columbia, 1969; interrogator, *Hustle,* Paramount, 1975; Jerry Jarvis, *Silver Streak,* Twentieth Century-Fox, 1976; Bob, *Fun with Dick and Jane,* Columbia, 1977; Van Der Hoff, *Americathon,* United Artists, 1979; Presidential Assistant Feebleman, *First Family,* Warner Brothers, 1980; Robert, *How to Beat the High Cost of Living,* American International, 1980; Lieutenant Hookstratten, *This Is Spinal Tap* (also known as *Spinal Tap*), Embassy, 1984; Terrence "Doc" Williams, *Moving Violations,* Twentieth Century-Fox, 1985; Mayor Deebs, *Roxanne,* Columbia, 1987. Also appeared in *Jenny* (also known as *And Jenny Makes Three*), Cinerama, 1969; as an F.B.I. agent, *Chesty Anderson, U.S. Navy* (also known as *Anderson's Angels*), 1976; in *Cracking Up,* American International, 1977; and in *National Lampoon Goes to the Movies* (also known as *National Lampoon's Movie Madness*), 1981.

PRINCIPAL TELEVISION APPEARANCES—Series: Regular, *The Burns and Schreiber Comedy Hour,* ABC, 1973; Bud Nugent, *Sirota's Court,* NBC, 1976-77; Jerry Hubbard, *Forever Fernwood,* syndicated, 1977; Jerry Hubbard, *Fernwood 2-Night,* syndicated, 1977, renamed *America 2-Night,* syndicated, 1977-78; regular, *Real People,* NBC, 1979, then 1981-83; regular, *D.C. Follies,* syndicated, 1987—. Pilots: Bower, *Operation Greasepaint,* CBS, 1968; Captain Thomas Woods, *Space Force,* NBC, 1978; Jack LaRosa, *Flatbed Annie and Sweetiepie: Lady Truckers,* CBS, 1979; Ralph, *Pen 'n' Inc.,* CBS, 1981. Episodic: Tobin, "Tobin's Back in Town," *The Bob Newhart Show,* CBS, 1975; *Thicke of the Night,* syndicated, 1983 and 1984; also *SCTV Network 90,* NBC. Movies: Lance Colson, *How to Break Up a Happy Divorce,* NBC, 1976; Pearson, *Escape from Bogen County,* CBS, 1977; Larry Crockett, *Salem's Lot,* CBS, 1979; A.J. Foley, *Lots of Luck,*

Disney Channel, 1985. Specials: *Gabriel Kaplan Presents the Small Event,* ABC, 1977; *Battle of the Network Stars,* ABC, 1981.

RELATED CAREER—Member, Second City (an improvisational comedy troupe), Chicago, IL; member, Ace Trucking Company (an improvisational comedy troupe), San Francisco, CA.

ADDRESSES: AGENT—William Morris Agency, 151 El Camino Drive, Beverly Hills, CA 90212.*

*   *   *

WILLIAMS, Clarence III   1939-

PERSONAL: Born August 21, 1939, in New York, NY; married Gloria Foster (an actress), November, 1967. MILITARY: U.S. Army, 101st Airborn Division.

VOCATION: Actor.

CAREER: STAGE DEBUT—*Dark of the Moon,* New York City. BROADWAY DEBUT—Chris, *The Long Dream,* Ambassador Theatre, 1960. PRINCIPAL STAGE APPEARANCES—Washington Roach, *Walk in Darkness,* Greenwich Mews Theatre, New York City, 1963; the Sax, "Sarah and the Sax" in *Doubletalk,* Theatre De Lys, New York City, 1964; Randall, *Slow Dance on the Killing Ground,* Plymouth Theatre, New York City, 1964; Hector Case, *The Great Indoors,* Eugene O'Neill Theatre, New York City, 1966; Roosevelt, *The Party on Greenwich Avenue,* Cherry Lane Theatre, New York City, 1967; Hubert de Burgh, *King John,* New York Shakespeare Festival, Delacorte Theatre, New York City, 1967; Ray, *Suspenders,* New Federal Theatre, New York City, 1979; President Mageeba, *Night and Day,* American National Theatre and Academy Theatre, New York City, 1979. Also appeared as the Sax, *Sarah and the Sax,* summer theatre production, Dobbs Ferry, NY, 1964; and in *Does a Tiger Wear a Necktie?,* Spingold Theatre, Brandeis University, Waltham, MA, 1967.

PRINCIPAL FILM APPEARANCES—Blood, *The Cool World,* Cinema V, 1963; Father, *Purple Rain,* Warner Brothers, 1984; Bobby Shy, *52 Pick-Up,* Cannon, 1986; Bolo, *Tough Guys Don't Dance,* Cannon, 1987; Lieutenant Kevin White, *Perfect Victims,* Academy Home Entertainment, 1988; Kalinga, *I'm Gonna Git You Sucka,* Metro-Goldwyn-Mayer, 1989. Also appeared in *King: A Filmed Record . . . Montgomery to Memphis* (documentary), Commonwealth United, 1970.

PRINCIPAL TELEVISION APPEARANCES—Series: Linc Hayes, *The Mod Squad,* ABC, 1968-73. Episodic: Legba, *Miami Vice,* NBC, 1985; also *Daktari,* CBS, 1967; *The Danny Thomas Show,* NBC, 1968; *Tarzan,* NBC. Movies: Linc Hayes, *The Return of Mod Squad,* ABC, 1979; D.J. Johnson, *The Last Innocent Man,* HBO, 1987. Specials: Mr. Simpson, "The Hero Who Couldn't Read," *ABC Afterschool Special,* ABC, 1984.

RELATED CAREER—Artist in residence, Brandeis University, Waltham, MA, 1966-67.

NON-RELATED CAREER—Cook, bartender, and office worker.

AWARDS: Theatre World Award, 1965, for *Slow Dance on the Killing Ground.*

MEMBER: Actors' Equity Association.

ADDRESSES: AGENT—O'Neil, Abbott and Associates 375 S. Third Street, Suite 307, Burbank, CA 91502.*

*   *   *

WILLIAMS, Kenneth   1926-1988

PERSONAL: Born February 22, 1926, in London, England; died of a heart attack, April 15, 1988, in London; son of Charles George and Louise Alexandra (Morgan) Williams.

VOCATION: Actor.

CAREER: STAGE DEBUT—*Seven Keys to Baldpate*, Vic Theatre, Singapore, 1946. LONDON DEBUT—Slightly, *Peter Pan*, Scala Theatre, 1952. PRINCIPAL STAGE APPEARANCES—Ninian, *The First Mrs. Fraser*, Newquay Repertory Theatre, Cornwall, U.K., 1948; Dauphin, *Saint Joan*, Arts Theatre, London, 1954, then St. Martin's Theatre, London, 1955; Elijah, *Moby Dick*, Duke of York's Theatre, London, 1955; Montgomery, *The Buccaneer*, Lyric Hammersmith Theatre, London, 1955, then Apollo Theatre, London, 1956; Maxime, *Hotel Paradiso*, Winter Garden Theatre, London, 1956; Kite, *The Wit to Woo*, Arts Theatre, 1957; Green, *Share My Lettuce* (revue), Lyric Hammersmith Theatre, then Comedy Theatre, London, both 1957, later Garrick Theatre, London, 1958; Portia, the Ugly Sister, *Cinderella*, Coliseum Theatre, London, 1958; ensemble, *Pieces of Eight* (revue), Apollo Theatre, 1959; ensemble, *One Over the Eight* (revue), Duke of York's Theatre, 1961; Julian, "The Public Eye" in *The Private Ear and the Public Eye*, Globe Theatre, London, 1961; Jack, *Gentle Jack*, Queen's Theatre, London, 1963; Truscott, *Loot*, Arts Theatre, Cambridge, U.K., 1965; Bernard, *The Platinum Cat*, Wyndham's Theatre, London, 1965; Drinkwater, *Captain Brassbound's Conversion*, Cambridge Theatre, London, 1971; Henry, *My Fat Friend*, Globe Theatre, 1972; Barillon, *Signed and Sealed*, Comedy Theatre, London, 1976; the Undertaker, *The Undertaking*, Greenwich Theatre, then Fortune Theatre, both London, 1979.

PRINCIPAL STAGE WORK—Director: *Loot*, Lyric Studio, London, 1980; *Entertaining Mr. Sloan*, Lyric Hammersmith Theatre, London, 1981.

PRINCIPAL FILM APPEARANCES—Lloyd Haulage, *Men Are Children Twice* (also known as *Valley of Song*), Associated British Films/Pathe, 1953; Peter Wishart, *Land of Fury* (also known as *The Seekers*), Universal, 1955; Oliver Reckitt, *Carry On Nurse*, Anglo-Amalgamated, 1959; James Bailey, *Carry On Sergeant*, Anglo-Amalgamated, 1959; Constable Benson, *Carry On Constable*, Anglo-Amalgamated, 1960; Honorable Fred Warrington, *Make Mine Mink*, Continental, 1960; vice-counsul, *Tommy the Toreador*, Warner Brothers/Pathe, 1960; Francis Courtenay, *Carry On Regardless*, Ango-Amalgamated, 1961; policeman, *His and Hers*, Eros, 1961; Leonard Majoribanks, *Carry On Cruising*, Anglo-Amalgamated, 1962; Edwin Milton, *Carry On Teacher*, Anglo-Amalgated, 1962; Harold, *Roommates* (also known as *Raising the Wind*), Herts-Lion International, 1962; Harry Halfpenny, *Twice Round the Daffodils*, Anglo-Amalgamated, 1962; Captain Fearless, *Carry On Jack* (also known as *Carry On Venus*), Warner Brothers/Pathe, 1963; Julius Caesar, *Carry On Cleo*, Warner Brothers/Pathe, 1964; Desmond Simkins, *Carry On Spying*, Warner Brothers/Pathe, 1964;

Judge Burke, *Carry On Cowboy*, Warner Brothers/Pathe, 1966; Doctor Watt, *Carry On Screaming*, Warner Brothers/Pathe, 1966; Citizen Camembert, *Don't Lose Your Head*, Rank, 1967; Commandant Burger, *Follow That Camel*, Rank, 1967; Doctor Tinkle, *Carry On Doctor*, Rank, 1968; Khasi of Kalabar, *Carry On, Up the Khyber*, Rank, 1968; Frederick Carver, *Carry On Again, Doctor*, Rank, 1969; Doctor Soper, *Carry On Camping*, Rank, 1969; Sir Thomas Cromwell, *Carry On Henry VIII* (also known as *Carry On Henry*), Rank/American International, 1970; Percy Snooper, *Carry On Loving*, Rank, 1970; Emile, *Carry On Emanuelle*, Hemdale International, 1978; Sir Henry Baskerville, *The Hound of the Baskervilles*, Atlantic, 1980. Also appeared in *The Beggar's Opera*, Warner Brothers, 1953; *Trent's Last Case*, British Lion, 1953; and *Innocents of Paris*, Tudor, 1955.

PRINCIPAL TELEVISION APPEARANCES—Series: *Hancock's Half Hour*, *International Cabaret*, *The Kenneth Williams Show*, and *Whizz Kids Guide*.

PRINCIPAL RADIO APPEARANCES—Series: *Round the Horne*, *Stop Messing About*, and *Just a Minute*.

NON-RELATED CAREER—Draftsman.

WRITINGS: Acid Drops, 1980; *Back Drops*, 1983.

OBITUARIES AND OTHER SOURCES: Variety, April 20, 1988.*

*   *   *

WILLIAMS, Steven

PERSONAL: Born in Memphis, TN; married Ann Geddes (a talent agent); children: two daughters. EDUCATION: Attended the GM Institute (engineering school of General Motors). MILITARY: U.S. Army.

VOCATION: Actor.

CAREER: PRINCIPAL STAGE APPEARANCES—*Don Juan*, Goodman Theatre, Chicago, IL, 1977; also appeared in productions of *Slow Dance on the Killing Ground*, *Joplin*, and *Cinderella Brown*, all in Chicago; and with the Milwaukee Repertory Theatre, Milwaukee, WI, 1977-78.

PRINCIPAL FILM APPEARANCES—Jimmy Lee, *Cooley High*, American International, 1975; bar patron, "Prolog" in *Twilight Zone—The Movie*, Warner Brothers, 1983; Trooper Mount, *The Blues Brothers*, Universal, 1980; tree trimmer, *Better Off Dead*, Warner Brothers, 1985; Nester, *Missing in Action 2—The Beginning*, Cannon, 1985; cop, *House*, New World, 1986. Also appeared in *Mahogany*, Paramount, 1975; *Dr. Detroit*, Universal, 1983; and in *Under the Gun*.

PRINCIPAL TELEVISION APPEARANCES—Series: Lieutenant Jefferson Burnett, *The Equalizer*, CBS, 1985-86; Captain Adam Fuller, *21 Jump Street*, Fox, 1987—. Pilots: National security agent, *Northstar*, ABC, 1986. Episodic: *Hill Street Blues*, NBC; *The A-Team*, NBC; *Remington Steele*, NBC; *Hunter*, NBC; *MacGyver*, ABC. Movies: Julius Lang, *Dummy*, CBS, 1979; Les Averback, *The Lost Honor of Kathryn Beck*, CBS, 1984; Ted Gunning, *Silent Witness*, NBC, 1985; Frazier, *International Airport*, ABC, 1985; Kyle Banks, *Triplecross*, ABC, 1986; Mo,

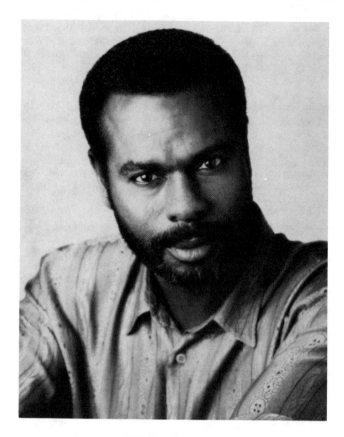

STEVEN WILLIAMS

Dreams of Gold: The Mel Fisher Story, CBS, 1986; also *The Marva Collins Story,* CBS, 1981; and *Murder Among Friends.*

RELATED CAREER—Model.

NON-RELATED CAREER—Salesman.

AWARDS: Joseph Jefferson Award nominations for *Joplin* and *Cinderella Brown.*

ADDRESSES: AGENT—Ann Geddes, Geddes Agency, 8457 Melrose Plaza, Suite 200, Los Angeles, CA 90069. PUBLICIST—The Garrett Company, 6922 Hollywood Boulevard, Los Angeles, CA 90028.

*　　*　　*

WILLIAMSON, Fred　1937-

PERSONAL: Born March 5, 1937 (some sources say 1938), in Gary, IN. EDUCATION: Attended Northwestern University.

VOCATION: Actor, director, and screenwriter.

CAREER: Also see *WRITINGS* below. FILM DEBUT—Spearchucker Jones, *M*A*S*H,* Twentieth Century-Fox, 1970. PRINCIPAL FILM APPEARANCES—Beach boy, *Tell Me That You Love Me, Junie Moon,* Paramount, 1970; B.J. Hammer, *Hammer,* United Artists, 1972; title role, *The Legend of Nigger Charley,* Paramount,

1972; Tommy Gibbs, *Black Caesar,* American International, 1973; Tommy Gibbs, *Hell Up in Harlem,* American International, 1973; title role, *The Soul of Nigger Charley,* Paramount, 1973; Jefferson Bolt, *That Man Bolt* (also known as *To Kill a Dragon* and *Thunderbolt*), Universal, 1973; Stone, *Black Eye,* Warner Brothers, 1974; title role, *Boss Nigger,* Dimension, 1974; Willy, *Crazy Joe,* Columbia, 1974; Jagger Daniels, *Three the Hard Way,* Allied Artists, 1974; Joe Snake, *Three Tough Guys,* Paramount, 1974; Ben, *Adios Amigo,* Atlas, 1975; Duke, *Bucktown,* American International, 1975; Tyree, *Take a Hard Ride,* Twentieth Century-Fox, 1975; title role, *Mean Johnny Barrows,* Atlas, 1976; Jess Crowder, *No Way Back,* Atlas, 1976; title role, *Joshua,* Lone Star, 1976.

As himself, *Fist of Fear, Touch of Death* (documentary), Aquarius, 1980; Fred, *Counterfeit Commandoes* (also known as *Inglorious Bastards*), Aquarius, 1981; Call, *One Down, Two to Go,* Almi, 1982; Frank Hooks, *The Big Score,* Almi, 1983; Jesse Crowder, *The Last Fight,* Best Film and Video, 1983; Nick, *Vigilante* (also known as *Street Gang*), Film Ventures, 1983; the Ogre, *1990: The Bronx Warriors* (also known as *1990: I guerrieri del Bronx* and *Bronx Warriors*), United Film Distribution, 1983; Nadir, *The New Barbarians* (also known as *I nuovi barbari* and *Warriors of the Wasteland*), Deaf International, 1983; Thomas Fox, *Foxtrap,* Snizzlefritz, 1986; Jake Sebastian Turner, *The Messenger,* Snizzlefritz, 1987; Curt Slate, *Deadly Intent,* Fries Distribution, 1988. Also appeared in *Darktown,* 1975; *Blind Rage,* 1978; *Deadly Impact,* 1983; *Vivre pour survivre,* 1984; and in *Warrior of the Lost World,* 1985.

PRINCIPAL FILM WORK—Co-producer (with Jack Arnold), *Boss Nigger,* Dimension, 1974; producer and director, *Adios Amigo,* Atlas, 1975; producer and director, *Mean Johnny Barrows,* Atlas, 1976; producer and director, *No Way Back,* Atlas, 1976; producer and director, *One Down, Two to Go,* Almi, 1982; director, *The Big Score,* Almi, 1983; director, *The Last Fight,* Best Film and Video, 1983; producer and director, *Foxtrap,* Snizzlefritz, 1986; producer (with Pier Luigi Ciriaci) and director, *The Messenger,* Snizzlefritz, 1987. Also producer and director, *Death Journey,* 1976.

PRINCIPAL TELEVISION APPEARANCES—Series: Steve Bruce, *Julia,* NBC, 1970-71; commentator, *Monday Night Football,* ABC, 1974; Chester Long, *Half Nelson,* NBC, 1985. Mini-Series: Leonard Wingate, *Wheels* (also known as *Arthur Hailey's "Wheels,"*), NBC, 1978. Episodic: Anka, "The Cloudminders," *Star Trek,* NBC, 1969. Movies: Williams, *Deadlock,* NBC, 1969.

NON-RELATED CAREER—Professional football player with the Kansas City Chiefs.

WRITINGS: FILMS—*Boss Nigger,* Dimension, 1974; *Adios Amigo,* Atlas, 1975; *No Way Back,* Atlas, 1976; *Joshua,* Lone Star, 1976; *The Last Fight,* Best Film and Video, 1983.

ADDRESSES: AGENT—H. David Moss and Associates, 8019 Melrose Avenue, Suite 3, Los Angeles, CA 90046.*

*　　*　　*

WILLIS, Gordon　1931-

PERSONAL: Born in 1931 in New York, NY; father, a motion picture makeup artist; wife's name, Helen; children: three. MILITARY: U.S. Air Force, photographer.

VOCATION: Cinematographer.

CAREER: PRINCIPAL STAGE WORK—Cinematographer of film sequences, *Singin' in the Rain,* Gershwin Theatre, New York City, 1985.

MAJOR TOURS—Cinematographer of film sequences, *Singin' in the Rain,* U.S. cities, 1987.

FIRST FILM WORK—Cinematographer, *End of the Road,* Allied Artists, 1970. PRINCIPAL FILM WORK—Cinematographer: *The Landlord,* United Artists, 1970; *Loving,* Columbia, 1970; *The People Next Door,* AVCO-Embassy, 1970; *Klute,* Warner Brothers, 1971; *Little Murders,* Twentieth Century-Fox, 1971; *Bad Company,* Paramount, 1972; *Corky* (also known as *Looking Good*), Metro-Goldwyn-Mayer (MGM), 1972; *The Godfather,* Paramount, 1972; *Up the Sandbox,* National General, 1972; *The Paper Chase,* Twentieth Century-Fox, 1973; *The Godfather, Part II,* Paramount, 1974; *The Parallax View,* Paramount, 1974; *The Drowning Pool,* Warner Brothers, 1975; *All the President's Men,* Warner Brothers, 1976; *Annie Hall,* United Artists, 1977; *9/30/55,* Universal, 1977; *Comes a Horseman,* United Artists, 1978; *Interiors,* United Artists, 1978; *Manhattan,* United Artists, 1979; *Stardust Memories,* United Artists, 1980; (also director) *Windows,* United Artists, 1980; *Pennies from Heaven,* MGM, 1981; *A Midsummer Night's Sex Comedy,* Warner Brothers, 1982; *Zelig,* Warner Brothers, 1983; *Broadway Danny Rose,* Orion, 1984; *Perfect,* Columbia, 1985; *The Purple Rose of Cairo,* Orion, 1985; *The Money Pit,* Universal, 1986; *The Pick-Up Artist,* Twentieth Century-Fox, 1987; *Bright Lights, Big City,* United Artists, 1988.

PRINCIPAL TELEVISION WORK—Movies: Cinematographer, *The Lost Honor of Kathryn Beck,* CBS, 1982.

RELATED CAREER—Actor, stage designer, and lighting designer for summer theatre productions, Gloucester, MA, for two seasons; assistant cameraman and photographer for documentaries; worked on television commercials.

AWARDS: Academy Award nomination and New York Film Critics Circle Award, both Best Cinematography, 1983, for *Zelig.*

ADDRESSES: OFFICE—c/o Ron Taft, 18 W. 55th Street, New York, NY 10019.*

*   *   *

WILLIS, Ted   1918-
(John Bishop, George Dixon—a joint pseudonym)

PERSONAL: Full name, Edward Henry Willis; born January 13, 1918, in Tottenham, England; son of Alfred John (a bus driver) and Maria Harriett (Meek) Willis; married Audrey Mary Hale (an actress), August 18, 1944; children: John Edward, Sally Ann Hale. MILITARY: British Army, Royal Fusiliers, then War Office and Ministry of Information, during World War II.

VOCATION: Writer and director.

CAREER: Also see *WRITINGS* below. PRINCIPAL STAGE WORK—Director, all at the Unity Theatre, London: *The Yellow Star,* 1945; *Boy Meets Girl* and *All God's Chillun Got Wings,* both 1946; *Golden Boy,* 1947; also *Anna Christie.*

RELATED CAREER—Artistic director, Unity Theatre, London, 1945-48; board of governors, Churchill Theatre Trust, Bromley, U.K., 1964—; director, World Wide Pictures; board of governors, National Film School; fellow, Royal Society of Arts; fellow, Royal Television Society; freelance journalist.

NON-RELATED CAREER—Member, Sports Council, 1971-73; also delivery boy, newsboy, farm hand.

WRITINGS: STAGE—*Buster,* Unity Players, Arts Theatre, London, 1943; (as John Bishop) *Sabotage,* first produced in London, 1943; *All Change Here,* first produced in London, 1944; *God Bless the Guv'nor: A Moral Melodrama in Which the Twin Evils of Trades Unionism and Strong Drink Are Exposed, "After Mrs. Henry Wood,"* first produced in London, 1945, published by New Theatre Publications, London, 1945; *The Yellow Star,* Unity Theatre, London, 1945; *What Happened to Love?,* first produced in London, 1947; *No Trees in the Street,* first produced in London, 1948; *The Lady Purrs,* first produced in London, 1950, published by Deane Publishers, 1950; *The Magnificent Moodies,* first produced in London, 1952; (with Jan Read) *The Blue Lamp,* first produced in London, 1952; (adaptor, with Talbot Strothwell) *A Kiss for Adele,* first produced in London, 1952; (with Allan Mackinnon) *Kid Kenyon Rides Again,* first produced in Bromley, U.K., 1954; *George Comes Home,* first produced in London, 1955, published by Samuel French, Inc., 1955; *Doctor in the House,* first produced in London, 1956, published by Evans, then Samuel French, Inc., both 1957; *Hot Summer Night,* first produced in Bournemouth, U.K., then in London, both 1958, published by Samuel French, Inc., 1959; (with Henry Cecil) *Brothers-in-Law,* first produced in Wimbledon, U.K., 1959, published by Samuel French, Inc., 1959; (book for musical with Ken Ferry) *When in Rome,* first produced in Oxford, U.K., then in London, both 1959; *Farewell Yesterday,* first produced in Worthing, U.K., 1959, then as *The Eyes of Youth,* produced in Bournemouth, 1959, published by Evans, 1960.

Mother, first produced in Croydon, U.K., 1961; *Doctor at Sea,* first produced in Bromley, 1961, then in London, 1966, published by Evans, then Samuel French, Inc., both 1961; *The Little Goldmine,* first produced in London, 1962, published by Samuel French, Inc., 1962; *Woman in a Dressing Gown,* first produced in Bromley, 1963, then London, 1964, published by Evans, 1964; *A Slow Roll of Drums,* first produced in Bromley, 1964; *A Murder of Crows,* first produced in Bromley, 1966; (lyrics for musical) *The Ballad of Queenie Swann,* first produced in Guildford, U.K., 1966, then as *Queenie,* London, 1967; *Dead on Saturday,* Thorndike Theatre, Leatherhead, U.K., 1972. Also wrote *A Fine Day for Murder,* 1970; *The History of Mr. Polly,* 1977; *Doctor on the Boil,* 1979; *Stardust,* 1983; and *Tommy Boy,* 1988.

FILMS—*It's Great to Be Young,* Columbia, 1946; *Holiday Camp,* Gainsborough Pictures, 1947; *The Huggets Abroad,* General Films Distributors, 1949; *A Boy, a Girl, and a Bike,* General Films Distributors, 1949; *Good Time Girl,* Sydney Box, 1950; *The Blue Lamp,* Ealing Studios, 1950; *Burnt Evidence,* Act Films, 1952; *The Wallet* (also known as *Blueprint for Danger*), Archway, 1952; *Trouble in Store,* Two Cities Films, 1953; *Top of the Form,* Rank, 1953; *The Large Rope,* United Artists, 1953; *Up to His Neck,* Rank, 1954; *One Good Turn,* General Films Distributors, 1954; *Woman in a Dressing Gown,* Godwin-Willis, 1957; *The Young and the Guilty,* Associated British/Pathe, 1958; *No Trees in the Street,* Associated British/Pathe, 1958; *The Horsemasters,* Buena Vista, 1961; *Flame in the Streets,* Atlantic, 1962; *Bitter Harvest,* Rank, 1963. Also *The Waves Roll On* (documentary), 1945; (with Gerard Bryant) *The Undefeated* (documentary), 1950; *The Skywalkers,*

1956; *Six Men and a Nightingale,* 1961; *Last Bus to Banjo Creek,* 1968; *Our Miss Fred,* 1972; and *Mrs. Harris Goes to Monte Carlo.*

TELEVISION—Series: *Dixon of Dock Green,* 1960; (with Edward J. Mason) *Flowers of Evil,* 1961; *Sergeant Cork,* 1963; *Mrs. Thursday,* 1966; *Virgin of the Secret Service,* 1968; *Crimes of Passion,* 1970-72; *Copper's End,* 1971; *Hunter's Walk,* 1973, then 1976; *Black Beauty,* 1975; also *Patterns of Marriage,* BBC; *Big City,* ITV; and *Taxi.* Pilots: *Dial 999* and *Lifeline.* Plays: *Woman in a Dressing Gown,* 1956, published in *Woman in a Dressing Gown and Other Television Plays,* Barrie and Rockcliffe, 1959; *The Young and the Guilty,* 1956, published in *Woman in a Dressing Gown and Other Television Plays,* 1959; *Look in Any Window,* 1958, published in *Woman in a Dressing Gown and Other Television Plays,* 1959; *Strictly for the Sparrows,* 1958; *Scent of Fear,* 1959; (with Mason) *Days of Vengeance,* 1960; (with Mason) *Outbreak of Murder,* 1962; *The Four Seasons of Rosie Carr,* 1964; *Dream of a Summer Night,* 1965; *The Ballad of Queenie Swann,* 1966; *Barney's Last Battle,* 1976; also *A Place for Animals* and *Racecourse,* both Phoenix Films, Germany; and *The Sullavan Brothers, Valley of the Kings, The Campbells in Canada,* and *The Handlebar.*

RADIO—Plays: *Big Bertha,* 1962.

OTHER—Novels: *The Blue Lamp,* Convoy, 1950; *The Devil's Churchyard,* Max Parrish, 1957; (with Charles Hatton under the joint pseudonym George Dixon) *Dixon of Dock Green: My Life,* William Kimber, 1960; (with Paul Graham) *Dixon of Dock Green: A Novel,* Mayflower, 1961; *Seven Gates to Nowhere,* Max Parrish, 1962; *Dead on Saturday,* Odanti Script Services, 1970; *Black Beauty,* Hamlyn, 1972; *Death May Surprise Us,* Macmillan, 1974, then as *Westminster One,* Putnam, 1975; *The Left-Handed Sleeper,* Macmillan, 1975, then Putnam, 1976; *Man-Eater,* Macmillan, 1976, then Morrow, 1977; also *A Problem for Mother Christmas,* Gollancz, then David and Charles. Non-Fiction: *Fighting Youth of Russia,* Russia Today Society, 1942; *Whatever Happened to Tom Mix? The Story of One of My Lives* (autobiography), Cassell, 1970.

AWARDS: Created Baron Willis of Chislehurst, 1963; Berlin Film Festival Award and London Picture-Goer Award, both 1957, for *Woman in a Dressing Gown;* Writers Guild awards, 1964 and 1967; Edinburgh Festival Award.

MEMBER: League of Dramatists (executive member, 1948-74), Writers Guild of Great Britain (chairor, 1958-63; president, 1963-68, then 1976—), International Writers Guild (president, 1967-69).

SIDELIGHTS: RECREATIONS—Tennis, badminton, football, traveling.

ADDRESSES: HOME—5 Shepherd's Green, Chislehurst, Kent, England. AGENT—ALS Management, 67 Brook Street, London W1, England.

*   *   *

WILSON, Hugh   1943-

PERSONAL: Born August 21, 1943, in Miami Beach, FL.

VOCATION: Producer, director, and screenwriter.

CAREER: Also see *WRITINGS* below. PRINCIPAL FILM APPEARANCES—Mayday customer, *Burglar,* Warner Brothers, 1987. PRINCIPAL FILM WORK—Director: *Police Academy,* Warner Brothers, 1984; *Rustler's Rhapsody,* Paramount, 1984; *Burglar,* Warner Brothers, 1987.

PRINCIPAL TELEVISION APPEARANCES—Episodic: D. Wayne Thomas, *Frank's Place,* CBS, 1987. PRINCIPAL TELEVISION WORK—Series: Producer (with Gary David Goldberg), *The Tony Randall Show,* CBS, 1976-77, then ABC, 1977-78; creator and executive producer, *WKRP in Cincinnati,* CBS, 1978-82; creator and supervising producer, *Easy Street,* NBC, 1986-87; creator and executive producer, *Frank's Place,* CBS, 1987-88; creator and executive producer, *The Famous Teddy Z.,* CBS, 1989—. Pilots: Director, *The Chopped Liver Brothers,* ABC, 1977. Episodic: Director, *The Tony Randall Show,* CBS, 1976-77, then ABC, 1977-78; director, *WKRP in Cincinnati,* CBS, 1978-82; director, *Easy Street,* NBC, 1986-87; director, *Frank's Place,* CBS, 1987-88; director, *The Famous Teddy Z.,* CBS, 1989—.

WRITINGS: FILM—*Stoker Ace,* Warner Brothers, 1983; *Police Academy,* Warner Brothers, 1984; *Rustler's Rhapsody,* Paramount, 1984; (with Joseph Loeb III and Matthew Weisman) *Burglar,* Warner Brothers, 1987.

TELEVISION—Pilots: (With Tom Patchett and Jay Tarses) *The Chopped Liver Brothers,* ABC, 1977. Episodic: *The Tony Randall Show,* CBS, 1976-77, then ABC, 1977-78; *WKRP in Cincinnati,* CBS, 1978-82; *Easy Street,* NBC, 1986-87; *Frank's Place,* CBS, 1987-88; *The Famous Teddy Z.,* CBS, 1989—; also *The Bob Newhart Show,* CBS.

AWARDS: Humanitas Award, 1988, for *Frank's Place.*

ADDRESSES: AGENT—William Morris Agency, 151 El Camino Drive, Beverly Hills, CA 90212. MANAGER—John Mucci and Associates, 9200 Sunset Boulevard, Suite 905, Los Angeles, CA 90069.*

*   *   *

WILSON, Lambert

PERSONAL: Born in Paris, France; son of Georges Wilson (a theatrical manager and director of the Theatre Nationale de Paris). EDUCATION: Studied acting at the Drama Center, London.

VOCATION: Actor.

CAREER: PRINCIPAL STAGE APPEARANCES—Cupid, *L'Amour de l'amour,* Paris, France, 1981; also appeared in *Leocadia,* France, 1985; and at the National Theatre, Marseilles, France.

PRINCIPAL FILM APPEARANCES—Boy with hatbox, *Julia,* Twentieth Century-Fox, 1977; Jean Charles, *New Generation,* Silenes/French Lollipop, 1978; Johann, *Five Days One Summer,* Universal, 1982; Jaffar, *Sahara,* Metro-Goldwyn-Mayer/United Artists, 1984; Milan Mliska, *La Femme publique* (also known as *The Public Woman*), Europex/Hachette-Fox, 1984; Villain, *L'Homme aux yeux d'argent* (also known as *The Man with the Silver Eyes*), AAA/Revcom/Michel Gue International, 1985; Stephane, *Rouge baiser* (also known as *Red Kiss*), Circle, 1985; Quentin, *Rendezvous,* Spectrafilm, 1985; Ned, *Bleu comme l'enfer* (also known as *Blue*

Like Hell), Union Generale Cinematographique, 1986; Michel Sauvage, *Corps et biens* (also known as *Lost with All Hands*), Films du Semaphore, 1986; Carlo/Davide, *La Storia* (also known as *The Story*), Sacis, 1986; Caspasian Speckler, *The Belly of an Architect*, Hemdale, 1987; Nikolas Stavrogin, *Les Possedes* (also known as *The Possessed*), Gaumont, 1988; Arsene, *La Vouivre*, Gaumont International, 1988; Pedro DeUrsua, *El Dorado*, Union Generale Cinematographique, 1988; Tarquin, *Chouans!*, Union Generale Cinematographique/World Marketing, 1988. Also appeared in *Chanel Solitaire*, United Film Distribution, 1981.

PRINCIPAL TELEVISION APPEARANCES—Movies: Paul Perrier, *The Blood of Others*, HBO, 1984.*

*   *   *

WILSON, Scott   1942-

PERSONAL: Born in 1942 in Atlanta, GA.

VOCATION: Actor.

CAREER: PRINCIPAL STAGE APPEARANCES—*Guys and Dolls*, Marriott's Lincolnshire Theatre, Lincolnshire, IL.

FILM DEBUT—Dick Hickock, *In Cold Blood*, Columbia, 1967. PRINCIPAL FILM APPEARANCES—Harvey Oberst, *In the Heat of the Night*, United Artists, 1967; Corporal Ralph Clearboy, *Castle Keep*, Columbia, 1969; Malcolm Webson, *The Gypsy Moths*, Metro-Goldwyn-Mayer (MGM), 1969; Slim Grissom, *The Grissom Gang*, Cinerama, 1971; Gus, *The New Centurions* (also known as *Precinct 45: Los Angeles Police*), Columbia, 1972; Thrush Feather, *Lolly-Madonna XXX* (also known as *The Lolly-Madonna War*), MGM, 1973; George Wilson, *The Great Gatsby*, Paramount, 1974; Judah, *The Passover Plot*, Atlas, 1976; Captain Cutshaw, *The Ninth Configuration* (also known as *Twinkle, Twinkle, Killer Kane*), Warner Brothers, 1980; Scott Crossfield, *The Right Stuff*, Warner Brothers, 1983; Mitch, *Rio Abajo* (also known as *On the Line* and *Beyond Good and Evil*), Miramax/Nelson Entertainment, 1984; Norman, *Rok Spokonjnego Slonca* (also known as *Year of the Quiet Sun*), Sandstar Releasing, 1984; Jerry Stiller, *The Aviator*, Metro-Goldwyn-Mayer/United Artists, 1985; Perry Kerch, *Blue City*, Paramount, 1986; Paul Barlow, *Malone*, Orion, 1987.

PRINCIPAL TELEVISION APPEARANCES—Episodic: Matthew Foreman, "Quarantine," *The Twilight Zone*, CBS, 1986. Movies: Red Jack Stillwell, *The Tracker*, HBO, 1988; Sam Maloney, *Jesse* (also known as *Desert Nurse*), CBS, 1988.

ADDRESSES: AGENT—Tom Korman, Agency for the Performing Arts, 9000 Sunset Boulevard, Suite 1200, Los Angeles, CA 90069.*

*   *   *

WILSON, Snoo   1948-

PERSONAL: Full name, Andrew Wilson; born August 2, 1948, in Reading, England; son of Leslie (a teacher) and Pamela (a teacher; maiden name, Boyle) Wilson; married Ann Patricia McFerran, 1976; children: two sons, one daughter. EDUCATION: University of East Anglia, B.A., 1969.

VOCATION: Playwright, director, and actor.

CAREER: Also see WRITINGS below. PRINCIPAL STAGE APPEARANCES—The Porpoise, *Freshwater*, London, 1983; also appeared in *Lay By*, London, 1971.

PRINCIPAL STAGE WORK—Director: *Pericles, the Mean Knight*, Oval House Theatre, London, 1970; *Pignight*, Civic Hall, Leeds, U.K., 1971; *Blowjob*, Other Pool Theatre, Edinburgh, Scotland, 1971; *Lay By*, Traverse Theatre, Edinburgh, 1971; *England's Ireland*, Mickeri Theatre, Amsterdam, Holland, 1972; *The Everest Hotel*, Bush Theatre, London, 1976; (with Simon Stokes) *More Light*, Bush Theatre, 1987; also *Bodyworks*, London, 1974; and (with Simon Callow) *Loving Reno*, London, 1983.

PRINCIPAL TELEVISION WORK—Series: Script editor, *Play for Today*, BBC, 1972.

RELATED CAREER—Founding director, Portable Theatre, Brighton, U.K., and London, 1968-75; dramaturge, Royal Shakespeare Company, Stratford-on-Avon, U.K., and London, 1975-76; director, Scrab Theatre, 1975-80.

WRITINGS: STAGE—*Girl Mad As Pigs*, University of East Anglia, Norwich, U.K., 1967; *Ella Daybellfesse's Machine*, University of East Anglia, 1967; *Between the Acts*, Canterbury, U.K., then Kent University, Kent, U.K., both 1969; *Device of Angels*, Traverse Theatre, Edinburgh, Scotland, 1970; *Pericles, the Mean Knight*, Oval House Theatre, London, 1970; *Pignight*, Civic Hall, Leeds, U.K., 1971, published by Calder and Boyers, 1972; *Blowjob*, Other Pool Theatre, Edinburgh, 1972, published in *Pignight*, Calder and Boyers, 1972; (with others) *Lay By*, Traverse Theatre, 1971, published by Calder and Boyers, 1972; *Reason* (also known as *Reason the Sun King* and *Reason: Boswell and Johnson on the Shores of the Eternal Sea*), Oval House Theatre, 1972, then in Chicago, IL, 1975, published in *Gambit* Volume 8, 1976; (with others), *England's Ireland*, Mickeri Theatre, Amsterdam, Holland, then Round House Theatre, London, both 1972; *The Pleasure Principle: The Politics of Love, the Capital of Emotion*, Royal Court Theatre, London, 1973, published by Methuen, 1974; *Vampire*, Oval House Theatre, 1973, published in *Plays and Players*, 1973; *The Beast*, Other Place Theatre, London, 1974, published by Calder and Boyers, then Riverrun Press, both 1983.

The Everest Hotel, Bush Theatre, London, published in *Plays and Players*, 1976; *England—England*, Jeannetta Cochrane Theatre, London, 1977; *The Glad Hand*, Royal Court Theatre, 1977, published by Pluto Press, 1979; *The Language of the Dead Is Tongued with Fire*, Etcetera, Bush Theatre, 1978; (libretto) *La Colombe* (opera), Buxton Festival, Buxton, U.K., then Sadler's Wells Opera, London, both 1982; *The Soul of the White Ant*, New York Theatre Studio, AMDA Studio, New York City, 1982; *Our Lord of Lynchville*, New York Theatre Studio, AMDA Studio, 1983, then Royal Shakespeare Company, U.K., 1986; *The Grass Widow*, first produced in Seattle WA, 1982, then Royal Court Theatre, 1983, published by Methuen, 1983; (with David Pountney) *Orpheus in the Underworld*, Coliseum Theatre, London, then Houston Grand Opera, Houston, TX, both 1985; *More Light*, Bush Theatre, 1987. Also wrote *Charles the Matyr*, first produced in Southampton, England, 1970; *The Number of the Beast*, first produced by the Royal Shakespeare Company, (RSC), 1974, published by Calder, 1982; *Elijah Disappearing*, first produced in London, 1977; (with others) *In at the Death*, first produced in London, 1978; *The Greenish Man*, first produced in London, 1978, published by Pluto Press, 1979; *Magic Rose*, first produced in London, 1979; *Flaming*

Bodies, first produced in London, 1979, published by Calder and Riverrun Press, 1983; *Spaceache,* first produced in Cheltenham, U.K., then London, both 1980; *Salvation Now,* first produced in Seattle, WA, 1981; *Hamlyn,* first produced in Loughborough, U.K., 1984.

FILM—*Shadey,* Film Four International/Skouras, 1986.

TELEVISION—Episodic: (With Trevor Griffiths) "Don't Make Waves," *Eleventh Hour,* 1975. Also *The Good Life,* 1971; *Swamp Music,* 1972; *More about the Universe,* 1972; *The Barium Meal,* 1974; *The Trip to Jerusalem,* 1975; *A Greenish Man,* 1975.

OTHER—*Spaceache,* Chatto and Windus, 1984; *Inside Babel,* Chatto and Windus, 1985.

AWARDS: John Whiting Award, 1978; U.S. Bicentennial fellowship, 1980.

SIDELIGHTS: RECREATIONS—Beekeeping and tennis.

ADDRESSES: HOME—41 the Chase, London SW4, England.

*   *   *

WINDOM, William   1923-

PERSONAL: Born September 28, 1923, in New York, NY; son of Paul (an architect) and Isobel Wells (Peckham) Windom; married Carol Keyser (a dancer), August 10, 1947 (divorced, December, 1955); married Barbara Joyce (an actress), June 30, 1958 (divorced, March, 1963); married Barbara G. Clare, April 12, 1963 (divorced); married Jacquylyne Dean Hopkins, August 8, 1969 (marriage ended); married Patricia Veronica Tunder (a writer), December 31, 1975; children: Rachel, Heather Juliet, Hope, Rebel Russell. EDUCATION: Attended Williams College, 1942, the Citadel, 1943, Antioch College, 1943, the University of Kentucky, 1943-44, Biarritz American University, 1945, Fordham University, 1946, and Columbia University, 1946. MILITARY: U.S. Army, 1943-46.

VOCATION: Actor.

CAREER: STAGE DEBUT—Duke of Gloucester, *Richard III,* Biarritz, France, 1937. LONDON DEBUT—*Thurber I* (one-man show), New London Theatre, 1975. PRINCIPAL STAGE APPEARANCES—Surrey, *Henry VIII,* Columbus Circle Theatre, New York City, 1940; Earl of Surrey, *Henry VIII,* Erhart Borkman, *John Gabriel Borkman,* townsman, *What Every Woman Knows,* and Retiarius, *Androcles and the Lion,* all American Repertory Theatre, International Theatre, New York City, 1946; McClelland, *Yellow Jack,* and the White Rabbit and Gentleman Dressed in White Paper, *Alice in Wonderland,* both American Repertory Theatre, International Theatre, 1947; the Poet, *Joan of Lorraine,* Cape Playhouse, Dennis, MA, 1947; janitor, *My Sister Eileen,* and Bill Page, *The Voice of the Turtle,* both Brookfield Center, Brookfield, CT, 1948; Doctor, *Blithe Spirit,* and the Author, *Light Up the Sky,* both Southbury Playhouse, Southbury, CT, 1950; telephone voice, *A Girl Can Tell,* Royale Theatre, New York City, 1953; Edouard, *Mademoiselle Colombe,* Longacre Theatre, New York City, 1954; David, *Claudia,* and Snake Man, *My Three Angels,* both Putnam Playhouse, Putnam, CT, 1954; the Frenchman, *Sabrina Fair,* Sacandaga Garden Theatre, Sacandaga Park, NY, 1954; John

Condon Mitchell, *The Grand Prize,* Plymouth Theatre, New York City, 1955; Morris Townsend, *The Heiress,* Tent Theatre, Philadelphia, PA, 1955; Frederick Starbuck, *Fallen Angels,* Playhouse Theatre, New York City, 1956; Mack Daniels, *Double in Hearts,* John Golden Theatre, New York City, 1956; Orsino, *Twelfth Night,* New York Shakespeare Festival, Belvedere Lake Theatre, New York City, 1958.

Jim Leary, *Viva Madison Avenue!,* Longacre Theatre, 1960; Adam and Cockney, *Drums under the Window,* Cherry Lane Theatre, New York City, 1960; Guida Venanzi, *The Rules of the Game,* Gramercy Arts Theatre, New York City, 1960; *Thurber* (one-man show), Tyrone Guthrie Theatre, Minneapolis, MN, then Cleveland Playhouse, Cleveland, OH, both 1978. Also appeared in *The Marquise* and *Dream Girl,* Cape Playhouse, 1947; *The Jailor's Wench,* Cape Playhouse, 1949; *The Vinegar Tree, The Three-Cornered Moon, It's a Wise Child, Your Uncle Dudley, Meet the Wife,* and *Charm,* all Southbury Playhouse, 1950; *The Automobile Man,* Bucks County Playhouse, New Hope, PA, 1954; *Private Lives, Affairs of State, I Am a Camera,* and *The Voice of the Turtle,* all Theatre in the Round, Glens Falls, NY, 1954; *You Never Can Tell,* Olney Theatre, Olney, MD, 1955; *The Shoemaker's Children* and *Mrs. Gibbon's Boys,* both Bucks County Playhouse, 1955; *Career,* Seventh Avenue South Playhouse, New York City, 1957; *Time Remembered,* Morosco Theatre, New York City, 1957; *Hotel Paradiso,* Henry Miller's Theatre, New York City, 1957; *The World of Suzie Wong,* Broadhurst Theatre, New York City, 1958; *U.S.A.,* Martinique Theatre, New York City, 1959; *Come Blow Your Horn,* Brooks Atkinson Theatre, New York City, 1961; *U.S.A., Period of Adjustment,* and *The Child Buyer,* all Theatre Group, University of California, Los Angeles, 1961-62; and *When the Bough Breaks,* in New York City.

PRINCIPAL STAGE WORK—Stage manager, *Double in Hearts,* John Golden Theatre, New York City, 1956; stage hand, *Candide,* Martin Beck Theatre, New York City, 1956; assistant stage manager, *The Greatest Man Alive,* Ethel Barrymore Theatre, New York City, 1957.

MAJOR TOURS—Title role, *Richard III,* U.S. Army bases, European cities, 1945-46; Nicky Holroyd, *Bell, Book, and Candle,* U.S. cities, 1957; *Thurber* (one-man show), U.S. cities, 1972; *Thurber II* (one-man show), U.S. cities, 1975; *Ernie Pyle I* (one-man show), U.S. cities, 1976; *Ernie Pyle II* (one-man show), U.S. cities, 1979; also in *Famous Poems Illustrated.*

PRINCIPAL FILM APPEARANCES—Gilmer, *To Kill a Mockingbird,* Universal, 1962; Harry Travers, *Cattle King* (also known as *Guns of Wyoming*), Metro-Goldwyn-Mayer (MGM), 1963; Sam Travis, *For Love or Money,* Universal, 1963; Captain Harry Spaulding, *The Americanization of Emily,* MGM, 1964; Reverend Clifford Peale, *One Man's Way,* United Artists, 1964; Texas Jack Vermillion, *Hour of the Gun,* United Artists, 1967; Colin MacIver, *The Detective,* Twentieth Century-Fox, 1968; Vance Patton, *The Angry Breed,* Commonwealth United, 1969; Allen Brandon, *The Gypsy Moths,* MGM, 1969; Sheriff Weeks, *Brewster McCloud,* MGM, 1970; the President, *Escape from the Planet of the Apes,* Twentieth Century-Fox, 1971; Roy K. Sizemore, *Fools' Parade* (also known as *Dynamite Man from Glory Jail*), Columbia, 1971; Dr. West, *The Mephisto Waltz,* Twentieth Century-Fox, 1971; Arthur Eaton, *The Man,* Paramount, 1972; Professor Lufkin, *Now You See Him, Now You Don't,* Buena Vista, 1972; Dr. Hallett, *Echoes of a Summer,* Cine Artists, 1976; Victor Lacey, *Mean Dog Blues,* American International, 1978; Huey, *Separate Ways,* Crown International, 1981; Bob Cody, *Grandview, U.S.A.,* Warner Brothers, 1984; Ferguson, *Prince Jack*, Castle Hill, 1985; voice of Puppetino, *Pinocchio and the Emperor of the Night* (animated), New World, 1987; Boss, *Planes, Trains, and Automobiles*, Paramount, 1987; Governor Tovah, *Space Rage*, Vestron, 1987; McWhorter, *Mace*, Double Helix, 1987; Burt, *Means and Ends*, Progressive, 1987; Funland owner, *Funland*, Double Helix, 1987; Russ Bainbridge, *She's Having a Baby*, Paramount, 1988. Also appeared in *Goodbye Franklin High*, Cal-Am, 1978; and as James Caldwell, *Last Plane Out*, 1983.

TELEVISION DEBUT—Title role, "Richard III," *Philco Television Playhouse*, NBC, 1950. PRINCIPAL TELEVISION APPEARANCES—Series: Congressman Glen Morley, *The Farmer's Daughter*, ABC, 1962-65; John Monroe, *My World and Welcome to It*, NBC, 1969-70; Stuart Kline, *The Girl with Something Extra*, NBC, 1973-74; Larry Krandall, *Brothers and Sisters*, NBC, 1979; voice characterization, *Pink Panther and Sons* (animated), NBC, 1984-85; voice characterization, *The New Jetsons* (animated), syndicated, 1985; Dr. Seth Hazlitt, *Murder, She Wrote*, CBS, 1985—; voice characterization, *Sky Commanders* (animated), syndicated, 1987. Mini-Series: John Meyers, *Seventh Avenue*, NBC, 1977; General Duke Pulleyne, *Once an Eagle*, NBC, 1976-77; Richard Kleindienst, *Blind Ambition*, CBS, 1979. Pilots: Burt Gordon, *Prescription: Murder*, NBC, 1968; Raymond Hanson, *U.M.C.*, CBS, 1969; Dr. Henry Walding, *Escape*, ABC, 1971; Charlie Snead, *The Homecoming—A Christmas Story*, CBS, 1971; Dr. Tim Newly, *Is There a Doctor in the House?*, NBC, 1971; Mr. Farrigan, *The New Healers*, ABC, 1972; Arnold Springfield, *Richie Brockelman: Missing 24 Hours*, NBC, 1976; Colonel Gregory Heck, *Heck's Angels*, CBS, 1976; Panama Cassidy, *Hunters of the Reef*, NBC, 1978; Ben Landon, *Landon, Landon, and Landon*, CBS, 1980; Thaddeus Clark "T.C." Cooper, *Quick and Quiet*, CBS, 1981; Bronco Mallory, *The Tom Swift and Linda Craig Mystery Hour*, ABC, 1983; government official, *Velvet*, ABC, 1984; Commander Leevanhoek, *Dirty Work*, CBS, 1985.

Episodic: The Major, "Five Characters in Search of an Exit," *The Twilight Zone*, CBS, 1961; Dr. Wallman, "Miniature," *The Twilight Zone*, CBS, 1963; Commodore Matthew Decker, "Doomsday Machine," *Star Trek*, NBC, 1967; Wayne Altfield, *Knight Rider*, NBC, 1985; Lou Stappleford, *Airwolf*, CBS, 1985; Henry, *Glitter*, ABC, 1985; Captain Lyle, *Magnum, P.I.*, CBS, 1986; Mr. Rooney, *Newhart*, CBS, 1987; Alex, *Have Faith*, ABC, 1989; also *Masterpiece Playhouse*, NBC, 1950; "Man of Mystery," *Thriller*, NBC, 1962; "Doomsday Minus One" and "Summit Meeting," *The Invaders*, ABC, 1967; "They're Tearing Down Tim Riley's Bar," *Rod Serling's Night Gallery* (also known as *Night Gallery*), NBC, 1970; "Success Story," *All in the Family*, CBS, 1971; "Little Girl Lost," *Rod Serling's Night Gallery*, NBC, 1971; "Doomsday," *Barney Miller*, ABC, 1975; "Contempt," *Barney Miller*, ABC, 1981; Charlie Banks, *Flamingo Road*, NBC; Mr. Halloran, *St. Elsewhere*, NBC.

Movies: Paul Durstine, *House on Greenapple Road*, ABC, 1970; Captain Frank Reardon, *Assault on the Wayne*, ABC, 1971; Warren Duden, *Marriage: Year One*, NBC, 1971; Harold Jannings, *A Taste of Evil*, ABC, 1971; Rob Stewart, *A Great American Tragedy*, ABC, 1972; Robert Phillips, *Pursuit*, ABC, 1972; Stan Petryk, *Second Chance*, ABC, 1972; Sam Dutton, *The Girls of Huntington House*, ABC, 1973; Judge Tom Backsler, *The Day the Earth Moved*, ABC, 1974; Ted Morrisey, *The Abduction of Saint Anne* (also known as *They've Kidnapped Anne Benedict*), ABC, 1975; Walt Adamson, *Guilty or Innocent: The Sam Sheppard Murder Case*, NBC, 1975; Dr. Cavaliere, *Journey from Darkness*, NBC, 1975; Daniel Webster, *Bridger*, ABC, 1976; Monseigneur Soldini,

Portrait of a Rebel: Margaret Sanger*, CBS, 1980; Smiley Jenkins, *Leave 'em Laughing*, CBS, 1981; Byron Gage, *Side Show*, NBC, 1981; Dr. Jarvis, *Desperate Lives*, CBS, 1982; George Olsen, *The Rules of Marriage*, CBS, 1982; Mayor Malcolm Wallwood, *Off Sides*, NBC, 1984; General, *Why Me?*, ABC, 1984; Dr. Madsen, *Surviving*, ABC, 1985; Lee Hertzig, *There Must Be a Pony*, ABC, 1986. Specials: Max Halliday, "Dial M for Murder," *Hallmark Hall of Fame*, NBC, 1958; *Robert Young and the Family*, CBS, 1971; Thomas Edison (host), *One Hundred Years of Golden Hits*, NBC, 1981; *The Screen Actors Guild Fiftieth Anniversary Celebration*, CBS, 1984; Herb Medlock, "Moscow Bureau," *ABC Comedy Specials*, ABC, 1986.

RELATED CAREER—As a child, appeared in minstrel show, Camp Overall, Virginia, 1932.

AWARDS: Actors Fund Citation of Merit, 1958; Emmy Award, Outstanding Continuing Performance by an Actor in a Leading Role in a Comedy Series, 1970, for *My World and Welcome to It*.

MEMBER: Actors' Equity Association, Screen Actors Guild, American Federation of Television and Radio Artists, Players Club, Friends of Richard III, Corinthians, Malibu Yacht Club, Catboat Association.

SIDELIGHTS: RECREATIONS—Sailing, tennis, and chess.

ADDRESSES: OFFICE—Howard Askenase, 6217 Glen Airy Drive, Los Angeles, CA 90068. AGENT—Mike Livingston, The Artists Agency, 10000 Santa Monica Boulevard, Los Angeles, CA 90067.*

*   *   *

WINSLOW, Michael

PERSONAL: EDUCATION: Attended the University of Colorado.

VOCATION: Actor.

CAREER: FILM DEBUT—*Cheech and Chong's Next Movie*, Universal, 1980. PRINCIPAL FILM APPEARANCES—Superspade, *Cheech and Chong's Nice Dreams*, Columbia, 1981; Gowdy, *T.A.G.: The Assassination Game*, New World, 1982; voice of the Mountain, *Heidi's Song* (animated), Paramount, 1982; Lippy, *Alphabet City*, Atlantic, 1984; Spencer, *Grandview, U.S.A.*, Warner Brothers, 1984; J.D., *Lovelines*, Tri-Star, 1984; Larvell Jones, *Police Academy*, Warner Brothers, 1984; voice characterization, *Starchaser: The Legend of Orin* (animated), Atlantic, 1985; Larvell Jones, *Police Academy 2: Their First Assignment*, Warner Brothers, 1985; Sergeant Larvell Jones, *Police Academy 3: Back in Training*, Warner Brothers, 1986; Sergeant Larvell Jones, *Police Academy 4: Citizens on Patrol*, Warner Brothers, 1987; radar technician, *Spaceballs*, Metro-Goldwyn-Mayer/United Artists, 1987; Ronny Walker, *Zartliche Chaoten* (also known as *Without You*), 1987; Sergeant Larvell Jones, *Police Academy 5: Assignment Miami Beach*, Warner Brothers, 1988; Sly, *Buy and Cell*, Empire Films, 1989; Sergeant Larvell Jones, *Police Academy 6: City under Siege*, Warner Brothers, 1989.

PRINCIPAL TELEVISION APPEARANCES—Pilots: Redlight, *Nightside*, ABC, 1980; Michael, *Irene*, NBC, 1981. Episodic: *The Gong Show*, syndicated; *Love Boat*, ABC.

ADDRESSES: AGENT—Camden Artists, 2121 Avenue of the Stars, Suite 410, Los Angeles, CA 90067. PUBLICIST—Guttman and Pam, 8500 Wilshire Boulevard, Suite 801, Beverley Hills, CA 90211.*

*   *   *

WINTER, Edward   1937-

PERSONAL: Born June 3, 1937, in Roseburg, OR.

VOCATION: Actor.

CAREER: PRINCIPAL STAGE APPEARANCES—Deputy from Lyons, soldier, and jailer, *Danton's Death,* Repertory Theatre of Lincoln Center, Vivian Beaumont Theatre, New York City, 1965; Werner, *The Condemned of Altona,* Mr. Dorilant, *The Country Wife,* and Simon Shashova and palace guard, *The Caucasian Chalk Circle,* all Repertory Theatre of Lincoln Center, Vivian Beaumont Theatre, 1966; Ernst Ludwig, *Cabaret,* Broadhurst Theatre, New York City, 1966; McCann, *The Birthday Party,* Booth Theatre, New York City, 1967; J.D. Sheldrake, *Promises, Promises,* Shubert Theatre, New York City, 1968; Benjamin Stone, *Follies,* Shubert Theatre, Century City, CA, 1972. Also appeared in *Night Watch,* Morosco Theatre, New York City, 1972; and *Angel City,* Center Theatre Group, Mark Taper Forum, Los Angeles, CA, 1977.

PRINCIPAL FILM APPEARANCES—Lorenzo Pierce, *Special Delivery,* American International, 1976; Steven Rutledge, *A Change of Seasons,* Twentieth Century-Fox, 1980; Gebhardt, *Porky's II: The Next Day,* Twentieth Century-Fox, 1983; Jim Parks, *The Buddy System,* Twentieth Century-Fox, 1984; Raymond Torkenson, *From the Hip,* De Laurentiis Entertainment, 1987.

PRINCIPAL TELEVISION APPEARANCES—Series: Attorney Kip Kipple, *Adam's Rib,* ABC, 1973; Captain Ben Ryan, *Project U.F.O.,* NBC, 1978-79; T. Howard Daniels, *Empire,* CBS, 1984; Captain Wes Biddle, *Hollywood Beat,* ABC, 1985; William "Bud" Coleman, *9 to 5,* syndicated, 1986-88; also Chuck Hillman, *Somerset,* NBC. Pilots: Staff sergeant, *Sam,* CBS, 1977; Dr. Peter Cabe, *The Girl in the Empty Grave,* NBC, 1977; J.C. Hadley, *Never Con a Killer* (also known as *The Feather and Father Gang: Never Con a Killer*), ABC, 1977; Daniel Frazier, *Woman on the Run,* CBS, 1977; Dr. David Norman, *The Second Time Around,* ABC, 1979; Jim Becker, *Rendezvous Hotel,* CBS, 1979; Lieutenant Colonel Hannibal, *Fly Away Home,* ABC, 1981; Jerrold Farrenpour, *The Big Black Pill* (also known as *Joe Dancer: The Big Black Pill*), NBC, 1981; Captain Mike Houston, *The 25th Man,* NBC, 1982; Herman Chilton, *The Adventures of Pollyanna,* CBS, 1982; Barney Hathaway, *Family in Blue,* CBS, 1982; also *Big Daddy,* CBS, 1973.

Episodic: Captain Halloran, *M*A*S*H,* CBS, 1973; Colonel Flagg, *M*A*S*H,* CBS, 1974-79; Senator Bob Hartford, *Karen,* ABC, 1975; J.C. Hadley, *The Feather and Father Gang,* ABC, 1977; also *The Bob Newhart Show,* CBS, 1974; *The Mary Tyler Moore Show,* CBS, 1976; Representative Walter McCallam, *Soap,* ABC; J. Benson Landale, *Falcon Crest,* CBS. Movies: McCheer, *The Disappearance of Flight 412,* NBC, 1974; Major Edward Fechet, *The Invasion of Johnson County,* NBC, 1976; Joe McCall, *Eleanor and Franklin,* ABC, 1976; Roger, *The Gathering,* ABC, 1977; Doug, *Mother and Daughter: The Loving War,* ABC, 1980; Clark Gable, *Moviola: The Scarlett O'Hara War,* NBC, 1980; Captain

Michael McKenzie, *The First Time,* ABC, 1982; Carl Macaluso, *The Lost Honor of Kathryn Beck,* CBS, 1984; Thomas A. Renfield, *The Christmas Gift,* CBS, 1986; Jonathan Eastman, *Perry Mason: The Case of the Notorious Nun,* NBC, 1986; Tommy Claybourne, *Stranded,* NBC, 1986; David Hollis, *There Must Be a Pony,* ABC, 1986. Specials: Sam Hendrix, *Wait Until Dark,* HBO, 1982.

MEMBER: San Francisco Actor's Workshop.

ADDRESSES: AGENT—Sam Gores, Gores/Fields Agency, 10100 Santa Monica Boulevard, Suite 700, Los Angeles, CA 90067.

*   *   *

WINTERS, Deborah

PERSONAL: Born in Los Angeles, CA. EDUCATION: Attended the Professional Children's School; studied acting with Stella Adler and Lee Strasberg.

VOCATION: Actress.

CAREER: PRINCIPAL FILM APPEARANCES—Becky, *Hail, Hero!,* National General, 1969; Betty Simon, *Me, Natalie,* National General, 1969; Maxie Mason, *The People Next Door,* AVCO-Embassy, 1970; Erica Herzenstiel, *Kotch,* Cinerama, 1971; Julie, *Class of '44,* Warner Brothers, 1973; Eve Farrell, *The Outing* (also known as *The Lamp*), Movie Store, 1987; Alicia Sweeney, *Blue Sunshine,* Cinema Shares, 1978.

PRINCIPAL FILM WORK—Associate producer and assistant casting director, *The Outing* (also known as *The Lamp*), Movie Store, 1987; casting director, *Aloha Summer* (also known as *Made in Hawaii* and *Hanuama Bay*), Spectrafilm/Lorimar Home Video, 1988; also associate producer, *Breakdancers from Mars.*

PRINCIPAL TELEVISION APPEARANCES—Mini-Series: Janice LaCouture, *The Winds of War,* ABC, 1983. Episodic: *Gemini Man,* NBC, 1976. Movies: Cindy Beck, *Tarantulas: The Deadly Cargo,* CBS, 1977; Sandy, *Crisis in Sun Valley,* NBC, 1978; also "Little Girl Lost," *General Foods Golden Showcase,* ABC, 1988. Plays: *Six Characters in Search of an Author.* Specials: Maxie, *The People Next Door,* CBS, 1968.

RELATED CAREER—Child actress in television commercials.*

*   *   *

WOHL, David   1953-

PERSONAL: Born September 22, 1953, in Brooklyn, NY.

VOCATION: Actor.

CAREER: OFF-BROADWAY DEBUT—Arthur "Gruely" Gruelbacher, *The Buddy System,* Circle in the Square Downtown, 1981. PRINCIPAL STAGE APPEARANCES—Gus, *Portrait of Jenny,* New Federal Theatre, Harry DeJur Playhouse, New York City, 1982; Harry, "Luna Park," and Walter, "Shenandoah," in *Delmore,* Jewish Repertory Theatre, New York City, 1982; G. Gordon Liddy,

Basement Tapes, Top of the Gate, New York City, 1983; Marty Sterling, *Isn't It Romantic?,* Lucille Lortel Theatre, 1985. Also appeared in *The Man Who Came to Dinner,* Cincinnati Playhouse, Cincinnati, OH, 1981; *Northern Lights,* Cricket Theatre, Minneapolis, MN, 1981; *Awake and Sing!,* Jewish Repertory Theatre, 1981; and *Ghetto,* Center Theatre Group, Mark Taper Forum, Los Angeles, CA, 1986.

PRINCIPAL FILM APPEARANCES—English teacher, *Sophie's Choice,* Universal, 1982; Phil, *Terms of Endearment,* Paramount, 1983; Dean Ulich, *Revenge of the Nerds,* Twentieth Century-Fox, 1984; Eugene Provost, *Brewster's Millions,* Universal, 1985; Mr. Nesbit, *D.A.R.Y.L.,* Paramount, 1985; Professor, *Gotcha!,* Universal, 1985; TV producer, *Turk 182!,* Twentieth Century-Fox, 1985; prosecutor, *Armed and Dangerous,* Columbia, 1986; Stanley Dickler, *Beer,* Orion, 1986; Dr. Roger Hartwood, *Like Father, Like Son,* Tri-Star, 1987.

PRINCIPAL TELEVISION APPEARANCES—Series: Eddie Kybo, *Once a Hero,* ABC, 1987. Pilots: Trumway's assistant, *A Doctor's Story,* NBC, 1984. Movies: Doctor, *Carpool,* CBS, 1983; meat handler, *Terrible Joe Moran,* CBS, 1984; Ken Klein, *Badge of the Assassin,* CBS, 1985; Loudon, *Hero in the Family,* ABC, 1986; Ira Handel, *Oceans of Fire,* CBS, 1986; also *Island Sons,* ABC, 1987.

ADDRESSES: AGENT—The Gage Group, 1650 Broadway, New York, NY 10019.*

*   *   *

WONG, B.D.

BRIEF ENTRY: Full name, Bradd Wong; born c. 1962 in San Francisco, CA. Actor B.D. Wong electrified critics in his Broadway debut in early 1988 with a portrayal of Song Liling, a female Chinese opera star who carries on a twenty year relationship with a French diplomat, in David Henry Hwang's drama *M. Butterfly.* In the course of the play the supposedly submissive, Madame Butterfly-like Song Liling is revealed to be a male spy. In the revelatory scene, according to Leslie Bennetts of the *New York Times,* "Mr. Wong undergoes a stunning metamorphosis: before the audience's eyes, he transforms himself from 'the perfect woman' into a brash, cocky, insolent man who thumbs his nose at authority and ridicules both racial sterotypes and conventional sex roles, as well as conventional sexuality."

Wong made his professional stage debut in a production of *Androcles and the Lion* at Town Hall in New York City in 1982 and later toured the United States with the road company of *La Cage aux Folles.* Settling in Los Angeles, he appeared in episodes of the television series *Blacke's Magic, Simon and Simon, Shell Game,* and *Hard Copy,* in the film *The Karate Kid II,* and in such stage productions as *See Below Middle Sea, Gifts of the Magi,* and *Mail,* as well as in the first Asian-American production of *A Chorus Line* presented by the East/West Players.

While in Los Angeles, he was given a copy of *M. Butterfly* and was asked to audition for the role of Song Liling. After reading the script he was convinced, he told Gerard Raymond of the [New York] *East Side Spirit,* that "this was a role that was going to change someone's life. It was going to be the unquestionable highlight of one's career—it was also an opportunity to fail miserably." Far from failing, Wong received the Antoinette Perry and Drama Desk

awards as Best Featured Actor, and the Clarence Derwent, Outer Critics Circle, and Theatre World awards, all for outstanding debut. "I knew what I could do," he told the *New York Times,* "but other people didn't. Now they do."

OTHER SOURCES: [New York] *East Side Spirit,* June 12, 1988; *New York Times,* March 25, 1988, September 16, 1988.*

*   *   *

WOPAT, Tom   1951-

PERSONAL: Born September 9, 1951, in Lodi, WI. EDUCATION: Attended the University of Wisconsin.

VOCATION: Actor.

CAREER: PRINCIPAL STAGE APPEARANCES—Wally, *I Love My Wife,* Ethel Barrymore Theatre, New York City, 1977; Dan, *A Bistro Car on the CNR,* Playhouse Theatre, New York City, 1978; ensemble, *Hey, Look Me Over* (revue), Avery Fisher Hall, New York City, 1981; Jupiter, Jove, and Zeus, *Olympus on My Mind,* Lambs Theatre, New York City, 1986; Billy, *Carousel,* Opera House, Kennedy Center for the Performing Arts, Washington, D.C., 1986. Also appeared in *The Robber Bridegroom,* Ford's Theatre, Washington, D.C., 1977; *Oklahoma!,* Equity Library Theatre, Master Theatre, New York City, 1978; and at the Barn Theatre, Augusta, MI.

PRINCIPAL TELEVISION APPEARANCES—Series: Luke Duke, *The Dukes of Hazzard,* CBS, 1979-85; voice of Luke Duke, *The Dukes* (animated), CBS, 1983; Frank Cobb, *Blue Skies,* CBS, 1988; also *A Peaceable Kingdom,* CBS, 1989—. Movies: Tom Silver, *Burning Rage,* CBS, 1984; Pete, *Christmas Comes to Willow Creek,* CBS, 1987. Specials: *Celebrity Challenge of the Sexes,* CBS, 1980; *Battle of the Network Stars,* ABC, 1982.

ADDRESSES: AGENT—J. Michael Bloom, Ltd., 9200 Sunset Boulevard, Suite 710, Los Angeles, CA, 90069. PUBLICIST—Sandy Brokaw, The Brokaw Company, 9255 Sunset Boulevard, Suite 706, Los Angeles, CA, 90069.*

*   *   *

WRIGHT, Garland

PERSONAL: Born in Texas; father, a building contractor. EDUCATION: Attended Southern Methodist University, 1969.

VOCATION: Director and set designer.

CAREER: PRINCIPAL STAGE APPEARANCES—Officer, attendant, Cypriot, and soldier, *Othello,* American National Theatre and Academy Theatre, New York City, 1970; also appeared with the American Shakespeare Festival, Stratford, CT, 1970.

PRINCIPAL STAGE WORK—Director: *Kingdom of Earth,* McCarter Theatre, Princeton, NJ, 1974; *The Tempest,* Lion Theatre Company, New York City, 1974; *Vanities,* Chelsea Westside Theatre, New York City, then Center Theatre Group, Mark Taper Forum,

Los Angeles, CA, both 1976, later Ford's Theatre Society, Washington, DC, then Seattle Repertory Theatre, Seattle, WA, both 1977; (also set designer) *Marathon '33,* Lion Theatre Company, 1976; (also set designer with John Arnone) *K—Impressions of Kafka's "The Trial,"* Lion Theatre Company, Westside Airlines Terminal, New York City, 1977; *Patio/Porch,* Century Theatre, New York City, 1978; *New Jerusalem,* New York Shakespeare Festival, Public Theatre, New York City, 1979; *Private Wars,* on a double-bill with *Lone Star,* Century Theatre, 1979.

The Duenna, Center Stage, Baltimore, MD, 1980; *Eli* and *Candida,* both Tyrone Guthrie Theatre, Minneapolis, MN, 1981; *The Country Wife,* American Place Theatre, New York City, 1982; *Guys and Dolls,* Tyrone Guthrie Theatre, 1983; *A New Approach to Human Sacrifice,* Circle Repertory Theatre, New York City, 1983; *The Misanthrope,* Seattle Repertory Theatre, 1983; *The Importance of Being Earnest,* Tyrone Guthrie Theatre, 1984; *Anteroom,* Playwrights Horizons, New York City, 1985; *The Good Person of Setzuan* and *Old Times,* both Arena Stage, 1985; *The Misanthrope* and *The Piggy Bank,* both Tyrone Guthrie Theatre, 1987; *On the Verge,* Acting Company, John Houseman Theatre, New York City, 1987; *The Imaginary Invalid* and *Hamlet,* both Tyrone Guthrie Theatre, 1989. Also assistant director, American Shakespeare Festival, 1971, then associate director, 1972; director, Milwaukee Repertory Theatre, Milwaukee, WI, 1979-80; director, Arena Stage, Washington, DC, 1982-87; director, Tyrone Guthrie Theatre, 1984; and director, Denver Center Theatre Company, Denver, CO, 1985-86.

PRINCIPAL TELEVISION APPEARANCES—Specials: *Onstage: Twenty-Five Years at the Guthrie,* syndicated, 1988.

RELATED CAREER—Co-founder, Lion Theatre Company, New York City, 1973; associate artistic director, Tyrone Guthrie Theatre, Minneapolis, MN, 1981-84, then artistic director, 1986—.

AWARDS: (With John Arnone) Obie Award from the *Village Voice,* Best Design, 1977, for *K—Impressions of Kafka's "The Trial,";* Obie Award, Best Director, 1987, for *On the Verge.*

MEMBER: Society of Stage Directors and Choreographers.

ADDRESSES: OFFICE—20 W. 84th Street, New York, NY 10036.*

*   *   *

WYLIE, John   1925-

PERSONAL: Born December 14, 1925, in Peacock, TX. EDUCATION: Graduated from North Texas State University.

VOCATION: Actor and director.

CAREER: PRINCIPAL STAGE APPEARANCES—Mr. Dussel, *The Diary of Anne Frank,* Hudson Guild Theatre, New York City, 1976; Sheridan Whiteside, *The Man Who Came to Dinner,* Alaska Repertory Theatre, Anchorage, AK, 1981; title role, *King Lear,* Antonio, *Much Ado about Nothing,* and Player King and Ghost, *Hamlet,* all Folger Theatre, Washington, DC, 1984-85; Friar Thomas, *Measure for Measure,* New York Shakespeare Festival, Delacorte Theatre, New York City, 1985; Danforth, *The Crucible,* Philadelphia Drama Guild, Philadelphia, PA, 1986; Sam, *The Lucky Spot,* Manhattan Theatre Club, New York City, 1987;

Senator Norval Hedges, *Born Yesterday,* 46th Street Theatre, New York City, 1989. Also appeared in *The Seagull,* Alley Theatre, Houston, TX, 1967; *The Man Who Came to Dinner,* Mummers Theatre, Oklahoma City, OK, 1971; *Summer,* Kennedy Center for the Performing Arts, Washington, DC, 1974; *The Real Inspector Hound,* Center Stage, Baltimore, MD, 1975; *Sherlock Holmes,* Repertory Company of the Virginia Museum of Fine Arts, Richmond, VA, 1975; *The Last Meeting of the Knights of the White Magnolia,* Seattle Repertory Theatre, Seattle, WA, 1975; *The Spelling Bee,* Playwrights Horizons, New York City, 1976; *Oliver!, A Month in the Country,* and *Heartbreak House,* all Playhouse in the Park, Cincinnati, OH, 1976-77; *The Caucasian Chalk Circle,* Arena Stage, Washington, DC, 1977; *Compulsion, Buried Child, The Gin Game,* and *A Life in the Theatre,* all Playhouse in the Park, 1980-81; *Death Defying Acts,* Long Island Stage, Rockville Centre, NY, 1986; *The Boys Next Door,* Lamb's Theatre, New York City, 1987; Harpagon, *The Miser;* Shylock, *The Merchant of Venice;* and with the Alley Theatre, 1965-67, 1968-69, and 1985-86; Actors Theatre of Louisville, Louisville, KY, 1972-73; Arena Stage, Washington, DC, 1978-79; and the Folger Theatre, 1982-83 and 1985-86.

PRINCIPAL STAGE WORK—Associate director, Alley Theatre, Houston, TX, 1966-67; associate artistic director, Mummers Theatre, Oklahoma City, OK, 1970-71, then artistic director, 1971-72.

MAJOR TOURS—Drumm, *Da,* U.S. and Canadian cities, 1979-80.

PRINCIPAL FILM APPEARANCES—Waiter in club, *Hanky-Panky,* Columbia, 1982; accountant, *Fletch Lives,* Universal, 1989.

PRINCIPAL TELEVISION APPEARANCES—Mini-Series: *The Adams Chronicles,* PBS, 1976. Episodic: *Hothouse,* ABC, 1988. Movies: Florist, *Daddy, I Don't Like It Like This,* CBS, 1978. Also appeared in *The Grimke Sisters.*

AWARDS: Helen Hayes Award nomination for *The Miser.*

SIDELIGHTS: FAVORITE ROLES—Sheridan Whiteside in *The Man Who Came to Dinner.*

ADDRESSES: AGENT—Bret Adams, Ltd., 448 W. 44th Street, New York, NY 10036.*

*   *   *

WYNER, George

VOCATION: Actor.

CAREER: PRINCIPAL STAGE APPEARANCES—*The Caine Mutiny Court Martial,* Centre Theatre Group, Ahmanson Theatre, Los Angeles, CA, 1971; also appeared with the Syracuse Repertory Theatre, Syracuse, NY, 1972.

PRINCIPAL FILM APPEARANCES—Attorney, *All the President's Men,* Warner Brothers, 1976; Michael Fitzgerald, *Dogs,* La Quinta Film Partners, 1976; network director, *The Bad News Bears Go to Japan,* Paramount, 1978; Dr. Jacobs, *Whose Life Is It, Anyway?,* Metro-Goldwyn-Mayer/United Artists (MGM/UA), 1981; Myron Fein, *My Favorite Year,* MGM/UA, 1982; Ratkowski, *To Be or Not to Be,* Twentieth Century-Fox, 1983; Gillet, *Fletch,* Universal,

1984; Principal Walker, *Wildcats,* Warner Brothers, 1986; Colonel Sandurz, *Spaceballs,* MGM/UA, 1987; Gillet, *Fletch Lives,* Universal, 1987. Also appeared in *Lady Sings the Blues,* Paramount, 1972.

PRINCIPAL TELEVISION APPEARANCES—Series: Assistant District Attorney Dorfman, *Delvecchio,* CBS, 1976-77; District Attorney Frank Revko, *Kaz,* CBS, 1978-79; George Korman, *Big Shamus, Little Shamus,* CBS, 1979; Saul Panzer, *Nero Wolfe,* NBC, 1981; Assistant District Attorney Irwin Bernstein, *Hill Street Blues,* NBC, 1982-87; Murray Chase, *Matt Houston,* ABC, 1982-85; Corporal Wessel, *At Ease,* ABC, 1983; Max Rubin, *She's the Sheriff,* syndicated, 1987. Mini-Series: Dr. McCabe, *Once an Eagle,* NBC, 1976-77. Pilots: Happy Jack, *Duffy,* CBS, 1977; Rantzen, *Lucan,* ABC, 1977; Stewart Rose, *Sheila,* CBS, 1977; Ray Banks, *The Sunshine Boys,* NBC, 1977; Mike, *Friends,* CBS, 1978; Arnie Simms, *The Islander,* CBS, 1978; Max Rosencrantz, *Cass Malloy,* CBS, 1982; Mike, *Man About Town,* ABC, 1986; Wes Bushnell, *Chameleon,* ABC, 1986. Episodic: Irving Metzman, *Hail to the Chief,* ABC, 1985; Henry Morris, *The Fall Guy,* ABC, 1986; Dr. Lewis, *Murder, She Wrote,* CBS, 1988; also *The Bob Newhart Show,* CBS, 1975; *M*A*S*H,* CBS, 1978; *All in the Family,* CBS, 1979. Movies: Deputy District Attorney Piper, *The Law,* NBC, 1974; Roy Cohn, *Tail Gunner Joe,* NBC, 1977; Blandings, *The Trial of Lee Harvey Oswald,* ABC, 1977; John Wiepert, *Reunion,* CBS, 1980; Dr. Irving Lefkowitz, *Drop-Out Father,* CBS, 1982; Joe Haley, *A Death in California,* ABC, 1985; Mr. Gladstone, *The Leftovers,* ABC, 1986; Victor Rigsby, *The Richest Cat in the World,* ABC, 1986.

ADDRESSES: AGENT—Mary Ellen White, 151 N. San Vicente Boulevard, Beverly Hills, CA 90211. PUBLICIST—Brad Lemack, Lemack and Company, 7060 Hollywood Boulevard, Suite 320, Los Angeles, CA 90028.*

*   *   *

WYNTER, Dana   1930-

PERSONAL: Born Dagmar Spencer-Marcus, June 8, 1930, in London, England; daughter of Peter and Frederique (Spencer) Winter; married Gregson Bautzer, June 10, 1956; children: Mark Ragan. EDUCATION: Attended North London Collegiate School and Rhodes University.

VOCATION: Actress and producer.

CAREER: PRINCIPAL STAGE APPEARANCES—*Black-Eyed Susan,* New York City, 1954.

PRINCIPAL FILM APPEARANCES—Dinah Higgins, *The View from Pompey's Head* (also known as *Secret Interlude*), Twentieth Century-Fox, 1955; Valerie, *D-Day, the Sixth of June* (also known as *The Sixth of June*), Twentieth Century-Fox, 1956; Becky Driscoll, *Invasion of the Body Snatchers,* Allied Artists, 1956; Holly Keith, *Something of Value,* Metro-Goldwyn-Mayer, 1957; Erika Angermann, *Fraulein,* Twentieth Century-Fox, 1958; Sue Trumbell, *In Love and War,* Twentieth Century-Fox, 1958; Jennifer Curtis, *Shake Hands with the Devil,* United Artists, 1959; Anne Davis, *Sink the Bismarck!,* Twentieth Century-Fox, 1960; Lady Margaret Mackenzie, *Smith, On the Double,* Paramount, 1961; Lady Jocelyn Brutenholm, *The List of Adrian Messenger,* Universal, 1963; Ellen Whitlock, *If He Hollers, Let Him Go,* Cinerama, 1968; Cindy, *Airport,* Universal, 1970; Valerie, *Santee,* Crown International, 1973; wife, *The Savage* (also known as *Le Sauvage* and *Lovers Like Us*), Gaumont, 1975.

PRINCIPAL TELEVISION APPEARANCES—Series: Eva Wainwright, *The Man Who Never Was,* ABC, 1966-67. Pilots: Lynn Oliver, *Owen Marshall: Counselor at Law,* ABC, 1971; Lady Helena Trimble, *The Questor Tapes,* NBC, 1974; Andrea Hardesty, *The Lives of Jenny Dolan,* NBC, 1975; Margaret Michaels, *M Station: Hawaii,* CBS, 1980. Mini-Series: Mrs. Colgate, *Backstairs at the White House,* NBC, 1979. Episodic: Harriet Whitney, *Tenspeed and Brownshoe,* ABC, 1980; also *Robert Montgomery Presents,* NBC, 1953; *Studio One,* CBS, 1953; *Bob Hope Presents the Chrysler Theater,* NBC, 1953; *Playhouse 90,* CBS, 1955; *Wagon Train,* ABC, 1961; *The Virginian,* NBC, 1962; *Ben Casey,* ABC, 1967; *My Three Sons,* CBS, 1968; *The Invaders,* ABC, 1968; *The Wild Wild West,* CBS, 1968; *Gunsmoke,* CBS, 1969; *Medical Center,* CBS, 1970; *Marcus Welby, M.D.,* ABC, 1970; *Ironside,* NBC, 1970; *To Rome with Love,* CBS, 1970; *It Takes a Thief,* ABC, 1970; *Burke's Law,* ABC; *Bob Hope Presents,* NBC; *Twelve O'Clock High,* ABC; *The Rogues,* NBC; *Cannon,* CBS; *McMillan and Wife,* NBC; *The Love Boat,* ABC; *Hawaii Five-O,* CBS; *Alfred Hitchcock Presents,* CBS; *Fantasy Island,* ABC; *Suspense; U.S. Steel Hour.* Movies: Julia Klanton, *Companions in Nightmare,* NBC, 1968; Jane Peterson, *Any Second Now,* NBC, 1969; Eleanor Warren, *The Connection,* ABC, 1973; Queen Elizabeth, *The Royal Romance of Charles and Diana,* CBS, 1982. Specials: Laura Hunt, *Laura,* CBS, 1955; also *Dana Wynter in Ireland,* 1976.

PRINCIPAL TELEVISION WORK—Producer, *Dana Wynter in Ireland,* 1976.

PRINCIPAL RADIO APPEARANCES—*The Private Lives of Harry Lime,* British radio, 1953.

ADDRESSES: AGENT—Charles Goldring, 9044 Melrose Avenue, Suite 101, Los Angeles, CA 90069.*

Y

YOUNG, Robert 1907-

PERSONAL: Full name, Robert George Young; born February 22, 1907, in Chicago, IL; married Elizabeth Louise Henderson, 1933; children: Carol Anne, Barbara Queen, Elizabeth Louise, Kathleen Joy. EDUCATION: Studied acting at the Pasadena Playhouse.

VOCATION: Actor.

CAREER: PRINCIPAL STAGE APPEARANCES—Appeared in productions with the Pasadena Playhouse, Los Angeles, CA, for four years.

MAJOR TOURS—Bolton, Generation, U.S. cities, 1966-67; also appeared in The Ship, U.S. cities, 1931-35.

FILM DEBUT—Jimmy Bradshaw, The Black Camel, Twentieth Century-Fox, 1931; PRINCIPAL FILM APPEARANCES—Marco Ricca, The Guilty Generation, Columbia, 1931; Dr. Claudet, The Sin of Madelon Claudet (also known as The Lullaby), Metro-Goldwyn-Mayer (MGM), 1931; young officer, Hell Divers, MGM, 1932; Ricardo, The Kid from Spain, United Artists, 1932; Ralph Thomas, New Morals for Old, MGM, 1932; Gordon, Strange Interlude (also known as Strange Interval), MGM, 1932; Dick Ogden, Unashamed, MGM, 1932; Kip Tarleton, The Wet Parade, MGM, 1932; Lieutenant Brick Walters, Hell Below, MGM, 1933; Geoffrey, Men Must Fight, MGM, 1933; Bob Preble, Right to Romance, RKO, 1933; Jim Fowler, Saturday's Millions, Universal, 1933; Claude, Today We Live, MGM, 1933; Alec Brennan, Tugboat Annie, MGM, 1933; Tony Ferrera, The Band Plays On, MGM, 1934; Will Connelly, Carolina (also known as House of Connelly), Twentieth Century-Fox, 1934; Larry Kelly, Death of the Diamond, MGM, 1934; as himself, Hollywood Party, MGM, 1934; Captain Fitzroy, The House of Rothschild, Twentieth Century-Fox, 1934; Bill Drexel, Lazy River, MGM, 1934; Pat Wells, Paris Interlude, MGM, 1934; John Stafford, Spitfire, RKO, 1934; Jack Forrester, Whom the Gods Destroy, Columbia, 1934.

Pat, Calm Yourself, MGM, 1935; Jeff, Red Salute (also known as Arms and the Girl, Runaway Daughter, and Her Enlisted Man), United Artists, 1935; Tony Milburn, Remember Last Night, Universal, 1935; Tony Spear, Vagabond Lady, MGM, 1935; Little Mike, West Point of the Air, MGM, 1935; Jack Bristow, The Bride Comes Home, Paramount, 1936; Hugh McKenzie, The Bride Walks Out, RKO, 1936; Peter Carlton, It's Love Again, Gaumont, 1936; Charley Phelps, The Longest Night, MGM, 1936; Robert Marvin, The Secret Agent, Gaumont, 1936; Tommy Randall, Stowaway, Twentieth Century-Fox, 1936; Hank Sherman, Sworn Enemy, MGM, 1936; Joe Hatcher, The Three Wise Guys, MGM, 1936; Rudi Pal, The Bride Wore Red, MGM, 1937; Hank Medhill, Dangerous Number, MGM, 1937; Grand Duke Peter, The Emper-

or's Candlesticks, MGM, 1937; Gene Anders, I Met Him in Paris, Paramount, 1937; Tom Wakefield, Married before Breakfast, MGM, 1937; Roger Ash, Navy Blue and Gold, MGM, 1937; Pierre Brossard, Josette, Twentieth Century-Fox, 1938; Fritz Hagedorn, Paradise for Three (also known as Romance for Three), MGM, 1938; Bill Harrison, Rich Man, Poor Girl, MGM, 1938; David Linden, The Shining Hour, MGM, 1938; Gottfried Lenz, Three Comrades, MGM, 1938; Andre Vallaire, The Toy Wife (also known as Frou-Frou), MGM, 1938; Neil McGill, Bridal Suite, MGM, 1939; Brooks Mason and George Smith, Honolulu, MGM, 1939; Slim Martin, Maisie, MGM, 1939; Michael Morgan, Miracles for Sale, MGM, 1939.

Douglas Lamont, Dr. Kildare's Crisis, MGM, 1940; Anton, Florian, MGM, 1940; Fritz Marlberg, The Mortal Storm, MGM, 1940; Langdon Towne, Northwest Passage, MGM, 1940; Myles Vanders, Sporting Blood, MGM, 1940; Harry Pulham, H.M. Pulham, Esq., MGM, 1941; Eddie Crane, Lady Be Good, MGM, 1941; Randolf Haven, Married Bachelor, MGM, 1941; Jimmy Blake, The Trial of Mary Dugan, MGM, 1941; Richard Blake, Western Union, Twentieth Century-Fox, 1941; Homer Smith, Cairo, MGM, 1942; title role, Joe Smith, American (also known as Highway to Freedom), MGM, 1942; John Davis, Journey for Margaret, MGM, 1942; David Naughton, Claudia, Twentieth Century-Fox, 1943; Bob Stuart, Slightly Dangerous, MGM, 1943; Sam Mackeever, Sweet Rosie O'Grady, Twentieth Century-Fox, 1943; Cuffy Williams, The Canterville Ghost, MGM, 1944; Oliver, The Enchanted Cottage, RKO, 1945; Hank, Those Endearing Young Charms, RKO, 1945; David Naughton, Claudia and David, Twentieth Century-Fox, 1946; Larry Scott, Lady Luck, RKO, 1946; Alex Hazen, The Searching Wind, Paramount, 1946; Captain Finlay, Crossfire, RKO, 1947; Larry Ballentine, They Won't Believe Me, RKO, 1947; Nick Buckley, Relentless, Columbia, 1948; Harry, Sitting Pretty, Twentieth Century-Fox, 1948; Dr. Sheldon, Adventure in Baltimore (also known as Bachelor Bait), RKO, 1949; Vernon Walsh, And Baby Makes Three, Columbia, 1949; Steve Adams, Bride for Sale, RKO, 1949; Philip Bosinney, That Forsyte Woman (also known as The Forsyte Saga), MGM, 1949; Dr. James Merrill, Goodbye, My Fancy, Warner Brothers, 1951; Jeff Cohalan, The Second Woman (also known as Here Lies Love and Ellen Twelve Miles Out), United Artists, 1951; Dan Craig, The Half-Breed, RKO, 1952; Dr. Stanley Moorehead, Secret of the Incas, Paramount, 1954.

PRINCIPAL TELEVISION APPEARANCES—Series: Jim Anderson, Father Knows Best, CBS, 1954-55, then NBC, 1955-58, later CBS, 1958-60; Cameron Garrett Brooks, Window on Main Street, CBS, 1961-62; title role, Marcus Welby, M.D., ABC, 1969-76; Mr. James Laurence, Little Women, NBC, 1979. Pilots: Nick Holloway, Holloway's Daughters, NBC, 1966; title role, Marcus Welby, M.D., ABC, 1969; James Lawrence, Little Women, NBC,

1978; title role, *The Return of Marcus Welby, M.D.*, ABC, 1984. Episodic: *Climax!*, CBS; *Dr. Kildare*, NBC; *Bob Hope Present the Chrysler Theatre*, NBC; *The Name of the Game*, NBC. Movies: Senator Earl Gannon, *Vanished*, NBC, 1971; Judge Charles Raleigh, *All My Darling Daughters*, ABC, 1972; Judge Charles Raleigh, *My Darling Daughters' Anniversary*, ABC, 1973; Jim Anderson, *Father Knows Best: The Father Knows Best Reunion*, NBC, 1977; Jim Anderson, *Father Knows Best: Home for Christmas*, NBC, 1977; Roswell Gilbert, *Mercy or Murder*, NBC, 1987; Grandpa Joe, *Conspiracy of Love*, CBS, 1987; title role, *Marcus Welby, M.D.—A Holiday Affair* (also known as *Dr. Marcus Welby in Paris*), ABC, 1988. Specials: Host, *Robert Young and the Family*, CBS, 1971; *A Salute to Television's Twenty-Fifth Anniversary*, ABC, 1972; host, *Robert Young with the Young*, ABC, 1973; *Celebration: The American Spirit*, ABC, 1976; *NBC's Sixtieth Anniversary Celebration*, NBC, 1986.

PRINCIPAL RADIO APPEARANCES—Series: Jim Anderson, *Father Knows Best*, 1949-54; also *Good News of 1938*, 1938; and *Maxwell House Coffee Time*, 1944.

RELATED CAREER—Founder (with Eugene Rodney) and president, Cavalier Productions, 1947—; actor in television commercials.

NON-RELATED CAREER—Clerk, salesman, reporter, and loan company collector.

AWARDS: Emmy Awards, Best Continuing Performance by an Actor in a Dramatic Series, 1957, and Best Continuing Performance by an Actor in a Leading Role in a Dramatic or Comedy Series, 1958, both for *Father Knows Best*; Emmy Award, Outstanding Continued Performance by an Actor in a Leading Role in a Dramatic Series, 1970, for *Marcus Welby, M.D.*; also Emmy Award nomination for *Vanished*.

ADDRESSES: AGENT—Herb Tobias and Associates, Inc., 1901 Avenue of the Stars, Suite 840, Los Angeles, CA 90067.*

*   *   *

YOUNG, Sean   1959-

PERSONAL: Full name, Mary Sean Young; born November 20, 1959, in Louisville, KY; daughter of Donald Young (a journalist) and Lee Guthrie (a public relations executive and writer). EDUCATION: Graduated from Interlochen Arts Academy, 1978.

VOCATION: Actress.

CAREER: FILM DEBUT—Ariadne Charlton, *Jane Austen in Manhattan*, Comtemporary, 1980. PRINCIPAL FILM APPEARANCES—Louise, *Stripes*, Columbia, 1981; Rachael, *Blade Runner*, Warner Brothers, 1982; Dr. Stephanie Brody, *Young Doctors in Love*, Twentieth Century-Fox, 1982; Chani, *Dune*, Universal, 1984; Susan Matthews-Loomis, *Baby: Secret of a Lost Legend*, Buena Vista, 1985; Susan Atwell, *No Way Out*, Orion, 1987; Kate Gekko, *Wall Street*, Twentieth Century-Fox, 1987; Linda Brown, *The Boost*, Hemdale, 1989; Tish, *Cousins*, Paramount, 1989. Also appeared as artist at party, *Arena Brains* (short film), 1987.

PRINCIPAL TELEVISION APPEARANCES—Mini-Series: Rosemary Hoyt, *Tender Is the Night*, CBS, 1986. Movies: Leonore,

Blood and Orchids, CBS, 1986. Specials: Myra Harper, *Under the Biltmore Clock*, PBS, 1985.

RELATED CAREER—Professional model; member, American Tap Dance Orchestra.

NON-RELATED CAREER—Research assistant, National Lung Program, New York City, 1978; secretary.

ADDRESSES: AGENT—David Schiff, Creative Artists Agency, 1888 Century Park E., Suite 1400, Los Angeles, CA, 90067.*

*   *   *

YOUNG, Terence   1915-

PERSONAL: Born June 20, 1915, in Shanghai, China; married Dosia Bennett (a novelist), June 24, 1944 (died, 1985); children: three. EDUCATION: Received B.A. in history from Cambridge University. MILITARY: British Army, Guards Armoured Division, major, during World War II.

VOCATION: Director and screenwriter.

CAREER: Also see WRITINGS below. PRINCIPAL FILM WORK—Director: *Corridor of Mirrors*, Apollo, 1948; (as Shaun Terence Young) *One Night with You*, Universal, 1948; *Woman Hater*, Universal, 1949; *They Were Not Divided*, United Artists/Rank, 1951; *The Frightened Bride* (also known as *Tall Headlines*), Grand National, 1952; *Valley of Eagles*, Lippert, 1952; *Paratrooper* (also known as *The Red Beret*), Columbia, 1954; (with Zoltan Korda) *Storm over the Nile*, Columbia, 1955; *That Lady*, Twentieth Century-Fox, 1955; *Safari*, Columbia, 1956; *Zarak*, Columbia, 1956; *Action of the Tiger*, Metro-Goldwyn-Mayer (MGM), 1957; (with Richard Maibaum) *Tank Force* (also known as *No Time to Die*), Columbia, 1958; *Too Hot to Handle* (also known as *Playgirl after Dark*), Topaz, 1961; *Black Tights*, Magna, 1962; *Dr. No*, United Artists, 1962; *Immoral Charge* (also known as *Serious Charge* and *A Touch of Hell*), Governor, 1962; *From Russia with Love*, United Artists, 1963; (with Ferdinando Baldi) *Duel of Champions* (also known as *Orazi e curiaz*), Medallion, 1964; *The Amorous Adventures of Moll Flanders*, Paramount, 1965; *Thunderball*, United Artists, 1965; *The Poppy Is Also a Flower*, Comet, 1966; (with Chistian-Jacque and Carlo Lizzani) *The Dirty Game*, American International, 1966; *The Rover* (also known as *L'Avventuriero* and *The Adventurer*), Cinerama, 1967; *Triple Cross*, Warner Brothers, 1967; *Wait until Dark*, Warner Brothers, 1967; (with Denis Cannan and Joseph Kessel) *Mayerling*, MGM, 1968; *The Christmas Tree*, Continental, 1969; *Red Sun* (also known as *Soleïl rouge*), National General, 1972; *The Valachi Papers* (also known as *Joe Valachi: I segretti di Cosa Nostra*), Columbia, 1972; *Cold Sweat* (also known as *L'uomo dalle due ombre*, and *De la part des copains*), Emerson, 1974; *The Klansman*, Paramount, 1974; *Bloodline* (also known as *Sidney Sheldon's "Bloodline"*), Paramount, 1979; *Inchon*, Metro-Goldwyn-Mayer/United Artists, 1981; *The Jigsaw Man*, United Film Distribution, 1984.

PRINCIPAL TELEVISION WORK—Specials: Director, *The Poppy Is Also a Flower* (also known as *Poppies Are Also Flowers*), ABC, 1966.

WRITINGS: FILM—(With Brian Desmond Hurst and Patrick Kirwan) *The Fugitive* (also known as *On the Night of the Fire*), Universal,

1940; (as Shaun Terence Young; with Hurst and Rodney Ackland) *Suicide Squadron* (also known as *Dangerous Moonlight*), RKO, 1942; (with Clive Brook) *On Approval*, English Films Incorporated, 1944; (with Daphne du Maurier) *Hungry Hill*, General Films Distributors, 1947; (with Anthony Thorne, Peter Quennell, Lawrence Kitchen, and Paul Holt) *The Bad Lord Byron*, General Films Distributors, 1949; *They Were Not Divided*, United Artists/Rank, 1951; *Valley of Eagles*, Lippert, 1952; (with Richard Maibaum) *Tank Force* (also known as *No Time to Die*), Columbia, 1958; (with Denis Cannan and Joseph Kessel) *Mayerling*, Metro-Goldwyn-Mayer, 1968; *The Christmas Tree*, Continental, 1969.

AWARDS: Gold Medal from the Venice Film Festival, 1961, for *Black Tights;* Prix Femina (European Critics Award), 1970, for *The Christmas Tree.*

MEMBER: Directors Guild of America, Travellers Club.

ADDRESSES: OFFICE—The Garden Suite, Pinewood Studios, Iver Heath, England. AGENT—Laurence Evans, International Creative Management, 388 Oxford Street, W1, England.

*   *   *

YOUNGS, Jim

PERSONAL: Born October 16, in Old Bethpage, NY; son of Robin Youngs (a journalist, producer, and director); mother, an opera singer. EDUCATION: Attended the University of Miami.

VOCATION: Actor.

CAREER: PRINCIPAL FILM APPEARANCES—Buddy, *The Wanderers*, Orion, 1979; Jim, *The Final Terror*, Comworld, 1981; Chuck, *Footloose*, Paramount, 1984; cowboy, *Out of Control*, New World, 1984; Kelly Youngblood, *Youngblood*, Metro-Goldwyn-Mayer/United Artists (MGM/UA), 1986; Billy, *Nobody's Fool*, Island, 1986; Jimmy Kristidis, *Hot Shot*, Arista, 1987; Bronson Green, *You Talkin' to Me?*, MGM/UA, 1987.

PRINCIPAL TELEVISION APPEARANCES—Series: John Grey, *The Secrets of Midland Heights*, CBS, 1980-81. Episodic: Billy Ray, *Private Eye*, NBC, 1987. Movies: Alan "Toots" Tuttle, *Splendor in the Grass*, NBC, 1981; Sterling Baker, *The Executioner's Song*, NBC, 1982; Ronnie Norton, *Roses Are for the Rich*, CBS, 1987.

NON-RELATED CAREER—Janitor; parking attendant, then manager, My Father's Place (nightclub), Roslyn, NY; doorman, Roxy Theatre, Los Angeles.

ADDRESSES: AGENT—Marion Rosenberg, The Lantz Office, 9255 Sunset Boulevard, Suite 505, Los Angeles, CA 90069.*

*   *   *

YULIN, Harris   1937-

PERSONAL: Born November 5, 1937, in California. EDUCATION: Attended the University of Southern California.

VOCATION: Actor and director.

CAREER: PRINCIPAL STAGE APPEARANCES—Dust, *Next Time I'll Sing to You*, Phoenix Theatre, New York City, 1963; Gabriele, *Troubled Waters, or The Brother Who Protects and Loves*, Gate Theatre, New York City, 1965; Lord Hastings, *King Richard III*, New York Shakespeare Festival (NYSF), Delacorte Theatre, New York City, 1966; title role, *King John*, NYSF, Delacorte Theatre, 1967; uncle, *The Cannibals*, American Place Theatre, New York City, 1968; Piet Bezuidenhout, *A Lesson from Aloes*, Yale Repertory Theatre, New Haven, CT, 1979, then Playhouse Theatre, New York City, 1980; Teck de Brancovis, *Watch on the Rhine*, Long Wharf Theatre, New Haven, CT, 1979, then John Golden Theatre, New York City, 1980; George Tesman, *Hedda Gabler*, Roundabout Theatre, New York City, 1981; P.T. Barnum, *Barnum's Last Life*, La Mama Experimental Theatre Club, New York City, 1983; Sir George Crofts, *Mrs. Warren's Profession*, Roundabout Theatre, 1985; Claudius, *Hamlet*, NYSF, Public Theatre, New York City, 1986; Gordon, "April Snow," *Marathon '87*, Ensemble Studio Theatre, New York City, 1987; Wallace Blossom, *Approaching Zanzibar*, Second Stage Theatre, New York City, 1989. Also appeared in *Iphigenia in Aulis*, Circle in the Square at Ford's Theatre, Washington, DC, 1969; *Henry V*, Hartford Stage Company, Hartford, CT, 1971; *Hamlet*, Center Theatre Group, Mark Taper Forum, Los Angeles, CA, 1973; *Uncle Vanya*, Yale Repertory Theatre, 1981; *The Doctor's Dilemma*, Long Wharf Theatre, 1982; *Tartuffe*, Tyrone Guthrie Theatre, Minneapolis, MN, 1984; *A Midsummer Night's Dream*, Off-Broadway production; with the Yale Repertory Theatre, 1967-68; Studio Arena Theatre, Buffalo, NY, 1968-69; and with Arena Stage, Washington, DC, 1984-85.

PRINCIPAL STAGE WORK—Director: *Cuba Si* and *The Guns of Carrar*, both American National Theatre Academy Matinee Series, Theatre De Lys, New York City, 1968; *The Guardsman*, Long Wharf Theatre, New Haven, CT, 1982; *Winterplay*, Second Stage Company, South Street Theatre, New York City, 1983; "Fine Line," *Marathon '84*, Ensemble Studio Theatre, New York City, 1984.

MAJOR TOURS—Mike Talman, *Wait until Dark*, U.S. cities, 1967.

PRINCIPAL FILM APPEARANCES—Joe Morgan, *End of the Road*, Allied Artists, 1970; Wyatt Earp, *Doc*, United Artists, 1971; Zebulon Yandro, *Who Fears the Devil* (also known as *The Legend of Hillbilly John* and *My Name Is John*), Jack H. Harris, 1972; Casey, *The Midnight Man*, Universal, 1974; Gordon Pankey, *Watched*, Penthouse, 1974; Marty Heller, *Night Moves*, Warner Brothers, 1975; Detective Oller, *St. Ives*, Warner Brothers, 1976; Eddie Cassidy, *Steel* (also known as *Look Down and Die* and *Men of Steel*), World Northal, 1980; Bernstein, *Scarface*, Universal, 1983; Detective Harrigan, *Good to Go*, Island, 1986; Donald Calder, *The Believers*, Orion, 1987; Elmore Silk, *Candy Mountain* (also known as *There Ain't No Candy Mountain*), Films Plain Chant/Metropolis/International Film Exchange, 1987; Conrad Kroll, *Fatal Beauty*, Metro-Goldwyn-Mayer/United Artists, 1987; Dr. Beresford, *Bad Dreams*, Twentieth Century-Fox, 1988; Bruno Ristau, *Judgment in Berlin* (also known as *Judgment over Berlin*), New Line Cinema/Vidmark Entertainment, 1988; Paul, *Another Woman*, Orion, 1988. Also appeared in *Maidstone*, Supreme Mix, 1970.

PRINCIPAL TELEVISION APPEARANCES—Mini-Series: Senator Joseph McCarthy, *Robert Kennedy and His Times*, CBS, 1985. Pilots: John Connors, *A Mask of Love* (broadcast as an episode of *ABC's Matinee Today*), ABC, 1973; Hog Yancy, *The Greatest Gift*, NBC, 1974; George "Machine Gun" Kelly, *Melvin Purvis: G-Man* (also known as *The Legend of Machine Gun Kelly*), ABC, 1974; John Blackwood, *James A. Michener's "Dynasty,"* (also known as *Dynasty*), NBC, 1976; Isaac Pratt, *Ransom for Alice!* NBC, 1977; Arthur Pennington, *Roger and Harry* (also known as *Roger and Harry: The Mitera Target* and *Love for Ransom*), ABC, 1977; Billy "Bowlegs" Baines, *The Night Rider*, ABC, 1979; Haman, *The Thirteenth Day: The Story of Esther*, ABC, 1979. Episodic: Ross O'Brien, *Cagney and Lacey*, CBS, 1986; also Deek Peasley, *How the West Was Won*, ABC. Movies: J. Edgar Hoover, *The F.B.I. Story: The F.B.I. versus Alvin Karpis, Public Enemy Number One* (also known as *The F.B.I. Story—Alvin Karpis*), CBS, 1974; Johnny Lazia, *The Kansas City Massacre*, ABC, 1975; Lieutenant Kastner, *The Trial of Chaplain Jensen*, ABC, 1975; General Dan Shomron, *Victory at Entebbe*, ABC, 1976; Joseph T. Antonelli, *When Every Day Was the Fourth of July*, NBC, 1978; Jesse James, *The Last Ride of the Dalton Gang*, NBC, 1979; U.S. Attorney Thomas Foran, *Conspiracy: The Trial of the Chicago Eight* (also known as *The Trial of the Chicago Eight* and *The Truth and Nothing but the Truth: The Chicago Conspiracy Trial*), HBO, 1987. Specials: Alexandr Fomin, *The Missiles of October*, ABC, 1974.

ADDRESSES: AGENT—The Artists Agency, 10000 Santa Monica Boulevard, Suite 305, Los Angeles, CA 90067.*

Z

ZABKA, William

PERSONAL: Born October 20, in New York, NY; son of Stan Zabka (an assistant director); mother, a production assistant. EDUCATION: Studied advanced guitar and music theory at California State University, Northridge.

VOCATION: Actor.

CAREER: FILM DEBUT—Johnny, *The Karate Kid*, Columbia, 1984. PRINCIPAL FILM APPEARANCES—Greg, *Just One of the Guys*, Columbia, 1985; Jack, *National Lampoon's European Vacation*, Warner Brothers, 1985; Chas, *Back to School*, Orion, 1986; Johnny, *The Karate Kid, Part II*, Columbia, 1986; Randy, *A Tiger's Tale*, Atlantic, 1987.

PRINCIPAL TELEVISION APPEARANCES—Series: Scott McCall, *The Equalizer*, CBS, 1986-89. Episodic: *Gimme a Break*, NBC; *The Love Boat*, ABC; *The Greatest American Hero*, ABC. Movies: Kim Fisher, *Dreams of Gold: The Mel Fisher Story*, CBS, 1986; also *Emergency Room*, syndicated, 1983. Specials: Rick Peterson, "Contract for Life: The S.A.D.D. Story," *CBS Schoolbreak Special*, CBS, 1984.

RELATED CAREER—Appeared in more than twenty television commercials from the age of twelve.

SIDELIGHTS: RECREATIONS—Surfing, backpacking, rafting, horseback riding, skiing, karate, soccer, swimming, and deep-sea diving.

ADDRESSES: MANAGER—Frank Campana Personal Management, 20121 Ventura Boulevard, Suite 343, Woodland Hills, CA 91364.*

*   *   *

ZANUCK, Richard D.   1934-

PERSONAL: Full name, Richard Darryl Zanuck; born December 13, 1934, in Los Angeles, CA; son of Darryl F. (a producer) and Virginia (Fox) Zanuck; married Lili Gentle (divorced); married Linda Harrison, October 26, 1969 (divorced); married Lili Fini, September 23, 1978; children: Virginia, Janet (first marriage). EDUCATION: Stanford University, B.A., 1956. MILITARY: U.S. Army, second lieutenant.

VOCATION: Producer and film executive.

CAREER: All as producer, unless indicated: Assistant to the producer, *The Sun Also Rises*, Twentieth Century-Fox, 1956; assistant to the producer, *Island in the Sun*, Twentieth Century-Fox, 1957; *Compulsion*, Twentieth Century-Fox, 1959; *Sanctuary*, Twentieth Century-Fox, 1961; *The Chapman Report*, Warner Brothers, 1962; assistant to the producer, *The Longest Day*, Twentieth Century-Fox, 1962; (with David Brown) *SSSSSSSS* (also known as *Sssnake*), Universal, 1973; executive producer (with Brown), *The Sting*, Universal, 1973; (with Brown) *Willie Dynamite*, Universal, 1973; (with Brown) *The Sugarland Express*, Universal, 1974; (with Brown) *The Black Windmill*, Universal, 1974; (with Brown) *The Girl from Petrovka*, Universal, 1974; (with Brown) *The Eiger Sanction*, Universal, 1975; (with Brown) *Jaws*, Universal, 1975; (with Brown) *MacArthur*, Universal, 1977; (with Brown) *Jaws 2*, Universal, 1978; (with Brown) *The Island*, Universal, 1980; (with Brown) *Neighbors*, Columbia, 1981; (with Brown) *The Verdict*, Twentieth Century-Fox, 1982; (with Brown and Lili Fini Zanuck) *Cocoon*, Twentieth Century-Fox, 1985; (with Brown) *Target*, Warner Brothers, 1985.

RELATED CAREER—Story department, Twentieth Century-Fox, Hollywood, CA, 1954; publicity department, Twentieth Century-Fox, New York City, 1955; vice-president, Darryl F. Zanuck Productions, 1958; president's production representative, Twentieth Century-Fox, 1963; executive vice-president in charge of production, Twentieth Century-Fox, 1967; president, Twentieth Century-Fox Television, 1967; chairman of the board, Twentieth Century-Fox Television, 1968; president, Twentieth Century-Fox, 1969; senior executive vice-president, Warner Brothers, 1971; founder (with David Brown), Zanuck/Brown Production Company, 1972; executive, Twentieth Century-Fox, 1980-83; executive, Warner Brothers, 1983-86; executive, Metro-Goldwyn-Mayer Entertainment, 1986-89.

NON-RELATED CAREER—National chairman, Cystic Fibrosis Association; member, Organizing Committee for 1984 Olympics, Los Angeles, CA.

MEMBER: Academy of Motion Picture Arts and Sciences (trustee and board member), Screen Producers Guild, Phi Gamma Delta.

AWARDS: Producer of the Year Award from the National Association of Theatre Owners, 1974; Academy Award, Best Picture, 1974, for *The Sting;* (with David Brown) Academy Award nomination, Best Picture, 1976, for *Jaws;* (with Brown) Academy Award nomination, Best Picture, 1983, for *The Verdict*.

ADDRESSES: OFFICE—202 N. Canon Drive, Beverly Hills, CA 90210.*

ZEMECKIS, Robert   1952-

PERSONAL: Born in 1952 in Chicago, IL; married Mary Ellen Trainor (an actress). EDUCATION: Received professional training at the University of Southern California (USC) Film School.

VOCATION: Director, screenwriter, and editor.

CAREER: Also see *WRITINGS* below. PRINCIPAL FILM WORK—Director: *I Wanna Hold Your Hand,* Universal, 1978; *Used Cars,* Columbia, 1980; *Romancing the Stone,* Twentieth Century-Fox, 1984; *Back to the Future,* Universal, 1985; *Who Framed Roger Rabbit?,* Buena Vista, 1988; *Back to the Future II,* Universal, 1990. Also producer and director, *A Field of Honor* (short film).

PRINCIPAL TELEVISION WORK—Specials: ''And All through the House,'' *Tales from the Crypt,* HBO, 1989.

RELATED CAREER—As a film editor, worked on television commercials and for NBC News, Chicago.

WRITINGS: FILM—(With Bob Gale) *I Wanna Hold Your Hand,* Universal, 1978; (with Gale) *1941,* 1979; (with Gale) *Used Cars,* Columbia, 1980; (with Gale) *Back to the Future,* Universal, 1985; also *A Field of Honor* (short film). TELEVISION—Episodic: (With Gale) *McCloud,* NBC.

AWARDS: Academy Award nomination, Best Original Screenplay, 1986, for *Back to the Future;* also special jury award from the Second Annual Student Film Awards of the Academy of Motion Picture Arts and Sciences and fifteen international honors, all for *A Field of Honor.*

ADDRESSES: AGENT—Jack Rapke, Creative Artists Agency, 1888 Century Park E., Suite 1400, Los Angeles, CA 90067.*

*   *   *

ZINNEMANN, Fred   1907-

PERSONAL: Born April 29, 1907, in Austria; son of Oskar (a doctor) and Anna (Feiwel) Zinnemann; came to the United States, 1929; naturalized U.S. citizen, 1937; married Renee Bartlett, October 9, 1936; children: Tim. EDUCATION: University of Vienna, B.A., law, 1927; attended the Technical School of Cinematography, Paris, France, 1927-28.

VOCATION: Producer and director.

CAREER: PRINCIPAL FILM APPEARANCES—*All Quiet on the Western Front,* Universal, 1930.

PRINCIPAL FILM WORK—All as director, unless indicated. *A Friend Indeed* (short film), Metro-Goldwyn-Mayer (MGM), 1938; *The Story of Dr. Carver* (short film), MGM, 1938; *That Mothers Might Live* (short film), MGM, 1938; *Tracking the Sleeping Death* (short film), MGM, 1938; *They Live Again* (short film), MGM, 1938; *Weather Wizards* (short film), MGM, 1939; *While America Sleeps* (short film), MGM, 1939; *Help Wanted!* (short film), MGM, 1939; *One against the World* (short film), MGM, 1939; *The Ash Can Fleet* (short film), MGM, 1939; *Forgotten Victory* (short film), MGM, 1939; *The Old South* (short film), MGM, 1940; *Stuffie* (short film), MGM, 1940; *The Way in the Wilderness* (short

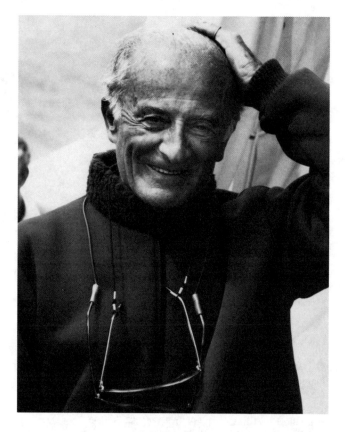

FRED ZINNEMANN

film), MGM, 1940; *The Great Meddler* (short film), MGM, 1940; *Forbidden Passage* (short film), MGM, 1941; *Your Last Act* (short film), MGM, 1941; *The Lady or the Tiger?* (short film), MGM, 1942; *Kid Glove Killer,* MGM, 1942; *Eyes in the Night,* MGM, 1942; *The Seventh Cross,* MGM, 1944; *Little Mister Jim,* MGM, 1946; *My Brother Talks to Horses,* MGM, 1946; *The Search,* MGM, 1948; *Act of Violence,* MGM, 1948.

The Men (also known as *Battle Stripe*), United Artists, 1950; *Teresa,* MGM, 1951; (also producer) *Benjy* (short documentary film), Paramount, 1951; *High Noon,* United Artists, 1952; *The Member of the Wedding,* Columbia, 1952; *From Here to Eternity,* Columbia, 1953; *Oklahoma,* Magna Corporation, 1955; *A Hatful of Rain,* Twentieth Century-Fox, 1957; *The Nun's Story,* Warner Brothers, 1959; (also producer with Gerry Blattner) *The Sundowners,* Warner Brothers, 1960; (also producer) *Behold a Pale Horse,* Columbia, 1964; (also producer) *A Man for All Seasons,* Columbia, 1966; *The Day of the Jackal,* Universal, 1973; *Julia,* Twentieth Century-Fox, 1977; (also producer) *Five Days One Summer,* Warner Brothers, 1981. Also assistant cameraman, *La Marche des machines,* 1927; assistant cameraman, *Ich Kusse Ihre Hand, Madame,* 1929; assistant cameraman, *Sprenbagger 10 10,* 1929; assistant cameraman, *Menschen am Sonntag* (also known as *People on Sunday*), 1929; assistant director, *Man Trouble,* 1930; assistant director, *The Spy,* 1931; assistant director, *The Wiser Sex,* 1932; assistant director, *The Man from Yesterday,* 1932; assistant director, *The Kid from Spain;* director, *The Wave* (also known as *Los redes;* documentary), 1935.

RELATED CAREER—Contributor to the *Encyclopaedia Britannica* entry on film directing.

AWARDS: Screen Directors Guild Award and Academy Award nomination, both Best Director, 1948, *The Search;* Academy Award, Best Documentary, 1951, for *Benjy;* New York Film Critics Award, Screen Directors Guild Award, and Academy Award nomination, all Best Director, 1952, for *High Noon;* Academy Award, Best Director, 1953, New York Film Critics Award, Best Director, 1953, Directors Guild of America Award, Best Director, 1953, and Golden Globe Award, Best Motion Picture Director, 1954, all for *From Here to Eternity;* New York Film Critics Award and Academy Award nomination, both Best Director, 1959, for *The Nun's Story;* Academy Award nomination, Best Director, 1960, for *The Sundowners;* Golden Thistle Award from the Edinburgh Film Festival, 1965, Moscow Film Festival Award, 1965, Academy Awards, Best Picture and Best Director, 1966, New York Film Critics Awards, Best Film and Best Director, 1966, Directors Guild of America Award, Best Director, 1966, and Golden Globe Awards, Best Motion Picture Director and Best Motion Picture—Drama, 1967, all for *A Man for All Seasons;* Gold Medal from the city of Vienna, Austria, 1967; D.W. Griffith Award from the Directors Guild of America, 1971; Academy Award nomination, Best Director, 1977, British Academy Award, Best Director, 1978, and David di Donatello Award, 1978, all for *Julia;* British Academy of Film and Television Arts Fellowship Award, 1978; Order of Arts and Letters (France), 1982; U.S. Congressional Award for Lifetime Achievement, 1987.

MEMBER: American Film Institute (co-founder, 1961), Academy of Motion Picture Arts and Sciences, Directors Guild of America (vice-president, 1961-64), Directors Guild of Britain (honorary president), British Academy of Film and Television Arts (honorary fellow), Sierra Club.

ADDRESSES: OFFICE—128 Mount Street, London W1Y 5HA, England. AGENT—Stan Kamen, William Morris Agency, 151 El Camino Drive, Beverly Hills, CA 90212.

*   *   *

ZIPPRODT, Patricia   1925-

PERSONAL: Born February 24, 1925, in Evanston, IL; daughter of Herbert Edward (an advertising executive) and Irene (Turpin) Zipprodt. EDUCATION: Wellesley College, A.B., sociology, 1946; attended the Art Institute of Chicago, 1935-49, and the Fashion Institute of Technology, 1952-53.

VOCATION: Costume designer.

CAREER: FIRST BROADWAY WORK—Costume designer, *The Potting Shed,* Bijou Theatre, 1957. PRINCIPAL STAGE WORK—Costume designer: *A Visit to a Small Planet,* Booth Theatre, New York City, 1957; *The Virtuous Island* and *The Apollo of Bellac* (double-bill), Carnegie Hall Playhouse, New York City, 1957; *Miss Lonelyhearts,* Music Box Theatre, New York City, 1957; *The Rope Dancers,* Cort Theatre, New York City, 1957; *The Crucible,* Martinique Theatre, New York City, 1958; *Back to Methusaleh,* Ambassador Theatre, New York City, 1958; *The Night Circus,* John Golden Theatre, New York City, 1958; *Our Town,* Circle in the Square, New York City, 1959; *The Gang's All Here,* Ambassador Theatre, 1959; *The Crucible* and *The Quare Fellow,* both Circle in the Square, 1959.

The Balcony, Circle in the Square, 1960; *Camino Real,* St. Mark's

Playhouse, New York City, 1960; *Period of Adjustment,* Helen Hayes Theatre, New York City, 1960; *The Blacks,* St. Mark's Playhouse, 1961; *The Garden of Sweets,* American National Theatre and Academy (ANTA) Theatre, New York City, 1961; *Sunday in New York,* Cort Theatre, 1961; *Madame Aphrodite,* Orpheum Theatre, New York City, 1961; *The Matchmaker, Next Time I'll Sing for You,* and *Oh Dad, Poor Dad, Mama's Hung You in the Closet and I'm Feeling So Sad,* all Phoenix Theatre, New York City, 1962; *Don Perlimplin,* Playhouse in the Park, Cincinnati, OH, 1962; *La Boheme* (opera), Boston Opera Company, Boston, MA, 1962; *A Man's a Man,* Masque Theatre, New York City, 1962; *Step on a Crack,* Ethel Barrymore Theatre, New York City, 1962; *Calvary,* Princeton Experimental Theatre, NJ, 1963; *The Dragon,* Phoenix Theatre, 1963; *She Loves Me,* Eugene O'Neill Theatre, New York City, 1963; *Oh Dad, Poor Dad, Mama's Hung You in the Closet and I'm Feeling So Sad,* Morosco Theatre, New York City, 1963; *Morning Sun* and *A Man's a Man,* both Phoenix Theatre, 1963; *Too Much Johnson* and *The Tragical Historie of Dr. Faustus,* both Phoenix Theatre, 1964; *Fiddler on the Roof,* Imperial Theatre, New York City, 1964; *Anya,* Ziegfeld Theatre, New York City, 1965; *La Sonnamnbula* (ballet), National Ballet of Washington, Washington, DC, 1965; *Pousse-Cafe,* 46th Street Theatre, New York City, 1966; *Cabaret,* Broadhurst Theatre, New York City, 1966; *Hippolyte e Aricie* (opera), Boston Opera Company, 1966; *Katerina Ismailova* (opera), New York City Opera Company, State Theatre, New York City, 1967; *The Little Foxes,* Vivian Beaumont Theatre, New York City, 1967; *The Flaming Angel* (opera), New York City Opera Company, State Theatre, 1968; *Plaza Suite,* Plymouth Theatre, New York City, 1968; *Zorba,* Imperial Theatre, 1968; *1776,* 46th Street Theatre, 1969; *Les noces* (ballet), American Ballet Theatre, New York City, 1969; *Tales of Kasane,* National Theatre of the Deaf, New York City, 1969.

Georgy, Winter Garden Theatre, New York City, 1970; *The Poppet* (ballet), Joffrey Ballet, New York City, 1970; *Scratch,* St. James Theatre, New York City, 1971; *Pippin,* Imperial Theatre, 1972; *Watermill* (ballet), New York City Ballet, State Theatre, 1972; *The Rise and Fall of the City of Mahagonny* (opera), Boston Opera Company, 1972; *The Mother of Us All* (opera), Guggenheim Museum, New York City, 1972; *Waiting for Godot,* Tyrone Guthrie Theatre, Minneapolis, MN, 1973; *Lord Byron* (opera), Juilliard Opera, New York City, 1973; *Lord Byron Ballet* (ballet), Alvin Ailey American Dance Theatre, New York City, 1973; *Dumbarton Oaks* (ballet), New York City Ballet, State Theatre, 1973; *Don Giovanni* (opera), Metropolitan Opera, New York City, 1973 (not produced); *Dear Nobody,* Cherry Lane Theatre, New York City, 1974; *Mack and Mabel,* Majestic Theatre, New York CIty, 1974; *Dybbuk Variations* (ballet), New York City Ballet, State Theatre, 1974; *The Leaves Are Fading* (ballet), American Ballet Theatre, 1975; *All God's Chillun Got Wings,* Circle in the Square, 1975; *Chicago,* 46th Street Theatre, 1975; *Poor Murderer,* Ethel Barrymore Theatre, 1976; *Four Saints in Three Acts,* National Theatre of the Deaf, 1976; *Tannhauser* (opera), Metropolitan Opera, 1977; *Naughty Marietta* (opera), New York City Opera, State Theatre, 1978; *Stages,* Belasco Theatre, New York City, 1978; *King of Hearts,* Minskoff Theatre, New York City, 1978.

Charlotte, Belasco Theatre, 1980; *Fools,* Eugene O'Neill Theatre, 1981; *One Night Stand,* Nederlander Theatre, New York City, 1980; *Kingdoms,* Cort Theatre, 1981; *Fiddler on the Roof,* State Theatre, 1981; *Don Juan,* Tyrone Guthrie Theatre, 1982; *Brighton Beach Memoirs,* Center Theatre Group, Ahmanson Theatre, Los Angeles, CA, 1982; *Alice in Wonderland,* Virginia Theatre, New York City, 1982; *Whodunnit,* Biltmore Theatre, New York City, 1982; *Don Juan,* New York Shakespeare Festival, Delacorte Theatre, New York City, 1982; *The Barber of Seville* (opera), Metropolitan Opera, 1982; *Brighton Beach Memoirs,* Alvin Theatre, New York City, 1983; *Sunday in the Park with George,* Playwrights Horizons, New York City, 1983; *Sunset,* Village Gate Downstairs, New York City, 1983; *Estuary* (ballet), American Ballet Theatre, 1983; *The Glass Menagerie,* Eugene O'Neill Theatre, 1983; *The Loves of Don Perlimplin* (opera), San Francisco Opera, and State University of New York, Purchase, NY, 1984; *Anna Christie,* Central Theatre Institute, Beijing, China, 1984; *Sunday in the Park with George,* Booth Theatre, 1984; *Accidental Death of an Anarchist,* Belasco Theatre, 1984; *Helgi Tommasen* (ballet), Houston Ballet Company, TX, 1985; *Big Deal,* Broadway Theatre, New York City, 1986; *Sweet Charity,* Minskoff Theatre, 1986; *Cabaret,* Imperial Theatre, 1987; *Macbeth,* Mark Hellinger Theatre, New York City, 1988. Also *Laurette,* New York City, 1961; *Madame Butterfly* (opera), 1962; *L'Histoire du soldat* (ballet), Israel Cultural Foundation, 1967; *Tres Cantos* (ballet) and *Caprichos* (ballet), both Ballet Hispanico, 1976; *Swing,* New York City, 1979; for the Tyrone Guthrie Theatre, 1981; *Smile,* New York City, 1983; *Llamada* (ballet), Ballet Hispanico, 1983; and *Tito on Tambales* (ballet), Ballet Hispanico, 1984.

MAJOR TOURS—All as costume designer, unless indicated: Assistant to the costume designer, *The Amazing Adele,* U.S. cities, 1955-56; *Fiddler on the Roof,* U.S. cities, 1966-67; *Pippin,* U.S. cities, 1977-78; *Chicago,* U.S. cities, 1977-78; *Brighton Beach Memoirs,* U.S. cities, 1983-85; *Pippin,* U.S. cities, 1986; *Cabaret,* U.S. cities, 1987; *Macbeth,* U.S. cities, 1988.

PRINCIPAL FILM WORK—Costume designer: *The Graduate,* Embassy, 1967; *The Last of the Mobile Hotshots,* Warner Brothers, 1969; *1776,* Columbia, 1972.

PRINCIPAL TELEVISION WORK—All as costume designer. Specials: *Annie, the Women in the Life of a Man,* CBS, 1970; *June Moon,* PBS, 1973; *The Glass Menagerie,* ABC, 1973; *Alice in Wonderland,* PBS, 1983; also *Pippin,* HBO.

RELATED CAREER—Costume designer for touring shows featuring Bette Midler, 1976, and Ben Vereen, 1983; assistant to the theatre designers Rouben Ter-Arutunian, William and Jean Eckart, Boris Aronson, Robert Fletcher, and Irene Sharaff; teacher and lecturer in design at Yale School of Drama, Harvard University, Wellesley College, Smith College, Northwestern University, University of Rhode Island, New York University School of the Arts, Pratt Institute, U.S. Institute of Theatre Technicians, Martha's Vineyard Sculpture Gallery series, and the Brooklyn Museum; visiting Joseph Siskind Professor of Theatre Arts, Brandeis University; adjunct professor of theatre design, University of Utah.

AWARDS: Antoinette Perry Award, Best Costume Design, 1965, for *Fiddler on the Roof;* Antoinette Perry Award and *Variety* New York Drama Critics Poll Award, both Best Costume Design, 1967, for *Cabaret;* Drama Desk Award, Outstanding Costume Design, 1969, for *Zorba* and *1776;* Antoinette Perry Award nomination, 1969, for *Zorba;* Joseph P. Maharam Award, 1969, and *Variety* New York Drama Critics Poll Award, Best Costume Design, 1970, both for *1776;* Emmy Award, Best Costume Design, 1970, for *Annie, the Women in the Life of a Man;* Wellesley College Alumnae Achievement Award, 1971; Drama Desk Award, Outstanding Costume Design, 1972, and Antoinette Perry Award nomination, Best Costume Design, 1973, for *Pippin;* special award for creative excellence from the New England Theatre Conference, 1973; Antoinette Perry Award nomination, Best Costume Design, 1975, for *Mack and Mabel;* Antoinette Perry Award nomination, Best Costume Design, 1976, for *Chicago;* Ritter Award from the Fashion Institute of Technology, 1977; Drama Desk Award, Outstanding Costume Design, 1978, for *King of Hearts.*

Joseph P. Maharam Award nomination, 1981, for *Fools;* Antoinette Perry Award nomination, Best Costume Design, and Joseph P. Maharam Award, both 1983, for *Alice in Wonderland;* Joseph P. Maharam Award, 1983, for *Don Juan;* Antoinette Perry Award nomination, Best Costume Design, and Joseph P. Maharam Award, both 1984, for *Sunday in the Park with George;* Distinguished Career Award from the Southeastern Theatre Conference, 1985; Antoinette Perry Award, Best Costume Design, 1986, for *Sweet Charity.*

MEMBER: United Scenic Artists, Costume Designers Guild, National Academy of Arts and Sciences.

SIDELIGHTS: Patricia Zipprodt's design sketches have been exhibited in the United States and Europe.

ADDRESSES: HOME—29 King Street, New York, NY 10014.*